BY THE EDITORS OF

CONSUMERGUIDE®

FAMILY MEDICAL & PRESCRIPTION DRUG GUIDE

With Ira J. Chasnoff, M.D.,
Jeffrey W. Ellis, M.D.,
Zachary S. Fainman, M.D.,
and Peggy Boucher Mullen, Pharm. D.

PUBLICATIONS INTERNATIONAL, LTD.

TABLE OF CONTENTS

Notice:
In this book, the authors and editors have done their best to outline the symptoms and general treatment for various conditions, injuries, and diseases. Also, recommendations are made regarding certain drugs, medications, and preparations; and descriptions of certain medical tests and procedures are offered. Different people react to the same treatment, medication, preparation, test, or procedure in different ways. This book does not attempt to answer all questions about all situations that you may encounter.
Neither the Editors of CONSUMER GUIDE® and Publications International, Ltd., nor the consultants, authors, or publisher take responsibility for any possible consequences from any treatment, procedure, test, action, or application of medication or preparation by any person reading or following the information in the book. The publication of this book does not constitute the practice of medicine, and this book does not attempt to replace your physician. The authors and the publisher advise the reader to check with a physician before administering any medication or undertaking any course of treatment.

Medical Consultants:
Ira J. Chasnoff, M.D., Pediatrics
Jeffrey W. Ellis, M.D., Obstetrics and Gynecology
Zachary S. Fainman, M.D., Internal Medicine

Consultant for Prescription Drugs:
Peggy Boucher Mullen, Pharm. D.

Illustrations: Teri J. McDermott, M.A., Medical Illustrator

INTRODUCTION

The objective of *The New Illustrated Family Medical & Health Guide* is to help you take charge of your family's health care. The best way to begin is to become a knowledgeable patient and an informed consumer of health services.

Health care in America is changing rapidly. Health-care providers increasingly view patients as consumers of their services, and each person is being called on to accept the responsibility of making informed decisions about his or her own health. Each day brings reports of sophisticated new diagnostic techniques and methods of treatment, but this outpouring of information can be more overwhelming than it is reassuring. To take full advantage of this new era in medicine, you owe it to yourself and your family to learn all you can about safeguarding your health. *The New Illustrated Family Medical & Health Guide* provides a wealth of information about medical care and health practices that will help you make crucial decisions for your family.

This book is designed to help the one person who is ultimately responsible for your health and the health of your family—you. After all, you are the one person who can closely monitor your physical well-being and regulate your personal health habits on a daily basis. You are the one who decides what you eat, how much you exercise, and where you go when a medical problem arises.

You are the one who wishes to avoid expensive trips to the doctor while at the same time being prudent about obtaining medical advice when it is truly necessary. You are the one who is most directly concerned with preserving your good health and preventing illness. *The New Illustrated Family Medical & Health Guide*, with its wide coverage of health and medical topics, will give you the information you need to protect the health and well-being of every member of your family.

This book offers important information on making the right decisions about nutrition and lifestyle changes and on recognizing and coping with common symptoms. You will also find advice on how to select the doctor who is the most appropriate for your family's medical needs, as well as explanations of the various specialties in medicine—from anesthesiology to urology.

To help you understand disease as a departure from the normal healthy state, *The New Illustrated Family Medical & Health Guide* offers a survey of the human body and how it works in sickness and in health. There are chapters on each of the various organ systems of the body, with clear explanations of how they function in the healthy body and what has gone wrong in various abnormal conditions. In those sections that describe a disease or disorder, the cause, the risk factors, the symptoms, the diagnosis, the treatment, and the prognosis are discussed, and pre-

ventive action (if available) is outlined. Each entry is as inclusive as possible, with language that is clear and understandable.

As you read on, you will learn about commonly administered clinical and laboratory tests and other diagnostic procedures. If you have to undergo tests, you will know what to expect, how to prepare yourself so that you'll experience as little discomfort as possible, and what the results may indicate.

If your doctor prescribes a medication, you will learn how to read the prescription and interpret the directions. There is also important information about saving money on prescriptions when you buy drugs and about storing your medications in order to preserve their effectiveness.

This book is intended as a home adviser about health and medical problems. However, it is not a substitute for your own doctor. If you suspect that you may need medical care, you should always consult a physician. The information in this book will help you to communicate with the doctor about your medical problems and concerns and to understand the basis for your doctor's treatment plan.

Remember that maintaining good health is a team effort between you and your doctor. With the help of *The New Illustrated Family Medical & Health Guide*, you can become a more active participant in protecting your family's health. Read it in good health!

STAYING HEALTHY

Medicine and health care today are based on the premise that definite physical factors are responsible for diseases and disorders. The discovery in the nineteenth century that micro-organisms (bacteria and viruses) cause infectious diseases led to remarkable advances in medical care. So for many years, the public relied on the miracles of medicine to cure illnesses and to prolong life as much as possible.

In this century, noninfectious disorders—cancer, heart disease, hypertension, birth defects—have become the major causes of sickness and death. Modern medical research shows more and more that it is what individuals do for themselves and how they take care of their bodies that make the greatest difference in the length and quality of their lives.

Most people are born healthy, with bodies meant to last a full lifetime. Many diseases and disorders can be prevented with a healthy lifestyle. That includes eating nutritious meals, exercising regularly, controlling weight, getting adequate sleep and rest, avoiding hazardous substances and harmful habits, and having regular physical examinations.

The effects of abusing our health by such practices as smoking cigarettes, consuming a high-fat diet, and overindulging in alcohol do not usually show up for years. By then, it is often too late to reverse the ill effects.

In contrast, following the simple guidelines for a healthy lifestyle produces much more immediate results—a better-looking body, more energy, and less need for expensive medical care. Even those who are born with an inherited tendency to suffer from a disorder can often decrease the risk of developing problems by taking care of themselves.

Good health in the future depends on taking care of your body today. Practicing preventive health care does not guarantee that a person will live past 100 years of age or run marathons at age 90, but neither does it mean living a life of constant denial or deprivation. It does involve changing some habits and learning new ways.

Be an active participant and take responsibility for your health. You have taken the first step by picking up this book. Read it and learn more about how the body functions. Be aware of the major warning signs of cancer and be attuned to the changes in your body that could be symptoms of illness. Think about the quality of your life and the ways that your family can practice preventive medicine.

A man who was celebrating his 100th birthday was asked what advice he could give about living a long life. The man replied, "Keep breathing!" Good advice, but as you will learn in this chapter, living a long, *healthy* life is not quite that simple. Nevertheless, practicing preventive health care is well worth your efforts.

EATING TO STAY HEALTHY: GOOD NUTRITION

Nutrition refers to the way the body uses food to maintain itself and grow. Planning good nutrition involves learning which nutrients the body needs and identifying and eating the foods that supply those nutrients.

Your body is made up of billions of cells—the basic building blocks of the body. To survive, each cell needs a continuous supply of fuel for energy, oxygen with which to burn the fuel, water, and a variety of other nutrients. The process of digestion breaks down food into nutrients that are small enough to pass through the wall of the small intestine and be absorbed into the bloodstream. The bloodstream carries the nutrients to each cell in the body, where they are broken down and utilized. Some nutrients provide energy, others help form new tissues, and still others enable the body to grow or restore itself.

Nutrients

There are six categories of nutrients, and all are present in many foods. In order of predominance, they are water, fats, carbohydrates, proteins, vitamins, and minerals. The body is composed of similar materials in about the same order of predominance. Thus, the body of a person who weighs 125 pounds contains about 75 pounds of water, 25 pounds of fat, and 25 pounds of protein, carbohydrates, vitamins, and minerals.

The body requires varying amounts of all six categories of nutrients to maintain body heat, to move, to build and restore bones and tissues—in short, for any function or activity.

Calories—body energy

Fuel supplied by nutrients is measured in calories. When a person consumes more calories than their body burns up during basic body functions or exercise, the excess is stored as fat. So good nutrition also involves consuming sufficient amounts of all the nutrients the body needs *without* adding extra fat.

To obtain all the essential nutrients without consuming too many calories, a person must learn to select foods wisely. Foods that provide more nutrients than calories are said to have a high nutrient density. For example, three ounces of steak and three ounces of sardines provide the same amount of iron, but the steak contains 330 calories, while the sardines have only 175 calories; with respect to iron, therefore, the sardines have a higher nutrient density than the steak.

In contrast, 12 ounces of beer has almost no nutritional value but provides 150 calories of energy that, if not used, is converted to fat. Thus, beer is not the wisest "food" choice.

Making wise choices

There is growing evidence that excessive amounts of cholesterol, animal fats, sugar, and salt are underlying and/or aggravating factors in such major disorders as heart attack, hypertension, diabetes, and cancer of the colon. Yet the average American diet is laden with these substances. How can you be sure that you are getting the nutrients you need to stay healthy without eating too much of those substances that may be harmful?

The federal government periodically publishes a list of Recommended Dietary Allowances (RDAs), or suggested intakes, of certain nutrients, based on the latest scientific information. It also sets guidelines for average caloric needs to maintain certain weights according to an individual's height and age. The RDAs are guidelines, not requirements, for healthy persons. The needs of

pregnant women, the elderly, and those with medical problems often differ from the RDA guidelines.

Labels on packaged goods usually list the nutritional values of the items and the percentages of the RDAs that they meet. In addition, many recipes now include nutritional and caloric data. All this information helps you keep tabs on, and control your intake of, calories and nutrients.

It's not necessary to count nutrients when making diet choices. Foods are grouped by their similarities in nutritional content. After learning to recognize the groups to which items belong, a person can maintain a well-balanced diet by eating from the four food groups each day: two servings of meat or fish protein; two servings of milk or dairy products; four servings of fruits or vegetables; and four servings of grains, breads, or cereals.

Those who prefer a vegetarian diet must select their nutrients from fewer food groups. The lacto-ovo-vegetarian (*lacto* means milk and *ovo* means egg) excludes meat, fish, and poultry but can substitute other protein-rich foods, such as milk, eggs, and legumes (beans and peas). The strict vegetarian, who also eliminates dairy products, must add other supplements to the diet or risk developing illnesses from certain nutrient deficiencies.

Keeping up-to-date about nutrition

In recent years, research has uncovered more and more information about nutrition. Although the volume of new facts may seem to complicate the choices,

the more knowledge you have access to, the more easily you can make decisions in your own best interests. To keep abreast of the most recent scientific data, read and listen to as many informed sources as possible and become aware of the differences in information.

For instance, some figures strongly suggest certain assumptions, but they do not scientifically prove them. Studies reveal that in cultures in which people consume foods containing a lot of fiber, there are virtually no colon disorders, in contrast to cultures in which people eat primarily low-fiber foods. These facts strongly suggest, but do not prove, that a high-fiber diet has beneficial effects.

The flood of new information has also spurred much debate. A prime example is the controversy that surrounds the nonsugar sweeteners. The government banned cyclamates in 1969 because some tests indicated that they might cause cancer. But when the government tried to prohibit saccharin eight years later for the same reason, consumers protested that the benefits were greater than the potential risks. The ban has been suspended, and consumers are free to use the product if they wish. Recently, a third sweetener, aspartame, came under scrutiny because of reported side effects. Other such sweeteners are surely forthcoming. Information on the known side effects of these sweeteners can be obtained from the manufacturer. In addition, check with the manufacturer and/or your personal physician to find out whether any medical condition you have precludes the use of the sugar substitutes.

Another source of controversy is the use of food additives. Most packaged foods contain additives—many of which are natural substances—considered safe by the government. The additives retard or prevent spoilage; maintain or add vitamins, minerals, and proteins; enhance the flavor and appearance; or help in the preparation of the food. Additives are listed on package labels, which is important for people with allergies to certain ingredients or for those who must follow strict sugar-free or salt-free diets.

Current data warns of the possible perils of excessive use of substances that are safe or even necessary when used in moderation. Two of these are salt (sodium chloride) and caffeine. The body requires small daily amounts of sodium to maintain the volume and constant flow of blood in the blood vessels. Excessive sodium intake, however, may lead to fluid retention (the holding in of extra body water) or elevation of blood pressure. People with high blood pressure, heart disease, kidney disease, or kidney disorders should be particularly alert to the sodium content of foods.

Caffeine—an ingredient in coffee, tea, cocoa, many cola drinks, and many nonprescription medicines—is a great pick-me-up in small doses. However, it is also a habit-forming stimulant that, in larger doses, may lead to nervousness, insomnia, and irregular heartbeat. Caffeine intake may aggravate symptoms in people with heart disease, high blood pressure, fibrocystic breasts, or anxiety disorder.

Be wary of the many health-food quacks. They promote gimmicks, worthless products, and megadoses of vitamins with claims of preventing and curing all sorts of nutritional deficiencies or problems, building muscles without exercise, and

melting away pounds without dieting. Large (mega) doses of vitamin or amino-acid preparations taken without the knowledge or supervision of a physician are usually of no health value and can even be hazardous to your health.

Reliable information about nutrition is available, often free of charge, from national and local health and medical associations and from the U.S. Department of Agriculture.

With so many discoveries being made in the field of nutrition, it often seems that what applies today may change tomorrow. However, one fact will not become outdated: it is less expensive and less time-consuming to prevent the diseases that result from nutritional deficiencies than it is to cure them.

Follow these nutritional rules to change bad eating habits.
• Eat well-balanced, nutritious meals, including breakfast.
• Limit calories sensibly to lose weight.
• Read labels to learn the ingredients of packaged foods.
• Drink plenty of water.
• Cut out or moderate intake of animal fats, caffeine, sugar, salt, alcohol, and other substances that add calories without nutritional benefit or that pose possible hazards.
• Learn as much as possible about how your body functions.
• Stay alert to new findings.

The following sections will explain in more detail some of the more important and interesting nutrition-related topics.

Amino acids

Amino acids are the main building blocks of proteins and are found in all living cells. There

are 20 or more different kinds of amino acids, each of which contains carbon, hydrogen, oxygen, and nitrogen. Each protein molecule is made up of thousands of amino acid molecules, linked to each other in chains.

Functions

In the body, food proteins are broken down to their amino acids in the small intestine. The amino acids are then transported through the bloodstream to form, maintain, and repair body protein. Sometimes they are also used as fuel. In the cells, enzymes (special proteins that cause or speed up chemical processes in the body) break down some amino acids into simpler compounds, use some for structure, and form others into chains of new proteins.

Types

Nutritionists divide amino acids into two groups:
• Nonessential amino acids, which can be manufactured by the body if not enough of them are supplied by the diet
• Essential amino acids, which must be included in our diets if we are to remain healthy

Rich sources of amino acids include meat, fish, fowl, eggs, milk, cheese, grains, nuts, and legumes (beans and peas). The proteins from animal sources are much more complete—that is, they contain more essential amino acids in the right proportions—than those from plant sources. Therefore, the person who avoids consuming meat and dairy products should be sure to include substantial amounts of two or more plant proteins in each day's meals.

Beriberi

Beriberi is a disease that is caused by an insufficiency of thiamin (vitamin B_1). It has been most common in those parts of the world where people's diets have been limited almost entirely to polished (white) rice. Milling removes the brown rice husks, which are rich in thiamin.

Other causes of beriberi include the following:

- Increased need for thiamin, such as occurs with fever, pregnancy, breast-feeding, or overactivity of the thyroid gland (which causes the body to increase the rate at which it uses nutrients)
- Failure of the body to absorb enough thiamin, such as may occur with long-lasting diarrhea
- Poor use of the vitamin by the body, as in severe liver disease

A combination of these factors occurs in alcoholism because of lowered food intake, poor vitamin absorption, increased need for thiamin, and poor use of it by the body.

Symptoms

Because thiamin is necessary for the proper use of fats, starches, and sugars and for the normal functioning of nervous tissue and of enzymes (which modulate body processes), symptoms of beriberi usually occur in the digestive and nervous systems. In severe cases, heart muscle is damaged. Early symptoms include fatigue, irritability, poor memory, loss of appetite, constipation, abdominal discomfort, and difficulty in rising from the squatting position. There may be burning of the feet, prickling of the soles, and tenderness and cramps in the calves. Certain muscle reflexes are lost. Mental confusion, paralysis of speech and eye muscles, coma, and death can occur in untreated beriberi affecting the brain. Heart damage from beriberi produces heart failure with buildup of body fluids, seen as swelling in the abdomen and legs, and difficulty in breathing.

Babies who are breast-fed by mothers deficient in thiamin may develop heart failure and loss of speech and certain muscle reflexes.

Treatment

Treatment for beriberi consists of daily doses of thiamin, at first by injection into a muscle or vein and later by mouth. Improvement usually begins in one or two days.

Prevention

Eating a well-balanced diet of fruits, vegetables, meat, and whole grains is the best way to prevent such B-vitamin deficiency diseases as beriberi. Beriberi itself is rare in the United States because breads, cereals, and flours are enriched with thiamin.

Carbohydrates

Carbohydrates are organic substances made up of carbon, hydrogen, and oxygen. Carbohydrates are a basic fuel source for the body. They come in the form of sugars, starches, and glycogen (a storage form of carbohydrate). Nonfood carbohydrates are gums and cellulose (plant fiber).

Sugars such as sucrose, glucose, fructose (fruit sugar), and lactose (milk sugar) can be used very quickly by the body. Starches must be turned into sugars by digestive enzymes before they can be used. Sugars travel through the bloodstream and are stored in the liver and muscles (as glycogen) or are incorporated into fat for longer storage.

Potatoes, rice, and wheat are rich sources of starch; they are made up of 90 percent starch, after the water has been removed. Fruits and vegetables generally have less starch and more fiber, which aids in digestion.

Starches and sugars are essential to life, but they have a poor reputation because many of them are refined before use and stripped of some of their vitamins, minerals, and fiber. The bran and the germ of wheat and the husk of rice—all rich in vitamins, minerals, and fiber—are often removed. Highly refined carbohydrates provide calories without some other food benefits. That is one reason why whole-grain breads and cereals are recommended.

Cholesterol

Cholesterol is a fatlike substance found in all animal fats and oils. It is manufactured by the liver from saturated fats and is a basic ingredient in the formation of normal male and female hormones, vitamin D, blood, bile, cell membranes, brain tissue, the sheaths that protect nerve fibers, and other body substances. After the first six months of life, the liver can make all the cholesterol the body needs—about 1,000 milligrams a day. However, the average American consumes an additional 400 to 600 milligrams of cholesterol a day from such sources as eggs and meat.

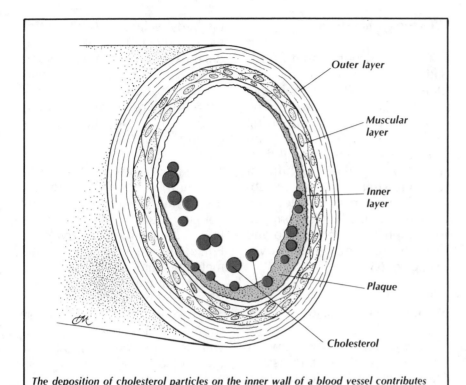

Outer layer

Muscular layer

Inner layer

Plaque

Cholesterol

The deposition of cholesterol particles on the inner wall of a blood vessel contributes to the formation of a plaque, which impedes blood flow.

High blood cholesterol level and disease

Eating foods containing cholesterol and saturated fats (found in dairy products, animal fat, and coconut and palm oils) can raise the level of cholesterol in the blood. When the blood contains too much cholesterol, or when there is an inherited defect that interferes with the body's ability to use or process cholesterol and fats, the risk of heart attack and blood-vessel disease rises.

Atherosclerosis (one type of hardening of the arteries), which causes most heart attacks, may begin with an injury to an artery wall. Normally, a blood clot would form over the injury and heal it. But when there is too much cholesterol in the blood, cholesterol is also deposited at the site of the wound, which promotes the formation of a plaque. The plaque—made up of choles-terol, dead and dying cells, connective tissue, and calcium—may eventually grow to obstruct the artery. If the blockage is in one of the arteries nourishing heart muscle, it can cause a heart attack.

In the United States, levels of cholesterol in the blood are generally found to be in the range of 100 to 280 milligrams per 100 milliliters. However, dietitians and doctors recommend keeping the cholesterol level below 180, and some researchers suggest that the healthiest range is 100 to 150. Studies show that heart attack risk rises in almost direct proportion to the amount of cholesterol in the blood.

Not all people with high blood cholesterol levels develop heart disease or atherosclerosis, however. This may, in part, be due to the level of a substance called high-density lipoprotein (HDL) in their blood. HDL transports ex-cess cholesterol to the liver, from which it is eliminated in the bile. Persons with high levels of HDL seem to have less risk of vascular (blood vessel) disease. Some people have high HDL levels because of heredity. Exercise raises HDL levels. Cigarette smoking lowers HDL levels.

Lowering the cholesterol level

Diet is the mainstay of therapy to lower blood cholesterol levels. Diets rich in saturated fats and cholesterol have been proven to contribute to atherosclerosis. A diet that lowers the intake of both saturated fats and cholesterol will lower the total level of blood cholesterol more than a diet that lowers either one alone.

You can reduce the cholesterol in your blood by avoiding fatty meats, cutting back on eggs, and eating more fish and poultry, which contain less cholesterol and saturated fat than meats. Olive oil and oils made from corn, sunflower, safflower, soybean, sesame, and cottonseed are better for cooking than is oil derived from animal fat. Reduction in the use of butter will also be helpful. Seafood, such as lobster, shrimp, crab, clams, oysters, scallops, and abalone, has little or no fat. Therefore, it can be eaten in reasonable amounts. It was previously thought that seafood elevated blood levels of cholesterol. This has since been disproved. There is some evidence to suggest that increasing dietary fiber is also a good idea. Raw fruits and vegetables and whole-grain breads and cereals are all good sources of dietary fiber.

If dietary therapy alone does not lower blood cholesterol sufficiently, then drugs must be added. There are multiple drug preparations available for this purpose. Since all drugs have side effects, these must never be taken unless prescribed by a licensed physician. It must also be remembered that drugs alone will not do the job. Diet modification must be continued. Taking off excess weight, exercising regularly, and quitting smoking also help to reduce blood cholesterol levels.

Fluoride

Fluoride is a compound of the chemical element fluorine. Fluoride is found in soil and is necessary to plant life and to the formation of teeth and bones in animals, including humans. In the human body, traces of fluoride are found in the bones, the teeth, the thyroid gland, and the skin.

Preventing tooth disease

It has been found that fluoride can help prevent or reduce tooth decay when taken in somewhat larger amounts than are naturally present in the teeth. The best source of fluoride for prevention of tooth decay is fluoridated drinking water. Water with a fluoride content of one part per million is considered safe and effective, especially if given to children while their teeth are developing. The maximum benefit is obtained when the child drinks fluoridated water daily until the permanent teeth are complete (between the ages of 10 and 13). However, if fluoride intake is excessive before the permanent teeth erupt (while the tooth enamel is still forming), the enamel may become stained and mottled. If the teeth have erupted, this staining and mottling cannot occur.

Effects on other diseases

There is evidence that fluoridation prevents dental problems other than cavities, such as periodontal diseases (diseases of the gums and the bones supporting the teeth). Many physicians and researchers have found that fluoride also may play a significant role in the treatment and prevention of osteoporosis (thinness and brittleness of the bones, common in women after menopause and in both men and women over the age of 65).

The fluoridation debate

Fluoridation of drinking water has been a controversial issue. Opponents of fluoridation are concerned about the unknown long-range effects of adding fluoride to the water supply and about what they see as the infringement on freedom of choice inherent in imposing this "compulsory medication" on the population. Supporters of fluoridation counter these charges by pointing out that fluoride is not a medication but a preventive, used in the same way that chlorine is used to kill bacteria in water supplies. They also assert that fluorides are normally found in teeth and bones as well as in water and that other methods of obtaining fluoride are more costly and less effective in the long run than fluoridation of the water supply. Most health scientists today believe that a fluoride level of about one part per million does not damage either teeth or other body tissues.

Obesity

Obesity is a term commonly applied to the condition in which the body weight is 20 percent or more above normal. It has been linked statistically to high blood pressure, diabetes, cardiovascular disease, and chronic back and joint pains, among other ailments. It is a potentially serious condition that shortens the life span.

The risk of disease and death among the obese is greater for men than for women, but for both it increases in direct proportion to the degree of overweight. For example, it has been estimated that among those who are 20 percent overweight, there are 25 percent more deaths for men and 21 percent more for women than among those of normal weight in a given age group; for those who are 30 percent overweight, there are 42 percent more deaths for men and 30 percent more for women.

Causes

Obesity tends to occur more frequently in some families than in others. This may indicate a hereditary tendency, or it may be due to shared food consumption patterns and attitudes toward food. Women tend to gain weight after menopause, and men gain in middle age. Overweight children often grow up to be overweight adults. This is particularly true when food is used as a reward for a child or is withheld as a punishment. Food may then come to represent security and love—an attitude toward food that often continues into adult life.

Obesity is most often the direct result of taking in more food than is "burned off" in activity. Certain glandular (endocrine) disturbances can affect the appetite or the distribution of fat in the body, but these conditions are uncommon. It is said that only one percent of all obesity is due to factors other than diet. The appetite for food is influenced by habit as well as by emotional factors, and it is not always prompted by hunger. The appetite control center, or feeding center, is thought to be located in the area of the brain called the hypothalamus. The term appestat (suggested by the word thermostat) has been coined to describe the mechanism of appetite control.

The connection between smoking, appetite, and weight gain is unclear. Because smoking has been said to decrease appetite, giving up smoking is often thought to be followed by increased appetite and weight gain. The gain in weight that *may* follow when smoking is stopped has also been attributed to the dependence of some smokers on oral satisfaction; when they stop smoking, they may be compelled to substitute the oral satisfaction of eating for that of smoking. Many smokers, however, gain no weight whatsoever after quitting.

Treatment

The treatment for obesity is twofold: eat less and exercise more. A low-calorie diet that is nutritionally well balanced and that can form the basis of permanent eating habits is the first step. Combined with a regular exercise program, such a diet can, in most cases, eliminate obesity. Anyone embarking on such a program, however, should consult a doctor for a checkup and for guidance.

Appetite-decreasing drugs can be harmful and should be taken only under medical supervision. Even physicians who prescribe

them in selected cases recognize that these drugs are, at best, only a temporary prop, not a long-term answer to the problem of obesity.

Crash diets and fad diets can lead to nutritional deficiencies; if they are effective at all, it is basically only because they furnish fewer calories. The quick weight loss that many such diets promise is often merely a loss of fluid from body tissues; weight lost will quickly be regained as fluid is replaced. Other complications, such as gallbladder disease, may be associated with these diets as well.

Massage is not effective in removing or redistributing local fat deposits. Hot baths and sweating serve only to remove water from the tissues—water that will soon be replaced.

In extreme cases, surgery is sometimes performed to remove excessive layers of fatty tissue. However, the expense of the operation and the inherent dangers of any surgery make this a treatment to be used only in very select cases. The same caution should be exercised with stomach-stapling surgery or intestinal bypass surgery.

Although there are a variety of medical and surgical treatments for obesity, these are mostly reserved for those individuals who are severely obese and have had no success with more conventional diets. In the vast majority of cases, a diet and exercise program prescribed and supervised by a qualified medical professional is all that is necessary.

Prevention

It is particularly important for parents to teach their children good eating habits and to control any tendency toward obesity be-

fore it becomes a serious problem. The old notions that children should have food urged on them and that a fat child is a healthy child should be recognized as not only false but harmful. Older people, too, need to take special care to avoid obesity. They tend to be less active than they were in their younger days yet may continue to follow their established eating patterns. Reduced activity may make it necessary for the elderly to seek out a form of regular exercise—whether it be calisthenics or sports, such as swimming, bicycling, or hiking—that is suited to their capacities and tastes.

One safeguard for those of all ages is to control weight strictly, at an early stage, by weighing daily and embarking on a program of diet and exercise as soon as the weight is three to five pounds above the norm for the individual's height and body type. It is far easier to take off a few pounds than to wait until massive obesity requires a protracted and difficult struggle. Increased life span and improved health and vigor—not to mention improved appearance—will be a satisfying reward.

Pellagra

Pellagra is a disorder caused by a deficiency of niacin (also known as nicotinic acid), a vitamin found in many foods. Niacin is vital to many of the important chemical reactions by which energy is generated in the body, as well as to maintenance of healthy skin and normal functioning of the nervous system. Since niacin is abundant in many foods, only those who seriously neglect their diets, such as alcoholics, are likely to lack the daily requirement of between 9 and

20 milligrams of niacin. At one time, pellagra was widespread in the United States, especially in the South, but today it occurs far less frequently.

Symptoms

Physical symptoms of pellagra include weakness; loss of appetite; sore, red, cracked skin with symmetrical spots that turn scaly and brownish; a painful scarlet mouth, tongue, and gums; a burning sensation throughout the digestive tract; diarrhea; and headaches. Psychological symptoms are anxiety, forgetfulness, insomnia (inability to sleep), irritability, and dementia (loss of intellectual abilities).

Treatment

The deficiency can be reversed by eating a balanced diet and taking niacin supplements.

Pica

Pica is an abnormal craving to eat substances not ordinarily considered to be foods.

Causes

The causes of pica are not completely understood. In the case of a pregnant woman who eats laundry starch, pica may be an almost instinctive effort to make up for deficiencies in the diet. In the case of a child who eats chips of lead-based paint (a common cause of lead poisoning in children), the cause is less clear: it could be a teething impulse, or it could be the result of unconscious drives that are not fully understood.

Common substances ingested

Although lead poisoning is the most serious pica problem with children, the effects of pica are as varied as the substances that are consumed. The substances most commonly eaten as a result of pica are those that are used as ingredients in the manufacture of such products as paints, matches, soaps, cleaners, and pesticides. Some doctors also include consumption of a variety of growing plants, such as mushrooms, century plants, and toxic (poisonous) plants (for example, poison ivy), as pica.

Some pica sufferers (especially children) eat nonfoods indiscriminately; others exhibit pica as a compulsion to consume only one or several specific inedible substances.

Treatment

The treatment for pica is not simple, since medical science has not yet pinned down the root of the compulsion. Obviously, if the craving is induced by a deficiency of an element such as iron, the treatment is to remedy the deficiency. Medical treatment for the effects of ingested nonfoods depends on the nature of the substance consumed. If a child is the pica sufferer, the first line of defense is to remove the material from his or her reach and to search the immediate area for other such substances.

Scurvy

Scurvy is a disease caused by vitamin C deficiency. It is characterized by anemia (deficiency of red blood cells), spongy gums, a tendency to bleed, and abnormal bone and tooth formation. The disease may be either acute (short-term) or chronic (long-term).

Causes

Vitamin C is essential for the formation and maintenance of connective tissue, bone tissue, and teeth. It is also essential for the healing of wounds and burns.

There are two forms of scurvy, infantile and adult. Vitamin C deficiency in infants is due simply to lack of sufficient quantities of vitamin C. In adults, scurvy is usually due to improper diet. Adult scurvy may also result from being on an "ulcer diet" for gastrointestinal disorders that limits citrus fruits and juices because of their acid content. Pregnancy and breast-feeding increase the vitamin C requirement; pregnant women and nursing mothers must be sure to include adequate vitamin C in the diet. In addition, diarrhea, inflammatory disease, burns, surgery, and exposure to intense cold all increase the vitamin C requirement.

Symptoms

Infantile scurvy usually appears between the ages of six months and one year. The earliest symptoms include irritability, loss of appetite, and failure to gain weight. Often the child screams or cries whenever he or she is moved and may hold his or her legs motionless because of the pain caused by internal bleeding of the bone surface. There may be abnormal enlargement or hardening of the joints or long bones (especially in the thighs) and a tendency toward gum hemorrhage as the teeth erupt. Fever, anemia, and increased pulse and respiration rates are also common signs.

Adult scurvy usually takes a long time to develop. Early symptoms include extreme fatigue, weakness, irritability, weight loss, loss of appetite, multiple splinter hemorrhages at the nails, failure of wounds to heal, loosening of teeth, and swollen, purplish, and spongy gums. Secondary infections, gangrene (death and decay of tissue, frequently due to inadequate blood supply), breaks in old scars, spontaneous hemorrhaging, muscle pain, pain in the joints, and small hemorrhagic spots on the skin of the legs are all symptoms of a more advanced stage of the disorder. In some cases there is edema (fluid retention) in the lower extremities and a form of arthritis that resembles rheumatoid arthritis. There may even be bleeding in the conjunctiva (the membrane that covers the front of the eye and lines the eyelids).

Diagnosis

In infantile scurvy, an X-ray study of the ends of the long bones of the legs will show areas of crosswise thickening and increased density, the so-called white lines. Also, a therapeutic dose of vitamin C given orally will stop pain due to infantile scurvy almost immediately and reduce swelling and bleeding of gums within 72 hours.

In adults, scurvy can mimic arthritis, hemorrhagic disease, and gingivitis (inflammation of the gums). The blood level of vitamin C is usually low, but this is not always an accurate diagnostic indication. The level of vitamin C in the urine will be low, and there may be anemia not caused by blood loss.

Treatment

Fortunately, scurvy is easy to treat. Vitamin C given orally for one week, supplemented with orange and tomato juice, is the remedy for infantile scurvy. If diarrhea or vomiting is present, half the recommended oral dose can be given intravenously (in a vein).

For adult scurvy, vitamin C is taken orally until symptoms have disappeared; the patient can then receive maintenance doses. Vitamin C is given for several months for chronic scurvy that appears in connection with gingivitis, hemorrhaging, or joint symptoms.

Prevention

A balanced diet with plenty of vitamin C is the best preventive measure for scurvy. Fortunately, natural sources of vitamin C are plentiful: besides citrus fruits and tomatoes, many green vegetables, such as green peppers, are rich in vitamin C. In the case of patients on bland diets or ulcer diets, a physician should be consulted about how to prevent vitamin C deficiency.

Vitamins and minerals

Vitamins and minerals are substances that are essential in small amounts to maintain good health, to promote growth, and to regulate body functions. Most vitamins and minerals are supplied by the diet, but sometimes (as in the case of vitamins D and K) they are formed in the body as well.

A balanced and varied diet usually provides all the necessary vitamins and minerals without the need for supplements. Dark-green vegetables, yellow fruits and vegetables, citrus fruits, whole-grain products, dairy products, meats, seafood, and dried beans and peas supply adequate quantities of vitamins and minerals, as well as other nutrients.

A carefully selected diet is essential for everyone, but is especially vital for those individuals with special needs. Pregnant and nursing women, newborns and growing children, and elderly and ill persons have special nutritional requirements. Most of these needs can be met by a varied diet. However, due to the special demands placed upon the body by these conditions, vitamin and mineral supplements in addition to diet are often necessary to ensure adequate nutrition. It is important to remember that during periods of physical growth and change or during illness, a nutritious diet is imperative.

Deficiency

Occasionally, a person may experience a vitamin or mineral deficiency (insufficient amounts in the body to maintain good health). There may be several reasons for such a deficiency of a vitamin or mineral, such as:
- An unbalanced diet that features too many vitamin- or mineral-deficient foods. For example, some vegetarians omit all animal protein sources and are either careless about or unaware of the proper balance of vegetable nutrients.
- An inadequate diet that lacks the proper amounts of nutritious foods. People on strict weight-reducing programs or those who restrict their diets

for religious reasons may be susceptible to deficiencies.

- An inability of the body to absorb or utilize vitamins or minerals despite a nutritious diet.
- An unusual need for vitamins or minerals (for example, during pregnancy or illness).
- An excessive intake of one vitamin, which may adversely affect the body's use of another vitamin, even though the second vitamin is present in normal amounts. For instance, large amounts of vitamin E may change the body's need for vitamin K to the point of causing a vitamin K deficiency.

All of these reasons point up the importance of careful attention to balance in the diet. In addition, it is necessary to understand that there are two categories of vitamins: fat-soluble (vitamins A, D, E, and K) and water-soluble (B vitamins, folic acid, niacin, and vitamin C). Fat-soluble vitamins are stored in the body, whereas water-soluble vitamins are eliminated daily. Therefore, vitamin deficiencies are more likely to involve water-soluble vitamins, which must be replenished often.

Toxicity

Vitamin toxicity is more likely to occur with fat-soluble vitamins, which can accumulate to toxic levels in the tissues where they are stored. In general, water-soluble vitamins, because they are excreted daily, are considered nontoxic, although large doses (especially of B_6 and niacin) may cause side effects.

Vitamin and mineral toxicity can be as dangerous as deficiency. Again, a balanced and adequate diet is the key to preventing any toxic effects of vitamins and minerals.

The use of so-called "megadoses" (very large doses) of vitamins without the knowledge or supervision of a physician is quite dangerous and can cause serious health problems. In the absence of vitamin deficiency, illness, or other change in the body, there is no health benefit to taking megadoses of vitamins.

The table in this section lists some of the most common vitamins and minerals, with their sources, their functions in the body, and the effects, if any, of having too little or too much of them in the body.

VITAMINS

A vitamin is any of a large group of organic substances often identified as "enzyme components," which are found in many foods in small amounts and are necessary for normal body functioning. Many vitamins help to regulate the rate at which chemical reactions take place in the body.

Vitamin supplementation

Vitamins are not themselves direct sources of energy. As enzyme components, they can act only in the presence of nutrients contained in food. Hence, taking massive doses of supplements in place of normal eating is useless and dangerous.

In general, vitamin megadoses (large doses far beyond daily requirements) are not needed. Many reputable nutritional guides suggest that for persons on restricted-calorie diets (containing less than 1,000 to 1,200 calories daily), a multivitamin preparation may be useful, but higher potency or "therapeutic" formulas are not generally necessary.

Recommended daily allowances

The Food and Drug Administration has developed a system of nutrition labeling for foods, the U.S. Recommended Daily Allowances (USRDAs). The USRDAs for selected vitamins for adults and children four years and older are as follows:

Vitamin A	5,000 international units
Vitamin B_1	1.5 milligrams
Vitamin B_2	1.7 milligrams
Vitamin B_6	2 milligrams
Vitamin C	60 milligrams
Vitamin D	400 international units
Vitamin E	30 international units
Folic acid	0.4 milligrams
Biotin	0.3 milligrams
Niacin	20 milligrams

Vitamin A

Vitamin A is found in fish-liver oils, liver, butter, egg yolks, cheese, dark-green vegetables, and yellow vegetables and fruits. Deficiency of this vitamin in the diet causes inadequate production of rhodopsin (a substance important in the functioning of the eye), resulting in night blindness. Vitamin A deficiency can also result in disorders of the skin and mucous membranes and decreased resistance to infection. Megadoses of this vitamin in the absence of deficiency may cause serious health problems.

Vitamin B

The name vitamin B may refer to any member of the vitamin B complex, including thiamin, riboflavin, niacin, the B_6 group, biotin, pantothenic acid, folic acid, and cyanocobalamin.

Vitamin B_1, or thiamin, helps maintain a healthy nervous system and aids heart function. It is found in enriched and whole-grain breads and cereals, meat (especially pork and liver), dried beans and peas, and nuts. A deficiency can result in beriberi, a disease marked by abnormal heart function, swelling, and inflammation of the nerves.

Vitamin B_2, or riboflavin, is found in milk, meats (especially liver), eggs, dark-green vegetables, and enriched cereal products. It acts as a catalyst in bodily processes that involve oxidation (use of oxygen). Deficiency may result in eye disorders and inflammation of the mucous membranes and lips.

Vitamin B_6 is a group of substances (pyridoxine, pyridoxal, and pyridoxamine) that are widely distributed in animal and plant tissues. These substances are involved in the metabolism of amino acids (the building blocks of protein) and in the breakdown of glycogen (a stored sugar). Vitamin B_6 is found in liver, pork, chicken, fish, and whole grains. A deficiency can result in functional disturbances of the nervous system.

Vitamin B_{12}, or cyanocobalamin, affects the formation of red blood cells and is found in all animal products, especially liver and other meats, fish, cheese, and eggs. When vitamin B_{12} is absent from the diet or is not absorbed by the body, anemia (deficiency of red blood cells) may result.

Niacin helps the body use oxygen to produce energy from foods and helps maintain the skin and other tissues. Foods that are good sources of niacin (or substances that the body can convert into niacin) are milk, eggs, and meats. Deficiency can result in pellagra, a disease marked by weakness; appetite loss; rough, red skin; diarrhea; and delirium.

Pantothenic acid plays a role in the synthesis of fat and in the release of energy from carbohydrates, fats, and proteins. All foods contain this vitamin in varying amounts. Good sources are eggs, salmon, liver, kidney, and wheat bran. Deficiency is not likely in people eating an ordinary, varied diet.

Biotin acts as a coenzyme in several metabolic reactions. Some of these are important for the manufacture of fatty acids; others are essential for the synthesis of glucose, a primary source of energy. Some biotin is normally produced in the intestinal tract by bacteria that live there. Because of the difficulty of measuring how much biotin these bacteria make, nutritionists have been unable to establish how much biotin the body needs each day. However, it has been found that ordinary mixed diets usually provide from 100 to 300 micrograms of biotin a day. This amount, plus the amount produced by bacteria, is apparently enough. Biotin deficiency is almost unheard of in humans.

Folic acid is found in dark-green vegetables, liver, and legumes. Folic acid functions as a coenzyme, or catalyst, in a number of biological reactions. One of the most important of these is the synthesis of the gene-containing material deoxyribonucleic acid (DNA). In adults, symptoms of folic acid deficiency—such as anemia, nerve damage, and sore, red, swollen tongue—may not appear for months because the body tends to hold on to its supply of the vitamin. In infants and children, however, symptoms may appear much more quickly. Because they are growing rapidly, infants and children need proportionally more folic acid than do adults; a deficiency slows and stunts growth.

Symptoms of folic acid deficiency may also occur rapidly in pregnant women. Pregnancy increases the need for folic acid because it is a time of rapid growth and manufacture of new cells. Anemia caused by folic acid deficiency is quite prevalent among pregnant women on restricted diets.

Vitamin C

Vitamin C, or ascorbic acid, is found in many vegetables and fruits, especially green peppers and most citrus fruits. It is an essential element in the human diet. A deficiency may result in a disease called scurvy, in which the victim suffers anemia, spongy gums, bleeding, and edema (excess fluid retention in the tissues). An overdose of vitamin C (such as may result from taking "megadoses") may cause gout, kidney stones, and decreased fertility.

Vitamin D

Vitamin D includes any of several related antirickets compounds. These compounds are present in fish-liver oils, liver, butter, cream, egg yolks, and fortified milk; they are also produced in the body on exposure to sunlight. A vitamin D deficiency may cause rickets in children and osteomalacia (softening of the bones) or osteoporosis (decreased bone mass) in adults. As with vitamin A, large doses of this vitamin in the absence of deficiency can be quite toxic, especially in young children.

(Continued on page 22)

Vitamin or Mineral	Primary Sources	Functions
Vitamin A	Liver, fish-liver oils, egg yolks, yellow and dark-green vegetables, butter, cream	• Aids vision, especially at night • Maintains healthy skin and mucous membranes • Promotes normal growth and reproduction
Vitamin B₁ (thiamin) *Can be destroyed by high temperatures and leached from foods in cooking water; prepare foods at lowest possible temperature in least amount of water for shortest period*	Whole-grain (or enriched) breads and cereals, meats (especially pork and liver), dried beans and peas, nuts	• Maintains healthy nervous system • Aids heart function
Vitamin B₂ (riboflavin) *Can be destroyed by light; cover food, and keep milk out of direct light*	Milk, milk products, meats (especially liver), eggs, dark-green vegetables, enriched cereal products	• Helps body use foods to produce energy • Maintains healthy skin and eyes
Niacin	Meats, eggs, milk	• Helps body use oxygen to produce energy from foods • Maintains healthy skin, mouth, tongue, and digestive tract • Aids health of nervous system
Vitamin B₆	Liver, pork, chicken, fish, whole-grain cereals, dried beans and peas	• Helps body use protein • Aids in manufacture of hormones and red blood cells • Maintains healthy nervous system
Folic acid	Dark-green vegetables, liver, dried beans and peas	• Promotes normal growth and development • Promotes red blood cell formation and prevents macrocytic anemia
Vitamin B₁₂ (cyanocobalamin)	Eggs, fish, cheese, meats (especially liver)	• Helps in production of red blood cells • Maintains healthy nervous system
Pantothenic acid	Eggs, beans, meat (especially liver and kidney), dairy products, cereals	• Helps body use food to produce energy • Helps body synthesize fat
Biotin *Produced by intestinal bacteria*	Bacteria and yeast in many foods make or retain it	• Helps body make fatty acids • Helps body synthesize glucose
Vitamin C (ascorbic acid) *Can be destroyed by cooking, air contact, fine mincing of food, and use of copper utensils*	Citrus fruit, tomatoes, potatoes, cabbage, green peppers, strawberries, cantaloupe	• Promotes tooth and bone formation • Strengthens walls of blood vessels • Aids in connective tissue formation • Helps in healing wounds and broken bones
Vitamin D *Sunlight on skin enables body to form vitamin D*	Vitamin D-fortified milk, fish-liver oils, liver, cream, butter, egg yolks	• Helps body absorb calcium and phosphorus for growth of bones and teeth

Symptoms of Deficiency	Symptoms of Toxicity
• Night blindness • Dry, rough skin • Dryness of outer layers of eyes • Decreased resistance to infection	• Excessive doses may cause headache, peeling skin, hair loss, enlarged liver and spleen, loss of appetite, vomiting, weight loss, vision problems, and liver disease
• Beriberi (muscle weakness, muscle cramps, loss of appetite, nervous system disorders, lack of coordination, edema, abnormal heart function)	• Shock, if given in large intravenous doses
• Cracks at corners of mouth • Inflamed and sore lips • Inflamed tongue • Itching and burning eyes	• No known toxicity
• Pellagra (muscle weakness; loss of appetite; rough, red skin; diarrhea; and, in advanced cases, delirium)	• May cause flushing and burning skin, dizziness, nausea, vomiting, diarrhea, and skin rash
• Decreased number of red blood cells (anemia) • Convulsions • Skin inflammation • Nervous system deterioration	• Excessive doses taken for extended periods have been reported to cause numbness and tingling in the hands and feet and an inability to walk
• Stunted growth (especially of fetus in pregnancy and of infants) • Macrocytic anemia • Abnormal white blood cell production • Sore, swollen tongue	• No known toxicity, but very high doses can interfere with drugs for treatment of epilepsy and can interfere with diagnosis of pernicious anemia
• Macrocytic anemia • Pernicious anemia • Numbness or tingling • Dementia • Problems in walking	• No known toxicity, but those with pernicious anemia should receive injections, not oral doses, of B_{12}
• Deficiency rare—Symptoms may include stomach ache, vomiting, leg cramps, fatigue, and reduced resistance to infection	• No known toxicity
• Deficiency almost unknown	• No known toxicity
• Scurvy (bleeding under skin, muscle weakness, loose teeth, bleeding gums, fatigue) • Poor or slow wound healing • Greater susceptibility to infection	• Diarrhea • Dependence • Kidney stones • Large doses may interfere with accuracy of some lab tests
• Rickets (poor bone and tooth development in children, causing bowlegs and decayed teeth) • Osteomalacia (loss of calcium from bones in adults, causing weak and easily fractured bones)	• Excessive doses cause large amounts of calcium to be absorbed, resulting in possible kidney damage because of accumulation of calcium in body tissues

(Continued on page 20)

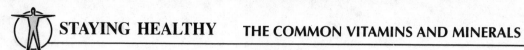

Vitamin or Mineral	Primary Sources	Functions
Vitamin E (tocopherol)	Vegetable oils, wheat germ, whole-grain products, egg yolks, liver, dark-green vegetables	Prevents oxygen in body from combining with wastes to form toxic substances (antioxidant)
Vitamin K *Formed in intestinal tract in healthy persons*	Leafy green vegetables, liver, milk products, bacon, coffee	• Maintains normal blood clotting
Calcium	Milk, milk products	• Helps bone and tooth formation • Aids in blood clotting • Maintains healthy muscle function • Helps transmission of nerve impulses
Phosphorus	Meats, poultry, fish, eggs, whole-grain products	• Works with calcium to ensure bone and tooth formation • Aids metabolism
Sodium	Table salt; salt used in food processing; natural salt occurring in meats, milk, milk products, eggs, fish	• Regulates body's water and acid-base balances • Helps transmission of nerve impulses • Maintains healthy muscles
Chloride	(Same as sodium)	• Helps maintain water balance in body • Helps form component of stomach acid
Potassium	Bananas, citrus fruits, carrots, leafy green vegetables, potatoes, tomatoes, milk, whole-grain products, meats	• Regulates acid-base balance of body • Helps transmission of nerve impulses • Promotes healthy muscle action
Magnesium	Dried beans and peas, whole-grain cereals, cocoa, dark-green vegetables, seafood, nuts	• Maintains healthy nerve and muscle functions • Helps bone and tooth formation • Helps regulate use of sugars for energy
Iron	Liver, seafood, meats, egg yolks, dried beans and peas, green vegetables	• Helps form hemoglobin, which helps carry oxygen in body • Aids metabolism
Iodine	Iodized salt, seafood	• Controls energy production • Regulates body heat • Maintains healthy connective tissue • Promotes physical and mental development
Fluoride	Seafood, meats, fluoridated water, tea	• Helps bone and tooth formation and protects against tooth decay
Zinc	Seafood, meats, dried beans and peas, milk, cheese, egg yolks	• Promotes normal growth and sexual maturity • May help wound healing • Aids protein digestion

Symptoms of Deficiency	Symptoms of Toxicity
• Rarely occurs, except in premature infants, in whom it can cause anemia	• Rarely occurs, but may cause nausea and diarrhea and may interfere with absorption of vitamins A and K and with absorption of drugs to prevent blood clots
• Hemorrhage • Delayed blood clotting	• Rupture of red blood cells and jaundice • Large doses can interfere with action of drugs used to prevent blood clots
• Rickets (poor bone and tooth development in children, causing bowlegs and decayed teeth) • Osteomalacia (loss of calcium from bones in adults, causing weak and easily fractured bones)	• Possible kidney damage due to accumulation of calcium in body tissues
• Weight loss • Anemia • Weakness • Bone pain	• May interfere with calcium absorption and may be a factor in bone loss in adults
• Deficiency rare—Sodium depletion can temporarily occur due to profuse sweating or chronic diarrhea or vomiting, causing muscle cramps, weakness, headache, and loss of appetite	• Edema • Elevated blood pressure in sensitive individuals • Confusion • Coma
• Extremely rare—Upset of acid-base balance when it occurs	• Extremely rare
• Usually occurs only with excessive loss of potassium due to use of diuretics or to extremely severe diarrhea or vomiting, causing weakness, paralysis, heart rhythm disturbances	• Nausea, vomiting • Heart disturbances, including death from cardiac standstill • Weakness • Paralysis
• Weakness • Muscle tremors • Behavior changes • Heartbeat irregularities • Muscle cramps	• If renal function is impaired, may cause confusion, heartbeat irregularities, and muscle twitching
• Iron deficiency anemia (lack of hemoglobin, causing shortness of breath, weakness, fatigue, rapid heartbeat)	• Most potentially toxic mineral, causing nausea, abdominal cramps, liver and intestinal damage, skin discoloration
• Malfunction of thyroid gland • Goiter (enlarged thyroid gland) • Cretinism (impaired mental and physical development) • Subnormal body temperature	• Symptoms of hypo- or hyperthyroidism • Enlarged thyroid gland
• Inclination toward dental cavities	• Mottled or pitted teeth • Brittle bones if taken without adequate calcium
• Retarded growth • Delayed sexual maturity Slow or poor wound healing	• Vomiting • Diarrhea • Kidney damage • Copper deficiency and iron deficiency anemias

Vitamin E

Vitamin E is necessary in human diets for normal muscular and reproductive functioning and development, normal red blood cell functioning, and other biochemical processes. Vitamin E is found in wheat germ oil, vegetable oils, whole-grain products, egg yolks, organ meats (especially liver), and dark-green vegetables.

Vitamin K

Vitamin K is a group of vitamins found in their natural state in spinach, cabbage, and other leafy green vegetables and in egg yolk and liver. These vitamins play a role in clotting of the blood by increasing the production of prothrombin, the clotting agent in the blood. A deficiency can result in blood coagulation abnormalities. Individuals who are on anticoagulant drugs, such as warfarin, should consult their physician about vitamin K, because too much of the vitamin will lessen the effect of the drug and too little of the vitamin will increase the drug's effect.

MINERALS

Minerals are natural, nonorganic substances with a specific chemical composition and characteristic crystalline structure. Minerals are essential for health and growth. They are important components of the bones and soft tissues, and they play a vital role in regulating the cardiovascular system, the internal pressure of body fluids, nerve responses, and oxygen conduction.

The body requires some minerals in relatively large amounts; these "macrominerals" are calcium, chloride, magnesium, phosphorus, potassium, sodium, and sulfur. Others are called trace minerals (or micronutrients) because they are needed only in minute quantities; these include iron, manganese, copper, iodine, zinc, chromium, cobalt, fluoride, and selenium. Large amounts of these minerals taken for nonmedical reasons can cause serious health problems. Still other minerals, such as lead, mercury, and cadmium, are toxic even in small amounts.

Mineral supplementation

Although minerals are essential, they are required only in specific amounts and can be harmful if taken in excess. Those who use mineral supplements should take care not to surpass the daily requirement. An overload can upset the balance of other minerals and block their performance, can result in decreased physical capabilities, and can contribute to such conditions as anemia, bone demineralization (mineral depletion) and brittleness, nervous system disease, and fetal abnormalities. With certain minerals, even consuming twice the daily requirement or taking one day's requirement all in one dose can lead to severe illness. Taking minerals in excessive quantities is especially risky for children, pregnant or nursing women, and the elderly.

Calcium

Calcium is the most prevalent mineral in the body; in fact, the bones and teeth together contain an average of two to three pounds of calcium. In addition to its role in the structure of bones and teeth, calcium regulates certain body processes—normal nerve function, muscle tone, and blood clotting. Major sources are milk and milk products.

Phosphorus

Phosphorus coexists with calcium in the bones and teeth but is also present in most body tissues. Phosphorus is present in so many foods that a deficiency is rare; it is most abundant in meat, poultry, fish, eggs, and whole-grain products.

Sodium chloride

Sodium and chlorine combine to form sodium chloride (table salt), yet each element functions separately. Sodium maintains regular water balance both inside and outside the cells and is found in blood plasma and fluids outside the cells. Foods rich in sodium include meat, fish, poultry, eggs, milk, and such processed foods as bacon, ham, bread, and crackers. Chloride is a constituent of hydrochloric acid, which is concentrated in gastric (stomach) juices and is necessary for the functioning of the digestive system. People who perspire heavily may have to add salt to their diet, but most people eat too much salt because of their high consumption of processed foods and added table salt. Surplus salt increases water retention and, in predisposed individuals, has been associated with edema (excess fluid retention in the tissues) and high blood pressure.

Potassium

Potassium, mainly present in the fluid in cells, regulates the balance and volume of body fluids in tandem with sodium. Because most foods (both plant and animal) are rich in potassium, a nutritional deficiency is very rare, although it may occur in conjunction with prolonged diarrhea, use of diuretics (medications that remove water from the body), or a diet that lacks protein. Use of potassium supplements without medical supervision is very dangerous.

Magnesium

Magnesium is contained mostly in bones, although it is present in all body tissues. It is vital to the enzymes that help convert food into energy. Magnesium deficiencies usually occur only in postsurgical patients, alcoholics, and others who do not eat a well-balanced diet. Magnesium-rich foods include whole-grain cereals, dried peas and beans, cocoa, nuts, seafood, and dark-green vegetables.

Sulfur

Sulfur, found in all tissues, is a part of several important amino acids and of the vitamins thiamin and biotin. It is not fully understood how it works in the body.

Iron

Iron is found throughout the body, chiefly in the blood, liver, spleen, and bone marrow. It is an integral part of the compounds that are necessary to transport oxygen to the cells and to regulate its use there. Foods that provide significant amounts of iron include liver, seafood, meats, egg yolks, fish, green vegetables, and dried peas and beans.

An inadequate supply of iron in the diet causes iron deficiency anemia, which most often affects women in their reproductive years (especially pregnant women), infants, and teenagers (particularly during the adolescent growth spurt).

Manganese

Manganese is fundamental for the normal building of tendons and bones and is part of some enzymes. Foods rich in this mineral include whole-grain breads and cereals, coffee, tea, nuts, peas, and beans. Deficiency in humans is virtually unknown.

Copper

Copper, an element involved in the storage and release of iron to form the oxygen-carrying hemoglobin in red blood cells, is most vital in the early months of life. If a pregnant woman's intake is sufficient, her baby will be born with enough copper. It is most available in processed foods, organ meats, shellfish, nuts, and dried peas and beans.

Iodine

Iodine is indispensable to the normal working of the thyroid gland. A shortage can result in goiter (thyroid enlargement). Before the introduction of iodized salt in the United States in 1924, iodine-deficiency goiter was common in inland areas. Foods from the sea are rich in iodine.

Zinc

Zinc is a fundamental part of the enzymes that move carbon dioxide in the red blood cells from the tissues to the lungs for exhalation. A deficiency of zinc may show up as a loss of the sense of taste or delayed healing of wounds. Associated with protein, zinc is found in meats (especially liver), cheese, dried beans and peas, seafood, egg yolks, and milk. Although it is available in whole-grain cereal, it is not likely to be absorbed because of the presence of other substances.

Cobalt

Cobalt is not needed in the body by itself, but is part of cyanocobalamin (vitamin B_{12}), which is available in meat, eggs, fish, and dairy products.

Chromium

Chromium acts with insulin in the use of glucose (a form of sugar). A shortage produces a condition that is similar to diabetes. Chromium is present in dried brewer's yeast, whole-grain cereals, and liver.

Selenium

Selenium appears to work in conjunction with vitamin E. Not much is known about selenium, except that it is important in the body and that it is found in animals and plants where it is accessible in the earth. A deficiency may cause muscle pain and impairment of heart function.

Fluoride

Fluoride is important in the formation of teeth and resistance to dental caries (cavities), especially in children, and may help maintain calcium in the bones of the elderly. It is available in fluoridated water, seafood, and meats.

AVOIDING HAZARDOUS SUBSTANCES TO STAY HEALTHY

The nation's leading recreational drugs are alcohol, tobacco, cocaine, and marijuana. All are used by both adults and minors, although only the first two are legal—and only for adults. All are powerful substances that can be addictive to young and old alike and that have the capacity to injure or destroy the body.

The perspective from which to view these hazardous substances when considering changes in your lifestyle is that this is one area of your life over which you can exercise control. There are many situations that threaten our good health that we cannot prevent or avoid—for example, aging, being exposed to microorganisms and environmental pollutants, and suffering from inherited disorders. But the risks posed by the substances discussed in this section can be controlled by limiting or avoiding their use.

Alcohol

In cultures around the world, drinking alcohol is generally a socially acceptable way for adults to relax and enjoy themselves. In moderation, drinking alcohol is a fairly harmless prac-

tice for most people. However, alcohol is a central nervous system depressant. The short-term effects can disrupt mental and motor-skills, resulting in bad judgment, poor coordination, and a tendency to have accidents. Consumed heavily on a regular basis, alcohol damages internal organs, especially the liver and the heart.

The fact that alcohol is so prevalent and acceptable in our society makes it easier to form a dependence on it—a good reason why those who drink should examine their drinking habits from time to time. It has been estimated that one American in ten suffers from alcoholism at some time in his or her life.

Alcoholism

Alcoholism is a disorder in which a person repeatedly drinks excessive amounts of alcoholic beverages, with resulting harm to health, relations with other people, and work performance. The person becomes physically and psychologically dependent on alcohol. There is a genuine craving for alcohol when it is withdrawn for one to three days, and unpleasant responses such as delirium tremens (characterized by a severe stress reaction, hallucinations, and tremors) and convulsions may be seen when alcohol is not available.

Causes of alcoholism

Various causes of alcoholism have been suggested. These include depression, self-hatred, and having a shy, lonely, immature, or dependent personality. Some societies and groups within those societies encourage overuse of alcohol as recreation

and as an escape from life's problems. There is also evidence that a tendency to alcoholism may be inherited or may be the result of a chemical defect. Whatever the cause, alcoholism is a self-damaging disease and an ineffective way to deal with life.

Symptoms of alcoholism

The fact that a person is an alcoholic is not always obvious. Alcoholics often do not recognize their own alcoholism, or they try to hide symptoms from spouses, other family members, friends, and employers. Signs of alcoholism include:
• Frequent drunkenness
• Tolerance to alcohol (A great deal of liquor is required before the person shows signs of intoxication; however, this is not true in all cases, especially if alcohol has damaged the liver.)
• Physical dependence, resulting in withdrawal symptoms a day or more after stopping drinking (Symptoms may range from tremors and physical pain to seizures and hallucinations.)
• Continued drinking even when it is harming the person's health and personal life
• Poor job performance
• Depression
Other signs may include an odor of liquor on the breath in the morning, stealthy drinking, suspicious work absences (to sleep off hangovers), and frequent falls, accidents, and cigarette burns on hands and body (caused by drunken carelessness).

Alcoholism can cause permanent damage to the liver, brain, heart, and nervous system. Moderate to heavy drinking by a pregnant woman can result in mental retardation in her baby, as well as low birth weight and birth defects.

If an alcoholic has been drinking as much as a gallon of beer or a pint of whiskey a day for several months, sudden withdrawal of alcohol may even result in death because of convulsions or delirium tremens.

Treatment of alcoholism

Alcoholism is not a cause for shame or embarrassment, nor is it a sign of failure or degeneracy. It is a disease that, like any other, requires professional treatment, not only for the alcoholic's sake but also for the sake of the others—family, friends, and coworkers—whose lives he or she affects.

Treatment of severe alcoholism involves two stages: immediate and long-term. Both require a physician's attention.

The first step is to stop the drinking while treating the symptoms of withdrawal. The drug disulfiram is sometimes prescribed, to be taken daily by mouth; it causes vomiting if the patient drinks anything alcoholic. It stops the person from drinking, but the patient may refuse to continue taking it because of its unpleasant effects.

In most situations, withdrawal is best done in a hospital alcoholic unit under a doctor's care. Psychological support and reassurance may be enough to comfort the patient during the withdrawal stage. Frequently, however, other measures are needed. The patient may be undernourished from drinking so much and eating so little and may need replacement doses of vitamins, particularly thiamin (vitamin B_1). Fluids containing glucose (a form of sugar) and salt water may be added to the blood, which has been robbed of water and glu-

cose by the effects of overuse of alcohol. Tranquilizing drugs are given to help ease withdrawal symptoms, which usually peak at 48 to 72 hours and may continue for days. In severe cases, withdrawal seizures can occur. If the individual is not in a hospital where these can be immediately treated, serious consequences—even death—can result.

Long-term treatment may include psychiatric help to treat the problem that caused the alcoholism in the first place, such as depression or mental illness. For many alcoholics, the solution is to join an organization known as Alcoholics Anonymous (AA). Members help each other overcome their drinking problems and vow to stay away from alcohol completely. In helping each other, they develop confidence and positive feelings about themselves.

Prevention of alcoholism

Alcoholism is a significant social and medical problem that cannot be easily stopped. However, its threat may be diminished by:

- Learning about the full extent of its dangers
- Finding more healthful ways to deal with life's problems and disappointments—by facing, rather than avoiding, them
- Learning to recognize the symptoms of alcoholism
- Seeking help from a physician or a group like Alcoholics Anonymous

Cocaine

Cocaine is prepared from the leaves of the plant *Erythroxylon coca*. The earliest known use of

the coca plant dates back to approximately A.D. 600. However, it was not until 1855 that cocaine was isolated from coca leaves.

Use

In recent years, there has been an enormous increase in cocaine use. At present, it is estimated that some ten million Americans have used cocaine and that about five million use it on a regular basis. Since the drug is relatively expensive, users often believe that it puts them in an elite group, and they frequently take the drug to boost their self-esteem. Multiple drug use is common among cocaine users, with most also using alcohol or marijuana.

Cocaine is usually used in one of four ways: nasal inhalation of the powdered form ("snorting"), intravenous injection, smoking the crystalline form ("crack"), or inhalation of the vapor ("freebasing"). Free-basing is an extremely dangerous technique, rapidly delivering high concentrations of cocaine into the central nervous system.

Effects

Cocaine is best known for its effect as a central nervous system stimulant. At lower doses, cocaine produces talkativeness, euphoria (a heightened sense of well-being), excitement, enormous self-confidence, and a deceptive sense of increased concentration. At higher doses, tremors, seizures, and severe mental disorders can develop. Cocaine also impairs the appetite; with chronic (long-term) use, poor nutritional intake results.

Cocaine also acts by impairing the control of neurologic hormones at nerve endings throughout the body. This causes the heart rate to increase rapidly, the heart to beat irregularly, and the blood vessels to constrict; this combination of events results in a rapid rise in blood pressure. There have been frequent reports of healthy young adults suffering a stroke or heart attack due to the acute effects of cocaine.

According to a number of recent studies, a pregnant woman who uses cocaine endangers not only her own health but also that of her unborn child. Associated with cocaine use in pregnancy is an increased risk of miscarriage, as well as a greater incidence of premature births. Infants have been born addicted to the drug and have suffered severe neurologic and behavioral consequences as a result of their mothers' drug habits.

Treatment

In the past, it was thought that cocaine is not addictive and does not produce dependence or a withdrawal syndrome. However, with the increasing use of cocaine (in particular, large amounts of free-base cocaine), it has become apparent that a withdrawal syndrome does exist. This syndrome usually consists of depression, irritability, sleep disturbance, gastrointestinal upset, and headaches. The onset of the syndrome begins approximately 24 to 48 hours after cessation of cocaine use and lasts seven to ten days. The emotional and psychological effects of cocaine addiction, however, can last indefinitely.

Because of the diversity of reasons for cocaine use, a multifaceted approach to the treatment of patients is required. The goals of treatment include the cessation of all chemical abuse, the restoration of normal patterns of behavior, and the development of new attitudes and more positive ways of coping with life's problems. Hospitalization is required for every patient for whom outpatient attempts to cease cocaine use have repeatedly failed or for whom severe complications in physical, psychological, or social functioning exist. Cocaine addiction, like any other addiction, is a long-term problem, with remissions (periods when the disorder seems to get better) and exacerbations (periods when it gets worse). As with any chronic disease, treatment must continue on a long-term basis.

Marijuana

Marijuana, or cannabis, is the dried flower clusters, stems, and leaves of the Indian hemp plant (*Cannabis sativa*). It looks like coarse tobacco. It is also known as "weed," "pot," "grass," "tea," and "Mary Jane," as well as a number of other slang equivalents.

Marijuana has been smoked, drunk, eaten, and sniffed throughout recorded history. When marijuana is rolled into a cigarette, it is called a "joint" or a "reefer." When it is smoked, it has a very distinctive odor.

Immediate effects

All of the effects of smoking or ingesting marijuana are not yet known because long-term studies are still under way. It is known that marijuana raises the heart rate by as much as 50 percent and lowers sex-hormone and fertility levels in both males and females.

Visible symptoms of marijuana use include reddened eyes, dilated pupils, and lack of physical coordination. Sometimes, users feel lethargic and nauseated. Reactions to marijuana differ: Some users feel happy, talkative, and silly; others may become withdrawn.

Marijuana relaxes the body and the mind. It gives a feeling of exhilaration and euphoria. In addition, marijuana alters perceptions—colors seem brighter, music more intense—and gives a sense of time being extended. However, these effects are often accompanied or followed by mood swings, panic, depression, hallucinations, and fear of death, particularly if marijuana is being used in combination with other drugs.

Marijuana does not increase intellectual functioning or creative capacity, although it may produce that impression during use. Actually, marijuana affects the brain by interfering with the ability to think, to make judgments, and to solve problems. Marijuana also slows reaction time and hinders coordination and visual perception. For these reasons, driving a car while under the influence of marijuana is dangerous.

Long-term effects

It is believed that use of marijuana may cause long-term physical effects, including damage to the brain, heart, lungs, and reproductive system.

Users of marijuana often experience a decrease in motivation and become psychologically dependent on the drug because it represents a way to avoid facing the problems and stresses of life.

Marijuana users do not, however, appear to become physically addicted to it and generally do not suffer serious physical withdrawal reactions when they abstain from its use. Most users of marijuana do not progress to use of hard drugs, such as heroin or cocaine, although that risk does exist.

Occasional use of marijuana does not appear to pose highly dangerous long-term effects. Nevertheless, there are several reasons for concern about the use of this substance. First, much of the marijuana used is smoked by young people in their formative years; they tend to use the drug more regularly than adults. Second, improved methods of cultivation have resulted in harvests of the plant that are increasingly more potent. Third, unlike alcohol, the mind-altering chemical in marijuana can remain in the body for a week or more. Fourth, because the substance is illegal, there are no quality controls over its content; large quantities of marijuana have been found to be contaminated with pesticides or laced with more dangerous or addictive narcotics. Fifth, because marijuana cigarettes do not have filters, their smoke irritates lung tissue much more than the smoke of regular filtered cigarettes. Marijuana cigarettes also contain more tar and benzopyrene (a cancer-causing agent) than do tobacco cigarettes.

Tobacco

Tobacco use usually begins as a social behavior and results in significant physical consequences to the body. Cigarette smoke is much more hazardous in this regard than pipe or cigar smoke. Cigarette smoking is habit-forming, and the accumulated effects of this habit increase the risks for the development of life-threatening disease.

The chemical makeup of cigarette smoke is complicated and still under scientific investigation. One of the chemicals in tobacco is tar, a powerful carcinogen (cancer-causing agent). Another chemical, nicotine, produces harmful effects on the nervous system. Various chemicals in tobacco interfere with other biochemical processes and body functions.

Links to cancer

Smoking cigarettes, pipes, and cigars and chewing smokeless tobacco have been linked to oral cancers. Oral cancers include those of the mouth, lips, salivary glands, tongue, and throat. Symptoms of oral cancers include a persistent sore, which may bleed; a thickened area; discoloration; difficulty in chewing or swallowing; and persistent sore throat. Such symptoms should be called to a physician's attention immediately.

Cigarette smoking has also been implicated in lung cancer. Initially, cigarette smoke may destroy the tiny hairs that normally function in clearing away mucus in the respiratory tract. The bronchial lining may then undergo changes that result in cancer-cell production. Early symptoms of lung cancer may include coughing, wheezing, and chest pain. Anyone with a history of smoking should be alert to these symptoms. If you have not smoked cigarettes, your chances of developing lung cancer are very greatly reduced. If you do have a history of smoking, stopping will decrease your risk of developing lung cancer.

Links to chronic respiratory diseases

Emphysema and chronic bronchitis are most often caused by cigarette smoking. Both of these diseases are considered chronic obstructive pulmonary diseases (COPDs), in which there is airway blockage. Emphysema and chronic bronchitis frequently co-exist. In emphysema, abnormally large amounts of air accumulate in the alveoli (the tiny air sacs of the lungs), making exhalation especially difficult. In chronic bronchitis, the bronchi (the large airways connecting the windpipe and the lungs) undergo changes that impede the flow of air into the lungs.

The initial symptom of emphysema is shortness of breath. This may be accompanied by a persistent cough. Progression of the disease, usually occurring over a course of years, results in severe breathing difficulty and restriction of activity. In chronic bronchitis, a persistent cough develops initially and is usually accompanied by excessive production of mucus. If you experience shortness of breath or develop a persistent cough, consult your physician. Stopping smoking will generally provide the best means of slowing the course of these diseases in smokers. Fortunately, emphysema and chronic bronchitis can usually be prevented by avoiding cigarette smoking.

Links to circulatory disorders

Stopping smoking can also significantly reduce the incidence of arteriosclerosis, in which the walls of the arteries thicken and lose elasticity. This condition is associated with heart attacks and strokes.

Interactions with medications

Smoking can also produce indirect adverse reactions in the body. Chemicals in smoke can interfere with the action of some medications by altering the absorption rate and duration of effect. Always mention your smoking habits to the physician when drugs are being prescribed. The physician will then be able to make the proper adjustments in dosage.

Effects on nonsmokers

Nonsmokers who continuously breathe the cigarette smoke of others are known as passive smokers. Research indicates that passive smokers suffer ill effects from exposure to cigarette smoke, including increased heart rates and blood pressure levels and constriction of the airways in the lungs. Children are especially vulnerable to the respiratory effects of breathing "second-hand" smoke.

Breaking the smoking habit

Stopping smoking is beneficial to yourself and to those around you, even if there are not yet any signs of disease. Unfortunately, despite the proved medical risks of tobacco use, many smokers who want to quit seem unable to break the habit. For those who cannot do it on their own, help is available from many sources, such as the American Cancer Society and the American Lung Association.

Nicotine in the form of gum has been on the market for several years. Since nicotine is a dangerous drug, the gum is available only by physician's prescription. The gum can ease the physical symptoms of withdrawal from nicotine while the individual removes cigarettes from his or her routine. However, certain people with medical conditions such as heart or blood pressure problems may not be able to use the preparation. Further, it must be remembered that nicotine is a drug, and directions for use of the gum must be strictly followed.

Many over-the-counter preparations are also available as nicotine substitutes. Check with your doctor prior to using one of these. The purpose of such items is to make quitting smoking less unpleasant, not to substitute one habit for another.

If you want to try quitting by yourself, it may help first to figure out why you smoke and then to substitute other activities or substances when you feel the urge to light up. The motivation for smoking may be addiction, habit, a response to anxiety, a need to have something to do with the mouth and hands, or a desire for stimulation or relaxation.

There is no single method for quitting smoking that is right for everyone. Ex-smokers have quit in a variety of ways. If one plan fails, try another; if you don't succeed the first time, keep trying. Remember, smoking is a learned behavior that can be changed.

YOU AND YOUR DOCTOR

Most people never think about how to choose a doctor until they need one in a hurry. When a person is injured or suddenly becomes ill, finding a good doctor is a necessity, and there is often no time to spare in the search.

If a person does not have a family doctor, injury or sudden illness often means a quick visit to the emergency room or outpatient section of the nearest hospital, where staff physicians who may know little about the patient's personal medical history must treat him or her symptomatically and, often, on an urgent basis. This is usually not a good way to establish a lasting physician-patient relationship.

A better way to assure yourself of medical care is to have a personal physician who is familiar with you and your family's medical history and who is available (or has associates who are available) when you need care. In this way, your health needs will be met by someone who knows you and whom you know.

The best time, then, to choose a doctor is when you don't need one. You should never wait until you have no choice about the doctor you see. How do you choose a doctor? Here are some guidelines for making an informed choice.

Choosing a family doctor

Many families want a doctor who is familiar both with family members as individuals and with the family as a group. Doctors who have specialized in family medicine are called family practitioners. Their education and training enable them not only to provide medical care but also to recognize and handle the social, emotional, and psychological factors that affect the health and well-being of patients and their families. Whereas a physician needs to have only one year of internship (postgraduate hospital training, usually divided among several branches of medicine) before entering general practice, today's family practitioner completes a one-year internship and a two-year residency in family practice. During that time, he or she receives more intensive training in general surgery, internal medicine, obstetrics/gynecology, and pediatrics, among other fields.

Family practitioners care for all the members of a family, so there is usually no need for a different specialist for each individual. A family practitioner is well equipped to handle most aspects of medical care, such as uncomplicated pregnancies, immunizations, and routine physicals. A family practitioner can generally diagnose and treat all of the common ailments, as well as many of the uncommon ones, and can guide you to the right specialist when you need one.

In addition to providing comprehensive medical care for all family members, today's family practitioner is as interested in *maintaining* your good health as in curing or treating illness. The family practitioner's overall goal is to treat each family member as an individual with physical, emotional, and social needs, as well as medical requirements.

How can you find a family practitioner who is right for your family? You can call the county medical society or your state medical society. These organizations have uniform requirements for physicians to be admitted to their membership (for example, completion of appropriate training and board certification). They also can tell you where you can find a specialist. However, these societies do not offer an opinion on the overall quality of a physician. This is something you must assess for yourself.

Another valuable source is the physician referral service of your local hospital. This service will give you the names of family physicians who are on staff and are accepting new patients.

You should also ask people in your neighborhood about their doctors. They may be able to offer suggestions based on personal experience with local physicians. In addition, if you live in a city, you may find that there is a local organization that evaluates the medical profession on behalf of the consumer. Neighborhood consumer groups often will make medical referral information available to you at no charge and will steer you toward physicians who have a record of treating their patients with respect and concern.

In the process of selecting a family physician, you should draw up a list of basic questions to ask the doctor, including:

- Will the doctor treat all family members?
- Does the doctor provide care during pregnancy and perform deliveries?
- Does the doctor have staff privileges at a nearby accredited hospital?
- Does the doctor perform surgery? If so, what kind?
- Does the doctor encourage preventive medicine, such as routine checkups, immunizations, and follow-up tests?
- Does the doctor make emergency house calls for bedridden family members?
- Does the doctor have office hours that are convenient for your family, especially for

those who work or attend school?

- What arrangement does the doctor have for a substitute when he or she is unavailable?
- What are the fees for the various services?
- Is the doctor certified by the American Board of Family Practice (or a specialty board of another area)?

The answers to these questions, along with the recommendations of friends and neighbors, will help you select the right doctor for you and your family.

How to choose a specialist

In approaching the problem of finding a specialist, you should remember that most specialists receive their patients through referrals from family doctors or from other specialists. Many have a policy of not accepting a patient who has not first been examined and referred by a family doctor. This is a method of making sure that those who really need specialists see them and that those who do not need them do not incur the expense that seeing a specialist entails.

Your family doctor will usually decide whether your medical complaint needs the attention of a specialist. For example, if you have a mild inflammation of the ear canal, your family doctor is quite capable of treating it. If there is chronic inflammation of the ear canal, however, or if you have suffered a partial loss of hearing, your doctor will probably refer you to an otorhinolaryngologist (ear, nose, and throat specialist).

You must also remember that difficulties in one area of the body affect other areas, so a spe-

cialist is not always needed to diagnose and treat a problem. For example, visual problems may be limited to abnormalities in the eye itself, but they may also be the result of a wide variety of causes, including diabetes, hardening of the arteries, a stroke, or a tumor in a part of the brain that controls vision. The human body is an organic system. Changes in one part of the system affect other parts, and no part of the system functions in isolation. Consequently, the first task in treating an illness is to discover the underlying primary cause of the ailment. When the culprit is found, you may then be referred to a specialist who deals with the specific area of the body most affected by that problem.

The first line of action in selecting a specialist is to follow your family doctor's advice. He or she will know whether you need a specialist. However, you can always ask for a second opinion or seek out a specialist on your own. If for no other reason than to know that you did all you were able to do, you should always try to get as much information as possible about your own or a family member's illness. You may even find something that the doctors missed.

If your family doctor refers you to a specialist, or if you seek one on your own, you should know what each specialty consists of and what to expect when you see each specialist. The following section gives you a brief description of more than 30 medical and surgical specialties. As you read about each one, remember that an internship is the period immediately after graduation from medical school, during which a doctor receives supervised practical experience in a hospital setting. A residency, also supervised in a hospital setting,

follows an internship; it is a period of advanced training in a doctor's chosen medical specialty. As noted in the following section, the length of residency varies, depending on the specialty. Even within a specialty, however, the length of residency may vary from one medical center to another and may change with time. Board certification means that a doctor has been certified as meeting the professional standards of a medical specialty organization called a board, which requires completion of a residency at an accredited institution, acceptable performance on a rigorous set of examinations, and, in some fields, a year or two of clinical experience.

Allergy and immunology

This branch of medicine is concerned with the study, diagnosis, and treatment of disorders related to immunity (the body's ability to resist disease or threatening substances). The body's immune system fights against the intrusion of outside forces, whether they are irritating substances that cause allergic reactions or microorganisms that cause infection. This is the system that helps us fight off illness every day of our lives. Modern immunological research indicates that many infections can be as much a result of defects in a person's immune system as they are a result of exposure to viruses or bacteria.

Immunologists are also studying the role of the immune system in cancer growth. It may someday be possible to prevent cancer by modifying the immune system to reject cancerous growths in the body. Immunologists are also interested in the opposite effect of the immune system—the rejection of foreign substances that are actually beneficial (the most obvious example is an organ transplant). Immunologists are seeking ways to make the immune system work selectively, so that the body would reject cancer cells but accept a new heart, kidney, or liver.

The best-known branch of immunology deals with allergies, which are responses of the body's immune system to irritating substances in the environment. Doctors who practice as allergists are involved in identifying environmental irritants that cause symptoms and in formulating a plan of treatment. Allergists may treat allergies by suggesting environmental modifications to eliminate the offending substance or by using drugs to relieve the symptoms. Another option is a program of desensitization, which involves injecting minute amounts of the offending agent to make the immune system less sensitive to it. Once such a program has been set up, your family doctor can often give the injections. Allergists also consult in the management of certain diseases, such as asthma.

An immunologist must complete a residency in internal medicine or pediatrics after graduating from medical school. After this residency, he or she completes a two-year fellowship program in allergy and immunology. Specialty board examinations are also required.

Anesthesiology

With the use of anesthetics, surgery may be done without pain during the procedure. Many minor procedures may be done with a local anesthetic (a pain-killer that is usually injected into or rubbed onto the affected area), but more complex procedures require that the patient be unconscious.

An anesthesiologist is a specialist in the use of those drugs that cause a cessation of the experience of pain. Anesthesiologists must complete medical school, an internship, and a residency in their specialty before starting their practice. They may also receive some training in a field other than anesthesiology, such as internal medicine, pediatrics, or obstetrics. Some of them also do tours of surgical residency to broaden and deepen their knowledge of surgical techniques and needs.

Bariatrics

Bariatrics is a relatively new field in medicine, brought into popularity by the public's keen interest in the problems of being overweight.

Bariatricians have been making advances in what is known about being overweight or underweight by dispelling myths and substituting hard scientific evidence. Their training usually includes an internship in internal medicine, with a special residency in bariatrics. Bariatricians are certified by their specialty group, the American Society of Bariatric Physicians.

Cardiology

Cardiology is a branch of internal medicine that deals with the diagnosis and treatment of disorders of the heart and circulatory system, including those that stem from birth abnormalities, childhood diseases, or advancing age. Cardiologists take care of a variety of heart conditions, such as rheumatic heart disease in children and congestive heart failure and heart attacks in adults.

Cardiology and cardiovascular surgery complement each other. Over the years, doctors in these fields have worked closely together in the treatment of heart diseases. For example, the cardiologist may determine that a child has been born with a hole between the chambers of the heart; the cardiovascular surgeon is the one who will repair this hole through open-heart surgery.

In the past few years, many advances in the medical and surgical treatment of heart disease have been made. A cardiologist must be acquainted not only with anatomy and physiology, but also with modern computerized diagnostic equipment. One special diagnostic procedure performed by cardiologists is cardiac catheterization, in which a catheter (a long, thin, flexible tube) is inserted into the heart and adjacent blood vessels, allowing the injection of a special dye that affords visualization of those structures. Angioplasty (the opening of a blocked artery by insertion of a balloon-tipped catheter) is a treatment procedure that is commonly performed by cardiologists.

Training in cardiology includes completion of a residency in internal medicine, followed by at least two years of specialized training in cardiology.

Cardiovascular surgery

The cardiovascular surgeon performs many different types of surgery on the heart and blood vessels, including replacement of heart valves and bypasses of blocked coronary arteries. Open-heart surgery came into its own during the 1950s and underwent further refinement in the 1960s and 1970s. Two decades have passed since the first human heart transplant. In 1982, the first implantation of an artificial heart took place.

Training in cardiovascular surgery includes the completion of a general surgery residency, followed by two or three years of specialized training.

Dentistry

Dentistry is concerned with the prevention, diagnosis, and treatment of diseases, disorders, and malformations of the teeth, mouth, and jaws. Most people select a dentist with a general practice who can provide routine dental care and, if necessary, recommend a dental specialist for those conditions needing specialized treatment. Some of the dental specialties include:
- Orthodontia (straightening of teeth)
- Periodontia (treatment of gums and underlying bone)
- Endodontia (root canal)
- Exodontia (extraction of teeth)

A dentist planning to establish a general practice will complete four years of dental school and perhaps an optional one-year general residency. Dental specialists have additional specific training in their specialty.

Finding a family dentist is much like finding a family doctor. You should ask friends and neighbors for recommendations or contact your local dental society. Your family doctor may also be able to suggest a dentist.

Dermatology

Dermatology is the study of diseases and disorders of the skin, ranging from acne to psoriasis to skin cancer.

The dermatologist must also be knowledgeable about diseases that primarily affect other parts of the body but that may have some bearing on the skin. In addition, dermatologists have training in allergies, since many skin conditions have been recognized as allergic reactions.

Dermatologists are required to do an internship, usually in internal medicine, followed by a three-year residency in dermatology.

Endocrinology

When we think of "messages" being sent throughout the body, we usually think of the nervous system. But there is another communication system in the body, called the endocrine system. It is made up of the ductless glands, including the pituitary gland, the adrenal glands, the thyroid gland, the parathyroid glands, the islet cells in the pancreas, the ovaries (in women), and the testes (in men). These glands secrete hormones that travel as messengers throughout the body to direct and integrate many bodily functions. Disorders of the system include diabetes, Cushing's syndrome, and growth abnormalities.

An endocrinologist is a specialist in the diagnosis and treatment of disorders of the endocrine system. He or she must complete an internship and a residency in internal medicine, followed by two years of training in endocrinology.

Epidemiology

Specialists in this medical field study the outbreak, frequency, distribution, and control of communicable diseases. The unofficial headquarters of this activity is the Centers for Disease Control (once the Communicable Disease Center) in Atlanta, Georgia.

Epidemiology deals not only with communication of disease in general, but also with the specific conditions under which certain diseases seem to flourish. For example, the relatively new field of urban epidemiology specifically addresses itself to those diseases and conditions peculiar to city settings. In addition, epidemiologists work to devise ways of preventing disease, such as developing vaccines.

Epidemiology is also concerned with causes of illness other than infectious diseases. For example, lead poisoning as a result of eating lead-based paint was a major cause of brain damage among children before epidemiologists discovered the connection. Epidemiologists have led the medical field in seeking environmental causes for a host of disorders once attributed to bacteria or other sources. Air and water pollution, toxic substances in foods, toxic substances used in the manufacture of a variety of products—all have come under the scrutiny of the epidemiologist.

Epidemiology attracts physicians not only from internal medicine but also from other fields, such as immunology, occupational medicine, and pediatrics. An epidemiologist will usually have completed three years of specialized training and a year of independent research or teaching.

Gastroenterology

A gastroenterologist specializes in the diagnosis and treatment of diseases and disorders of the stomach and the intestines, as well as related organs that help in the digestive process, such as the esophagus, liver, and pancreas. Gastritis (inflammation of the stomach), enteritis (inflammation of the intestinal tract), ulcers, inability to digest certain foods, constipation, diarrhea, hyperacidity, and heartburn are among the disorders treated by the gastroenterologist.

Gastroenterologists often use the procedure called endoscopy, in which a flexible tubelike instrument is used to directly view hollow organs, such as the esophagus, stomach, and colon. Diagnosis and treatment of many conditions, such as ulcers and polyps, may be done with this procedure. Biopsies (in which tissue samples are gathered for testing) are also carried out with endoscopy.

These specialists are trained as internists or pediatricians with an additional two-year fellowship in gastroenterology.

Hematology

Hematology is the study of diseases and disorders of the blood and the blood-forming tissues, such as the bone marrow and the spleen. A hematologist is proficient in a wide range of diagnostic techniques in which blood and bone marrow samples are used to shed light on disease processes. Blood analyses can aid in developing treatment for a patient. The hematologist's primary concern, however, is the host of diseases and disorders relative to the blood itself, including inability of the red blood cells to carry sufficient oxygen, inability of the white blood cells to fight against invading microorganisms, and inability of the

bone marrow to manufacture enough red blood cells. The hematologist is also an expert on cancer of the blood (leukemia) and on blood clotting problems, such as hemophilia.

The hematologist must be firmly grounded not only in internal medicine, anatomy, and physiology, but also in biochemistry. Knowledge of computerized diagnostic equipment and sophisticated biochemical analyses is also necessary.

A hematologist completes an internship and a residency in internal medicine plus two years of training in hematology. Hematologists are also trained as oncologists (cancer specialists).

Internal medicine

Internal medicine is the branch of medicine that deals with the diagnosis and treatment of diseases of adults, except for those conditions that require management by a surgeon or an obstetrician. Like the family practitioner, the internist is trained to handle a wide range of illnesses; in fact, many people select an internist as their family doctor. The internist is specifically trained to deal with chronic (long-term) illnesses, such as diabetes and high blood pressure, and acute (short-term) diseases, such as infections. In addition, an internist has both the range and the depth to diagnose illnesses that might escape detection by a specialist if they lie outside his or her special field. For this reason, internists are often called diagnosticians.

After graduating from medical school, an internist completes one year of internship, followed by two years of residency in internal medicine. Internal medicine is also the basis for many other

specialties, such as cardiology, endocrinology, gastroenterology, hematology, and nephrology. That is why these branches are often referred to as subspecialties, and the doctors who practice them as subspecialists. In order to become a subspecialist, an internist must complete at least two years of additional training, referred to as a fellowship, in his or her chosen subspecialty before becoming eligible for subspecialty board certification.

Nephrology

Nephrologists treat kidney disorders. Their patients are usually referred to them by internists when kidney problems are diagnosed as needing special care. In treating kidney disorders, the nephrologist may make use of medications or dialysis (removal of wastes and other undesirable substances from the blood by means of a special machine). Referral for surgery (for example, if a transplant is indicated) is also initiated by a nephrologist. Nephrologists also perform kidney biopsies, which are used to diagnose and follow up a number of kidney diseases.

Nephrologists are thoroughly grounded in internal medicine, with special attention to the physiological processes performed by the kidneys. Because of the complex nature of kidney function, they must be equally well grounded in biochemistry and the tools of modern biochemical analysis. A nephrologist must also be familiar with all of the latest computerized diagnostic equipment, as well as the latest in dialysis machines.

Training includes internship and a residency in internal medicine, followed by a two-year fellowship in nephrology, after which the specialty board examinations may be taken.

Neurology

Neurology is the field of medical science that is concerned with the nervous system—the brain, the spinal cord, and the complex network of nerves. Clinical neurology concerns itself specifically with the diagnosis and treatment of diseases of the nervous system, but the neurologist must be familiar with the total functioning of the body because disorders of other systems can affect the nervous system and vice versa.

Training in neurology includes a one-year internal medicine internship, followed by a three-year residency in neurology.

Obstetrics/gynecology

The fields of obstetrics and gynecology are closely related, and physicians generally practice these specialties together. While gynecology encompasses the diagnosis and treatment of disorders of the female reproductive system, obstetrics deals specifically with pregnancy, childbirth, and related conditions.

Many obstetricians are members of a group practice. Most obstetric groups make sure that every doctor in the group either has seen or is familiar with each patient during her pregnancy. Thus, when it comes time for delivery, the mother will generally be taken care of by a doctor whom she knows.

After medical school, an obstetrician/gynecologist completes a four-year residency. During this time, he or she will also receive some training in internal medi-

cine, general surgery, and care of the newborn infant.

The obstetrician/gynecologist often acts as the primary caregiver for women. He or she will also work closely with other medical specialists if specific problems occur that do not directly involve the reproductive system.

Occupational medicine

Occupational medicine began with industrial and business clinics, which were usually staffed by a physician and an industrial nurse (one who has specialized in the care of patients within a working environment). Occupational medicine has grown to include the study, diagnosis, and treatment of a vast range of illnesses caused by the industrial environment itself. Asbestos-induced cancer, "black lung" (in which coal dust literally turns the inside of the lungs black, with accompanying damage to the lungs), allergic reactions to industrial fibers, eye damage from welding arcs, and injury to the feet from jobs that require standing are but a few of the hundreds of disorders treated by occupational medicine physicians.

Specialists in occupational medicine generally have a strong background in internal medicine, with special training in the causes of industry-related illnesses. Often these doctors complete a public health program before going on to their specialty residency.

Oncology

Oncology is the study of tumors, particularly cancer. This relatively new field is often associated with hematology (the

study of the blood). Strictly speaking, oncology deals only with solid tumors and not with cancers of the blood. Today, however, hematologist-oncologists are certified to deal with both types of cancer.

Oncology requires expertise in a large number of medical and technical disciplines, from surgery to nutrition, from immunology to biochemistry, from diagnosis of symptoms to treatment of tumors with nuclear radiation.

There are subspecialties within the field of oncology. The medical oncologist is primarily responsible for prescribing and implementing chemotherapy, along with diagnosing and treating complications unique to cancer and coordinating the total treatment plan for cancer patients. Surgical oncologists perform cancer surgery. Pediatric oncologists diagnose and treat cancer in children. Gynecologic oncologists deal with cancer that occurs in the female reproductive system.

After graduating from medical school, a medical oncologist completes an internship and residency in internal medicine, followed by an additional training program in oncology, which includes training in hematology and chemotherapy. Surgical oncologists are usually general surgeons who have completed a fellowship in cancer surgery. Pediatric and gynecologic oncologists are first certified in their respective fields and then go on to oncology fellowships.

Ophthalmology

An ophthalmologist is a medical doctor who diagnoses and treats diseases and injuries of the eyes. Most ophthalmologists are also eye surgeons. They perform a variety of operations, such as reattaching retinas, removing cataracts, relieving pressure caused by glaucoma, and repairing blood vessel ruptures and other injuries.

Ophthalmologists have a background in both internal medicine and surgery. This specialty requires an additional three- or four-year residency in ophthalmology after a one-year general internship before specialty board examinations may be taken.

There are allied health-care workers who are often referred to as "eye doctors," but who are not medical doctors and therefore are not permitted to treat diseases of the eyes or to prescribe drugs. An optometrist tests the eyes for the purpose of fitting a person with glasses or contact lenses. An optician makes and fits glasses according to the ophthalmologist's or the optometrist's specifications. An ocularist fits artificial eyes.

Orthopedics

Orthopedics is the branch of surgery that is concerned with the diagnosis and treatment of disorders of the bones and joints. The orthopedist treats broken bones, disorders of the bones and joints that can be corrected surgically, and bone tumors, as well as other problems of the skeletal system. Because of his or her knowledge of the functioning of the musculoskeletal system, the orthopedist often treats sports injuries and may serve as the physician for amateur and professional athletic teams.

The orthopedist is required to complete a one-year internship in general surgery, four years of training in orthopedic surgery,

and a year of medical practice before taking specialty board examinations.

Otorhinolaryngology

This specialty combines the study of the ear, nose, and throat into a single discipline commonly referred to as ENT. The more formal term "otorhinolaryngology" is derived from the Greek roots ot- ("ear"), rhin- ("nose"), laryng- ("voice box"), and logos ("study").

The ears and throat are connected by the eustachian tubes, which lead from the middle ear to the throat. The nose leads directly into the part of the throat referred to as the nasopharynx. Inflammations of the nose may spread to the throat, and vice versa. Inflammations of the throat often spread through the eustachian tubes to the ears. Consequently, infection in any of these areas could result in infection in all of them.

Ear, nose, and throat specialists are primarily surgeons. They perform such varied procedures as rhinoplasty (reconstructive nose surgery); removal of tumors from the oral, nasal, and neck areas; reconstructive ear surgery; and sinus surgery. They also function as diagnosticians of diseases of the head and neck, excluding the brain and eyes.

This specialty requires a one-year residency in general surgery and a four-year residency in otorhinolaryngology.

Pathology

Pathology is the study of the changes in body tissues brought about by disease and the ways in which these changes provide clues not only to the causes of

disease and death, but also to ways in which the spread of disease may be checked.

There are a variety of subspecialties within pathology, including the following:
- Cellular pathology, in which cells are the focus of study
- Clinical pathology, in which laboratory methods are used to aid clinical diagnosis
- Comparative pathology, in which diseases in humans are compared with those in other animals
- General pathology, which is the study of the processes that may occur in various diseases
- Forensic pathology, in which the results of pathologic examinations (such as autopsies and analyses samples) are used as evidence in legal proceedings

Much of the pathologist's work is done with the microscope, preparing and examining biopsy specimens (tissue samples). Pathologists are charged with deciding whether a tissue specimen indicates the presence of a disease. They also perform autopsies to determine the cause or causes of death. The pathologist must be knowledgeable about both the cause and the course of disease processes.

Pathologists ordinarily do work in both internal medicine and surgery during their training. A strong laboratory background is a necessity, with extensive training in modern instrumentation. Three- to four-year residencies in pathology are required, depending on the subspecialty.

Pediatrics

Pediatricians specialize in the diagnosis and treatment of diseases of children from birth through adolescence. They administer the appropriate immunizations to prevent disease and watch for any abnormalities that may appear. They also advise parents about the child's social and psychological needs.

After completion of medical school, pediatricians must have at least three years of training in general pediatrics. This is followed by an examination by the specialty board.

Peripheral vascular diseases

While cardiovascular surgeons treat disorders that affect the heart and its blood vessels specifically, surgeons who specialize in peripheral vascular diseases treat conditions that affect the rest of the circulatory system. Among these are the following:
- Arteriosclerosis, in which the artery walls become abnormally thickened or hardened (in advanced cases, the arteries may become partially or completely blocked)
- Arterial occlusion and embolism, in which undissolved material in the bloodstream (such as clumps of clotted blood, bacteria, or tissue fragments) blocks the flow of blood in the artery, causing a loss of blood to tissue beyond the blockade and sometimes necrosis (death of tissue)
- Carotid occlusive disease, in which the carotid arteries (the arteries in the neck that supply the brain with blood) become blocked
- Aortic or femoral artery occlusive disease, in which the aorta (the main artery from the heart going through the chest and abdomen) or one of the femoral arteries (the main arteries that carry blood to the legs) becomes blocked
- Venous thrombosis, in which the veins become clogged, usually with blood clots, with resulting pain and swelling of the affected extremity
- Pulmonary embolism, in which blood clots travel to the lungs

Specialists in this area can be internists with extensive cardiovascular training. For the most part, however, they are surgeons.

Physical medicine and rehabilitation

The field of physical medicine and rehabilitation is concerned with the diseases and disorders of the neuromuscular system (the nerves and muscles). Specialists in this field are skilled in using heat, cold, water, electricity, massage, and exercise to help patients regain use and function of parts of the body that have been damaged by stroke, severe arthritis, or spinal or other injury.

After completion of medical school, the physical medicine and rehabilitation specialist is required to complete at least three additional years of training, followed by two years of specialty practice. Specialty board examinations are required.

Podiatry

Podiatrists treat diseases and injuries of the feet. Only recently have all the states recognized podiatry as a legitimate healing field. Doctors in this area have degrees in podiatric medicine, but not M.D. degrees; they have not attended medical school. Many podiatrists have joined the ranks of sports medicine practitioners, since many foot injuries result from sports activities.

Many podiatrists are qualified to perform surgery on the feet when it is indicated. They also fit orthotic devices (inserted into shoes) to correct foot problems. The fitness movement has increased the demand for podiatric services.

Preventive medicine

Specialists in this relatively new field seek to prevent illnesses from happening. Physicians from every field have made contributions to preventive medicine. Practitioners range from immunologists (who seek to prevent illness with inoculations) to urban epidemiologists (who search out the causes of widespread illnesses, such as childhood lead poisoning, and try to alter the environment so that illnesses can be prevented).

Preventive medicine advocates often recommend regular or periodic physical examinations, prescribe certain regimens, and warn against toxic environments. Critics of the field claim that there are no safeguards against some types of illnesses. Advocates of the field point out that the same was said of infections before antibiotics.

Occupational medicine and public health specialists are important members of this field of medicine. In addition, preventive medicine is concerned with reviewing present health services and anticipating and planning to meet future medical needs.

Preventive medicine specialists complete at least three years of specialized training, one year of research or teaching, and examinations by their specialty board.

Proctology

The proctologist specializes in diseases and disorders of the anus and rectum. The rectum is the last portion of the large intestine; the anus is the opening to the outside from the rectum. Some of the conditions a proctologist treats include hemorrhoids (enlarged blood vessels around the anus) and rectal cancer.

Proctologists complete a residency in general surgery plus one or two years of training in colon and rectal surgery.

Psychiatry

A psychiatrist is a medical doctor—with the authority to prescribe medications and make medical decisions—who deals with mental disorders. (Psychologists do not have a medical degree and therefore cannot prescribe drugs.) Many psychiatrists use psychoanalysis as part of their therapeutic or diagnostic method, and all psychiatrists have intensive training in psychology.

There are four chief branches of psychiatry: (1) descriptive psychiatry, which is based on the observation of external factors that may be the cause of mental illness; (2) dynamic psychiatry, which is the study of the processes, origins, and mechanisms of emotional states; (3) forensic psychiatry, which deals with the legal aspects of mental illness; and (4) orthomolecular psychiatry, which is the study of the molecular bases of mental illnesses. Areas such as psychopharmacology (the study of the effects of drugs on a person's emotional and mental state) and psychophysiology (the study of the physiology of mental illness) are offshoots of orthomolecular psychiatry.

Psychiatrists go through the usual medical sequence: medical school, internship, and residency. The psychiatrist may spend five years or more in specialized training in psychiatry and neurology.

Pulmonary medicine

This field deals with the study, diagnosis, and treatment of diseases and disorders of the lungs and related passageways. Among the diseases included are:
- Lung cancer
- Tuberculosis
- Pneumonia (inflammation of the lungs)
- Bronchitis (inflammation of the passageways from the windpipe into the lungs)
- Tracheitis (inflammation of the windpipe)
- Black lung (in which the lungs become clogged with coal dust)
- Pleurisy (inflammation of the lining of the lungs and the chest cavity)
- Emphysema (in which lung tissue is destroyed, causing air to become trapped within the lungs)

These specialists also perform bronchoscopy (examination of the trachea and bronchial passages directly with a flexible, lighted, tubelike instrument) and specialize in managing ventilators (artificial breathing machines).

The pulmonary specialist's training is in internal medicine, followed by two years of specialized training in the diagnosis and treatment of pulmonary diseases and disorders.

Radiology/radiation oncology/nuclear medicine

A radiologist is a physician who uses X rays to diagnose and treat disorders. Radiologists have training in physics and instrumentation, as well as in biochemistry and the effects of radiation on human tissues.

Diagnostic radiology is primarily concerned with the administration of radiation to produce images of the body and the interpretation of the resultant X-ray films. Some procedures involve the injection of special dyes, called contrast media. Other procedures also performed by radiologists use sound waves or magnetic impulses, rather than radiation, to create images.

A specialist in diagnostic radiology must complete a four-year residency in that field, which is often preceded by a year of internship in another medical field. Some diagnostic radiologists then subspecialize by completing a fellowship in a branch of radiology, such as neuroradiology (imaging of the nervous system) or uroradiology (imaging of the urinary tract).

Radiation oncology is concerned with the application of radiation in the treatment of cancer. A specialist in radiation oncology must have completed a one-year internship, either rotating among specialties or in internal medicine, followed by a three-year residency in the specialty.

Nuclear medicine is the field in which radioactive substances, called isotopes, are used to diagnose and treat diseases, such as an overactive thyroid gland. A nuclear medicine specialist must have completed a three-year residency in diagnostic radiology, plus a one-year residency in nuclear radiology.

Rheumatology

Rheumatology is the field of medicine concerned with the

study, diagnosis, and medical treatment of diseases and disorders of bones, joints, and muscles. These disorders are often characterized by inflammation or degeneration and include such conditions as arthritis, gout, lupus erythematosus, and other connective tissue diseases.

A rheumatologist has completed an internship and residency in internal medicine, followed by two or more years of training and experience in rheumatology.

Sports medicine

This is one of the newest fields in medicine and has come into its own largely as a result of two factors: the training and rehabilitation needs of both amateur and professional athletes and the tremendous growth in fitness and sports-related activities among members of the public. Doctors from a variety of fields now list themselves as sports medicine practitioners. Many of them have trained as orthopedists, since that specialty field is concerned with the mechanics of muscular and skeletal function. Orthopedists are surgeons and thus are qualified to diagnose and surgically treat many sports injuries. They also apply casts, splints, and many other aids. Since most sprains, fractures, and muscle strains do not require surgery, many nonsurgical physicians also practice sports medicine. Exercise physiology has become an integral part of medical and sports training programs, and what was once a collection of lore on how to get the most out of your body in a game has become a field of medical research and practice.

Sports medicine has made great contributions to the general public welfare by producing hard evidence of the benefits of healthful exercise. As a consequence, information about subjects such as nutrition, kinesiology (the study of body movement), and biomechanics (the study of lever systems and their effect on performance) has become available to the average weekend athlete. Training need no longer be haphazard or hazardous; by using information available from sports medicine practitioners, you can train for strength, power, endurance, or speed and minimize your chances of becoming injured. Each goal calls for a different kind of training method. Sports medicine and exercise physiology have made a science out of athletic training.

In a sense, with the advent of sports medicine as a medical field, athletics serves the same function for ordinary people that auto racing serves for the development of new ways to make the family car better: The desire for high performance calls for research and ingenuity in converting research findings into practical applications. Sports medicine converts the lessons learned on the playing field and in the laboratory to insights into the medical problems of ordinary people who want to play a little golf, tone up, or trim down.

Surgery

Surgery is the branch of medicine that uses surgical operations to treat disease, injury, or deformity. Surgeons go into the human body by way of incisions through the skin and muscles to alter, correct, remove, or replace the offending organ or tissue. There are many surgical specialties, among them the following:

- General surgery (including surgery of the abdomen and breasts)
- Thoracic (chest) surgery
- Cardiac (heart) surgery
- Oral (mouth) surgery (usually performed by dentists with a subspecialty in oral surgery)
- Neurosurgery (surgery of the nervous system, particularly the brain and spinal cord)
- Plastic surgery (to correct damage caused by injury or to improve appearance)
- Orthopedic surgery (to correct disorders of the bones, joints, ligaments, and tendons)

Surgeons work closely with internists, pathologists, radiologists, anesthesiologists, and other specialists. In a very real sense, everything that physicians know about diagnosing and treating illnesses is relevant in an operating room.

After the usual four years of medical school, surgeons complete a general surgery internship and a general surgery residency, followed by additional training in their specific field of surgery.

Urology

Urology deals with diseases and disorders of the kidneys, the urinary tract, the prostate gland, and the male sex organs. The urologist's skills include knowledge of diagnostic procedures and surgical techniques, as well as the ability to treat infections of the urinary tract and the male reproductive system.

After completion of medical school, the urologist has two years of training in general surgery, followed by a three-year training period in urology and urologic surgery and an 18-month period of clinical practice before specialty board examinations may be taken.

COPING WITH SYMPTOMS

Most of us are aware of what we need to do to promote good health; choosing a proper diet, getting appropriate exercise and adequate rest, and dealing with stress effectively are only a few of the good health habits that contribute to fitness and vigor. However, many of us forget that understanding illness is also important to maintaining health. By learning to recognize the symptoms of illness, we can better prevent and treat problems that threaten our health.

A symptom is an abnormal physical or psychological condition that accompanies or results from a disease or disorder. It indicates a departure from the normal well-being of the body. Sometimes a symptom is a disorder in and of itself. For example, indigestion may simply be the temporary result of eating too much or too fast or of eating fatty or spicy foods. However, indigestion may also be a sign of a more serious disorder, such as an ulcer, a heart attack, or cancer; if that is the case, indigestion is more than a temporary inconvenience, and you need to be able to tell the difference.

At other times, a symptom is a defensive reaction of the body— an attempt to restore the body to normal functioning. Falling into a faint in an overheated room, for instance, is the body's method of restoring adequate blood supply to the brain by lowering the head to the same level as the heart. However, fainting may be a sign of a serious illness, and you need to know when to report it to your doctor.

Observing symptoms

Your ability to recognize and understand symptoms of illness is important in helping your doc-tor diagnose and treat disorders. When you go to the doctor with a medical problem, you should be prepared to describe your symptoms exactly. You should note the time of their onset and the nature of your activity when they occur (for example, after eating, upon awakening, after strenuous exercise like shoveling snow, or when lying down). Be prepared to describe the rapidity with which your symptoms appear. Sometimes the symptoms themselves provide fewer clues than does the manner in which they occur.

To do all of this well, you must learn to be observant of your body. The following descriptions of some of the more common symptoms will help you become alert to changes in your body. This section also offers some guidance on when to seek medical attention for symptoms. As an additional aid, you may want to read the introductions to the chapters in this book that discuss the various systems of the body. Those introductions explain the normal functioning of the body systems and may help you recognize when your body is not working the way it should.

Chest pain

Chest pain is a major symptom in many disorders, including heart disease, indigestion, and pleurisy. It is important that you report to your doctor any prolonged or severe chest pain, since prompt evaluation and treatment may be lifesaving.

Heart disease

In heart disease, chest pains may be the temporary discomfort of angina pectoris or the similar, but more severe and long-lasting, signs of a heart attack. In both cases, the discomfort is usually felt as an aching, tight, crushing sensation beneath the breastbone that may radiate to the left shoulder and arm. It may also be felt in the back, throat, jaws, and teeth, or it may spread to the abdomen. In angina, the discomfort typically is brought on by exertion and disappears in a few minutes with rest or with the taking of nitroglycerin. In a heart attack, the pain is usually much more intense and deep and is most often not relieved by nitroglycerin; in addition, the patient is restless, pale, and perspiring. Nausea and vomiting also often accompany a heart attack.

When the chest pains of angina or a heart attack spread to the abdomen, they are often mistaken for the discomfort of indigestion. Conversely, severe indigestion, ulcer pains, and gallbladder attacks can be mistaken for a heart attack. If there is any possibility that the symptoms might be those of a heart attack, the only recommended plan of action is to obtain emergency medical assistance immediately. The diagnosis must always be left to a physician.

Indigestion

Indigestion is a sign of failure of proper digestion and absorption of food. Among the signs of indigestion may be discomfort in the chest, whether perceived as the burning sensation of heartburn or as sharp, dull, or gnawing pains in the chest area. If chest pain or discomfort occurs only in relation to eating, it is probably due to simple indigestion. Any change in severity or frequency of symptoms, however, should always be reported to a physician.

Pleurisy

The chest pains of pleurisy, which may be sharp and stabbing or merely uncomfortable, may occur with every breath or only when the patient breathes deeply or coughs. The pains are caused by inflammation of the pleurae (the membranes that surround the lungs and line the chest cavity). The pains may appear only over the site of the infection or may radiate to the lower chest and abdomen.

Other causes

Among other causes of chest pain are rib injuries, pneumonia, a blood clot in the lung, endocarditis (inflammation of the tissues surrounding the heart), inflammation of the nerves supplying the chest wall, and tenderness of the chest muscles after injury or exertion.

Constipation

Constipation is a condition in which the stool (feces) is hard and its elimination from the bowels is infrequent and difficult. This condition is often more uncomfortable than harmful, although occasionally a change in the bowel movements, (for example, prolonged constipation or extreme discomfort when eliminating) may be a symptom of a serious illness, such as cancer, intestinal obstruction, or a nervous system or endocrine gland disorder.

It is important to remember, however, that it is not necessary to have a bowel movement every day. From three bowel movements per day to three per week is considered in the normal range.

Causes

Common causes of constipation are physical inactivity; lack of fiber or roughage in the diet; inadequate fluid intake; emotional stress, particularly depression; drug side effects; and the habit of postponing bowel movements.

Symptoms

Conditions that often accompany constipation are difficulty and strain in producing a bowel movement, a bloated feeling, abdominal cramps, headache, gassiness, and hemorrhoids.

Treatment

The treatment of constipation usually depends on its cause. In mild cases that are not related to other disorders, simple methods of recommended treatment include adding more fiber-rich foods (such as bran, whole-grain breads and cereals, fruits, vegetables, and other forms of roughage) to the diet; drinking eight to ten glasses of water daily; increasing exercise; and developing good bathroom habits. This last recommendation may involve an attempt to have a bowel movement at the same time every day, usually 30 to 60 minutes after breakfast. Early morning is a good time, because the entry of food into an empty stomach activates and increases normal intestinal contractions; also, residue from the previous day's meals has moved by this time to the rectal area for elimination.

Laxatives and enemas are usually not recommended for treating simple constipation. Laxatives should be used only when absolutely necessary; overuse can lead to irritation of the rectal lining, and the intestine can become so dependent on the stimulation of laxatives that it cannot function properly without them. Frequent enemas can also lead to dependence.

Prevention

Drinking plenty of water, getting adequate exercise, eating fiber-rich foods, and recognizing the urge for a bowel movement as soon as it is felt should be beneficial in promoting regular elimination and preventing constipation.

Cough

A cough is a normal reflex of the body to clear the airways. Coughing can result from inhaling dust, dirt, or irritating fumes; from breathing icy air; or from drawing food into the airways. It can also be caused by mucus and other secretions from such respiratory disorders as the common cold, influenza, pneumonia, and tuberculosis. Persistent coughs (those that last several weeks) without other respiratory symptoms may, on occasion, suggest diseases of other organs, such as the heart. For example, a cough may be an early sign of congestive heart failure.

Types

The type of cough—productive or nonproductive—partially

determines how it should be treated. Productive coughs (those that produce fluid or mucus) are often caused by a lung infection. When microorganisms attack the lungs, the lung tissue produces large amounts of secretions in defense. These accumulated secretions irritate the lungs, resulting in coughing that brings up fluid or mucus. A yellowish or reddish fluid in particular may indicate infection or other serious problems that require a doctor's attention.

Nonproductive coughing does not bring up fluid. It occurs when secretions from nasal passages drip into the throat or when smoke, dust, pollen, or other irritants enter the respiratory tract. Irritations and tumors may also cause a nonproductive cough, as can any inflammation of the airways or lung tissue, infectious or not. Another cause of nonproductive coughing is insufficient moisture in the air. The airways become dry and irritated, and coughing develops. This is particularly common in winter, when humidity is lowest. By adding moisture to the air, a humidifier or vaporizer may provide more relief than any cough-suppressing drug.

Treatment

Because coughing has the vital function of clearing the airways, it should never be totally suppressed. In fact, suppressing a cough in an individual with chronic lung disease may be dangerous. Furthermore, indiscriminate use of cough suppressants may mask important symptoms. However, controlling a cough that disrupts sleep or aggravates other conditions may sometimes be necessary. This may be accomplished by using a cough suppressant or an expectorant. A suppressant helps to inhibit the cough by depressing the coughing center in the brain. An expectorant promotes the discharge of mucus from the respiratory tract.

For all but the mildest coughs with obvious causes, and certainly for persistent coughs, a doctor should be consulted to determine the cause and to suggest appropriate treatment.

Dehydration

Dehydration is a condition in which the body in general or certain body tissues in particular suffer from lack of water.

Causes

Tissue dehydration may occur in dry climates and during the winter heating season: extremely dry air causes rapid evaporation of water from the skin and from the mucous linings of the respiratory (breathing) system. The results are discomfort and sometimes cracking of the skin, unless it is protected by lotions, and increased susceptibility of the respiratory system to infections.

Dehydration of the entire body can be life-threatening. Illnesses that produce diarrhea and vomiting are common causes of dehydration, since both of these conditions cause loss of body fluids. Cholera, which results in extreme diarrhea and vomiting, can kill through dehydration. Other causes of dehydration include diabetes, kidney disease, excessive use of diuretics (drugs that stimulate production of urine), liver disease, and inflammation of the abdominal cavity.

Burns may also be a cause of dehydration. Tissue beneath a burn swells with body fluid. If the burn covers much of the body, the buildup of fluid in burn tissue draws considerable water from the blood. This can decrease the blood volume so much that shock (general collapse of the circulatory system) occurs.

Symptoms

Symptoms of dehydration include thirst; sudden weight loss; rough, dry skin; dry mucous membranes; rapid heartbeat and low blood pressure; lack of energy; and weakness. In an extreme case, the patient goes into shock, which is characterized by pale skin; bluish lips and fingertips; rapid, shallow breathing; and a weak, rapid, irregular pulse. Blood tests reveal thickening of the blood because of decreased water content.

Treatment

The treatment of mild to moderate dehydration is to have the patient drink water with some salts added. However, if the individual has been vomiting, suffers from diarrhea, or is unconscious, it may be necessary for medical personnel to administer saline (saltwater) solution intravenously (through a vein). The intravenous method is always used in severe cases of dehydration. The goal is to totally replace the lost fluid within 48 to 72 hours, together with the valuable mineral salts that have also been lost.

Diarrhea

Diarrhea is abnormally frequent and excessively liquid bowel movements. This is often the body's defensive attempt to rid itself of irritating or toxic substances. It is a symptom that accompanies many disorders, both mild and serious.

Types

There are two basic types of diarrhea, acute (short-term) and chronic (long-term). Acute diarrhea, the more common form, comes on quickly and usually lasts no more than two or three days, although it can last as long as two weeks. Chronic diarrhea may also appear suddenly, but it lingers for many weeks or months, either being constantly present or alternately appearing and disappearing.

Both acute and chronic diarrhea can become a serious problem because of the danger of dehydration (excessive loss of body fluids), as well as loss of nutrients. Diarrhea may also be a symptom of an inflammatory bowel disease (for example, Crohn's disease).

Causes

The reasons for the consistency of the stool (feces) in diarrhea are complex. In an infection, the intestine may pour out massive quantities of fluids and salts in response to a bacterial toxin (poison) or other irritant. In inflammatory bowel disease, protein, blood, and mucus are lost through the inflamed lining of the colon, taking large quantities of water with them. Other disorders speed up the normal movement of the colon, thereby not allowing time for absorption of fluids. Yet another type of diarrhea is caused by poor absorption of a type of sugar called lactose, which draws fluid out of

the colon. In many cases, diarrhea is caused by a combination of these mechanisms.

Other causes of diarrhea include changes in the diet, drugs taken for other disorders (particularly antibiotics, which upset the bacterial balance in the intestines), stress, infection, and food allergies.

Symptoms

The symptoms often experienced with the characteristic loose and frequent stools are nausea, cramps or pain in the abdomen, gassiness, fatigue, and fever.

Diagnosis

Diagnostic evaluation will include assessment of the patient's normal diet and emotional state, as well as recent changes in daily habits. In addition, a sample of the stool may be examined for color, consistency, odor, chemical content, and presence of blood. Stool cultures are often done to identify the causative agent if infection is suspected.

Treatment

Treatment for diarrhea usually involves removing or correcting the cause of the condition. If diarrhea lasts for more than three days or is a recurring problem, a doctor should be consulted, as this may be a warning sign of a more serious illness. Antidiarrheal medications can be prescribed for particularly bothersome or persistent diarrhea, but these should be used only with caution; in the case of some infections, they may actually prolong the course of the illness.

The discomfort of occasional bouts of acute diarrhea, however, is usually treated with simple remedies, such as adequate rest and increased intake of liquids to replace lost fluids. The diet should consist of light meals, perhaps soup or broth at first; as solid food is added to the diet, irritating substances, such as bran, fruits and vegetables, fried foods, coffee, and alcoholic beverages should be avoided.

Dizziness and vertigo

Dizziness and vertigo are sensations of disorientation and distorted perception. Occasional episodes are not serious, but recurrent dizziness or vertigo can be a symptom of a variety of disorders, particularly those involving the eyes, ears, or nervous system.

Dizziness and vertigo are sometimes confused with each other. Dizziness is characterized by unsteadiness and a distorted sense of the environment; the word *dizziness* is often used to describe a sensation of light-headedness or faintness. Vertigo is a false sense of movement, often the perception that one is spinning or that one's environment is whirling around. Vertigo is often accompanied by nausea.

Causes

Dizziness and vertigo can be caused by a malfunction in one of the parts of the body that is responsible for giving the brain information on balance, position, and movement. These parts include the eye, the inner ear, and certain areas of the brain. Thus, balance can be disturbed by any injury, impairment, or disorder involving the eyes, ears, and certain areas of the brain, as well as the nerves leading to and from these areas. A wide variety of problems, such as injury to the head, ear infections, and migraine headaches, can include dizziness or vertigo as a symptom. Also, occasional mild upsets to the body can cause dizziness (but usually not vertigo), including such harmless factors as being overheated, overtired, or tense. Standing up too quickly after reclining or sitting for some time is another harmless cause of dizziness.

Symptoms

Dizziness is characterized by feelings of unsteadiness, swaying, light-headedness, weakness, and faintness and may be accompanied by nausea and vomiting. Vertigo is marked by a feeling of spinning and may be associated with unsteady walking, a tendency to fall or to veer to one side while walking, paleness, sweating, nausea and vomiting, and continuous rapid eye movement.

Prevention and treatment

Simple dizziness can easily be avoided. Getting up slowly after reclining or sitting, leaving overheated rooms to get some fresh air, eating a balanced diet, and getting adequate rest should all help to prevent dizziness. Recurrent dizziness, however, should be brought to the attention of a physician.

True vertigo, on the other hand, may be a sign of physical disease, such as labyrinthitis (inflammation of the inner ear) or a brain disorder. Frequently, how-ever, no cause is found, and the vertigo is treated symptomatically with drugs. In all cases, any episode of true vertigo should be reported to a physician.

Edema

Edema is the accumulation of excessive amounts of fluid within the body's tissues. It is a symptom of many conditions, both minor and serious.

The fluid that accumulates comes from the blood. Normally, there is a constant exchange of fluid between the blood vessels and other body tissues. The blood removes any extra fluids and carries them to the kidneys, from which they are excreted via the urinary tract. Edema occurs when that exchange does not take place properly, either allowing too much liquid to leave the blood vessels or too little fluid to enter the blood vessels.

Causes

A change in pressure within the blood vessels because of heart disease, high blood pressure, blocked or damaged vessels, or a kidney disorder can cause an imbalance in fluid exchange.

Mild edema is common before menstruation and during pregnancy, when the blood volume increases. Being overweight, wearing tight clothing, and becoming overheated can also lead to edema.

Forms of edema

Edema can be confined to a small area of the body or can become generalized. Some forms are more noticeable than others. For example, the swelling that appears around a splinter in the skin is edema. However, generalized edema results in widespread swelling and puffiness, usually first noticed in the fingers and feet. The most serious forms of edema occur within the internal organs. Heart disease, for example, may cause the lungs to fill with fluid, creating severe difficulty in breathing.

Treatment

Simple or temporary edema can be relieved by decreasing salt intake, since the sodium in salt causes the body to retain fluid. More severe or internal edema can be treated with a diuretic (a drug that stimulates production of urine). Edema that is symptomatic of an underlying disorder will often disappear with management of that condition.

Prevention

Controlling weight gain, eating a balanced low-salt diet, and wearing loose clothing may prevent milder forms of edema. Any prolonged edema not attributable to causes such as hot weather or menstruation should be investigated by a physician.

Fainting

Fainting is a temporary loss of consciousness and is often the result when the body attempts to supply extra blood to the brain. Fainting can be a symptom of a relatively mild condition, such as hunger, or a serious disorder, such as heartbeat irregularity.

When the brain experiences a temporary reduction of its blood supply, the body reacts defensively; in effect, it causes itself to fall down, bringing the head to the level of the heart and thereby minimizing the effect of gravity, which favors pooling of blood in the legs. The net effect is an increase in the amount of blood coming back to the heart, which allows the heart to pump blood to the brain more easily.

Causes

Fainting can be caused by interference with any one of several internal mechanisms that protect and maintain the brain's blood supply. These mechanisms work against gravity and its tendency to allow blood to pool in the lower parts of the body. One of these mechanisms is the "muscle pump." The muscles of the legs act to squeeze the veins in the legs, thereby forcing blood up toward the heart. If a person stands motionless for a long period of time without using these muscles, blood pools in the legs, reducing the amount available to the brain. This reduction frequently causes fainting or loss of consciousness. The ability of the heart to increase its rate and force of contraction when under stress is another built-in protective mechanism.

These protective functions can be impaired by a variety of conditions, such as an overheated or crowded environment, emotional stress, hunger, extreme fatigue, various medications (particularly some high blood pressure medications), and certain circulatory disorders.

Symptoms

The symptoms that usually precede fainting are light-head-edness, confusion, spots before the eyes, white or grayish coloring of the face, and cold, moist skin. Nausea and vomiting may also be present.

Treatment

Fainting is treated by taking several simple steps to make the person more comfortable. The patient should be lying down, preferably with the feet higher than the head (to help blood return to the brain), and the clothing should be loosened. The patient should have plenty of fresh air to breathe. Recovery should occur within a few seconds of fainting, but a sense of disorientation may linger for several minutes. Spirits of ammonia and smelling salts are not usually recommended for fainting, as they may be ineffective or may cause vomiting. Recurrent fainting should be reported to a doctor.

Prevention

Fainting can often be prevented by lying down, preferably with the legs up, as soon as any of the warning symptoms is noticed. This precaution lowers the brain to the level of the heart, increasing the blood supply to the brain.

Fatigue

Fatigue may be physical or mental exhaustion, an overwhelming feeling of weariness, or a lack of energy and enthusiasm for even pleasant activities. It is a symptom of a vast number of diseases and disorders.

Fatigue should not be confused with weakness, which is an actual loss of physical strength.

Causes

Feeling fatigued and tiring rapidly with minimal activity are often among the early signs of an approaching illness. Fatigue is a warning signal of a variety of diseases and disorders, among them the common cold, influenza, hepatitis, infectious mononucleosis, and other infectious diseases; heart disease; lung disorders, such as emphysema; some glandular diseases, such as diabetes; anemia and nutritional deficiencies; and some diseases of the nervous system. Overwork, either physical or mental, can also cause fatigue, as can psychological disorders or emotional stress.

Symptoms

In addition to the general feeling of being more tired than usual, fatigue can be accompanied by nervousness, anxiety, depression, and feelings of irritability, as well as by headache, diminished sexual function, and difficulty in concentrating. When fatigue is due to psychological problems, sleep disorders, including insomnia, and a pattern of frequent nighttime and early morning awakening are often present as well.

Treatment

Fatigue is best dealt with by treating the physical disorder or psychological problem that is causing it. Some types of fatigue, particularly those due to physical overexertion, can probably be prevented by getting adequate exercise and rest, as well as by eating well-balanced meals and reducing stress, tension, and overwork.

Before taking someone's temperature, shake down the mercury in the thermometer so that the top of the column is below 96°F. Then place the thermometer under the person's tongue and have her hold it there (with her mouth closed) for three minutes. The average normal temperature taken by mouth is 98.6°F to 99.6°F. A false reading will be obtained if the person drinks a hot or cold beverage immediately before measurement.

Fever

Fever is an abnormally high body temperature. A fever is present when the body temperature rises above the normal range of 98.6°F to 99.6°F. Generally, if the body temperature is more than 101.5°F when measured with a rectal thermometer, 100.5°F when measured with an oral thermometer, or 99.5°F when measured under the arm, it is considered abnormal.

Fever is a symptom of illness and often appears to be an undesirable condition, but many researchers believe that fever acts as a defense mechanism for the body when it is being attacked by bacteria or viruses. There is a regulatory center in the brain that acts to maintain a constant body temperature regardless of the surrounding environment. Fever occurs when this center responds to an illness or infection, such as a common cold or influenza, by setting the body temperature higher. This mechanism is thought to work because infectious microorganisms cannot survive the higher-than-normal temperatures.

Causes

Infections are the most common cause of fever, but a fever can also be a symptom of heart attack, some forms of cancer, and disorders in the portion of the brain that regulates temperature (such as stroke, brain tumor, or brain injury).

Symptoms

The early signs of fever include chills or hot flashes, flushed skin, increased pulse and breathing rates, headache, and aching of muscles or joints. A slight fever, however, may produce none of these symptoms. A high fever may result in delirium or convulsions, and a prolonged fever may cause weakness and dehydration (excess loss of body fluids).

Treatment

Treatment of fever depends on its severity, duration, and cause. Immediate emergency medical treatment should be sought if the temperature is more than 105°F or if convulsions have occurred. A doctor should be consulted if a child has a fever higher than 101°F for more than 24 hours; if a child with a fever acts extremely ill; if an adult has a high fever (103°F to 104°F) that lasts for 12 to 24 hours; if a moderate fever (101°F to 102°F) in an adult lasts for several days; if the body temperature fluctuates widely; or if the fever disappears and then returns several days later, which usually signals a new infection.

The goal in treating a patient with a fever is actually to diagnose and treat the cause of the fever, rather than the fever itself. Merely lowering a mild fever may do more harm than good, because it reduces the protection that the fever may be providing in fighting off the infection; it may also mask the underlying cause or disturb the natural course that the disease would have taken, thus hindering diagnosis. Therefore, treating a fever should never be confused with treating its cause.

At times, however, fever should be lowered to keep the patient comfortable and to prevent the weakness and dehydration that can result from prolonged fever. Increasing fluid intake and taking aspirin or an aspirin substitute (such as acetaminophen) will usually lower a fever; taking tepid, not cold, baths and using comfortable, but not overly warm, clothing and blankets will help to lower the fever and also keep the patient from feeling chilled.

It should be noted that any drug treatment for fever, especially for children, should be undertaken only after consulting with a doctor. An association between the use of aspirin in children with viral illnesses (particularly chicken pox and influenza) and the often fatal Reye's syndrome (a condition characterized by severe, sudden deterioration of liver and brain function) has been demonstrated. It is therefore recommended that the use of aspirin be avoided in children with viral illnesses unless the aspirin has been prescribed by a physician.

Heartburn

Heartburn is an uncomfortable, burning sensation felt behind the lower part of the breastbone, sometimes extending up into the upper chest or lower neck. Despite its name, it is not caused by pain in the heart or by a heart attack. In fact, heartburn is often triggered by simple digestive upsets, although occasionally a severe case may be a symptom of a more serious disorder.

Causes

Heartburn occurs when the acidic digestive juices and partially digested food from the stomach back up into the lower esophagus (the passageway between the mouth and the stomach) and irritate its tissues.

Heartburn most often develops ten minutes to one hour after eating. It may be caused by overeating, smoking, lying down or bending over after eating (which allows the backup of stomach acids and food into the esophagus), taking aspirin, or consuming alcoholic drinks, coffee, spicy or highly seasoned foods, or acidic fruits or fruit juices. Heartburn is a common problem during pregnancy because the expanding uterus exerts pressure on the stomach and esophagus, encouraging digestive juices to move up toward the throat; this disappears after childbirth.

Symptoms

The major symptom of heartburn is the characteristic burning sensation behind the breastbone and up toward the throat. It may be accompanied by gassiness, belching, and an uncomfortable, tight feeling in the chest.

Heartburn can usually be relieved by merely standing or sitting upright or by drinking milk or something soothing and nonacidic. Nonprescription antacids may also be helpful in more severe cases. Any case of persistent, uncontrollable, or severe heartburn should be reported to a doctor because it may be a sign of a more severe condition, such as peptic ulcer.

Prevention

Heartburn can often be prevented by avoiding spicy, acidic, or other troublesome foods, as well as coffee and alcoholic beverages, if they seem to trigger it. Eating smaller meals more fre-quently and refraining from smoking at mealtimes are also beneficial in avoiding heartburn. Sleeping with the back and head propped up on pillows may prevent the stomach contents from flowing upward and into the esophagus.

Hypothermia

Hypothermia is a condition in which the body temperature falls well below the normal temperature of 98.6°F. The lowering of the temperature can occur accidentally, or it can be induced intentionally as part of a medical treatment plan.

When hypothermia happens accidentally, the person's condition can become serious if the symptoms or signs are ignored. Among the causes of accidental hypothermia are immersion in cold water, use of certain drugs, and long periods of being exposed to the cold without appropriate clothing. Hypothermia can easily occur in newborns and infants, because their heat-retaining mechanisms are not fully developed. Elderly persons are also at risk, because their heat-retaining mechanisms are easily overtaxed.

Symptoms

The signs and symptoms of hypothermia include an altered level of consciousness, slow breathing, low pulse rate, listlessness, and mental confusion. The hands, feet, and abdomen are cold to the touch.

Treatment

Basic treatment for hypothermia is gradual rewarming of the

body. The rewarming must be gradual to prevent the sudden enlargement of blood vessels at the surface of the body, which may divert too much blood from some of the body's vital internal organs. Medical help should always be obtained for a person with hypothermia. While waiting for help to arrive, the cold person should be covered with blankets and, if alert, should be offered a warm, nonalcoholic beverage. Alcoholic drinks do not help because they tend to reduce body heat. Also, briskly rubbing hands or feet to restore warmth is *not* recommended. Any other type of treatment depends on the underlying cause of the drop in body temperature. In severe cases in which body temperature is critically reduced, warm fluids may be given intravenously. Peritoneal dialysis (a process by which warm fluids are injected into and withdrawn from the abdominal cavity) is sometimes used to restore normal temperature, as is immersion in a specially designed tank filled with warm water.

Indigestion

Indigestion (also called dyspepsia) is the discomfort caused by difficulty in digesting food. It is an uncomfortable feeling of fullness, pressure, slight pain, or gassiness and is usually related to eating. (Constipation, diarrhea, heartburn, and nausea are *not* indigestion, although they may be related to the problem.)

Causes

Indigestion is usually caused by an eating problem, such as eating too fast or too much; chewing insufficiently; eating in an emotionally upsetting environment; eating particularly bothersome foods, such as spicy, fatty, or oily foods, or those that may cause an allergic reaction; or smoking, especially immediately before or after a meal. Indigestion can also be caused by serious disorders, such as cancer, ulcers, and diseases involving the organs associated with digestion (the esophagus, intestines, gallbladder, liver, stomach, and pancreas). In addition, heart attack, tumors, and emotional problems may be accompanied by symptoms that are similar to those of indigestion.

Any case of indigestion that lingers for some time or that cannot be controlled in any way should be reported to a doctor for diagnosis and treatment.

Diagnosis

The cause of indigestion is diagnosed primarily by observing the symptoms and the conditions under which they occur. A doctor will want a description of the symptoms and of the patient's dietary habits; of the time, length, and location of the discomfort, as well as the circumstances surrounding it and the foods eaten preceding it; and of the emotional environment that usually exists during meals and snacks. X-ray studies of the gastrointestinal tract or analysis of stool (feces) may also be used to make a diagnosis of the cause of indigestion.

Treatment

Antacids often relieve indigestion, but they should not be used without the advice of a physician by people who have kidney disease.

Prevention

The best treatment consists of preventing indigestion in the first place. Eating balanced meals in a relaxed setting, eliminating foods that can cause indigestion, and refraining from smoking, especially at mealtimes, should help to prevent indigestion.

Insomnia

Insomnia is the inability to sleep during normal sleeping hours when there is no apparent reason for wakefulness. Insomnia may vary from simple restlessness, to wakefulness on and off throughout the night, to total sleeplessness.

Causes

Although the condition is most often associated with psychological or emotional problems, it can also be related to physical disorders or to conditions in the immediate environment.

Depression and anxiety are often the cause of insomnia. Among physical disorders that can lead to insomnia are urination problems, heart trouble, high blood pressure, infection, hardening of the arteries, spastic colon, and leg cramps. Less serious causes of insomnia can be found in the immediate environment—bright lights, noise, excessive heat or cold, lack of ventilation. Insomnia may also be caused by having too many or too few bedclothes, by being constipated or hungry, or by having consumed too much coffee, tea, cola, or other beverage containing caffeine, which is a stimulant.

Strangely, drugs to promote sleep can cause insomnia. The

careless or inappropriate use of tranquilizers and sedatives can disrupt sleep patterns. If high doses of tranquilizers or sedatives are taken, the waking-sleeping pattern can be reversed, and sleep can become irregular. The person may doze throughout the day and then be unable to sleep at night.

Treatment

A person who has persistent insomnia should consult a physician so that the underlying cause—emotional or physical—can be diagnosed and treated.

Prevention

Ways of preventing or coping with simple insomnia include taking a 10- or 15-minute walk before bedtime, taking a warm bath, drinking warm milk (milk contains a substance called tryptophan, which promotes drowsiness), reading, or watching television. Taking sleep-promoting medications should be discussed with a doctor.

Itching

Itching is an uncomfortable or irritating sensation on the surface of the skin, accompanied by an urge to scratch. It has been described as a pricking, stinging, burning, or crawling feeling.

Causes

The biological reactions that lead to itching are not clearly understood, but it is known that this stimulation of the nerve endings can be caused by physical and psychological factors.

Itching can be caused by insect bites; small cuts or scrapes; hives and other allergic reactions; a fungal infection; the rash that often accompanies infectious diseases, such as chicken pox; dry skin, often stemming from bathing or showering too frequently or using harsh soaps; reactions to drugs; and psychological stress.

Symptoms

Itching is characterized by a feeling of discomfort, the urge to scratch, and possibly redness, peeling, and other irritations of the skin as a result of scratching. Itching of just the scalp and forearms with no obvious cause may be triggered by psychological stress.

Treatment

Treatment of itching depends on its cause. Itching from dry skin is usually treated by applying skin lotions or creams to small areas and using body lotions or bath oils for larger areas; reducing the frequency of showers and baths to only twice weekly (because water tends to dry the skin); and trying a new brand of soap or shampoo.

If itching seems to be a reaction to a drug, the doctor should be consulted before making any changes in medication. (A patient should *never* stop taking a prescription drug without the approval of his or her doctor.) Generally, the doctor will either lower the dosage to relieve the itching or give advice on treatment of the itching while maintaining the original dosage.

If no outside substances seem to be triggering itching, psychological or emotional stress may

be the cause. Treatment of itching in this situation will center on removing the stress or learning how to deal with it.

If itching persists for more than a week after attempts at self-treatment, a doctor should be consulted because persistent itching with no visible cause may be a symptom of diabetes, thyroid disease, kidney failure, liver disease, or cancer.

Prevention

Limiting bathing to twice weekly and using humidifiers to keep the air moist should help prevent the itching caused by dry skin.

Loss of appetite

Loss of appetite (also known as anorexia) is a lack of interest in or desire for food. Simple loss of appetite should not be confused with the illness called anorexia nervosa, which occurs most often in young women. Rather, loss of appetite is a common symptom that accompanies many illnesses.

Causes

Appetite is controlled by two areas of the brain—the "feeding" center and the "fullness" center—that work to regulate feelings of hunger depending on the body's need for food. In rare cases, appetite loss can be caused by damage to these areas of the brain. More commonly, it results from fatigue, the common cold, and psychological problems, such as anxiety and depression. Serious disorders that can lead to longer periods of appetite loss include certain types of cancers, as well as glandular and intestinal diseases.

Symptoms

Loss of appetite is indicated by a general lack of interest in food or eating, reduced food intake, and, in severe cases, weakness and a decrease in the body's natural resistance to disease.

Treatment

A doctor's advice should be sought if appetite loss stems from emotional or psychological problems, if it lasts for long periods, or if it seems to have no obvious cause. Counseling may be beneficial if emotional problems are connected to loss of appetite.

Nasal congestion

Nasal congestion occurs when the blood vessels in the nose enlarge. These enlarged blood vessels leak fluid into the surrounding tissues, which fills the nasal cavity and impairs breathing.

Nasal congestion is not a serious problem in itself, although it may be bothersome enough to interfere with daily activities and sleep. Persistent cases should be reported to a doctor, as nasal congestion may be a symptom of mild infections or more serious disorders.

Causes

The common cold, influenza, allergy, and bronchitis are the most frequent causes of nasal congestion. Persistent cases may be caused by structural abnormalities in the nose or by the daily use of certain drugs, particularly those often prescribed for high blood pressure, which act to enlarge all blood vessels, including those in the nose.

Treatment

Occasional nasal congestion is often treated with over-the-counter (nonprescription) decongestants, such as nasal sprays, nose drops, and nasal inhalers, all of which act to shrink swollen blood vessels in the nose and stop fluid secretion. However, they can also shrink blood vessels elsewhere in the body, resulting in increased blood pressure and heart rate, as well as nervousness and insomnia. For this reason, over-the-counter decongestants should not be used without the advice of a physician by those with high blood pressure, heart disease, diabetes, or thyroid disorders.

Those who do use decongestants for nasal congestion should use them only for brief periods, perhaps three days at the most. Since they act to constrict the blood vessels, their overuse tends to tire the blood vessels, relaxing them completely and making the nose more congested than it was before decongestants were used. This is called rebound congestion.

In addition, specific medicine that is inserted in the nose may be prescribed by a doctor. Also, the use of vaporizers or humidifiers is often beneficial in relieving some of the discomfort of nasal congestion.

Nausea and vomiting

Nausea is an extremely uncomfortable or queasy feeling in the stomach area, often accompanied by an urge to vomit. Vomiting is the forceful ejection of the contents of the stomach through the mouth.

Both nausea and vomiting can be symptoms of relatively mild upsets in the body, such as motion sickness, or of more serious disorders, such as peptic ulcer.

The sensation of nausea and the urge to vomit originate in an area of the brain called the vomiting center. In response to certain messages from nerves in the digestive system or the inner ear (part of which controls balance) or to direct stimulation by certain drugs, the vomiting center can trigger the muscular actions that result in vomiting.

Nausea and vomiting are usually temporary conditions and may be beneficial if they result in the expulsion of something potentially harmful to the body. However, persistent or recurring vomiting can lead to a dangerous loss of fluids and salts (called dehydration) and of nutrients, and can also damage the esophagus (the passageway from the mouth to the stomach) and the upper portion of the stomach.

Causes

Several relatively mild conditions and disorders may cause nausea and vomiting, including motion sickness, the "morning sickness" of pregnancy, excessive alcohol intake, emotional upset, and drug side effects. Eating too much, eating especially bothersome foods (such as oily or greasy foods), and eating spoiled food may also be responsible. More serious conditions that may be accompanied by nausea and vomiting are severe injury or pain, serious disorders of the digestive system (such as peptic ulcer or gastritis), heart disease, and certain glandular disorders. Vomiting without a preceding feeling of nausea may be a symptom of brain injury or brain tumor.

Symptoms

The symptoms that accompany nausea include a "sour" or queasy stomach, chills, perspiration, drowsiness, headache, rapid heartbeat and breathing, and excessive production of saliva.

Treatment

In most cases, nausea and vomiting require little or no treatment—they will subside when the cause is removed or corrected. However, if vomiting occurs regularly or frequently without an obvious cause, or if blood or red or dark brown spots appear in the vomitus (the material discharged during vomiting), medical treatment should be sought immediately. (The physician may want to examine a sample of the vomitus.)

Home remedies will often help to relieve the discomfort of occasional bouts of nausea and vomiting. Drinking tea, noncola beverages (especially ginger ale), and soup or broth is often suggested to replace the fluids that are lost due to vomiting. Solid food usually is not recommended during bouts of vomiting, but when vomiting subsides, toast or crackers may be tried before returning to a normal diet.

Several medications can successfully control the urge to vomit, but they need to be prescribed by a doctor and should be used only with caution. Any woman who is pregnant or thinks she may be pregnant should consult her doctor before taking this (or any other) type of medication.

Pain

Pain is an unpleasant or uncomfortable sensation that can range from mild irritation to excruciating agony. It is probably the most commonly reported symptom and may be associated with innumerable disorders and diseases.

Causes

Pain occurs when specialized nerve endings are stimulated; within a fraction of a second this pain "signal" travels through a network of nerves to the brain. Pain can be a warning sign, indicating impending damage to the body, or it can be a protective mechanism, causing a person to remove the cause of the pain or to reflexively draw away from the source. Most healthy people have occasional, brief twinges of pain that have no specific cause and are usually harmless. However, bothersome, recurring, or persistent pain can be caused by thousands of factors. Most commonly, pain is a symptom of disease, injury, or abnormal changes in the body.

Types

There are many types of pain. Pain can be dull and constant, sharp and sudden, crushing, burning, piercing, or aching. When it is felt in areas other than the location of the disorder (for example, when the pain of heart attack is felt in the arm), it is called referred pain.

Diagnosis

Unexplainable pain should be reported promptly to a doctor for investigation and possible treatment. It is best to observe any accompanying symptoms and to be prepared to answer two questions that the doctor will almost certainly ask in trying to identify the cause of the pain: "What brings on the pain?" and "What brings relief?"

Treatment

The ideal treatment for pain consists of finding and correcting its source. In some cases, however, such as in widespread cancer, this would be impossible, so the pain itself needs to be treated, most commonly with analgesic drugs (painkilling medications). Aspirin and acetaminophen are probably the most common painkillers that can be obtained without a prescription. More potent painkillers, such as narcotics, must be prescribed by a doctor. Other drugs, both prescription and nonprescription, are designed to treat and relieve the pain of a specific disorder (for example, antacids treat the discomfort of heartburn).

If the pain comes from the muscles (such as that from overexertion or from a bruising injury), adequate rest of the affected area may bring relief. Surface treatment of this type of pain is often very beneficial; this consists of massage or application of heat or cold (depending on the injury and the time elapsed since incurring it).

Rash

A rash is an eruption on the surface of the skin, covering either small areas of the body or extensive areas, in the form of red spots, patches, or blisters. A rash often causes itching, but this is not always the case. A rash is usually a temporary condition, appearing and disappearing within a few days, if not sooner. If so, there is little need for worry; however, a rash can also be a symptom of infectious diseases or other disorders.

Causes

Allergic rashes may be caused by exposure to the sun, heat, cold, the chemicals in household cleansers or detergents, fabrics, or certain foods. A rash may also be a symptom of certain diseases, such as measles, rubella (German measles), chicken pox, and shingles.

Rashes that appear regularly with no other symptoms may indicate the presence of an allergy; if a rash is accompanied by other symptoms, such as fever, it is more likely that the cause is an infectious disease.

Treatment

Any rash that lasts for more than a few days should be examined by a doctor. A rash will usually disappear when its cause is treated. In the case of an allergy, the only treatment may be something to relieve itching and irritation, but allergy testing may indicate which irritant to avoid in the future.

Sore throat

A sore throat is a painful irritation in the throat, often a symptom of the common cold. A sore throat can range from mild scratchiness to severe pain and difficulty in swallowing.

Causes

A sore throat is most frequently seen as a symptom of the common cold, when the nasal passages are congested and the person is forced to breath through the mouth, leaving the throat dry and irritated. Coughing may also irritate the throat, as will the secretions that drain into the throat from the back of the nose during a cold.

Irritating environmental substances, such as smoke, pollen, pollution, and dust, can cause a sore throat when inhaled; also, soreness of the throat may result when hot liquids or foods are swallowed.

A severe sore throat may be caused by a bacterial (frequently streptococcal) infection of the throat, middle ear, nose, or sinuses. Left untreated, a certain type of strep throat can lead to rheumatic fever (a disease that can affect the heart valves) or to glomerulonephritis (a disease of the kidneys).

Symptoms

A sore throat is characterized by dryness and scratchiness in the throat and pain when swallowing. A doctor should be notified if a sore throat lasts more than several days, if it occurs without a cold, or if no obvious irritant can be found; these circumstances may indicate a serious disease, a blood disorder, or a severe infection. If a sore throat is accompanied by fever, achiness, and fatigue, or if the throat and mouth are very red or covered with yellow or white spots, a bacterial infection may be present, and appropriate cultures should be obtained. A recently developed screening test allows the physician to diagnose a streptococcal infection (strep throat) within minutes.

Treatment

A simple sore throat accompanying a cold is treated by relieving the other cold symptoms. A nasal decongestant may be used if the nose is congested. A cough suppressant may be used if coughing is irritating the throat; cough suppressants are not always recommended, however, because they allow mucus to accumulate and thus may trigger further complications. Sour, hard candy can stimulate saliva production, which will moisten the throat. Frequent gargling with warm salt water soothes the irritated tissues of the throat by reducing swelling.

If a strep infection is the cause of the sore throat, antibiotics are prescribed to prevent rheumatic fever and to fight the infection, and aspirin or an aspirin substitute, such as acetaminophen, is prescribed to relieve pain and fever.

Vital signs

Vital signs is a term used in diagnostic medicine for four easily observed variables—body temperature, pulse rate, respiratory rate, and blood pressure. Although evaluation of the vital signs is not sufficient to arrive at a clear diagnosis of a patient's condition, these four items taken together serve as important indicators of the presence of disease or injury. A check of the vital signs is usually the first step in a diagnostic evaluation.

Temperature

Temperature is a useful index of a patient's condition, since a fever (an abnormal rise in body temperature) is usually a significant indicator of disease. Fever is generally a sign of infection, but it can be present whenever there is tissue destruction (from a severe sunburn, for example).

Pulse rate

The pulse rate reflects the heart rate. The heart rate varies with a person's level of physical activity; for example, the heart beats faster during exercise and more slowly during rest. An inappropriate heart rate may indicate disease. A feverish patient will have an increased heart rate, while a weak but rapid pulse is characteristic of severe blood loss or diseases of the heart itself. An irregular pulse rate may also indicate a reaction to stress or to overconsumption of caffeine.

Respiratory rate

The respiratory rate is the rate of breathing. Patients with fever hyperventilate (have an increased respiratory rate), which lowers body temperature. Hyperventilation is a common response to pain or stress, as well. Any condition that leads to acidosis (the presence of abnormally high acid levels in the body) drives the respiratory rate upward. Diseases of the lungs, such as emphysema, also increase respiratory rate.

Blood pressure

The blood pressure is an indicator of the amount of blood in circulation and the pumping force of the heart. A decrease in circulating blood volume, such as occurs in cases of severe bleeding, lowers blood pressure and deprives the tissues of adequate blood flow. Reflexes then are initiated that compensate, in part, for the reduced blood volume and pressure. For example, the heart rate increases in an attempt to make up for the reduction in blood volume, and the blood vessels supplying the digestive organs narrow, which diverts blood to more vital areas, such as the brain. Sustained elevation of blood pressure constitutes a disorder in its own right—hypertension.

INFECTIOUS DISEASES

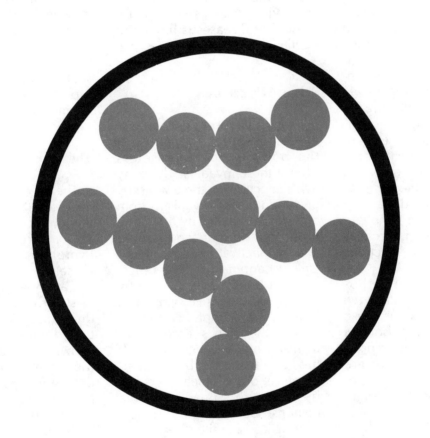

The human body is both surrounded and inhabited by billions of microorganisms (living organisms that are so small that they can be seen only with a microscope). Most microorganisms are harmless or even beneficial; for example, certain bacteria that normally live in the digestive system help digest food. Occasionally, however, a microorganism capable of causing a disease invades the body. Diseases caused by such microorganisms are called infectious diseases.

Infectious diseases are contagious; that is, they can be passed from one person to another. They can be transmitted by skin contact, through body fluids, in contaminated food or drink, or via airborne particles containing the microorganisms. Animal or insect bites are another means of transmission. (If an insect, for example, bites an infected person, the insect can carry the microorganism and pass the disease by biting another person.) The two most common types of infectious diseases are bacterial infections and viral infections.

Disease-causing, or pathogenic, bacteria either attack the body's tissues directly or cause damage by secreting poisonous substances called toxins. Fortunately, bacterial infections are frequently curable; certain bacteria can be killed by drugs. Other bacterial diseases can be prevented by vaccination. (Bacteria will be discussed later in this chapter.)

Viruses are the smallest known microorganisms. They are responsible for diseases as relatively harmless as the common cold and as serious as meningitis. Viruses live and reproduce only within living cells, and only certain cells are susceptible to a specific virus. You can be host to many viruses without suffer-

ing any adverse effects, but if enough cells are attacked, you will become sick.

There is no effective medical treatment for most viral infections. Because a virus lives inside a cell, any treatment designed to kill the virus is also likely to harm the cell. In addition, there are thousands of different viruses—each with different properties—and an agent effective against one virus probably will not affect the others. Although there are vaccinations for some viral diseases, therapy for most viral diseases is limited to treating the symptoms.

The body's defenses

Despite the prevalence of disease-causing microorganisms, the body is not defenseless against these invaders. The body fights infections in three ways: by preventing these organisms from entering the body, by attacking those that do manage to enter, and by inactivating those organisms it cannot kill. Sometimes, too, the body fights disease by developing defensive symptoms. Fever is an example. During an illness, the body's temperature regulator may respond to the illness by raising the body's temperature. Some researchers believe that this is an effective response because the microorganisms causing the disease may not be able to survive the higher body temperature.

The skin is the first barrier that guards the underlying tissues of the body. Where there are natural openings in the skin, there are also defenses. For example, tear glands in the eyes secrete and bathe the eyes with fluid that contains bacteria-fighting components. The salivary glands in the mouth and the tonsils in the

throat help prevent microorganisms from attacking the mouth and throat. Many openings, as well as internal passages, in the body are lined with mucous membranes. These delicate layers produce mucus, a slippery secretion that moistens and protects by repelling or trapping microorganisms. Internally, certain body organs fight infection. For instance, the liver and the spleen (a large glandlike organ located in the abdomen) filter out harmful substances from the blood flowing through them. The lining of the stomach produces acids that attack germs in food that has been eaten. The body's lymph system manufactures white blood cells, which attack and kill invading organisms.

The lymph system

The lymph system is a network of vessels that carry lymph, a watery fluid containing white blood cells, throughout the body. Lymph drains from the blood vessels and body tissues, carrying away waste products. The waste products are filtered out of the lymph by small structures called lymph nodes (popularly known as lymph glands). Within the lymph nodes, harmful microorganisms are trapped, attacked, and destroyed by white blood cells. This is one of the body's primary and most efficient lines of defense.

Antibodies are manufactured in the lymph system. Antibodies are protective substances that the body produces in response to invasion by a hostile organism or the presence of a foreign substance. Antibodies counteract some invading bacteria and viruses by inactivating them so that they are powerless. Antibodies that neutralize toxins (poisons) produced by bacteria are called antitoxins.

The body's production of white blood cells and antibodies in response to an invading disease organism is called the immune reaction. Immunity is the body's ability to resist an invasion of disease-causing bacteria or viruses. Once antibodies have been made to fight a certain type of microorganism, that type usually no longer poses a threat to the body. That is why one attack of a disease often prevents the recurrence of that disease. The first attack causes antibodies to be produced, and these antibodies protect the system against subsequent attacks.

Immunization

Immunity can be provided artificially by vaccination and other forms of immunization. A vaccine is a preparation containing the offending organism—usually in a weakened form that will not cause the actual disease. When introduced into the body, the vaccine stimulates the body to produce antibodies against the disease. These antibodies remain in the system for a long time (often for life), and the body is thus prepared to resist the actual disease.

A number of viral diseases can be prevented by immunization. Currently there are vaccines for polio, measles, rubella (German measles), mumps, and some strains of influenza. Researchers are working on a vaccine against chicken pox and shingles; however, this vaccine is not yet available to the public. A new vaccine against Hemophilus influenza type B is now available to prevent the most common cause of bacterial meningitis in children.

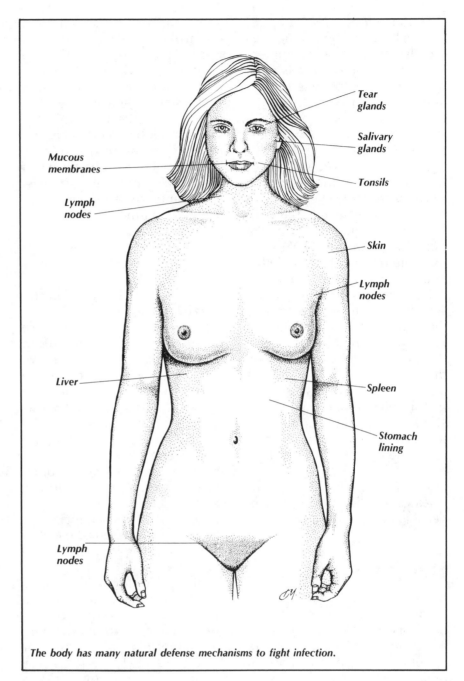

The body has many natural defense mechanisms to fight infection.

Tear glands

Salivary glands

Mucous membranes

Tonsils

Lymph nodes

Skin

Lymph nodes

Liver

Spleen

Stomach lining

Lymph nodes

Medications

Besides vaccination, there are other measures that can be used to help the body's natural defenses fight off infectious diseases. Bacterial infections can often be conquered by medications called antibiotics. These are substances derived from living microorganisms that kill other microorganisms. Penicillin, for example, comes from a living mold called *Penicillium*. Penicillin is one of the most commonly used antibiotics, along with streptomycin, tetracycline, and erythromycin. Each of these is effective against specific diseases. Antibiotics work either by destroying bacteria or by preventing their reproduction.

Sulfonamides, or sulfa drugs, are synthetic antibiotic drugs that are also effective against infections. This type of drug is often prescribed for localized infections in the urinary tract.

Unfortunately, these medications do not attack viruses. Viruses, therefore, are responsible for many of the serious or fatal infectious illnesses today, since no generally effective cures have been developed. The virus that causes acquired immune deficiency syndrome (AIDS) is an example of a particularly lethal virus for which there is no cure.

Researchers are continually searching for new ways to help the body combat infectious diseases. Medical advances against these diseases have already been dramatic; not too many years ago infectious diseases were uncontrollable and thus a constant danger. The control of many infections has been one of medicine's greatest accomplishments.

The more common infectious diseases are discussed in greater detail in the following pages.

Bacteria

Bacteria are one-celled microscopic organisms. Some kinds of bacteria cause disease in humans and animals, but many others are beneficial. Bacteria dispose of organic waste, enrich the soil, and are used to make wine, beer, vinegar, cheese, and yogurt. In human beings, certain beneficial bacteria live in the intestines, where they assist in digestion.

Bacteria are different from viruses in that they are able to multiply outside a living cell, whereas viruses can grow and multiply only in living cells. Bacteria are different from other causes of infection—protozoa

(one-celled animals) and fungi (plantlike organisms)—in two ways: They have a primitive nucleus (center where genetic material is located), rather than a well-defined one with an enclosing membrane and chromosomes; and they reproduce simply by splitting in two (binary fission), rather than by means of the more complex process, called mitosis, that is seen in higher organisms.

Types

One way of classifying bacteria is by shape:

Rod-shaped bacteria are known as bacilli. They often have waving projections known as flagella, which they use to propel themselves. Some form thick-walled cells known as spores, which can survive for long periods even after the parent bacteria have been killed by freezing, disinfectants, or other harsh forces. When conditions are favorable, the spores are able to generate new bacteria. Typhoid fever is caused by bacilli.

Round or egg-shaped bacteria are known as cocci. They occur singly (micrococci), in chains (streptococci—the cause of strep throat), in pairs (diplococci—the cause of a common type of pneumonia), or in irregular bunches (staphylococci—a cause of many skin infections). Cocci do not form spores, nor do they usually move about.

Bacteria also exist as comma-shaped organisms called vibrios (the organisms responsible for cholera) and as spiral-shaped organisms, such as the spirochete that causes syphilis.

Another way to classify bacteria is by whether they can live in the presence of air. Those that can are called *aerobic;* those that

cannot are called *anaerobic.* Some can live either with or without air and are called *facultative anaerobes.* Tetanus (lockjaw) is an example of a disease caused by anaerobic bacteria that are commonly found in the soil. They pose no danger to humans unless they enter the body through a wound, particularly a puncture wound (such as one made by a nail). The air then cannot get to the organisms to destroy them, and so they multiply within the body, unless the infected person has been vaccinated against tetanus.

How bacteria are transmitted

Disease-causing bacteria enter the body in many different ways. Those that cause pneumonia and sore throat are carried in droplets that an infected person sneezes or coughs into the air; the bacteria are then inhaled and deposited on the mucous membranes of the throat or lungs of a healthy person, where they multiply and eventually cause disease, unless checked by the body's immune system. The bacteria that cause intestinal diseases like cholera and typhoid can be transmitted in foods that have been handled by an infected person or in water tainted by body wastes from an infected individual. Another important route for infection is any break in the skin, which is why it is important to clean any cut in the skin as soon as possible.

Bacteria and the body's defenses

Once inside the body, bacteria do their damage in two main ways: by direct destruction of tissue and by producing toxins (poisons). Certain white blood cells, known as lymphocytes, produce substances called antitoxins, which neutralize the toxins of the bacteria, and substances called antibodies, which destroy the invading bacteria themselves. Once created, the antibodies against a specific disease can persist in the body or be reproduced when needed, providing continuous immunity—sometimes for life. Still other white blood cells, known as phagocytes, entrap and destroy bacteria.

Candida albicans

Candida albicans is a fungus that is normally present on the skin and on membranes of the mouth, throat, intestines, and vagina. It becomes an infecting agent only when there is some change in the body environment that allows it to grow out of control.

Causes

The most common cause of infection may be the use of antibiotics that destroy beneficial as well as harmful microorganisms in the body and permit *Candida* to multiply in their place. The resulting condition is known as candidiasis, candidosis, moniliasis, or a "yeast" infection. In the mouth, it is thrush; on the skin, an inflamed rash such as diaper rash; in the vagina, vaginitis, moniliasis, or yeast infection; and in or next to the nails, candidal onychomycosis or paronychia, respectively. Candidal infection can also affect the esophagus (food tube) and the digestive tract. In rare instances, when body resistance is low, *Candida albicans* enters the bloodstream and causes serious infection of the vital organs.

Those at risk

Drug addicts, diabetics, people with AIDS, and patients receiving chemotherapy are especially at risk. So are those whose natural defenses are weakened by drugs that suppress the immune system (such as those given to recipients of organ transplants). Pregnant women are often susceptible to moniliasis, and thrush may develop in babies who passed through an infected birth canal.

Symptoms and treatment

The symptoms and treatment for the various forms of *Candida* infection are as follows:
• Vaginitis is characterized by a white or yellow discharge, with inflammation of the walls of the vagina and of the vulva (external genital area). A white, curdlike substance may cling to the walls of the vagina. Treatment is with an antifungal drug, such as nystatin, which is inserted deep in the vagina and, if necessary, applied to the entire region around the entrance to the vagina. The infection is often passed to the woman's sexual partner, causing irritation, redness, and soreness of the head of the penis and sometimes a slight discharge. Both partners should use the medication when one has a recurring infection. Otherwise, the disease may pass back and forth between them. Recurrent *Candida* vaginitis or vaginitis that does not respond to treatment may indicate that another illness, such as diabetes, is present or that a different microorganism is responsible.
• Thrush appears as creamy-white or bluish-white patches on the tongue, which is inflamed and sometimes beefy red; on the lining of the mouth; or in the throat. This is especially common in young infants. Treatment is usually with nystatin oral solution or drops five times a day until a few days after all of the patches have disappeared.
• Diaper rash caused by *Candida* can be treated by keeping the baby's diaper area as dry as possible with frequent diaper changes. In severe cases, an antifungal ointment may be prescribed.
• Infections of the fingernails and toenails appear as red, painful swelling around the nail; later, pus develops. After the area has been treated with hot compresses and drainage (if necessary), and the nail has been cut back, an antifungal lotion is applied. The nail itself may be involved (appearing hard, yellow, and dull), making treatment more difficult and perhaps necessitating long-term use of oral drugs. Newer oral drugs, such as ketoconazole, are reserved for more severe or resistant infections.
• Systemic infection (when infection enters the bloodstream and affects the kidneys, heart, lungs, eyes, or other organs) can result in high fever, chills, anemia, and sometimes a rash or shock. Disease in the lungs can cause bloody sputum (mucus discharge); in the kidneys, blood in the urine; in the brain, seizures; in the heart, murmurs and valve damage; in the eye, pain and blurred vision. An antifungal medicine is usually given intravenously.

In all cases, the underlying condition that caused the outbreak of *Candida* must be removed, if possible. This may mean stopping the use of antibiotics or controlling diabetes. The same approach is used to prevent future infections.

Chicken pox

Chicken pox is an extremely contagious disease that is characterized by a blistery rash. It occurs most frequently in children between the ages of five and eight; less than 20 percent of the cases in the United States affect people over 15 years old. Chicken pox is transmitted so easily that almost everyone gets the disease at some time.

Causes

Chicken pox is caused by infection with the varicella zoster virus.

Chicken pox is contracted by touching an infected person's blisters or anything that has been contaminated by contact with them. The virus is also thought by some researchers to be airborne, since it may be caught from an infected person before the rash develops. Another way to get chicken pox is by exposure to shingles, a localized rash caused by the same virus.

The incubation period (the time between exposure to the illness and the appearance of symptoms) of chicken pox is 10 to 21 days. It is contagious for about six to eight days after the rash appears or until all of the blisters have dried out.

Symptoms

The first symptom of chicken pox is usually a rash, which can be very itchy. It begins as small, red spots on the trunk. Within hours, the spots become larger,

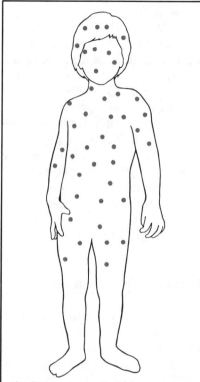

The first symptom of chicken pox is usually an itchy rash that begins as small red spots on the trunk. Within hours, the spots become larger, fluid-filled blisters and begin spreading out from the trunk to the face, scalp, arms, and legs.

fluid-filled blisters on a red base that begin to spread out from the trunk to the face, scalp, arms, and legs. Over the next few days, the blisters continue to fill with pus, burst, and then form a scab or crust. New spots appear periodically during a two- to six-day period. They may spread to the soles and palms. The rash may even affect the eyes, mouth, throat, vagina, and rectum.

Another main symptom is a mild fever (101°F to 103°F) that rises and disappears as the rash comes and goes. Some children have a slight fever and feel sluggish a few days before the rash begins; however, this warning is more common in adults.

Adults usually have higher fevers, a more severe rash, head-

aches, and muscle aches, and they take longer to recuperate than children. Recovery from all symptoms takes ten days to two weeks.

Complications

Complications of chicken pox seldom develop in otherwise healthy people. The most common complication is bacterial infection of the blisters, which may occur if the blister is scratched and the skin is broken. In some instances, the rash spreads to the eyes and causes pain and possible damage. Generally, the chicken pox rash heals without leaving scars, unless the blisters have been scratched and become infected. A rare but serious complication of chicken pox in children is Reye's syndrome (brain inflammation accompanied by liver deterioration). A doctor should be consulted if breathing problems, high fever, extreme drowsiness, severe headache, vomiting, or unsteadiness occurs within the course of the disease or within several weeks of recovery. It may indicate further complications.

Treatment

Since there is no known cure for chicken pox, treatment consists of reducing the effects of the symptoms. A soothing lotion, such as calamine lotion, lessens itchiness. Baths in warm (not hot) water sometimes mixed with a special oatmeal solution keep the skin clean, reduce the risk of infection in the rash, and reduce itching. It is important to gently yet thoroughly dry the skin after bathing. If itching is severe, the fingernails should be trimmed and gloves should be worn at night to minimize unconscious scratching. Children may need to wear mittens and socks all day for the duration of the rash.

Since an association has been established between aspirin use during a viral infection and Reye's syndrome in children, it is recommended that aspirin not be given to a child with chicken pox. A doctor can suggest an aspirin substitute if needed for discomfort or fever.

Prevention

Although almost everyone contracts chicken pox once, most people do not get it again because the body manufactures antibodies to combat the virus. Nevertheless, the same virus may cause shingles later in life. Researchers are working on a vaccine against chicken pox and shingles; however, this vaccine is not yet available to the public. There is a substance known as zoster immune globulin, which is human antibody against the virus. It must be used shortly after a known exposure to the virus, and there are no guarantees of disease prevention. Because of limited supplies and possible side effects, its use is limited to special cases of exposure, such as in pregnant women or individuals for whom chicken pox could be fatal.

Diphtheria

Diphtheria is a sudden, severe, and highly contagious disease that primarily affects the tonsils, upper airways, and larynx (voice box). Diphtheria bacteria destroy the outer layer of the mucous membrane of the throat or larynx; the slush of dead cells, bacteria, and white blood cells that

remains forms the grayish membrane covering the tonsils and throat that is the chief sign of the disease. Complications may include inflammation of the heart muscle (myocarditis), which sometimes results in heart failure, and temporary neuritis (nerve inflammation). Diphtheria bacteria also infect skin wounds but cannot invade intact skin.

Cause

Diphtheria is caused by the bacterium known as *Corynebacterium diphtheriae,* which is transmitted via droplets of moisture from the throat and nose of an infected person. It is most common during the colder months, when schools are in session and people are in closer contact. Frequently, the bacteria are transmitted by carriers—people who have no symptoms and do not even know that they harbor the disease. The incubation period (the time between exposure to the infection and appearance of the first symptom) is one to seven days.

Symptoms

Early symptoms include a mild sore throat, hoarseness, a rasping croupy cough, pain when swallowing, and a mild fever. Children may be nauseated, may vomit, and may have chills and headache as well as fever and other symptoms. The membrane that forms typically is tough, adheres tightly, and causes bleeding if removed. It appears in patches and can vary from yellowish to grayish green or dirty gray (the most common color). Some people have little or no characteristic membrane. If the membrane extends from the

throat to the trachea (windpipe), larynx, or bronchi (air tubes in the lungs), it can become detached and obstruct the passage partially or completely, choking off the air supply. Signs of this life-threatening emergency are rapid breathing, high-pitched breathing sounds, and blue lips and fingertips. Narrowing of the air passage may also be caused by edema (swelling of fluid-filled tissue) of the lining of the larynx and throat.

Treatment

Treatment is with diphtheria antitoxin (a solution of refined and concentrated protective antibodies obtained from the blood of horses that have been immunized against the poisons created by the diphtheria bacteria). This should be done at once, after a skin test to determine that the patient is not allergic to horse serum (blood fluid). (A patient who is found to be allergic is desensitized with a series of diluted doses of antitoxin.) After the antitoxin has been administered, antibiotics, such as penicillin or erythromycin, are given for at least a week to eliminate the diphtheria organisms. The patient is isolated until two cultures obtained 24 hours apart indicate that the infection is gone.

Because of the possible severe or even fatal complications of diphtheria, patients with symptoms need to be placed in a hospital intensive care unit for complete rest and careful observation. If signs of airway obstruction occur, a tracheotomy (surgical creation of a hole in the neck) will be performed immediately so that a tube can be passed into the lungs to supply oxygen. Frequent checking of the heart and nervous system is needed to identify complications. In severe cases, these can include heart irregularities, heart stoppage, and nervous system disorders, such as swallowing difficulty caused by paralysis of swallowing muscles.

Those who have been in close contact with the patient and who have not been immunized should receive throat cultures and be immunized with vaccine. These people should be watched carefully for the development of symptoms and be given antitoxin should symptoms occur. Another approach is to give antitoxin immediately (after allergy has been ruled out). In people who have been immunized, a booster of vaccine will be sufficient. Cultures of the nose, throat, and any open wounds should be obtained from all contacts of patients with diphtheria. Carriers of diphtheria should be given seven to ten days of treatment with an appropriate antibiotic. If the organism is still present, another course of drug therapy should be given. If this fails, tonsillectomy may be needed.

Prevention

Fortunately, widespread immunization has made diphtheria a rare disease. To maintain this status, children should be immunized beginning in infancy. The diphtheria vaccine is usually given in combination with the vaccines against tetanus and pertussis (whooping cough)—the DTP immunization.

Enteroviral infections

The enteroviruses are a group of viruses that cause a wide variety of usually brief, but occasionally serious, illnesses that are particularly common in children. Included in the group are the coxsackieviruses, the echoviruses, and the polioviruses.

Enteroviral infections occur most often in the summer and fall and can be spread by contact with infected human feces or respiratory secretions. Although they produce a great deal of temporary discomfort, most of the enteroviral infections generally do not cause lasting illness. Often, the only treatment possible is to make the patient comfortable, with plenty of liquids, bed rest, lukewarm sponge baths, and nonaspirin pain relievers, such as acetaminophen, to control fever until the illness has passed. Careful hand washing and proper disposal of human wastes can help prevent the spread of infection.

The following diseases are among those caused by the enteroviruses.

Aseptic meningitis

This inflammation of the membrane covering the brain causes headache, pain and stiffness in the neck and back, fever, nausea, vomiting, drowsiness, and a general sick feeling. Most patients recover in a week or so, but the disease may be fatal for newborns.

Hand, foot, and mouth disease

In this disease, which is common in young children, little blisters erupt all over the mucous membranes in the mouth, on the hands and feet (including the palms and soles), and sometimes in the diaper area. A low-grade fever is common.

Herpangina

An epidemic disease in infants and young children, herpangina is marked by sudden high fever, headache, sore throat, vomiting, and the appearance of grayish spots on the soft palate (rear roof of the mouth), tonsils, or throat. The spots become shallow ulcers and heal in three to six days.

Myocarditis and pericarditis

Possibly fatal heart failure in newborns may result from myocarditis (inflammation of the heart muscle) caused by coxsackieviruses or echoviruses transmitted to the baby by the mother. Myocarditis and pericarditis (inflammation of the sac around the heart) in older children and in adults may also be caused by a coxsackievirus; patients usually make a complete recovery, although congestive heart failure can occur.

Paralytic disease

Various echoviruses, coxsackieviruses, and polioviruses produce muscle weakness or paralysis that is similar to the paralysis of poliomyelitis and is treated in the same manner.

Pleurodynia (Bornholm disease)

Sudden, recurrent pains in the lower chest or abdomen signal the onset of this illness, which is often accompanied by fever, headache, nausea, abdominal tenderness, and sore throat. The disease may spread to cause pleuritis (inflammation of the tissue surrounding the lungs and lining the chest), pericarditis, or aseptic meningitis.

Poliomyelitis

Poliomyelitis (also known as polio and infantile paralysis), caused by the three types of polioviruses, is a serious infection of the spinal cord, which can result in paralysis of all of the muscles. The symptoms include muscle soreness and stiffness of the neck and spine. With the development of the polio vaccine, polio has been virtually eradicated in the United States, but the threat of polio epidemics remains if children are not routinely immunized.

Respiratory disease

The enteroviruses cause respiratory illnesses accompanied by head cold, fever, sore throat, and sometimes vomiting and diarrhea.

Rubellalike rash

A mild rash like that of rubella (German measles), but lasting longer, this usually occurs in epidemic form and only on the face, neck, and chest. Fever is common, and meningitis can develop, but usually this is a mild disease.

Histoplasmosis

Histoplasmosis is an infection that follows the inhalation of spores from the fungus *Histoplasma capsulatum*. The parts of the body principally affected are the lungs, liver, and spleen.

Cause

The *Histoplasma capsulatum* spore is found in soil and in the air. There is no practical defense against breathing the spores. Development of symptoms seems to be a matter of individual immune system response.

Symptoms

In most instances, histoplasmosis does not reach the point at which symptoms appear. People may have the disease but, because of the action of their immune system, never have enough damage to make the symptoms noticeable, much less to create an acute condition. However, if symptoms do appear, they can be serious, especially when left untreated. The most common symptoms are as follows:
- Acute pneumonia (inflammation of the lungs)
- Influenzalike illnesses, with lethargy, cough, fever, and lung involvement
- Enlargement of the liver and the spleen, with accompanying interruption of their normal functioning
- The development of fibrous scar tissue in affected organs, particularly the lungs

Histoplasmosis can become inactive and then be reactivated at a later date. In cases of reactivated histoplasmosis, the lungs, meninges (coverings of the brain and spinal cord), heart, peritoneum (lining of the abdominal cavity), and adrenal glands can be involved.

Most affected people probably have histoplasmosis in a dormant form (present within their bodies, but not at the stage at which symptoms are evident). Fatalities occur only in cases of massive infection (which also implies massive breakdown or malfunctioning of the body's immune system).

Diagnosis

Treatment for histoplasmosis begins with diagnosis. The best procedure is to cultivate growths of *Histoplasma capsulatum* organisms from tissue or fluid samples. Another method is to note the rise in the body's production of antibodies (the protective substances produced by the body).

Treatment

An antifungal medication, such as ketoconazole or amphotericin B, is usually used to treat chronic cases. These drugs help control the disease but appear to have little effect on the fibrous scarring that often occurs in advanced cases.

Influenza

Influenza, more commonly called the flu, is a contagious disease that is accompanied by respiratory problems and fever. A bout of influenza is unpleasant, but it is usually not dangerous to otherwise healthy people.

Causes

Two types of viruses cause influenza: influenza A virus and influenza B virus. Each type encompasses several different strains, which are named for the place where they were first identified, for example, Hong Kong flu virus and Russian flu virus.

The unusual characteristic of the flu viruses is that once a strain has spread throughout a population, it changes in structure, becoming capable of causing a new form of influenza. The antibodies produced by the body to combat the virus are no longer effective because the virus has taken on different qualities. Scientists are generally able to predict what type of altered virus to expect each year, but about every ten years an entirely new strain appears.

Because influenza is thought to be transmitted by airborne particles from an infected person's respiratory tract, large numbers of people in a community or even in a country can easily contract the disease in a relatively short period of time. Overcrowded living conditions promote the transmission of the virus. Since flu spreads most easily when temperatures and humidity are low, most cases occur in the fall and winter.

Symptoms

Flu symptoms usually develop one to three days after exposure to the virus. Some people experience symptoms in as short a time as 18 hours. Fever, chills, headache, muscle aches, and total exhaustion can occur suddenly. Fevers generally do not exceed 104°F, but they may rise to 106°F.

Frequently, people experience a dry cough and a runny or congested nose as their initial symptoms begin to subside. These respiratory symptoms worsen and remain for three to four days. The cough and fatigue may persist for two weeks or more after the other symptoms have disappeared.

Complications

The most common complications are those that involve parts of the respiratory system—for example, pneumonia (inflammation of the lungs), which affects both adults and children, and croup (infection of the larynx), which affects young children. If the patient has extreme difficulty in breathing, blood in the coughed-up mucus, bluish skin, or a bark-like cough, a physician should be consulted immediately.

One life-threatening complication of influenza that affects children and adolescents between the ages of 2 and 16 years is Reye's syndrome. It is a type of encephalitis (inflammation of the brain) that is accompanied by deterioration of the liver.

Treatment

In most cases, influenza cannot be cured and is treated only by relieving symptoms. Amantadine, a drug used in the treatment of Parkinson's disease, can be used to prevent and treat some forms of influenza A infection. This drug can produce unpleasant side effects, however, so physicians usually prescribe it only when a patient is susceptible to additional complications.

Treatment for flu is generally the same as treatment for a bad cold or fever. Physicians recommend bed rest, extra fluids, and an aspirin substitute to reduce fever and muscle aches. Because an association has been established between aspirin use during a viral infection and Reye's syndrome in children, it is recommended that aspirin not be given to a child with influenza. Acetaminophen, however, has not been linked to Reye's syndrome and can be used. Nasal sprays or drops, when used sparingly so that nasal tissues are not damaged, and cough medicines can help relieve coldlike symptoms. Using a vaporizer in the patient's room to add moisture to the air relieves congestion.

Prevention

Each year, researchers prepare an influenza vaccine in an attempt to prevent spread of the virus. The vaccine is composed of inactivated organisms from several virus strains and provides protection against influenza caused by these strains. Unfortunately, protection is not necessarily afforded against new or different strains. Vaccines are typically between 67 percent and 92 percent effective. It is important for the elderly; people with lung disease, heart disease, or other chronic diseases; and those with immune system disorders to have this vaccine. Influenza can be devastating in these individuals.

Some people have reactions to the influenza vaccine. These reactions range from inflammation at the injection site to mild flu symptoms. On very rare occasions, nervous system disorders result. These vaccines are commonly prepared using eggs. Therefore, individuals with a known allergy to eggs should inform their physician before having the influenza vaccine. Vaccination is not usually recommended for children unless they are in a high risk group, such as those with heart or lung conditions.

Measles

Measles (also called rubeola) is a contagious disease that mainly affects the respiratory system, skin, and eyes. It was once considered one of the more dangerous childhood diseases because the threat of serious complications was so great. Fortunately, development of a vaccine to prevent measles has drastically reduced its occurrence.

Causes

Measles is caused by a virus. The virus is transmitted via droplets of moisture from the respiratory tract of an infected person that travel through the air. Some researchers contend that the virus enters the body through the eyes.

The incubation period (the time between exposure and the appearance of symptoms) for measles is 8 to 12 days. An infected person is contagious for up to four days before symptoms appear and for up to six days after the rash develops.

Symptoms

Measles usually begins much like a cold, with a runny nose, nasal congestion, sneezing, a dry cough, and a fever of 102°F to 104°F. After three or four days, the eyes may become sensitive to bright light as they grow red and swollen. Then the fever drops, and red spots with tiny white centers (called Koplik's spots after the physician who first identified them) appear in the cheek pouches of the mouth.

By the fourth or fifth day, the fever increases again, and a rash appears. The rash usually starts on the face and neck and behind the ears, and then spreads to the rest of the body. As the spots multiply, they grow larger, become raised, and sometimes blend together. They turn dark red and then brown before the skin begins to peel in small flakes. This process takes about one week after the rash first emerges, although skin discoloration can last as long as two weeks. Other symptoms usually disappear within seven to ten days after the appearance of the first symptoms.

The measles rash usually starts on the face and neck and behind the ears and then spreads to the rest of the body.

Complications

Breathing problems, increased coughing, earache, or extreme drowsiness may indicate complications that warrant consulting a doctor immediately. The more serious complications that may develop are pneumonia (inflammation of the lungs) and encephalitis (an inflammation of the brain). Subacute sclerosing panencephalitis, a rare but often fatal disease of the brain, has also been linked to measles. Severe ear infections can occur, particularly in young children. In addition, bronchitis, laryngitis, and swelling of the lymph nodes in the neck can prolong the course of the illness or make it appear to return.

Diagnosis

Generally, physicians diagnose measles by the initial symptoms. To confirm diagnosis, nasal discharge, blood, or urine can be tested for signs of the virus.

Treatment

Since measles is caused by a virus, it does not respond to antibiotics, and treatment must focus on relieving the patient's discomfort. A vaporizer in the patient's room will ease coldlike symptoms by adding moisture to the air. If the eyes are irritated, warm compresses may relieve the inflammation. Also, dim lights are easier on the eyes. Soaps that may irritate the skin should not be used. The doctor may suggest adding baking soda to bath water or applying a soothing lotion, such as calamine lotion, to the rash to relieve itching.

An association has been established between aspirin use during or immediately after a viral infection and Reye's syndrome (inflammation of the brain accompanied by deterioration of the liver). It is recommended that aspirin not be given to a child with measles. A doctor can suggest an aspirin substitute, such as acetaminophen, if needed for relief of discomfort or fever.

Prevention

Until recently, measles had been almost eliminated through childhood immunization. Unfortunately, over the last few years, the number of measles cases in the United States has increased dramatically due to low rates of immunization. This new epidemic has occurred in young children and older adolescents. The newest recommendation is that children receive the initial measles vaccine by injection at 15 months of age; a measles booster vaccine should be given at 11 or 12 years of age. If a measles outbreak occurs, anyone between 4 years and 21 years of age should receive a booster. If measles or vaccine history is unknown in an adult, it is best to check with your doctor. Blood tests that can show immunity are available. The vaccine, which is prepared from measles virus, stimulates production of antibodies (protective substances) in the body. Because the vaccine effectiveness rate is very low in young infants, babies are not vaccinated before 15 months of age unless measles cases have been reported in the area. The infants of women who are immune to measles (either because they have had measles or have been immunized) acquire temporary natural immunity that lasts for about the first six months of life. If a baby is exposed to measles, however, a doctor should be consulted. Measles is dangerous for anyone under three years of age and for anyone with a chronic illness.

Mononucleosis

Infectious mononucleosis, or "mono," is a contagious viral illness that initially attacks the lymph nodes in the neck and the throat. When these tissues become less effective in fighting infection, sore throat, swelling of the nodes, and fever result.

Cause

Mono is caused by the Epstein-Barr virus, which is named

Swelling of the lymph nodes in the neck and throat is often an early sign of mononucleosis.

after the scientists who first identified it in the mid-1960s. The virus enters the lymph nodes and attacks the lymphocytes (the white blood cells manufactured there). As the white blood cells come into contact with the virus, they change shape and multiply. At first there are no symptoms, because it takes several weeks before enough of the altered cells can accumulate to generate a reaction. Gradually, however, symptoms appear. First, there is a mild sore throat, sluggishness, and fever. The symptoms worsen as the body tries to fight the infection by creating more white blood cells. The symptoms usually diminish and disappear about six to eight weeks later.

Mononucleosis spreads by contact with moisture from the mouth and throat of a person who is infected with the virus. Kissing; sharing drinking glasses, eating utensils, and toothbrushes; or touching anything that has been near the mouth of an infected person may result in transmission of the disease.

Those at risk

Teenagers and young adults seem to be the most susceptible to acquiring mono. However, even children who are less than one year old can develop mono. The disease is uncommon in persons over the age of 35.

Symptoms

In all cases, the infection develops so slowly with such mild symptoms that it may be initially indistinguishable from a cold or the flu. However, a sore throat that lasts two weeks or more; swollen lymph nodes in the neck, throat, armpits, and groin; a persistent fever (usually about 102°F); and tiredness and malaise (a vague feeling of discomfort) may indicate mono. Mono symptoms can be mild or so severe that throat pain impedes swallowing and fever reaches 105°F. Some people also experience a rash, eye pain, and photophobia (discomfort in bright light).

Complications

Most cases of mono run an uncomplicated course. Occasionally, however, the infection spreads to other parts of the body besides the throat and lymph nodes. For example, mono may lead to monohepatitis (an inflammation of the liver that is not the same as hepatitis A, B, or non-A, non-B). Jaundice, a symptom of this complication, appears as a yellow discoloration of the skin and whites of the eyes. A much more serious problem is pain or tenderness in the abdomen. This discomfort may mean a swollen spleen (an organ in the lymph system), which could burst. Any of these symptoms should be reported to a physician for immediate attention.

Diagnosis

To diagnose infectious mononucleosis, blood samples are analyzed to detect the presence of antibodies to the Epstein-Barr virus and to determine overall blood cell count. Inflammation of the liver can also be detected and followed up with blood tests.

Treatment

As long as there are no complications, the best treatment is to rest, drink plenty of liquids until the temperature returns to normal, and then gradually resume normal activities as strength returns. If the patient feels well enough, complete bed rest is probably not necessary or beneficial.

Antibiotics are ineffective against mono, since it is a viral infection and viruses do not respond to antibiotics. However, mono can be accompanied by a streptococcal infection of the throat, in which case an antibiotic will be prescribed to treat that condition. In severe cases, corticosteroid drugs that reduce swelling are prescribed. If the spleen is swollen, the doctor may recommend avoiding strenuous activities, such as lifting and pushing, which may cause sudden rupture of the spleen. Hospitalization is necessary if there is a serious complication, such as rupture of the spleen.

Most people recover in six to eight weeks, but some cases take as long as six months for complete recovery. A tired feeling, which may include depression, is the last symptom to disappear. Mono may return in a milder form within a few months. Fortunately, mono almost never reappears in its full-blown form after a year.

In a related condition, chronic Epstein-Barr virus infection, symptoms of mono recur periodically over a period of years. This illness, among others, is often referred to as "chronic fatigue syndrome." Symptoms are similar to acute mono in that the individual notices severe fatigue, aches and pains in the muscles and joints, and low-grade fevers (less than 100°F). These symptoms generally tend to flare and subside chronically. There is no specific treatment for this illness, but analgesics, low doses of antidepressants, and rest during acute flare-ups are often helpful. It is important that these symptoms be differentiated from other diseases, such as malignancies of the lymph system. There is no specific diagnostic test for "chronic mono," but persistent high blood levels of antibody to the E-B virus can be found with a simple blood test and is helpful in establishing the diagnosis. Other than feeling miserable at times and perhaps losing work days, there are generally no serious complications of this condition.

Mumps

Mumps is a contagious viral disease that is usually contracted during childhood. More than 85 percent of the cases occur before the age of 15, especially between the ages of six and ten years.

Cause

Mumps is caused by a virus that attacks cells of the parotid salivary glands. This invasion results in painful swelling of the face beneath the ear along the jawline. Mumps virus spreads by contact with airborne moisture from an infected person's nose or throat. Sometimes, the infection comes from someone who has the disease without symptoms or who is not yet aware of the symptoms. The disease occurs most often during the spring months, although it can happen at any time of the year.

Symptoms

Symptoms can be so mild that they are almost nonexistent, or they can be very severe. Fever (101°F to 103°F), headache, and loss of appetite usually develop first, followed by earache; then the characteristic swelling of the salivary glands appears. Swelling may start on one side of the face and then appear on the other side within a few days. Sometimes, however, only one side swells. The inflammation may cause soreness and difficulty in eating or swallowing.

The sex glands may become swollen as well. Orchitis (inflammation of one or both testes) can cause considerable pain. Affected testes may shrink some-

what, but contrary to popular belief, it is not common for mumps to lead to sterility in males. Girls may have swelling in the ovaries, but there is seldom any severe discomfort. In addition, swelling may occur in other glands and organs, including the breasts, other salivary glands, the liver, and the brain.

Complications

Although mumps can be unpleasant, it rarely has long-term complications. Encephalitis (inflammation of the brain) is the most dangerous complication of mumps because it carries the risk of death. Another possible consequence of mumps encephalitis is hearing loss or even deafness. Hearing may return to normal after several months, however. A milder complication is meningoencephalitis (inflammation of the brain and its covering, the meninges). This disease causes a

stiff neck, headache, high fever, drowsiness, sensitivity to bright light, and sometimes delirium; these symptoms usually disappear without brain damage.

Pancreatitis (inflammation of the pancreas) can also result from mumps. Symptoms of pancreatitis include stomach pain, vomiting, chills, fever, and extreme weakness. Although these signs usually vanish and leave no damage, diabetes can result in rare cases. Other complications of mumps include nerve inflammation, heart problems, and nervous system disorders—all usually temporary. Symptoms of any of these should be brought to the attention of a doctor.

Diagnosis

A doctor diagnoses mumps on the basis of the characteristic form and texture of the swollen parotid glands. Boys may have swelling and tenderness in the testes. Exposure to the disease is also a clue. The incubation time (the time between exposure to the virus and the appearance of signs and symptoms) is 14 to 21 days. If mumps is suspected, secretions from the salivary glands can be tested for mumps virus.

Treatment

Treatment for mumps involves relieving the discomfort of the symptoms, since there is no cure for the disease. Bed rest is usually not necessary. Soft foods and liquids may be easier to swallow. However, fruit juices with a high acid content, like orange juice, may sting the mouth.

If the glands are severely swollen, a physician may prescribe painkilling drugs. Steroid drugs may be recommended for

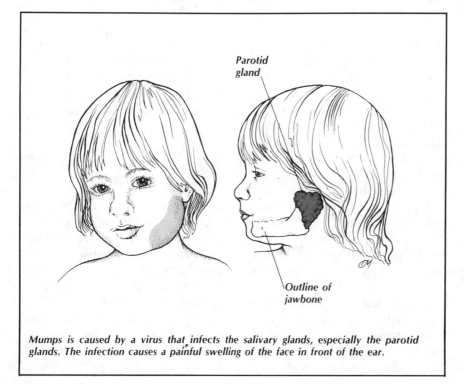

Parotid gland

Outline of jawbone

Mumps is caused by a virus that infects the salivary glands, especially the parotid glands. The infection causes a painful swelling of the face in front of the ear.

men or boys with extremely swollen testes, but these drugs may prove ineffective. Warm or cold compresses or an ice pack may relieve some pain. Most mumps symptoms disappear within about ten days.

Prevention

There is a vaccine that is 95 percent effective in preventing mumps. The vaccine stimulates the production of antibodies to resist the disease. Mumps vaccine is usually combined with measles and rubella (German measles) vaccines and given to children by injection when they are 15 months of age. There are usually no side effects from the mumps vaccine.

Reiter's syndrome

Reiter's syndrome is characterized by the occurrence of urethritis (inflammation of the urethra, which is the tube from the bladder to the outside of the body), conjunctivitis (inflammation of the membrane that covers the front of the eyeball and the insides of the eyelids), and arthritis (joint inflammation). It affects males more often than females.

Cause

It is thought that Reiter's syndrome is caused by a bacterial infection that is often sexually transmitted.

Symptoms

Reiter's syndrome exhibits multiple symptoms, any one of which might be mistaken for a sign of another disease. The conjunctivas become inflamed, with corresponding discomfort around the eyes. Urethritis causes discomfort during urination. Arthritic symptoms appear, with joint swelling and pain. Many victims also have a fever; diarrhea; sores on the palms of the hands, the soles of the feet, the trunk, the mouth, and the penis; and inflammation of the iris (the colored part of the eye).

Treatment

Treatment for Reiter's syndrome is similar to that for rheumatoid arthritis—aspirin or, if aspirin is ineffective, another nonsteroidal anti-inflammatory drug, such as ibuprofen, indomethacin, or naproxen. An antibiotic may help control the urethritis. Conjunctivitis can be treated with eye drops.

Rubella

Rubella, or German measles, is a relatively mild viral infection with coldlike symptoms and a short-lived rash. The disease is contagious; however, rubella outbreaks have become infrequent since the development of a vaccine to prevent the illness. Rubella is usually not dangerous, unless it occurs during pregnancy, when it can cause serious birth defects.

Cause

Rubella is caused by a virus. The virus spreads from one person to another via airborne droplets from an infected person's respiratory system. The incubation period (the time be-

The rubella rash usually first appears on the face and neck and then gradually spreads over most of the body.

tween exposure to the infection and appearance of symptoms) is usually 14 to 21 days. An infected person can spread the virus as early as one week before the rash appears and as late as five days after the rash has faded. A child with congenital (present at birth) rubella syndrome can transmit the virus until he or she is about 12 to 18 months old. Second infections have been reported, but they are rare.

Complications

Although rubella is generally a mild infection, some complications can arise. Encephalitis (inflammation of the brain) occurs in one in 5,000 cases. Thrombocytopenic purpura, a blood disease characterized by a lowered platelet count, can prove fatal when it accompanies rubella. High or prolonged fever and extreme fatigue should be reported to a physician to prevent further complications.

Congenital rubella syndrome occurs when the disease is transmitted to the fetus during pregnancy. Rubella virus may cause one or more serious organic and growth disorders of the fetus, particularly if contracted during the first three months of pregnancy. The most common problems include congenital heart defects, hearing and vision problems, blood disorders, and mental retardation and other brain disorders.

Symptoms

The first symptoms of rubella are a runny nose, swollen lymph nodes in the neck, and a low-grade fever (up to 101°F). About two days later, a rash of very small red or pink spots appears on the face and neck. The spots are flat initially. They then become slightly raised and fade within a day or two. As the first spots fade, more spots develop until the rash has spread over most of the body. The rash lasts only two to three days, but swelling of the lymph nodes may persist for as long as a week. All other symptoms have usually disappeared by then. When there is joint pain, as is common with older women, discomfort may last another week.

Diagnosis

Under normal circumstances, rubella is difficult to diagnose because the symptoms are so mild and variable. Sometimes there is no rash, and the disease resembles a cold. Other cases may be so severe that the infection may be confused with measles. A doctor can identify the virus by testing a blood sample. Tracing a history of exposure to the disease also helps to establish the diagnosis.

Treatment

Most patients require little or no treatment for rubella because the symptoms are so mild. An aspirin substitute may afford relief from joint pain. Otherwise, drugs are not needed. Some patients may want bed rest, but most people feel well enough to be somewhat active.

Prevention

Rubella rarely occurs now because children routinely receive rubella vaccine at about 15 months of age. The vaccine is usually combined with measles and mumps vaccines in one injection, but it can be given alone. The rubella vaccine can cause some mild muscle or joint aches, but they are rarely significant. The rubella vaccine works in the body to stimulate the production of antibodies (protective substances) that fight the disease.

Women who want to become pregnant should have a blood test to determine whether they are already immune to rubella; if not, they can be vaccinated. Vaccination is not recommended during pregnancy because of the possible risk to the fetus. Doctors also caution women to wait at least three months after rubella vaccination before trying to become pregnant.

Scarlet fever

Scarlet fever (also known as scarlatina) is a highly contagious illness caused by *Streptococcus* bacteria and is almost always accompanied by a strep throat.

Symptoms

The symptoms of scarlet fever include fever; sore throat; widespread scarlet rash beginning in the armpits and groin and spreading to the neck, chest, back, extremities, and even the tongue; and peeling and scaling of the skin, even on the palms and the soles. The incubation period (the time between exposure and appearance of symptoms) is two to four days.

Treatment

In the past, scarlet fever was often fatal, but today it is easily treated with penicillin, and complications are rare. Bed rest and a nourishing diet with plenty of fluids help speed recuperation.

Shingles

Shingles, or herpes zoster, is a painful viral infection of one or more nerves. The infection produces a blistery, itchy skin rash on the area of skin supplied by the affected nerve. Shingles rash looks identical to the rash of chicken pox, since shingles and chicken pox are both caused by the varicella zoster virus.

Causes

Shingles usually occurs only in persons who have already had chicken pox. Some scientists believe that after a case of chicken pox has run its course, the varicella zoster virus lies dormant in the body, but can be reactivated by injury to the affected area or after emotional or physical upset. Others believe that the number and strength of antibodies produced by the body to fight the varicella zoster virus diminish with time, making the person susceptible to another attack of the virus; because some antibodies endure, the person gets shingles rather than chicken pox. If an adult who has not had chicken pox is exposed to the virus, he or she will get chicken pox, not shingles.

The incidence of shingles increases with age. It rarely occurs in people under the age of 15. More than 50 percent of those who get shingles are over 45.

Symptoms

Shingles begins with prickling or tenderness in the skin over the affected nerve. Burning or shooting pain in the same area is also an early symptom. Within two to four days, a rash of small, red spots appears over the affected part of the body. As the spots enlarge, they blister and sometimes blend together. Eventually they fill with pus, burst, and crust over, much the same as with chicken pox rash. With shingles, however, the process takes longer and is confined to the skin area above the affected nerve.

The shingles rash is very itchy. Pain increases as the area beneath the rash becomes redder and more swollen. Shingles most often attacks nerves of the chest, back, neck, arms, and legs; however, facial nerves are frequently involved. The rash appears in a band or strip following the distribution of the nerve, usually on

Shingles is an infection of a nerve characterized by a blistering skin rash following the path of the affected underlying nerve. The rash itself is identical to that of chicken pox, since both diseases are caused by the same virus.

one side of the body. The rash persists for two to three weeks; the pain continues for three or four weeks. In persons over age 60, pain may persist for months to years after the rash has disappeared; this condition is called postherpetic neuralgia. This condition is difficult to treat. Antidepressants, antiseizure medications, electrical stimulation of the affected areas, and analgesics have been helpful in reducing the pain.

Complications

Occasionally, the shingles rash spreads over the entire body.

This develops most often in people who have some underlying disease, such as Hodgkin's disease (cancer of the lymph system) or leukemia (cancer of the blood). When these serious disorders already exist, shingles can cause death, but this is rare. A signal that other illness may be present is recurrence of shingles, since the condition seldom occurs more than once.

The most common complication of shingles is bacterial infection of the rash. This can prolong the rash and cause scarring of the skin.

Less common complications may follow a shingles attack on facial nerves. Eye disorders and

Bell's palsy (a disorder that temporarily paralyzes one side of the face) can result. Shingles in other parts of the body can cause similar temporary paralysis of the area over the affected nerve.

Treatment

Since there is no known cure for shingles, treatment focuses on reducing pain. An analgesic (pain-killing drug) may relieve the burning sensation. Some physicians prescribe steroid drugs to reduce nerve inflammation in older patients. To be effective, steroids must be taken soon after shingles begins. Steroid treatment is usually not recommended for persons with underlying disease because steroids can interfere with resistance to infection. Acyclovir, an antiviral drug given in ointment, oral, and intravenous forms, has been shown to shorten the course and decrease the severity of the illness in many cases.

Preventing infection is also important. Baths in warm (not hot) water soothe and clean the skin. If itching is severe, patients should cut their fingernails and wear gloves when asleep to control unconscious scratching.

Tetanus

Tetanus is an infectious disease, commonly associated with improperly cleaned deep wounds, that causes severe muscle contractions.

Cause

Tetanus is caused by toxins (poisonous substances) that are produced by *Clostridium tetani* bacteria. These bacteria may be present on the skin at the time of the injury or may enter the body through a wound caused by an object that has been in contact with material, such as soil, in which bacterial spores are present. Puncture wounds and animal bites, because of their depth, are especially vulnerable to tetanus infection since they are difficult to clean and medicate.

Symptoms

Symptoms are varied, depending on the extent of infection and the body part affected. A common symptom is lockjaw, in which the jaw muscles go into severe, continuous contraction, rendering the jaw immobile. Other symptoms include bowing or arching of the body (rare) because of contraction of lower back muscles, back muscle spasms, and throat spasms, which can block the airway. The affected body parts become immobile because of the simultaneous and continuous contraction of opposing muscles.

In severe cases, the contractions involve most of the fibers in an affected muscle, similar to what would be required to lift a heavy weight or to marshal all the potential force of a muscle against a great resistance. Such violent and prolonged muscle contractions can be very painful.

Treatment

Treatment includes muscle relaxant drugs, such as diazepam, to ease the contractions. Antimicrobial drugs, such as penicillin, are used to fight the infection. Antitoxin is injected into a muscle in the hope of lessening the severity of the disease. However, the antitoxin does not counteract the toxin already in the nervous system, nor does it relieve symptoms already present.

Prevention

Immunization with the tetanus vaccine is the best preventive. Infants begin at two months of age to receive the initial series of tetanus shots combined with diphtheria and whooping cough. Boosters are given at 18 months and five years and then every ten years after that through adulthood. Also, wounds should be attended to immediately, especially puncture wounds and animal bites. It is especially important that the tetanus booster be administered periodically if small skin wounds are common.

ALLERGIES AND THE IMMUNE SYSTEM

Immunity is the body's ability to defend itself against harmful organisms and substances. Essentially, it is a resistance to infection that may be inherited or acquired naturally or artificially.

Immunity develops when foreign organisms or substances, called antigens, enter the body, causing particular specialized cells to react either by attacking the antigen directly or by producing special proteins (microscopic molecules essential to living cells) that neutralize the foreign agents. The most common types of antigens are forms of bacteria (one-celled organisms that have the potential to attack body tissues or secrete poisonous substances called toxins) and viruses (the smallest infective agents, responsible for a variety of diseases).

Lymph system

The lymph system is the body's drainage system. It is composed of a network of vessels and small structures called lymph nodes. The lymph vessels convey excess fluid collected from all over the body back into the blood circulation. Along the way, however, these fluids are forced to percolate through the lymph nodes so that they can be filtered. Harmful organisms are trapped and destroyed by the specialized white blood cells, called lymphocytes, that are present in these nodes. Lymphocytes are also added to the lymph that flows out of nodes and back to the bloodstream.

Antibodies

Antibodies are manufactured by the lymph system. Antibodies are specialized proteins that the body produces in response to invasion by a foreign substance. The process of antibody formation begins when an antigen stimulates specialized lymphocytes, called B cells, into action. Antibodies then counteract invading antigens by combining with the antigen to ultimately render it harmless to the body. Some antibodies coat the harmful organisms so that the body's scavenger cells can destroy them more easily. The antibody molecule combines with the antigen molecule by matching combining sites; they fit together like the pieces of a jigsaw puzzle. Other antibodies that neutralize toxins produced by bacteria are called antitoxins.

During periods of active antibody production, lymph nodes often enlarge and become tender to the touch. For example, a vaccination (injection of a natural or artificial antigen to stimulate the body to produce protective antibodies) in the arm can cause swelling of the nodes in the armpit, while mononucleosis causes enlargement of nodes that can be felt under the skin of the armpits, groin, and neck. The spleen (an organ located in the upper left part of the abdomen) is also important in the production of antibodies.

Immune response

Production of white blood cells and antibodies in reaction to an invading disease organism is called an immune response. This response is one of the body's primary and most efficient lines of defense. In most cases, once antibodies have been produced to fight a certain organism, it no longer poses a great threat to the body. That is why one attack of a disease often pre-

vents that same disease from infecting the body again—the first attack causes production of antibodies that protect the body against subsequent attacks. With measles, for example, antibodies are produced as a result of having the disease or of being immunized with the measles vaccine. These antibodies are able to resist a second attack of the disease, providing protection against recurrence.

Antibodies are not always beneficial. For example, when tissue from another body, such as a transplanted heart, is introduced, antibodies are produced to destroy the "invader." Transplants usually are made possible only by means of drugs that act against the body's natural immune response. Also, when blood is transfused from one person to another, it must be of a matching type; otherwise, the recipient's immune system will manufacture antibodies to destroy the transfused blood.

Sometimes, the immune system causes reactions that make the body unusually sensitive to foreign material. When the immune response is disruptive to the body in this way, it is called an allergic reaction.

Allergic reaction

An allergy is a state of special sensitivity to a particular environmental substance, or allergen. An allergic reaction is the body's response, directed by the immune system, to exposure to an allergen.

Although an allergy can be present almost immediately after exposure to an allergen, it usually develops over time, as the immune system forms antibodies against the foreign substance. Under normal conditions, such

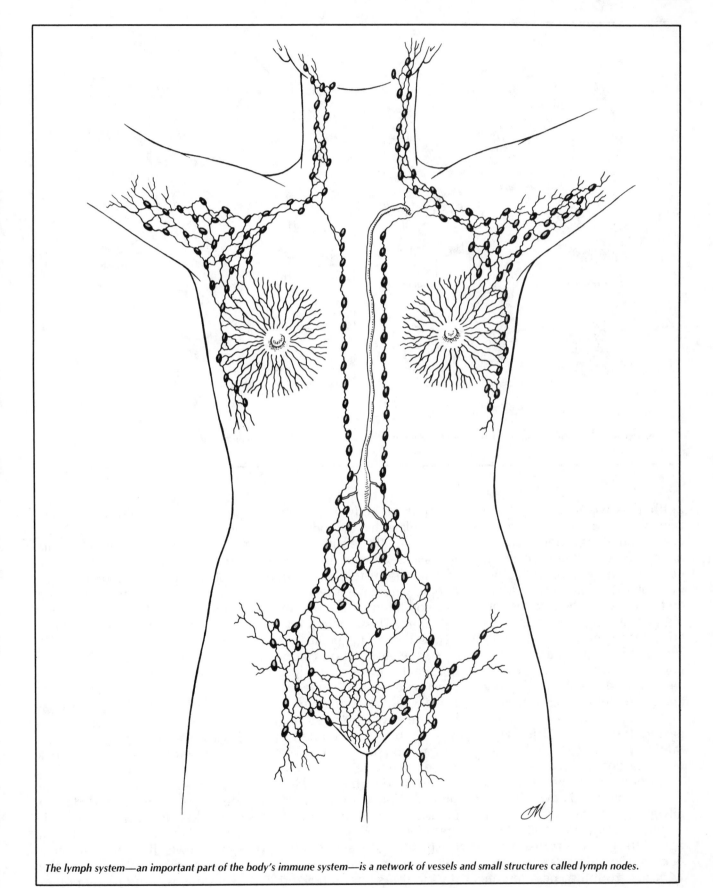

The lymph system—an important part of the body's immune system—is a network of vessels and small structures called lymph nodes.

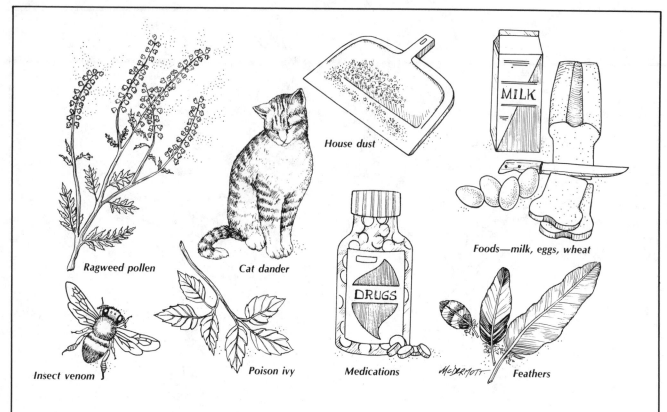

An allergy is an increased sensitivity to an environmental substance. Some of the more common offending substances, or allergens, are shown here.

antibodies work to protect the body from further attack. In the case of an allergy, however, the antibodies and other specialized cells involved in this protective function trigger an unusual sensitivity, or overreaction, to the foreign substance. The antibodies stimulate specialized cells to produce histamine, a powerful chemical. Histamine causes the small blood vessels to enlarge and the smooth muscles (such as those in the airways and the digestive tract) to constrict. Histamine release can also cause other reactions, such as hives.

No one knows why allergies develop, but it is known that an allergy can appear, disappear, or reappear at any time and at any age. Allergic reactions rarely occur during the first encounter with the troublesome allergen because the body needs time to accumulate the antibodies. Also, an individual's sensitivity to certain allergens seems to be related to a family history of allergies. People who have a tendency to develop allergies are referred to as atopic. This atopic tendency frequently runs in families.

An allergic reaction can be so mild that it is barely noticeable or so severe that it is life-threatening. Common symptoms of allergy are watery eyes, runny nose, itching or inflamed skin, and a swollen mouth or throat. Some allergic reactions may be accompanied by headaches, sinus stuffiness, a reduced sense of taste or smell, or difficulty in breathing.

An extremely severe allergic reaction, called anaphylactic shock, is characterized by breathing difficulties (caused by swelling of the throat and larynx and narrowing of the bronchial tubes), itching skin, hives, and collapse of the blood vessels, as well as by vomiting, diarrhea, and cramps. This condition can be fatal if not properly treated.

Types of allergens

There are four categories of allergens: inhalants, contactants, ingestants, and injectants.

Inhalant allergens are those that are breathed in, including such substances as dust, pollen, feathers, and animal dander (small scales from an animal's skin). Hay fever is an inhalant allergy in which the mucous membranes react to various inhaled substances, usually the pollens associated with the changing seasons. Year-round "hay fever" may actually be a reaction to pet dander, feathers, mold, or dust. (For additional information on hay fever, see page 82.)

Contactant allergens are those that are touched, including such substances as poison ivy, poison oak, cosmetics, detergents, fabrics, and dyes. Contact dermatitis is an example of an allergic reaction to a contactant allergen. (For additional information on contact dermatitis, see pages 80-81.)

Ingestant allergens are those that are swallowed. A variety of foods and medications can act as ingestant allergens. Food allergies occur more frequently in children than in adults. Some common ingestant allergens are milk, eggs, shellfish, fish, peanuts, chocolate, strawberries, tomatoes, and citrus fruits. (For additional information on food allergies, see page 81.)

Injectant allergens are substances that penetrate the skin, such as insect venom and drugs that are injected. For example, people who have severe allergic reactions to insect bites or stings are suffering from a reaction to an injectant allergen. (For additional information on insect bites and stings, see page 84.)

Diagnosis

Identifying an offending allergen may be uncomfortable, time-consuming, and expensive, but it is sometimes necessary in order to avoid future allergic reactions. A medical history, a record of any recent changes in daily habits, skin-scratch tests (in which small amounts of suspected allergens are applied to tiny scratches in the skin), and intracutaneous skin tests (in which allergens are injected

under the skin) are used to help identify the troublesome foreign substance. A special study called radioallergosorbent testing (RAST) is sometimes performed to detect and measure antibodies in the blood that have been manufactured in response to invading substances.

Treatment

Once the allergen has been identified, half the battle is won. Avoiding the troublesome substance is the first step toward relieving an allergy problem. If the allergen cannot be avoided or removed, medication or immunotherapy may be recommended. Three types of medications are commonly prescribed: antihistamines, which combat the effect of the histamines in the body; corticosteroids, which reduce inflammation and swelling; and bronchodilators, which ease breathing by opening bronchial tubes.

Allergy immunotherapy, or "desensitization," consists of injections of an allergen in gradually increasing quantities. This allows the body to build up a tolerance to the offending substance. Immunotherapy works best in controlling allergies to pollen, insect venom, and house dust.

A little common sense goes a long way toward controlling allergies. Obviously, the offending allergen needs to be avoided. Natural fibers in the home can be replaced with synthetics. Air conditioners or air filters can be installed for hay fever sufferers. Those susceptible to insect bites can wear protective clothes and avoid wearing bright clothing and perfumes, both of which attract insects. Babies born into allergy-prone families should be

breast-fed as long as possible to delay exposure to cow's milk, eggs, and citrus fruits.

Prevention

In most cases, allergies cannot be prevented, but much can be done to help control or diminish their effects on overly sensitive individuals.

AIDS

Acquired immune deficiency syndrome (AIDS) is a disease in which the body's natural defense system is disabled, allowing organisms that are normally fought off to become deadly.

Causes

This disease, discovered in 1979, is caused by a microorganism called the human immunodeficiency virus. This virus is carried and transmitted in bodily fluids (mainly blood, semen, and vaginal secretions). Sexual intercourse (heterosexual or homosexual), use of nonsterile hypodermic needles (a common practice among drug addicts), and infected blood transfusions have all been implicated as means of transmission of the AIDS virus. Transmission from a pregnant woman to her infant or from a mother to her nursing infant may occur. There is currently a great deal of controversy as to whether an infected physician or dentist can infect a patient. There have been isolated reports of transmission by being splashed with infected blood.

In Western countries, male homosexuals, prostitutes, drug addicts who inject drugs, and hemophiliacs who receive multiple blood transfusions for their disorder are all at high risk of contracting AIDS. In Africa (where the disease seems to have originated), heterosexual transmission is apparently the most common route.

A widespread misconception has been that AIDS can be contracted by *giving* blood—this notion is not true. In addition, since the introduction of a blood screening test for use in blood banks and hospital laboratories, acquisition of the AIDS virus by *receiving* blood transfusions is now extremely unlikely. Furthermore, the evidence to date indicates that casual contacts—such as would occur in school or in the workplace—are not responsible for transmission of the virus.

Symptoms

Clinical illness from AIDS can have its onset as long as ten years after initial infection with the virus. Initial symptoms include low-grade fever, swollen lymph nodes, weight loss, fatigue, night sweats, and long-standing diarrhea. (These symptoms can also be present in many less serious illnesses.) Because of immune system impairment, people with AIDS easily fall prey to many diseases, including cancer, skin infections, fungal infections, and tuberculosis. About one third of people with AIDS develop Kaposi's sarcoma, a previously rare cancer that often appears as purplish bumps on the skin. Many suffer *Pneumocystis carinii* pneumonia (an often fatal lung infection).

Diagnosis

The blood of people with AIDS contains an abnormally small number of specialized white blood cells called lymphocytes. Lymphocytes play an important role in combating infectious diseases and may also be instrumental in destroying malignant growths in their early stages. There are two types of lymphocytes actively engaged in coping with infection: T cells, which directly kill invaders, and B cells, which are involved in the production of infection-fighting antibodies. The finding that people with AIDS have decreased numbers of T cells, particularly a subtype called "helper" T cells, has proved useful in diagnosis.

A person may be a carrier of the disease without being aware of the fact and without having any of the symptoms. Blood tests for the detection of antibodies to the AIDS virus have recently been developed. The implications of a positive blood test are controversial, however. Although a positive blood test definitely indicates exposure to the disease, it is not known whether all individuals with positive test results will subsequently develop full-blown AIDS. Newborns whose mothers are infected with the AIDS virus will initially test positive for the antibody to AIDS. However, in only about half of those infants will this positive test persist after 15 to 18 months of age, and these are the infants who will eventually develop the disease.

Treatment

No cure for AIDS has been found yet. The drug zidovudine (formerly called azidothymidine or AZT) acts by preventing replication of the AIDS virus in human cells. Although this drug has been shown to prolong survival and improve the quality of life for people with AIDS, it cannot be considered a cure.

Until a cure for AIDS is found, treatment is limited to countering the effects of the disease (for example, surgery to remove skin cancer, chemotherapy, and use of drugs to raise the body's resistance to diseases).

Prevention

Since there is no cure for AIDS, prevention is critical. Limiting the number of one's sexual partners and using condoms decrease the risk of sexual exposure to the AIDS virus. Avoiding contact with potentially contaminated hypodermic needles and with blood and blood products is also important.

If a person has tested positive for the presence of the AIDS antibody, a number of precautions should be taken to promote the effectiveness of the immune system and to prevent the spread of infection. Substances that will burden the immune system should be avoided. These include live-virus vaccines, such as those against measles, mumps, rubella, and polio; alcohol, tobacco products, and illicit drugs, such as marijuana and heroin; and possible sources of salmonella and other food-borne infections, such as unpasteurized milk and inadequately cooked meats. A physician may also recommend avoidance of immunosuppressive drugs, such as corticosteroids, some antibiotics, and certain anticancer drugs, as well as aspirin and other painkillers, which may be immunosuppressive.

Among the activities that may increase risk of infections in a person with AIDS are changing cat litter (cats transmit toxoplasmosis), cleaning bird cages (birds transmit histoplasmosis and psittacosis), sharing razor blades and toothbrushes, and engaging in sexual activity without a condom or with a partner who might transmit cytomegalovirus, Epstein-Barr virus, syphilis, or AIDS virus. Pregnancy is also somewhat immunosuppressive. It is important that the immune system be bolstered by maintaining general health—the person should choose a balanced diet, get regular exercise and adequate rest, and avoid stress.

Needless to say, the infected person should inform all sex partners and medical and dental personnel with whom he or she comes into contact of his or her immune status and should not donate blood, sperm, organs, or any other body tissues.

Anaphylaxis

Anaphylaxis is said to be present if a person is extremely sensitive to a substance on first exposure. If the person is exposed to the substance again, the result may be anaphylactic shock, an explosive overreaction of the body's immune system. Anaphylactic shock is a violent allergic reaction characterized by itching skin, hives, breathing trouble, collapse of the circulatory system, and sometimes vomiting, diarrhea, and abdominal cramps.

Causes

Anaphylaxis may be triggered by an insect sting, such as that of a bee or wasp; by animal serum used in a vaccine; by desensitizing injections; or by one of various drugs. The allergen (the substance that sets off the reaction) is usually a protein, called an antigen. When it first enters the body, certain body cells treat it like an invading microorganism and create antibodies, which are protective substances that fight infection. On subsequent exposures to the same antigen, the antibodies are ready for the "invader" and stimulate the release of certain chemicals. One of these chemicals, histamine, causes contraction of muscles in the digestive and respiratory tracts, resulting in abdominal cramps and wheezing. Histamine also causes the small blood vessels to enlarge and lose plasma (blood fluid) to surrounding tissues. The decrease in the volume of blood in the vessels results in a drop in blood pressure, which may lead to shock (circulatory system collapse).

Symptoms

Symptoms develop rapidly. Within 15 minutes, the victim becomes uneasy, upset, and red in the face. Rapid heartbeat, prickling and itching sensations in the skin, throbbing in the ears, sneezing, coughing, and breathing difficulty are also likely. Vomiting, incontinence (involuntary release of urine and bowel contents), and even convulsions may occur. In another one or two minutes, shock may result, in which blood vessels collapse, the pulse becomes weak and rapid, and the person becomes cold, clammy, and faint. Without immediate medical aid, death may result.

Treatment

In cases of anaphylactic shock, medical aid should be obtained as quickly as possible—call an emergency squad. Keep the pa-

tient's airway open. Have the patient lie down, with legs elevated. Immediate treatment with the drug epinephrine is critical. It counteracts the action of the histamine released in the blood, which is causing the symptoms of anaphylactic shock. If a drug injection has caused the reaction, a tourniquet is applied above the site of the injection, and epinephrine is often injected into the site. Antihistamine drugs are also given. In extreme cases, especially when shock has occurred or there is great breathing difficulty, intravenous solutions are given to restore blood volume and raise blood pressure. Anyone with a severe reaction is usually hospitalized for at least 24 hours to guard against a recurrence of the condition.

Prevention

A preventive measure against anaphylactic shock is routine allergy skin testing before the use of substances that may cause sensitivity or that have been known to cause anaphylaxis, such as animal serums in vaccines. In addition, anyone who has had an allergic reaction to an insect sting should carry a kit containing a syringe of epinephrine and an epinephrine-filled nasal sprayer for prompt self-treatment if stung again. Desensitizing injections of the insect venom should also be considered to allow the body to build up a resistance to the venom, if the doctor feels that such injections will not trigger an anaphylactic reaction.

Anaphylactoid reactions

Similar to anaphylaxis in effect (but not in cause) are anaphylactoid reactions, which can occur on the first injection of certain drugs, such as morphine, and of contrast media (special solutions used when performing certain X-ray studies). These are not allergic reactions in the pure sense, but they may be just as serious nevertheless.

Autoimmune diseases

Autoimmune diseases are disorders in which the body's immune system reacts against some of its own tissue and produces antibodies to it.

Examples

Ailments believed to be autoimmune diseases include Hashimoto's thyroiditis and Graves' disease, which are disorders of the thyroid gland; systemic lupus erythematosus, which attacks multiple organ systems; myasthenia gravis, a neuromuscular disease; and autoimmune hemolytic anemia, in which red blood cells are destroyed before the end of their normal 120-day life span.

Diseases that are, at least in part, autoimmune disorders include rheumatoid arthritis, a connective tissue disease; pernicious anemia, a serious blood disorder; glomerulonephritis, a disorder that affects the kidneys; and Addison's disease, which attacks the adrenal glands.

Other diseases that have autoimmune features are chronic active hepatitis (a liver disorder), some forms of vasculitis (inflammation of blood vessel walls), and many other diseases that produce inflammation, or wasting away of body tissues.

Causes

An autoimmune disease can begin in several ways:
- A body substance that ordinarily never enters the bloodstream may do so because of injury. For example, a disease known as sympathetic ophthalmia occurs when tissue from the inside of an injured eye is released into the bloodstream. The tissue is recognized as "out of place" or "foreign" by the body's immune system, and antibodies attack it, causing irritation in both the injured eye and in the noninjured eye. The reaction may be severe enough to cause blindness.
- A body substance may be altered by chemicals, sunlight, or a virus so that it seems foreign to the body's immune system. The substance is then attacked by antibodies. An example of this process occurs when the metal in a bracelet causes chemical changes in the skin on one's wrist. The body reacts against the "different" skin and attacks it, causing the rash of contact dermatitis.
- Infection may cause an immune response so strong that the body reacts against some of its own normal tissues.
- Genetic factors may play a role.

Treatment

Treatment is dependent on the particular autoimmune disease that is present. Many treatments involve decreasing the patient's immune response. Other cases, however, require more aggressive therapy to allow repair of the damage that is caused by the body's attack on itself.

Contact dermatitis

Contact dermatitis is a type of allergy in which the skin becomes inflamed in the area where it has come in contact with an irritating substance.

Causes

Contact dermatitis can be caused by a virtually limitless array of substances, among them soaps, detergents, metals, shaving materials, shampoos, hair colorings or sprays, solvents in household cleaners, chemicals in foods and cosmetics, dyes in household products, and certain plants, such as poison ivy and poison oak. Photodermatitis (a skin inflammation caused by light) is a type of dermatitis that develops when certain ingested drugs, such as some antibiotics, sensitize the skin so that a rash develops on skin that is exposed to the sun.

Symptoms

The major symptoms of contact dermatitis are burning, swelling, severe itching, and stinging sensations on the area of the skin that has been exposed to the allergen. Blisters that ooze a clear fluid may form (a cloudy or yellow, foul-smelling fluid indicates that a bacterial infection, rather than contact dermatitis, is present).

Diagnosis

Contact dermatitis is diagnosed by first identifying the allergen causing the trouble. The location of the rash often gives an important clue to the identity of the allergen. For instance, if the inflammation is on the scalp, the disorder may be assumed to be triggered by a shampoo, hair spray, or hair coloring. More specific identification of the allergen may be obtained with one of several available tests, including scratch tests, in which a small amount of the suspected allergen is applied to a scratch on the skin; intracutaneous tests, in which a small amount of the allergen is injected into or under the skin; and radioallergosorbent testing, a blood test in which antibodies produced in response to the allergen are measured.

Treatment

Once the allergen has been identified, the best treatment for contact dermatitis is for the patient to avoid the allergen or to remove it from his or her environment. It is often possible to do this by switching brands of soaps or shampoos, wearing rubber gloves when using harsh detergents, and using unscented or hypoallergenic cosmetics. If the use of a drug cannot be discontinued despite a case of photodermatitis, sunscreens should be used and adequate clothing should be worn to shield the skin when outdoors.

Oral steroid drugs (such as cortisone) help to relieve the itching of contact dermatitis; however, these are reserved only for the most serious cases. Topical (applied directly to the skin) steroids and antihistamines are more commonly used.

Prevention

There is no preventive treatment for contact dermatitis, but those susceptible to one or more contactant allergens can usually prevent outbreaks by avoiding exposure as much as possible.

Food allergy

A food allergy is an unusual sensitivity to a specific food. A food allergy is not a food intolerance, which exists when the body lacks the enzymes that are needed to digest a certain food. A food allergy exists when the body's immune system manufactures antibodies as a reaction to the food. This food then becomes an ingestant allergen (an allergy-causing substance that is swallowed or eaten). Any food can become an allergen, but the foods most commonly found to cause allergic reactions are milk, eggs, shellfish, fish, peanuts, chocolate, tomatoes, strawberries, and citrus fruits.

Symptoms

The symptoms of a food allergy most commonly arise in the digestive tract and include cramps, nausea, vomiting, and diarrhea. Other signs that may also be present include hives, rash, headache, nasal congestion, and anaphylactic shock (a very serious reaction that can be fatal, characterized by breathing problems due to swelling of the larynx and collapse of blood vessels). Food allergies occur more often in children than in adults.

Diagnosis

Food allergy is diagnosed by having the patient maintain a detailed record of all foods eaten, as well as of the times when symptoms appear. Elimination trials may also help identify the allergen; the patient eliminates one food at a time from the diet to see if the symptoms disappear. In addition, several tests are used to detect various types of allergens: scratch tests, in which a small amount of the suspected allergen is applied to a scratch on the skin; intracutaneous tests, in which a small amount of the allergen is injected in or under the skin; and radioallergosorbent testing, in which antibodies developed in response to specific allergens are measured in a blood sample.

Treatment

There is no way to treat a food allergy other than to avoid eating the food and to treat the symptoms of a reaction should one develop. Fortunately, children usually outgrow these allergies.

Some doctors feel that infants who are breast-fed for up to a year are less likely to develop food allergies than babies who are formula-fed or who are breast-fed for only a couple of months. This continues to be a controversial issue.

Gamma globulin

Gamma globulin preparations are derived from the blood of a person or animal and contain antibodies made by that person or animal in response to invasion by harmful agents, such as bacteria and viruses. These preparations are widely used for the prevention, modification, diagnosis, and treatment of many kinds of infectious diseases.

Gamma globulin is usually injected. Since it contains almost all the antibodies circulating in the blood, it can provide passive (borrowed) immunity that lasts for about six weeks.

Gamma globulin injections may be useful in preventing infectious hepatitis when given—within about two weeks of exposure—to individuals who have been in intimate contact with someone with hepatitis. Many physicians recommend that persons traveling to underdeveloped countries, particularly rural areas, receive doses of gamma globulin before departure and during an extended stay.

Measles can often be prevented by the administration of gamma globulin injections within five days of exposure. The injections are especially important for children under three years of age, for pregnant women, for tuberculosis patients, and for those with impaired immune mechanisms. Even if measles is not prevented, a less serious case may result; however, gamma globulin is of no use once the symptoms have appeared.

Gamma globulin level in the body can also be used as a diagnostic tool. For example, one symptom of multiple sclerosis is an elevated level of gamma globulin in the cerebrospinal fluid.

Hay fever

Hay fever is the name for acute (short-lived), seasonal attacks that are allergic reactions to pollen. Most often, spring attacks are reactions to tree pollen; summer attacks are reactions to grass pollen; and autumn attacks are reactions to weed pollen.

Symptoms

The symptoms of hay fever are usually the same, regardless of the allergen (irritating substance). Common symptoms include itching of the nose and roof of the mouth; a thin, watery discharge constantly draining from the nose; itchy, watery eyes; sneezing; headache; irritability; a feeling of exhaustion; insomnia; loss of appetite; and, in advanced cases, coughing and wheezing.

Diagnosis

Hay fever, as with other allergies, is diagnosed by identifying the allergen. This is done by taking a medical history and reviewing the patient's environment, daily habits, and recent changes in lifestyle. Skin tests and blood tests may also be performed. These include scratch tests, in which a small amount of the suspected allergen is applied to a scratch on the skin; intracutaneous tests, in which a small amount of the allergen is injected in or under the skin; and occasionally radioallergosorbent testing, in which antibodies developed in response to specific allergens are measured in a blood sample.

Treatment

A severe case of hay fever may be best treated by changing the environment, that is, by removing the allergen causing the trouble or reducing the patient's exposure to it. Those who react to weed pollen may need to move to a more urban location with a lower concentration of pollen in the air. Many hay fever sufferers will benefit from using an air conditioner, which filters the air and thus keeps pollen levels in the home to a minimum.

Several medications are available for the hay fever sufferer: oral antihistamines, which counteract the histamine that is released by the body in reaction to the allergen; corticosteroids, which reduce inflammation; eye drops, which relieve itching and redness; and desensitization shots, which cause the body to develop tolerance to the allergen.

Prevention

There is no way to prevent hay fever, but avoiding the allergen as much as possible may help relieve some of the discomfort.

Hives

Hives (also called urticaria) is a reaction of the skin marked by intense itching and by the rapid development of raised, smooth patches, or welts (also called wheals). Hives is most often a sign of an allergic reaction.

Causes

Hives is often caused by an allergy to certain foods, particularly shellfish, tomatoes, strawberries, eggs, milk, and chocolate. It can also be a reaction to drugs, food dyes, molds, bacteria, and animal skin or hair. In a susceptible person, cold, sunlight, and vigorous exercise have been known to cause hives.

Symptoms

Hives is characterized by an outbreak of red and white welts that vary in size and appear suddenly either in small areas or all over the body. They often appear and disappear, lasting anywhere from a few minutes to a day or two, but the outbreak can last for weeks. Accompanying symptoms may include intense itching, fatigue, fever, nausea, and difficulty in breathing if the allergic reaction has led to swelling of the mucous membrane lining the respiratory tract.

Diagnosis

Diagnosing the allergy and pinpointing the allergen can require extensive testing, especially when a food may be involved. Eliminating many suspected foods and then reintroducing them one at a time sometimes helps to diagnose the cause of hives. This must be done under professional supervision and with caution.

Treatment

Hives can be treated immediately by taking antihistamines. When taken several times a day at a prescribed dosage, the correct type of antihistamine will help control swelling by preventing the released histamine from triggering the hives. Drowsiness and dry mouth are common side effects of antihistamines, so the type and dosage may need to be adjusted periodically. Concurrent medical problems, such as glaucoma, enlarged prostate, or heart disease, may preclude the use of antihistamines. It is best to consult your doctor before taking an antihistamine. Other drugs (such as corticosteroids, which reduce inflammation) may be used to treat serious hives.

Prevention

Hives can be prevented by avoiding contact with the aller-gen or stimulus once it has been identified. Sometimes, no stimulus or disease process can be identified, and the hives are called idiopathic (of unknown cause). This condition can result in chronic episodes of hives and may require chronic treatment with antihistamines and/or corticosteroids.

Immunization

Immunization is the means of producing immunity (resistance by the body) to a specific disease. There are two types of immunization—active and passive.

Active immunization

Active immunization is accomplished by injecting weakened or killed viruses or bacteria into the body. This stimulates the body's natural defense system. Certain specialized white blood cells produce substances known as antibodies, which are carried in the bloodstream and are tailormade to fight invading organisms. These antibodies remain in the body for years—sometimes a lifetime—to protect it against that particular disease.

Passive immunization

Passive immunization involves injecting ready-made antibodies into the body. These antibodies are usually extracted from the blood of humans who are immune to a certain disease or of animals that have been immunized solely for the purpose of producing antibodies to be used in passive immunization. Passive immunization is borrowed immunity and is only temporary, but it serves to protect a person who may already be infected until the body has time to create sufficient quantities of its own antibodies.

Immunization can protect against diphtheria, measles, mumps, pertussis (whooping cough), polio, rubella (German measles), and tetanus.

Children's immunizations

Every child should receive injections of the combined diphtheria-tetanus-pertussis (DTP) vaccine at 2, 4, 6, and 18 months of age. The child should also receive a dose of the oral polio vaccine (OPV) at 2, 4, and 18 months of age. Every child should also receive injections of the vaccine against *Hemophilus influenzae* type B (HiB), the most common cause of bacterial meningitis in children. The recommended schedule for Hib vaccination depends upon the brand of vaccine used. For example, one brand of the vaccine should be given at 2, 4, and 12 months of age; another should be given at 2, 4, 6, and 15 months of age. The physician who performs the initial vaccination can tell you which schedule applies to your child. At 15 months, a child should receive the combined measles, mumps, and rubella (MMR) vaccine and a test for tuberculosis (TB). DTP and OPV boosters should be given around the time of school entry (when your child is four to five years old). A measles booster should be given when your child is eleven or twelve years of age, and anyone between 4 and 21 years of age should receive a measles booster during a measles outbreak. A diphtheria and tetanus toxoids (DT) booster shot should be given between 14 and 16 years of age.

Immunization and testing schedule

2 months	DTP, OPV, HiB*
4 months	DTP, OPV, HiB*
6 months	DTP, HiB*
12 months	HiB*
15 months	MMR, TB test, HiB*
18 months	DTP and OPV
4-5 years	DTP and OPV
11-12 years	Measles booster**
14-16 years	DT booster

* The schedule for HiB depends on the brand of vaccine. Injections should be given either at 2, 4, 6, and 15 months or at 2, 4, and 12 months. Check with your doctor.
** If there is a measles outbreak, anyone between the ages of 4 years and 21 years of age should receive a booster.

If the family does not have a physician, immunizations can usually be obtained through the local public health department. If a child has an acute illness with fever, immunization should be delayed.

Adult immunizations

Adults need a tetanus shot once every ten years. Otherwise, there are no routine immunizations necessary for adults in the United States, with the possible exception of influenza shots given annually (usually in the fall) to the aged and to patients with heart, lung, or other chronic diseases. A vaccine that would protect against 80 percent of serious cases of pneumonia is available. Immunization against rabies is possible both before and after exposure.

There are precautions to consider. Immunizations should not be given routinely to pregnant women, nor in general to anyone whose immune system has been weakened by leukemia, cancer, AIDS, or prolonged X-ray or corticosteroid treatment.

Vaccinations for foreign travel

Most persons traveling abroad in developed countries need no additional vaccinations. In general, in the United States, Canada, Australia, New Zealand, Japan, and Europe, the traveler is safe without vaccinations. Travel in Mexico and the less-developed countries of Africa, Asia, South America, Central America, the South Pacific, the Middle East, and the Far East may hold more risks, particularly in small villages and rural areas not usually visited by tourists.

In recent years, no vaccination has been necessary for *direct* travel from the United States to most countries or for return to the United States. However, some countries require proof of vaccination from travelers who have passed through infected areas, and it is best to get the necessary vaccinations before leaving home.

Any physician can give immunizations except for yellow-fever vaccinations, which must be given at an official "Yellow Fever Vaccination Center." Weeks before you plan to leave on your trip, call your local health department for the latest information about vaccination requirements and recommendations for all of the countries you plan to visit. The vaccinating physician must fill out and sign an "International Certificate of Vaccination," which must be validated by a health department or by an authorized physician.

Insect bites and stings

Insect bites and stings are minor inconveniences to most people, but to those who have an allergy to insect venom, the consequences can be serious.

Symptoms

Reactions to insect venom show themselves in various symptoms—shortness of breath, rapid heartbeat, coughing, wheezing, and light-headedness. The affected area swells and becomes tender or numb. In extreme cases, anaphylaxis (see pages 79-80) can occur.

Treatment

Serious reactions to bites and stings are treated by slowing the spread of the venom throughout the body and getting emergency medical treatment as soon as possible. The progress of the venom can be slowed somewhat by applying an ice pack or a tourniquet (but not so tightly as to stop the blood flow) to the affected area. Emergency medical treatment will usually consist of an epinephrine injection and an injection of antihistamine. In some cases, a corticosteroid may be given as well. These serve to lessen existing symptoms and to halt progression of the reaction.

Prevention

Prevention of recurrent reactions may be accomplished with desensitization shots; starting with an initially weak solution of insect extract, doses are gradually increased with each shot. This allows the body to build up tolerance to the effects of the insect venom.

Persons with known sensitivity to insect bites should carry kits with injectable epinephrine (available by prescription).

THE BRAIN AND NERVOUS SYSTEM

The nervous system is a complex network of specialized tissues that regulates thoughts, emotions, actions, sensations, and basic body functions.

Nerve cells

The basic element of the nervous system is the nerve cell, or neuron. In combination, neurons form nerves, which transmit impulses throughout the body. A protective covering of myelin, a fatty substance, insulates parts of those fibers.

The action of nerve cells is both electrical and chemical. At the ends of each nerve cell there are specialized regions called synaptic terminals, which contain large numbers of tiny membranous sacs that hold neurotransmitter chemicals. These chemicals transmit nerve impulses from one nerve cell to another. After an electrical nerve impulse has traveled along a neuron, it reaches the terminal and stimulates the release of neurotransmitters from their sacs. The neurotransmitters travel across the synapse (the junction between the neighboring neurons) and stimulate the production of an electrical charge, which carries the nerve impulse forward. This process is repeated over and over again until a muscle is moved or relaxed or a sensory impression is noted by the brain. These electrochemical events can be considered the "language" of the nervous system, by which information is transmitted from one part of the body to another.

Nervous system

There are two major divisions of the nervous system: the cen-

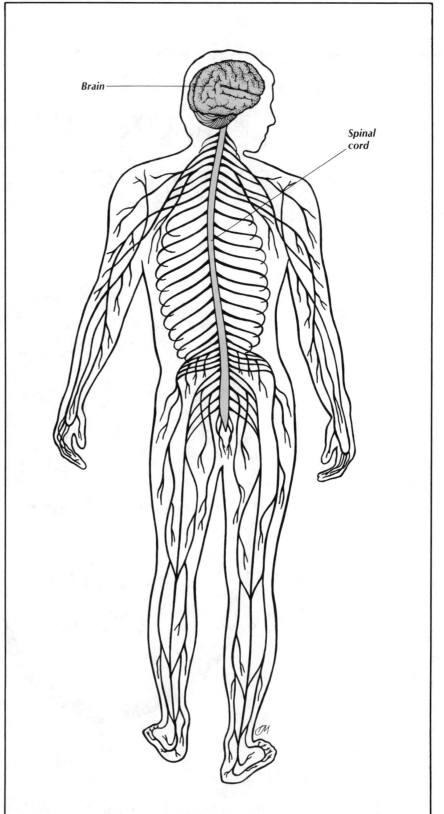

The nervous system has two major divisions: the central nervous system (brain and spinal cord) and the peripheral nervous system (nerves that branch out from the brain and spinal cord).

tral nervous system and the peripheral nervous system. The *central nervous system* consists of the brain and the spinal cord. The brain lies within the skull (the bony framework of the head). It governs body functions by sending and receiving messages through the spinal cord. Protecting the brain and spinal cord are bones, layers of tissue, and cerebrospinal fluid.

Once messages leave the central nervous system, they are carried by the *peripheral nervous system.* The peripheral system includes the cranial nerves (nerves branching from the brain) and the spinal nerves (nerves branching from the spinal cord). These nerves convey sensory messages from receptor cells in the body to the central nervous system. They also transport motor impulses from the central system out to the body, where muscles and glands can respond to the impulses.

The *autonomic nervous system,* which is part of the peripheral nervous system, regulates all activity that is involuntary but necessary for life, including activity of the internal organs and glands.

Working together, these divisions coordinate adjustment and reaction of the body to internal and external environmental conditions.

Brain

The brain is the control center for the entire body. The brain sends messages to and receives stimulation from all parts of the body. More than ten billion interlinked brain cells regulate the functioning of the body during sleep and wakefulness.

Different areas of the brain control different body functions.

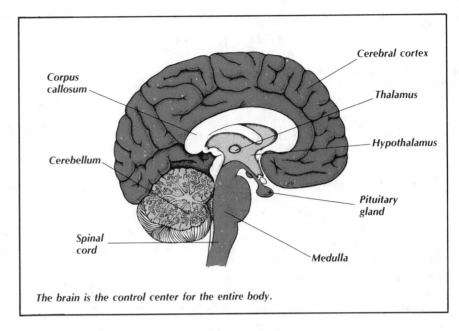

The brain is the control center for the entire body.

At the back of the skull is the cerebellum, which controls coordination of movements, balance, and posture. Deep inside the brain is the thalamus, which is the relay station for incoming impulses from the rest of the body, conveying sensations of pain, touch, and temperature to other parts of the brain. Around the thalamus is the hypothalamus, which governs involuntary (automatic) body operations, such as heartbeat and blood circulation. The pituitary gland is attached to the hypothalamus by a thin stalk. Because the pituitary gland controls most of the hormones in the body, the hypothalamus is considered a major influence on primary drives governed by hormones, such as sexual desire, hunger, and thirst.

Covering the inner parts of the brain is the cerebral cortex, which consists of two cerebral hemispheres. In these hemispheres are the nerve centers that regulate thought and voluntary action. Connecting the left and right cerebral hemispheres is a broad band of fibers called the corpus callosum. Because nerve fibers from the two hemispheres cross one another in a structure called the medulla at the base of the brain before progressing down the spinal cord, each hemisphere generally controls functions in the opposite side of the body. For example, a region in the left hemisphere governs movement of the right arm.

The brain is the most complex organ in the body. Although research has identified many of its capabilities in memory, reasoning, and creative thought processes, many functions of the brain remain a mystery.

Cerebrospinal fluid

Cerebrospinal fluid (CSF) is a clear, colorless fluid that surrounds the brain and spinal cord, cushioning them against injury.

The CSF is made of water containing small amounts of minerals and organic substances (especially protein). It is continually being produced by a specialized network of capillaries (tiny blood vessels) known as the choroid plexus, located in the ventricles (chambers) of the brain. About one pint is produced every 24 hours, and about five ounces is circulating at any one time. From the two side ventricles, the CSF flows into the third and fourth ventricles of the brain. It then passes into the space between the innermost and second layers of tissue covering the brain, bathing the entire outer surface of the brain before passing downward around the spinal cord. Eventually the fluid returns upward, is absorbed into special tissue between the linings of the brain, and passes into the blood vessels.

Samples of CSF, drawn from around the spinal cord in a procedure called a lumbar puncture (see page 405), can be valuable in diagnosing disorders of the brain and spinal cord. The samples may indicate a hemorrhage or blood clot in the brain, various types of meningitis, a brain abscess, or a tumor of the brain or spinal cord.

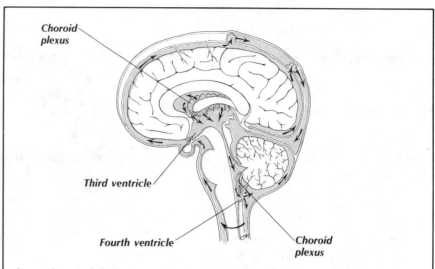

The cerebrospinal fluid is produced by a network of tiny blood vessels called the choroid plexus, located in the ventricles of the brain. From the two side ventricles, the fluid flows into the third and fourth ventricles and then passes into the space between the innermost and second layers of tissue covering the brain. The fluid bathes the outer surface of the brain and the spinal cord.

Alzheimer's disease

Alzheimer's disease is a disorder in which there is a steady deterioration of brain function resulting in progressive loss of memory, recognition, personality, and mental powers. Although Alzheimer's may begin as early as age 40, it is most prevalent in the aged. It accounts for about half of all serious mental impairment in persons over age 65.

Changes in the brain

In Alzheimer's disease, as in any senile (characteristic of old age) mental disorder, there is atrophy (shrinkage or wasting) of the cerebral cortex (the outer layer of the brain, which is mostly concerned with intellectual and social functioning). There are also more specific abnormalities, such as the presence of tangles of fibers within the nerve cells and of senile plaques, which are probably deposits of amyloid (a semisolid protein complex seen in many degenerative diseases). These abnormal changes are scattered throughout the cortex of a person with Alzheimer's and serve to distinguish the disease from other forms of senility. Because brain biopsy specimens (tissue samples taken from the brain for laboratory examination) are not obtained without very specific reasons and without intention of specific treatment, these changes are usually seen only after death.

Causes

Theories abound as to the possible causes of Alzheimer's disease. So-called slow viruses (viruses acquired early in life that take many years to do their damage) have been considered, as have environmental factors and damage from previous diseases. Recently, a diminished amount of the enzyme choline-acetyl-transferase (which is necessary to manufacture the neurotransmitter acetylcholine) has been found in some patients, and theories about replacement of the enzyme or neurotransmitter are being formulated. Deficiencies of other neurotransmitters are constantly being discovered. Heredity seems to play some part, since a family member of an Alzheimer's victim is more likely than others to develop the condition. It is generally agreed that hardening of the arteries is not a cause. The disease does not appear to be contagious, nor is it caused by emotional stress.

Symptoms

Symptoms vary considerably from one person to another and

may occur days or months apart. They begin with small memory lapses, almost always first involving loss of recall for recent events. Such lapses can happen to anyone, but in Alzheimer's disease they grow more serious with time. A person may forget a close relative's name, get lost coming home from the office, forget to turn off the oven, misplace articles, recheck to see if a task was done, or repeatedly ask questions that have already been answered.

Eventually, the gaps in memory and the failure to recognize friends and family members interfere with the individual's normal work and social life. The individual starts having trouble with figures when working on bills, with understanding what is being read, and with organizing the day's work.

As the disease progresses, the victim of Alzheimer's disease becomes confused, frustrated, and irritable. Although at first the person seems physically unaffected by the disease, as the condition advances the patient becomes restless, always moving about, and must be watched so that he or she does not wander away or into danger. Endless repetition of unnecessary actions, such as the opening and closing of drawers, is another characteristic of the disease. Some victims of Alzheimer's disease may become extremely agitated with little or no provocation.

The course of the disease, which eventually can result in deterioration of the rest of the nervous system and other parts of the body and in loss of control over bladder and bowels, may range from 1 to 20 years. It may cut life expectancy by contributing to death from another cause, such as pneumonia or heart or kidney failure.

Diagnosis

Other conditions can cause many of the symptoms of Alzheimer's disease, and many of these conditions are treatable. Therefore, it is very important for the patient to undergo a thorough medical evaluation, which may include extensive neurological and psychological examinations and other diagnostic studies, such as computed tomography (a special X-ray technique for obtaining cross-sectional images), electroencephalography (a study of brain waves), blood tests, and sampling of cerebrospinal fluid. These procedures can rule out or identify possible causes of nervous system malfunctioning, such as a series of "little strokes," brain tumors or infections, pernicious anemia (curable with vitamin B_{12}), overmedication with barbiturates or bromides, alcoholism, drug side effects, abnormal thyroid function, or hydrocephalus (blockage of cerebrospinal fluid in the head). Psychological depression is also an important—and treatable—cause of senile symptoms, such as apathy, slowness of thought, inattention, and poor concentration. Death of a spouse or a shock, such as moving to a nursing home, could cause such symptoms temporarily.

Treatment

Medical science does not yet know how to prevent or treat Alzheimer's disease. However, it is important to find a physician who is able to help the patient and his or her family handle the many problems that are bound to arise. At times, tranquilizers can lessen agitation and anxiety and reduce the incidence of undesirable behavior. Medication may

also help to improve sleeping patterns and treat depression caused by the disease.

It is important that the patient continue the daily routine, exercise as usual, and keep in touch with friends. Memory aids, such as lists of daily chores, reminders about safety, and a large calendar, can help in day-to-day living. As care of the patient becomes more difficult, it may be best (for the patient and family alike) to move the patient to a health facility where a professional staff can provide around-the-clock care.

Amnesia

Amnesia is the loss of memory and the inability to form new memories. It can be either temporary or permanent. The causes may range from brain damage to a psychological reason.

Retrograde amnesia

This type of amnesia usually follows any severe head injury that produces unconsciousness. The patient is not able to recall what happened immediately before the accident that caused the injury, the accident itself, or some of the events of the recovery period. In most cases, this type of amnesia is not significant because no other memory is affected, and no treatment is needed.

Korsakoff's syndrome

An inability to record new memory along with a defect in recent memory, usually accompanied by confabulation (storytelling of fabricated events), is known as Korsakoff's syndrome.

It may be caused by head injury, stroke, encephalitis (inflammation of the lining of the brain), deficiency of vitamin B_{12}, cancer of the brain, or poor blood supply to memory tissue or pathways in the brain. However, heavy drinking of alcohol, with resultant brain damage, is commonly the cause.

Although there may be little or no loss of memory or skills that were acquired before the disease began, the person with Korsakoff's syndrome cannot effectively learn new skills or remember recent events. To hide this loss, from himself or herself as well as from others, the patient may describe imaginary or confused experiences to take the place of the missing experiences. Sometimes the stories are so convincing that the patient appears normal.

Treatment of Korsakoff's syndrome is limited to treating the condition that caused it. Permanent brain damage may make it incurable. Frequently, however, the condition will disappear with time, especially if it was caused by a concussion (a swelling in the head that puts pressure on the brain).

Psychological amnesia

Amnesia of psychological origin is less common but more dramatic and newsworthy than other forms of amnesia. A man disappears from home, job, and family; he travels to a new place and assumes a new identity—all without being aware that anything has changed. After days or weeks, he "awakens," becomes his old self, and wonders what happened. There is no memory of the period of amnesia.

Anxiety is the cause of this type of amnesia. The person is faced with an intolerable situation of high emotional stress or pain. To protect itself, the mind forgets the anxieties and everything related, including the person's identity.

Treatment may not be necessary, since most affected persons recover without help. However, if the problem that caused the amnesia still remains, it must be faced and solved. Family therapy and change of work or activities may help. Hypnosis may be used to bring back the memory of the "lost days" and unlock the ideas and feelings that caused the original flight from home and self.

Ataxia

Ataxia is a condition characterized by muscular incoordination, producing irregular and inaccurate movements of the body. The result may be a clumsy manner of walking, with feet wide apart; a lack of balance; tremor (shakiness) of the arms; and slurring of speech.

Causes

Ataxia may be caused by anything that affects the motor control centers of the brain or the nerve pathways leading from them. Drunkenness can produce a temporary staggering ataxia. Permanent ataxia is caused by damage to the brain, spinal cord, or spinal nerves.

Locomotor ataxia may be a late result of untreated syphilis. Its symptoms include sharp, stabbing pains, usually in the legs; an unsteady walk; and a feeling of walking on foam rubber. There may be an increased sensitivity of the skin, sometimes with burning, prickling, creeping, or crawling sensations.

Ataxia occurs in one case in ten of cerebral palsy, which is a movement disorder caused by damage to the brain or nerve pathways before or around the time of birth. Weakness, unsteadiness, clumsy walking, and difficulty with fine or rapid movements are typical. Physical and occupational therapy can help patients handle daily life.

Ataxia may also be caused by any one of a group of hereditary diseases that attack the central nervous system. They cause degeneration of the spinal cord and cerebellum (the portion of the brain responsible for fine control of muscle movements) and also frequently damage the brain stem (the portion of the brain that controls the most basic body functions, such as breathing and circulation) and various nerves. Inherited disorders of body chemistry are believed to be involved, but little is known about them. Only one of these disorders—Refsum's syndrome—can be treated, by reducing the excessive level of a body chemical known as phytanic acid.

Symptoms

Symptoms of the hereditary ataxias include unsteadiness in walking, tremor of the arms, muscle weakness, and wasting away of muscles. Various other abnormalities may be present, depending on the disease. For example, Friedreich's ataxia causes curvature of the spine and damages heart tissue.

Treatment

All of these diseases continue throughout life. With the exception of Refsum's syndrome, none can be treated effectively.

Bell's palsy

Bell's palsy is total or partial paralysis (loss of function or movement) of one side of the face. It is believed to be due to inflammation of the nerve that controls the facial muscles. The inflammation, often of unknown cause but suspected to be the result of viral infection, causes the nerve to swell and to be compressed inside its bony passage in the skull. This compression reduces the blood supply to the nerve and thus its ability to function.

Symptoms

This disorder can occur in someone of any age, but is most common from ages 20 to 50. The first sign may be an aching pain behind or below the ear. Paralysis may develop in a few hours or more slowly, causing the entire side of the face to be flat and without expression (this is different from the facial paralysis caused by stroke or brain tumor, in which the weakness is mostly below the forehead). The mouth droops on the weak side, with saliva drooling from the corner. The sense of taste may be impaired. The eyebrow cannot be raised. In most cases, the eye cannot be shut. When the patient tries to close the affected eye, it can be seen to roll upward (which also happens in a healthy person, but is not seen because the eyelid normally closes). Unprovoked tears may come from the affected eye.

Diagnosis

In making a diagnosis, the doctor must determine if the paralysis might be caused by

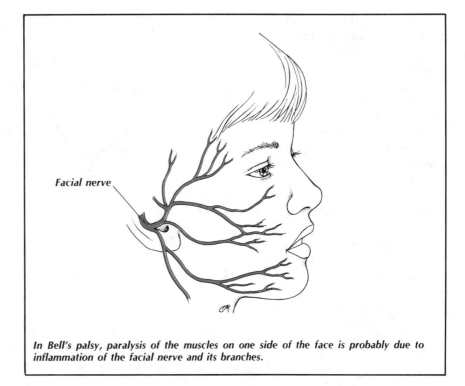

Facial nerve

In Bell's palsy, paralysis of the muscles on one side of the face is probably due to inflammation of the facial nerve and its branches.

other disorders affecting the facial nerve, including ear infections, cancer, or a skull fracture. In such disorders, there is usually involvement of other nerves as well, and distinctive signs and symptoms are frequently present. X-ray studies of the head may be performed.

Treatment

Primary treatment is aimed at reducing the inflammation of the nerve before any permanent damage is done to it. An oral corticosteroid, such as prednisone, may be given for this purpose. However, in many (if not most) uncomplicated cases, treatment with medication is unnecessary. After two weeks, if there has been no improvement in the ability of the muscles to move, the muscles of the weak side of the face may be stimulated electrically to maintain muscle tone.

The affected eye should be covered with an eye patch, especially when the patient is outdoors, and protected from dirt and wind. Application of moist, moderate heat on the affected side of the face can reduce pain. Brief periods of upward facial massage help maintain muscle tone, as do specific facial exercises.

Fortunately, most Bell's palsy patients recover in one to eight weeks. Elderly patients may take much longer—up to two years. Complete recovery usually follows within several months if the paralysis is partial.

Carpal tunnel syndrome

Carpal tunnel syndrome is characterized by weakness, pain, tingling, numbness, or burning in the palm, the thumb, the index finger, the middle finger, and the ring finger, caused by entrapment of the median nerve in the wrist. (This condition, like any syndrome, is not a disease in itself but rather a collection of symptoms.) The condition most often affects women in their 30s, 40s, and 50s. It may develop or become worse because of work that requires repeated grasping, twisting, or turning of the hand and wrist, especially against resistance or while using vibrating tools.

The carpal tunnel is formed by the bones of the wrist (*carpal* means wrist) and the tough band of connective tissue known as the transverse carpal ligament. Among the structures inside the tunnel are the median nerve and the tendons that flex the fingers and thumb. Any swelling or thickening of tissue within the tunnel can cause the median nerve to be compressed between the transverse carpal ligament and the tendons and other contents of the tunnel. The squeezed nerve, which controls the thumb, index finger, and third finger, cannot work as it should, and the symptoms of carpal tunnel syndrome result.

Causes

Pregnancy and other conditions that produce generalized swelling of body tissues may be a cause of carpal tunnel syndrome, as can localized swelling caused by a dislocation, sprain, or fracture of the wrist. Rheumatoid arthritis can cause inflammation of the coverings of the tendons, causing compression. Other possible causes include an inflamed wrist joint, a noncancerous tumor, myxedema (tissue swelling due to lack of thyroid hormone), tuberculosis, amyloidosis (a disease character-

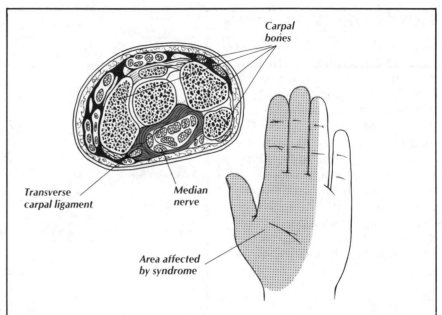

Carpal tunnel syndrome is characterized by weakness, pain, tingling, numbness, or burning in the palm, the thumb, the index finger, the middle finger, and the ring finger. These symptoms are caused by entrapment of the median nerve within the carpal tunnel of the wrist. The carpal tunnel is formed by the carpal bones of the wrist and the tough band of connective tissue called the transverse carpal ligament.

ized by abnormal deposits of the protein amyloid), acromegaly (overgrowth of connective tissue), and diabetes mellitus.

Symptoms

Aching pain may travel up the forearm and even into the shoulder joint, neck, and chest. (This type of pain can usually be relieved by shaking the hand vigorously or dangling the arm loosely from its socket; occasionally, however, such pains are caused by compression of the median nerve in the forearm or upper arm.) Other (late) signs include an inability to make a fist, deterioration of the nails, and dryness and shininess of the skin over the involved surfaces. The pains may occur in both hands at the same time. They may be constant or may come and go, and are increased by manual work or movement that flexes the wrist or

palm. Weakness of the fingers occurs later than other symptoms and accompanies atrophy (wasting away) of the muscles. Symptoms are usually worse at night and in the morning.

Diagnosis

Preliminary diagnostic tests include tapping the wrist, which causes tingling in the area of pain if carpal tunnel syndrome is present, and forced flexion of the wrist, which may also reproduce the pain. An X-ray examination may reveal abnormalities of the wrist bones. Testing of the conduction of nerve impulses is the most specific means of diagnosing carpal tunnel syndrome.

Treatment

Treatment is aimed first at relieving pressure on the median nerve. If soft-tissue swelling is a cause, elevating the hand may eliminate the symptoms. It may help to place the forearm in a splint at night, which keeps the hand turned upward, extending the wrist. If an inflammation inside the wrist is at fault, cortisone may be injected into the carpal tunnel. Other causes or aggravating factors are treated appropriately.

If conservative forms of treatment prove ineffective, which they frequently do, surgery to release the transverse carpal ligament may be necessary to relieve the pressure on the nerve and prevent permanent damage. Usually, muscle strength gradually returns after such surgery, but if surgery has been delayed too long and muscles have severely deteriorated, full strength does not return. Symptoms usually disappear shortly after the operation, and recurrence is possible.

Concussion

Concussion is an injury to the brain, caused by a violent jar or shock, such as a blow to the head. The force of the shock causes the brain to strike against the inside of the skull, producing temporary brain swelling and malfunctioning and often loss of consciousness. The shock may even be strong enough to cause cerebral contusion (bruising of brain tissue), cerebral hemorrhage (bleeding between the covering of the brain and the skull or inside the brain covering), or formation of a hematoma (collection of clotted blood).

Symptoms

Unconsciousness is a common symptom of concussion. Uncon-

sciousness may last only a few minutes or as long as a few hours, but rarely more than 24 hours (a longer period of unconsciousness or a deep coma indicates more serious brain damage). The patient may then feel nauseated, irritable, "dragged out," or dizzy, or may have a severe headache; these symptoms may continue for days or weeks (or longer) after the accident. Frequently, the individual cannot remember what happened just before the injury and later may not be able to recall anything that happened in the first few hours or on the day following the concussion.

A person who suffers an accident serious enough to cause a cerebral contusion; laceration (cutting and tearing) of nerve tissue, blood vessels, and brain covering; or edema (fluid buildup) within or around the brain often shows symptoms other than those accompanying a simple concussion. Signs of serious damage to the brain include partial paralysis of the body, posture with the arms and legs extended and with the jaws clenched, and

unequal or pinpoint pupils of the eye.

Diagnosis

A simple concussion usually requires no special care. The purpose of the doctor's examination is to determine if any more serious injury may have occurred. The patient is observed for level of consciousness, mental sharpness (if awake), and proper nerve and muscle functions and reflexes. An X-ray study of the head may be performed to rule out a skull fracture (although most simple undepressed skull fractures are allowed to heal without treatment). If the patient acts strange or out of character or does not respond correctly to the tests, hospitalization and evaluation by a neurologist or neurosurgeon may be necessary.

Treatment

Once a doctor has determined that a patient has had only a sim-

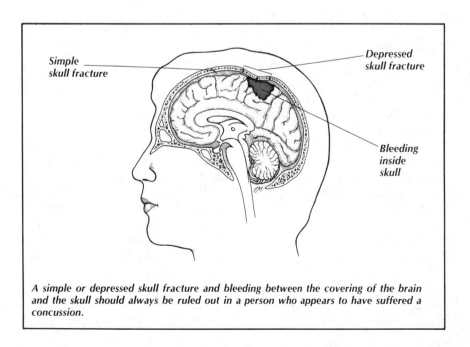

A simple or depressed skull fracture and bleeding between the covering of the brain and the skull should always be ruled out in a person who appears to have suffered a concussion.

ple concussion, the patient may be allowed to return home without hospitalization. For the next 24 hours, the person is advised to relax and to take no medication stronger than an aspirin substitute (acetaminophen). It is best not to eat solid foods following any vomiting (which is common after concussion). A parent, roommate, or spouse is usually asked to wake the patient every two hours during the night and ask three questions: What is your name? Where are you? What is my name? If the patient cannot answer these questions, will not awaken, or has convulsions, he or she should be rushed to the hospital. The patient should return to the hospital immediately if any of the following danger signals is noted: a continuing or worsening headache, blurring vision, extreme or constant vomiting, unusual eye movements, twitching, a staggering way of walking, or any change in personality. If none of these symptoms develops, the patient can resume normal activities after a day or so of rest.

Encephalitis

Encephalitis is an inflammation of the brain. The term is usually used to describe an infectious process caused by bacteria, parasites, vaccines, or, most often, viruses. Noninfectious agents such as poisons, metabolic abnormalities due to liver or kidney failure, and tumors can cause conditions that closely resemble encephalitis.

Causes

Viruses may cause encephalitis either as a primary disease or as a complication of an infection.

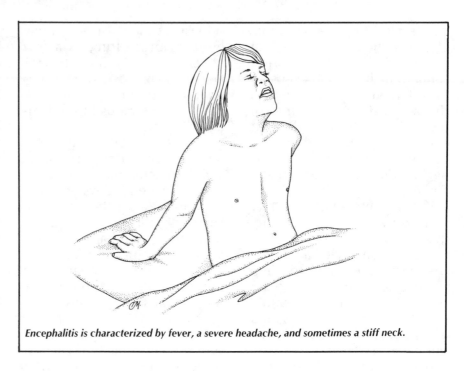

Encephalitis is characterized by fever, a severe headache, and sometimes a stiff neck.

Some of these viruses are mosquito-borne and afflict humans only in warm weather, when mosquitoes are in season. Many cases of encephalitis occur as complications of viral infections, such as measles, mumps, chicken pox, and rubella (German measles). These cases usually develop five to ten days after the onset of the original illness, but can develop as long as six weeks afterward.

Symptoms

Encephalitis may be associated with meningitis (infection of the layers of tissue that cover the brain and spinal cord). There may be evidence of brain disturbances, such as alterations in mental state, personality changes, seizures, and paralysis. Edema (fluid buildup) in the brain is present, and there may be petechial hemorrhages (small, red spots that indicate bleeding) scattered throughout parts of the brain and spinal cord. Fever, headache, vomiting, a general feeling of ill-

ness, and a stiff neck may be the first symptoms to appear.

Diagnosis

Prompt diagnosis and supportive treatment are essential in any case of encephalitis or suspected encephalitis. Even patients who have been seriously or critically ill with encephalitis often recover. One diagnostic problem is differentiating encephalitis from bacterial meningitis and other similar ailments. Even with ideal circumstances for diagnosis, the encephalitis virus is often not identified. Viruses can sometimes be isolated directly from cerebrospinal fluid or from the tissues. Since many forms of encephalitis, such as the mosquito-borne forms, have important public health implications, blood is often drawn whenever encephalitis is suspected; the sample is sent to the local department of health, which can provide a more precise diagnosis.

Treatment

With a form of encephalitis called herpes simplex encephalitis, early recognition and treatment with a medication that inhibits the reproduction of viruses reduce the chances of death and neurologic impairment significantly. However, for maximal effectiveness, the drug should be given before coma or paralysis occurs. Supportive therapy involves bed rest and maintaining fluid balance to avoid dehydration (loss of body fluids).

Epilepsy

Epilepsy is a disorder characterized by sudden surges of disorganized electrical impulses in the brain, which lead to seizures.

There are several categories of seizures; they can be so mild as to go almost unnoticed or so severe that, if untreated, they can cause serious harm.

Causes

Epilepsy is usually divided into two categories: idiopathic (of unknown cause) and acquired (caused by some known factor, such as a brain tumor or an injury). Until the age of 25, idiopathic epilepsy is a very common cause of seizures. Seizures beginning after the age of 25 are more often a sign of acquired epilepsy due to injury, tumors, or other brain disorders (such as cerebral palsy, infection, or malformations of blood vessels).

Idiopathic epilepsy, although by definition of unknown cause, has several consistent attributes. It occurs with highest frequency between the ages of two and five years and again at puberty and tends to run in families.

Symptoms

The symptoms of epilepsy vary according to the type of seizure experienced. Not all seizures are convulsions. A convulsion involves the nerves that control movement and is characterized by jerking, spastic muscle movements. It is also marked by alterations in sensation and consciousness; loss of consciousness is common.

Seizures are classified according to the symptoms present. In the past, classifications were grand mal (French for "big sickness"), petit mal (French for "little sickness"), psychomotor, and focal. The current classification separates seizures into partial and generalized types, depending on the extent of brain involvement.

The four currently used categories (and their symptoms) are as follows:

- Simple partial seizures, confined to small areas of the brain, may be accompanied by feeling a tingling sensation in the arm, finger, or foot; perceiving a bad odor; seeing flashing lights; or speaking unintelligibly. The patient remains conscious.
- Complex partial seizures include episodes of "automatic behavior," in which the patient remains conscious but sits motionless or moves or behaves in a strange, repetitive, or somehow inappropriate way.
- Generalized convulsive seizures have a number of symptoms: the patient may cry out, stiffen and fall to the ground unconscious, lose urinary and bowel control, and have muscle spasms or thrashing movements that cause the limbs to jerk. Spasm of the jaw muscles can cause the victim to bite his or her tongue. After the con-

vulsion, the patient falls into a deep sleep and then awakens dazed, often with a headache and no recollection of the seizure. A warning sensation, called an aura, may precede the seizure; this may be a headache, sleepiness, yawning, or tingling in arms or legs.
- Generalized nonconvulsive, or absence, seizures are characterized by periods of staring into space, rhythmic blinking, and what appears to be daydreaming. The patient remains conscious but is totally unaware of the seizure. This type of seizure, which is most common in children, may be mistaken for a short attention span or a learning disability.

Diagnosis

Epilepsy is diagnosed by observing the symptoms and by obtaining an electroencephalogram (EEG), which is a visual record of the electrical activity of the brain. Abnormal electrical discharges can be detected if they are present in the brain. However, an abnormal EEG in the absence of symptoms is by no means proof of epilepsy, nor does a normal EEG rule it out.

Treatment

Nonmedical treatment of an epileptic seizure should be limited to preventing injury and keeping the patient comfortable by loosening clothing or placing a pillow under the head. The patient should not be left in any position in which vomit can be swallowed or inhaled or in any position in which he or she might suffocate. *Never* should an attempt be made to pry open the mouth or insert any object into the mouth of a person who is having a convulsion.

Epilepsy cannot be cured, but it can usually be controlled with a program of anticonvulsant drug therapy. Patients who tend to have seizures following emotional or physical stress may also benefit from tranquilizers. After two to five years of drug control of idiopathic epilepsy, the dosage is sometimes decreased and, occasionally, when enough time has elapsed during which no seizures have occurred, medication can be discontinued.

Epilepsy cannot be prevented, but once the seizures have been controlled by medication, epileptic persons can lead normal lives.

Headaches

A headache is a symptom, not a disease. A headache is rarely the symptom of a serious illness, but severe or frequent headaches can be exhausting and can affect daily life.

There are three basic types of headaches. The *vascular headache* occurs when blood vessels in the head enlarge and press on nerves, causing pain. The most common vascular headache is the migraine. The second type of headache is the *muscle contraction headache,* which results when the muscles of the face, neck, or scalp contract and tighten. A tension headache is an example of a muscle contraction headache. The third kind of headache is the *inflammatory headache.* Such a headache is the result of pressure within the head. The causes range from relatively minor conditions, such as sinusitis, to more serious problems, such as brain tumors.

A more detailed description of each type of headache follows.

MIGRAINE HEADACHE

One theory about migraine headaches is that they occur when the blood vessels in the head expand and press on the nerves, causing pain. However, another theory is that they result when the blood vessels first overreact to outside stimuli by constricting and thus blocking blood flow to parts of the brain; this may cause the visual impairment and numbness that often accompany or precede a migraine headache. The blood vessels then become full of blood and press on surrounding nerves, causing pain.

Women are more prone to migraines than are men, and a certain personality type—compulsive, perfectionist, excessively neat, and very success-oriented—seems to be more susceptible to this kind of headache.

Causes

A number of physical and emotional factors may contribute to migraine headaches. Migraines may be triggered by a sharp reduction in caffeine intake or by allergies to certain foods or food additives (among them chocolate, coffee, fatty foods, alcohol, citrus fruits, monosodium glutamate, and nitrates). Emotional stress can also cause migraine headaches, as

A migraine headache occurs when the blood vessels in the head expand and press on nerves, causing pain.

can drinking, smoking, or an interruption in routine eating and sleeping habits (all of which may be responsible for "weekend" headaches suffered by some patients). Cyclical, seasonal, or emotional factors, such as menstruation, for instance, may be associated with migraine. A tendency toward having this type of headache may also be inherited.

Symptoms

The predominant symptom of a migraine headache is a sharp, pulsating, incapacitating pain on one or both sides of the head. Paleness, sweating, nausea, and sensitivity to light may accompany the pain.

A warning sensation (called an aura) may indicate an approaching migraine headache. Before the pain begins, some individuals may see flashing lights or "shooting stars," hear noises, smell fragrances or odors, or feel a tingling sensation in the arms or legs.

Cluster headaches, a form of migraine most commonly experienced by men, occur in groups of up to six a day, lasting for weeks or months. Their chief symptom is intense pain on one side of the head, accompanied by tearing of the eye and a runny nose on the same side. Drinking and smoking may aggravate these headaches.

Diagnosis

Vascular headaches are diagnosed by a careful review of the circumstances surrounding the headaches as well as by a physical examination to rule out any other disorder that might be causing them. Elimination tests may be done to identify the

exact cause of migraines suffered by people who seem to react to certain foods or changes in eating and sleeping habits. In an elimination test, all the substances that are suspected of causing the trouble are eliminated and then reintroduced one at a time to identify the cause.

Treatment

Treatment of a migraine already in progress usually consists of a drug therapy program chosen from a variety of painkillers, sedatives, and special drugs to combat migraine. For the occasional migraine sufferer, tranquilizers and sedatives may relieve some of the symptoms.

Prevention

Prevention of migraines is possible with several types of medication. One commonly prescribed is ergotamine, which constricts the blood vessels and thus prevents the swelling that causes pressure on the surrounding nerves. This drug is usually taken to stop an approaching migraine; it may have no effect on the aura symptoms some patients experience. Antidepressant drugs, taken in small doses, may prevent migraines in a patient who experiences them regularly.

A recent development in migraine treatment is the use of the beta-blocking drugs. These drugs work in the body to block what are called the beta effects, one of which is dilation (enlargement) of the blood vessels. Because these drugs block the dilation of blood vessels, they have been used to prevent, but not treat, acute attacks of migraine headaches. New drugs known as calcium-channel blockers, such as

verapamil, nifedipine, and diltiazem, are also effective in prevention of migraine headaches. These drugs probably act by preventing the initial constriction of blood vessels.

MUSCLE CONTRACTION HEADACHE

A muscle contraction headache occurs when muscles of the face, neck, or scalp remain contracted (tightened) for long periods. These muscles are then said to be in spasm.

Causes

A muscle contraction headache usually occurs following a specific event that has caused the muscles to tense. The tension is then translated into physical discomfort in the form of a clenched jaw, aching neck, and tightened muscles of the face and head.

Muscle contraction headaches can also be brought about by abnormalities in the eyes, neck, teeth, or jaws or by poor posture—especially by holding the head at an awkward angle while reading, driving, or watching television, for example.

Symptoms

The major symptom is a tight, squeezing pain in the forehead or jaws or around the back of the head or neck. This constant, dull pain usually occurs on both sides of the head.

Diagnosis

Diagnostic evaluation involves a review of the events that usu-

A muscle contraction headache occurs when muscles of the face, neck, or scalp contract (tighten) for long periods.

lined with mucous membranes, within the facial bones. When mucus, which normally flows freely through the sinuses and drains down the nasopharynx or out the nose, cannot drain properly, it collects in the sinuses and causes excess pressure on the surrounding tissues, leading to headache.

Other causes of inflammatory headaches include an aneurysm (a bulge in a blood vessel) in the head and a brain tumor. Aneurysms may not cause pain until they rupture or enlarge rapidly. Brain tumors are usually associated with swelling in the surrounding tissues, which causes increased pressure within the skull and, as a result, a dull, constant headache and sensation of pressing.

High blood pressure, which causes blood to rush through the vessels with too great a force; infections, which inflame sensitive tissue; and fever, which may enlarge the blood vessels, can also cause headache due to excess pressure within the skull.

ally precede the headaches, as well as a physical examination to rule out any other disorder that might be causing them. A psychological examination may also be conducted to detect any emotional problems that may be contributing to the headaches.

Treatment

Eliminating the tension or correcting the physical problem that is causing the headaches is a good start in treating them. Painkillers, muscle relaxants, and tranquilizers may be used occasionally (although not on an everyday basis) to treat muscle contraction headaches. Also,

antidepressant drugs may be effective in preventing these headaches in those persons who suffer from them regularly.

INFLAMMATORY HEADACHE

An inflammatory, or traction, headache is caused by pressure within the head, due to any of a variety of disorders.

Causes

Clogged sinuses and sinus infections are probably the chief cause of this type of headache. The sinuses are the cavities,

Symptoms

The symptoms of an inflammatory headache are a dull, aching pain, often occurring early in the day, accompanied by a feeling of pressure in the head. The pain is heightened by sneezing, coughing, bending over, or doing anything that increases the amount of blood in the head.

Diagnosis

This type of headache is diagnosed by determining first whether sinus problems are causing it. If not, the doctor may order an electroencephalogram (EEG), which is a visual record of electrical activity in the brain; X-ray studies; a computed tomographic (CT) scan, which provides a cross-sectional picture of the brain; or a magnetic resonance imaging (MRI) study, which yields images comparable to those obtained with CT but without the use of X rays. These tests may detect the presence of a tumor, an aneurysm, or another abnormality in the brain.

Treatment

Inflammatory headaches are treated according to their cause. Those triggered by a sinus infection can be treated with pain-killers; antibiotics, which fight the infection; or antihistamines and decongestants, which dry out and help drain the sinuses. Headaches resulting from more serious disorders, such as a brain tumor or aneurysm, will almost certainly require surgery.

Prevention

Prevention of these headaches is sometimes possible if the cause is as simple as a sinus infection. Of course, the correction of a more serious disorder that has caused the pain should also prevent future problems with inflammatory headaches.

Meningitis

Meningitis occurs when bacteria or viruses enter the spinal fluid and infect the meninges, the three layers of membrane that surround the brain and spinal cord. Meningitis can be fatal, although this is becoming less common because of the increased use of effective medications.

Meningitis seems to strike males more often than females and is most commonly seen in children up to the age of four years and in adults over the age of 60. Swelling of the brain, as well as epilepsy, blindness, amnesia, and deafness, can result

The meninges are the three membranes that cover the brain and spinal cord: the dura mater (outer layer), the arachnoid (middle layer), and the pia mater (inner layer). Between the pia mater and the arachnoid is the subarachnoid space, which is filled with cerebrospinal fluid. Meningitis results when infection is spread from the cerebrospinal fluid to the meninges.

when meningitis is not properly and promptly treated.

The three layers of meninges are the dura mater (the outermost layer), the arachnoid (the middle layer), and the pia mater (the innermost layer). The space between the inner two layers, called the subarachnoid space, is filled with clear cerebrospinal fluid, which is produced in the brain. When bacteria or viruses invade this fluid and form pus, the surrounding membranes soon become infected, resulting in meningitis.

Causes

Meningitis is caused by an infection that enters the system through a serious head wound or through the bloodstream from a source of infection in another part of the body. The bacteria may also reach the meninges from an abscess (localized infection) of the brain itself, but this is quite rare.

A deficiency in the immune system, which can be either inherited or acquired over time, may lead to a greater chance of contracting this disease. Also, newborns may be at a greater risk if the mother had a genital infection, such as herpes, during the last week of pregnancy; if the membranes of the uterus ruptured prematurely; or if labor was prolonged.

Symptoms

The symptoms of meningitis are a "bursting" headache, high fever, rising pulse rate, irregular breathing, vomiting, and sensitivity to light. Pain extends down the neck, into the back and lower limbs; the neck may be stiff, and it will be difficult for the patient to bend forward. As the disease progresses, convulsions or coma may occur.

Diagnosis

Unless increased pressure in the brain is suspected, meningitis is diagnosed with a test called a lumbar puncture, or spinal tap, in which a sample of the cerebrospinal fluid is withdrawn and examined to see if it is clear (normal) or cloudy (pus-filled) and to identify the bacteria causing the infection. A physical examination, blood cultures, and cultures from the secretions of the respiratory tract may also be useful in determining the type of bacteria present. A viral infection is much harder to diagnose; it may not show up on any tests.

Treatment

Because immediate treatment is so important, medication may be prescribed before the specific infecting agent has been identified. Once the cause has been determined, a more appropriate medication, most often an antibiotic, can then be administered. The patient will be admitted to the hospital, where measures can be taken to reduce fever and control brain swelling.

Viral infections are much more difficult to treat. Fortunately, most cases run their course without causing serious consequences. Treatment is generally limited to hospitalization, so that supportive therapy can be administered.

Prevention

Prevention of meningitis caused by certain strains of bacteria may be possible with some vaccines that are now available. Research continues on vaccines against other bacterial strains.

Rifampin, an antituberculosis drug, is used for prevention of meningococcal meningitis (a bacteria known as meningococcus is the causative agent). The drug is given orally to individuals who have been in close contact with a person who has a documented case of meningococcal meningitis.

Multiple sclerosis

Multiple sclerosis is a chronic disease of the central nervous system (the brain and spinal cord) in which the protective myelin sheath (the insulating covering) of the nerve fibers degenerates. When this protection disappears, body functions may become impaired. In some cases, the patient ultimately becomes wheelchair-bound or even dies. In other cases, the disease may flare up only once in a lifetime and leave the individual with no or only minimal disabilities.

Causes

Researchers have not yet determined the exact cause of multiple sclerosis. Some studies indicate that the disease follows exposure to a virus that may lie dormant (inactive) until some factor, such as stress or a second exposure to the virus, triggers the disease.

Another theory suggests that multiple sclerosis affects people who have some defect in their immune system (the body system responsible for protection from foreign substances or infective agents). It is thought that following viral exposure, the immune

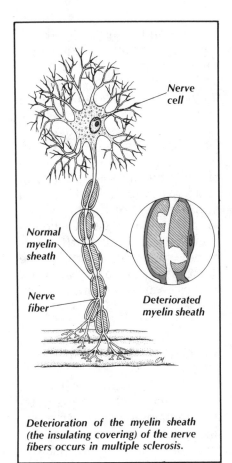

Deterioration of the myelin sheath (the insulating covering) of the nerve fibers occurs in multiple sclerosis.

Labels in figure: Nerve cell; Normal myelin sheath; Nerve fiber; Deteriorated myelin sheath

system mistakenly identifies the myelin covering of the nerves as foreign tissue and tries to destroy it. The symptoms of multiple sclerosis may be the consequence of this destructive process.

Symptoms

Initial attacks of multiple sclerosis are most common in people in their late 20s and early 30s. The disease begins with one or more of the following symptoms: tingling and numbness in the arms and legs, muscle spasms, partial loss of vision, difficulty in walking, and impaired bladder control. After the first attack, there is usually a period of remission (a time without symptoms) for as long as two to three years.

Subsequent attacks occur at irregular intervals and cause gradually increasing disability. Frequent episodes cause weakness, general incoordination, impaired speech, and burning sensations. Sexual function deteriorates, and mood swings are common.

More extensive nerve damage may result in loss of muscle control and may necessitate the use of a wheelchair. Usually, the earlier the onset of disease, the more slowly it progresses. Ten years after onset, fewer than half of patients with multiple sclerosis can continue regular daily activity. After 20 years, fewer than one fourth are able to function normally. Often, however, an individual may suffer one attack and never have another.

Diagnosis

Physicians diagnose multiple sclerosis through physical examination and observation of symptoms. Often, diagnosis remains unconfirmed until a second attack occurs. Analysis of the spinal fluid in conjunction with magnetic resonance imaging (MRI) studies is very useful in establishing the diagnosis.

Treatment

Since there is no cure for multiple sclerosis, treatment concentrates on relieving the symptoms. Muscle relaxants may ease muscle spasms and corticosteroid drugs may shorten attacks by reducing nerve tissue inflammation. Many patients are more comfortable if they are well rested; afternoon naps and adequate sleep at night are advised. Cold temperatures sometimes relieve symptoms, whereas heat makes them worse.

Myasthenia gravis

Myasthenia gravis is an uncommon disease of the nerves and muscles, characterized by great fatigue and weakness in the muscular system, most notably in the face and throat. Although the muscles do not atrophy (wither or waste away), there is slow and progressive paralysis. The disease is most likely to strike adults, especially women between the ages of 18 and 25 and men older than 40, but it can affect persons of any age.

Causes

Myasthenia gravis is sometimes associated with thyroid disease, excessive growth of the thymus (a gland in the chest that is an essential part of the immune system), or tumors in the thymus.

The condition is a neuromuscular disorder; the muscles fail to receive messages from the nerves because of a lack of the important neurotransmitting chemical acetylcholine. Experts believe that the disorder originates in the immune system and causes the body to destroy or block the sites responsible for receiving acetylcholine.

Symptoms

The muscular weakness first shows up in the face: the eyelids droop, often causing squinting and double vision; there is an inability to move the mouth and lips, with subsequent difficulty in talking, chewing, and swallowing; and the cheeks generally droop or sag. Sometimes the arms and legs are afflicted, affecting basic motor movements, like walking and standing, and the performance of simple tasks, like lifting a cup. The progressive muscular weakness can also impair breathing. The degree of paralysis or weakness varies from hour to hour and day to day, although it tends to be least severe in the morning and worst at night. Blood tests and chest X rays aid in the diagnosis.

Treatment

Myasthenia gravis is usually not curable, but drugs are available that restore nerve transmission to the muscles. The drugs neostigmine and pyridostigmine help to reestablish muscle strength and enable the patient with myasthenia gravis to live a more normal life. If a disorder of the thymus gland is found to be the underlying problem, the gland can be surgically removed. Corticosteroids are used to help regulate the immune system.

Narcolepsy

Narcolepsy is a disorder in which a person is recurrently subject to an irresistible, uncontrollable desire to sleep.

Causes

Narcolepsy is not necessarily related to any other abnormal condition, although it may be the result of an abnormality in the hypothalamus that causes a disorder in the endocrine system.

Symptoms

The most obvious symptom is the pattern of uncontrollable lapses into deep sleep during waking hours, often at inopportune times. These episodes of sleep last only a few minutes; the person wakes up feeling refreshed but is likely to fall asleep again a few hours later. The condition may be associated with cataplexy, a disorder in which stress or an unexpected emotional reaction causes collapse due to sudden muscle weakness.

Diagnosis

The diagnosis is confirmed by observation in a sleep laboratory or by special electroencephalographic (EEG) studies.

Treatment

Central nervous system stimulants are often prescribed.

Neuralgia

Neuralgia is pain that runs along the course of a damaged nerve. The condition ranges from mild and temporary to severe and chronic. The pain itself is sharp and extreme, lasting only a few seconds but tending to recur. There are various types of neuralgia. These include carpal tunnel syndrome (see pages 91-93), sciatica (see page 106), and the three types listed below.

Peripheral neuropathy

In peripheral neuropathy, impairment of the peripheral nerves (those outside the brain and spinal cord) occurs as a complication of another disorder, such as diabetes mellitus, alcoholism, certain vitamin deficiencies, anemia, or a tumor, or as a result of overexposure to particular chemicals or drugs (the typical cause for farm and industrial workers). The first symptom is frequently a tingling sensation in the hands and feet, which slowly spreads up the limbs to the trunk; numbness follows in the same pattern, the skin becomes sensitive, and neuralgic pain ensues. Numbness in the hands leads to a loss of dexterity and susceptibility to accidents. A special risk is that a numbed part of the body can sustain an injury without the patient's awareness until it becomes infected or ulcerated. The muscles gradually atrophy (wither away), and paralysis may set in.

Shingles

Shingles, or herpes zoster, is a viral infection characterized by intense pain and skin rash along the course of a nerve. Red blisters appear in a band, usually along one side of the chest, trunk, or abdomen. Shingles occurs almost exclusively in persons who have already had chicken pox (which is caused by the same virus) and appears during times of stress or after a subsequent exposure to the chicken pox virus. Shingles can often be diagnosed by sight. (For additional information on shingles, see pages 70-72.)

Trigeminal neuralgia

Trigeminal neuralgia, or tic douloureux, primarily affects elderly persons (most commonly, those over age 70), although it may also occur in younger persons with multiple sclerosis. The pain arises from the trigeminal nerve, which controls sensation in the face, teeth, mouth, and nasal cavity and movement of the jaw. The pain, usually excru-

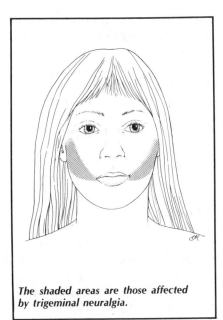

The shaded areas are those affected by trigeminal neuralgia.

ciating, covers one side of the face and can be set off by eating, by washing, or even by being exposed to a gust of air. With time, the stabbing pains occur more and more frequently, until they become constant. The cause is unknown. Although the condition is not life-threatening, it can become very disabling.

Treatment

Treatment for the various types of neuralgia depends on the location of the damaged nerves, the severity of the pain, and the reason behind the impairment. Therapy may vary from cold or hot packs and aspirin to stronger prescription painkillers. For shingles, ointments may soothe and dry up blisters, and the antiviral drug acyclovir may shorten the course of the illness. A physician may refer a patient with neuralgia to a neurologist (a specialist in problems of the nervous system). In rare instances, neurosurgery to sever a damaged nerve is necessary to eliminate the pain.

Prevention

There is virtually no way to prevent neuralgia, except to treat underlying diseases that may precipitate nerve damage and to avoid overexposure to chemicals and drugs.

Paralysis

Paralysis is the loss of the ability to move a part of the body, usually brought on by damage to either the muscles or to the nervous system. The condition can vary in severity and degree from paralysis of one small muscle to paralysis of almost the entire body. Irreversible and permanent paralysis results when a nerve is completely severed and destroyed, whereas paralysis caused by some diseases that cause inflammation without actual destruction of nerve tissue may diminish as the condition is treated and the body recuperates.

Causes

There are numerous causes of paralysis. Brain damage resulting from disease or a stroke can lead to partial or total paralysis of various parts of the body. Such damage interferes with the transmission of nerve impulses from the brain to the muscles. Certain other diseases (for example, poliomyelitis, a viral infection of the central nervous system, and myasthenia gravis, a severe muscular disorder of the neurochemical transmission system) and poisons (such as nerve gas and the toxin that causes botulism) also prevent nerve impulses from making contact with muscles, but do not necessarily cause complete loss of movement.

Damage to the spinal cord at the level of the middle or lower back can cause paralysis of the legs and the structures in the lower part of the body, including the bladder and rectum; this condition is called paraplegia. Injury to the spinal cord at the level of the neck affects both arms and both legs; this is known as quadriplegia.

Diabetes, cancer, alcoholism, vitamin deficiency, and drug reactions, among other conditions, can injure peripheral nerves (those outside the brain and spinal cord), occasionally weakening or totally immobilizing the muscles they control, as well as causing loss of sensation in the areas they serve.

Treatment

Well-being and survival depend on the cause and extent of the paralysis. Obviously, paralysis that affects the muscles involved in breathing is life-threatening, and the job of breathing must be taken over by machines until the paralysis improves or disappears.

Patients whose paralysis does not require artificial measures for survival may benefit from physical or occupational therapy. These patients can learn to reuse a muscle or to develop other muscles to compensate for a disabled muscle. All patients with disabled muscles require special attention to prevent muscle atrophy (withering away) and ulcers (pressure sores or bed sores).

Parkinson's disease

Parkinson's disease is a progressive disorder characterized primarily by uncontrollable tremors in the limbs, a shuffling gait, and generalized muscular rigidity. It most often strikes people over the age of 60.

Parkinson's disease is usually not fatal, but it leads to changes in the entire body, making the patient more susceptible to other diseases. It can be present in a mild form for 20 or 30 years, but a severe form can lead to serious disability within five to ten years.

Cause

The cause of Parkinson's disease is unknown. No inherited, physiological, or environmental factors have been identified as causes of the disease. It is known, however, that Parkinson's disease is a reflection of a chemical imbalance in the brain. Those with the disease have been shown to have low levels of a neurotransmitter called dopamine. (Neurotransmitters are chemicals in the brain that transmit impulses across junctions between neurons; the delicate balance of neurotransmitters

in the brain is responsible for brain function and muscular control.) To date, no cause for this chemical deficiency has been found.

Symptoms

The symptoms of Parkinson's disease are uncontrollable shaking of the limbs, stiff muscles, drooling, reduced blinking, an expressionless face, stooping posture, and a shuffling walk. Tremors may worsen during rest periods and times of increased anxiety, but they may decrease when the patient makes a conscious effort to perform an action.

As the disease progresses, speech slurs and sentences trail off into unintelligible muttering. Small muscle movements become increasingly difficult—reducing the ability to write, eat, chew, and swallow—and all movements seem overly stiff and slow. The term "cogwheel rigidity" is often used to describe the typical arm motion these patients display; when the arm is pulled straight from a flexed position, it

seems to jerk up and down as if controlled by a ratchet in a cogwheel.

Excitement and tension can cause these symptoms to worsen, as can depression. Depression is common among Parkinson's disease victims, who are understandably upset by their loss of muscle control.

Diagnosis

Diagnostic evaluation involves a history, physical examination, and observation of the symptoms. If tremors are the only symptom displayed, tests may be done to rule out the possibility that other disorders are causing the tremors, such as liver disease, multiple sclerosis, chronic alcoholism, or overactivity of the thyroid gland.

Treatment

Treatment of Parkinson's disease consists of correcting the dopamine deficiency. Dopamine itself cannot be absorbed directly into the brain from the bloodstream, so a substance called levodopa is prescribed to help the brain manufacture more of its own dopamine.

Levodopa has several undesirable side effects, among them nausea (which is decreased if the drug is taken with meals), an uneven "on-off" effect (causing symptoms to disappear and then reappear), and a loss of effectiveness over time. Levodopa preparations are often given in combination with anticholinergic drugs, which decrease nerve-to-muscle transmission, thereby reducing tremor and rigidity, and also decrease drooling. Levodopa is most often prescribed in combination with carbidopa, a

"Cogwheel rigidity" is noted in a patient with Parkinson's disease when the arm moves in a jerky fashion (as if controlled by a ratchet in a cogwheel) after being pulled straight from a flexed position.

substance that prevents destruction of levodopa in the body before it reaches the brain, thus allowing the use of smaller amounts of levodopa. Bromocriptine, a drug that enhances the effects of dopamine, has also been successful, as have other drugs.

Surgery to halt the tremor of Parkinson's has been helpful in select groups of patients. Physical therapy and exercise are important in a treatment program for patients with Parkinson's disease. Emotional support and understanding are also critical.

Rabies

Rabies is an acute infectious viral disease of mammals, especially carnivores (meat eaters), characterized by central nervous system irritation followed by paralysis and, in some cases, death. Human infection usually follows the bite of a rabid animal (dogs, skunks, cats, bats, foxes, and coyotes are among those that may be affected). In the later stages of the disease, it is marked by paralysis of the swallowing muscles and by throat spasms, which are set off by drinking or even the sight of liquids. Convulsions, tetanus (a condition characterized by severe muscular contractions), and paralysis of the respiratory (breathing) muscles are other symptoms of the last stages. Fortunately, because of animal immunization programs, only a handful of cases are reported in the United States each year.

Cause

Rabies is caused by a virus that is present in the saliva and respiratory secretions of rabid animals. Rabid animals transmit the infection by biting other animals or human beings. Rabies can be acquired by exposure of a mucous membrane or an open skin wound to infected animal saliva or by inhalation of the virus.

The rabies virus travels from the site of entry to the spinal cord and brain, where it multiplies. It then spreads to the salivary glands and into the saliva itself. In human beings, the incubation period (the time between exposure to the virus and development of symptoms) may extend from ten days to one year, but the average incubation period is 30 to 50 days. The incubation period is shortest in persons who have been bitten on the head or trunk and in those who have multiple bites.

Symptoms

The first symptom is a short period of mental depression, restlessness, and fever. In the next stage of the disease, the restlessness increases to uncontrollable excitement and hyperactivity. There is excessive salivation ("foaming at the mouth") and painful spasms of the throat muscles. The spasms can be easily initiated—by a breath of air, a slight breeze, an attempt to drink water. Generally, the patient experiences overwhelming thirst but cannot drink. In untreated cases, death occurs within three to ten days. However, patients often survive the disease if diagnosis and treatment are prompt.

Diagnosis

In human patients, rabies is usually suspected if there has been a report of an animal bite or exposure to the saliva of a rabid animal. The diagnosis is confirmed by testing for the virus once the symptoms appear. A domestic animal with no symptoms that suddenly bites a human should be confined and observed by a veterinarian for ten days. If the animal still shows no symptoms, it was most likely not infectious at the time of the bite and is usually released. However, if the animal is apparently rabid or is a wild animal, it should be captured. The police or local health department should be notified so that they can capture and examine the animal. Only an experienced professional should attempt to capture the animal.

Treatment

The contaminated area should be cleansed thoroughly with soap and water or an antiseptic as soon as possible.

The next step is administration of antirabies serum or human rabies immune globulin for passive immunization. This is followed immediately by vaccine for active immunization. A new active immunization, called HDCV, is said to have only mild side effects for most people. Subsequent HDCV injections are given on days 3, 7, 14, and 28 after exposure. The World Health Organization recommends that a sixth injection be given routinely 90 days after the first injection.

Prevention

The best preventive measure for rabies is to minimize contact with animals that may be rabid. In many cases, persons with a high occupational risk of animal bites receive preexposure injections. This is especially helpful for zoo personnel and persons whose work or hobbies take them into areas where they might encounter rabid animals.

As for domestic animals, restraining dogs and cats from contact with wild animals and impounding stray animals are important preventive measures. Immunizing 70 percent or more of the dog population of major cities has helped to restrict transmission of rabies, even in areas where wild animals have it.

Controlling rabies in wildlife areas is more difficult, although rabies as a disease is self-limiting, because it tends to kill off susceptible hosts in an area. Expensive control efforts are generally limited to areas where humans are apt to be exposed to wildlife (as in campgrounds).

Sciatica

Sciatica is characterized by pain that extends along the entire length of the sciatic nerve (which runs down the lower back and outer side of the thigh, leg, and foot), radiating across the back of the pelvis through the buttocks and into the leg.

Cause

Sciatica is commonly associated with injury to or rupture of a lumbar disk, located between the lumbar (lower back) vertebrae. When the injured disk exerts pressure against the sciatic nerve, pain radiates down the nerve.

Symptoms

The symptoms of sciatica vary in intensity, depending on the

Area of lumbar vertebrae

Path of sciatic nerve

Sciatica occurs when pressure on the sciatic nerve in the area of the lumbar vertebrae causes pain to radiate along the path of the sciatic nerve.

extent to which the injured disk presses on the sciatic nerve and on the individual's susceptibility to pain. In mild cases, the pain may be a slight discomfort in the lower back and along the leg. In severe cases, the pain is excruciating and often completely immobilizes the victim. Since the cause is frequently a ruptured ("slipped") disk, it is difficult to know when an attack will begin. A sudden cough may cause the disk to move and press on the sciatic nerve, resulting in the pain that such pressure causes. It is common for patients to be free

of pain one moment and in agony the next.

Repeated problems with a ruptured lumbar disk can cause general inflammation of the sciatic nerve. In these cases, it is not a matter of pain that comes and goes. Instead, it is a matter of having somewhat less pain at one time than at another.

Treatment

The primary treatment of sciatica is rest, to allow the inflammation of the nerve to subside. In an effort to alleviate the pain, various medications, such as analgesics and muscle relaxants, may be prescribed, or anesthetic agents may be injected into the area around the spinal cord. In cases that do not respond to such conservative measures, surgery may be necessary. Recently, new surgical techniques, such as microsurgery and percutaneous (through the skin without cutting, as with a needle) removal of disk fragments, have been developed. These techniques have considerably decreased hospital stays and loss of work time. So far, success at relieving pain and neurologic symptoms has been good. Not all individuals with disk problems, however, are suitable for this surgery.

Physical therapy (under a doctor's supervision or according to a doctor's prescription) is often used to relieve the pain of sciatica. This treatment includes hydrotherapy, in which a stream of water is directed at the affected area. Many therapists advise their patients to overcome the effects of a ruptured disk by developing the core muscles (the four muscle groups that form the waist) in order to provide a supportive column of muscle that will help keep the disk in place.

THE SKIN

The skin is the largest organ of the body, covering 18 square feet and weighing about seven pounds in an average adult. This waterproof barrier affords protection from invasion by dirt, bacteria, and other harmful substances and helps to regulate body temperature.

The skin is composed of three layers—the epidermis, the dermis, and the subcutaneous layer.

Epidermis

The outermost layer of skin is the epidermis. The epidermis contains pigment cells that determine skin color and help to shield the skin against damaging sun rays. Specialized cells within this layer manufacture keratin, a tough substance also found in hair and nails.

Epidermal cells are continuously being worn away and replaced. This reconstruction process is usually invisible, except when skin becomes irritated, as in psoriasis, a disease that appears as scaly red patches. Since the outer skin layer repairs itself quickly, any injury to the epidermis rarely causes injury to the body as a whole.

Dermis

The dermis contains blood vessels, nerve endings, hair follicles, sweat glands, and sebaceous (oil) glands. Damage at this level can send infection into the bloodstream and throughout the body.

Within the dermis, blood vessels and sweat glands help the body regulate heat. If the temperature of blood rises, the brain stimulates secretion by the sweat glands. Sweat then flows to the surface skin through ducts and

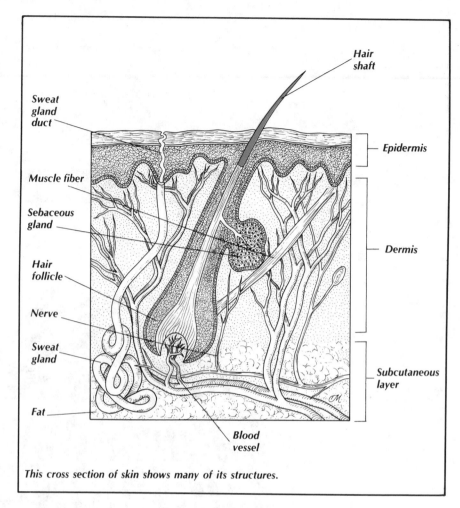

This cross section of skin shows many of its structures.

Labels: Sweat gland duct; Muscle fiber; Sebaceous gland; Hair follicle; Nerve; Sweat gland; Fat; Hair shaft; Epidermis; Dermis; Subcutaneous layer; Blood vessel

cools the skin by evaporating. The sebaceous glands prevent excessive evaporation by coating the skin surface with an oily substance called sebum.

Subcutaneous layer

Beneath the dermis is the subcutaneous layer, in which the sweat glands originate and fat is stored. This layer also supports the blood vessels and nerves that supply the outer layers of the skin.

Because the dermis and the subcutaneous layer are rich with nerve endings, the skin is also a sensory organ. Nerves throughout these layers transmit tactile perceptions to the brain.

Acne

Acne is a condition of the skin that ranges in appearance from small raised bumps to pustules (large cysts and pimples). Acne is so common that more than 80 percent of the population will have some form of it at some time in their lives.

Causes

Although there are several theories about what causes acne, authorities generally believe that acne is a by-product of hormonal changes in the body during puberty—that period of life when a child develops the secondary sex characteristics (such as facial and body hair, deepened voice, and increased muscle mass in boys and breast development and menstruation in girls). At this time, production of hormones (particularly the male hormone testosterone) increases and stimulates the sebaceous glands in the skin to produce sebum (an oily secretion). Most excess oil produced by these glands leaves the skin through the hair follicles (the tubelike structures from which hairs develop). Sometimes, oil clogs these tubes and creates comedones (blocked hair follicles). Comedones are what form the initial lumps in acne.

If comedones are open to the surface of the skin, they are called blackheads. They contain sebum from the sebaceous glands, bacteria, and any skin tissue that accumulates near the surface. Comedones that are closed at the surface are called whiteheads. Plugged follicles can rupture internally, resulting in a discharge of their contents into the surrounding tissues. This process begins an inflammatory response that sets the stage for the development of acne.

The role of bacteria in acne is unclear. Bacteria may act by causing chemical reactions in the sebaceous fluid, leading to the release of very irritating compounds called fatty acids. These in turn may cause inflammation that increases susceptibility to infection.

Authorities disagree about the role of diet as a cause of acne. Diet alone does not cure acne, nor does acne stem from an allergic reaction to a specific food. However, some cases of acne appear to improve after eliminating certain foods, particularly chocolates and fats. In addition, emotional stress seems to increase the severity of acne in certain cases.

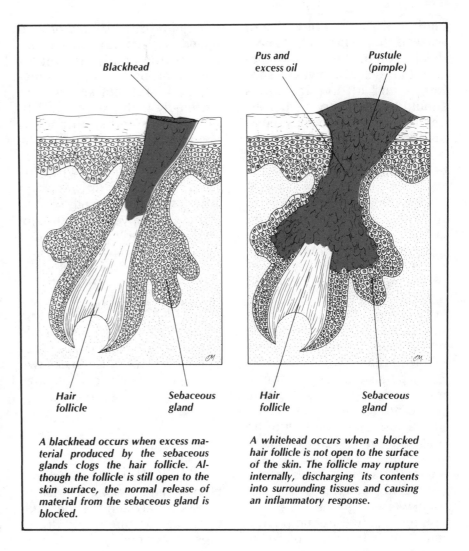

A blackhead occurs when excess material produced by the sebaceous glands clogs the hair follicle. Although the follicle is still open to the skin surface, the normal release of material from the sebaceous gland is blocked.

A whitehead occurs when a blocked hair follicle is not open to the surface of the skin. The follicle may rupture internally, discharging its contents into surrounding tissues and causing an inflammatory response.

Symptoms

Acne causes raised swellings, most frequently on the face, neck, back, chest, and shoulders. In severe cases, there may be pus-filled sacs that break open and discharge fluid. Soreness, pain, and itching may accompany the bumps. These symptoms could be acne, or they could indicate other skin reactions to such substances as cosmetics, medications, and grooming or cleaning products.

Since puberty plays a role in the onset of acne, the condition usually appears during the teenage years. However, it can extend to age 25 and over, particularly in women. Although acne is not life threatening, it can be problematic. If untreated, acne lesions can leave permanent scars, which can cause embarrassment and emotional stress.

Treatment

Acne has no prevention or cure, but there are several treatments. The simplest home remedy is to wash the affected areas thoroughly at least twice a day with warm water and mild soap. Washing gently will not dry or irritate sensitive skin. Regular shampooing also helps, especially if the hair is oily. Use of makeup should be limited. In addition, skin may heal with exposure to the sun. However, sunlamps and ultraviolet lamps should be used very cautiously, and only under a doctor's supervision.

One form of treatment not recommended is picking or squeezing pimples, since more inflammation and scarring may result. Also, the risk of infection is increased.

Some over-the-counter acne medications, particularly lotions or creams containing benzoyl peroxide, can help troubled skin. However, most of these preparations tend to dry the skin if the manufacturer's directions are not followed carefully.

For persistent acne, a doctor may prescribe an antibiotic preparation that can be applied to the surface of the skin or an oral antibiotic, such as tetracycline and erythromycin. These antibiotics act to suppress bacterial growth, which may be a factor in worsening acne.

Another drug, tretinoin (vitamin A acid), has reduced acne in more than 50 percent of the persons who have tried it. This drug can be used independently or in combination with an antibiotic, and must be used under a doctor's supervision. A newer drug, isotretinoin, is related to tretinoin and is used to treat severe cystic acne. It is usually not prescribed, however, unless all other acne treatments have failed. This drug works by temporarily suppressing the production of secretions by the sebaceous glands. It is important to note that this drug can have very serious side effects and should never be used without the knowledge and supervision of an experienced medical doctor. In addition, isotretinoin should not be used by any woman who is,

who thinks she may be, or who intends to become pregnant. Use of this drug in any amount for even short periods during pregnancy is associated with an extremely high risk of fetal abnormalities and spontaneous abortion. Women of childbearing potential should use contraception during therapy with this drug; use of contraception should begin one month prior to starting therapy and should not be discontinued until at least one month after therapy is complete.

Athlete's foot

Athlete's foot (known medically as *tinea pedis*) is a fungal infection of the foot. It is also known as ringworm of the foot, although it is not caused by a worm.

Symptoms

Athlete's foot causes itching, burning, and stinging sensations. The skin between the toes reddens, cracks open, and crumbles. In extremely long-lasting cases, the toenails may become infected, discolored, and overgrown. The fungus may spread to the underside of the foot, beneath the arch, producing groups of itching blisters and peeling of the skin.

Diagnosis

It is important to rule out other causes of similar symptoms. For example, hot, tight shoes may make the feet sweaty in warm weather; the moisture and friction may cause softening and peeling of the skin on the soles. Dyes, adhesive cements, and other substances inside the shoes may cause irritation, as may

powders and nail polishes. Eczema, psoriasis, and scabies are other possible causes of similar symptoms.

Treatment

Most people can treat athlete's foot at home using one of several good salves, powders, or liquids obtainable without a prescription from the drugstore. These include undecylenic acid ointment, tolnaftate, and miconazole. Clotrimazole is another effective medication, but it must be prescribed by a physician. Directions usually call for application morning and night, to continue until one week after all symptoms have vanished. As long as loose skin remains, the feet should be soaked before the ointment is applied, and the loose skin removed carefully.

If sweaty feet are the cause, athlete's foot ointments should not be used. Instead, you should ask your doctor for suggestions about controlling the excessive sweating. Changing shoes may eliminate the problem if the feet are sensitive to chemicals inside the shoes.

Severe cases of athlete's foot call for treatment by a physician. To relieve symptoms, the doctor may prescribe soaking the feet three times a day in a solution of aluminum sulfate and calcium acetate (often called Burow's solution), with an antiseptic solution added if a secondary infection is present.

Prevention

Athlete's foot can recur despite any treatment, especially during hot weather. The organisms that cause athlete's foot thrive in a hot, moist setting. However, there are several things you can do to help prevent the disease. You can keep your feet clean, dry between your toes after bathing, and change socks frequently. Use dusting and drying powders to keep the feet dry. Separate your toes with small wads of cotton when you are sleeping. Wear clogs in motel and community showers and wear sandals, open-toed shoes, or no shoes at all (when safe and practical) in hot weather.

Baldness

Baldness (known medically as alopecia) is partial or complete loss of hair on the head. This may be caused by an inherited tendency, aging, fever, drugs, radiation, or disease.

Male-pattern baldness

Male-pattern baldness is the most common form. There seems to be an inherited tendency toward it, and androgen (a male hormone) contributes to it. However, the exact mechanism by which it occurs is not known. Hair loss is gradual, occurring at the forehead, on either side of the front (sometimes leaving a center tuft known as a "widow's peak"), and on top of the head. It can begin as early as age 15 or 16, in which case it may indicate that considerable baldness is likely later (however, male-pattern baldness does not usually advance at a steady or predictable rate).

Female-pattern baldness

Female-pattern baldness is fairly common in menopausal women and usually involves

Hair loss in male-pattern baldness is gradual, beginning at the forehead on either side of the front and continuing to the top of the head.

only the area around the crown of the head. Like male-pattern baldness, it is believed to be due to hormonal causes.

Temporary baldness

Temporary baldness sometimes occurs up to three or four months following a severe illness, especially one with fever, such as scarlet fever. It can result from decreased activity of the pituitary or thyroid gland, early stages of syphilis, pregnancy, use of birth control pills and certain other medications, "crash" dieting or malnutrition, or a diet containing too much vitamin A. When the cause is removed, the missing hair usually returns.

Spotty baldness

Spotty baldness, or alopecia areata, may affect areas of the head and beard. The cause is unknown. It often clears up after a few months if there are just a few spots and if it first occurs in adulthood; it may recur, however. The outlook is less favorable if it begins in childhood or if hair loss is widespread. Occasionally, all body hair is lost. If there is no apparent cause, such as fever or severe illness, the hair is not likely to return.

Permanent baldness

Permanent baldness occurs when the scalp is scarred as a result of burns, other injury, or disease. Conditions that can cause scarring baldness include severe bacterial and fungal infections, tuberculosis, ulcers, lupus erythematosus, and certain slow-growing tumors.

Treatment

There is no totally satisfactory medical treatment at this time to cure or prevent baldness. However, hair transplants can be effective. Scalp plugs containing active hair follicles are taken from the back of the head, which is not affected by male-pattern baldness. The transplanted follicles continue to produce hair just as before, despite the new location.

A topical form of the antihypertensive drug minoxidil has recently been released for use in treating baldness. This preparation has been shown to stimulate hair growth in some individuals; however, it must be applied on a continuous basis and is available only by prescription.

Boils

A boil, or furuncle, is caused by a bacterial infection and irritation of the skin and its underlying structures. It is a painful swelling in the skin that is easily detected by touch. When a group of boils interconnects below the surface of the skin, a carbuncle forms.

Causes

Boils develop when *Staphylococcus* bacteria enter the skin through a hair follicle and multiply in its warm, moist environment. Bacteria continue to grow while producing substances that invade surrounding cells. White blood cells (which attack and kill invading organisms) travel to the infected hair follicle and enclose bacteria. As more white blood cells gather, they eventually consume the bacteria and eliminate the infection. This buildup by the white blood cells is what produces the pustule in the center of the boil. When the pustule ruptures, pus and dead skin cells killed by the bacteria drain out, and the boil heals.

Staphylococcus bacteria are often found in the nose and throat, where washing cannot reach them. They can spread to a hair follicle from there or from another site on the body. They can also be transmitted by contact with an infected person or by contact with an infected article, such as a washcloth or towel. In most cases, however, other persons who come in contact with the bacteria do not get boils.

Those at risk

Persons who are run-down or who suffer diseases such as anemia (deficiency of red blood cells), diabetes, or infections that weaken their natural defenses against bacteria seem to be more susceptible to developing boils. Those who work with greasy or oily substances are also more likely to develop boils because these materials tend to trap bacteria against the skin. Poor bathing habits, especially in the summer months, when sweaty skin provides the moist climate conducive to bacterial growth, also invite infection.

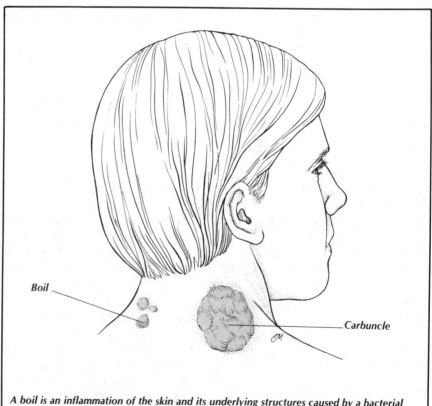

A boil is an inflammation of the skin and its underlying structures caused by a bacterial infection. When a group of boils interconnects below the surface of the skin, a carbuncle forms.

Boil

Carbuncle

Symptoms

Boils can develop anywhere on the skin. They appear most frequently on the neck, face, and back, and they can erupt in several places at once. Although boils vary in size, they characteristically form white or yellow pustules. As the infection progresses, the pustule becomes red and hot. Excess fluid in the boil produces pressure on the nerves underneath, which can result in considerable pain. When boils contain little pus, they are called blind boils; the inflammation recedes slowly without rupturing, but sometimes it leaves a scar.

If boils are large or extensive, the person may also experience fever and a general feeling of weakness. Sometimes, the infection gets into the bloodstream and spreads throughout the body. The same bacteria that cause the boil may also produce a toxin (poison) that causes blood clots, usually in the blood vessels around the boil.

Treatment

Any treatment plan for boils and carbuncles emphasizes that they should *never* be squeezed, particularly if they are on the face. Squeezing may force the infection deeper into the skin and possibly into the bloodstream. Only a physician should lance a boil to encourage drainage. Afterward, the doctor may prescribe an oral antibiotic, such as penicillin or erythromycin, to fight further infection.

Many boils will rupture and heal on their own. However, holding a soft cloth soaked with warm water against the boil for 15 to 20 minutes at least four times a day will speed the process. These warm compresses increase blood flow to the area and encourage pustule formation. Since bacteria from the boil are contagious, the cloth should be disinfected in boiling water or in the hot cycle of a washing machine.

When a boil bursts, the infected area should be washed thoroughly and covered with an antibiotic cream and sterile gauze. If the boil does not heal within a few days, or if the boil is located on or near the face, a physician should be consulted.

Prevention

To prevent new eruptions, the skin needs to be kept cool and dry. Sometimes, physicians advise washing the entire body with an antiseptic soap twice a day. If boils frequently recur, underclothing and bed linen should be changed daily.

Calluses

Calluses are thickened areas of the skin. They develop most often on the balls and heels of the feet and on the hands.

Causes

Skin buildup is the result of excessive friction or pressure against the surface of the skin. As pressure mounts, dead skin cells accumulate, and the skin thickens. Wearing shoes that fit improperly or holding pencils too tightly can create the problem. Since calluses often follow blisters on the same site, they are considered to be the body's way of shielding the area against further injury.

Flat-footed persons have a greater incidence of calluses. Because of the abnormal shape of the foot, the small bones in the front portion of the foot are forced downward against the skin of the sole with great pressure during walking, creating pressure points. Those who wear high heels promote growth of calluses by increasing pressure on the balls of their feet.

Symptoms

Calluses vary in size and shape depending on where they grow and how much skin is affected. Sometimes, calluses grow so thick and irregular in shape that the skin becomes inflexible and cracks.

When pressure is relieved, calluses usually produce no pain. However, continued irritation, especially involving areas where the skin is split, can cause enough discomfort to interfere with physical activities.

Treatment

Immediate treatment involves removal of the pressure that caused the callus in the first place. Extremely persistent or painful calluses should be examined by a doctor. In rare instances, surgery may be necessary to alleviate intense pressure. In milder cases, calluses can often be eased by padding the exposed area to reduce further friction.

There are over-the-counter remedies that soften the callused tissue, making it easier to remove. Salicylic acid plasters, which are sold in medicated sheets, can be placed over the callus after bathing and secured with tape. The pad should be removed just before the next bath so that the softened skin can be gently removed with a pumice stone or a special implement with a rough surface designed for that purpose.

Home remedies should not be used by persons who have diabetes, atherosclerosis, or other disorders affecting circulation because their risk of infection is greater. They should consult their doctor before attempting any form of treatment.

Canker sores

Canker sores (medically known as aphthous ulcers) are inflamed tissue cavities, usually found in the mouth. They can be quite painful, often inhibiting eating ability. Even though up to one out of every four persons develops canker sores, they are not contagious.

Causes

Researchers disagree about the cause of canker sores. One unconfirmed theory suggests that the sores are the result of an autoimmune response, whereby the body develops antibodies to its own tissue. Other factors that have been said to trigger canker sores include fever, menstruation, fatigue, tension, and allergies. Some people get canker sores after eating certain foods. Poor dental hygiene, ill-fitting dentures, and injuries from stiff toothbrushes may also lead to the condition. All of the above may be contributing factors; however, the true cause of canker sores is unknown.

Symptoms

Canker sores may occur singly or in groups. They can be found

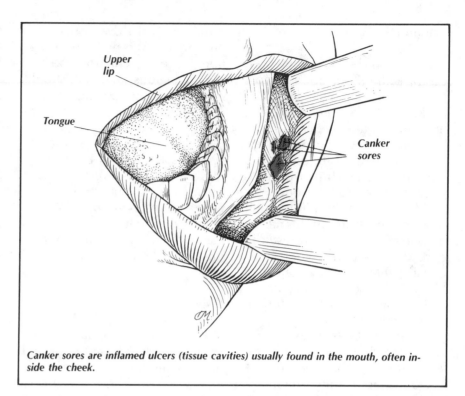

Canker sores are inflamed ulcers (tissue cavities) usually found in the mouth, often inside the cheek.

almost anywhere in the mouth—inside the cheek and on the tongue, lips, or gums.

A canker sore begins as a small blister. After the blister breaks, a small ulcer develops and enlarges until there is a bright red sore surrounding the whitish-yellow cavity. This sore can last about 10 to 14 days before healing. Canker sores leave no scars. However, they often recur, sometimes every few weeks or months.

Treatment

Canker sores have no cure, but there are several treatments that may relieve pain. Some physicians prescribe the antibiotic tetracycline for canker sores. Treatment involves dissolving the capsule in an ounce of warm water and swishing the mixture in the mouth for five to ten minutes, three or four times a day for five to seven days. Sometimes,

therapy includes soaking a cotton wad in the solution and applying it directly to the sores.

There are also various over-the-counter preparations designed to reduce discomfort. However, they are of uncertain value, and you should always check with your doctor before using them.

Prevention

Persons who have repeated attacks of canker sores should see a physician or dentist. Recurrence may be lessened by improving oral hygiene or by avoiding certain foods or other substances.

Corns

Corns are small, round mounds of firm, dead skin that form on or between the toes. Their hard, waxy core, which bore down into the skin and press on the underlying tissue and nerves, can cause extreme pain. Corns sometimes are associated with bursae (fluid-filled sacs that cushion the juncture of two or more bones), which can become irritated, resulting in bursitis.

Causes

Corns are caused by a great deal of pressure or friction on the toes (as are calluses, their basis), usually from ill-fitting shoes or high heels. Since the skin acts as the body's protector from the outside environment, corns form when the body attempts to protect the troubled area from more pressure by building up a mass of dead skin cells and secreting a hard substance called keratin. Persons who have abnormal bone structure in their feet or certain types of arthritis tend to develop corns. Generally, however, those who avoid wearing high-heeled or tight-fitting shoes should be able to avoid corns.

Symptoms

Corns are usually regular in shape, and can be white, gray, or yellow. They most often form on the outside of the first or fifth toes, since that is where pressure most often occurs. Corns that form between the toes are called soft corns; they are not as firm as other corns because of the moistness between the toes.

Treatment

Corns are best treated by first eliminating the cause of the pressure. Over-the-counter preparations are available. These include padding to reduce the

A corn is a small mound of dead skin that forms on or between the toes. Its core, formed in the epidermis, bores down into underlying tissue and nerves in the dermis, causing pain.

friction on the area, ointments, and medicated pads, which will soften and blister the skin layers, making them easier to remove and reducing the pain. Severe or persistent corns must be treated by a doctor, but only rarely do they necessitate surgery. Persons with diabetes, atherosclerosis, or other circulatory diseases should *never* treat a corn themselves, as the risk of infection is much greater for them.

Cyst

A cyst is an abnormal sac or membrane containing a fluid or semisolid material.

Cysts may develop virtually anywhere in the body. They may form around a foreign body, such as a particle in the lung or beneath the skin, or around a parasite. They may entrap an escaping body liquid, such as blood hemorrhaging into tissue or fluid leaking from a bursa (a fluid-filled sac that cushions the juncture of two or more bones).

Types and treatment

Perhaps the most common cysts are those of the skin and mucous membranes.

A *sebaceous cyst* occurs when a sebaceous gland (the tiny oil gland at the base of each hair root) becomes plugged. Ordinarily, this plugging results in a blackhead or, if the blackhead becomes infected, a pus-filled pimple. Occasionally, however, the pimple does not break, and the swelling becomes entrapped beneath the surface of the skin. Sebum (oil from the sebaceous gland) continues to flow into the sac that forms in the cavity, and the cyst grows to the size of a marble or larger. Sebaceous cysts—which can occur in any part of the body where there is hair, including the neck, scalp, and back—can easily be removed surgically if bothersome; if they become infected, they must be drained and removed. A type of tiny cyst known as *milium,* which usually occurs on the face and scrotum, can simply be opened and drained. Larger cysts must be removed completely, or they will recur.

Mucous cysts that occur in the mouth, on the tongue, or on the lower lip are caused by plugged mucous glands and may grow to the size of a pea or larger. They may be removed in the same manner as sebaceous cysts.

Traumatic epithelial cysts usually result from the trapping of a piece of skin, a blood clot, or foreign material beneath the skin because of some injury. In some cases, they may not need to be removed.

Dermatitis

Dermatitis is an inflammation of the skin. There are many different kinds of dermatitis and a great variety of causes.

Chronic dermatitis

This often occurs on the hands or feet, and may simply be the result of continued irritation, especially by contact dermatitis. It is marked by thickened skin, inflammation, and scaling. It is sometimes caused by excessive hand washing or by accumulation of soaps or detergents under rings. Occasionally, a fungal infection is the cause.

Contact dermatitis

This is a skin inflammation caused by a substance that has touched the skin. This may be a harsh chemical or a detergent or soap that irritates directly, or it may be a substance that produces an allergic reaction that does not appear until five or six days after the contact. Less commonly, the reaction appears only after years of repeated use. Common causes of allergic contact dermatitis are poison ivy, chemicals in shoes and clothing, metal watchbands and rings, antibiotic salves, and cosmetics. There are also cases in which a substance, such as a shaving lotion or cosmetic, produces a "photoallergic" reaction—that is, a rash develops when the skin under the substance is exposed to sunlight.

Eczema

This inflammation of the skin is marked by small blisters (when severe), redness, fluid in the tissue, oozing, scales, crusts or scabs, burning or itching, and sometimes dryness. The skin of flexor surfaces (those subject to bending movements, such as the back of the knee and the top of the elbow) is most commonly affected. There are several different forms of eczema. One of the more common types is atopic dermatitis, which is an itching skin inflammation due to an allergy. Susceptible persons often have a family history of allergic diseases, such as asthma or hay fever. Typically, it begins in infancy, subsides by age three, and may reappear by age 10 or 12. Certain foods (such as wheat, milk, and eggs) and other substances (such as pollen and fur) often bring on symptoms; if so, they must be avoided.

Exfoliative dermatitis

This condition produces shedding of skin all over the body, together with hair loss. The entire skin surface is red, scaly, and thickened. The cause is unknown in most cases, but it sometimes occurs following a less severe case of dermatitis or as a side effect of a drug. Hospitalization is frequently necessary because the condition can be life threatening. A first step is to consult a doctor about any medications and to ask about stopping or changing them.

Localized neurodermatitis

This condition is characterized by thick, sharp-bordered, scaly breaks in the skin, occasionally with little blisters. This condition is caused by habitual scratching of an insect bite or other real or imagined irritation of the skin and is corrected by covering the area and stopping the scratching. In the case of an itch in the area around the openings of the vagina and colon, however, warts, pinworms, hemorrhoids, infections, or certain diseases may be the cause.

Nummular dermatitis

Coin-shaped patches of blisters that later ooze and crust over mark this condition, which usually is accompanied by dry skin and itching. Most often, it appears on the legs and sometimes the buttocks and trunk of middle-aged persons.

Seborrheic dermatitis

This is a scaling and inflammation of the scalp and sometimes the face and other parts of the body. This is the cause of dandruff in adults and cradle cap in infants.

Stasis dermatitis

This stubborn skin inflammation of the lower legs is usually the result of poor blood return from the area. There is redness, mild scaling, and brown discoloration of the skin. If the condition is neglected, the skin swells and may become infected, or ulcers (eroded skin sores) may develop.

Treatment

Because there is such a bewildering variety of skin diseases and because some can be dangerous if neglected, it is important to seek medical care for any dermatitis. In general, this care usually begins with very simple measures. Dry skin needs lubricating agents, while moist or oily skin may require powders or other drying substances. Inflamed skin is commonly treated with cortisone-type creams; cool, wet dressings; or baths.

Hardened, dried skin may be peeled off with strong substances available only by prescription. If possible, the cause of the dermatitis is sought (with the patient's help) and eliminated. Cortisone creams are often used to make the patient more comfortable by reducing inflammation, although continuous use is not usually recommended. Antibiotics are employed promptly to eliminate any infections before they can spread to other parts of the body. Patients must resist the constant temptation to scratch itchy areas or remove scabs, because that will simply prolong and even worsen the problem. In addition, while cleanliness is desirable, some patients need to be told to reduce hand washing and the number of baths they take, because they may be washing away natural oils that protect the skin. Along the same lines, patients should not use any medication that has not been recom-

mended by a doctor or use it more frequently than directed. Overmedication of skin diseases may be worse than undermedication in some cases.

Fever blisters

Fever blisters, also called cold sores, are fluid-filled blisters that appear on the border of the lips and on or around the nose. They are the result of a very contagious virus that affects most of the population at some time.

Causes

Fever blisters are caused by a type of herpes simplex virus. It enters the body most often through the mouth or nose areas, where the skin is easier to penetrate.

At first, characteristic blisters may not result. Antibodies (protective substances) in the body defend against the invading virus. The inactivated virus withdraws to a nearby nerve, where it remains until stress to the body or a diminished capacity to fight off infection triggers a recurrence. When the virus is reactivated, it overruns the body's protective system and progresses back along the nerve to the general area of original infection. Factors that seem to favor the appearance of blisters include fever, colds, menstruation, skin injury from dental work, excessive sun and wind exposure, and emotional stress. Cold sores can return every few weeks for several weeks or not at all.

Symptoms

Initially, the virus may present no symptoms, so some people

are unaware of infection. For others, the infection begins with numbness or tenderness in the affected area. Then small, fluid-filled blisters appear. These blisters break, encrust, and heal within one to two weeks.

Complications

Occasionally, excessive pain or swelling of lymph nodes develops. These symptoms may indicate a secondary bacterial infection that needs a doctor's attention.

Other complications can be more serious. Herpes simplex keratitis is a painful viral infection of the cornea that can result in blindness if not treated. When inflammation of the eyes accompanies fever blisters, a physician should be consulted immediately. Steroid (cortisone-type) medications should not be used near the eyes during a herpes attack without consulting a doctor, since these preparations can encourage spread of the virus to the eye.

Other serious complications can occur in infants and extremely ill patients who contract herpes virus if the infection travels to the lungs, brain, or other internal organs.

Treatment

Treatment involves relieving symptoms, since there is no known cure for fever blisters. Some over-the-counter remedies may relieve pain and help dry blisters. Topical corticosteroid creams, however, should not be applied unless prescribed by a physician; the possibility of spreading infection increases because the corticosteroid can depress the immune response.

Healing time may be shortened by certain newer prescription drugs, such as acyclovir, but these drugs should not be used for routine fever blisters.

Frostbite

Frostbite is damage to skin tissue resulting from exposure to low environmental temperatures. The condition can affect any part of the body, but the areas most often involved (such as the face, hands, and feet) are those with the poorest blood circulation and the greatest exposure to cold.

If the person must remain outdoors for a time, the frostbitten area should be wrapped in a warm, dry blanket.

Causes

When exposed to cold, the body tries to protect vital organs. Blood vessels near the surface of the skin constrict to preserve internal body heat. This tightening causes blood to be diverted from the outside of the body, reducing the supply of blood to skin tissues. As a result, skin tissue freezes from the lack of a warm blood supply and dies. Frequently, frostbite develops after prolonged exposure to cold. Extremely low temperatures or forceful winds can also cause the condition. Wearing insufficient or improper clothing increases susceptibility to frostbite. Skin can freeze to the surface of a metal object and block circulation to the area. In addition, any health problem that weakens the body or reduces circulation increases the likelihood of frostbite.

Stages of frostbite

Frostbite develops in three stages, and each stage can produce varying degrees of pain.

First-degree frostbite appears as whiteness or slight yellowness of the skin along with burning or itching sensations. In this stage, symptoms can be reversed if the area is gradually rewarmed.

Should exposure continue, sensation in the area ceases. Disappearance of pain and reddening and swelling of the tissue signals second-degree frostbite. At this stage, warming the area may produce blisters and skin peeling. The blisters may persist for weeks; tenderness may linger for months.

Skin with third-degree frostbite becomes waxy and hard. At this stage, skin tissue dies and edema (excess fluid retention in the tissues) may occur. Severe frostbite can damage muscles, tendons, and nerves. Blood clots may form in small blood vessels and inhibit or block circulation, which can lead to gangrene.

Treatment

Initial treatment focuses on what *not* to do, since there are many misconceptions about the proper course of action. Frostbitten tissue should not be rubbed with snow. In fact, the affected part should not be rubbed at all, because further damage to tissue can result. Exercising the frostbitten area will aggravate the condition.

To reduce tissue loss and avoid complications, frostbitten tissue should be immersed in lukewarm water rather than exposed to the extreme heat of a radiator, stove, or fire. Ideally, water temperature should be between 100°F and 110°F. Any temperature above 110°F can burn skin that lacks sensation, and thawing that is too rapid may produce pain, redness, and blisters. Gently patting (but not rubbing) the skin dry helps prevent additional injury.

If the patient remains outdoors, affected areas can be warmed by placing them in contact with warm portions of the body, such as under the armpits or between the thighs. The area can also be wrapped in a warm, dry blanket. Frozen areas should be kept clean to prevent infection. Warm, nonalcoholic drinks aid circulation. Smoking should be avoided because it causes constriction of blood vessels.

Once frozen tissue has been rewarmed, the affected area should be elevated to promote increased blood circulation and maintain the skin at room temperature. All cases of frostbite should be examined by a physician, who may prescribe medication to prevent infection or formation of clots in blood vessels.

Prevention

The best prevention is to wear adequate clothing to protect the skin. Feet, hands, and parts of the face need covering since these areas are likely to have the poorest blood circulation and are the most exposed. When weather is unusually cold or windy, remaining indoors or keeping outside trips short is recommended.

Head lice

Infestation with head lice (or pediculosis capitis, as it is known medically) has become a relatively common occurrence among school-age children; however, persons in all age groups are susceptible. Sometimes erroneously thought to be an indication of an unsanitary lifestyle, lice infestation can actually afflict anyone, without regard for distinctions of social status or personal hygiene.

Cause

Head lice are tiny parasites, less than one-eighth inch long. They are grayish-white, almost transparent, six-legged creatures that live exclusively on humans. Lice can be passed easily from one person to another (for example, by using the comb or wearing the hat of an infested person). Head lice live on or close to the scalp, where they bite and suck blood. Their eggs, which are called nits, are milk-white and about the size of a flake of dandruff.

Symptoms

Head lice cause itching of the scalp and sometimes a red, scaly rash on the back of the neck at the hairline. Scratching may cause sores on the scalp. The lymph nodes at the base of the skull may be enlarged.

Diagnosis

Unless hundreds are present, it is difficult to see lice in the hair. However, the nits attached to the shafts of the hairs are usually clearly visible. Although nits are about the same color and size as flakes of dandruff, they can be easily distinguished from dandruff: flakes of dandruff can be blown or brushed away; nits can be removed with the fingernails only with difficulty.

Treatment

Both prescription and nonprescription medicated shampoos (called pediculicides) are used to combat lice infestations. It is important to remember that these substances can be poisonous if swallowed or absorbed through the skin or if they come in contact with the eyes. Care must be taken to use them exactly as directed and neither more nor less

often than recommended, especially in pregnant women and young children. Sometimes a vinegar rinse is recommended to loosen the nits after using the special shampoo. The nits can then be removed with a fine-tooth comb.

If infected sores on the scalp or enlarged lymph nodes at the base of the skull accompany a lice infestation, this must be called to the attention of a physician.

Prevention

The best preventive measure is to avoid sharing combs, brushes, towels, and hats with others.

If one member of the family has head lice, it is usually necessary to treat the rest of the family as well (a physician may have special recommendations for infants and pregnant women). Lice cannot be transmitted by pets, however. Combs and hairbrushes should be discarded or thoroughly cleaned in boiling water. Pillowcases, hats, and clothing that may have been in contact with an infested person should be cleaned by washing in very hot water.

Heat rash

Heat rash, or prickly heat, is a mild skin condition that produces an itchy, burning sensation. Heat rash is found most often in infants and in overweight persons who have overlapping folds of fat.

Causes

The sweat glands in the skin normally work along with blood vessels to regulate the body's

Sweat gland duct

Skin surface

Sweat gland

Normal

Heat rash

A sweat gland normally releases sweat through its duct onto the skin surface. When perspiration cannot reach the surface, the sweat may break through the duct wall and become trapped beneath the skin, causing inflammation and a rash.

heat. When the blood temperature rises, the brain triggers a reflex in the sweat glands to encourage secretion of sweat. Sweating reduces body temperature by releasing sweat to the surface of the skin, where it evaporates and cools the skin. However, when skin surfaces press together, the sweat ducts, which carry secretions from the sweat glands to the skin's surface, become temporarily blocked. If sweat cannot reach the skin's surface, it may break through the duct wall and remain trapped in an inner layer of the skin, where it can cause inflammation and a rash.

Heat rash can result any time the body is unable to perspire adequately. Most often, hot weather or exertion triggers it. Wearing tight clothing or overdressing, even in cold weather, may compound the problem.

Heat rash in infants occurs primarily because their sweat glands cannot transport large amounts of perspiration to the surface of the skin. The sweat remains trapped within the skin, which causes the characteristic inflammation and irritation.

Symptoms

Usually, heat rash (known medically as miliaria) appears on moist parts of the body where skin surfaces can touch, such as on the neck, under the arms, and between the legs. An infant can have the rash under a tight-fitting diaper. The rash looks like tiny, pinhead-sized red pimples, and it can cause itching and a prickling or burning sensation.

Heat rash is sometimes confused with a condition called chafing because the symptoms are similar. However, chafing is caused by friction between two skin surfaces rubbing together and not by obstructed sweat ducts. Under extreme conditions, the warm, moist areas where heat rash develops can become breeding grounds for microorganisms that cause secondary infection.

Treatment and prevention

Treatment and prevention of heat rash involve reducing or eliminating the stimulus for sweating. The affected person needs to stay in a cool environment and refrain from exertion. Cool showers followed by thorough drying can also help, as can wearing light, loose-fitting clothes. Once sweating stops, the rash may disappear in a few hours.

Babies who suffer from heat rash should be bathed in clear water and dried thoroughly. Cloth diapers are more likely to allow the natural evaporation process to occur than are disposable diapers. If discomfort becomes prolonged or extreme, a doctor should be consulted in order to rule out the possibility that some other disorder is causing the symptoms.

Leukoplakia

Leukoplakia is a tough, fibrous lesion that occurs on a mucous membrane. When it occurs in the mouth, it is often referred to as a smoker's patch or smoker's tongue. Although these oral lesions are generally not painful, they may cause difficulty and discomfort when the person talks or swallows.

Causes

The oral condition may be caused by badly fitted dentures, excessive smoking, overconsumption of alcohol, or a diet of highly spiced foods. Leukoplakia may also be a symptom of syphilis and may develop into a cancerous growth.

Symptoms

Leukoplakia most often appears in the form of a white patch on the lips, tongue, or gums or in other areas that are lined by mucous membranes, such as the female genitals.

Diagnosis

If a person notices these persistent white patches, a physician should be seen immediately. A biopsy specimen (a small sample of tissue) is often obtained because the presence of cancer cannot be determined by merely looking at the lesion.

Treatment

One should never attempt to self-treat leukoplakia. After a physician has examined the lesion, he or she may advise having dentures refitted or cutting down on smoking and the consumption of alcohol and excessive amounts of spicy foods. These patches should be examined by a physician frequently, since cancer may develop in the future. In most cases, however, the physician will probably advise that the lesion be entirely removed surgically.

Mole

A mole is a cluster of cells, usually pigmented (colored), that appears on the skin. Moles are sometimes present at birth, but more often they appear during childhood, adolescence, or pregnancy. Although moles, which are commonplace, can become cancerous, they seldom do.

Symptoms

Moles vary in size, shape, and color. They may be large or small, flat or raised, smooth or warty. They may be the same color as the skin, or their color may vary from yellow-brown to black. Some moles have one or more hairs in them.

The most common type of mole is the intradermal nevus, which forms in the lower layer of skin. It is a raised cluster of cells that ranges in color from skin-tone to black. Other types of moles include the lentigo nevus (a flat, uniformly pigmented brown or black spot), the junctional nevus (a flat or slightly raised blemish that ranges in color from light brown to nearly black), the compound nevus (a raised mole that is usually dark in color), and the halo nevus (a pigmented mole in the middle of a ring of skin from which the pigment has been lost).

Treatment

Moles are often removed for cosmetic reasons. However, any mole that enlarges suddenly, becomes darker, begins to bleed, or changes in any other unexplained way should be removed by a physician and examined microscopically.

Onychogryphosis

Onychogryphosis (or onychogryposis) is unusual growth of the fingernails or toenails, to the extent that they begin to resemble claws or horns.

Causes

Injuries due to going barefoot or wearing tight shoes are the usual cause of onychogryphosis, but the condition can be hereditary. It may also be related to congestive heart failure, in which there may be a shortage of blood circulation to the feet; peripheral neuritis, which affects nerves in the legs, causing decreased sensation in the feet and thereby increasing the chance that the foot will be injured; dry, scaly skin; hormonal disorders; syphilis; and stroke.

Symptoms

The nail becomes thick, long, raised, and green or black in color with an opaque surface. This condition occurs most often in toenails, especially on the big toes.

Treatment

Properly fitting shoes, hot baths, massage with warm oil or hydrogen peroxide, or treatment of underlying disease may clear up the condition. Trimming or removal of an abnormal nail should be done only by a physician or podiatrist; serious complications can arise if this is done improperly.

Onychomycosis

The most common of inflammatory nail disorders, onychomycosis is a fungal infection of the nails that is prevalent among persons with a low resistance to infection (diabetics and patients taking corticosteroid or other hormonal drugs), those who work with their hands in water and are prone to paronychia (inflammation of the skin around the nail), and those with ingrown toenails. Onychomycosis is caused by a number of fungi and is often associated with paronychia.

Symptoms

The condition is chronic but painless. The affected nails look dull, opaque, and brittle; are marked with grooves or ridges; and appear flaky. The surrounding cuticle may become red, tender, and swollen and may ooze pus if a bacterial infection ac-

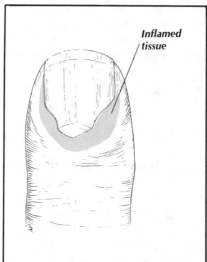

Paronychia (inflammation of the skin around the nail) often sets the stage for onychomycosis, a fungal infection of the nail.

companies the disorder. The fungi can be identified by examining nail scrapings in the laboratory.

Treatment

The condition is sometimes treated with griseofulvin, an antifungal medication that can either be taken orally or applied topically. However, the condition may take months to cure. Furthermore, the condition may never clear up at all, especially if the toenails are affected. Cutting the nails short or having the entire nail removed by a physician can help the healing process.

Prevention

In order to prevent onychomycosis, fingernails and toenails should always be dried thoroughly after bathing, showering, or swimming, because fungi thrive in a moist environment. Footwear should be changed often if the feet tend to perspire.

Photosensitivity

Photosensitivity is an abnormally increased sensitivity of the skin to the rays of the sun.

Causes

The causes of this condition are not fully understood, although it is known that certain substances, when combined with ultraviolet light, produce the reaction. Among those substances are contraceptive pills, hexachlorophene (a skin antiseptic), sandalwood oil, coal tar, certain perfumes and soaps, certain sunscreen agents, and a variety of orally administered drugs, including chlorothiazides, phenothiazines, sulfonamides, and tetracyclines.

Symptoms

The symptoms of photosensitivity include burning reactions similar to those ordinarily suffered after prolonged exposure to the sun, rashes, scaling, welts (raised areas) on the skin, dizziness, nausea, and vomiting. The most common symptom is a rash.

Treatment

The most effective treatment is to discover the basic cause of the heightened sensitivity and to eliminate it. If, for example, photosensitivity is a reaction to a contraceptive pill, a different kind of pill or form of contraception could be prescribed. Treatment of photosensitivity symptoms is similar to that used for sunburn: ointments, topical anesthetics, and creams. It should be remembered that these treatments are standard topical therapy for the skin but do not eliminate the underlying causes of photosensitivity.

If it is impossible to isolate the cause of photosensitivity, the next best step is to avoid exposure to sunlight by wearing light-colored clothing, white gloves, and broad-brimmed hats. Commercial sunscreen products are also helpful. Contact with the substances already listed should be avoided.

Psoriasis

Psoriasis is a persistent skin disease characterized by thick, red eruptions, often covered by silvery scales, either in small patches or over large areas of the body. Psoriasis is fairly common, affecting one to two percent of the population. The condition often first appears between the ages of 15 and 30 years and usually requires lifelong treatment.

Cause

Psoriasis is not contagious. The cause of psoriasis is unknown, but researchers believe that the condition is related to a malfunction in the process of skin growth and regeneration (cell replacement). With normal skin, old cells are continuously being shed from the epidermis and replaced by new cells formed in the deeper layers. Cells live for about one month before they die and flake off. With psoriasis, the rate of cell growth accelerates. Skin cells may move to the surface and die in as short a time as four or five days. Increased cell growth causes buildup that can be extremely dry and irritating. The normal shedding process is usu-

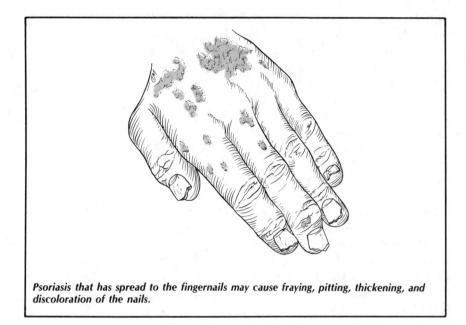

Psoriasis that has spread to the fingernails may cause fraying, pitting, thickening, and discoloration of the nails.

ally unnoticeable, but psoriasis can produce very obvious blemishes.

Psoriasis seems to involve a strong hereditary factor, although only one third of its victims can recall having a relative with the disease. There also seems to be some relationship between the condition and a type of arthritis.

Once psoriasis develops, outbreaks of the disorder can be triggered in several ways. Injury to the skin, such as a cut or burn, may provoke a flare-up, usually 8 to 18 days after the trauma. Seasonal changes may also affect psoriasis, with the disease worsening during winter months. Many patients have greater problems during periods of physical and emotional stress. Infections, particularly upper respiratory tract infections, may aggravate psoriasis.

Symptoms

Psoriasis is characterized by reddened, raised patches of skin with silvery scales called plaques. These clearly defined

plaques appear most commonly on the elbows, knees, trunk, and scalp, although the underarm and genital areas may also be involved. Patches on the scalp shed large, silver-white scales at the hairline that resemble severe dandruff. Those patches found in moist areas, such as the underarms, are usually less scaly and less red. All patches may itch. If fingernails are involved, they may be pitted, frayed, thickened, or discolored; in more advanced cases, the nails may be separated from the nail beds.

Usually, psoriasis produces no general health problems. Sometimes, however, the disease becomes so severe that chills, painful reddening of the skin, cracking of the skin around the joints, and shedding of large areas of scaled skin result. This condition, called exfoliative psoriasis, may necessitate hospitalization for intensive therapy.

Treatment

As yet, there is no known cure for psoriasis, and treatment offers only temporary relief from symptoms. Normal cleaning of the skin around the affected areas is important to prevent infection. Over-the-counter lotions and creams can cleanse irritated skin and reduce itching as well. These preparations often contain small amounts of coal tar and other ingredients designed to remove scales. If the skin becomes sensitive after application, use of these preparations should be discontinued. Many patients find regular and controlled exposure to sunlight helpful. Where sunlight is scarce, a special sunlamp may be used, but only under a doctor's supervision.

Various drugs have recently been shown to be effective in relieving the symptoms of psoriasis. Cortisone and newer steroids (hormonally based medications) can clear plaques in about 50 percent of the cases when applied directly to the affected skin. Many physicians recommend covering the treated areas with a thin plastic wrapping in addition to the cream. This is called occlusive therapy.

Some drugs slow the growth rate of cells. The most commonly used of these drugs, methotrexate, reduces symptoms in severe cases. Because its side effects may be severe, the drug is prescribed for use only under close medical supervision.

Another form of treatment is called PUVA therapy, which combines medication and ultraviolet light treatments. The benefits of this form of therapy should be carefully weighed against the premature skin aging and skin cancer that it may cause.

Purpura

The term purpura refers to a group of bleeding disorders that

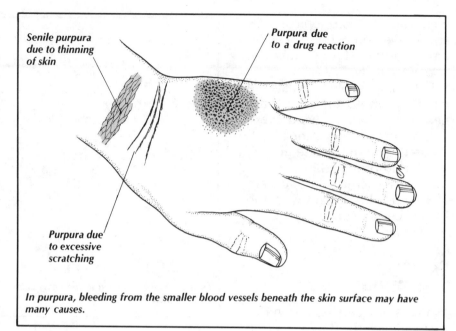

In purpura, bleeding from the smaller blood vessels beneath the skin surface may have many causes.

are all characterized by purplish or brownish-red discolorations, easily visible through the skin's outer layer, that are caused by hemorrhaging (internal bleeding) into the tissues.

Common purpura

Common purpura (also called simple purpura or senile purpura) is the most widespread of such disorders and is marked by easy bruising and increased blood vessel fragility. It is an inherited condition that occurs mostly in women, particularly following menopause. The condition often affects thigh tissue and produces large bruises rather than hemorrhages. The bleeding is usually under the skin and may be intensified by surgery or injury.

Henoch-Schönlein purpura

Henoch-Schonlein purpura (also known as allergic purpura and anaphylactoid purpura) most

often affects children. The condition may be associated with arthritis, gastrointestinal disorders, kidney failure, and erythema (redness of the skin).

Purpura fulminans

Purpura fulminans is most often seen in children, mainly after an infectious disease. It is marked by fever, shock (collapse of the circulatory system), anemia, and rapidly spreading symmetrical skin hemorrhages in the lower limbs, as well as by intravascular thrombosis (blockage of a blood vessel by a solid mass) and gangrene.

Thrombocytopenic purpura

Thrombocytopenic purpura is a disorder in which the number of platelets (the tiny elements in the blood that are vital to clotting) is decreased, whether because of a primary disease or as a consequence of another blood disorder. This form of purpura is characterized by anemia, side effects in the nervous system, and blood clots in tiny blood vessels.

Causes

Causes vary with the type of purpura. Common purpura in postmenopausal women appears to result from decreased estrogen (female hormone) levels and thinning of the deep layers of the skin. Henoch-Schönlein purpura may result from the development of sensitivities following an infection or allergic reaction. Purpura in the elderly is often due to the fragility of their skin. There are also temporary forms of purpura in which vascular bleeding occurs as a result of fever, hypothyroidism, generalized illness, defects in the small blood vessels, or a drug reaction to certain medications, such as aspirin. Purpura can sometimes stem from wearing overly tight clothing or from sustaining an injury, such as a black eye.

Diagnosis

Laboratory testing is essential in all cases of possible purpura in order to exclude other causes. Perhaps the most difficult of the forms of purpura to diagnose is Henoch-Schönlein purpura. Joint pain and bouts of abdominal pain in this disorder may mimic acute abdominal conditions or forms of arthritis. Later, kidney involvement during the course of this form of purpura may cause a misdiagnosis of kidney disease.

Treatment

In the case of allergic purpura, it is advisable to eliminate the possible allergic cause. Corticosteroid medications (artificial hormones) are often prescribed, but may produce disappointing results. Immunosuppressive therapy (suppression of the immune system by means of drugs) is sometimes useful. If the purpura is thrombocytopenic, the spleen (an abdominal organ that is a component of the circulatory system) may be removed if it is hoarding too many platelets. Milder cases of purpura often improve spontaneously.

Prevention

Estrogen therapy has proved helpful in preventing or relieving common purpura in postmenopausal women. Other than preventive measures to avoid infections or allergic reactions, there is little that can be done to prevent purpura.

Ringworm

Ringworm is a skin infection caused by a fungus, not a worm. The name originated because the infection is often characterized by round patches that enlarge as healing proceeds from the center, leaving red rings that persist on the skin for a few months.

Types

There are several different types of ringworm, each caused by a different type of fungus. Ringworm of the scalp, or *tinea capitis,* appears as scaly patches with stubs of broken-off hairs or as bald areas. Ringworm of the body, or *tinea corporis,* appears as round or oval, scaly, red patches on the torso. Ringworm of the groin, or *tinea cruris* (pop-ularly referred to as "jock itch"), is characterized by a scaly, red or brown rash in the crotch and genital area. Ringworm of the feet, or *tinea pedis,* is more commonly called athlete's foot (see pages 110-111).

Cause

Ringworm spreads by direct contact with an infected person or pet or by contact with contaminated objects, such as combs, pillows, towels, and clothing. Tight-fitting clothing, obesity, and heavy perspiration may be contributing factors in the development of ringworm of the body and the groin.

Diagnosis

Ringworm infections are generally unsightly rather than threatening to health. However, several other skin infections resemble ringworm, so a physician must make the diagnosis. The doctor may want to examine the rash under ultraviolet light and obtain a skin scraping to be examined microscopically.

Treatment

An antifungal ointment to be applied to the skin may be prescribed for ringworm of the body or the groin. Special medicated shampoos are available to treat ringworm of the scalp. In some especially resistant cases, an oral medication called griseofulvin may be necessary as well.

Prevention

To prevent spread of the infection, personal articles that have been in contact with infected areas, such as hats, combs, and bed linen, should be discarded or laundered in very hot water.

Sunburn

Sunburn is an inflammation of the cells of the skin caused by overexposure to the ultraviolet radiation of the sun or a sunlamp. Damage to the skin can be either insignificant or serious, depending on the intensity of the light source, the length of exposure, and the sensitivity of the individual to ultraviolet radiation.

Causes

Sunburn is caused by overexposure to ultraviolet radiation. Certain substances (such as deodorants, soaps, perfumes, cosmetics, and certain medications) may produce heightened sensitivity to ultraviolet radiation, with a corresponding increase in the severity of the burn. While light-skinned people usually burn more easily than dark-skinned people, skin color is not always a dependable guide to individual susceptibility.

Symptoms

Irritation of the skin and a prickling sensation mark the onset of sunburn; the skin also feels hot to the touch. Capillaries (tiny blood vessels) in the skin become congested because of the release of certain inflammatory agents, thus producing the characteristic redness. Oral contraceptive users may develop irregularly shaped dark splotches, and some sensitive individuals may have allergic reactions in the form of rashes or welts.

As the burn progresses in severity, the skin will feel tight, swollen, and dry or brittle and may become hypersensitive to touch. Overheating and loss of fluids through the damaged skin may also produce dizziness, nausea, vomiting, hyperventilation (abnormally rapid, deep breathing), impaired vision and hearing, irregular heartbeat, and loss of consciousness.

The aftermath of severe sunburn often includes blistering and peeling, as well as permanent freckling, splotching, or scarring of the skin. Long-term effects may include premature skin aging, marked by chronic dryness, wrinkling, leathery texture, and loss of elasticity. In some cases, melanoma (a form of skin cancer) may be induced by chronic overexposure to sunlight.

Treatment

Minor sunburn can be effectively treated by a wide variety of nonprescription ointments, oils, powders, creams, and sprays that restore fluids and prevent further drying, relieve discomfort, and promote healing. Many over-the-counter medications contain mild anesthetics to relieve stinging and suppress the desire to scratch itching areas. One of the most common complications is the infection of blistered and peeling areas of the skin. This condition should be treated by a physician.

In the case of severe sunburn, overheating and dehydration (loss of too much fluid) must be avoided. The victim should be taken out of the sun immediately and placed in a cool, shaded area until medical attention can be obtained. Cool (but not cold), wet cloths can be applied to the

arms, the head, and the legs. Chills should be avoided. Ice water and other cold drinks may trigger unwanted responses. If the victim is perspiring profusely, a fan may help evaporate the water on the skin's surface, thus aiding a natural cooling process.

Prevention

The best prevention of sunburn is simply to avoid prolonged exposure to the direct rays of the sun or a sunlamp. When this is not possible, the first line of defense is to cover the skin completely, preferably with loose-fitting, light-colored clothes made of loose-weave fabrics. Wearing a wide-brimmed hat will also help.

The second line of defense is a sunscreen, available as an oil, cream, paste, or liquid. Most sunscreens are intended to block ultraviolet rays. Many contain para-aminobenzoic acid (PABA). This compound may affect some individuals adversely, particularly those with photosensitivity (abnormal sensitivity of the skin to light) who are taking certain drugs. For these people, opaque (light-blocking) creams, pastes, and lotions are available, as well as other chemical sunscreens known as benzophenones. Anyone who is uncertain about a possible interaction between sunlight and a medication that has been prescribed should contact his or her doctor before exposure to sunlight.

Warts

Warts are infectious growths in the outer layers of the skin. Because they are contagious, they can spread from person to person or from one site to another on the same person. Most frequently, warts appear on the hands and fingers and on the soles of the feet. However, they can emerge anywhere on the skin, including the genital and anal areas.

Causes

Common warts are caused by exposure to a virus called the human papilloma virus. The virus can remain inactive for up to six months after contact before causing the eruption of abnormal skin masses.

The virus is transmitted to another person or another site on the body by direct contact. For example, brushing or combing the hair can spread the virus from a wart on the scalp. Shaving or scratching a given area on the body and then touching another area will also transmit the virus. In addition, moist parts of the body, such as the soles of the feet, provide a breeding ground for growth of the virus.

As people become older, they seem to develop an immunity or resistance to the wart virus. For this reason, children tend to acquire warts more frequently than adults. Nevertheless, warts can occur at any age.

Symptoms

Usually, warts appear as firm gray masses that feel tender or itchy. Their size and shape vary depending on the location and severity of the viral infection. Children are most likely to have flat warts, particularly on the face. This variety looks smooth, flat, and yellowish brown.

Plantar warts grow on the soles of the feet, where they can become as large as two inches in

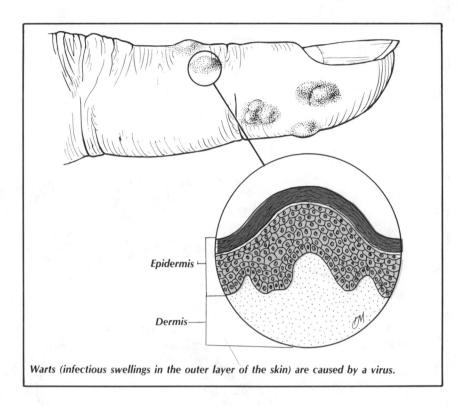

Warts (infectious swellings in the outer layer of the skin) are caused by a virus.

diameter. They cause considerable pain because the tissue swelling pushes inward with each step; the discomfort from plantar warts feels like walking with a pebble in your shoe.

Most warts are not health threatening. However, they can be so extensive in number as to cause extreme sensitivity or pain.

Treatment

Studies have shown that two out of every three warts disappear on their own, usually within two years. Consequently, physicians usually recommend leaving warts alone unless they cause discomfort or obstruction.

Doctors sometimes treat one or two warts and find that the patient's other warts also clear up. A possible explanation is that the original treatment stimulates manufacture of antibodies (protective substances) that fight the virus in other warts.

There are over-the-counter (nonprescription) preparations to aid removal of warts. Most of these remedies contain a form of acid, which is dangerous if not used according to directions. Although some of these drugs are effective, only a doctor should remove a wart.

Physicians may try a variety of topical preparations to loosen the warts. A solution containing cantharidin, a substance that causes blistering, may be applied directly to the wart. About one week after application, the doctor should be able to remove the wart with a surgical knife or scissors. Corn plasters containing salicylic acid soften the wart so that it can be scraped away.

When a wart persists, physicians may advise surgery to remove affected tissue. Electrosurgery dissolves wart tissue with electric current. Cryotherapy freezes the area with dry ice or liquid nitrogen; freezing allows the wart to be lifted off easily.

BONES AND
MUSCLES

The musculoskeletal system is an intricate structure of interconnecting parts. Every movement of the body is the result of the coordination of bones, muscles, tendons, and ligaments.

Bones

Bones are hardened masses of living tissue that have several functions. They collect calcium for the entire body, storing 99 percent of this mineral, which is required to keep all bones firm and strong. Within some bones is a substance called marrow, which produces red and white blood cells and platelets.

There are 206 bones in the human skeleton. The skeleton maintains the body's shape and protects internal organs. For example, the bones in the skull shield the brain, and the bones in the rib cage encircle the lungs and heart.

The place where two or more bones meet is called a joint. This juncture usually allows movement of the bones that are involved. However, movement is governed by ligaments (bands of fibrous tissue) attached to the bones and by cartilage (elastic tissue) covering the ends of the bones. Ligaments connect one bone with another. Cartilage cushions and protects bones with the aid of various joint fluids and bursae (small sacs containing lubricating fluid that encompass the joints). Other bands of connective tissue called tendons attach bones to muscles. Muscles are specific kinds of tissues that have the ability to contract. It is this contraction that pulls on the tendons and makes movement possible. To move any part of the skeleton, coordination of ligaments, tendons, and muscles is necessary.

Muscles

There are three types of muscle: striated, smooth, and cardiac. Striated, or striped, muscle consists of layers of tissue divided into bundles of interwoven fibers that run parallel to one another. These layers are attached to the skeleton, and they aid the body in voluntary movement.

Smooth, or organic, muscle is present in several of the internal organs, including the intestines and the bladder, and in the larger blood vessels. This type of muscle functions under involuntary control by the autonomic nervous system. Among its functions, smooth muscle helps circulate blood and glandular secretions throughout the body, move material through the digestive tract, and regulate breathing. Smooth muscle contains elongated, spindly cells arranged parallel to one another that are often grouped into bundles.

Cardiac muscle is the muscle of the heart, and its job is to pump blood within and from the heart. The unique characteristic of this muscle is that although it is striated (like the muscles of the

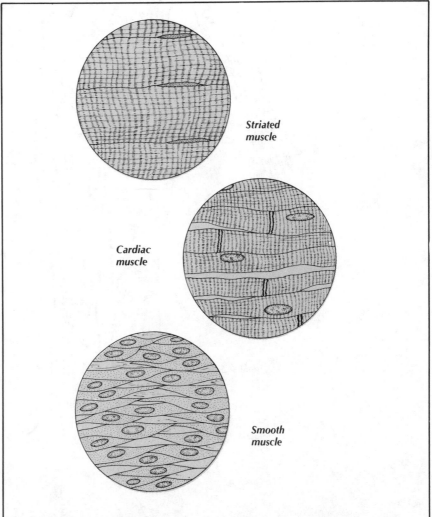

Striated muscle

Cardiac muscle

Smooth muscle

Muscles are connective tissues that have the ability to contract. There are three types of muscles: striated muscle, which is involved in voluntary movement; smooth muscle, which is involved in functions under involuntary control; and cardiac (heart) muscle.

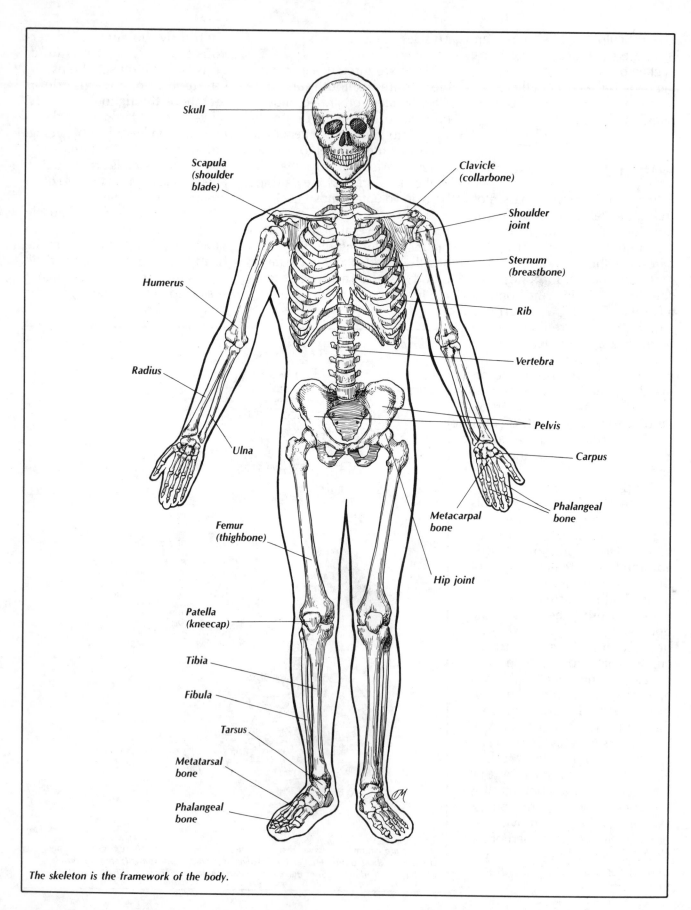

Skull

Scapula
(shoulder
blade)

Clavicle
(collarbone)

Shoulder
joint

Sternum
(breastbone)

Humerus

Rib

Radius

Vertebra

Ulna

Pelvis

Carpus

Phalangeal
bone

Metacarpal
bone

Femur
(thighbone)

Hip joint

Patella
(kneecap)

Tibia

Fibula

Tarsus

Metatarsal
bone

Phalangeal
bone

The skeleton is the framework of the body.

skeleton), it is controlled by the autonomic nervous system (like the muscles of the internal organs).

Ankylosing spondylitis

Ankylosing spondylitis is a form of arthritis, mainly affecting the sacroiliac joints, the spine, and nearby structures. Joints become inflamed and eventually stiff and immovable. The elastic cartilage disks between the vertebrae (bones of the spine) become dense, as does adjacent connective tissue. Bony connections form between the vertebrae. The lower vertebrae may become fused together, creating a straight "poker spine," frequently accompanied by a curve in the upper spine.

Causes

The cause of ankylosing spondylitis is unknown, but there appears to be an inherited tendency toward the disease. The disease affects men ten times more often than women, and many are born with a certain trait, called HLA-B27, in their blood. Persons carrying this trait are more likely to suffer the disease.

Ankylosing spondylitis is predominantly a disease of young men, occurring most commonly between the ages of 15 and 40. The disease may progress slowly for 10 to 20 years and then stop or slow down.

Symptoms

Chronic low back pain and stiffness in a young man is a

Area of fusion

Vertebra

Ankylosing spondylitis is a form of arthritis in which there is fusion of the vertebrae (bones of the spine), often accompanied by curvature of the upper spine.

chief sign of the disease; hip pain is also quite common, as is an inflammation of the eye known as anterior uveitis. Symptoms begin gradually, usually as low backaches. There may be morning stiffness and pain extending down the leg along the sciatic nerve, commonly alternating from one side to the other. The back pain and stiffness eventually affect the upper spine and sometimes the neck. In up to a third of the cases, large joints (such as those of the hips and shoulders) are affected. Knees and other smaller joints are affected less often, with symptoms

matching those of rheumatoid arthritis. The heart is eventually affected in up to three percent of cases, and inflammation of the lining of the eye occurs in about 25 percent of the cases. As the disease progresses, it is more difficult for the patient to flex the back and expand the chest, and neck movements may be limited. X rays of the back-related joints —especially those between the upper portion of the hip bone and the sacrum (the bony structure at the base of the spine)— reveal changes typical of ankylosing spondylitis. A sign of advanced disease is "bamboo spine," in which bony bands around the disks cement the vertebrae together.

Treatment

Although there is no cure for ankylosing spondylitis, certain measures can lessen the effects of the disease. These include rest; breathing exercises; and exercises to maintain posture, help with curvature of the upper spine, and keep the back as flexible as possible. To prevent curvature of the upper spine, sleeping on the back on a firm mattress with a small pillow or no pillow is advised. Locking the fingers behind the head and pushing the elbows back as far as possible is a good way to straighten the upper back and stretch the chest muscles. Painkillers and anti-inflammatory drugs may be given. Corticosteroid drugs are generally not prescribed because of their many side effects. Surgery is rarely needed.

Arthritis

Arthritis is an inflammation of the joints (the junctures where

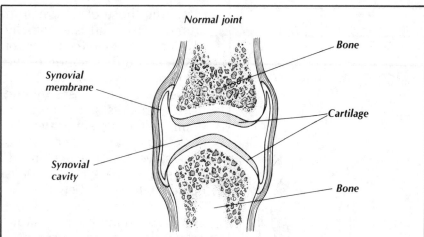

Normal joint

Synovial membrane

Bone

Cartilage

Synovial cavity

Bone

The normal joint is lined by a synovial membrane, which produces the lubricating synovial fluid that fills the synovial cavity. The bone ends are covered by cartilage.

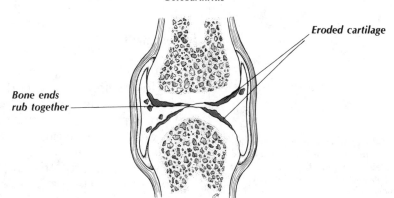

Osteoarthritis

Eroded cartilage

Bone ends rub together

In osteoarthritis, the cushioning cartilage at the bone ends is eroded (worn away), allowing the bone ends to rub together, which causes swelling and pain.

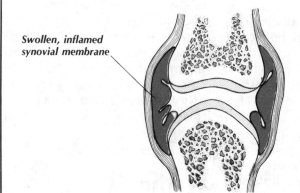

Rheumatoid arthritis

Swollen, inflamed synovial membrane

Rheumatoid arthritis is characterized by swelling and inflammation of the synovial membrane.

the ends of two or more bones meet).

Types

Inflammation develops in various ways. With *osteoarthritis,* there is gradual wearing away of cartilage. Healthy cartilage is the elastic tissue that lines and cushions the joints and allows bones to move smoothly against one another. When it deteriorates, the bones rub together, causing pain and swelling. Permanent damage and stiffness of the joints are possible. Although osteoarthritis can result from direct injury, it commonly occurs in adults over 55 due to long-term wear and tear on the joints.

Rheumatoid arthritis can attack at any age. This form of arthritis affects all the connective tissues, as well as other organs, in the body. The precise cause is unknown. Some researchers believe that a virus triggers the disease, causing an autoimmune response whereby the body develops an allergy to its own tissues. However, evidence for this theory is inconclusive as yet. What is confirmed is the progression of the condition. First, the synovium (the thin membrane lining and lubricating the joint) becomes inflamed. The inflammation eventually destroys the cartilage. As scar tissue replaces damaged cartilage, the joint becomes misshapen and rigid.

Rheumatoid arthritis may damage the heart, lungs, nerves, and eyes. Osteoarthritis can cause permanent damage, stiffness, and deformity of the joints.

Those at risk

Arthritis is not an inherited disease. Nonetheless, people who have a family history of arthritis are more likely to develop the disease. Women are at greater risk than men, although the reason for this is unclear. Excess body weight may promote osteoarthritis because of increased load on the joints. Constant sports- or job-related joint abuse may encourage arthritis, but inactivity can also aggravate the problem.

Symptoms

Symptoms of arthritis include swelling, tenderness, pain, stiffness, and redness in one or more joints. For many patients, pain is greatest in the morning and subsides as the day progresses. Damp weather and emotional stress do not cause arthritis, but they can make symptoms worse.

With rheumatoid arthritis, these symptoms may be accompanied by more generalized feelings of fatigue and fever. This form of arthritis may go into periods of remission, when symptoms disappear. When symptoms return, however, they are often more severe.

Diagnosis

To diagnose arthritis, a physician observes the symptoms and administers a standard physical examination. X-ray studies and laboratory tests may be recommended for confirmation of joint swelling and determination of the extent of damage.

Treatment

The most effective treatment program for arthritis consists of drug therapy, exercise, and rest. Treatment should begin early after diagnosis to prevent permanent damage.

Aspirin is the drug most commonly administered for arthritis. Taking two or three tablets several times a day is often recommended to reduce inflammation and relieve pain. If stomach irritation is a problem, aspirin may be taken after meals or in a coated tablet form. Nonaspirin pain relievers and nonsteroidal anti-inflammatory drugs (such as ibuprofen, naproxen, tolmetin, and sulindac) may also be prescribed. Corticosteroids relieve inflammation, but they can cause adverse side effects. Sometimes, a doctor needs to try several different drugs before finding an effective one that produces few side effects. Oral or injectable gold, when determined to be indicated by a physician, may prove helpful in treating rheumatoid arthritis. Some drugs usually used for cancer chemotherapy, such as methotrexate, may also be helpful.

Moderate daily exercise, such as swimming, walking, or physical therapy, is critical to maintaining mobility. A supervised exercise program interspersed with rest periods helps reduce joint inflammation. To lessen pain while increasing movement, moist heat often helps. In addition, maintaining correct posture and body weight reduces extra burden on joints.

Some severe cases of rheumatoid arthritis may require surgery to remove inflamed synovial tissue. With either form of arthritis, artificial joints may be implanted to replace those damaged beyond repair.

Backache

A backache is generally a gripping pain near the inward curve

Wrong

Right

Bending at the knees, rather than from the waist, when lifting large, heavy objects places the stress on the legs and helps prevent back injury.

of the back above the base of the spine. It is one of the most common physical ailments, affecting about 80 percent of the population at some time in their lives.

Causes

Pain results from a variety of causes. Strains are especially common when overworked or underexercised back muscles perform beyond their normal capacity. The muscles will then contract or go into spasm and become a tight mass of tissue. Meanwhile, the body transmits a sharp pain signal as nearby muscles tighten in an effort to protect strained muscles and prevent further damage. Strain of back muscles can be due to participation in a sport, a sudden jerking motion (such as a car braking), or reflex actions like sneezing.

Overweight is a leading factor in backache because it increases the stress on back muscles. Similarly, pregnancy can produce back pain because of the weight or position of the fetus. For some women, menstruation is also associated with back discomfort.

Many people experience back pain as they age and their joint tissues deteriorate or shift. Psychological tension, stress, or anxiety about everyday problems can also lead to backache. In addition, back pain can result from diseases of the kidneys, heart, lungs, intestinal tract, or reproductive organs.

Backache occasionally stems from a congenital (present from birth) malformation. In such cases, pain generally results from the unusual stresses that the deformity imposes on surrounding muscular structures rather than from the abnormality itself. For example, if one leg is shorter than the other, the muscles in the lower part of the body are forced out of alignment, causing back pain.

Symptoms

Backaches can appear abruptly after physical activity or may develop slowly. The pain may feel like a sharp jab or a dull ache. The pain sometimes becomes so piercing that a person who is bending over may not be able to straighten up. Severe back pain may also be accompanied by pain or numbness radiating down one or both legs. Most muscular back pains disappear within a week or two of their onset, while some will last one to two months. Pain may recur

unless preventive measures are taken.

Diagnosis

Prolonged back pain (lasting for more than one or two weeks) should be brought to the attention of a physician, who will check for underlying disorders, such as kidney, bone, or lung problems, that may be causing the backache. Once other medical causes have been ruled out, an orthopedic surgeon (a physician who specializes in bone and muscle conditions) may be able to determine the cause of the discomfort.

During the examination, the physician asks questions about the type of pain and its location, general health, previous illnesses, and physical activity routines. The patient walks, sits, stands, and performs exercises while being observed. An X-ray study may reveal adverse changes in the spine.

Treatment

If there are no apparent physical causes for the backache, physicians usually recommend an exercise program to strengthen weak muscles. Losing weight can also relieve pressure on the back.

For immediate treatment of symptoms, using a heating pad or, better yet, ice at the site of the pain will usually reduce soreness. Nonprescription analgesic creams containing methyl salicylate (oil of wintergreen) or a similar ingredient produce a soothing warm sensation when applied to the pain site. Muscle relaxants and/or anti-inflammatory drugs may also be prescribed.

When backache is the result of some deformity or damage to a

disk (the soft material that lies between the bones of the spine), surgery may be necessary to correct the problem. Braces, corsets, or shoe lifts sometimes improve the condition. Exercises to strengthen affected muscles and counter stress caused by the deformity may be prescribed.

Almost all types of musculoskeletal backaches respond well to rest, which allows muscles to relax and inflammation to subside. Time is often the best healer.

Prevention

To prevent back pain, stress to the spine should be avoided. Good posture, when awake and asleep, relieves tension on the spinal column. Wearing properly fitted shoes encourages good posture, as does sleeping on a semifirm bed. Contrary to popular belief, a hard mattress distorts alignment of the spine and causes back problems as much as a soft mattress does. A semifirm mattress is recommended because it conforms to the arch of the back and maintains spinal alignment.

Good posture is also important when performing daily activities. Bending at the knees, rather than from the waist, when lifting large, heavy objects places the stress on the legs and helps prevent back injury. One should avoid looking down for long periods of time while seated.

Bunion

A bunion is a swelling on the foot, usually at the joint of the big toe. Often, a bony protuberance is present at the joint of the big toe, which gives the bunion its bulging appearance.

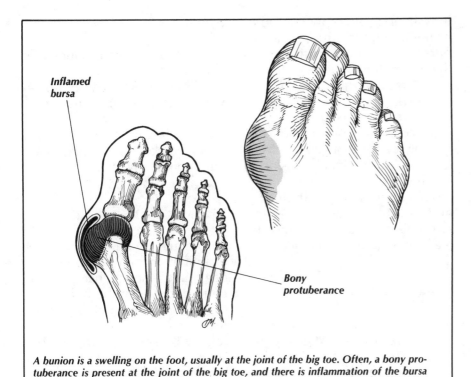

Inflamed bursa

Bony protuberance

A bunion is a swelling on the foot, usually at the joint of the big toe. Often, a bony protuberance is present at the joint of the big toe, and there is inflammation of the bursa (the fluid-filled sac that acts as a cushion for the joint). A bunion is most often caused by friction or pressure on the joint.

Causes

Bunions are most often caused by wearing poorly fitting footwear, but they can also be the result of inherited deformities in bone structure. In a normal foot, the two main bones of the big toe must align to fit together. However, some people have loose joints in the foot that allow their big toes to point toward the other toes. This inherited condition causes problems when footwear encloses the foot. The shoe forces the big toe inward and the big-toe joint outward so that the joint rubs against the inner surface of the shoe. Friction from such rubbing produces a bunion. The same action results when a tight or pointed-toe shoe puts pressure on the joint—regardless of whether the person has the predisposing inherited tendency to have loose joints in the foot.

Symptoms

A bunion is characterized by swelling at the big-toe joint, which may be accompanied by pain and tenderness. Bunion formations can be acute or chronic. Acute bunions are a type of bursitis, which is an inflammation of a bursa (a fluid-filled sac that cushions the juncture of two or more bones). With an acute bunion, the bursa covering the big-toe joint becomes inflamed from friction at the joint, often producing considerable pain. Chronic (long-term) bunions develop into inflexible bony protrusions.

Complications

Complications can occur if the bunion grows and increases pressure on the big toe. This pressure may force the other toes to overlap, encouraging the development of corns (mounds of dead skin found on toes) or other problems that could result from friction on the skin of the distorted toes.

Diagnosis

A physician diagnoses a bunion by general physical examination. To identify bone problems, an X-ray examination may be necessary.

Treatment

Surgery is the only permanent cure for bunions. It can entail simple removal of the excess bone or more complex realignment of the affected bones, muscles, and tendons. A doctor can sometimes remove a bony protrusion in the office. Local anesthetic can be used, the incision is often only about an inch long, and pain is minimal. With this treatment, the patient has full use of the foot in about six weeks.

For more extensive surgery, the patient is admitted to the hospital, and recuperation time is longer. Usually, an orthopedic surgeon performs this type of surgery.

Nonsurgical devices can often relieve the pain and discomfort of bunions. Padding can be used to shift the weight of the foot in the shoe, lessening friction. Protective shields can also prevent contact between the bunion and the inside of the shoe.

Prevention

Wearing properly fitting footwear is the best preventive measure. A child's first shoes should be wide enough to accommodate all the toes without cramping, since early childhood is when many foot problems begin.

When buying shoes, the width and length of each foot need to be measured separately. If one foot is larger than the other, the shoe size should correspond to the size of the larger foot. A one-inch gap between the big toe and the tip of the shoe allows enough space for movement. Even more room is needed with pointed-toe shoes. Shoes should be comfortable from the first wearing—no breaking-in period should be necessary. People who wear high-heel or pointed-toe shoes may be damaging their feet. Heels about one inch in height are actually best for feet. However, if higher heels are chosen, open-toe styles cause fewer problems.

Bursitis

Bursitis is an inflammation of a bursa (a fluid-filled sac that cush-ions the juncture of two or more bones). Bursae (the plural of bursa) contain lubricating fluid that normally eliminates friction in the area and maintains smooth muscle movement over the bones.

Bursitis seems to be more common in men than in women, possibly because of greater physical activity. Continual stress on a particular joint increases the probability of injury and inflammation. In advanced cases, swelling and calcium deposits may render a joint immobile.

Causes

The inflammation can result from either sudden extreme pressure or from continual strain. Some occupations and sports that require constant use of certain joints contribute to bursitis. For example, "typist's shoulder" and "baseball pitcher's elbow" are forms of chronic bursitis. Acute bursitis can develop suddenly and may be triggered by physical stress or injury.

Symptoms

Inflamed bursae produce tenderness and swelling near the affected joints. Pain can be so severe that movement becomes impossible. Any joint in the body can be the site of bursitis, but shoulders, knees, and elbows are most commonly affected.

Diagnosis

To diagnose bursitis, an X-ray examination may be ordered to determine whether there are calcium deposits in the bursa or if other problems, such as a fracture, exist. In the case of stress-related bursitis, however, such a study will show only swelling of the bursa.

Treatment

Acute bursitis may heal with time if the joint is immobilized. Complete bed rest or use of a sling or crutches may be recom-

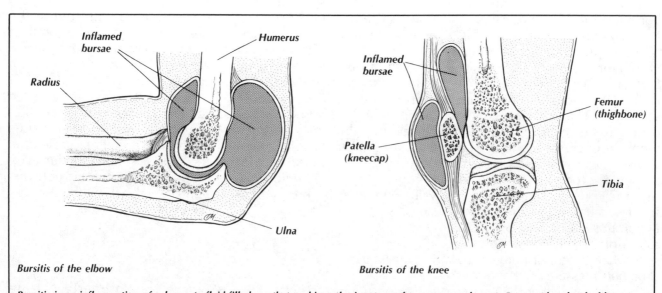

Bursitis of the elbow

Bursitis of the knee

Bursitis is an inflammation of a bursa (a fluid-filled sac that cushions the juncture of two or more bones). Bursae (the plural of bursa) contain lubricating fluid that normally eliminates friction and maintains smooth muscle movement over the bones. The elbow and the knee are common sites of bursitis.

mended to relieve pressure on the affected area.

Applying moist heat to the area of the inflamed joint frequently reduces the discomfort of bursitis, although some patients find cold compresses more effective. Aspirin and other over-the-counter pain relievers may also help. In some cases, anti-inflammatory corticosteroid drugs may be injected directly into the inflamed area, but they must be used judiciously since they have been known to cause adverse side effects.

For severe cases of bursitis, a doctor may recommend surgery to remove calcium deposits or free the area from chronic inflammation by removing all or part of the bursa.

Fracture

A fracture is a break in a bone or a cartilage. Among the possible consequences of a fracture are infection and damage to nearby nerves, blood vessels, and internal organs.

Causes

Most often, fractures are caused by direct stress, such as a blow from a heavy object, or a severe strain, such as a violent twist. They can, however, be the result of an indirect cause. A fall on a hand, for example, may result in a fracture of the collarbone. There are also pathological fractures, in which disease softens the bone, making it more vulnerable to a break.

Types

There are many different types of fractures including:

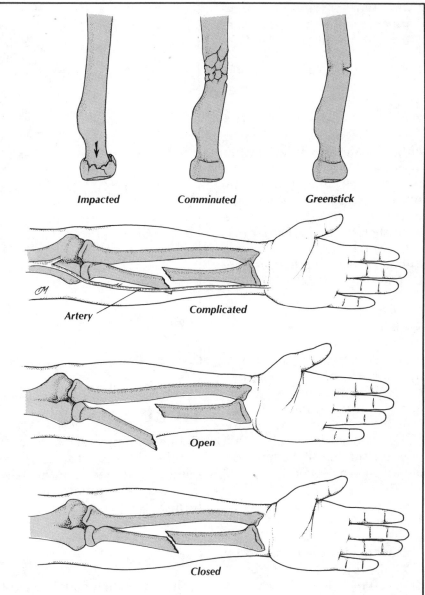

There are several major categories of fractures, depending on the site and extent of injury.

- Closed fracture—one in which the skin is not broken
- Comminuted fracture—one in which the bone is broken into several pieces
- Complicated fracture—one in which significant injury has been done to internal organs, blood vessels, or nerves
- Greenstick fracture—one in which only one side of the bone is broken

- Impacted fracture—one in which the ends or fragments of bone are jammed together
- Open fracture—one in which one or more of the broken ends of the bone actually pierce the skin
- Stress fracture—one in which there is a tiny crack (or cracks) in a bone; the crack causes severe pain but may be undetectable by conventional X ray.

This type of fracture is commonly seen in the small bones of the foot due to athletic activity.

Those at risk

Fractures are common among children and the elderly. Children have relatively soft, elastic bones; breaks in their bones are often incomplete, affecting only one side of the bone (called greenstick fractures). Elderly persons have brittle bones that tend to break easily; hip fractures are particularly common.

Symptoms

Among the symptoms of a fracture are pain, swelling, loss of strength, abnormal movement, and a grating sound when the pieces of broken bone rub together. Shock may occur with a severe fracture if large amounts of blood have been lost.

Treatment

Bone fractures are treated by closed (nonsurgical) or open (surgical) reduction. Reduction is a procedure in which the broken bone is manipulated (for example, by pulling or bending) so that its ends will be in the best position for healing. Most fractures are treated through closed reduction. However, open reduction may be necessary when damage to bones, joints, ligaments, tendons, or other internal parts is severe or extensive. In open reduction, the pieces of bone are often held together by pins, metal plates, or rods; some are left in the body, and others are removed after healing has taken place.

Gout is an extremely painful condition in which deposition of uric acid crystals around a joint triggers an inflammatory response and can ultimately cause degeneration of the bone.

Gout

Gout is a form of recurrent acute arthritis. Most gout victims are middle-aged men. Gout usually appears in women only after menopause.

Cause

The underlying cause of gout is a defect in the body's processing of uric acid, a chemical normally found in the blood and urine. If the body does not properly process uric acid, the level of uric acid in the blood becomes elevated. The excess uric acid may crystallize and become deposited in and around the joints and their tendons. An acute attack of gout is caused by the body's inflammatory response to the deposits of uric acid crystals.

The high levels of uric acid can also lead to deposition of crystals in areas of the body other than the joints, most notably the skin and the kidneys. Uric acid deposits in the kidneys may form kidney stones. About 20 percent of patients with chronic gout also have kidney stones. If the kidneys become blocked by stones, kidney failure may result.

Symptoms

Gout usually first appears as a sudden and extremely painful attack in a single joint, usually the big toe. Later attacks can involve several joints, such as the ankle, knee, wrist, and elbow. The pain, which commonly begins at night during sleep, may occur without warning or may be preceded by excessive alcohol consumption or unusual exercise earlier in the day. The pain grows in intensity and is often described as throbbing or crushing. Inflammation follows, with swelling, warmth, redness, and tenderness over the affected joint. The pain is sometimes so severe that the individual cannot tolerate the weight of a bed sheet over the joint. Other symptoms that may accompany the joint pain and swelling include fever, rapid heartbeat, chills, and an overall feeling of being unwell. Uric acid deposits in the skin may be noted as white lumps under the skin, most often appearing in the hands, the feet, the elbows, and the rims of the outer ears.

The first attacks usually last only a few days, but if the disorder goes untreated, later attacks may last for weeks. Symptoms eventually disappear, and joint function returns to normal between attacks. As the disease progresses, the periods of remission become shorter and shorter as more and more attacks occur each year.

Treatment

The treatment of gout is twofold—to relieve the symptoms of an acute attack and to prevent recurrences. The drug colchicine has traditionally been used to relieve a gout attack, but nonsteroidal anti-inflammatory drugs are now more often prescribed to relieve the inflammation and pain. These drugs are quite effective. However, they do have side effects, so they should be used only under close and continuous medical supervision.

Once the acute attack is under control, prevention of future attacks is the main goal. This can be done with the drug allopurinol, which interferes with the production of uric acid and thus prevents the deposition of uric acid crystals in the body. Allopurinol usually has to be taken for long periods of time to maintain normal blood levels of uric

acid. There are also other drugs, called uricosurics, that speed up the excretion of uric acid by the kidneys. These drugs, however, may not be used if there is known kidney damage or if the uric acid content of the urine is high.

Hernia

A hernia is an abnormal protrusion of part of an organ through the tissues that normally contain it. In this condition, a weak spot or opening in a body wall, often due to laxity of the muscles, allows part of the organ to protrude. A hernia may develop in almost any part of the body; however, the muscles of the abdominal wall are most commonly affected.

Types of hernias

A hernia can be congenital (present at birth) or acquired (often the result of stress or strain on the body wall). Although there are many types of hernias, the following are common:
- Umbilical hernia—protrusion of part of the intestine at the umbilicus (navel). This type is seen mostly in infants.
- Inguinal hernia—protrusion of a loop of intestine into the groin (where the folds of abdominal flesh meet the thighs). This type of hernia, which accounts for about 75 percent of all abdominal hernias, is often the result of increased pressure in the abdomen because of lifting, coughing, or straining.
- Scrotal hernia—an inguinal hernia that has passed into the scrotum (the sac containing the testes).
- Femoral hernia—protrusion of a loop of tissue into the

femoral canal, which carries nerves and blood vessels from the abdomen into the upper thigh/groin area. This type of hernia is more common in women than in men.
- Incisional hernia—a hernia that occurs at the site of a surgical incision. This type of hernia is often due to strain on healing tissues due to excessive muscular effort, lifting, coughing, or extreme pressure.
- Hiatal hernia—protrusion of part of the stomach through the diaphragm and into the chest (for more information, see pages 242-243).

Symptoms

The symptoms vary slightly, depending on the cause and the structures involved. Most hernias begin as small breakthroughs that are hardly noticeable. At first, they may be soft lumps under the skin, a little larger than a marble; there is usually no pain. As time goes by, the pressure of the internal contents against the weak wall increases, and the size of the lump increases.

In the early stages, the hernia may be reducible, in other words, the protruding structures can be pushed gently back into their normal places. If those protruding structures, however, cannot be returned to their normal locations through manipulation, the hernia is said to be irreducible, or incarcerated.

If an incarcerated hernia progresses, bulging out farther through the weakest points in its containing wall, the opening in the wall will close behind it, forming a narrow neck. If the neck is pinched enough to cut off the blood supply to the protruding tissue, the hernia will swell quickly and become strangulated—that is, the blood supply will be totally cut off. Unless treated, a strangulated hernia can cause tissue death. Fortunately, the symptoms of strangulation of a hernia are usually detectable. When a hernia suddenly grows larger, becomes tense, will not go back into place, and is accompanied by pain and nausea, the hernia is most likely strangulated. Sometimes, however, there is no pain or tenderness when this happens, especially in elderly patients.

Diagnosis

Diagnosis of a hernia can usually be made by thorough examination and by studying the patient's medical history and symptoms.

Treatment

For small nonstrangulated and nonincarcerated hernias, various supports and trusses may offer temporary, symptomatic relief. However, the best treatment is herniorrhaphy (surgical closure or repair of the muscle wall through which the hernia protrudes). When the weakened area is very large, some strong synthetic material may be sewn over the defect to reinforce the weak area. Postoperative care involves protecting the patient from respiratory infections that might cause coughing or sneezing, which would strain the suture line. Recovery is usually quick and complete.

Prevention

Avoiding strain or pressure on any body wall, especially the ab-

dominal wall in men, is the only real preventive measure against hernias.

Lupus erythematosus

Lupus erythematosus is a disorder that frequently affects the skin and the connective tissues (particularly the joints and muscles) but that can affect every tissue and organ in the body. The disorder occurs in two different forms—discoid lupus erythematosus and systemic lupus erythematosus.

Discoid lupus erythematosus

Discoid lupus erythematosus is a chronic disease of the skin that is characterized by a red rash that appears on the cheeks and nose, as well as on other parts of the body. It often appears for the first time after the skin has been exposed to sunlight. Discoid lupus erythematosus is usually treated with drugs commonly used in the treatment of malaria (even though the two conditions are not at all related).

Systemic lupus erythematosus

Systemic lupus erythematosus is a widespread autoimmune inflammatory disease of the blood vessels and connective tissues. The condition affects the joints, skin, and numerous other organs in the body, including the heart, lungs, liver, intestines, and kidneys. A red patch that resembles an open-winged butterfly may appear on the cheeks and nose. Symptoms may also include severe pain in the joints, intermittent fever, and unusual fatigue.

The inflammation may cause severe and irreversible damage to the blood vessels and to the kidneys.

Cortisone and other steroids are used to control the inflammation in the joints and in other parts of the body; aspirin and other analgesics are used to control the pain. As with discoid lupus erythematosus, antimalarial drugs are used in the treatment of the rash.

This disease may be mild, or it may progress rapidly to seriously affect many organs. Death may result in severe cases.

Osteoporosis

Osteoporosis is a relatively common disorder characterized by a decrease in the calcium content of the bones, which leaves them thin and susceptible to fracture.

Causes

The causes of osteoporosis are largely unknown. However, chances of acquiring the condition seem to increase dramatically with age, especially for women. One prevailing theory maintains that osteoporosis results from a loss of the female hormone estrogen, which affects the calcium content of the bones. Menopause (cessation of menstruation) may lead to osteoporosis because the body's production of estrogen is reduced at that time. Almost one third of all women over 60 years of age have the condition to some extent.

For reasons that are not entirely known, osteoporosis is more likely to affect white and Oriental women than black women. In addition, slender women, especially those who have fair skin,

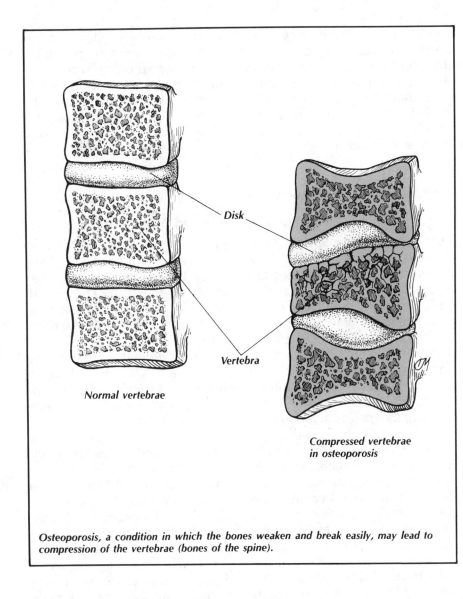

Disk

Vertebra

Normal vertebrae

Compressed vertebrae in osteoporosis

Osteoporosis, a condition in which the bones weaken and break easily, may lead to compression of the vertebrae (bones of the spine).

ity, which may weaken additional vertebrae. Hence, a vicious cycle develops whereby pain leading to inactivity encourages osteoporosis, which in turn increases bone fragility.

As the disease progresses, the spinal column may decrease in length, causing a height loss of as much as several inches, or may become curved, producing the characteristic "dowager's hump." These changes are the result of successive fractures due to the pressure of body weight on the deteriorating vertebrae.

Diagnosis

Often, osteoporosis progresses undetected until a bone is fractured and an X ray is taken. At that time, a physician may notice that bone thinning has become a generalized condition throughout the body.

Treatment

Physicians urge patients with osteoporosis to follow an exercise program that will strengthen the muscles supporting weakened bones. To protect bones in the spinal column, however, lifting heavy objects should be avoided. For advanced cases, a back brace may be necessary to help support body weight while sitting or standing. Crutches, walkers, or a cane may assist walking.

Physicians often prescribe estrogen or estrogen-progesterone combinations to women who are no longer menstruating in order to decrease bone loss. Women taking this medication need careful supervision because the hormone may cause adverse side effects. Anyone receiving estrogen therapy should have a physical

run a higher risk of developing this disorder than do stouter, darker-skinned women.

Osteoporosis can also occur as a result of other conditions. Surgical removal of both ovaries (the female sex glands, which produce estrogen) and chronic arthritis (inflammation of the joints) may lead to osteoporosis. People who are inactive, either by choice or due to confinement because of illness, seem more susceptible to the disorder. A diet deficient in nutrients, especially calcium (which promotes bone development), may also contribute to osteoporosis.

Symptoms

Depending on the strength of the bones, osteoporosis may initially cause either no symptoms or extreme pain. If there is pain, it is most commonly in the lower back. The disease is not life-threatening, but it may lead to fractures, which, for the elderly, can result in serious complications. Initially, sudden back pain may follow fracture of the vertebrae (the bones of the spine). Pain from the fracture itself may subside but discomfort from osteoporosis may continue. This pain may lead to further inactivexamination and a Pap test (examination of cells scraped from the vagina and cervix to detect cancer) every six months because of a suspected link between estrogen supplements and uterine and breast cancer. Men may be given the male hormone testosterone, which stimulates growth of body tissues, to treat osteoporosis.

For people prone to injury from osteoporosis, a balanced diet is an important factor in preventing or controlling the disease. Foods rich in vitamins and minerals, particularly calcium and vitamin D, encourage bone formation. When the diet is deficient in these nutrients, supplements may be prescribed.

Paget's disease

Paget's disease (known medically as osteitis deformans) is a disorder in which the normal process of breakdown and replacement of bone tissue is greatly accelerated. The disease develops in three stages. In the first, or destructive, stage, bone tissue breaks down and is replaced with blood vessels and dense fibrous tissue, making the bones very vascular (having a greater-than-normal number of blood vessels). During the second, or mixed, stage, new bone formation takes place at a rate geared to the breakdown process. In the third, or sclerotic, stage, the breakdown process slows, allowing the hardening of new bone, which becomes quite dense.

Although any bone can be affected, Paget's disease most commonly invades the pelvis, skull, thighbones, shinbones, vertebrae (the bones of the spine), collarbones, and ribs.

The condition affects one percent to three percent of the adult population. Men are more commonly afflicted than women. The incidence of the condition is higher in some European countries than in others. Paget's disease is rare in Asia, Africa, and South America. The cause of the disease is unknown.

Symptoms and complications

Bone pain is one of the most prevalent symptoms. Complications sometimes develop. The thickened, enlarged bones are susceptible to fracture, particularly during the destructive phase of the disease. When the disease attacks the skull bones, the auditory nerve, which relays signals from the ear to the brain, is often compressed, causing deafness. Heart failure can result from the stress of the increased blood flow through the bones. Malignant bone tumors are another complication, but fortunately they are uncommon. The disease can affect appearance if it enlarges the head, bends the back, or bows the legs. In some severe cases, particularly if the person is immobile, calcium levels in the blood and urine increase and may lead to formation of kidney stones.

Diagnosis

A history and physical examination, blood tests, and particularly X-ray studies are used to confirm the diagnosis.

Treatment

Although there is no cure, analgesics (painkillers) like aspirin offer some relief. Severe pain and other complications are sometimes managed with drug therapy. Injections of calcitonin (a hormone normally produced in the thyroid gland, which promotes calcification of bone) may help block excessive breakdown of bone. Oral drug therapy is now also available. In most cases, however, medication (oral or injectable) is not necessary.

Slipped disk

A slipped disk is a back problem involving the disks of soft elastic tissue located between the vertebrae (bones of the spinal column). The vertebrae are loosely strung together by bands of tissue called ligaments, which allow body movement and flexibility. The main function of each disk is to prevent friction and trauma between adjacent vertebrae as the body moves.

When this intricate spinal structure experiences strain and overexertion, the rim of a disk may weaken and tear, causing part of the gelatinous center of the disk to be forced out of position ("slip" or "herniate"). In its new location, the protruding material often presses against an adjacent spinal nerve, which causes pain along the path of the affected nerve.

Causes

Often, a slipped disk occurs when there is strain or injury to the spinal structure resulting from bending and straightening the back to lift heavy objects. Damage to the disk may not be realized for many months. More often, low back pain radiating into the buttock(s) and/or thigh(s) occurs soon after the injury.

Disks also seem to deteriorate with age. They lose some fluidity and become more compressed.

This form of degeneration usually results in only mild pain and intermittent backache and stiffness.

Symptoms

Symptoms may vary with the location of the disk. The most common site for a slipped disk is the lowest movable disk in the small of the back. Injury to this disk causes pain along the sciatic nerve, a condition called sciatica. Mild or disabling pain and tenderness may result. Any straining, such as coughing or moving, can aggravate the discomfort. Weakness, tingling, or numbness in parts of the arms, legs, or feet may also result from damage to a particular disk in the neck or back.

Diagnosis

To determine the source of back pain, a physician obtains a medical history; observes the patient sitting, walking, and bending; and explores for sensitive areas by maneuvering the patient's legs in different positions, checking ankle and knee reflexes, and testing muscle strength. Structural changes in bones, joints, or disk spaces (but not the disks themselves) can be seen on an ordinary X-ray study.

To locate a particularly problematic disk or to prepare for a surgical procedure, special tests are necessary. A myelogram is an X-ray study obtained after the injection of dye directly into the space surrounding the spinal cord and nerve roots. Discography gives much the same information as myelography; before this X-ray study, dye is injected directly into the disks. Computed tomography (page 407) and magnetic resonance imaging (pages 405-406) are also highly accurate in the diagnosis of disk problems. However, prior to surgery, most orthopedic neurosurgeons prefer to do a myelogram to best visualize the area.

Treatment

The first course of treatment for a slipped disk involves bed rest on a firm mattress. Rest relieves pressure exerted by the disk on the nerve. Some form of back support may improve comfort when moving about. Under no circumstances should a patient lift heavy objects.

For severe pain, a physician may prescribe an analgesic or anti-inflammatory drug. Frequently, direct injection of a steroid (cortisone) drug and local anesthetic into the area around the spinal cord (epidural space) will break the cycle of pain and nerve-root swelling and provide long-lasting relief. After the pain has completely subsided, an exercise program may be recommended to gradually strengthen muscles in the region.

Partial or complete relief from the pain of a slipped disk can usually be obtained without surgery. However, in some cases,

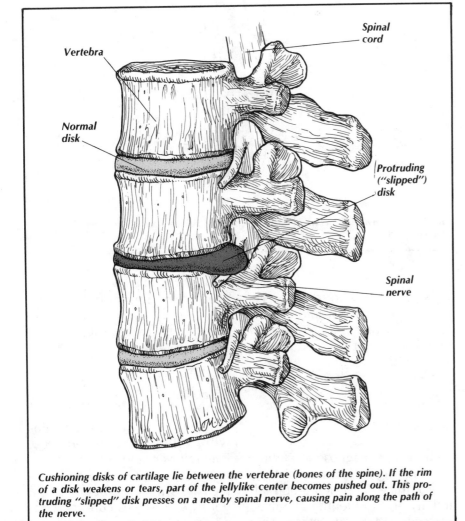

Cushioning disks of cartilage lie between the vertebrae (bones of the spine). If the rim of a disk weakens or tears, part of the jellylike center becomes pushed out. This protruding "slipped" disk presses on a nearby spinal nerve, causing pain along the path of the nerve.

Labels on figure: Vertebra; Normal disk; Spinal cord; Protruding ("slipped") disk; Spinal nerve surgical removal of the disk provides the only remedy. Newer microscopic techniques and percutaneous (through the skin without cutting) disk removal have greatly shortened recovery time and reduced surgical complications.

Tendinitis

Tendinitis is an inflammation of a tendon (a band of fibrous tissue connecting muscle to bone). The condition appears most often as a result of physical activity. It can also, however, be a symptom of a more generalized inflammatory disease, such as rheumatoid arthritis.

Causes

Improper activity, lack of conditioning, and poor athletic equipment encourage the development of tendinitis. Nonathletes who suddenly begin long-distance jogging or another athletic activity and athletes who resume strenuous sports after a period of inactivity are especially susceptible. In addition, people who wear shoes with run-down heels put needless tension on the Achilles tendon, which joins the two major muscles on the back of the leg to the back of the heel bone. Similarly, women who wear high-heel shoes may have problems with inflamed Achilles tendons because the stress created by the shoes considerably strains the tendons.

Symptoms

Tendinitis causes pain in the affected tendon, which is worsened by activity. The tendon may grow thicker than normal and

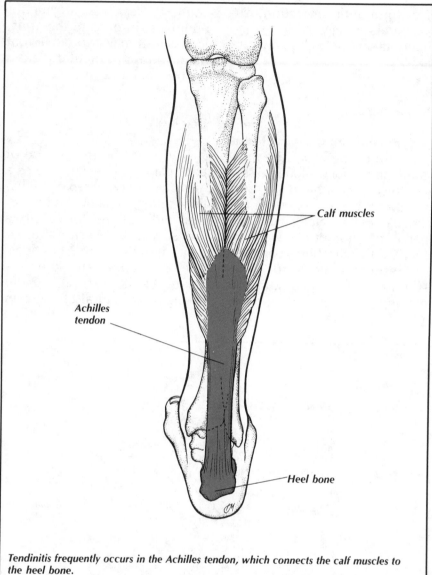

Tendinitis frequently occurs in the Achilles tendon, which connects the calf muscles to the heel bone.

be tender to the touch or very painful. When minor injuries are continually placed under stress, an already inflamed tendon can rupture and become a greater problem.

Diagnosis

Physicians diagnose tendinitis by acquiring an exercise history to determine the patient's normal activity and to identify changes in routine. Muscle lengths in the area of inflammation are also evaluated because unusually short or inflexible muscles are often the cause of tendinitis.

Treatment

Treatment for tendinitis begins with resting the affected area. Pain relievers and anti-inflammatory drugs are used to ease immediate symptoms, but they will not by themselves cure the condition or keep it from recurring.

Injecting cortisone and a local anesthetic into the area surrounding the tendon usually provides substantial relief within 24 to 72 hours. In rare cases, surgery is necessary to repair damaged tendons.

Prevention

People participating in sports can prevent tendinitis by warming up prior to exercise. For example, stretching the leg and calf muscles before and after running may help prevent inflammation of the Achilles tendon.

Wearing supports in shoes during physical activity can correct instability of the foot and lessen pain when tendinitis does occur.

Trichinosis

Trichinosis is a condition caused by the infestation of the body by *Trichinella spiralis,* a parasitic worm sometimes found in pork.

Cause

Trichinosis is most commonly caused by eating pork that has not been cooked for a sufficient length of time or at a sufficiently high temperature to kill the *Trichinella spiralis* worms. The worms are encapsulated in the meat itself. When the meat is eaten, the worms emerge from it and begin their life cycle in the human host. This begins in the small intestine, where the larvae (an immature form of the worms) mature within two days after they emerge from the meat. The adults breed, the males die, and the females produce more larvae, which invade the tissues of the bowel and are then dispersed to muscles throughout the body, where they lodge. The muscles around the eyes, the tongue, and the diaphragm (the muscle separating the chest cavity from the abdomen) and the muscles between the ribs are the most commonly affected.

Symptoms

Quite often, the infested patient is entirely unaware of the presence of trichinosis. When large infestations do occur, however, they are accompanied by symptoms. One to two days after consumption of the contaminated meat, a severe flulike illness consisting of fever, nausea, vomiting, diarrhea, and abdominal pain occurs. Tenderness and swelling around the infested muscles are common. After about a week, rash, swelling of the eyelids, and neurologic disorders may develop. Myocarditis (inflammation of the heart muscle) can also occur at this stage. Eventually the larvae in the muscles die and become calcified. Symptoms gradually disappear within a few months.

Treatment

Since there is no way to get the larvae out of the muscles, treatment is aimed at relief of discomfort. Analgesics, such as aspirin, are administered for pain, and anti-inflammatory steroids (cortisone drugs, such as prednisone) are administered for allergic symptoms, myocarditis, and central nervous system involvement. Thiabendazole (which tends to kill worms such as the *Trichinella*) is often given with good results. A close watch is kept for fever, abdominal pain, vomiting, and dermatitis (skin inflammation).

Prevention

The only preventive is to make sure that pork is sufficiently cooked (to an internal temperature of at least 170°F) to kill the larvae.

THE EYES AND VISION

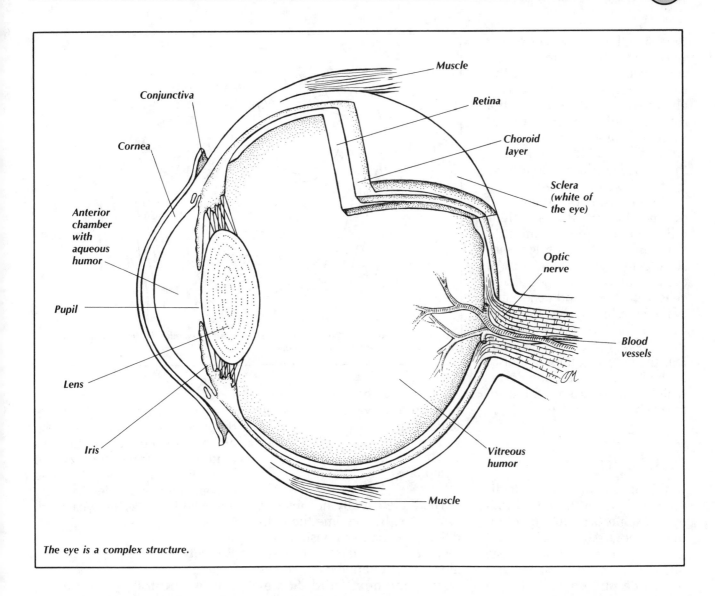

The eye is a complex structure.

The eye is the organ of sight. This complex structure works by capturing light and transforming it into impulses that the brain can interpret as images.

To understand visual perception, it is important to know the functions of the parts of the eye. The eye includes the eyeball and all structures within and surrounding its almost spherical mass. This delicate organ is nestled within the bony socket of the skull. A layer of fat cushions the socket; and the eyebrow, eyelashes, and eyelid provide a barrier against incoming irritants. Lining the inside of the eyelid

and continuing over the exposed surface of the eyeball is the conjunctiva, a thin protective membrane. Tears released from the lacrimal glands in the upper eyelid moisten the conjunctiva and keep the eye clean. The sclera is the tough, white, outer layer of the eyeball. The sclera covers the entire eyeball, except for the circular area in front that admits light, which is covered by the transparent cornea. The choroid layer contains blood vessels that nourish the eye.

Light enters the eye through the cornea. The curved cornea helps to focus the light inward.

Behind the cornea is a pigmented (colored) structure called the iris. The iris surrounds an opening known as the pupil. The iris changes the size of the pupil, depending on the amount of light present in the environment: If the surroundings are relatively dark, the pupil is enlarged to admit more light; if the environment is bright, the pupil is made smaller. Behind the iris is the lens, a transparent structure held in place by elastic, muscular-type tissue. The tissue can change the shape of the lens to accommodate the available light and to finely focus the incoming light rays onto the light-sensitive cells that line the back of the eye.

Between the cornea and the lens is a space, the anterior chamber, which is filled with a fluid called aqueous humor. Aqueous humor contains nutrients that nourish the cornea and the lens. The fluid also allows light rays to pass through easily.

The chamber of the eyeball behind the lens holds a clear jelly called vitreous humor. In the retina (the layer of light-sensitive cells that lines the back of the eyeball) are the specialized cells, called rods and cones, that convert light focused from the cornea and lens into electrical impulses. Sensitive nerve endings then transmit these impulses to the brain via the optic nerve, which extends from the rear of the eyeball to the brain.

Amblyopia

Amblyopia is the name for diminished vision in one or both eyes, usually without any obvious defect. (Amblyopia is not the same as nearsightedness, farsightedness, or astigmatism, which can be corrected with eyeglasses or contact lenses.)

There are two main types of amblyopia: "lazy-eye" amblyopia and toxic amblyopia.

LAZY-EYE AMBLYOPIA

Lazy-eye amblyopia occurs frequently in young children whose eyes do not line up correctly (a condition known as strabismus). To prevent double vision (in which the patient sees two images of everything), the brain suppresses the sight of one eye; the other eye does all the work. The brain structures dependent on the eye that is not working

Lazy-eye amblyopia may be corrected by using a patch to hinder the vision in the good eye, thus forcing the lazy eye to work.

may atrophy (waste away) or fail to develop.

Symptoms

There are usually no obvious symptoms. By the time the condition is recognized, vision may be permanently damaged. Usually, the child appears to see as well as the next child. Sometimes, however, the condition that causes the amblyopia is very noticeable: the eyes may turn either inward or outward, or one eye may be looking up while the other is looking down.

Treatment

To fully restore sight in the lazy eye, treatment must begin before the child is four to six years of age. If the eyes are out of focus because some of the muscles of the eye are weaker than others, the condition may be corrected by wearing special glasses or contact lenses, by

doing eye exercises, by using eye drops or a patch to diminish the ability of the normal eye to focus (and thereby force the lazy eye to work), or by surgery. Periodic reexaminations are needed until the child is at least ten years old.

Prevention

Prevention can begin soon after birth. If the eyes of a baby are continually out of alignment in the first weeks of life or are still out of alignment from time to time at six months of age, the condition should be investigated. A simple eye test given in the doctor's office should show whether one eye is not working properly. Evaluation should not be delayed. The child will not "grow out" of either strabismus or amblyopia.

TOXIC AMBLYOPIA

Toxic amblyopia, which usually occurs in both eyes, can result from excessive drinking of alcoholic beverages over a long period of time (and may be due mainly to the poor nutrition of heavy drinkers, who get most of their calories from alcohol and so do not eat enough nourishing food). It may also be found in heavy cigarette smokers and in people exposed to various chemicals and drugs, including lead, methanol (wood alcohol), digitalis, chloramphenicol, and arsenic. The toxic substance causes swelling and irritation of the optic nerve around the site where it leaves the eyeball. If the irritation continues, it can cause lasting damage to the nerve and even total blindness.

Symptoms

Symptoms include pain on moving the eyeball and an increasing area of poor eyesight in or near the center of the field of vision.

Treatment

Treatment is to stop exposure to the poison, if it can be discovered. In the case of lead poisoning, the patient is given medicine that combines with the lead and draws it out of the body tissues (this treatment is known as chelation therapy). If the cause is removed at once, vision may improve—unless there has been permanent damage to the optic nerve.

Astigmatism

Astigmatism is a type of distorted vision caused by a defect in the curvature of the cornea or lens of the eye. This prevents the rays of light entering the eye

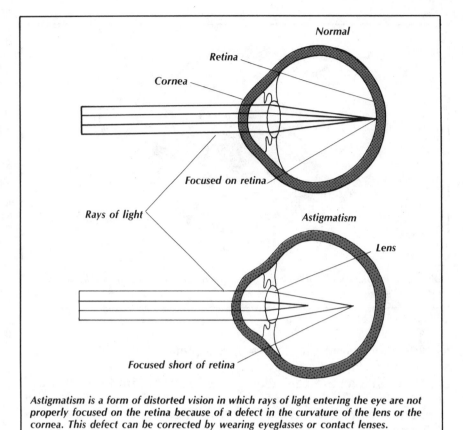

Astigmatism is a form of distorted vision in which rays of light entering the eye are not properly focused on the retina because of a defect in the curvature of the lens or the cornea. This defect can be corrected by wearing eyeglasses or contact lenses.

from being properly focused onto the retina at the back of the eyeball. Some rays are misplaced, causing the image to be partially out of focus.

Types

Most people with astigmatism can see clearly those objects that are directly in front of them, but their peripheral vision is defective. They may have vertical astigmatism, in which the areas that are above and below their direct gaze are imperfectly visualized. They may have horizontal astigmatism, in which the right and left sides of their field of vision are warped (for example, a straight horizontal line may appear to be curved to the right and to the left). The astigmatism may also be diagonal.

Treatment

Fortunately, a defect in the curvature of the cornea or lens is usually uniform and can be easily corrected by eyeglasses or contact lenses. The fault is usually in the shape of the cornea (the clear "window" in front of the iris and pupil of the eye), which may be slightly flattened vertically or horizontally. The eyeglass lenses or contact lenses are curved to adjust the angle of rays entering regions of the eye that are defective; they do not bend the rays entering the areas of clear vision.

Although most people with astigmatism were born with a tendency toward the condition, a few cases are caused by eye disease or injury. These may be more difficult to correct. Regardless of the cause, astigmatism—

Blepharitis is inflammation of the edges of the eyelids. Scales, crusts, or shallow ulcers may develop.

as with any vision problem—should be corrected as early as possible. Children, in particular, are at risk for development of permanently defective vision if astigmatism goes uncorrected.

Blepharitis

Blepharitis is an inflammation of the edges of the eyelids, with redness and thickening. Scales and crusts or shallow ulcers may also appear. The disease is common, especially in children, and often affects the upper and lower lids of both eyes.

Causes

Infection of eyelash follicles and oil glands by *Staphylococcus* bacteria causes blepharitis with ulcers. The nonulcerous variety may be due to an allergic reaction, or it may be linked to seborrheic dermatitis, an inflammatory scaling of the scalp, eyebrows, and sometimes ears. The nonulcerous form is occasionally caused by lice, which irritate lid margins.

Symptoms

Symptoms include itching, burning, "red-rimmed" eyes; lid swelling; loss of eyelashes; and irritation of the underside of the lid, as if sand were underneath. The eyes may tear and be sensitive to light. In ulcerous blepharitis, the tough, dry crusts that form leave a bleeding surface when removed. In nonulcerous blepharitis, greasy, easily removed scales appear on the edges of the lids.

Treatment

Blepharitis caused by a bacterial infection can be treated with an antibiotic ointment, such as erythromycin or bacitracin, that is specially formulated for use around the eyes. The medication is usually applied three times a day to the eyelash margins with a cotton-tipped swab, after the margins have been softened with warm compresses for ten minutes and the crusts have been removed. Medicated eye drops may also be used to combat irritation or other types of infection.

If an allergy to a cosmetic is the cause, its use should be discontinued. If there is scaling on the eyebrows and scalp due to seborrheic dermatitis, the doctor is likely to recommend a special shampoo, such as a sulfur or tar shampoo, for control of dandruff and to prescribe a cortisone lotion or cream to be rubbed into hairy areas. Careful attention to cleanliness of hair, scalp, eyebrows, and eyelid margins is necessary during treatment.

If the blepharitis is caused by head lice, the nits (lice eggs) should be carefully removed with tweezers, and steps should be taken to keep the patient free of lice (see page 119).

Both of the principal varieties are difficult to cure and often recur. Nonulcerous blepharitis causes no permanent damage. However, ulcerous blepharitis, if it recurs often enough, can cause scarring of eyelids, loss of eyelashes, and even ulcers of the cornea.

Prevention

Meticulous cleanliness may help prevent the disease. If it is treated promptly when it occurs, permanent damage can probably be prevented.

Cataract

A cataract is a clouding of the lens of the eye that results in obscured vision. People with this defect see their environment as if they were looking through a waterfall.

Normally, the lens is clear. Its function is to focus light onto the retina (the layer of light-sensitive cells lining the back of the eye), so that objects at various distances can be seen clearly. If the

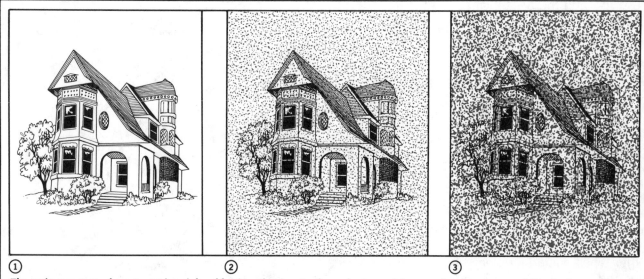

The main symptom of a cataract is painless blurring of vision. In the early stage, vision may be close to normal (1). As the condition progresses, vision gradually worsens (2) and eventually becomes extremely blurred (3).

lens becomes hazy, however, incoming light is scattered, and vision blurs.

Causes

The exact cause of cataracts is unknown. Aging may play a role, but the condition also occurs in newborns whose mothers contracted German measles during pregnancy and in other young persons.

Diabetes, glaucoma, and detachment of the retina may lead to cataracts. Injury to the lens, prolonged use of certain drugs, and high doses of radiation (for example, from prolonged exposure to X rays) may also trigger the condition.

Although the condition is usually curable, cataracts can cause blindness. In addition, the shadowy lens prohibits a clear view of the interior of the eye. Because of this obstruction, a physician may not be able to detect other potentially serious eye disorders, such as changes in the retina and damage to the optic nerve (which

transmits information from the eye to the brain).

Symptoms

The main symptom of cataracts is painless blurring of vision, occurring most often in only one eye. During the initial stages of development, cataracts can cause the person to experience glare in bright light, since the clouded lens scatters, rather than focuses, incoming light. As the condition progresses, the lens becomes milky white, and vision worsens.

Treatment

Successful treatment begins with surgical removal of the affected lens. With the aid of a microscope, the surgeon opens an area in the front of the eye and removes the lens. The use of local anesthetic eye drops makes the procedure relatively painless.

After the patient has recuperated for a few weeks, special

cataract eyeglasses or a contact lens can be prescribed to help correct the vision. These aids are by no means perfect and require an adjustment period. Another option, one that most doctors now recommend, is the implantation of an intraocular lens in the eye after cataract removal. The lightweight plastic lens is relatively free of distortion. It affords vision that is closer to normal than cataract eyeglasses or contact lenses can provide because it occupies the exact position of the natural lens. This lens allows vision without the use of special cataract lenses, although eyeglasses may still be necessary. Not everyone, however, can benefit from an intraocular lens.

In the vast majority of cases, surgery for cataracts is without complications. Restoration or substantial improvement of vision results after surgery in the majority of cases. If vision remains unimproved, a disorder that was not detected due to the presence of the cataract may be the cause. Generally, however, cataracts can be removed successfully, and the patient can resume a normal life.

Color blindness

Color blindness is an inability to distinguish certain colors. By far the most common type is inherited red-green color blindness, which affects 8 percent of men and boys but only 0.5 percent of women and girls. Total color blindness, which is very rare, and pastel-shade color blindness are believed to be inherited. Other types, including blue-yellow and red-green color blindness, can be either inherited or acquired. Disease or injury affecting the retina sometimes causes color blindness.

Description

Color blindness results from a defect in the cone-shaped light-sensitive cells of the fovea (the tiny pit in the macula, or central part of the retina, that is the center for perceiving color). The 7 million cone cells differ from the 130 million rod-shaped cells in the rest of the retina in that, while the rod cells register only black and white, the cone cells contain pigments for red, green, and blue—the colors that can combine to produce all the colors of the spectrum. The pigments become more vivid or fade in response to colors that the eye sees. The changes in pigmentation produce tiny flashes of electricity, which are carried by means of the optic nerve to the visual center of the brain. There, the electrical signals are combined into a full-color picture. In the color-blind person, for unknown reasons, cones are missing or defective. No cure is known.

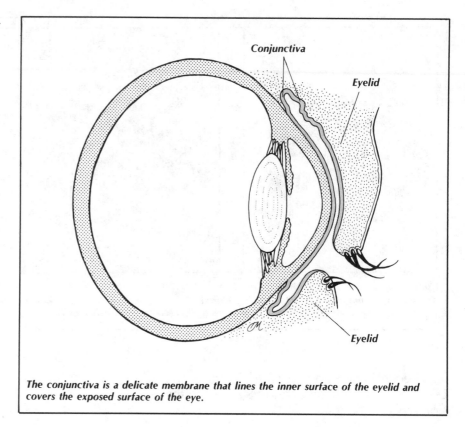

The conjunctiva is a delicate membrane that lines the inner surface of the eyelid and covers the exposed surface of the eye.

Inheriting red-green color blindness

Why is red-green color blindness inherited by boys more often than by girls? The reason is that the defective gene, which directs production of the defective pigment, is carried on the X sex chromosome. In a female child (who has two X sex chromosomes), a defective gene on one X chromosome is almost always counteracted by a normal gene on the other X chromosome; as a result, the girl is born with normal color vision. In a male child (who has an X and a Y sex chromosome), there is no matching normal gene to block the defect on the only X chromosome the boy has; the boy is, therefore, born color-blind.

Red-green color blindness cannot be passed from a father to his sons, nor will his daughters be color-blind, unless the mother carries the defective gene. However, his daughters will all be carriers of the defective gene, and the daughters' sons will have a 50 percent chance of being color-blind.

Conjunctivitis

Conjunctivitis, or pinkeye, is an inflammation of the conjunctiva. The conjunctiva is a delicate membrane that lines the inner surface of the eyelid and covers the exposed surface of the eye.

Causes

Most cases of conjunctivitis result from disease-causing microorganisms such as bacteria and viruses. Allergies, chemicals, dust, smoke, and foreign objects that irritate the conjunctiva may also lead to conjunctivitis. Swimming may also be associated with conjunctivitis, due to exposure to chlorine in a pool or to contaminated water. Occasionally, a sexually transmitted disease can cause pinkeye if the eyes are rubbed after the hands have touched infected genital organs.

Children are most often affected by conjunctivitis. Measles, a viral disease, may be accompanied by this eye inflammation. In addition, those people, both children and adults, who have allergies, such as hay fever, or who work and live in areas where they are exposed to chemicals or other irritants are more susceptible to noninfectious conjunctivitis.

If fluid collects between the retina and the underlying choroid, the retina may become partially or totally detached. Fluid from the vitreous cavity may penetrate beneath the retina through a small hole in the retina.

Symptoms

Conjunctivitis may cause redness, a grating sensation, burning, itching, and light sensitivity. Occasionally, tearing occurs, or a discharge containing pus will be present. Symptoms can last a few days or up to two weeks.

Conjunctivitis usually produces no permanent damage. However, if left untreated, the infection may lead to more serious eye problems. Ulcers (eroded areas) may form on the cornea (the clear "window" in front of the iris and pupil of the eye). If these ulcers persist, they can scar the eye and interfere with vision.

Treatment

Treatment depends on the cause and resulting symptoms of the conjunctivitis. If the inflammation is environmentally caused, simply removing the irritant may be sufficient to eliminate the condition. For more difficult cases, a physician may prescribe antibiotic, steroid, or combination eye drops to be used several times a day as directed. Frequent use is necessary because the drops tend to be washed away by the natural cleansing action of the tears.

Sensitive eyes should be rested and shielded from bright lights. When the discharge glues the eyelids closed, bathing them with warm water and wiping with a clean cloth will loosen them.

A most important fact about conjunctivitis is that its infectious form is highly contagious. Individuals with infectious conjunctivitis should not share handkerchiefs, towels, or washcloths and should be careful to avoid touching the unaffected eye after contact with the infected eye.

Detached retina

Normally, the retina is firmly attached to the choroid, an underlying layer of tissue that is rich in blood vessels. If blood or other fluid collects between the retina and the choroid, the retina may become partially or totally detached. Fluid from the vitreous cavity (the fluid-filled space behind the lens) may penetrate beneath the retina because of a small hole in the retina. Fluid leaking out of certain blood vessels in the eye may also penetrate beneath the retina to cause detachment.

Causes

Cataract surgery, severe myopia (nearsightedness), and injury can cause retinal detachment. Although injury can be the primary cause of this condition, it is more likely to accelerate a detachment that has already begun. Conditions that increase an individual's susceptibility to retinal detachment are inflammation or tumors of the eye, hypertension (high blood pressure); and vitreous hemorrhaging.

Symptoms

Initial symptoms include seeing floating dark spots or flashes or streaks of light and experiencing blurring of vision. As the condition progresses, a curtain or veil seems to fall over part or all of the field of vision.

Treatment

A detached retina can be treated by using a laser to fuse the retina to the choroid. It can also be treated by diathermy (repair using heat), cryotherapy (repair using extreme cold), or microsurgery. Left untreated, the detachment may increase and lead to the loss of sight.

Glaucoma

Glaucoma is an eye disorder caused by increased pressure within the eyeball, which builds up because fluids are unable to drain normally.

Cause

Although glaucoma is understood to be a problem with the fluid-regulating mechanism of the eye, its precise cause is unknown. In the healthy eye, aqueous fluid in the chamber between the lens and cornea is under a slight degree of pressure. If the fluid balance changes, internal pressure rises in the eye. This buildup produces damage to the structures and nerve endings within the eye.

Forms of glaucoma

Depending on the type of defect in the fluid-regulating system, one of two primary forms of glaucoma results. *Chronic,* or *open angle, glaucoma* develops when pressure is elevated gradually, and normal fluid drainage slows but is not obstructed at the drainage angle (the network of tissue between the iris and the cornea, through which fluid can normally pass). *Acute,* or *closed angle, glaucoma* occurs when pressure mounts suddenly and forces the iris into contact with the cornea, thereby blocking fluid drainage from the anterior chamber of the eye.

Those at risk

Both forms of glaucoma are more common in adults over 40 years of age. Statistics indicate that people with a family history of glaucoma have a greater risk of acquiring the condition, but inheritance has not been proved. Some evidence suggests that glaucoma may be linked to long-term use of certain drugs, especially steroids, which can alter body fluid levels. Glaucoma can also follow other eye disorders, such as infections and cataracts.

Symptoms

Chronic glaucoma begins with no noticeable symptoms. Vision deterioration is so gradual and painless that this form of glaucoma has been termed the "sneak thief of sight." Sometimes, loss of peripheral vision slowly progresses as central vision remains normal. As the disorder advances, other symptoms (which may be intermittent or constant) include foggy or

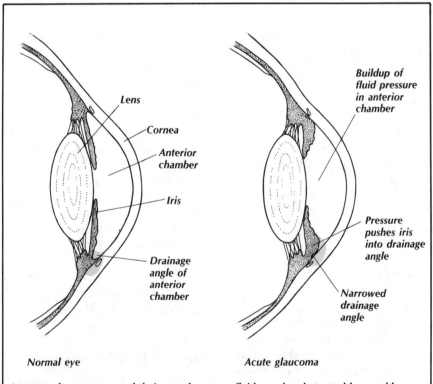

Lens

Cornea

Anterior chamber

Iris

Drainage angle of anterior chamber

Buildup of fluid pressure in anterior chamber

Pressure pushes iris into drainage angle

Narrowed drainage angle

Normal eye

Acute glaucoma

In acute glaucoma, normal drainage of aqueous fluid may be obstructed by a sudden elevation of pressure within the anterior chamber of the eye, which pushes the iris into the angle where the iris meets the cornea.

①　②　③

Normal vision (1) will deteriorate gradually if glaucoma is not treated. Loss of peripheral vision may slowly progress as central vision remains normal (2). Untreated glaucoma can lead to partial or complete vision loss (3).

blurred vision, difficulty in adjusting to brightness and darkness, and slight pain in or around the eye, usually on one side. The one symptom indicative of chronic glaucoma is the perception of a halo surrounding a light, which is most easily visible when looking at a distant light while in the dark.

Acute glaucoma brings sudden and severe symptoms of extreme eye pain and abrupt vision blurring. Frequently, the pain can be so intense that it causes nausea and vomiting. Acute glaucoma is rare, but when it occurs, medical attention is needed immediately to prevent permanent blindness. Usually the symptoms are so severe that medical help is promptly sought.

Diagnosis

If left untreated, glaucoma can lead to partial or complete vision loss. However, if diagnosed early, treatment can usually halt the process. Because chronic glaucoma has no warning signs,

it is particularly important that persons over the age of 40 be tested for glaucoma every two or three years. In addition, physicians recommend that persons with a family history of the disease be screened every year beginning even before the age of 40.

Glaucoma testing is a relatively simple office procedure. The doctor uses a special device called a tonometer to measure the amount of pressure within the eyeball. The doctor also inspects the interior of the eye through an instrument that allows a view of the angle where the iris and the cornea meet. This part of the examination shows whether there is blockage in the drainage system or damage to the optic nerve. Peripheral vision is also tested by measuring the point at which objects enter the patient's field of vision.

Treatment

Glaucoma treatment is usually effective if started early in the

course of the disease. Oral drugs work by decreasing production of eye fluid, while daily applications of eye drops promote fluid drainage. Because some medications cause constriction of the pupils of the eyes, which can be misconstrued as a symptom of drug overdose, many glaucoma patients carry an identification card that describes their medical history in case of emergency.

Beta-blocker eye drops reduce production of eye fluid without altering the size of the pupil. However, beta blockers can affect the heart rate and cause narrowing of the breathing passages, which may make these drugs unsuitable for patients with heart or respiratory disease. Other antiglaucoma medications are available.

Although chronic glaucoma responds to medication, some patients (fewer than five percent) require surgery to open new pathways for fluid drainage. Laser therapy is a relatively new surgical technique under investigation. The laser uses an intense light beam to slightly modify tissues in the region in order to allow better fluid drainage.

Prevention

The best way to prevent serious complications of glaucoma is to undergo periodic screening for early diagnosis.

Keratitis

Keratitis is an inflammation of the cornea (the clear "window" in front of the iris and pupil of the eye), which commonly produces redness, tearing, tenderness, sensitivity to light, and blurred vision.

Interstitial keratitis

Interstitial keratitis is often caused by congenital (present at birth) syphilis in children or by tuberculosis. This type of keratitis produces deep deposits of scar tissue, which cause the cornea to become hazy and give it a ground-glass appearance. There is little that can be done for this condition, although the inflammation and redness usually diminish after a month or two. Vision may or may not be impaired thereafter.

Herpes simplex keratitis

A common type of keratitis is caused by the herpes simplex virus, the same virus that produces cold sores. Herpes simplex keratitis is usually not painful, although at first there is a sensation that foreign matter may be present. If the infection is left untreated, all feeling in the cornea will eventually be lost. Like a cold sore, the infection tends to

come and go, but it should be taken care of when the first sign—a whitish lesion on the cornea—appears. Treatment usually consists of applying eye drops or ointment, but some specialists prefer to scrape the cornea, after which they cover the affected eye temporarily.

Traumatic keratitis

Traumatic keratitis occurs when scar tissue remains after a corneal injury has healed. If a considerable amount of scar tissue covers the pupil, blindness may result. This condition can generally be cured by corrective surgery or corneal transplantation.

Macular degeneration

Macular degeneration is the deterioration of the macula (the yellowish depression in the central part of the retina of the eye). The macula is the part of the eye with the greatest density

of visual receptor cells. As light enters the eye, the image that is focused on the macula is the one that is most clearly perceived in the brain. The function of the macula is to distinguish fine detail in the central visual field. Consequently, degeneration of the macula leads to blurring of central vision; peripheral (side) vision remains intact.

Causes

The exact cause of macular degeneration is unknown. In many cases, the deterioration of the cells in the macula may be a result of another disorder, atherosclerosis, which causes a narrowing of the blood vessels, including those that supply the macula with blood. In these cases, the macula "wastes away." This form is often referred to as the "dry" form. In another less common form of the disease, tiny blood vessels proliferate around the macula and leak blood or fluid, causing blurred or distorted central vision. This is often called the "wet" form of macular degeneration.

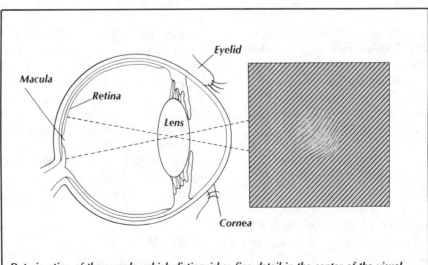

Deterioration of the macula, which distinguishes fine detail in the center of the visual field, causes blurring of central vision.

Symptoms

Macular degeneration, in its dry form, usually develops slowly and painlessly; the blurring of central vision is gradual. In the wet form, the blurring and loss of central vision may occur much more rapidly.

If both eyes are affected—as is almost always the case—activities requiring sharp vision, such as driving, usually have to be curtailed. Eventually, all central vision disappears, although side vision is unaffected.

Treatment

There was no treatment for macular degeneration until recently. It has been found that some individuals who have the wet form may be helped by treatment with laser beams if the treatment is initiated early in the disease process, before significant damage to the eyesight has occurred. There is no treatment for the dry form, although early in the course of the condition, vision may be improved by special powerful eyeglasses.

Myopia

Myopia, or nearsightedness, is a common optical defect in which close objects can be seen clearly but faraway objects look blurred. About one in every five persons is myopic. The condition tends to be hereditary, developing around age 12 and progressing until about age 20.

Cause

The optical defect occurs if the eyeball is too long from front to back. Normally, the cornea (the

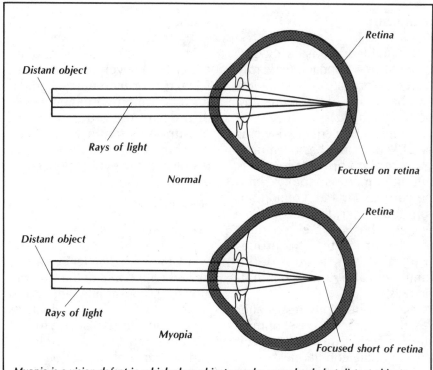

Myopia is a vision defect in which close objects can be seen clearly but distant objects appear blurred. This defect occurs if the eyeball is too long from front to back, which causes incoming light from distant objects to fall short of the retina.

clear "window" in front of the iris and pupil of the eye) and the lens (the disk-shaped structure just behind the front of the eye) refract (bend) light coming from a viewed distant object so that the image of the object is focused on the retina (the layer of specialized, light-sensitive cells that line the back of the eyeball). In myopia, however, the focused image falls short of the retina because of the greater length of the eyeball, resulting in a fuzzy image.

Types

There are several kinds of myopia. *Curvature myopia* occurs when there is an excessive curve of the refractive (light-bending) surfaces of the eye, which causes light to enter the eye in an abnormal path. The curvature is in

the front surface of either the cornea or the lens. In *index myopia,* there is an increase in the light-refracting properties of the lens. It is sometimes associated with future development of cataracts or iritis (inflammation of the iris). *Progressive myopia* is an uncommon form in which the eyeball continues to elongate throughout a person's life, eventually leading to degeneration or detachment of the retina.

Diagnosis

Blurred or fuzzy vision should be evaluated by an ophthalmologist (a physician who specializes in eye disorders), who will look inside the eyes with a special instrument called an ophthalmoscope, diagnose any disorders, and test the acuity (sharpness) of vision.

Treatment

Nearsightedness is easily corrected with a concave (inwardly curved) lens that pushes the images back toward the retina and focuses them clearly.

A surgical procedure known as radial keratotomy has been used to correct myopia. It involves cutting numerous "spokes" into the corneal surface, coming out from the center; the cornea flattens as it heals, which counteracts the problem. This procedure, however, is considered controversial by many ophthalmologists.

Myopia rarely progresses after age 30. In fact, the onset of middle age sometimes lessens the severity of the condition.

Night blindness

Night blindness, or nyctalopia, is a condition in which a person can see well in good light but not in dim or fading light.

The retina contains a layer of photoreceptors (specialized, light-sensitive cells) that lines the interior of the eyeball. These photoreceptors make the adjustments that are responsible for adaptation to varying degrees of light. There are two types of photoreceptors—cones and rods. Cones, concentrated in the center of the retina (the region called the macula), distinguish fine detail and color, while rods, which predominate around the edges of the retina, are sensitive to the intensity of light and do most of the work of seeing in dim light. Rods contain the pigment rhodopsin, or visual purple, which becomes temporarily bleached by bright light. The speed at which rhodopsin adjusts to darkness depends on a sufficient supply of vitamin A in the body.

Causes

Night blindness is caused either by a severe deficiency of vitamin A or by retinitis pigmentosa, an inherited degenerative disorder of the retina. In cases of extreme vitamin A shortage, the cornea may soften or start to dissolve or the eyes may become excessively dry.

Treatment

A vitamin A deficiency can be treated with doses of the vitamin. However, consuming large doses of vitamin A without a doctor's recommendation and without documentation of a deficiency can be extremely dangerous.

Prevention

The only preventive step is to obtain enough dietary vitamin A (for example, from liver, egg yolks, yellow and dark green vegetables, butter, and cream).

Nystagmus

Nystagmus is the involuntary, rhythmic, and rapid movement of the eyeballs in a horizontal, vertical, or rotary direction. The eye movements of a person who sits in a moving vehicle and watches the scenery flashing by are an example of normal nystagmus.

Abnormal nystagmus

Abnormal nystagmus is brought on by one of three problems: defective vision, such that the eye does not receive enough stimulation to concentrate on one object; disturbances in the elaborate mechanisms in the inner ear responsible for balance; and diseases of the nervous system, especially those affecting the parts of the brain responsible for eye movement and coordination. Generally, the only symptoms of abnormal nystagmus are double vision, vertigo, and dizziness. Treatment depends on the underlying cause.

Retinitis

Retinitis is an inflammation of the retina, the light-sensitive innermost lining of the eye.

Types and causes

There are several types of retinitis. *Toxoplasmic retinitis,* which may be either acquired or congenital (present at birth), is caused by a microorganism. If the condition is congenital, the microorganism was passed to the fetus through the placenta (the temporary organ in the uterus that nourishes the fetus during development). A similar type of retinitis is caused by a blood-borne infection that settles in the eye. *Exudative retinitis* stems from unknown causes, but may result in detachment of the retina from the internal surface of the eyeball. *Retinitis pigmentosa* is an inherited disorder in which excessive amounts of a substance called phytanic acid accumulate and cause extensive damage to the retina. This form of retinitis also usually accompanies a disorder called Refsum's syndrome (see page 90).

Symptoms

The symptoms of retinitis pigmentosa are night blindness, inflammation of the retina, marked limitation of the field of vision (tunnel vision), loss of kinesthetic sense (sense of body movement), shrinkage of the retina, clumping of retinal pigment, and dislodging of the blood vessels of the retina. Many of the same symptoms are found in the other forms of retinitis. They are sometimes accompanied by cloudiness of the vitreous humor (the liquid that fills the cavity behind the lens of the eyeball). This can be detected by a physician examining the interior of the eye with a special lighted instrument called an ophthalmoscope.

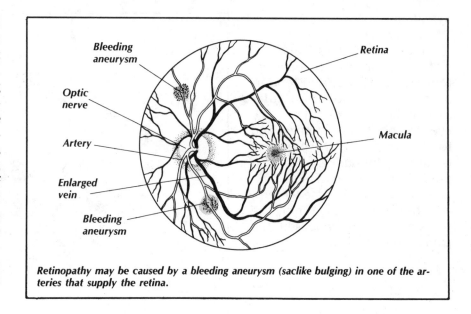

Retinopathy may be caused by a bleeding aneurysm (saclike bulging) in one of the arteries that supply the retina.

Treatment

In the case of retinitis pigmentosa, there is little that can be done. If the retina is detached (a condition often caused when a hole in the retina allows fluid to seep into the eye and create a pocket), surgery is usually the treatment. The pocket is eliminated either by freezing or by heat, sometimes with a laser. If retinitis is the result of blood-borne infection, that condition must be treated first.

Prevention

Other than genetic counseling for persons who have a family history of retinitis pigmentosa, there are no clear-cut preventive measures that can be taken to prevent retinitis.

Retinopathy

Retinopathy is a condition in which deterioration of the retina is caused by damage to or over-production of the blood vessels in that structure.

Causes

The vast majority of cases of retinopathy are due to diabetes. Although fewer than five percent of all diabetics completely lose their sight because of retinopathy, diabetes is one of the leading causes of irreversible blindness today. Other conditions that increase susceptibility to retinopathy include high blood pressure; hemorrhaging due to sudden vessel blockage by a blood clot, fat globule, or cholesterol plaque; and chronic kidney failure.

If a sudden hemorrhage is triggered, total blindness in the eye can strike swiftly; immediate medical attention is necessary. In cases of retinopathy due to hypertension (high blood pressure) or diabetes, vision usually worsens over time.

Treatment

Hypertensive retinopathy is primarily treated by strict control of the blood pressure through diet and, in many cases, through the use of medication (depending on the severity of the condition). Diabetic retinopathy is also treated through diet and medication; if diabetic patients continually allow their glucose levels to exceed normal bounds, retinal damage can be extensive and may require laser treatments in order to seal off the leaking blood vessels of the retina.

Sty

A sty is an inflamed or infected swelling of the sebaceous (oil-producing) glands on the inner or outer surface in the eyelid.

Causes

The infection is commonly caused by *Staphylococcus* bacteria. An external sty appears on the surface of the skin at the edge of the eyelid. An internal sty is due to inflammation, infection, or obstruction of a sebaceous gland on the inner surface of the eyelid. This type of sty is often seen as a protrusion or lump on the eyelid without visible pus or redness.

Symptoms

Initially, a sty feels like a foreign object in the eye. Tearing, redness, swelling, and tenderness in or around a particular area of the eye soon follow. The eye may be sensitive to light and touch. In addition, pustules (small, yellow bumps filled with pus) may develop. These pustules often burst, release the pus, and begin to heal. Once the pressure has been released, the pain usually subsides.

Treatment

Treatment for a sty often involves antibiotic eye drops or ointments. Applying warm, moist compresses to the eye for about ten minutes three or four times a day may encourage the sty to burst. In some cases, particularly if there is an internal sty, surgical opening may be needed to cure the condition. One should never attempt to open a sty on his or her own, as the risks of spreading and worsening the infection are quite high.

A sty is an inflamed or infected swelling of the sebaceous (oil-producing) glands of the eyelid. An external sty appears on the surface of the skin at the edge of the eyelid.

EARS, NOSE, AND THROAT

The ear, nose, and throat are interconnected, and for this reason they are usually grouped together. Because they are joined, infection in one structure often spreads into one of the others.

Ears

The ear consists of three parts: the outer ear, the middle ear, and the inner ear.

The outer ear consists of the pinna, or external ear, which captures sound waves and directs them inward, and the ear canal, which leads to the eardrum. In the middle ear, sound waves vibrate through three tiny bones commonly called the hammer (malleus), the anvil (incus), and the stirrup (stapes). The vibrations continue into the inner ear, where a spiral structure called the cochlea transforms them into nerve impulses. These impulses are conveyed to the brain via the auditory nerve.

The eustachian tube in the middle ear connects the ear with the nasopharynx (the upper part of the throat). This tube allows the air pressure in the middle ear to equalize with the pressure outside the body, thus helping to prevent rupture of the eardrum. However, it also provides a passageway for infecting microorganisms to enter the middle ear from the nose or throat.

The semicircular canals (also called the labyrinth) within the inner ear serve as the organ of balance by detecting motion of the head and conveying this information to the brain.

Nose

The nose is a specialized structure that serves dual func-

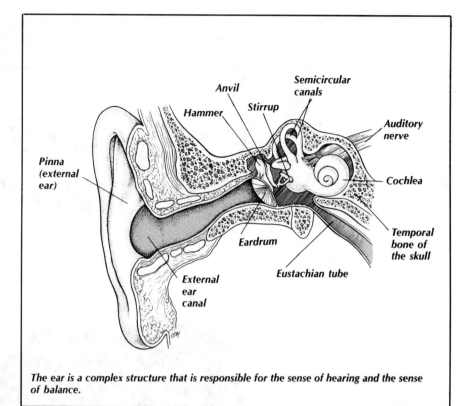

The ear is a complex structure that is responsible for the sense of hearing and the sense of balance.

tions as the organ for the sense of smell and as an entry to the respiratory tract.

Nerve receptor cells within the nose detect odors that enter via the nostrils and transmit signals to the brain through the olfactory nerve. The sense of smell also enhances the sense of taste. The ability to smell is more refined than the ability to taste; therefore, when a cold blocks nasal passages, food may seem bland and tasteless.

As part of the respiratory tract, the nose moisturizes and warms incoming air and filters out foreign materials. Small glands within the lining of the nose secrete mucus, a sticky substance that lubricates the walls of the nose and throat. Mucus humidifies the incoming air and traps bacteria, dust, and other particles entering the nose. Many bacteria are either dissolved by chemical elements in the mucus or trans-

ported to the entrance of the throat by tiny, hairlike structures called cilia. In the throat, bacteria are then swallowed and killed by acids and other chemicals produced in the stomach. This efficient line of defense protects the body against the billions of bacteria that continually enter the nose.

Connected to the nose are the sinuses—air-filled cavities lined with mucus-secreting glands that are located within certain facial bones. There are four groups of sinuses—frontal, sphenoidal, ethmoidal, and maxillary.

Throat

The throat, or pharynx, is a passageway connecting the back of the mouth and nose to the esophagus (the tube between the mouth and the stomach) and to the trachea, or windpipe (the tube between the mouth and the lungs). Because air and food pass through the throat, the throat is considered to be a part of both the respiratory and the digestive systems.

Three sections make up the five-inch throat tube. The nasopharynx is the upper part of the throat, which opens into the nose. The oropharynx is the middle portion, which opens into the mouth. The lower section of the throat, or laryngopharynx, connects the other sections with the larynx, or voice box.

Within the throat are two small, almond-shaped masses of lymphoid tissue called tonsils. Tonsils help fight disease by destroying bacteria that enter the throat.

Adenoids

Adenoids are masses of protective lymphoid tissue located in the lining of the nasopharynx. Like the tonsils located below them, the adenoids (technically known as the nasopharyngeal tonsils) are lymph nodes containing the specialized white blood cells that help localize and destroy harmful bacteria and viruses. They thus provide an important defense against diseases of the respiratory system.

Enlarged adenoids

It is normal for adenoids to become enlarged during throat infections, just as the tonsils do, and then to diminish in size after the infection has passed. Sometimes, however, as a result of continuing infection or allergies, the adenoids remain enlarged. The resulting obstruction of the nasal passage may cause mouth breathing, the characteristic

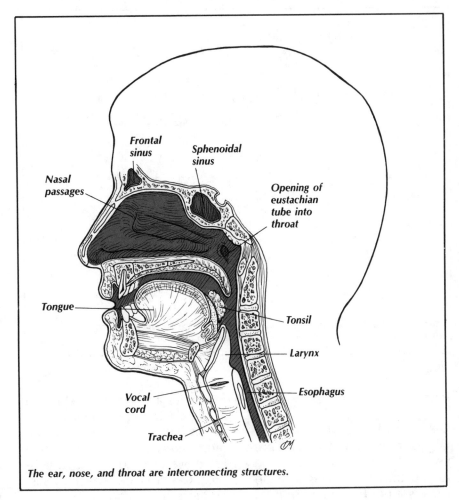

The ear, nose, and throat are interconnecting structures.

"nasal" voice, and continuing drainage of pus-filled mucus down the throat. It may also cause a blockage of the eustachian tubes, which connect the throat to the ears, resulting in retention of fluid in the middle ear, impaired hearing, earache, and recurring ear infections.

Treatment

Treatment is with antibiotics, taken by mouth. Surgery may be recommended when the infected or enlarged adenoids themselves are the source of the disease (usually the tonsils beneath are infected as well and are removed in the same operation). This would be the case if recurrent or continuing infection of the adenoids could not be eliminated with antibiotics, if the adenoids caused repeated ear infections, or if cancer or an abscess (a mass of pus in a cavity) was present. If chronically infected adenoids increase susceptibility to a serious condition, such as rheumatic fever or nephritis (a kidney disease), surgical removal of the adenoids may be recommended. However, surgery is generally not performed during an acute attack of tonsillitis, because it may worsen the infection.

Surgery may not be the answer to prevent snoring, mouth breathing, or the nasal voice caused by enlarged adenoids, since the enlargement usually diminishes after childhood.

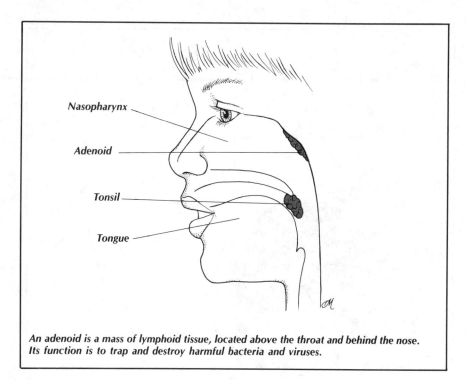

An adenoid is a mass of lymphoid tissue, located above the throat and behind the nose. Its function is to trap and destroy harmful bacteria and viruses.

Prevention

Adenoid infection and enlargement cannot always be prevented. In fact, enlarging in order to trap and fight infectious organisms is a normal function of the adenoids. Good general health measures can help, however, as can the use of antibiotics prescribed by a physician when the adenoids become infected and enlarged.

Common cold

A simple common cold is a collection of familiar symptoms signaling an infection of the upper respiratory tract, which includes the nose, throat, and sinuses.

Colds are self-limiting diseases, meaning that their symptoms last a certain length of time (or "run their course") and then disappear without leaving lasting ill effects. A cold is a mild but commonplace disease, contracted by adults about two to four times a year and by children about six to eight times a year. Adults with children at home are more likely to catch colds than are those who do not have children. Children are especially susceptible to colds because they have not yet developed immunity or resistance to the many viruses that can cause colds. Small children gradually build up immunity to the viruses in their homes; when they go to school and have close contact with many other children, they are exposed to new viruses. Similarly, adults who travel frequently or have a high number of close contacts outside their community are more likely to contract colds or encounter new cold viruses to which they are not immune than those leading more isolated lives.

Complications

A cold can be a minor irritation, but it can increase suscepti-bility to more serious conditions, especially in the very young, the very old, and the very weak. Pneumonia, an inflammation of the lungs, is probably the most serious. Ear infections, sinus infections, and bronchitis are other possible complications. A few days after a cold, children sometimes develop croup, recognized by a harsh, barking cough that signals swelling of the airways to the lungs.

Causes

At least five major categories of viruses cause colds. One of these groups, the rhinoviruses, includes a minimum of 100 different types of viruses. Various combinations of symptoms and possible complications can develop from each of these viruses. It is not known exactly how the viruses spread, but it seems to be a combination of physical contact and the presence of both virus particles and moisture in the air. A virus can be spread by hand-to-hand contact, for example, or by the passage of droplets from an infected person's nasal passages and throat into the air. Colds have an incubation period of 48 to 72 hours, meaning that it takes that long after the virus enters the body for early symptoms to appear.

Symptoms

Early symptoms of the common cold include a stuffy or runny nose, sneezing, a sore or scratchy throat, a cough, and occasionally a mild fever. Usually, as the cold progresses, other symptoms—burning or watery eyes, loss of the senses of taste or smell, pressure in the ears or sinuses, nasal voice, and ten-

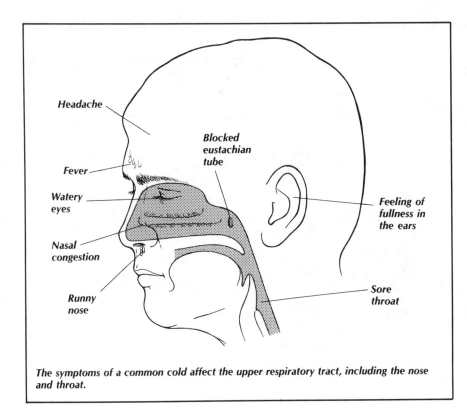

Headache

Blocked
eustachian
tube

Fever

Watery
eyes

Nasal
congestion

Runny
nose

Feeling of
fullness in
the ears

Sore
throat

The symptoms of a common cold affect the upper respiratory tract, including the nose and throat.

derness around the nose—may appear.

Symptoms vary in type and severity from one viral infection to another, so a cold can begin with any symptom or combination of symptoms. Most colds last about a week, but about 25 percent of all colds last two weeks. Smokers and those with chronic respiratory diseases tend to have more severe symptoms and longer-lasting colds and to experience complications more readily than do those who do not fall into these categories.

Diagnosis

Since common colds are mild diseases, the physician, in diagnosing a cold, will actually be looking for symptoms indicating a condition more serious than a common cold. Material from the patient's throat or nasal passages may be tested for bacterial infec-

tions. A blood test may be recommended to check for mononucleosis, a disease characterized by a long-lasting sore throat and swollen lymph nodes. An X-ray examination of the sinuses may be necessary if sinusitis (an infection of the sinuses) is suspected.

Treatment

Getting plenty of rest, drinking lots of fluids to prevent dehydration, and using a humidifier or vaporizer can help relieve the irritating symptoms of a cold. Nevertheless, the common cold cannot be cured, and no known treatment will actually hasten recovery. Many over-the-counter (nonprescription) medicines and preparations are available that will at least ease the discomfort of a cold. However, it is best to take specific medications only for the symptoms actually pre-

sent and to carefully follow directions on the medication package. Overuse of an otherwise effective remedy can backfire and actually make the symptoms worse, and treating symptoms that are not there can complicate matters. For example, the overuse of an antihistamine for nasal congestion can make a cough more uncomfortable, and the use of a nasal decongestant for more than three days can actually increase congestion (because the blood vessels tire and relax, causing rebound congestion). Anyone who is pregnant or has a chronic disease should check with a doctor before using cold preparations, even seemingly harmless over-the-counter drugs.

Prevention

There is no known preventive for the common cold. Vitamin C has been said to help prevent colds, but many studies have shown that it has no measurable effect in this regard. Avoiding exposure to viruses, when possible, may be the only means of avoiding the common cold.

Deafness

Deafness is a term used to describe complete or partial loss or absence of the ability to hear.

Types

There are three major types of deafness:

Conductive deafness is caused by a defect in the outer or middle ear, which prevents normal transmission of sound. It may be present at birth as the result of an inherited defect, an abnormality in development, or an infection

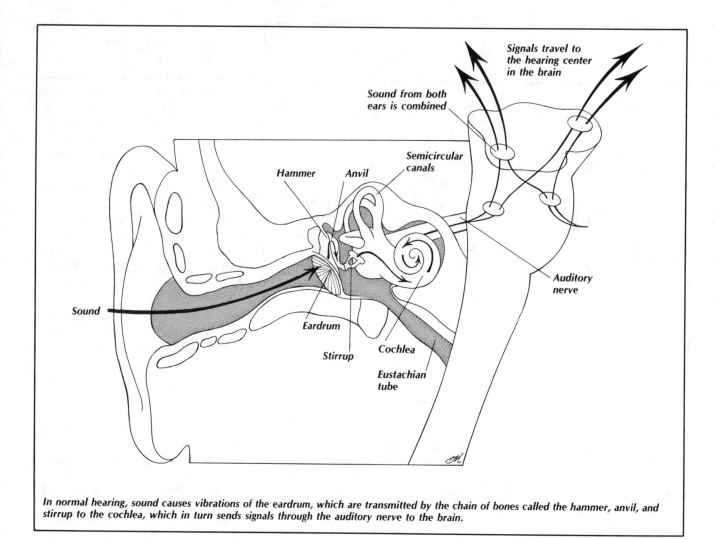

In normal hearing, sound causes vibrations of the eardrum, which are transmitted by the chain of bones called the hammer, anvil, and stirrup to the cochlea, which in turn sends signals through the auditory nerve to the brain.

of the fetus in the womb. It may be produced by an injury that perforates the eardrum or that breaks up the linkage of the three tiny bones—hammer, anvil, and stirrup—that normally transmit sound from the eardrum through the middle ear to the inner ear. Inflammation of the middle ear, a condition known as otitis media, is another important cause of conductive deafness. Infection from an upper respiratory tract ailment, such as strep throat or the flu, can produce a buildup of pus in the middle ear so great that it ruptures the eardrum. Also, a plugged eustachian tube (the tube leading from the back of the throat to the ear) may trap fluid in the middle ear, creating temporary deafness. Conductive deafness in the middle and later years is most often caused by otosclerosis. In this inherited condition, new spongy bone grows over the stirrup bone, preventing it from vibrating when sound travels to it through the hammer and anvil bones.

Sensorineural deafness is a type of hearing loss that occurs because of damage to the structures of the inner ear, to the auditory nerve carrying sound messages to the brain, or to the hearing center of the brain itself, located in the temporal lobe. It may be due to a head injury during birth, the effects of a woman's rubella infection on her unborn baby, a skull fracture affecting the inner ear or the auditory nerve, fever, bacterial or viral infections (such as mumps or meningitis), tertiary (final stage) syphilis, Meniere's disease, tumors, multiple sclerosis, a hemorrhage or blood clot in the inner ear, drug side effects, normal aging, prolonged or repeated exposure to intense noise, or edema (fluid buildup) caused by a thyroid deficiency. Most sensorineural deafness is not nerve deafness, the popular term for it. It is usually sensory deafness, caused by defects in the structure of the inner ear, especially in the cochlea and its organ of

Corti. The cochlea contains sensory cells that convert sound waves into electrical impulses, which are transmitted via the auditory nerve to the brain.

Mixed deafness is a relatively common condition. It is a combination of conductive and sensorineural deafness.

People with pure conductive deafness simply need louder volume to hear all sounds. Those with defects in the inner ear usually can hear low-pitched sounds more easily than high-pitched sounds, and some sounds may be distorted. When there is damage to the hearing center in the brain, the person may be able to hear sounds, but has trouble recognizing them and understanding words (this problem can also occur with the other types of deafness).

Diagnosis

When hearing loss is suspected, a complete examination of the ears, nose, and throat is necessary to identify infections or abnormalities that may be present. Infections of the adenoids or tonsils, as well as sinus or nasal infections, may be linked to ear infections.

Testing of hearing is important for all ages, but especially for infants. Many times, partial deafness in a baby is not discovered until the child fails to learn to talk, a direct result of the hearing loss. Babies who were born prematurely or ill or whose mothers had certain viral infections, such as rubella, during pregnancy are in special need of testing.

Treatment

Although inborn hearing defects usually cannot be cor- rected, deaf children can be helped to deal with their handicap. Starting very early, they can be fitted with hearing aids and can be instructed in lipreading, speaking, and sign language.

Surgery to correct conductive hearing loss includes operations to replace the stirrup bone or all three tiny bones with tissue or synthetic material, to repair a punctured eardrum, and to clean a chronically infected middle ear.

A hearing aid can often help to restore hearing. However, one should be purchased only after thorough testing by a specialist in audiometry, who can suggest the most appropriate type. Classes in lipreading and listening can also be helpful.

Prevention

It is far easier to prevent deafness than to cure it. Antibiotics have made it possible to eradicate most of the middle ear infections that have been the major source of conductive hearing loss in children. Middle ear problems are also sometimes eliminated by treating allergies that cause the eustachian tubes to close up or by removing infected adenoids. Nerve deafness caused by continued exposure to intense industrial noise, gunshots, rock music, or aircraft engines may be avoided by wearing earplugs or other ear protectors. Some lost hearing may return after several months of relief from intense sound. Medications that can cause hearing loss, including some antibiotics and certain diuretics (drugs that stimulate the production of urine), need to be used with caution, and signs of hearing loss should be brought to a doctor's attention as soon as they are noticed.

Glossitis

Glossitis is an acute (short-term) or chronic (long-term) inflammation of the tongue. It may exist either as a primary disease or as a symptom of another disease or disorder.

Causes

The causes of glossitis can be either local or systemic (affecting the entire body). Local causes include immediate irritants, such as jagged or broken teeth, badly fitting dentures, poor oral hygiene habits, biting of the tongue (such as during convulsions), and external irritants, such as alcohol, tobacco, hot or spicy foods, and even mouthwashes, toothpastes, and breath fresheners. Local infections, burns, and injuries may also produce symptoms of glossitis. Systemic causes may include certain vitamin deficiencies (especially vitamin B deficiencies, such as pellagra), anemia, syphilis, and generalized skin diseases.

Symptoms

Symptoms vary widely, ranging from simple redness of the tip and edges of the tongue (if the cause is pellagra, anemia, or irritation from smoking or a tooth with a rough surface) to painful ulcers and whitish patches. In the later stages of pellagra, the entire tongue may be fiery red, swollen, and ulcerated. In iron deficiency and pernicious anemia, the tongue is pale and smooth. Painful ulcers on the tongue may indicate a number of diseases, including herpes, tuberculosis, and streptococcal infection. White patches suggest candidiasis (a type of yeast infection), syphilis, or simple mouth breathing (which dries out the mucous membrane of the tongue). Very smooth and painless areas may be what is called geographic tongue, or benign (harmless) glossitis. So-called hairy tongue often follows antibiotic therapy, a high fever, excessive use of certain mouthwashes, or a simple reduction in saliva secretion.

Severe acute glossitis, which can result from local infection, burns, and injury, can cause tenderness, pain, and swelling sufficient to make the tongue protrude from the mouth into the back of the throat—creating the danger of airway obstruction and even suffocation. In severe cases, the patient may not be able to chew, swallow, or speak. Steroid drug treatment usually reduces the swelling and helps relieve symptoms.

Patients may also complain of a painful burning tongue without other symptoms of inflammation. This is a common complaint among postmenopausal women. Diabetes, anemia, nutritional deficiencies, and malignant conditions should all be considered as possible primary causes.

Treatment

The patient should be reassured that redness and most lesions of the tongue are usually harmless and respond well to treatment. Such complaints as ulcers and hairy tongue often recur periodically; however, if an ulcer does not respond to treatment after several weeks, a biopsy (removal of a tissue sample for examination under a microscope) may be performed.

In treating glossitis, specific causes, such as jagged teeth and ill-fitting dentures, should be cor-

rected. Irritants, including hot or spicy foods, tobacco, alcohol, mouthwashes, and toothpastes, should be avoided if they are the source of the trouble. A bland or liquid diet, preferably cool or cold, may have a soothing effect. Good oral hygiene is necessary in all cases.

Tiny brown growths on the tongue are usually caused by contact with tobacco or certain bacteria; the treatment is to stop smoking or otherwise correct the cause and also to brush the tongue with a toothbrush.

Symptomatic relief for large lesions includes rinsing the mouth with a medicated mouthwash before meals. Application of topical anesthetics, such as lidocaine and benzocaine, can also bring relief. Patients with complaints of painful burning should be tested to rule out vitamin B_{12} deficiency, diabetes, and some types of anemia.

Prevention

Prevention of glossitis involves avoiding irritants, correcting nu-

tritional and vitamin deficiencies, and treating primary infections that produce glossitis as a secondary symptom.

Laryngitis

Laryngitis is an inflammation of the mucous membrane lining the larynx (voice box), which is located in the upper part of the respiratory tract. It causes hoarseness and possibly a temporary loss of speech.

Causes

Laryngitis may result from a bacterial or viral infection, such as a cold or the flu; from an irritation of the mucous membrane of the larynx, such as that caused by smoking; or from overuse of the voice.

Chronic or persistent laryngitis is most often caused by smoking, air pollution, dust, or smoke. It may also stem from tonsillitis, tuberculosis, the early stages of some forms of cancer, or paralysis of the vocal cords. Because

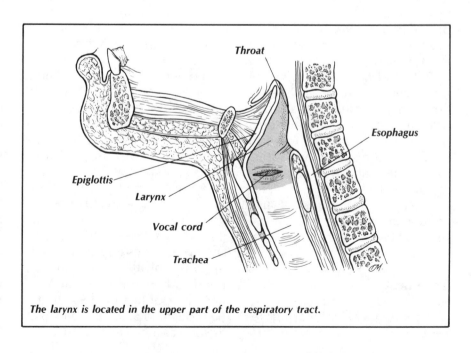

The larynx is located in the upper part of the respiratory tract.

laryngitis may be a symptom of a more serious condition, persons who consistently suffer from it should consult a physician.

Symptoms

Hoarseness, loss of the voice, dryness and scratchiness of the throat, coughing, and pain on speaking are common symptoms.

Treatment

Laryngitis is best treated by totally resting the vocal cords. Pain may be eased with throat sprays, steam inhalations, and mild pain relievers, such as aspirin and acetaminophen.

Mastoiditis

Mastoiditis is a bacterial infection of the mastoid air cells (small, air-filled cavities located in the mastoid process, which is the bulge in the skull behind the ear). Mastoiditis is most often a complication of a middle ear infection.

Symptoms

Mastoiditis is characterized by ringing in the ear, a discharge of pus from the ear canal, and fever. Other indications include swelling and tenderness over the mastoid process.

Complications

In severe cases, an abscess (a mass of pus in a body cavity) may develop in the mastoid process. This is a serious complication because it carries the risk

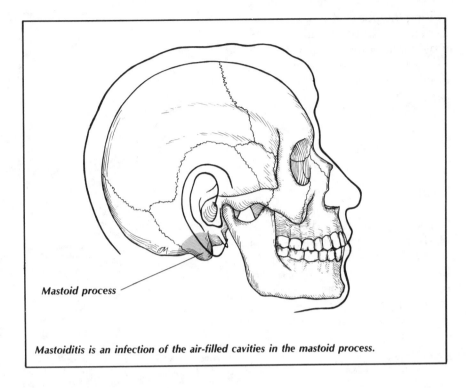

Mastoid process

Mastoiditis is an infection of the air-filled cavities in the mastoid process.

that infection will spread to the interior of the skull and cause meningitis (inflammation of the membranes covering the brain and spinal cord).

Treatment

Because antibiotics are so effective against ear infections and mastoid infections, mastoiditis is fortunately now rare. Sometimes, however, surgery is required to remove the infected cells if antibiotic treatment is started too late or is not effective.

Meniere's disease

Meniere's disease is the result of an increase in pressure in the inner ear because of a buildup of fluid in the semicircular canals of the inner ear, which control balance and equilibrium. This buildup of pressure distorts and sometimes ruptures the lining of the walls of the canals.

Causes

The cause of Meniere's disease is unknown, although it is thought that the pressure changes may be brought on by an infection, a small hemorrhage in the ear, or an allergic response. It occurs most commonly in men aged 40 to 60.

Symptoms

The symptoms of Meniere's disease include recurring and violent attacks of vertigo or dizziness, ringing in the ears, muffling or distortion of noises, and nausea that is sometimes accompanied by vomiting. Deafness in one or both ears may eventually develop.

Mild attacks of Meniere's disease may last from a half hour to several days before fading away naturally. They may recur regularly at intervals of weeks, months, or years. Severe attacks may last for several weeks, requiring the person to be confined to bed. In such cases, almost any movement of the head will result in bizarre and disturbing sensations that the floor and the furniture in the room are spinning around. Severe cases may also be accompanied by anxiety attacks and migraine headaches.

Treatment

The use of certain drugs, such as diuretics, tranquilizers, and antihistamines, may help to relieve severe and recurrent attacks. In severe cases, surgery may be necessary.

Middle ear infections

The ear can become infected in any one of its three parts—the inner ear, the middle ear, or the outer ear. However, ear infections most commonly settle in the middle ear. The medical term for middle ear infection is otitis media.

Ear infections are much more likely to affect children than adults; children are most susceptible between the ages of six months and six years. Children who contract ear infections in their first year are more likely to have chronic (long-term) ear infections later in life. By the age of eight, almost every child has had at least one ear infection.

Causes

Middle ear infections develop when viruses or bacteria in the nose or throat travel to the ear through the eustachian tube, which connects the middle ear to the nose and throat. The mid-

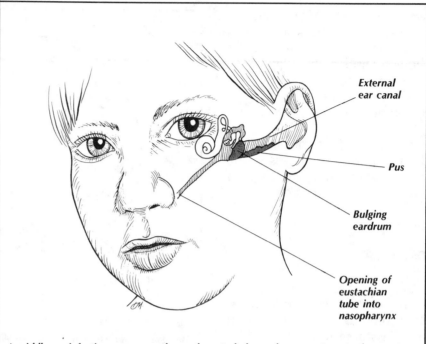

A middle ear infection may cause the eardrum to bulge and even rupture. In the event of a rupture, pus may leak into the external ear canal. A middle ear infection may follow a nose or throat infection that travels to the middle ear through the eustachian tube.

External
ear canal

Pus

Bulging
eardrum

Opening of
eustachian
tube into
nasopharynx

dle ear also can become infected when infection spreads from a severe outer ear infection or injury.

Symptoms

Middle ear infections can be recognized by severe throbbing pain in the ear, fever as high as 105°F (102°F in adults), hearing loss, and possibly dizziness, nausea, vomiting, or sore throat. The eardrum may bulge out or may even burst, oozing blood and pus into the outer ear and relieving the pain. Symptoms may worsen over a period of hours or days. A child too young to talk may seem ill or feverish or may pull on an ear.

Diagnosis

Ear infections are diagnosed by an inspection of the eardrum.

If it is red and swollen or bulging, middle ear infection can usually be confirmed.

Treatment

Middle ear infections are usually quickly eliminated by treatment with an antibiotic, often a form of penicillin. Decongestants may also be used. If a viral infection is present, however, antibiotics are not used, since viruses do not respond to antibiotics. If the eardrum is bulging and the pain is severe, the doctor may make a small cut in the eardrum (called a myringotomy) to relieve the pressure. If the eardrum bursts, the outer ear must be kept clean to prevent the infection from spreading.

The development of more effective antibiotics has lessened the need for surgery. In rare cases, however, the infected tissue may have to be surgically removed.

Middle ear infections usually clear up quickly, but the more severe or persistent infections can lead to a variety of serious complications, including temporary or permanent hearing loss, infection of the semicircular canals in the inner ear, facial paralysis, brain abscess, meningitis (inflammation of the membranes covering the brain and spinal cord), and infection of the mastoid process (the bulge in the skull behind the ear).

Nosebleeds

A nosebleed occurs when there is a break in the blood vessels in the inner lining of the nose, causing bleeding from the nose. Nosebleeds seldom require medical attention, but it is possible, although relatively rare, for nosebleeds to be a symptom of serious illness.

Causes

Nosebleeds can be caused by an injury to the nose, breathing dry air for prolonged periods, repeated blowing or picking of the nose, tumors in the nose, high blood pressure, and certain blood diseases.

Treatment

Very persistent or frequently recurring nosebleeds will require the attention of a doctor, who may cauterize (use heat or the chemical silver nitrate to seal off) the blood vessels in the back of the nose.

However, occasional nosebleeds can be treated simply by sitting up and leaning forward,

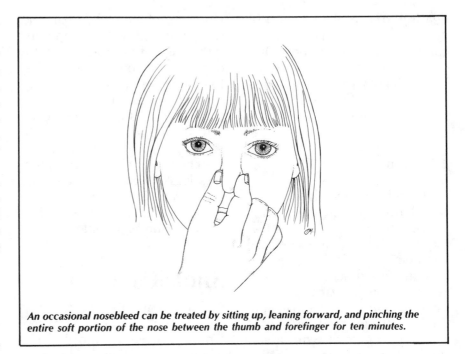

An occasional nosebleed can be treated by sitting up, leaning forward, and pinching the entire soft portion of the nose between the thumb and forefinger for ten minutes.

so as not to swallow the blood, and pinching the entire soft portion of the nose between the thumb and forefinger for ten minutes. If the bleeding does not stop, cold packs can be applied to the bridge of the nose for 15 to 20 minutes. If bleeding still persists, a doctor should be notified.

Frequent nosebleeds from breathing dry air may be relieved by the use of a humidifier. Also, those who have frequent nosebleeds should not blow the nose too harshly nor blow through one nostril.

When nosebleeds occur along with colds or other respiratory infections, a nasal decongestant may help to temporarily shrink the blood vessels in the nose. However, these decongestants should not be used by anyone with high blood pressure, heart disease, diabetes, or thyroid disorders, because decongestants also shrink blood vessels in parts of the body other than the nose, which can lead to complications for these patients.

Otosclerosis

Otosclerosis is a condition in which an abnormal spongy overgrowth of bone in the middle ear leads to totally or partially muffled hearing or deafness. The excess bone grows at the entrance to the middle ear, where it immobilizes the base of the stirrup, or stapes (one of the three tiny bones that transmit sound waves to the inner ear). As a result, sound-conducting vibrations are diminished, and hearing is impaired. In most cases, both ears are eventually affected. The cause is unknown, but the condition tends to be hereditary.

Symptoms

Hearing loss generally begins in the late teens or early 20s; the rate of deafness may accelerate and stabilize several times, but ordinarily the loss is complete within 10 to 15 years of onset— sooner if the disease began in childhood. In some cases, the hearing loss stops just short of deafness, and the affected person can still hear loud sounds. Otosclerosis usually affects one ear before the other and is preceded by ringing in the ear. Special hearing tests aid in diagnosis.

Treatment

The only way to halt or reverse otosclerosis is surgery, which is successful about 70 percent of the time. Although a hearing aid can help, most doctors prefer to operate. In a procedure called a stapedectomy, a surgeon folds back the eardrum, removes the affected stirrup, and replaces it with a synthetic or wire substitute that restores the conductive

vibrations of the middle ear. The surgery is very delicate and entails a risk of failure. It may be done on only one ear at a time, to reduce risk.

After surgery, the hearing of most patients is greatly improved within two to three weeks. In some cases, a residual blood clot temporarily blocks hearing until it dissolves. Patients with advanced otosclerosis in both ears are usually advised to undergo stapedectomy as soon as possible.

Sinusitis

Sinusitis is an infection (usually bacterial) of one or more of the sinuses. It occurs more commonly in adults than in children.

The sinuses are air-filled cavities located within the facial bone structure and connected to the nose. There are four major groups: frontal, ethmoidal, sphenoidal, and maxillary.

The sinuses are lined with mucous membrane and are normally kept clear when mucus drains through them into the nasal passages. If they are obstructed, normal drainage cannot occur, and infection of the sinuses can result.

Complications

It is rare but possible for chronic sinusitis to lead to more serious disorders. A persistent infection may travel to the brain,

Ethmoidal sinus

Frontal sinus

Nasal passage

Maxillary sinus

The sinuses are air-filled cavities within the facial bone structure, which are connected to the nasal passages. The four major groups are the frontal, ethmoidal, sphenoidal, and maxillary. The sphenoidal sinuses (not shown here) are located behind the ethmoidal sinuses.

causing meningitis (inflammation of the covering the brain and spinal cord), or to the bone, causing osteomyelitis (inflammation of a bone and its marrow).

Causes

A sinus infection may be triggered by anything that prevents the mucus in the sinuses from draining properly. Possible causes include swimming and diving, injuries, abnormal structure of the facial bones, congestion from the flu or a cold, allergies, or an abscess (inflamed pocket of pus) in a tooth, which may penetrate the sinuses and allow bacteria to enter them. Many different types of bacteria can cause sinusitis, including some of the same strains that lead to pneumonia, laryngitis, and middle ear infections.

Symptoms

Sinusitis is characterized by pain and tenderness above the infected sinus, which is felt in the face and forehead, behind the eyes, in the eyes, near the upper part of the nose, and even in the upper teeth (but not in a single tooth). This facial pain may be accompanied by headache, slight fever, chills, sore throat, nasal obstruction, and a discharge of pus from the nose.

Sinusitis usually lasts about two weeks, with the pain often subsiding in the morning and worsening as the day goes on, or fluctuating as the patient moves about and changes positions.

Diagnosis

The sinuses cannot be seen directly by a doctor, so diagnostic evaluation may include an X-ray examination to check for the presence of fluid or abnormalities in the sinuses and to determine which sinuses are infected. Computed tomography (see page 407) is an excellent tool for evaluating serious sinus problems.

Treatment

Sinusitis is treated by encouraging drainage of the sinuses. Nasal decongestants and moist heat work to aid sinus drainage. The doctor will usually prescribe an antibiotic that will kill the bacteria that most commonly trigger sinusitis.

If these treatments bring no relief, the doctor may perform a sinus puncture to determine exactly which bacteria are present. In this procedure, a needle is inserted into the sinus, and a sample of the fluid is removed. (This is necessary because the nasal discharge may contain bacteria different from those in the sinuses.) On the basis of analysis of the fluid sample, a more specific antibiotic may be prescribed.

In severe cases, codeine may be prescribed to dull the pain, and the doctor may clear the sinuses by injecting a solution through the nose to flush out the sinus cavities.

In some cases, surgery may be necessary to remove a nasal polyp (a mass of swollen tissue), repair abnormal bone structures, or remove infected sinus tissue.

Prevention

There is some evidence that smokers are more likely to suffer from sinusitis than are non-smokers. Those who often have colds are also more susceptible. Avoiding smoking and exposure to persons with colds may help prevent sinusitis.

Tonsillitis

Tonsillitis is an inflammation or infection of the tonsils. It occurs most commonly in children from 5 to 15 years old and only rarely in those under the age of two.

The tonsils are two small, almond-shaped lumps of specialized lymph node tissue located in the throat at the back of the mouth. They are barely visible in infants, increase in size during the preschool and early school years, and shrink by adulthood.

The function of the tonsils has not been pinpointed, but scientists believe that they perform at least two vital jobs: they release antibodies (protective agents) into the throat to prevent infection from spreading into the lungs (a useful service to children, who are highly susceptible to ear, nose, and throat infections); and they attract bacterial infection, thereby stimulating the production of antibodies, which accumulate in the body and are then available to prevent future, and potentially much more serious, infections. (Antibodies normally do not develop unless infection is present.) If the tonsils do indeed perform these two functions, then each attack of tonsillitis may help immunize a child against disease; once resistance has been developed, the function of the tonsils is complete.

There are two types of tonsillitis: acute tonsillitis, in which the infection flares up and then disappears in a short time; and chronic tonsillitis, in which the tonsils seem to be permanently inflamed and have abscesses (pus-filled cavities) on them.

Causes

Tonsillitis is caused by many different infectious agents, both viral and bacterial. *Streptococcus* bacterium is the most common bacterial cause; acute tonsillitis is usually a "strep" infection. Chronic tonsillitis, however, is more of a mystery; it is not known why chronic tonsillitis occurs in certain people or what causes it.

Symptoms

The symptoms of acute tonsillitis are a sore throat, fever (up to about 101°F), chills, headache, and muscle aches. These symptoms worsen for one to three days and then subside. Nausea, vomiting, stomachache, and swelling of lymph nodes in the neck may also occur and may last for about a week.

The symptoms of chronic tonsillitis include a persistent or recurrent sore throat, difficulty in swallowing or breathing, and foul breath.

Diagnosis

Tonsillitis is diagnosed by examination of the tonsils for redness, swelling, and the presence of gray or yellow infectious material. The doctor will take a sample of this material with a cotton swab in order to identify the organism causing the infection.

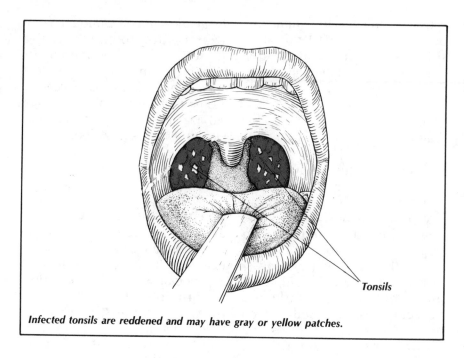

Tonsils

Infected tonsils are reddened and may have gray or yellow patches.

Treatment

Bed rest or reduced activity and the use of antibiotics, often penicillin, are recommended to treat tonsillitis if the inflammation is due to bacteria. Gargling with warm salt water can help relieve sore throat.

Surgical removal of the tonsils (called a tonsillectomy) is performed only if the tonsils are abscessed (filled with pus) or so enlarged that they are blocking the air passages. Tonsillectomies are seldom performed today, because research has found that even when tonsils are enlarged, they almost always shrink over time. Furthermore, removing the tonsils does not necessarily prevent recurrent sore throats and colds, as was once believed.

Complications

Complications resulting from tonsillitis seldom occur today because of effective, fast-acting antibiotics; rheumatic fever and infections of the sinuses, ears, and kidneys are rare but possible complications.

Prevention

Since it is not yet known why some people suffer from chronic tonsillitis, preventive measures have not been established. Because episodes of acute tonsillitis may be useful in the development of immunities in the body, prevention of such episodes may not be appropriate. More research is needed in this area.

THE LUNGS AND
RESPIRATORY SYSTEM

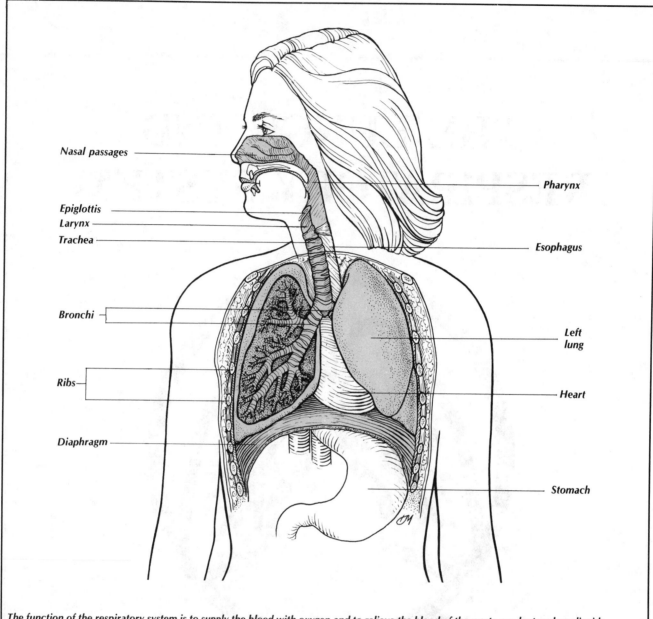

Nasal passages

Pharynx

Epiglottis
Larynx
Trachea

Esophagus

Bronchi

Left
lung

Ribs

Heart

Diaphragm

Stomach

The function of the respiratory system is to supply the blood with oxygen and to relieve the blood of the waste product carbon dioxide.

The respiratory system includes the nose, throat, larynx, trachea, bronchi, and lungs. The function of the respiratory system is to supply the blood with necessary oxygen and to relieve the blood of the waste product carbon dioxide. This exchange of oxygen and carbon dioxide occurs in the lungs. Air from the outside enters through the nose, where it is warmed, moistened, and fil-

tered before it passes through the throat and past the larynx (voice box) into the trachea (windpipe). The trachea divides into two main bronchi (the airways connecting the windpipe and the lungs). Within each lung, the bronchi divide and subdivide, forming progressively smaller passageways called bronchioles. The smallest bronchioles end in small, cup-shaped sacs called

alveoli. It is in the alveoli that the exchange of gas takes place. Each alveolus is served by numerous tiny blood vessels called capillaries. Oxygen in the alveolus crosses the thin alveolar and capillary walls to enter the blood, while carbon dioxide passes from the blood through the capillary walls into the alveolus. The oxygen is then carried by the blood to cells throughout the body, and the carbon dioxide is exhaled.

During inhalation and exhalation, the lungs are expanded and contracted by movements of the rib cage and the diaphragm (the large muscle separating the chest and abdominal cavities). During inhalation, the diaphragm contracts. This causes the diaphragm to descend and the chest cavity to expand. At this point, the air pressure inside the chest cavity is less than that of the air outside the body; consequently, air from the outside rushes into the lungs. During exhalation, the diaphragm relaxes and moves upward, reducing the chest capacity and pushing air out of the lungs. The friction caused by expansion and contraction of the lungs is eased by the pleurae (thin, moist membranes that cover the lungs and line the chest cavity), so that the surfaces of the lungs and chest cavity can move past each other smoothly.

Apnea

Apnea is strictly defined as the absence of breathing. The term is also used to refer to an interruption in breathing that occurs in some premature babies and also during the sleep of some children and adults.

Apnea in infants

The usual cause of apnea in infants is immaturity of the brain centers that regulate breathing. From time to time, the infant suddenly stops breathing completely and turns blue. If the baby is stimulated in some way (for example, by a flick of the finger on the bottom of the foot), he or she will usually start breathing normally at once. Seldom is it

necessary to use first-aid measures or a mechanical respirator to restart breathing. However, because a history of apnea is one of the factors that may be associated with sudden infant death syndrome (SIDS), physicians sometimes recommend monitoring high-risk infants with equipment that sounds an alarm if any stoppage of breathing is detected (for more on SIDS, see pages 359-360). In some cases, the tendency toward apnea disappears a few weeks after birth, when the breathing control centers have matured.

Apnea in children and adults

Apnea in children and adults is generally less immediately life threatening than apnea in infants, but it can be exhausting and, in a severe form, can cause cardiovascular and respiratory problems. In some patients, episodes of apnea can cause the blood concentration of carbon dioxide to build up to a dangerously high level.

Recognition of the problem generally cannot be made by the patient. A spouse or parent may be the first to notice an abnormal sleep pattern—for example, loud snoring, followed by silence (when the breathing stops), and then a loud choke or gasp as the sleeper partially awakens, clears the air passage, and resumes breathing. Such a pattern may be repeated many times during the night. As a result, persons with sleep apnea are likely to be drowsy during the day and irritable due to lack of sleep, with decreased memory and attention span. A definitive diagnosis can be made after observation in a hospital sleep laboratory.

In children and adults, apnea may occur because of a disorder

in the breathing control centers in the brain, or it may be a result of physical abnormalities of the chest, neck, and back due to obesity; the presence of a disease process; or an inborn structural defect. If apnea is due to an abnormality of the breathing control centers, drugs may be prescribed, or stimulation of the diaphragm (the large muscle separating the chest and abdominal cavities, which is instrumental in breathing) with an electronic pacemaker may be tried. Obesity is a common cause of sleep apnea in adults because the presence of excess tissue may block the airway in certain sleeping positions; the disorder may disappear after weight loss. If a physical abnormality due to disease or a structural defect is the cause, surgical treatment may be necessary; for example, enlarged tonsils and adenoids that are partially obstructing the upper airway may be removed. In extreme cases of airway obstruction, the only solution may be tracheostomy (surgical creation of a hole in the trachea and neck, through which the patient can breathe).

Asthma

Asthma is a respiratory disorder marked by unpredictable periods of acute breathlessness and wheezing. Asthma attacks can last from less than an hour to a week or more and can strike frequently or only every few years. Attacks may be mild or severe and can occur at any time, even during sleep.

The difficult breathing occurs when the small respiratory tubes called bronchioles constrict or become clogged with mucus or when the membranes lining the bronchioles become swollen.

When this happens, stale air cannot be fully exhaled but stays trapped in the lungs, so that less fresh air can be inhaled.

Causes

Asthma attacks can result from oversensitivity of the bronchial system to a variety of outside substances or conditions. About half of all attacks are triggered by allergies to such substances as dust, smoke, pollen, feathers, pet hair, insects, mold spores, and a variety of foods and drugs. Attacks not related to allergies can be set off by strenuous exercise, breathing cold air, emotional stress, and infections, particularly those of the respiratory tract. Heredity may play a part; if one or both of a child's parents are asthmatic, he or she has up to a 50 percent chance of developing the condition.

Asthma is rarely fatal, but it can be a very serious condition, especially in young children. Attacks often become less frequent and less severe as a child grows.

Symptoms

Common symptoms of an asthma attack include tightness in the chest, difficulty in breathing, coughing, and wheezing, which is caused by the effort to push air through the narrowed bronchioles. As the attack progresses, muscles surrounding the bronchioles constrict further, breathing becomes even more difficult, and mucus collects in the airways.

Diagnosis

Diagnostic procedures may include a complete physical exam-

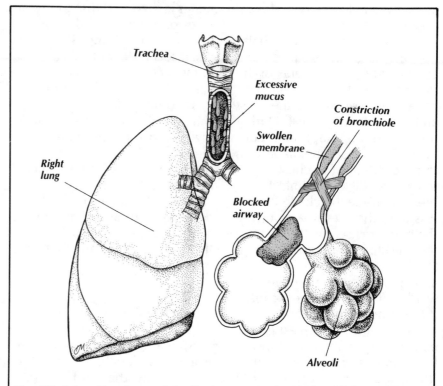

The difficult breathing characteristic of asthma occurs when the bronchioles constrict or become clogged with mucus or when the membranes lining the bronchioles become swollen. Stale air is trapped in the alveoli, and less fresh air can be inhaled.

ination and medical history, chest X ray, and allergy testing.

Treatment

Asthma, for the most part, cannot be cured, but it can be controlled with a variety of drugs. Epinephrine or isoproterenol may be given by injection or inhaled as an aerosol during an acute attack in order to enlarge the bronchioles; however, these drugs may overstimulate the heart and so cannot be used for long periods or by many people with heart conditions. (Individuals on beta-blocking drugs, such as propranolol, are also susceptible to complications from the use of epinephrine and should inform the treating physician that they are taking a beta blocker.) Similar drugs, such as metapro-

terenol, albuterol, and terbutaline, exert much less of a stimulating effect on the heart and can, therefore, be administered to a larger group of individuals. These drugs can be taken in an oral tablet form but are more commonly used in their aerosol form, which delivers the greatest effect in the bronchial system itself. They act by dilating or relieving the spasm of the bronchial tubes. A new aerosol form of an older drug, atropine, which blocks certain nerve impulses, probably acts in a similar fashion.

For long-term therapy, the drug theophylline can be used to help keep the bronchioles open. Its dosage, however, must be closely supervised because its rate of absorption into the body varies widely among patients: some persons eliminate the drug so quickly that it is almost ineffective; in others, the drug accumulates in the body, at times to toxic levels. Nausea, vomiting, and agitation are common side effects.

Corticosteroids can control asthma very effectively, but patients may experience such undesirable side effects as weight gain, ulcers, and high blood pressure. Stunting of growth has been reported in children. Consequently, corticosteroids such as prednisone are usually used in large doses in an acute attack and then are tapered as rapidly as possible. Some individuals, however, need relatively low doses chronically. Frequently, aerosol forms of corticosteroids are used to keep the asthmatic as "attack-free" as possible. Since there is less absorption of cortisone into the body with these forms, the likelihood of side effects is lessened.

Cromolyn, a drug that actually prevents attacks, acts to inhibit the release of histamines (the substances produced by the body during an allergic reaction). Cromolyn, however, cannot relieve an attack already in progress.

If an allergy is causing the attacks, the troublesome substance (called an allergen) must be removed from the patient's environment. If this cannot be done or if there are multiple allergies, injections of minute amounts of the allergen may help the body build tolerance to the allergen.

Prevention

Although there is no way to prevent asthma, several precautions can be taken to reduce the possibility that asthma attacks will occur. Allergy testing to determine sensitivity to common environmental agents such as dust, mold, pet hair, and pollen can be done by a physician. Once allergy is determined, desensitization injections can be tried. Rapid treatment of upper respiratory tract infections can help prevent severe attacks. Chronic preventative medication in known asthmatics will at least lessen the frequency and severity of attacks. With proper medical therapy and supervision, most asthmatics can lead normal lives.

Bronchiectasis

Bronchiectasis is a lung condition in which some of the bronchi and bronchioles have lost their elasticity and have expanded and filled with fluid.

Causes

Most often, bronchiectasis follows pneumonia, whooping cough, tuberculosis, or another lung disease. (Fortunately, the use of antibiotics has reduced the number of cases due to lung infection.) Other causes include obstruction; clogging of the airways by the thick, mucous secretions of cystic fibrosis; and Kartagener syndrome, which is a condition in which the cilia (hairlike projections that line the bronchial walls and wave mucus, pus, and dirt upward) do not work properly.

Symptoms

Bronchiectasis is a chronic condition that persists for life. The individual almost always has some symptoms, which will worsen if an acute infection occurs. The most typical symptom is a chronic cough that produces thick, white or green sputum (discharge). The sputum may be foul-smelling and abundant and may also contain blood. The individual generally coughs up large amounts of sputum after changing position (for example, after rising from bed).

Diagnosis

The doctor, listening to the chest with a stethoscope, can hear abnormal sounds inside the lungs as the patient breathes. An X ray obtained after the injection of dye into the bloodstream or directly into the bronchi will show the characteristic appearance of the disease. Chronic bronchitis must be ruled out as a cause, along with tuberculosis, certain fungal infections, a tumor, and the presence of an inhaled object that is lodged in a bronchi.

Treatment

Treatment of an active case of bronchiectasis includes fighting the infection with an antibiotic, such as penicillin or tetracycline, and eliminating the fluid with postural drainage. In the latter procedure, the patient lies face down in bed, with pillows elevating the hips, and a therapist strikes the back over the lungs with cupped hands to loosen mucus. The treatment, which can be taught to a family member, requires two to four ten-minute sessions a day. Inhaling warm mists may also help to moisten the thick mucus clogging the airways, so that it can be more easily expelled. The patient should avoid anything that can irritate the lungs, such as tobacco smoke, fumes, and dust.

In the relatively few cases in which the infection is confined to a small part of the lung and is progressing despite antibiotics and other forms of therapy, it may be best to surgically remove the affected portion of the lung.

Prevention

You can prevent progression of the disease by being immunized against flu and pneumonia, avoiding anyone with a cold or cough, and stopping smoking. Prompt treatment with antibiotics can help to control new infections.

Bronchitis

Bronchitis is a respiratory illness characterized by inflammation and swelling of the bronchi (the main airways connecting the windpipe and the lungs). When the mucous membranes lining these tubes become inflamed, the mucous glands in the membranes expand and release more mucus. The bronchi, already narrowed by the swelling, become further clogged by the excess mucus. This mucus must then be coughed up to keep the breathing tubes free for normal airflow into the lungs. This illness is characterized by frequent coughing, production of sputum (mucus), and, commonly, shortness of breath.

When the condition is of short duration, it is called acute bronchitis and is often accompanied by fever and production of thick, foul-smelling sputum. This condition is difficult to distinguish from pneumonia, and chest X rays are frequently obtained to establish diagnosis. When the symptoms linger for months or years, it is called chronic bronchitis. In either case, the coughing stops only when the source

To perform postural drainage, the therapist positions the patient head down with pillows elevating the hips and then strikes the patient's back over the lungs with cupped hands.

of inflammation has been removed or overcome and the inner linings of the bronchi have returned to normal.

Complications

Bronchitis alone is rarely fatal, but it may lead to another condition that proves fatal. For example, the functioning of lungs that have been severely damaged by chronic bronchitis may be so limited that the heart is deprived of adequate oxygen, ultimately resulting in death. Also, bronchitis can be very serious when combined with other respiratory diseases. Such is the case for people who suffer from a cate-

gory of respiratory conditions called chronic obstructive pulmonary disease (COPD). Bronchitis, emphysema, and several other diseases are included in this category. Patients may suffer from two or three of the COPD conditions, or one may lead to another.

Causes

Bronchitis occurs when the bronchial tubes are infected or irritated. A cold or the flu may lead to acute or, less often, chronic bronchitis. Chronic bronchitis is more commonly triggered by the constant irritation of environmental substances such as cigarette smoke, air pollutants, and occupational dusts.

Cigarette smoking is the predominant cause of chronic bronchitis. Seventy-five percent of all those who suffer from bronchitis are cigarette smokers. When tobacco smoke reaches the bronchial linings, it stops the action of the cilia (the hairlike projections that line the bronchial walls and wave mucus, pus, and dirt upward). When the cilia are stilled by smoke, particles remain trapped in the stagnant mucus, irritating the delicate bronchial tubes and eventually creating a breeding ground for infection.

Some degree of bronchitis occurs in about 90 percent of all smokers who live in polluted environments or who are exposed to occupational dusts. Babies and young children with chronic bronchitis usually overcome the condition. People who are undernourished, inadequately housed, or often fatigued are more likely to contract bronchitis. This disorder tends to occur within certain families, but the reason is not yet known.

Symptoms

Bronchitis can be recognized by its major symptom, the persistent cough in an effort to bring up the excess mucus. Acute bronchitis may be accompanied by hoarseness, chest discomfort, slight fever, wheezing, and shortness of breath. In children, chronic bronchitis may establish itself after several short-term infections. In adults, the beginning of chronic bronchitis is signaled by regular coughing and clearing of the throat the first thing each morning; the coughing will become more persistent and the mucus more plentiful as the dis-

Bronchitis is an inflammation of the mucous membranes lining the bronchial tubes. Airflow into the lungs is reduced as the membranes swell and secrete more mucus, which clogs the bronchial tubes.

ease progresses, and these symptoms may be accompanied by wheezing, shortness of breath, chest infections, and heavy panting after exercise.

As the years pass, chronic bronchitis may cause the bronchial tubes to become severely obstructed and the breathing to be irreversibly impaired. The heart sometimes becomes enlarged because it must pump harder than normal to deliver needed oxygen to the rest of the body. The nails, lips, and skin may develop a blue tinge due to lack of oxygen.

Diagnosis

To diagnose bronchitis, the doctor will obtain the medical history, do a physical examination of the chest with a stethoscope, and perhaps order a chest X ray. Special machines can measure the amount of air flowing in and out of the lungs and can measure how well oxygen is

being transported from the lungs to the bloodstream.

Treatment

Bronchitis is treated by removing the irritants from the patient's surroundings, clearing the lungs of mucus, and trying to prevent infections. A patient with chronic bronchitis will need to quit smoking and to avoid constant exposure to pollutants or hazardous dusts. Humidity plays a large part in treating bronchitis; patients should drink plenty of liquids and breathe warmed, humidified air from a vaporizer or humidifier. Humidity acts to moisten mucus trapped in the airways, allowing it to be brought up from the lungs and thereby promoting what is known as a productive cough. A bronchodilator drug, which relaxes the walls of the air passages, may be prescribed. The use of antibiotics to treat bronchitis is somewhat controversial but appears to be helpful, particularly in acute cases.

Prevention

Bronchitis can best be prevented by avoiding the irritants that cause it, namely cigarette smoke, air pollutants, and dusts. Patients with chronic bronchitis can prevent further irritation by maintaining good health habits to avoid infections. Other lung disorders may precipitate the condition; therefore, antibiotics may be prescribed to treat bacterial infections, and vaccinations against influenza and pneumonia are strongly recommended in those with chronic bronchitis.

Dyspnea

Dyspnea is a sensation of "air hunger." It is usually accompanied by difficult, labored breathing and discomfort. Dyspnea is a symptom that may occur in a variety of diseases and conditions, ranging from congestive heart failure to emotional upset.

Causes

Dyspnea may be caused by inadequate delivery of oxygen to the tissues, as in severe anemia; by failure of the heart to keep up with the needs of the body, as in congestive heart failure; by overexertion; by obstruction of the airways; by narrowing of air passages, such as occurs in asthma; or by restriction of lung capacity, which may be caused by a chest deformity. Emphysema is commonly associated with dyspnea. It can also occur if there is fluid in the lungs, as in pneumonia or congestive heart failure, because the entry of oxygen into the alveoli (the tiny air sacs in the lungs, where gas exchange takes place) is blocked by the fluid, thereby preventing oxygenation of the blood.

In a nighttime form of dyspnea called paroxysmal nocturnal dyspnea, the patient awakens gasping for breath and can breathe only by sitting up or standing. Usually this is caused by congestive heart failure.

Another type of dyspnea, called psychogenic or hysterical hyperventilation, is a physical response to stress, anxiety, or emotional upset. In this condition, excessive breathing results in exhalation of too much carbon dioxide, which causes light-headedness, numbness and tingling of the hands and toes, and fainting.

Symptoms

Signs of dyspnea include noisy breathing; an anxious, distressed expression; dilated nostrils; gasping; a protruding abdomen; an expanded chest; and blue lips and fingertips.

Treatment

Treatment involves controlling whatever condition is causing the dyspnea.

Emphysema

Emphysema is a chronic, progressive lung disease. Emphysema develops when the small air passages leading to the alveoli (the tiny air sacs in the lungs, where gas exchange takes place) become distended and the walls dividing the alveoli are injured or destroyed. Spaces form where alveoli had been, and lung tissue becomes nonfunctional and stiff rather than elastic. Emphysema is commonly associated with chronic bronchitis, in which the airways become inflamed, causing specialized cells within them to secrete abnormally large amounts of mucus. The inflammation, swelling, and excessive mucus production result in obstruction of airflow and entrapment of air within the lungs.

Effect on the body

As the disease progresses, many complex changes take place, ultimately leading to diminishment of the amount of oxygen in the blood, frequently associated with an increased amount of carbon dioxide. As the lung tissue deteriorates and loses its elasticity, changes also occur in the blood vessels carrying deoxygenated blood to the lungs for a fresh supply of oxygen. The net effect is that the right side of the heart, which is responsible for collecting deoxygenated blood from the veins and pumping it through the lungs, must work much harder. As the process continues, the muscle of the right side of the heart is weakened by this extra work and becomes less able to pump blood into the lungs. The blood "backs up," causing increased pressure in the veins. This causes fluid to recede into the tissues, resulting in severe swelling of the feet, ankles, and legs. If this right-sided heart failure (called cor pulmonale) is very severe, the abdomen will become distended with fluid.

Causes

External factors that irritate the lungs, such as tobacco smoke

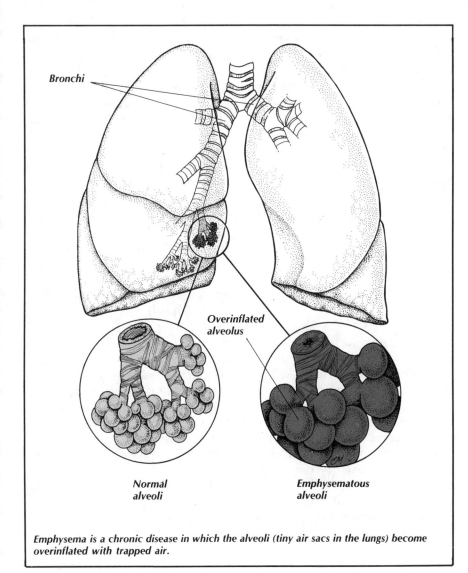

Emphysema is a chronic disease in which the alveoli (tiny air sacs in the lungs) become overinflated with trapped air.

and air pollutants, are commonly linked to emphysema. Unlike many respiratory diseases, emphysema is not caused by a viral or bacterial infection. However, it is often aggravated by bronchitis or another lung infection.

In a minority of cases, emphysema is a result of a genetic deficiency or an inherited lack of a blood protein, which leads to loss of elasticity in the alveoli.

Those afflicted with emphysema are most likely to be white men over the age of 50, although women are becoming equally susceptible because of an increase in smoking among women during recent years. The overwhelming majority of emphysema cases are directly linked to cigarette smoking.

Symptoms

Emphysema is characterized by one major symptom—shortness of breath. Patients may also have a persistent, racking cough, which either brings up mucus or is overly dry. Patients experience difficulty in breathing, often taking twice as many breaths as others to get enough oxygen. It has been found that advanced em-

physema sufferers exert tremendous amounts of energy just to breathe. They also tire quite easily and require more calories to maintain their weight than healthy individuals do. An enlarged, rounded "barrel" chest often develops due to overinflation of the lungs and excessive growth of the chest muscles due to the increased stress placed upon them to inflate stiff lungs. Lips, ear lobes, skin, and fingernails may be tinged blue from lack of oxygen in the blood.

Diagnosis

With the exception of the minority of cases caused by genetic disorder, no single test can pinpoint the condition. Breathing tests to measure the amount of air being inhaled and exhaled will not reveal the disease in its early stages. A blood test may be done to determine the red blood cell count (when emphysema causes diminished oxygenation of blood, more red blood cells are produced in an effort to increase oxygen transport; because of this, the red blood cell count is elevated). A chest X ray may be taken to search for specific changes in the lungs that may point to advanced stages of the disease; however, a chest X ray is not diagnostic of early emphysema. Thus, emphysema is diagnosed through a collection of findings.

Treatment

There is no known cure for emphysema, nor is it reversible. However, the progress of the disease can be checked by removing irritants, particularly tobacco smoke, from the patient's environment. Patients are encouraged to drink large amounts of fluids to help thin out the mucus that may block the airways. Adequate rest, a balanced diet, and moderate regular exercise are recommended. Vaporizers, humidifiers, and air conditioners help to moisturize and filter the air. A respiratory therapist can teach a patient how to use the chest and abdominal muscles to breathe more efficiently.

Several drugs may aid the patient. They act to loosen mucus or to relax and expand the air passages. Antibiotics are sometimes prescribed if infection exists. Cortisone drugs (corticosteroids) are often prescribed chronically. Drugs such as albuterol and terbutaline are also used both in inhalation aerosol and oral forms. In advanced cases, oxygen may have to be administered continuously. However, an emphysema patient must be particularly careful to use only the amount of oxygen prescribed. Too much oxygen can suppress the drive to breathe, causing respiratory failure and possibly death. In addition, sedatives and sleeping pills should be avoided by those with severe emphysema, as these can also lead to a dangerous slowing of breathing.

Emphysema is a very serious condition. However, with the help of modern treatments, breathing aids, and medications, patients can lead a reasonably comfortable life. It is, however, necessary for these individuals to stop smoking and avoid air pollutants as much as possible.

Legionnaires' disease

Legionnaires' disease is a severe bacterial infection of the respiratory tract. The first identifiable outbreak occurred in 1976 in Philadelphia. More than 180 people at the state convention of the American Legion became afflicted with the disease, and 29 of them died. Other outbreaks have since occurred in the United States and Europe. Studies have also shown that outbreaks of respiratory diseases later identified as Legionnaires' disease occurred as early as 1947.

Cause

Legionnaire's disease is caused by the *Legionella pneumophila* bacterium, which was not identified until the 1976 outbreak. The major environmental source of the infection is water from reservoirs and cooling units of air-conditioning systems. Lakes, creeks, and areas of excavation also may harbor the bacteria. Transmission is by breathing in droplets of contaminated water. Person-to-person transmission has not been documented.

Those at risk

Cigarette smokers, the elderly, and persons receiving drugs that depress the immune system are more likely to contract the disease than are other people. Persons who have another medical problem—heart trouble, cancer, respiratory illness, or kidney disease—are also believed to be particularly susceptible.

Symptoms

Legionnaires' disease has symptoms similar to those of many other respiratory diseases, making it difficult to differentiate

and diagnose. Symptoms include dry coughing, high fever, chills, diarrhea, shortness of breath, chest pains, headaches, excessive sweating, nausea, vomiting, and abdominal pain. Occasionally, bloody sputum is produced. Lethargy and confusion may occur in progressive, serious cases.

Although Legionnaires' disease is uncommon, it should be considered in the case of anyone (particularly an elderly or chronically ill person) who has a respiratory tract infection that worsens over a period of about four days. The disease can initially be mild and appear to be an episode of the flu. The diagnosis is made from the history and physical examination, chest X rays, and special tests of the blood and sputum that determine the presence and changing numbers of antibodies (protective substances that fight off infection).

Treatment

If an antibiotic (usually erythromycin) is given early in the course of the illness, the outlook for recovery is excellent.

Prevention

There is as yet no preventive vaccine against Legionnaires' disease. If an outbreak is suspected, public health officials may search for and attempt to eliminate the source of infection.

Pleurisy

Pleurisy, or pleuritis, is an inflammation of the pleurae (thin, moist membranes that cover the lungs and line the chest cavity). The pleurae normally reduce the friction between the chest structures as the lungs expand and contract. Inflammation of the pleurae causes breathing to become painful and less effective.

Types and causes

There are two types of pleurisy: dry pleurisy and wet pleurisy. In dry pleurisy, the more common condition, the inflamed pleurae rub directly against each other. In wet pleurisy, fluid oozes from the inflamed tissue into the space between the lungs and the chest wall. This fluid may compress the lungs, making breathing difficult.

Both types of pleurisy often occur as complications of respiratory tract infections, such as pneumonia, viral infections, and tuberculosis, and are more likely to develop in persons who are highly susceptible to such infections. They can also be caused by a tumor or an injury. Some cases are due to certain gastrointestinal tract diseases, particularly of the liver and pancreas, which can inflame the diaphragm (the large muscle separating the chest and abdominal cavities) and the portions of the pleurae that cover the diaphragm.

Symptoms

The major symptom of dry pleurisy is a sharp, stabbing pain toward the side and lower part of the chest. The pain may also be felt along the shoulders, neck, and abdomen. Any movement involving the chest, such as breathing or coughing, will aggravate the pain, which may be accompanied by shortness of breath, a dry cough, and fever.

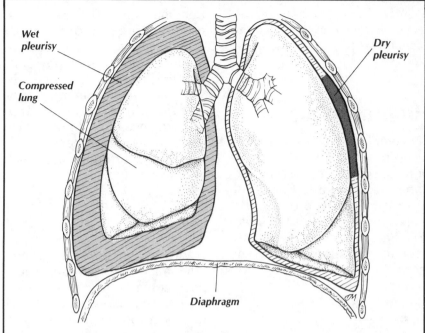

Pleurisy is an inflammation of the pleurae (the membranes that cover the lungs and line the chest cavity). In dry pleurisy, the inflamed pleurae rub directly against each other, causing painful breathing. In wet pleurisy, fluid oozes from the inflamed tissue into the space between the lungs and the chest wall, compressing the lung.

Wet pleurisy is characterized by similar symptoms, but there may also be difficulty in breathing.

Diagnosis

A diagnosis of pleurisy usually begins with a physical examination, during which the doctor listens to the chest with a stethoscope for the low-pitched, grating sound that occurs with each breath in a case of dry pleurisy. If fluid in the lungs is suspected, the physician may percuss, or tap on, the chest wall (usually on the back) to determine the level or amount. The skin near the affected area is often found to be tender. If wet pleurisy is suspected, a sample of the fluid oozing from the pleurae will usually be obtained (by inserting a needle directly into the pleura) and analyzed. A tuberculin skin test may be done to

learn whether tuberculosis is a factor. An X-ray study is very helpful in detecting the presence of pleural fluid.

Treatment

To treat pleurisy, the doctor will first need to treat the underlying infection or disease, often with antibiotics. The symptoms of pleurisy can be relieved somewhat by resting. Strapping the chest firmly with a nonadhesive elastic bandage is sometimes recommended; however, it may prevent deep breathing and coughing up of mucus, both of which are necessary to clear the respiratory tract. Painkillers may help to relieve chest discomfort at least enough so that the patient will not need to stifle the painful coughing that is necessary to loosen the mucus. Anti-inflammatory medications and even cortisone drugs are very effective in relieving the inflammation and pain, particularly in dry pleurisy.

Pneumonia

Pneumonia is an infection of the lungs in which the alveoli in one or more sections of the lungs become inflamed and filled with fluid and white blood cells, which try to fight off the infection. Pneumonia can be fatal, especially in the very young and the very old.

Types

There are several types of pneumonia, distinguished by the location, causative agent, and extent of infection. Lobar pneumonia is an infection in only one lobe (section) of the lungs. Double pneumonia is an infection in all or parts of both lungs. Bronchial pneumonia is an infection in the areas of the lungs near the bronchi (the main airways connecting the windpipe and the lungs). Walking pneumonia is a general term often used to describe a form of pneumonia that an individual may have for a week or more with no symptoms other than cough. When eventually seen by a physician, the individual is sent for a chest X ray, which shows pneumonia. This type of pneumonia is often caused by an organism known as *mycoplasma pneumoniae*. Although often mild, it can be quite serious if left unrecognized.

Pneumonia most often strikes the person whose resistance is lowered, frequently by an upper respiratory tract infection or a systemic (affecting the body generally) disease. It is commonly a secondary disease stemming from inadequate defense mechanisms, from a cold or the flu, or from long-term diseases, such as chronic bronchitis, emphysema, asthma, diabetes, cancer, or sickle cell anemia. In the elderly, pneumonia is a much-feared consequence of being bedridden for long periods, especially following injuries due to falls (such as broken bones).

Causes

Viruses, bacteria, fungi, and other microorganisms may cause pneumonia. It may also develop if a person inhales certain chemicals or if food, vomit, or a foreign object passes through the trachea (the windpipe) instead of the esophagus (food tube) and settles in a lung ("aspiration pneumonia"). Smoking, excessive drinking, a prolonged period of being bedridden, anesthesia, and use of sedatives and drugs that suppress the immune system may make an individual more susceptible to pneumonia if he or she is exposed to an infectious organism. Pneumonia is most common during flu and cold epidemics and during the winter months, when people are more likely to be indoors, where bacteria and viruses are easily spread.

Symptoms

Pneumonia is generally characterized by four major symptoms: chest pain, a sudden rise in

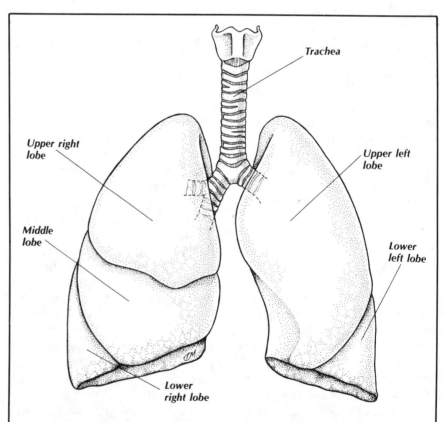

The lungs consist of five sections, called lobes. If there is an infection in only one lobe, the condition is called lobar pneumonia; if at least one lobe in each lung is affected, it is called double pneumonia.

body temperature, coughing, and difficulty in breathing. Viral pneumonia is signaled by coughing and other cold symptoms, as well as by general fatigue. Bacterial pneumonia generally comes on suddenly with shaking chills; a rapid, steep rise in temperature; shallow breathing; and a cough that brings up bloody, dark yellow, or rust-colored sputum. An oxygen shortage that is sometimes a result of fluid and debris blocking small airways in the lungs will be indicated by other symptoms, such as headache, nausea, vomiting, and bluish discoloration of the lips and fingertips.

Diagnosis

Pneumonia is diagnosed by listening to the chest with a stethoscope to detect the presence of fluid in the lungs. An analysis of the sputum and an X-ray examination are also done to identify the type and location of the infection.

Treatment

Viral pneumonia is generally treated by staying in bed, drinking lots of fluids, maintaining a light diet, and using painkillers to combat discomfort. Hospitalization is not usually necessary. Viral pneumonia, however, can be quite serious and even fatal, particularly in those with underlying diseases affecting the immune system and in premature newborns. Newer antiviral drugs, in both intravenous and aerosol form, have been extremely helpful in select cases.

Bacterial pneumonia is treated with antibiotics, such as penicillin. Patients also need to rest or, in severe cases, to enter the hospital for care, supervision, and intravenous drug therapy. If breathing is difficult, oxygen may be administered.

Prevention

There are vaccines that may help in preventing some types of pneumonia. Pneumonia caused by certain bacteria may be prevented with a vaccine, which is especially recommended for the elderly or for those with chronic diseases that may weaken the respiratory system. Pneumonia caused by one type of influenza virus may also be prevented with a vaccination.

The very young, the very old, and the chronically ill are the most likely to contract pneumonia, so care must be taken to protect them from respiratory infections.

Psittacosis

Psittacosis is a rare form of pneumonia caused by a microorganism called *Chlamydia psittaci,* which may be transmitted to humans by certain birds. It is often called parrot fever because it was first found to be transmitted by members of the parrot family, including parakeets and lovebirds. It may also be transmitted by other birds, such as sea gulls, pigeons, canaries, and poultry, in which case it is called ornithosis.

Causes

Infection usually takes place when a person inhales dust from the feathers or droppings of infected birds. It can also be transmitted directly to a person by a bite from an infected bird. Person-to-person transmission is rare. Eating poultry has not been reported as a source of infection.

Symptoms

The incubation period (the time between exposure to the illness and the appearance of symptoms) is one to two weeks. The disease usually begins with fever, chills, headache, muscle aches, and loss of appetite. Nausea, vomiting, and enlargement of the spleen may also be present. The patient's temperature continues to rise, and a dry cough develops. Coughing brings up mucus and pus in the later stages. Chest X rays made during the first week of noticeable symptoms often show inflammation of the lungs. During the second week, the typical symptoms of pneumonia develop. The temperature will remain above normal for at least two weeks and then begin to fall slowly. A steady increase in the pulse and breathing rate may be serious. About 30 percent of untreated cases end in death. Recovery of those who receive treatment may be gradual.

Treatment

The drug most commonly used to treat psittacosis is oral tetracycline, an antibiotic. Complete bed rest is necessary in most cases. Cough preparations with codeine are also advised. In severe cases, tetracycline may be given intravenously.

Prevention

Flocks of pigeons or other birds, dust from feathers, birdcage contents, and sick domestic birds or fowl should be avoided.

Special feed is often used to prevent spread of infection among imported parrots, parakeets, and lovebirds and among turkeys raised for market.

Pulmonary embolism

Pulmonary embolism is a serious and potentially fatal condition that occurs when an embolus (a clump of matter originating elsewhere in the body and traveling via the circulation) blocks a blood vessel in the lungs.

Causes

Emboli (the plural of *embolus*) may be solid (detached blood clots, clumps of tumor cells, or bits of foreign objects); liquid (globules of fat); or gaseous (air). Pulmonary emboli are venous thrombi (blood clots that form in the veins) that have originated most often in the lower extremities and pelvis, usually as the result of injury, surgery, or blood vessel diseases. Such thrombi are common in persons on prolonged bed rest, particularly after surgery, due to the lack of movement of blood in the legs.

Symptoms

The presence of a pulmonary embolus is indicated by the sudden development of wheezing, dyspnea (labored or difficult breathing), chest pains, and hemoptysis (spitting up of blood).

Diagnosis

Diagnostic procedures may include an electrocardiogram (see

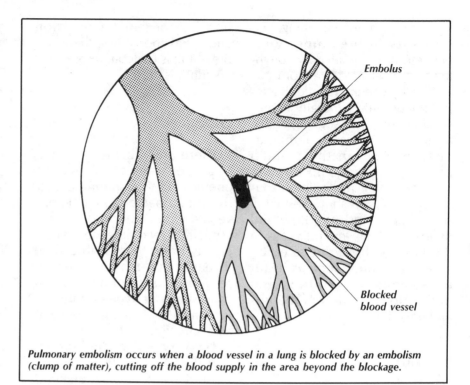

Pulmonary embolism occurs when a blood vessel in a lung is blocked by an embolism (clump of matter), cutting off the blood supply in the area beyond the blockage.

page 399) and analysis of arterial blood obtained from the wrist, arm, or groin. Nuclear medicine scanning (see pages 406-407) is very helpful. The definitive diagnostic procedure is pulmonary angiography, which is an X-ray scan of the lungs done after the introduction of a special dye into the pulmonary circulation (via a catheter inserted into the groin and floated up to the right side of the heart).

Treatment

Initial treatment may include administration of oxygen, pain relievers, and medication to maintain cardiovascular functions. An anticoagulant (usually intravenous heparin or oral warfarin) is given to prevent the development of additional emboli.

If it is determined that the embolism was caused by a venous thrombus, and there is some reason why anticoagulants should

not be used, the inferior vena cava (the main vein draining blood from the lower limbs and the pelvis) may be deliberately blocked with an "umbrella filter" or a clip to keep other venous thrombi from traveling to the lungs. Surgical removal of the embolus is done only in rare cases for large clots that can be removed immediately after detection. Clot dissolvers have been helpful in occasional cases.

Prevention

The best prevention of pulmonary embolism is prevention of venous thrombosis. Persons predisposed to embolism may be given injections of heparin or low doses of oral warfarin to prevent the formation of thrombi. Recently, "compression boots," soft plastic bags wrapped around the legs and rapidly inflated and deflated, have been shown to prevent clot formation in postoperative and bedridden individuals. Early ambulation—walking—after surgery is probably the best preventive measure.

Tuberculosis

Tuberculosis is a bacterial infection caused by *Mycobacterium tuberculosis* organisms. Because the body has difficulty fighting this type of bacterium, it attempts to wall off the organisms within small nodules, called granulomas or tubercles, which contain both the bacteria and the tissue produced by the body in reaction to them.

Of all persons who are infected by the tuberculosis bacteria, 80 percent will never experience the symptoms of the disease. Usually, the body is able to surround the offending bacteria with granulomas; the tuberculosis bacteria then lie dormant in the body, and active disease does not develop. However, because the body cannot kill the bacteria—only contain them—the infection can become active at a later time, often when some other disease has weakened the body's defenses.

Of the 20 percent of infected persons in whom an active case does develop, only half will become sick within three months of contracting the infection; the other half will suffer from the disease at some time in their lives, perhaps years later. Tuberculosis usually affects the lungs, but it can also involve other parts of the body, such as the spine, the kidneys, the digestive tract, and the lining of the heart.

Causes

Tuberculosis is contracted when a person breathes in droplets containing *Mycobacterium tuberculosis* organisms that have been coughed or sneezed into the air by a person who is infected with the bacterium. Tuberculosis is contagious, especially for persons living in crowded conditions. Also highly susceptible to this disease are those who are undernourished, in poor health, or living in poor urban areas, as well as the very young, the very old, and those in the medical professions. Anyone who has been in close contact with a tuberculosis patient should be tested for the disease.

Symptoms

Early signs include fever, fatigue, loss of appetite, and weight loss. Later signs include coughing up of blood-tinged sputum, chest pain, and shortness of breath.

Diagnosis

The symptoms of tuberculosis are similar to those of many other diseases, and its characteristic symptoms do not appear until the disease is in its advanced stages. For these reasons, coupled with the fact that the incidence of tuberculosis has been declining in recent years in the United States, this disorder often remains untreated or misdiagnosed for some time before the patient is finally tested for it. Tuberculosis may be accompanied by an infection due to *Streptococcus* bacteria, which often further complicates diagnosis.

Patients can be tested for tuberculosis with a tuberculin skin test. If the bacteria are present, whether active or inactive, the patch of skin that has been treated with dead tuberculosis bacteria will swell. Chest X rays or sputum analysis may also help to identify the site of infection.

Treatment

Tuberculosis is treated with a variety of antibacterial drugs simultaneously. Each medication acts on a different portion of the tuberculosis bacterium; only in combination do these drugs have the greatest probability of eliminating the infection. The drugs are usually prescribed for a long period of time, perhaps 9 to 18 months, but usually after two weeks the patient is no longer contagious and can resume normal activities. With this type of treatment, the disease is rarely fatal. Severe side effects, such as liver or hearing damage, can result from certain antituberculosis drugs.

Prevention

An active case of tuberculosis can be prevented in some high-risk persons by the administration of certain antituberculosis drugs, but these drugs are likely to have undesirable side effects. (High-risk persons include those under the age of 35, especially children, who have been exposed to the disease, as well as those with chronic diseases that have weakened their respiratory systems.) Liver damage resulting from use of antituberculosis medications is more likely to occur in those over the age of 35, so people in this age group seldom receive these drugs.

Regardless of age or physical condition, anyone who has been in close contact with a person who has an active case of tuberculosis should be tested for the disease.

THE HEART AND CIRCULATORY SYSTEM

The circulatory system, which includes the heart, the blood vessels, and the blood, brings nutrients and oxygen to every part of the body and carries away wastes.

Heart

The heart is a hollow, muscular organ that maintains blood circulation throughout the body. It lies behind the sternum (breastbone), between the lungs. Its size in most adults approximates that of the clenched fist. A heartbeat is a rhythmic contraction of the heart muscle as it pumps blood. A normal heart usually beats 60 to 90 times per minute when the person is at rest.

The heart has four chambers, through which the blood passes. Valves control the movement of blood between these compartments. The blood flows from two large veins (the superior vena cava and the inferior vena cava) into the right atrium (upper chamber). The blood continues down to the right ventricle (lower chamber). From this chamber, the blood is pumped to the lungs, where carbon dioxide (a waste product from the cells) is exchanged for oxygen (an element necessary for cell life). The rejuvenated blood then returns to the left atrium. From there, the blood passes to the left ventricle, which forces the blood away from the heart through the aorta (the main artery of the body, which extends through the chest and abdomen) to the other arteries, which carry the blood to all the tissues of the body.

Blood vessels

Blood vessels form the network of passageways that trans-

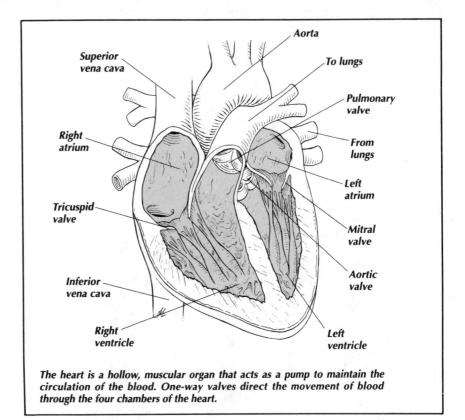

The heart is a hollow, muscular organ that acts as a pump to maintain the circulation of the blood. One-way valves direct the movement of blood through the four chambers of the heart.

port blood throughout the body. The blood leaves the heart and passes through arteries of progressively smaller diameter. When the blood reaches the smallest blood vessels, called capillaries, oxygen and nutrients are exchanged for carbon dioxide and other waste products. The "used" blood then continues on its journey back toward the heart through veins of progressively greater diameter.

Blood

Blood is the fluid that courses through the blood vessels of the body. It consists of plasma (a yellowish liquid composed of water, proteins, salts, and other substances) and three formed elements—red blood cells, white blood cells, and platelets—that are visible only under a microscope. These elements are manu-

factured by the bone marrow (the soft tissue in the center of some bones).

Red blood cells carry oxygen from the lungs to body tissues. Oxygen travels attached to hemoglobin, a pigmented substance in red blood cells that contains iron. When the amount of hemoglobin in each red blood cell or the total number of red blood cells falls below a certain level, anemia is said to be present. Normally, there are about 25 billion red blood cells in a teaspoon of blood.

The white blood cells protect the body from invasive organisms. When the body is wounded or infected, white blood cells attack and kill disease-causing agents in the affected area. In addition, certain white blood cells produce antibodies, which counteract harmful agents by destroying or inactivating them. Because the body produces more white

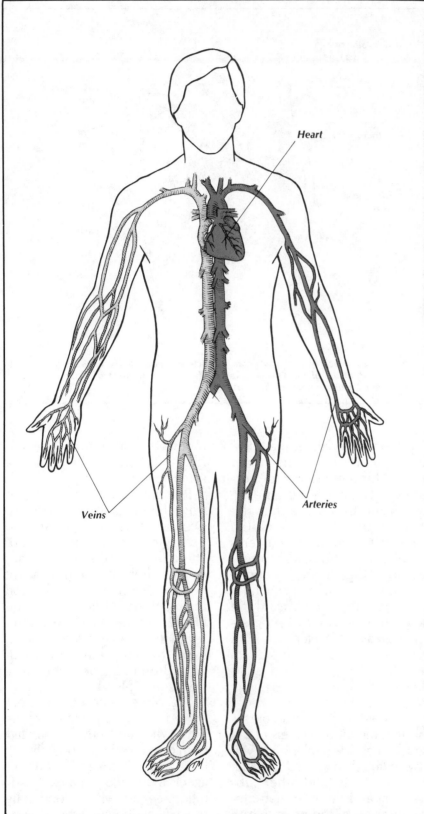

The circulatory system includes the heart, the blood vessels, and the blood. For purposes of illustration, only the major arteries are shown on the left side of the body, and only the major veins are shown on the right side.

blood cells than usual in response to infection, an increase in their number signals disease. From 25 million to 45 million white blood cells are normally present in one teaspoon of blood.

Platelets are small, colorless disks numbering approximately one and a half billion in a single teaspoon of blood. They work to help the blood form clots.

Antigens and blood types

An antigen is a substance that can provoke an immune (protective) response by the body. An antigen promotes the manufacture of antibodies that will interact only with that antigen. On the surfaces of all cells are numerous antigens, which cause production of different antibodies. The major blood groups (types A, B, AB, and O) are differentiated on the basis of the presence on the red blood cells of two of those surface antigens: type A blood has antigen A, type B has antigen B, type AB has both antigen A and antigen B, and type O has neither antigen A nor antigen B. A person's blood type must be identified before a blood transfusion can be given because his or her blood may reject transfused blood of the wrong type. Type A blood plasma, for example, does not contain any anti-A antibodies. It does, however, contain anti-B antibodies. If type B blood is transfused, the anti-B antibodies in the plasma will destroy the type B red cells, which have type B antigens.

Anemia

Anemia is a general term referring to a shortage of red blood cells or a reduction in their hemoglobin content. (Hemoglobin is the pigment in the blood that carries oxygen in the red blood cells.) A shortage of red blood cells or hemoglobin means that the blood is unable to carry adequate amounts of oxygen to all parts of the body.

Causes

Anemia can be caused by vitamin or mineral deficiencies or inability to absorb certain vitamins, the destruction of red blood cells, inherited abnormalities in the blood, or the failure of the bone marrow to manufacture enough red blood cells. Such diverse conditions as bleeding ulcers, drug allergies, cancer, and exposure to radioactivity can also lead to anemia. People with a poor diet or a history of alcoholism are likely to suffer from one of the types of anemia caused by vitamin and mineral deficiencies. A tendency toward certain types of anemia (for example, sickle cell anemia) can also be inherited.

Symptoms

Among the many symptoms of anemia are fatigue, shortness of breath, pounding heartbeat, rapid heart rate, headaches, loss of appetite, dizziness, ringing in the ears, weakness, and faintness. Burning of the tongue or a change in its appearance may also be a clue. Another sign of anemia may be paleness in the creases of the palms, under the fingernails, and in the lining of the eye. Very severe cases may be signaled by swollen ankles; rapid, weak pulse; pale, clammy skin; and a feeling of fullness in the neck or abdomen.

Diagnosis

Diagnosis is based on the findings from a physical examination and tests of the blood (and sometimes the bone marrow) to detect shortages of red blood cells or hemoglobin. A specific diagnosis is necessary because each type of anemia has a different cause and, therefore, a different treatment.

Iron deficiency anemia

Iron deficiency anemia is caused by a shortage of the mineral iron, which is necessary to produce hemoglobin. This shortage can be caused by a variety of conditions, among them a drastic blood loss, such as from an accident; a chronic blood loss, such as from a bleeding ulcer; hookworm infestation; and choosing a diet lacking in good sources of iron, such as dark green vegetables, egg yolks, meats (especially liver), fish, seafood, and dried peas and beans. Women are particularly susceptible to iron deficiency anemia because of regular loss of blood during menstruation as well as depletion of iron by the fetus during pregnancy. This type of anemia can be treated with iron supplements (ferrous sulfate or ferrous gluconate tablets).

Folic acid deficiency anemia

Folic acid deficiency is caused by insufficient dietary folic acid, which is necessary for hemoglobin production. This deficiency may be caused or aggravated by malnourishment or alcoholism. Some disorders of the small intestine, such as inflammatory bowel disease, may also cause it. It is treated with folic acid and sometimes additional supplements.

Pernicious anemia

Pernicious anemia arises if the body is unable to absorb vitamin B_{12}, which is necessary for the production of red blood cells in the bone marrow. A substance called intrinsic factor, which helps to absorb vitamin B_{12}, is lacking in the stomach of a person suffering from this condition. Inability to absorb vitamin B_{12} can also be caused by some parasites, inflammatory bowel disease, and diseases of the small intestine. Pernicious anemia is treated with vitamin B_{12} injections directly into the bloodstream, bypassing the stomach completely.

Aplastic anemia

Aplastic anemia is a serious condition caused by the inability of the bone marrow to produce white and red blood cells and platelets. Bone marrow function can be inhibited by cancer or exposure to radioactivity, hazardous chemicals, or some drugs. This variety of anemia is treated with blood transfusions and bone marrow transplants.

Hemolytic anemias

Hemolytic anemias are caused by the destruction of red blood cells. These anemias can be either acquired (developed over time) or congenital (present at birth).

Acquired hemolytic anemias can be caused by mismatched blood transfusions, a drug allergy, cancer, or a serious infection. Treatment of the primary condition is necessary to treat the resulting anemia. Blood transfusions can treat the condition temporarily.

Congenital hemolytic anemias are caused by an inherited abnormality in the red blood cells. The most common type is sickle cell anemia, a disorder that predominantly affects black persons. In this form of anemia, the red blood cells, which are sickle-shaped instead of disklike, cannot carry enough oxygen throughout the body. These cells are also very fragile and hemolyze (break down) easily. This disease is characterized by crisis periods of severe joint or abdominal pain and can lead to complications, such as kidney disease, gallstones, and heart failure. Sickle cell anemia is treated with painkillers, oxygen, and transfusions. Avoiding situations in which oxygen may be scarce, such as high altitudes, is advisable. (For more information on sickle cell anemia, see pages 383-385.)

Prevention

There are no specific methods to prevent anemias other than selecting a balanced diet to prevent those anemias caused by vitamin and mineral deficiencies and obtaining genetic counseling if a hereditary condition is a possibility.

Aneurysm

An aneurysm is a bulge in a blood vessel, usually an artery, due to a weakness in the vessel wall, particularly in the elastic, muscular middle layer of the artery wall. An artery has three layers: the intima, which is the smooth inner layer; the media, or

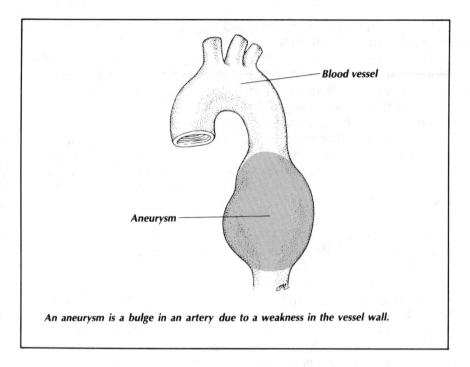

An aneurysm is a bulge in an artery due to a weakness in the vessel wall.

middle layer; and the adventitia, which is the tough outer layer. A true aneurysm involves all three layers, whereas a false aneurysm is a disruption or clot in one or two of the layers, causing a bulge in the vessel. A dissecting aneurysm occurs when blood separates the layers, thereby creating an extra channel, sometimes extending the full length of the artery, through which blood flow is diverted from the organs or tissues served by the blood vessel. This dangerous condition can develop in a matter of hours or days.

The main danger of most untreated aneurysms is that they may rupture, causing death due to loss of blood. Even if death does not occur, blood loss may so decrease blood flow to the heart that it cannot work properly.

Causes

There are various causes of aneurysms. Those occurring in

the arteries of the brain are often due to an inherited defect—a weakness or lack of elastic tissue in the media. If an aneurysm in the brain ruptures, a stroke can result. Aneurysms in the small arteries may be caused by blood vessel infections that weaken the vessel wall. Penetrating wounds occasionally can cause aneurysms.

The sexually transmitted disease syphilis may also be a cause of aneurysms. Syphilis can cause vasculitis (inflammation of the smaller arteries that feed a large one). When this occurs, these small arteries are lost, thereby denying nourishment to parts of the large arterial wall and causing scarring and death of tissue. This process leads to weakness of the wall and consequent formation of an aneurysm.

Dissecting aneurysms usually occur in the aorta. Atherosclerosis (hardening of the arteries) is the most common cause, especially in the elderly. If a young person is affected, the cause is usually an inherited defect.

Symptoms

Symptoms of dissecting aneurysms of the aorta, if in the chest, include sudden, severe pain in the area of the aneurysm, often resembling a heart attack. There may be pain under the breastbone or in the back of the neck, difficulty in swallowing, shortness of breath, hoarseness, or a heavy cough. An aneurysm in a neck artery may create a pulsating, swishing sound that the patient can detect.

Evidence of an aneurysm can be a tender, pulsating mass in the abdomen or a painful, tender mass at the back of the knee (the latter can lead to blood clots that can travel downward and may result in death of tissue in the toes). Symptoms of a dissecting aneurysm in the abdomen can include sudden, severe central or low abdominal pain radiating to the back; a loss of blood flow to the legs; and shock (collapse of circulation). Death can result quickly.

Diagnosis

Computed tomography (see page 407) and ultrasound studies (see pages 407-408) of affected areas are used to locate aneurysms and determine their extent. The most reliable and definitive test is an angiogram (also called an arteriogram). In this procedure, a thin catheter is inserted into an artery in the arm or leg and advanced to the site to be studied; a special dye is then injected to outline the area so that X rays may be taken.

Treatment

Treatment of most aneurysms, especially dissecting aneurysms,

should begin as soon as possible. Patients with dissecting aneurysms belong in an intensive care unit. Drugs are given to lower high blood pressure (which worsens a dissecting aneurysm) and thus reduce the chances of rupture. Occasionally, a dissecting aneurysm heals itself if pressure is lessened. Long-term medication that keeps blood pressure low is standard treatment for those who cannot undergo surgery. Surgery, however, is by far the most satisfactory solution when it is possible. The damaged portion of the blood vessel is removed and replaced with a synthetic vessel or a natural vessel taken from elsewhere in the body. Patients with ruptured aortic aneurysms need emergency surgery, as do most patients with dissecting aneurysms. Rapid replacement of blood is necessary, as is intensive monitoring. The surgery is usually long and difficult. However, with newer methods of diagnosis, many more people are being spared the risks of surgery by correction of the aneurysm before it becomes life threatening.

Angina pectoris

Angina pectoris, usually referred to simply as angina, is a dull constricting pain usually in the center of the chest that indicates that the heart muscle is not getting enough blood and, as a result, is not getting sufficient oxygen. When, during a period of stress or exertion, the oxygen needs of the heart muscle are greater than its blood supply from the coronary arteries can meet, angina occurs. Angina, therefore, is a mechanism for warning the body.

An angina attack is not a heart attack. Its pain is usually not as

severe or as long-lasting as that experienced during a heart attack, and it does not destroy heart muscle, as does a heart attack. However, those who suffer from this condition are probably more prone to heart attack than are those who do not.

Causes

Angina can be caused by any number of factors that prevent the heart muscle from getting enough blood. By far the most common cause of angina is coronary artery narrowing due to atherosclerosis. The coronary arteries supply the heart muscle itself with blood. When an increased demand is placed on the heart by the body, for instance, by exercise, the heart must work harder to supply blood (and thereby oxygen) to keep the muscles and organs nourished. This increased work effort causes the heart muscle itself to require more blood. When narrowing of a coronary artery is present, the areas of heart muscle supplied by that artery cannot get enough blood to keep up with the demand. When this occurs, the muscle reacts by causing the sensation of angina. Exercise, stress, and even cold weather can trigger an attack.

This sensation usually occurs during or after physical exertion or emotional stress, lasts only three to five minutes, and is relieved by resting or relaxing. If the pain does not go away within five minutes or if the pain increases, the condition causing it may not be angina. It may be another disorder unrelated to the heart, or it may be a heart attack.

Overeating and smoking can also trigger and aggravate angina—overeating, by drawing blood to the full stomach to aid in digestion; smoking, by causing the coronary arteries to constrict, reducing their capacity for carrying blood.

Risk factors

Several risk factors are associated with the development of coronary artery disease and angina. A family history of heart disease, smoking, high blood cholesterol levels, and high blood pressure are among the best known. There is much controversy in medicine regarding the degree of impact these factors have. It has not yet been clearly established whether alteration of the last three factors will definitely prevent or delay the onset of heart disease. However, there is much evidence favoring their reduction. Furthermore, common sense would dictate that one attempt to do so.

Symptoms

The major symptom of angina is the sensation of pressure, squeezing, or burning in the center of the chest behind the breastbone. This discomfort is often compared to that accompanying indigestion. Angina pain may also be felt along the neck, in the jaw or gums, in the upper part of the abdomen, or extending down the arm (most often the left) and hand to the little finger. The location and severity of the pain vary among angina sufferers, but in a given patient the same symptoms usually recur with each episode.

Diagnosis

Angina is diagnosed by first eliminating the possibility that

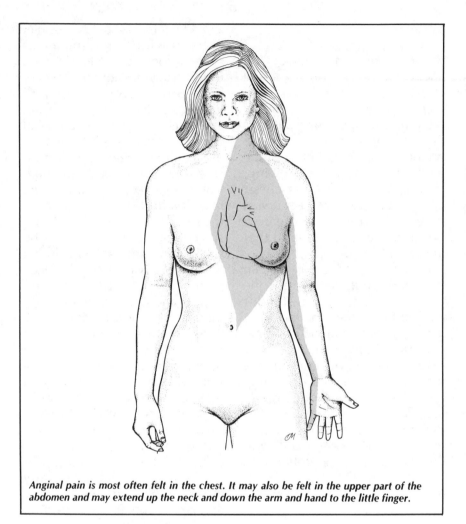

Anginal pain is most often felt in the chest. It may also be felt in the upper part of the abdomen and may extend up the neck and down the arm and hand to the little finger.

the pain is originating from some other disorder, such as gallbladder disease, rib injury, muscle spasm, or pleurisy (an inflammation of the membrane surrounding the lungs and lining the chest cavity). The doctor will take a complete medical history and perform a physical exam and probably a stress test, in which an electrocardiograph (an instrument that records the electrical impulses generated in the heart) is used to evaluate heart function during exercise. This test can indicate abnormalities in the blood supply to the heart.

The most definitive test for the diagnosis of coronary artery disease is coronary angiography (also called coronary arteriogra-

phy or cardiac catheterization). In this test, a radiopaque (able to be seen on X rays) dye is injected through a catheter (tube) placed into the heart through an artery in the leg or arm. Once the dye has been injected, X-ray films are taken, and areas of obstruction to the dye within the coronary arteries can be clearly seen. During this procedure, other important information, such as the overall condition of the heart muscle and its chambers, can also be obtained.

Treatment

Angina is often treated by recommending changes in the patient's lifestyle to reduce the strain on the heart and by administering medication to modify the relationship of the heart muscle and its blood supply.

A change in lifestyle will be necessary for patients who smoke, overeat, or overexert themselves. Certain types of exercise may be too stressful, but regular exercise is necessary to improve collateral circulation (a system of smaller blood vessels that bypass a blocked artery and increase the blood supply to the area served by that artery).

The medication most often used to treat angina attacks is nitroglycerin, which may act by expanding blood vessels to increase blood flow or by altering the volume of blood in the heart. Nitroglycerin is taken as a sublingual tablet that dissolves under the tongue or as an oral spray. Pain should stop within three or four minutes; if it does not, the pain may not be due to simple angina. Nitroglycerin can also be prescribed as a sustained release tablet or capsule, as an ointment, or as a patch applied to the skin. These forms are used for the prevention of attacks, not for the treatment of an acute episode.

Surgery to bypass the obstructions in the coronary arteries is performed only in specific circumstances. (For more on coronary bypass surgery, see pages 200-201.)

In recent years, the technique of angioplasty has become widely used to treat obstructions that are causing angina pectoris. This procedure consists of inserting a balloon-tipped catheter (tube) into an artery and inflating the balloon at the site of narrowing, thereby decreasing the obstruction (the balloon is then deflated and removed). The advantage of this technique is that it saves the patient from having to undergo surgery. Unfortunately, it is not useful in all types of coronary artery disease and can be associated with complications that necessitate emergency surgery. Also, the artery frequently becomes obstructed again, and another angioplasty or surgery must be performed.

Prevention

Incidents of angina can be prevented with several drugs: nitrates (such as nitroglycerin); calcium antagonists (such as diltiazem, nifedipine, and verapamil), which act by blocking the constricting action of calcium on arterial muscle; and beta blockers (such as metoprolol and propranolol), which decrease the work of the heart, thereby lessening its oxygen needs.

Atherosclerosis

Atherosclerosis is a slow, progressive disease of the arteries in which fatty deposits partially clog or totally block blood flow. Atherosclerosis is the most common form of arteriosclerosis (hardening of the arteries) and a major cause of coronary artery disease.

Atherosclerosis occurs when the normally smooth, firm linings of the arteries become roughened, thickened, and clogged by deposits of fat, fibrin (a protein involved in blood clotting), calcium, and cellular debris. The condition develops gradually. Lipids (fats), necessary for the production of certain hormones and tissues and as an energy reserve, are constantly present in the bloodstream. When the lipid concentration is greatly in-creased, however, fatty streaks form along the artery walls. These streaks can cause the development of small nodules of fatty deposits of cholesterol to jut out from the normally smooth linings of the artery walls. Fibrous scar tissue grows under these nodules and attracts calcium deposits. Accumulated calcium develops into a hard, chalky film (called plaque) that cannot be removed. This lining inside the arteries hampers their ability to expand and contract properly and slows the blood flow through the narrowed channels. Clots may then form easily, hindering or preventing the blood from traveling through the artery.

Causes

The exact cause of this process has not been pinpointed, but major risk factors have been identified: hyperlipidemia (abnormally elevated concentrations of fats in the blood), hypertension (high blood pressure), a history of smoking, and a family history of atherosclerosis (occurring before the age of 60) or diabetes mellitus. Hyperlipidemia, which promotes the formation of fatty streaks, seems to result from choosing a diet high in saturated fats (fats that are usually solid at room temperature, including all animal fats, such as those found in butter and meats) and cholesterol. Hypertension increases the risk of atherosclerosis because it puts constant strain on the arteries, which speeds up the clogging and hardening process. Smoking narrows the arteries, thus restricting blood flow and setting the stage for atherosclerosis. Diabetes is associated with accelerated atherosclerosis, particularly of small arteries.

Normal artery

Beginning of plaque formation

Blocked artery

Atherosclerosis occurs when the normally smooth, firm linings of the arteries become roughened, thickened, and clogged by deposits of fat, calcium, and cellular debris, which develop into a hard film called plaque. As the plaque accumulates, the artery becomes blocked.

Symptoms and complications

Atherosclerosis alone has no visible symptoms. The disease often remains undetected until the arteries leading to a vital organ are blocked. The symptoms that then become apparent are those of the specific condition caused by arterial blockage in that organ. For example, if an artery supplying the heart is partially blocked, angina (chest pain) may be felt; if the artery is totally blocked, heart attack (the death of heart tissue that is supplied by the artery) can result. If atherosclerosis affects an artery in the head, the person may ex- perience dizziness, blurred vision, and faintness or may suffer a stroke (death of brain tissue supplied by the blocked artery). Kidney failure can develop from obstruction in the arteries leading to the kidneys. Blindness can result from obstruction of vessels leading to the eyes. Diseases of the extremities can result from blockage of their arteries.

Diagnosis

Diagnostic evaluation begins with a medical history, physical examination, and analysis of the blood. An exercise tolerance test, or stress test, using an electrocardiograph (an instrument that records the electrical impulses generated in the heart) may indicate whether areas of the heart muscle are damaged or have inadequate blood supply. Nuclear medicine studies and angiography may pinpoint obstructions in blood vessels or areas of the body that are insufficiently supplied with blood. Nuclear medicine studies are X rays taken after the injection of radioisotopes into the bloodstream. Angiography is a procedure in which a thin catheter is inserted into an artery in the arm or leg and advanced to the site to be studied; a special dye is then injected through the catheter to outline the area so that X rays may be taken.

Treatment

Treatment of this disorder is aimed at reducing the strain on the heart and increasing blood flow to affected organs. Medications, changes in lifestyle and eating habits, and surgery may each be helpful.

Anticoagulants may be prescribed to prevent clotting of the blood. If atherosclerosis has led to angina, nitrates (such as nitroglycerin) and calcium-channel blockers (such as diltiazem, nifedipine, and verapamil) may provide relief by expanding the arteries and increasing blood flow. If high blood pressure contributes to the problem, antihypertensive medication is prescribed. There are not yet any medications that will actually dissolve deposits that are clogging arteries.

Lifestyle changes include quitting smoking, reducing saturated fat and cholesterol intake, losing weight (obesity puts a strain on the heart), and maintaining a moderate (but not strenuous) exercise program (exercise helps develop the collateral circulation, a system of smaller blood vessels that bypass a blocked artery and increase the blood supply to the area served by that artery).

Delicate surgical procedures, called endarterectomies, may be performed to remove deposits that are blocking arteries to vital organs. These procedures can be performed on relatively large vessels entering the brain, heart, kidneys, and legs, but cannot remove deposits in small blood vessels of these structures. If the patient suffers from severe and recurrent chest pain that is not relieved by medication, surgery may be performed to bypass major obstructions in arteries.

Recently, angioplasty (the opening of a vessel via inflation of a tiny balloon at the end of a catheter) has been quite successful in opening arteries to the kidneys and legs. Prior to this procedure, an angiogram must be performed to determine if the individual is an appropriate candidate.

Congestive heart failure

Congestive heart failure (also called left ventricular failure or, simply, heart failure) is a condition in which the heart weakens and fails to keep the blood moving adequately. As a result, the supply of blood to the body's tissues decreases, lowering efficiency and endurance. With poor circulation, the kidneys fail to remove enough water, salt, and wastes from the blood. In addition, the kidneys, because of the decreased blood flow pre-

sented to them, retain even more salt and water in an effort to increase blood volume. The increased blood volume makes more work for the already overworked heart, which may enlarge and beat faster in an attempt to satisfy the body's hunger for oxygen-rich blood. The veins distend with fluid, and the balance of pressures between fluids inside and outside the veins shifts, which causes fluid that normally stays in the bloodstream to leak into surrounding tissue. This fluid leakage, the reduction of forward blood flow, and the backflow of blood are primary factors responsible for the pulmonary edema (accumulation of fluid in the lungs) and the swelling of the abdomen and legs that often accompany this condition.

Causes

The usual cause of congestive heart failure is a diseased heart that cannot pump enough blood. The most common reason is severe coronary artery disease, which decreases blood flow to the heart muscle. If the person has suffered a heart attack, the resultant nonworking scar tissue further reduces the efficiency of the heart as a pump. Leaky or narrowed heart valves, due to a birth defect or rheumatic fever, are another cause of heart failure. A large cardiac aneurysm (a bulge caused by the thinning of the wall of the left ventricle of the heart) may also decrease the pumping ability of the heart.

Less frequently, the root of the problem is one of several heart muscle diseases; some are caused by poisons like excessive alcohol, some by a viral infection, and others by the deposition in the heart tissue of iron or

a protein called amyloid. Cardiac arrhythmias (disturbances of the normal rhythm of the heart) can also lead to heart failure.

Symptoms

Early signs of congestive heart failure include unexplained rapid heartbeat, unusual fatigue during exertion, shortness of breath during stair climbing or other mild exercise, and inability to withstand cold. Attacks of shortness of breath and coughing when lying in bed that are relieved by sleeping with pillows under the back to tilt the chest are also early symptoms. Sometimes, a person is actually awakened by a sensation of "air hunger" and must sit or stand to breathe more easily. These symptoms are caused by increased fluid pressure in the lung circulation. The relief obtained by assuming a more erect position is due to a shift of blood volume to the lower half of the body, easing the burden of the heart. In advanced congestive heart failure, shortness of breath and a severe cough with reddish-brown or brownish sputum are common. There may also be swelling of the legs and ankles and a feeling of fullness in the neck or abdomen.

Diagnosis

Usually, congestive heart failure can be diagnosed after a physical examination, on the basis of symptoms. However, a chest X ray is commonly taken to determine how much the heart has become enlarged by its overload and to see if fluid has accumulated within the lungs. An electrocardiogram (a recording of the electrical impulses generated in the heart) may reveal damage due to a previous heart attack and irregularities in the heart rhythm.

Treatment

Treatment for congestive heart failure includes rest, oxygen, medication (such as digitalis) to strengthen the pumping ability of the heart, and medication to prevent irregular heart rhythms. Diuretic medications are given to help the kidneys remove more salt and water from the blood and thus decrease the volume of blood the heart must pump. A low-salt diet is prescribed to prevent water buildup in the blood and tissues (salt tends to cause fluid to accumulate in the body). In more severe or chronic cases, a drug may be given to expand the blood vessels and thus make it easier for the heart to pump blood through them. Newer drugs known as angiotensin converting enzyme (ACE) inhibitors have been very effective in treating congestive heart failure.

In some cases, the original cause of the congestive heart failure can be corrected. For example, bypass surgery may be performed on the coronary arteries to improve blood supply to the heart muscle. Surgery may also be done to replace or correct a faulty heart valve or to repair an aneurysm. Contributing factors to be controlled or eliminated include high blood pressure, anemia, excess salt or alcohol intake, fever, an overactive thyroid gland, and stress due to overexertion.

Prevention

The prevention of congestive heart failure rests on those good health habits that help prevent heart disease in general: choosing a well-balanced diet with moderate or low intake of fats; maintaining appropriate body weight; getting plenty of exercise, rest, and sleep; avoiding tobacco and excess alcohol intake; and having periodic medical checkups to detect conditions, such as high blood pressure, that might eventually overload or injure the heart. Salt restriction in those suffering from mild congestive heart failure is also very important.

Coronary bypass surgery

Coronary bypass surgery is performed on one or more of the coronary arteries, which lie on the outer surface of the heart and supply the heart muscle with the oxygen and nutrients it needs. In coronary artery disease, a section or sections of the arteries gradually become obstructed by a buildup of cholesterol, calcium, and scar tissue. The purpose of the operation is to bypass the obstructed area in order to permit free blood flow. Without the procedure, heart muscle beyond the obstruction is starved for blood and oxygen, especially during periods of exercise or stress. This condition causes the chest pains known as angina. If one or more of the coronary arteries become completely obstructed, the result may be a heart attack, in which a portion of heart muscle becomes so starved for blood that it dies.

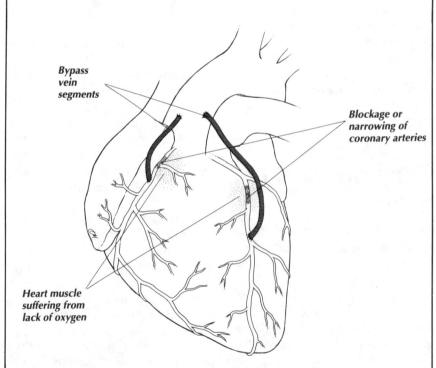

Coronary bypass surgery is performed if a section of one of the coronary arteries has become obstructed by a buildup of cholesterol, calcium, and scar tissue. A section of a blood vessel (usually a vein taken from the leg) is sewn into a small hole in the aorta and then attached to the affected vessel. The operation permits the return of free blood flow.

Indications and alternatives

Bypass surgery is usually considered when a person suffers frequent, severe chest pains from angina. However, not all persons with angina need bypass surgery. Advances are being made in using medication to control angina. Furthermore, some angina is caused by spasms (sudden, violent contractions) of the coronary arteries, which bypass surgery may not prevent or ease.

Obstructions in the coronary arteries can now sometimes be eliminated by methods that do not require cutting open the chest, such as percutaneous transluminal coronary angioplasty (also called balloon angioplasty), which consists of threading a long, balloon-tipped catheter (tube) through the arteries to the site of obstruction and inflating the balloon to open a clogged vessel (the balloon is then deflated and removed). Even without outside help, and given enough time, the heart may create its own partial bypass via collateral circulation (a system of smaller blood vessels that bypass a blocked artery and increase the blood supply to the area served by that artery).

If a patient often has severe chest pains that cannot be controlled by medication, the doctor may decide to order coronary angiography (also called coronary arteriography or cardiac catheterization). Through a thin, woven plastic catheter inserted into an artery in the arm or leg and passed through large blood vessels to the heart, X-ray contrast medium is injected so that it flows into the coronary arteries, outlining them on an X-ray screen. The pictures show exactly where and to what extent the blood vessels are narrowed or blocked. Thus, the doctor can determine whether bypasses are needed and, if so, where. The most urgent reason to operate is significant obstruction of the left main coronary artery, which supplies blood to about forty percent or more of the left ventricle.

Procedure

First, the surgeon makes several incisions in one leg to obtain a long section of a large vein for use as bypass tubing. Next, the surgeon makes an incision down the middle of the chest, divides the breastbone with an electric saw, and separates the two sides of the rib cage enough to expose the beating heart. The heartbeat is then stopped using electric shock, ice water, or certain drugs. A heart-lung machine is connected to the large vessels that carry blood to and from the heart and takes over the job of adding oxygen, removing carbon dioxide, and pumping the blood through the body.

The surgeon then cuts through the pericardial sac (a thin bag of tissue that surrounds the heart) to expose the coronary arteries, which lie on the surface of the heart. A small hole is made in the aorta, and one end of the vein segment to be used as bypass tubing is sewn to it. The other end is attached to the affected vessel beyond the obstruction. Thereafter, blood will flow freely around the obstructed portion of the artery to nourish the heart muscle, which should decrease the patient's chest pains and risk of heart attack.

The bypass surgery operation takes about four or five hours, depending on the number of bypasses. A double bypass operation is one in which portions of two vessels are bypassed, a triple bypass means that portions of three vessels are bypassed, and so forth. Usually the patient can walk about three or four days following the operation and return home in little more than a week.

Results

Considering that the procedure is such a major operation, the death rate is very low—less than one percent in most hospitals in which it is performed. In 80 percent of cases, angina pains are eliminated, and the patient can return to a normal life. Life expectancy may improve, but it cannot be guaranteed in all cases. There has been much controversy surrounding coronary bypass surgery, mainly centering on the question of whether this procedure can increase life expectancy for those with coronary artery disease and angina. At present, there is no question that the surgery relieves pain and allows for greater exercise tolerance in the majority of patients who undergo it for severe angina. In certain patterns of disease, such as obstruction of the left main coronary artery, the operation definitely prolongs life expectancy. In other patterns, such as triple vessel disease, in which branches of the coronary arteries (except for the left main coronary artery) are involved, the procedure most likely allows a longer life. In still other patterns, the question remains unsettled. Whether the surgery will prevent a heart attack has also not been determined.

Cyanosis

Cyanosis is a bluish discoloration of the skin and mucous membranes due to inadequate oxygenation of the blood. The abnormal coloration is easily seen in these areas because of both their rich blood supply and their relative transparency.

Blood rich in oxygen from the lungs is bright red. This is because of the red, iron-containing pigment known as hemoglobin, which is found in the erythrocytes (the disk-shaped red blood cells). When blood passes through the blood vessels of the lungs, oxygen from the air in the lungs combines with the hemoglobin, which causes it (and consequently the blood) to turn a very bright red. After the blood releases its oxygen to the cells of the body and picks up carbon dioxide and other waste products, the hemoglobin fades and the blood turns dark. However, if the lungs are not working well or if for some other reason the red blood cells are not being oxygenated, the blood appears bluish.

Cyanosis can be due to asthma, choking, pneumonia, or lung collapse. It can also be a sign of certain inborn heart defects, of severe cor pulmonale (right heart failure), or of abnormally excessive production of red blood cells. It is seen most frequently in cold weather when lips, toes, and fingers turn blue from extreme cold, the result of sluggish surface circulation of the blood (in this case, it may be a normal phenomenon).

Defibrillation

Defibrillation is a technique to correct fibrillation of the heart, an abnormal condition marked by very rapid, disorganized twitching or trembling of the heart muscle in place of the normal rhythmic beat. Ventricular fibrillation produces cardiac arrest, in which no heartbeat,

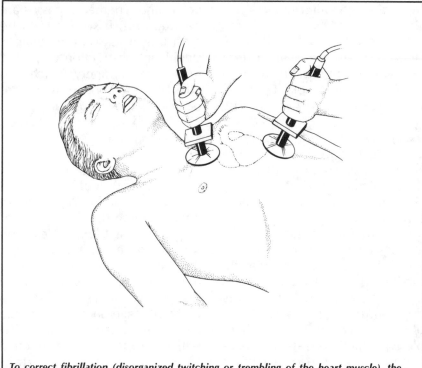

To correct fibrillation (disorganized twitching or trembling of the heart muscle), the metal paddles of the defibrillator are placed on the chest, and a jolt of electricity is directed through them into the heart to shock it back into its normal rhythm.

pulse, or blood pressure can be detected. Death or permanent brain damage follows within a few minutes unless this condition is corrected or unless first-aid measures maintain blood circulation and breathing until medical treatment is available.

Causes of fibrillation

The most common cause of fibrillation is a heart attack. When this happens, certain parts of the heart will start contracting independently of the normal heartbeat. Other causes of fibrillation are severe electrical shock and prolonged exposure to cold.

Defibrillation treatment

An electrical device called a defibrillator is used to correct fib-

rillation. A pair of metal paddles are placed on the patient's chest, and a jolt of direct-current electricity from the defibrillator is directed through them into the heart to shock it back into its regular rhythm. The shock stops the independent action of individual muscle fibers and allows the natural pacemaker of the heart to take over again.

Once the normal heartbeat has been restored, other measures are taken. A drug such as lidocaine is injected to prevent further fibrillation. An intravenous tube is inserted to administer sodium bicarbonate (to neutralize acids in the blood) and other medication. A breathing tube may be passed into the trachea (windpipe); it is attached to a mechanical pump that forces air in and out of the lungs. Then the patient is taken to a hospital cardiac intensive care unit, where monitoring devices constantly keep track of the patient's condition and sound an alarm if danger threatens. An electrical defibrillator is close at hand if needed in an emergency.

Electrical defibrillation is also used to restart a heart that has been stopped for purposes of heart surgery.

Embolism

An embolism occurs when some part of the circulatory system is either partially or completely blocked by some obstructing mass that has traveled through the system. The occurrence of such an obstruction is called an embolism, while the mass causing the embolism is called an embolus.

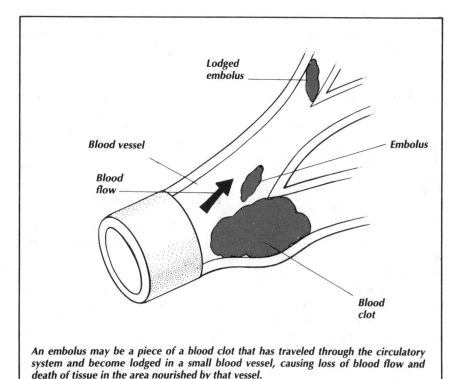

An embolus may be a piece of a blood clot that has traveled through the circulatory system and become lodged in a small blood vessel, causing loss of blood flow and death of tissue in the area nourished by that vessel.

Types

Emboli (the plural of *embolus*) are classified into three major groups:
- Solid emboli, which are made up of a variety of substances, such as clumps of tissue, tumor cells, or pieces of blood clots
- Liquid emboli, which are made up of globules of fat or amniotic fluid (fluid that surrounds the fetus in the uterus)
- Gaseous emboli, which are made up of the various constituents of air

Emboli may be further categorized according to their origin and the location of the blockage that they cause:
- Arterial emboli, which originate either from the heart or the artery itself, travel downstream, and become lodged in a smaller blood vessel, preventing the flow of fresh blood to whatever area or organ is normally supplied

- Paradoxical emboli, which originate in the venous system, pass into the arterial system (usually through a defect in the walls separating the chambers of the heart), and block an artery anywhere in the body
- Pulmonary emboli, which block vessels in the lungs (for more on pulmonary embolism, see pages 188-189)
- Coronary artery emboli, which block the coronary arteries of the heart
- Cerebral emboli, which block vessels in the brain but usually originate in the heart or the carotid arteries in the neck, which lead to the brain

Causes

The most common cause of emboli is blood clots from within the heart or blood vessels. Arterial emboli also commonly originate from plaques or other accu-

mulations on the valves of the heart, from aneurysms, and from plaques or clots within arteries. Fat emboli can result from injury to the bones (particularly the long bones of the legs) or from damage to cells in fat tissue. Air emboli can develop if a very large amount of air is admitted during an intravenous infusion or during surgery, especially in operations on the neck or chest (in the latter cases, air enters vessels that are open because of the surgery). However, the oxygen in air is not the only gas involved in gaseous emboli. When divers ascend from high-pressure levels in deep water to normal-pressure levels too quickly, or when pilots in planes without cabin pressurization climb from normal-pressure levels to low-pressure levels, there is always the possibility that nitrogen bubbles will arise in the bloodstream because of too rapid decompression. If any of these gaseous emboli find their way into the central nervous system, the results can be catastrophic.

Symptoms

The symptoms produced by an embolism vary according to the site at which the embolism occurs. An embolism deprives the affected area of its blood supply, which can cause damage or death of tissue in the area. An embolism in a brain artery may produce the symptoms of a stroke, such as unsteadiness, slurring of speech, and numbness or weakness in the face, arm, or leg on one side. If an embolism occurs in the leg, the area beyond the blockage may become white and painful. Pain may be the first symptom of embolism in other areas.

Treatment

Emboli resulting from blood clots are often treated with a variety of anticoagulants (agents that inhibit normal clotting mechanisms in the blood). Common anticoagulants, such as heparin and warfarin, do not dissolve clots, but instead prevent additional clots from forming and embolizing. There are newer drugs that do dissolve clots, but their use is restricted to special situations. If an embolism is in an accessible location, such as an artery in a limb, and tissue is threatened, surgery to remove the clot is the preferred method of treatment to save the limb. In cases of massive embolism in the lung in which life is threatened, surgery can also be attempted. If an individual has clots in the deep venous system of the lower half of the body and anticoagulants cannot be prescribed (for

example, because of a recent hemorrhage in the brain or other vital organ), blocking devices, such as clips, can be placed on or in the inferior vena cava (the main vein receiving blood from the lower part of the body) to prevent emboli from reaching the lungs.

Endocarditis

The heart is made up of three cellular layers: the epicardium (outermost layer), the myocardium (middle, muscular layer), and the endocardium (innermost layer). The endocardium lines all of the chambers and valves of the heart, and its cells are continuous with those of blood vessels leaving the heart. Endocarditis is an inflammation of the endocardial layer of the heart.

Causes

The most common form of endocarditis, infectious endocarditis, is caused by microorganisms. *Staphylococcus* and *Streptococcus* bacteria are most often the infectious agents, but viruses, fungi, and other bacteria may also be responsible.

Infective endocarditis usually occurs in persons with congenital (inborn) or acquired defects in the walls or valves of the heart. An example of a congenital defect would be a hole in the wall between two chambers of the heart. An example of an acquired defect would be damage of the heart valves caused by rheumatic fever or calcium deposition. Such abnormalities make the heart more susceptible to infection.

Bacteria probably circulate through the bloodstream of all people at some time or another.

However, certain procedures, such as dental work and surgery, may lead to bacteremia (the presence of large numbers of bacteria in the bloodstream). The bacteria accumulate on these abnormal areas in the heart and cause inflammation or infection that serves as a foundation for the collection of platelets, strands of fibrin (clotting material), and other debris of the circulatory system. The clump of material that forms is referred to as a vegetation.

Symptoms

Infectious endocarditis is a serious systemic disease with a wide spectrum of symptoms and signs. Patients may complain of fevers, weakness, and weight loss. Anemia (deficiency of red blood cells) may also be present. Pieces of vegetations may break off and travel through the bloodstream to other areas of the body, causing symptoms of obstruction (for example, a stroke if the brain is affected, or blood in the urine if a kidney is affected).

Diagnosis

The diagnosis is made on the basis of the history, the physical examination, and the results of laboratory studies, such as blood cultures, to identify the microorganisms present.

Treatment

Once the infectious agent has been isolated, appropriate antibiotics can be administered. Antibiotic administration is by the intravenous route, at least at first, and usually continues for long periods (up to eight weeks).

If infection of a heart valve is particularly severe or if a prosthetic (artificial) valve is involved, the valve may have to be replaced.

Prevention

Persons with abnormal heart valves, prosthetic valves, and other structural abnormalities must be given antibiotics before and after any procedure likely to disperse bacteria (for example, dental work, surgery of the urogenital tract or large intestine, or opening of an abscess). The antibiotics serve either to prevent the passage of microorganisms through the bloodstream or to lessen their number, thereby decreasing the chance that endocarditis will develop.

Extrasystole

An extrasystole is a contraction of the heart caused by a stimulus or impulse somewhere in the heart other than in the sinoatrial node, the natural pacemaker of the heart.

While physicians have for years debated the importance of extrasystoles, recent thought on the subject has led to a reassessment of the seriousness of the phenomenon. In many cases of sudden death attributed to severe cardiac arrhythmia (a disturbance of the normal rhythm of the heartbeat) in patients with severe underlying heart disease, the arrhythmia may have actually been triggered by ventricular extrasystoles.

Causes

While the immediate cause of an extrasystole is an accidental signal telling the heart muscle to contract, the real causes lie elsewhere. For example, strenuous activity, especially if there are existing heart problems, can trigger extrasystoles, which, in turn, may trigger an episode of heart arrhythmia that leads to more serious complications. Coffee, nicotine, and certain drugs, as well as anxiety and sudden shocks or frights, are thought to play a role in extrasystoles. It is important to note, however, that extrasystoles also occur in normal hearts and, in these cases, are quite harmless and do not necessarily indicate underlying heart disease.

Symptoms

The symptoms of extrasystoles are familiar to anyone who has ever been startled and felt his or her heart had "skipped a beat." The extrasystole sometimes presents itself as one or two extra heartbeats. On other occasions, there will be a beat followed by a long silence, then a couple of quick beats. Some people experience a feeling of giddiness, shortness of breath, and weakness, with momentary feelings of blacking out. These symptoms, if prolonged (particularly if associated with loss of consciousness), usually indicate that a sustained arrhythmia is occurring, which should be reported to a doctor.

Diagnosis

The primary tool used to diagnose extrasystole is the electrocardiograph (an instrument that records the electrical impulses generated in the heart). One method of documenting the occurrence and nature of extrasystoles is a technique called continuous ambulatory electrocardiographic monitoring, which employs a device called a Holter monitor. The monitor, which is like a combination tape recorder-electrocardiograph, is worn by the patient for as long as 24 hours. A diary is furnished so that the patient can record his or her activities and symptoms during the test period. The patient goes about his or her routine during the test. After the specified time period, the monitor is taken off, and the tape is translated into a continuous electrocardiographic record. Comparison of this record with the diary allows a diagnosis to be made as to the presence and type of arrhythmia.

Treatment

Any treatment program must be based on the underlying cause of the extrasystoles, as revealed by electrocardiographic studies. Treatment may involve medications to regulate the heartbeat, lifestyle changes (such as restriction of tobacco use and caffeine intake), or implantation of an artificial cardiac pacemaker. If the electrocardiographic studies indicate that the extrasystoles do not reflect any disease process, no medical treatment is necessary.

Gangrene

Gangrene is a term that refers to the death of body tissue due to diminishment or loss of blood supply, leading to nutrient and oxygen deprivation. There are three major types of gangrene: moist, dry, and gas gangrene. Although gangrene usually affects the extremities, it can sometimes affect the internal organs.

Causes

Moist gangrene is generally caused by a sudden stoppage of blood flow to a body site, usually resulting from burning by heat or by acid, from severe freezing, from a physical accident that destroys the tissues, from keeping a tourniquet in place too long, or from a blood clot or other blockage. The tissue death that results from loss of blood supply is accompanied by decomposition due to bacterial action. The gangrenous infection is likely to spread rapidly as toxins (poisons) are formed in the affected tissues and absorbed.

Dry gangrene usually occurs gradually and results from a slow, progressive reduction of blood flow in the arteries. There is generally no bacterial decomposition; the tissues simply become dry and shriveled. This type of gangrene occurs only in the extremities. It may occur as a secondary effect of arteriosclerosis in the elderly, of advanced stages of diabetes, or of Buerger's disease (an inflammatory condition that affects the blood vessels of the limbs, primarily the legs).

Gas gangrene is often caused by infection of a wound by anaerobic (able to live without air) bacteria, which are commonly found in soil. It can follow rapidly after contamination of deep wounds. The bacteria break down tissues, giving off gas and toxic by-products.

Gangrene in an internal organ can be caused by any condition that cuts off blood supply to an area. For example, if a loop of intestine is caught in an opening in the abdominal wall, the blood supply to that part of the intestine may be cut off (causing what is called a strangulated hernia), and gangrene may then occur in that section of the tissue. In acute

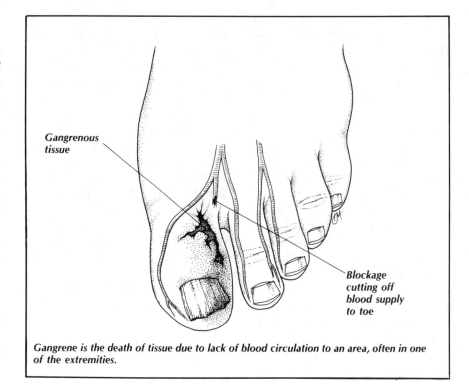

Gangrene is the death of tissue due to lack of blood circulation to an area, often in one of the extremities.

appendicitis, areas of gangrene may occur in the walls of the appendix, with rupture of the appendix through the gangrenous area. In severe cholecystitis (inflammation of the gallbladder, usually associated with gallstones), gangrene can develop in areas where the stones compress the mucous membrane, cutting off the blood supply.

Symptoms

Moist gangrene is characterized by a purplish-red, bruised appearance; by swelling; and, often, by blisters.

Dry gangrene is marked by gradual shrinking of the tissues, which first grow cold and lack a pulse, then turn brown, then black. Usually there is a sharp line of demarcation where the gangrene stops because the unaffected tissue nearby is continuing to receive blood. This type of gangrene is sometimes called

mummification of tissue because of the dry, shriveled, and dark appearance.

The initial symptoms of gas gangrene are swelling, paleness of skin, and a thin, bloody (but not foul) discharge. The characteristic foul smell comes later in the progression of this form of the disorder. It is an acute, painful condition in which the muscles and tissues under the skin become filled with gas and a thin, brownish-black fluid.

Symptoms of gangrene in an internal organ may include pain, tenderness over the organ, and fever.

Diagnosis

The appearance of the affected area usually suggests the diagnosis to the physician. Laboratory analysis of a tissue specimen will allow the identification of the infective microorganism, which is necessary for selection of an appropriate antibiotic. Areas of gas gangrene may be seen on X ray.

Treatment

Treatment of gangrene generally involves cleaning of the area and administration of antibiotics. The effectiveness of antibiotic therapy seems to depend on the time elapsed between injury or infection and the beginning of treatment.

In the case of gangrene caused by deterioration in the blood supply of the elderly or gangrene associated with appendicitis, hernia, diabetes, or Buerger's disease, the treatment begins with the diagnosis and treatment of the underlying condition.

Prevention

Preventing gangrene in an open wound begins with cleanliness. All dirt and particles in an open wound should be removed as soon as possible, and the wound should be cleansed with a soap solution and water. Burned skin requires careful, antiseptic handling to avoid infection. Frostbite also is dangerous because freezing impairs the circulation of the skin, making it tender and easily damaged. Frostbitten skin, especially on the fingers, toes, and earlobes, must be handled with great care.

Heart attack

A heart attack, or myocardial infarction, occurs when an area of the heart muscle is damaged or dies because a coronary artery (an artery that delivers blood to the heart muscle itself) has been blocked and the oxygen-rich blood supply to that area of the

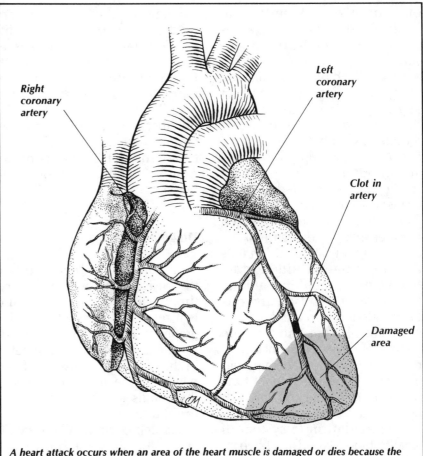

A heart attack occurs when an area of the heart muscle is damaged or dies because the coronary artery supplying the area has been blocked by a blood clot or advanced atherosclerosis.

heart has been drastically reduced. The damaged muscle tissue of the heart is replaced with scar tissue, which does not function as muscle, but rather as a kind of patch. If the area of damage is large enough, the ability of the heart to pump blood is seriously diminished.

Although the chances of surviving a heart attack are now better than ever and complete recovery is common, heart attack is still the number one cause of death in the United States. Heart attacks that do not result in death may lead to serious complications, including shock, cardiac arrhythmia (irregularity of the heartbeat), and congestive heart failure.

Causes

Heart attack is caused by the blockage of a coronary artery by a thrombus (blood clot) or by atherosclerosis, a disease in which the arteries become clogged by deposits of fat, fibrin (a protein involved in blood clotting), calcium, and celluar debris. Damage to the heart muscle occurs when the narrowed coronary arteries are unable to deliver the oxygenated blood needed by the heart.

Risk factors

A number of factors have been associated with an increased risk of heart attack. Hypertension (high blood pressure) increases the resistance in the blood vessels, forcing the heart to pump harder to push blood through the body. Smoking acts to constrict and damage the arteries and reduce blood flow to the heart muscle. Use of birth control pills, especially by women over the age of 35 and by women who smoke, has been linked to an increased incidence of heart attack. Stress increases the oxygen requirement of the heart muscle. A diet high in saturated fats (fats that are usually solid at room temperature, including animal fats in butter and meats) has been found to increase the blood cholesterol level and thus the chance of developing atherosclerosis. The lack of moderate, regular exercise results in poor tone of the heart muscle and may also prevent development of collateral circulation (a system of smaller blood vessels that bypass a blocked artery and increase blood supply to the area served by that artery).

Symptoms

The major symptom of a heart attack is a crushing pain in the middle of the chest, behind the breastbone; the pain can also extend down one or both arms and into the neck, back, teeth, or jaws. Fatigue, heavy perspiration, dizziness, difficulty in breathing, and fever may accompany this pain. The pain may be somewhat similar to that due to angina pectoris, but the pain of a heart attack is more intense, will not be relieved by nitroglycerin, and will not go away within a few minutes, as angina pain will. Also, a heart attack may take place during sleep, which is uncommon for angina pain.

Heart attacks may be very mild, signaled only by slight discomfort, faintness, and nausea. In very serious cases, a heart attack may be accompanied by cardiac arrest (cessation of the heartbeat) or ventricular fibrillation (degeneration of the normal, steady heartbeat to a useless quivering that prevents blood from being pumped through the body).

Diagnosis

Heart attack is diagnosed on the basis of the medical history, the physical examination, and test results. The electrocardiograph (an instrument that records the electrical impulses generated in the heart) will show disturbed patterns of heart activity because the impulses must travel around the damaged area. The white blood cell count may also be elevated because the body's immune system increases the number of white blood cells to remove damaged tissue from the heart. Measurements of certain enzymes (special proteins) in the blood may signal that heart muscle has been damaged, although these tests may not confirm that a heart attack has taken place until 24 to 72 hours after the event.

Treatment

There is no home treatment other than emergency first-aid measures—cardiopulmonary resuscitation (CPR)—if the patient loses consciousness. The only recommended plan of action is to summon emergency medical assistance as soon as a heart attack is suspected. Until help arrives, keep the patient warm and comfortable.

Many deaths could be prevented if heart attack victims or their families, acting on their behalf, did not delay seeking medical attention. Studies have shown that, on the average, heart attack victims wait three hours before seeing a doctor.

In almost every case, hospitalization will be necessary following a heart attack. Treatment in the hospital will probably begin in the cardiac care unit, with limited physical activity at first and a gradual return to normal activities.

A variety of medications are used to treat heart attack patients: antiarrhythmics, which inhibit irregularities in the heartbeat; diuretics, which reduce strain on the heart by removing excess water from the blood; antianginals, which diminish chest pain; sedatives, which relax the body; and beta blockers, which ease the strain on the heart by decreasing its work. Another category of drugs, calcium-channel blockers, also appear to be effective in reducing injury to the heart muscle and risk of death due to a heart attack.

Interventional therapy during the first few hours following a heart attack has become common. Usually, an angiogram (also called an arteriogram or cardiac catheterization) is performed first. In this procedure, a thin catheter is inserted into an artery in the arm or leg and advanced through the large blood vessels to the heart; a special dye is then injected through the catheter into the coronary arteries, outlining them on an X-ray screen. Once the area of obstruction has been localized, it may be possible to inject drugs to dissolve an obstruction. In other cases, percutaneous transluminal coronary angioplasty (also called balloon angioplasty) may be performed. In this procedure, a long tube with a balloon tip is threaded through the arteries to the site of the obstruction, and the balloon is inflated to open a clogged vessel (the balloon is then deflated and removed).

Prevention

Prevention of heart attack begins with sensible health and dietary habits. Those who do not smoke and do not overeat or overindulge in saturated fats, but who do exercise regularly and eliminate as much stress as possible from their lives, are much less likely to become heart attack victims. Those who have already suffered one or more heart attacks may be able to prevent further attacks by changing their living habits along these lines.

Heartbeat irregularities

Heartbeat irregularities (also called cardiac arrhythmias) are deviations from the normal, steady beating of the heart.

Minor irregularities in the heartbeat are common, but more serious arrhythmias can lead to fainting, angina pectoris, or heart attack. The most devastating heartbeat irregularity is called ventricular fibrillation, which occurs when the normally steady pumping action of the heart is reduced to a useless quivering.

Causes

Serious arrhythmias are usually caused by damage to the heart muscle or to specialized heart tissue called the conduction system. The first part of the

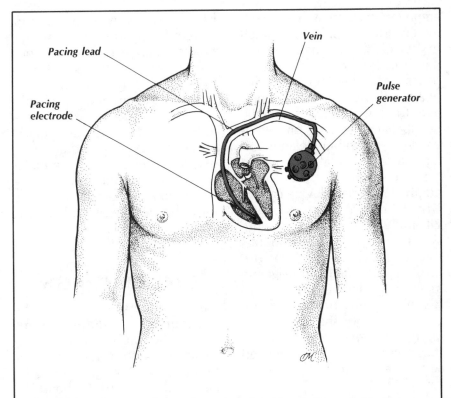

Pacing lead

Vein

Pacing electrode

Pulse generator

An artificial cardiac pacemaker can be used to correct heartbeat irregularities in persons whose natural conduction system is defective. The pacing lead is threaded through a vein until the pacing electrode at the tip of the lead rests within the heart. The electrical pulse generator is then sewn in place under the skin.

conduction system, called the sinus node, serves as the natural pacemaker of the heart; it is responsible for establishing and maintaining a healthy, steady heartbeat.

Heartbeat irregularities can also be caused by improper use of certain drugs (among them, drugs for arrhythmia, which can actually cause arrhythmia if the dosage is too high), excessive smoking (the nicotine alters the heartbeat), or consumption of large quantities of caffeine (the amounts found in coffee, tea, chocolate, cola, and some cold medicines may overstimulate the heart).

Irregularities may also develop as a result of congenital (present at birth) damage to the heart, a poorly functioning left ventricle, high blood pressure, or a previ-

ous heart attack (the resulting scar tissue may interfere with transmission of nerve impulses governing heartbeat).

Ventricular fibrillation often occurs after a myocardial infarction (heart attack) or some other serious injury, such as a severe electrical shock.

Symptoms

Some irregularities have no noticeable symptoms. Others are signaled by light-headedness, fainting, pounding of the heart, dizziness, and chest pain.

Diagnosis

Arrhythmias are diagnosed primarily with the electrocardiograph (an instrument that records the electrical impulses generated in the heart). A normal heart will produce a record of regular peaks and valleys; an arrhythmic heart will show an uneven pattern. Continuous recording of the heartbeat can be done on an outpatient basis with a Holter monitor, which is like a combination tape recorder-electrocardiograph. This small device can be worn by the patient for as long as 24 hours. Electrocardiographic wires are taped to the patient's chest, and recordings of the heartbeat are made on magnetic tape. The patient makes a note of his or her activities and of any symptoms he or she experiences during the testing period, and these reports are later correlated with the recorded heartbeat rhythm.

Treatment

Occasionally, cardiac arrhythmias are so mild that no particular treatment is required. However, more serious irregularities are treated with medication, defibrillation, or implantation of an artificial pacemaker. All of these methods act to steady the heart rhythm and to maintain a healthy, steady heartbeat.

Medications commonly used include digitalis, beta blockers, and antiarrhythmics, such as quinidine.

A defibrillator is a device applied to the chest that electrically jolts a quivering heart in a state of ventricular fibrillation back into a normal pattern of beating.

For those whose arrhythmia is caused by a faulty conduction system, an artificial cardiac pacemaker may be implanted in the chest. The pacemaker incorporates a small electrical generator, which causes the heart to beat when its own conduction system fails and steadies an abnormal heartbeat by sending out electrical impulses similar to those emitted by the heart.

Lifestyle changes will probably be recommended to patients suffering from heartbeat irregularities; they may need to quit smoking, lose weight, exercise more regularly, and reduce their caffeine intake. These precautions may also be taken in an effort to prevent arrhythmias.

Heart murmurs

Heart murmurs are extra whishing sounds—in addition to the regular "lub-dub" sounds of the heartbeat—that are made as blood flows through the chambers and valves of the heart. In most cases, heart murmurs are quite harmless and represent no cause for concern. In other cases, however, heart murmurs can be a symptom that first alerts a doctor to the presence of heart disease or a structural abnormality in the heart.

Causes

Heart murmurs can be heard in many healthy persons, especially children, teenagers, and pregnant women. These murmurs are normal sounds caused by the blood rushing through the heart and do not indicate a heart condition. They are called innocent, functional, or insignificant heart murmurs.

In contrast, organic, or structural, heart murmurs are caused by narrowing or obstruction of the heart valves or by incomplete closure of the valves, which allows blood to seep back into the upper or lower heart chambers. Such heart murmurs can be congenital (existing at birth) or acquired, due to damage to the heart valves caused by rheumatic fever, atherosclerosis, syphilis, or other ailments. Heart murmurs also occur when there are holes in the walls separating the chambers of the heart.

Symptoms

Heart murmurs can be detected only by physical examination. By listening to the heart through a stethoscope, a doctor can usually distinguish any extra sounds and judge (by their quality, intensity, location, and timing) whether they signify a serious problem.

Diagnosis

If the heart murmur is considered to be organic, the doctor will order special studies—for example, chest X ray, electrocardiography (see page 399), and angiography (see page 403) in order to evaluate the cause and extent of the condition.

Treatment

An innocent heart murmur does not require any medical treatment or special care, and a person with such a murmur can live a completely normal life. In fact, it is very important that a child with an innocent murmur be treated as the normal, healthy child that he or she is. Parents are sometimes frightened by the idea of a heart murmur and overprotect a child unnecessarily, which is not good for the child's emotional well-being. Most innocent murmurs detected in children disappear or become undetectable by adolescence; only 15 percent to 20 percent of such murmurs continue into adulthood.

If a murmur is organic, the underlying condition can usually be corrected surgically. In cases of heart murmur due to actual diseased valves, it is important to discuss with your physician or dentist the taking of antibiotics prior to dental work or surgery. This simple technique may prevent bacterial endocarditis (for more on endocarditis, see pages 204-205).

Hemoglobin

The role of the red blood cells is to carry oxygen throughout the body. The red blood cells can perform this task because of the presence of hemoglobin, the pigment (coloring agent) that is formed when the red blood cells develop in the bone marrow.

Each hemoglobin molecule is made up of a protein molecule called globin and four pigmented molecules of a compound called heme. Each heme molecule has one atom of iron, and there are four heme molecules in a single molecule of hemoglobin; hence, a single molecule of hemoglobin has four atoms of iron. This structure makes it possible for one hemoglobin molecule to join with four oxygen molecules to form a substance called oxyhemoglobin. This reaction is reversible, enabling hemoglobin to pick up oxygen when the blood is in the lungs and enabling it to release oxygen in the cells when the blood is pumped to the tissues of the body.

In general, the blood of men usually has a greater concentration of hemoglobin than that of women. Men have about 14 to 16 grams of hemoglobin per 100 milliliters of blood, whereas women have only about 12 to 14 grams per 100 milliliters of blood. (One hundred milliliters is approximately equal to three and one-half ounces.)

A number of blood disorders have to do with hemoglobin abnormalities. In many forms of anemia, there is not enough hemoglobin in the red blood cells (for more on anemia, see pages 192-194). In polycythemia, there is too much hemoglobin in the blood (for more on polycythemia, see page 216). In other conditions, such as thalassemia, the abnormal chemical composition or production of hemoglobin molecules reduces the oxygen-carrying or oxygen-releasing capability of the red blood cells.

Hemorrhage

Hemorrhage is the technical term for bleeding, often referring to substantial blood loss or uncontrollable bleeding, either externally or internally. The effects of hemorrhage depend on the part of the body that is bleeding and the total amount of blood that is lost. Hemorrhage can be a symptom of a number of serious, sometimes fatal, disorders.

Causes

Hemorrhage occurs when blood vessels are torn or broken. Normally, blood will clot within seconds or minutes, stopping the blood flow. However, when serious injuries or other disorders (such as hemophilia, peptic ulcer, or cancer) are involved, the body's normal blood-clotting mechanism may be inadequate or may malfunction. If blood loss is not quickly stopped, death may result.

Symptoms

Severe external hemorrhage is associated with the following symptoms: rapid pulse; dizziness or faintness; collapse; a drop in blood pressure; a rise in pulse rate; and pale, cold, clammy, or sweaty skin.

Internal hemorrhage may also show symptoms, even if the bleeding is slight. Black, tarry stools may signal bleeding in the intestinal tract from a peptic ulcer; blood in the vomitus indicates bleeding in the stomach; and blood in the urine means that bleeding is occurring in the kidneys or urinary tract.

Blood in the stool, urine, or vomitus should always be reported to a doctor at once, as should external bleeding that occurs frequently or that cannot be stopped within minutes.

Treatment

Treatment for internal hemorrhage involves correcting the cause of the bleeding, possibly with surgery. External hemorrhage is treated by applying pressure to the wound with a sterile bandage (or, in an emergency, just pressing it with the fingers) until the bleeding stops. If bleeding cannot be stopped, the patient will almost certainly have to be hospitalized, so that lost blood can be replaced with transfusions of blood products and, in some cases, so that damaged blood vessels can be surgically tied off and sealed.

Hypertension

Hypertension, or high blood pressure, refers to persistently elevated pressure of blood within the arteries, which carry blood

Manometer

Inflatable cuff

Main artery in arm

Bulb to inflate cuff

Stethoscope

Blood pressure is measured by using a sphygmomanometer, which consists of an inflatable arm cuff and a manometer (a pressure-measuring instrument). The pulse is listened to with a stethoscope while the blood flow in a main artery of the arm is shut off by inflating the cuff and then released by deflating the cuff.

from the heart through the body. The exertion of excessive force on the artery walls may cause damage to the arteries themselves and thereby to the heart, kidneys, and brain, leading to heart attack, kidney failure, and stroke.

Causes

Although many people believe that hypertension is caused by extreme activity or tension, this theory has not been proved. When no underlying cause is discovered, the disease is called primary, or essential, hypertension. If another disease, such as kidney or heart disease, causes the elevated blood pressure, the condition is labeled secondary hypertension.

Risk factors

Contrary to popular belief, there is no typical hypertensive person. However, some people are more susceptible to developing high blood pressure than others. Heredity appears to play a role; persons whose parents are hypertensive are at greater risk of becoming hypertensive themselves. In the past, hypertension was attributed to aging, but current evidence indicates that age is not a primary factor. The incidence of hypertension in black persons, both children and adults, is about twice that in white persons.

Overweight, prolonged stress, smoking, drinking, and excessive sodium in the diet (which causes fluid retention) may increase blood pressure, especially in per-

sons prone to hypertension. There are also indications that use of oral contraceptives may contribute to increased blood pressure; however, this is more likely to occur in women who are overweight, whose parents are hypertensive, or who have other hypertensive risk factors.

Symptoms

Hypertension has been called the "silent disease" because it often has no obvious symptoms. A person may have high blood pressure for years without noticing any symptoms. Symptoms may include headache, fatigue, dizziness, flushing of the face, ringing in the ears, thumping in the chest, and frequent nosebleeds. However, these symptoms may also result from other conditions.

Diagnosis

To diagnose hypertension, a simple, risk-free, painless test using a stethoscope and a sphygmomanometer is used. Blood pressure is measured in a main artery of the arm by shutting off and then releasing the flow of blood in the artery with the inflatable cuff of the sphygmomanometer while listening to the arterial pulse with the stethoscope.

The blood pressure measurements are given as the systolic pressure (the pressure at which the first beat of the pulse can be heard as gradual deflation of the cuff begins) over the diastolic pressure (the pressure at which steady flow through the artery can be heard as the cuff is deflated)—for example, 150/95. The systolic pressure essentially measures the pressure of the heart during a contraction. The diastolic pressure is that which exists when the heart is filling between beats. Although diastolic pressure is lower than systolic, there is still pressure in the body when the heart is filling. Both values are important. An unusually high systolic pressure may mean that the heart is pumping too hard or the arteries are stiff; a high diastolic pressure means that the arteries have abnormally high muscular tone or resistance.

Normal blood pressure is about 80/46 at birth and climbs as age increases. The normal adult pressure is about 120/80.

Treatment

Fortunately, hypertension responds well to treatment, although female hypertensive patients seem to do better than male patients. When the condition is mild (a blood pressure of about 140/90) and there is no indication of other disease, a doctor may suggest lifestyle changes before prescribing medication. These changes may include weight loss, a regular exercise program, and strict limitation of sodium intake, which affects fluid balance and volume and therefore blood pressure. Controlling sodium in the diet requires restriction of table salt as well as careful scrutiny of all food and drug labels.

If medication is indicated, a physician may prescribe one or several drugs. There is no "cookbook" approach to treating hypertension. The choice of therapy is governed by multiple factors, including the patient's age, sex, and any coexisting illnesses, as well as by the severity of the hypertension.

While tension and stress do not directly cause hypertension, these factors do affect the condition. Persons with hypertension, therefore, are urged to avoid high-pressure situations and to learn to deal with stress. Biofeedback, self-hypnosis, and meditation have proved useful for reducing stress and may help someone with hypertension.

Blood pressure can be monitored at home with a special kit. If three separate elevated readings (above 140/90 in adults) are obtained, a trip to the doctor is in order. Furthermore, everyone should have his or her blood pressure measured by a health-care professional at least once a year. Persons with a history of hypertension or with any of the risk factors for hypertension should carefully follow their physician's recommendations for periodic blood pressure checks.

It is also recommended that children of hypertensive parents begin to receive regular blood pressure measurements early in life.

Hypotension

Hypotension is low blood pressure. Unlike chronic high blood pressure, which can be a serious health problem, low blood pressure usually need not be a cause for concern or even treatment.

Blood pressures vary, depending on such factors as age, race, sex, and environment. On rare occasions, individuals may have medical problems that cause low blood pressure. Among such conditions are some types of heart disease, hormonal deficiencies, and malnutrition. In these cases, the hypotension will be corrected by the treatment of the medical problem.

Postural hypotension

Postural hypotension, or orthostatic hypotension, is a form of low blood pressure in which dizziness or faintness occurs when a person stands up abruptly from a sitting or reclining position. Normally, when an individual stands up, the blood vessels contract to maintain normal blood pressure in the new position. However, in persons with postural hypotension, this mechanism probably does not work properly, and on standing, a temporary reduction in the blood flow to the brain leads to feeling faint. Rising slowly from a sitting or reclining position will usually prevent the symptoms in this situation.

Sometimes, postural hypotension results from taking a medication for high blood pressure; in these cases, the physician may reduce the dosage or change the medication.

Fluids, including blood, lost from the body may also cause postural hypotension, as may many diseases. Consequently, although postural hypotension is a benign condition in most individuals, it should be reported to a physician.

Ischemia

Ischemia is a deficiency of blood in a specific part of the body caused by an obstruction of the blood vessels supplying that area. The obstruction may be due to narrowing, compression, or destruction of arteries caused by such conditions as blood clots and atherosclerosis (clogging of the arteries). The resultant oxygen deprivation, if prolonged, leads to tissue death in the affected area.

Ischemia in the brain

An ischemic attack in the brain occurs when the supply of blood to the brain is temporarily reduced. This type of attack resembles a stroke. If the brain is deprived of blood for more than several minutes, the result is irreversible brain damage and often death.

Ischemia in the heart

When the blood supply to the heart is reduced, angina pectoris results. When the blood supply to a region of the heart is cut off, a heart attack occurs. The lower the blood supply that gets through to the heart, the greater the severity of the attack. If a weakened heart is unable to

pump an adequate supply of blood to the rest of the body, the other organs will also work at less than capacity.

Treatment

Ischemic attacks can be controlled by vasodilator medications, which widen blood vessels. Angina pectoris is often managed in this way. In many cases, surgery to remove or to bypass the obstruction is recommended.

Lymphocytes

Lymphocytes are a type of white blood cell. They are produced in the bone marrow and lymph nodes and stored in the thymus gland, spleen, and lymph nodes.

Lymphocytes play an important role in the body's immune system. Lymphocytes make their way through the lymph channels into the bloodstream, where they identify and "memorize" the characteristics of foreign elements called antigens. There are two types of lymphocytes—B cells and T cells. B cells manufacture antibodies (highly specialized proteins that destroy the antigens by combining with them). T cells, which make up 70 percent of the lymphocyte total, regulate antibody production and oversee immune responses.

Lymphocytes are the second most numerous type of white blood cell, normally constituting between 22 percent and 28 percent of the white blood cells in an adult's circulation. In cases of infection, especially those caused by viruses, the percentage of lymphocytes in the blood may increase to above 50 percent.

Pericarditis

Pericarditis is an inflammation of the pericardium (the membranous sac surrounding the heart). The inflammation is often accompanied by development of an effusion (a collection of fluid) between the membrane and the heart, which may lead to complications.

Causes

The inflammation commonly stems from an infection, such as bacterial pneumonia, tuberculosis, or a viral infection. Pericarditis can also occur in noninfectious diseases, such as connective tissue disorders and chronic kidney failure. Pericarditis sometimes follows a heart attack or chest injury.

Occasionally, long-term pericarditis arises from a chronic condition, most notably tuberculosis. The chronic inflammation causes thickening and contraction of the pericardium to the point that it restricts the heartbeat. Called constrictive pericarditis, this condition is no longer common because of the decrease in the incidence of tuberculosis, but it is a severe condition calling for immediate attention.

Symptoms

Pain in the center of the chest (and possibly the shoulders, neck, and upper arms) that worsens with coughing, lying flat, or breathing and is relieved by leaning forward may signify pericarditis. Since this type of pain is a symptom of a number of serious illnesses, a doctor should be consulted about any severe chest pain.

Constrictive pericarditis is signaled by difficulty in breathing, swelling of the veins in the neck, and edema (fluid retention) in the legs and abdomen.

Diagnosis

A chest X ray, electrocardiogram (see page 399), and blood tests, along with the medical history and a physical examination, are used to diagnose pericarditis. If an effusion is present, a sample of the fluid may be obtained in order to identify any infectious agent.

Treatment

When a large effusion exists, the motion of the heart may be restricted, thereby preventing it from filling and pumping effectively. This life-threatening condition must be corrected as soon as possible. The fluid may be drained by inserting a needle through the chest into the pericardial sac.

Once the underlying cause of pericarditis has been identified, the doctor can treat it (for example, by using dialysis in kidney failure or antibiotics for bacterial infection).

Constrictive pericarditis cannot be corrected without surgery to remove scarred tissue (called pericardiectomy).

Platelets

Platelets (also called thrombocytes) are tiny, disk-shaped, cell-like structures that play a critical role in the process of blood coagulation (clotting). They are manufactured in the bone marrow and usually survive for about ten days.

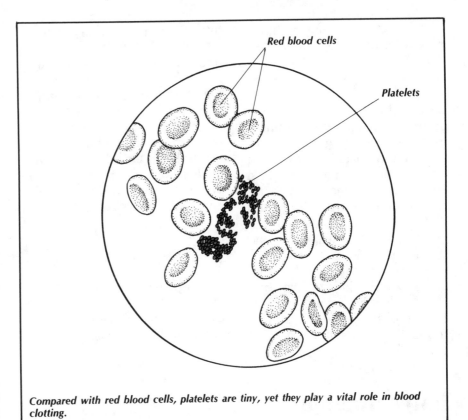

Compared with red blood cells, platelets are tiny, yet they play a vital role in blood clotting.

Role in coagulation

Blood coagulation is a complex process requiring the presence of many substances in the blood besides platelets. However, without platelets, coagulation would be impossible. Platelets initiate the coagulation process by aggregating (clumping together). The usual amount of time for adequate coagulation is five minutes or less.

The number of platelets per unit volume of blood plays an important role in proper platelet function. The normal number ranges between 200,000 and 500,000 platelets per cubic millimeter of blood.

Low platelet count

A low platelet count may be seen with many different diseases, including certain liver diseases, uncommon forms of anemia caused by vitamin deficiencies, and certain cancers (such as leukemia) of the blood-forming organs. Use of certain drugs also may cause a low platelet count.

The most common cause of a low platelet count is destruction of platelets by the body's immune system. For some unknown reason, the immune system mistakenly identifies the platelets as foreign and forms antibodies to destroy them.

When a lack of platelets prolongs bleeding time, several types of treatment may be attempted, depending on the cause of the low platelet count. The usual way to immediately increase the number of platelets is by transfusion (this is generally reserved for patients with severe platelet deficiencies). Care must be taken to avoid increasing the platelet count too much, however, because emboli (clots that obstruct blood vessels) may develop.

Care should be taken by any patient whose platelet count is low, since bleeding will be prolonged and coagulation will not occur within normal time limits. For this reason, many physicians recommend that until normal platelet counts are attained, patients should not take aspirin and should avoid doing anything that may cause bleeding, such as vigorous toothbrushing, eating abrasive foods, and having enemas. They should also avoid contact sports and use caution regarding personal injury.

Polycythemia vera

Polycythemia vera is a relatively rare chronic disorder characterized by an increase in red blood cell mass and in the concentration of hemoglobin (the substance in red blood cells that carries oxygen).

Cause

The immediate cause of polycythemia is excessive production of red blood cells by the bone marrow, but the underlying cause remains unknown. The condition is most often seen in the elderly and in persons of Jewish descent.

Symptoms

The initial symptoms include fatigue, difficulty in concentration, headache, drowsiness, forgetfulness, and dizziness. About

half of the patients with polycythemia vera complain of itching, especially after a hot bath. Reddish skin color, or flushing, may be observed; however, patients may have completely normal skin color, with redness only of the mucous membranes, especially the inner lids of the eyes. Patients may complain of blurred vision, ringing in the ears, and circulatory disturbances.

Diagnosis

Diagnosis can usually be made on the basis of a physical examination and medical history and analysis of the blood.

Treatment

Phlebotomy (withdrawal of blood from a vein) to counterbalance the overproduction of red blood cells is probably the safest treatment since it does not interfere with the functioning of the bone marrow. Radiation therapy to suppress bone marrow activity may also be useful.

Raynaud's disease

Raynaud's disease involves spasm of the arterioles (small artery branches), especially in the fingers and hands and occasionally in other parts of the body, such as the nose and tongue. It is often accompanied by intermittent paleness or bluish discoloration of the skin.

Causes

Attacks of Raynaud's disease are most often precipitated by

exposure to cold temperatures or by emotional stress. When the symptoms are caused by another condition, such as scleroderma (a connective tissue disorder), a nerve disorder, a drug reaction, or pulmonary hypertension, the condition is called Raynaud's phenomenon. Raynaud's disease is most common in young women.

Symptoms

The color changes in the skin in the classic form of the disease come in three stages—pallor (extreme paleness), cyanosis, and then extreme redness, called reactive hyperemia. Sometimes the color changes may go through only two stages, cyanosis and then redness. Normal color and sensation are restored when the hands are warmed. Color changes in the hands do not affect the joints and seldom affect the thumb. Pain is usually not present, but numbness, tingling, and burning are common complaints. Ulcers (open sores) may appear on the tips of the fingers. Raynaud's disease differs from Raynaud's phenomenon in that both sides of the body are involved.

A wide range of other symptoms may be associated with Raynaud's phenomenon, depending on the underlying disease process.

Treatment

Mild cases of Raynaud's disease can be relieved substantially by protecting the body and extremities from exposure to cold. This is extremely important because prolonged spasm of the small arteries leads to severe tissue injury. Mild sedatives, taken orally, can sometimes be of help. The patient is strongly advised to stop smoking, since nicotine acts as a constrictor of blood vessels. Drugs known as calcium-channel blockers, such as nifedipine, verapamil, and diltiazem, are of great benefit in relieving symptoms but do not cure the condition.

A more extreme measure, which is not often used, is regional sympathectomy (an interruption of certain portions of the nerve pathways). This operation is reserved for patients with progressive disability; while it abolishes the symptoms, the relief may last only for a year or two. Results of the surgical procedure are usually better in patients with Raynaud's disease than in those with Raynaud's phenomenon.

Therapy for Raynaud's phenomenon depends chiefly on correctly diagnosing and then treating the underlying disorder.

Restless legs syndrome

Restless legs syndrome (also called Ekbom syndrome, "jimmy legs," and "jitter legs") is a feeling of uneasiness, shakiness, twitching, and restlessness that affects the legs after a patient has gone to bed for the night. Insomnia is almost always a result of the syndrome.

Causes

The precise cause of the syndrome is not known, although some authorities consider it to be brought about, or intensified, by poor blood circulation. Some physicians believe that it is more common in hyperactive patients; others say that it can be brought

about by intense activity, especially physical activity, just before bedtime.

Symptoms

The patient often has difficulty falling asleep in the evening because of an uncomfortable feeling or a jerking sensation within the legs, usually in the thighs and calves. The discomfort is often relieved by moving about, but as a result, normal sleep is largely prevented. Consequently, the person may be excessively tired the next day. The condition most commonly affects middle-aged women.

Diagnosis

Diagnosis can generally be made on the basis of the medical history and reported symptoms. The doctor will perform a physical examination to rule out more serious disorders.

Treatment

Since the syndrome has been connected with circulatory disorders, drugs that increase the circulation to the lower extremities may prove helpful. A mild sedative at bedtime may also help.

Rheumatic fever

Rheumatic fever is the result of a bacterial disease characterized by inflammation, swelling, and soreness of the joints—especially the ankles, knees, and wrists—and inflammation of the heart. Occurring most commonly in children and adolescents, it is a serious illness that can result in permanent damage to the heart.

The attacks of fever may recur over a period of years and last from a few weeks to several months.

Cause

The disease is considered to be a late stage of a streptococcal infection, such as strep throat; however, not all species of *Streptococcus* bacteria cause rheumatic fever. In some cases, the earlier infection may have been so minor that it cannot be recalled. Some researchers believe that rheumatic fever is an autoimmune disorder, in which the immune system forms antibodies to attack the body's own healthy tissues, such as those of the joints and the heart. The disease is more prevalent in some families than in others, but whether this indicates a hereditary factor or is due simply to sharing the same environment and living habits is not clear. Because only one percent of all cases of streptococcal infection in children and adolescents are followed by rheumatic fever, it is believed that a special susceptibility may be involved.

Symptoms

Rheumatic fever should be immediately suspected when a child or teenager develops an unexplained fever with joint inflammation a few weeks after a throat infection or tonsillitis, even if that preceding condition was very mild. The joints then become inflamed one after another. A peculiar skin rash of large, reddened, nonitchy areas with irregular borders develops, lasting a day or two. Nodules may emerge over the elbows, kneecaps, and other bony prominences; they may also form within the heart. Chorea (involuntary movement of the limbs and facial features) may occur if the infection spreads to involve the brain. Fortunately, chorea leaves no lasting brain damage and passes after some time, even without specific treatment.

Effects on the heart

The acute stage of joint involvement leaves no permanent deformity or crippling, but damage to the heart is permanent when it involves destruction of heart valve tissue. Scar tissue is then eventually formed on the valves, so that they cannot open and close properly. The heart, unable to efficiently carry out its function of pumping blood through the circulatory system, must work harder and becomes enlarged. Blood clots may form on its inner lining and may be carried in the blood throughout the body, often lodging in a blood vessel and blocking it.

Diagnosis

Joint inflammation, heart abnormalities, chorea, and the appearance of the rash and the nodules are the most common manifestations of rheumatic fever, but these signs may appear alone or in different combinations. Because no single laboratory finding or symptom is common to all cases, the diagnosis is made presumptively on the basis of the total clinical picture.

Treatment

The chief treatment for rheumatic fever is the use of antibiotics for an extended period

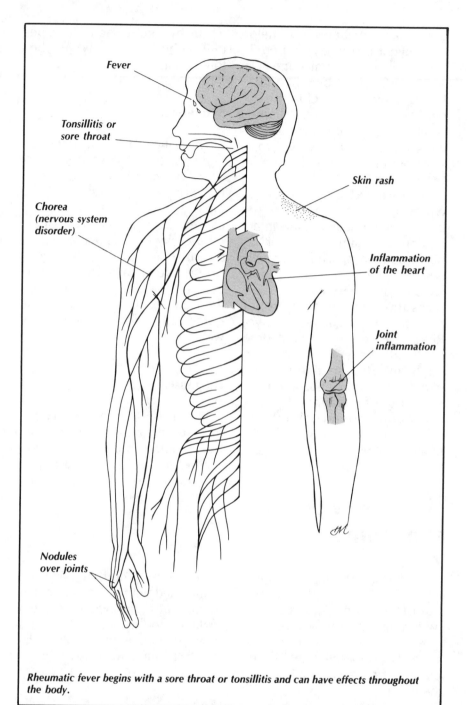

Rheumatic fever begins with a sore throat or tonsillitis and can have effects throughout the body.

of time to eliminate any remaining *Streptococcus* bacteria. Aspirin is commonly used to bring down fever and relieve inflammation and pain. Corticosteroid drugs are sometimes given if there are signs of heart involvement, and sedatives may be prescribed if chorea becomes se-

vere. The long periods of immobilization in bed that were once recommended are now believed to be unnecessary, although bed rest during acute attacks may be prescribed. Seriously damaged heart valves can often be repaired surgically or replaced by prosthetic (artificial) valves.

Prevention

The only preventive measure is prompt diagnosis and adequate treatment of all streptococcal infections, especially those involving the throat and ears. Since dental procedures can sometimes be a source of bacterial infection, special precautions (such as the administration of antibiotics) may be recommended for persons whose heart valves have been injured.

Rheumatic heart disease

Rheumatic heart disease consists of a variety of abnormal cardiac conditions, including heart valve scarring and endocarditis (inflammation of the lining of the heart).

Cause

This disease is a potential aftermath of rheumatic fever, once one of the prime killers of children. Rheumatic fever may cause inflammation of the heart valves and scarring of the valve leaflets. This scarring can result in valve leakage, allowing blood to flow backward, or severe narrowing of the valve, restricting blood flow out of the heart.

Symptoms

The most common symptom is a heart murmur, caused by abnormal blood flow across a scarred valve. There may be hemorrhaging (excessive bleeding) and impairment of vision if microscopic blood clots that have formed in the heart block tiny blood vessels in the eye.

Kidney function may deteriorate in middle or later life. Muscle shrinkage due to inactivity may be accompanied by lack of muscular and cardiovascular endurance. Irregular pulse, shortness of breath, and fainting spells are also common.

Treatment

Many persons who have suffered rheumatic heart disease have gone on to live extremely active lives, despite heart murmurs, heart enlargement, and damaged valves. Although rheumatic heart disease is a serious matter, regular exercise, a sensible diet, and determination can mean the difference between a sedentary and an active life.

Supervision by a physician is a necessity for anyone who suffers from rheumatic heart disease and wants to embark on a regular exercise program. In some cases, however, it may be impossible for a patient to participate in vigorous physical activity, especially if the heart damage is advanced or severe. For some of these individuals, surgery to implant an artificial valve can offer relief.

Persons with rheumatic heart disease must consult their physicians about antibiotic treatment before undergoing any dental or surgical procedures.

Rh factor

Rh factor refers to a specific antigen present in the blood. ("Rh" is derived from the name of the rhesus monkey, in which the factor was discovered.) An antigen is a substance that can induce the production of antibodies, which are crucial to the functioning of the body's immune system. Rh-positive blood has the antigen on its red cells; Rh-negative blood does not. An estimated 85 percent of the population has Rh-positive blood (they possess Rh antigens).

Dangers of anti-Rh antibodies

Blood normally has no anti-Rh antibodies. Anti-Rh antibodies can develop in Rh-negative blood, however, if Rh-positive blood is introduced into the bloodstream. This can come about in two ways: if a person with Rh-negative blood receives a transfusion of Rh-positive blood or if a woman with Rh-negative blood conceives a child with Rh-positive blood (inherited from the father) and some of the Rh-positive cells from the fetus find their way into the bloodstream of the mother. In either case, the Rh-positive red blood cells will stimulate the person's body to form anti-Rh antibodies. If this happens, the blood will form clumps, and a potentially lethal situation will develop—the clumps may block the blood vessels, leading to death.

If difficulties do not appear with the formation of these antibodies during the first transfusion or the first pregnancy, they will surely appear if Rh-positive blood is ever again introduced into the person's bloodstream. The antibodies are already present, and the introduction of additional Rh-positive blood will result in a mobilization of existing antibodies and the production of even more. In addition to clumping of blood, other problems will arise. For example, hemolysis (the breakdown of red blood cells and release of their hemoglobin) will make it impossible for those cells to carry oxygen, resulting in anemia.

There are potential dangers to the fetus if the mother's blood contains anti-Rh antibodies. If the fetus has Rh-positive cells, anti-Rh antibodies may pass through the placenta from the mother's bloodstream to cause hemolysis of the child's blood cells. Once born, the baby may need to have massive, possibly even total, transfusions of Rh-negative blood to prevent clumping of the red blood cells and hemolytic anemia. This situation is now relatively rare because injections of gammaglobulin are routinely given to an Rh-negative mother after every pregnancy. These injections inhibit the formation of the potentially dangerous antibodies.

A stroke is caused by an interruption in the blood supply to the brain. A stroke may be caused by a blood clot blocking an artery leading to the brain.

Cross section of the brain

Blood clot

Area of damage

Blocked artery

Stroke

Stroke is a nervous system disorder of abrupt onset caused by interruption of the blood supply to an area of the brain, resulting in malfunction or loss of function in those parts of the body that the damaged area controls. Generally speaking, each side of the brain controls the motor and sensory functions of the opposite side of the body (for example, damage to cells on the left side of the brain will impair function on the right side of the body). Stroke can have a wide range of consequences, among them temporary or permanent loss of memory and difficulty in speaking, walking, and controlling emotions.

Causes

Stroke can be caused by several conditions. One is called cerebrovascular embolism, which occurs when a blood clot formed elsewhere in the body (usually in the heart or in one of the carotid arteries in the neck) lodges itself in an artery in the brain or leading to the brain. Interruption of blood flow also occurs when a clot is formed in the arteries that supply blood to the brain, usually due to a condition called atherosclerosis (clogging of the arteries).

Stroke can also be caused by cerebral hemorrhage, in which a diseased artery in the brain bursts, depriving the cells that are normally nourished by that artery and flooding the surrounding tissue with blood. This accumulation of blood forms a clot, which displaces and compresses brain tissue and thus interferes with brain function. This type of stroke often afflicts people who have both hypertension (high blood pressure) and atherosclerosis.

A third condition that can lead to stroke is rupture of an aneurysm (a bulge in an artery because of a defect in its wall), which interrupts blood flow to an area of the brain and floods the area with blood. The formation of aneurysms is sometimes associated with hypertension. Congenital (present at birth) aneurysms are often the cause of cerebral hemorrhage in young people.

Those at risk

People who have both hypertension and atherosclerosis are the most likely to suffer a stroke, since both diseases weaken and damage the arteries. Hypertension probably also encourages hemorrhage. Heredity may play a role in stroke, since the tendencies to develop both hypertension and atherosclerosis appear to be inherited. Black persons are more susceptible to stroke because high blood pressure is about twice as common in the black population as in the white population.

Smoking, diabetes, and high blood cholesterol levels may also contribute to stroke. Stroke is more likely to occur if there is a history of mild strokelike episodes called transient ischemic attacks (TIAs), which are like mild strokes that clear up within 24 hours, leaving no residual effects.

Symptoms

A stroke can present itself in many ways, but some of the more common symptoms are sudden weakness or numbness in the face, arm, and leg on one side of the body; loss or slurring of speech or difficulty in understanding others; unexplained unsteadiness; and persistent falling to one side. It is possible to suffer a mild stroke and experience minor degrees of these symptoms.

Diagnosis

Stroke is diagnosed mostly from the history and physical examination. Sophisticated X-ray techniques are also employed. For example, angiography will show damage or clots in the arteries in the brain or leading to the brain. In this procedure, a thin catheter is inserted into an artery in the arm or leg and advanced to the site to be studied; a special dye is then injected through the catheter to outline the area so that X rays may be taken. Computed tomography (see page 407) will provide cross-sectional images that may indicate whether the stroke was caused by a hemorrhage or by blockage of blood flow. Tumors, which can cause symptoms identical to those of stroke, are also often diagnosed this way.

Treatment

Treatment of stroke begins with immediate hospitalization. Blood pressure is normalized, and drug therapy to prevent further damage, as well as to reduce swelling of the brain tissue, is often begun. Anticoagulants (drugs that inhibit the normal clotting of blood) are sometimes administered in the hope of limiting the progress of the stroke or preventing additional strokes. After the acute period, rehabilitation is begun by speech, physical, and occupational therapists.

Prevention

For those who have experienced TIAs or other warning signs of stroke, precautions can be taken to prevent an actual stroke. After a TIA, some form of angiography (also called arteriography) is usually performed to locate obstructions or ulcerated areas of the arteries supplying blood to the head. Depending on the results of the angiogram, the general condition of the patient, and many other factors, surgery to "clean out" the arteries or treatment with anticoagulants or other drugs may be elected.

Prevention of stroke mainly involves control of high blood pressure and other risk factors, such as smoking and high cholesterol intake.

Thrombocytopenia

Thrombocytopenia is a disorder characterized by a decrease in the number of platelets in the blood. Platelets are tiny components of the blood that act to promote clotting when there is an injury or another problem that requires bleeding to be stopped.

Normally, about five to ten times the number of platelets needed for clotting circulate in the bloodstream; this amounts to about 200,000 to 500,000 per cubic millimeter. In general, thrombocytopenia is considered to be present when the platelet count is less than 100,000. Abnormal bleeding commonly does not occur, however, until the count is less than 50,000, and serious or unprovoked bleeding usually does not occur with counts above 20,000.

Causes

There are basically two mechanisms whereby thrombocytopenia occurs: decreased production of platelets and increased destruction of platelets. In the former, the elements in the bone marrow responsible for the production of platelets may malfunction or be severely diminished. Increased destruction of platelets occurs in essential, or idiopathic (of unknown cause), thrombocytopenia. In this disorder, which is most common in children, antibodies are made against the person's own platelets, thereby causing their destruction. Thrombocytopenia can also be due to the use of some medications. Severe, overwhelming infection can also cause increased destruction of platelets. In pregnancy, platelets from the fetus can sometimes enter the circulation of the mother, causing antibody formation and the consequent destruction of fetal platelets, with abnormal bleeding at birth.

Symptoms

An obvious sign of thrombocytopenia is a rash of reddish to

reddish-purple spots. These are due to bleeding within and underneath the skin. Abnormal or easily provoked bleeding is the most dangerous symptom. This bleeding may be minor, such as oozing from the gums while brushing the teeth or bruising caused by leaning on or brushing up against something. The bleeding can be much more serious, however, as in spontaneous internal bleeding, which may go unrecognized until the person goes into shock (collapse of the circulatory system).

Diagnosis

Laboratory evaluation of the blood is the basis of a diagnosis of thrombocytopenia. Examination of a sample of bone marrow may also be performed.

Treatment

Treatment depends on the cause. If infection is present, this must be remedied; usually, the platelet count will then return to normal on its own. In essential thrombocytopenia, corticosteroids (cortisone or prednisone) are the initial treatment. In drug-induced thrombocytopenia, the first step is generally to discontinue the drug. This will usually result in improvement; if not, corticosteroids may be helpful. In severe immune thrombocytopenia of the newborn, exchange transfusion (whereby all or most of the blood is exchanged with transfused blood) may be necessary. If the platelet count in any of these conditions is dangerously low (around 20,000 per cubic millimeter), transfusion of platelets may be indicated until the disease process has been controlled.

Prevention

Thrombocytopenia may not be preventable in most cases, but early recognition of symptoms, such as rash and easy bleeding, may lead to prevention of serious complications.

Thrombophlebitis

Thrombophlebitis is a condition in which both inflammation and blood clots exist in a vein. This can be caused by a number of factors. Commonly, when a person is immobilized, blood stagnates in the veins of the legs; this induces clotting, which in turn prevents blood from returning to the heart. The blood below the clot remains there, causing a buildup of pressure that forces fluid into the tissues, resulting in swelling. Simultaneously, the veins and surrounding area may become quite inflamed and tender. This condition is most often found in the deep veins of the legs, but it can also occur in veins of the pelvis and arms.

Thrombophlebitis itself may not be too serious, but it can lead to a life-threatening condition called pulmonary embolism if a blood clot formed in a deep leg vein breaks loose, travels through the bloodstream, and becomes lodged in a blood vessel in the lung. Pulmonary embolism can lead to chest pain, shortness of breath, coughing up of blood, and even death.

Causes

The development of thrombophlebitis is favored by any condition that inhibits the free flow of blood through the veins, such as prolonged bed rest or inactivity, perhaps following illness or surgery; congestive heart failure, which affects the ability of the heart to pump blood throughout the body; and injury or infection that damages a vein. Other factors that may lead to an increased tendency toward thrombophlebitis are pregnancy, the use of birth control pills by susceptible individuals, occupations that require long periods of standing or sitting, obesity, old age, and chronic infections. In some cases, thrombophlebitis may indicate the presence of a blood disorder or a tumor in the pancreas or lung.

Symptoms

Symptoms of deep-vein thrombophlebitis (which often appear only in advanced cases) are swelling, aching, and a feeling of heaviness in the leg or affected area. The skin may appear white and will be painful to the touch. If the veins of the leg are affected, the condition is characterized by increased pain when walking or when the foot is flexed backward or forward.

Diagnosis

Thrombophlebitis of a surface vein (superficial thrombophlebitis) can be diagnosed by physical examination, which usually reveals a red, warm, tender cordlike vein.

Diagnostic tests for thrombophlebitis include Doppler imaging (a technique used to detect obstructions by changes in the sounds made by flowing blood), nuclear medicine scans (see pages 406-407), plethysmography (a test to measure the resistance to blood flow in the veins), and venography. Venography involves the injection of a special dye into the veins so that a clot, if present, will be visualized on an X ray. This is the most sensitive and specific test for thrombophlebitis.

Treatment

Treatment of the superficial form of thrombophlebitis begins with bed rest with elevation of the leg. Warm compresses are also helpful, as are anti-inflammatory drugs. Superficial thrombophlebitis rarely, if ever, leads to pulmonary embolism.

Deep-vein thrombophlebitis, because of the potential for pulmonary embolism, is treated much more aggressively. The patient is usually hospitalized and put on bed rest with the leg elevated. Heparin (an anticoagulant, which inhibits the normal clotting mechanism of the blood) is given intravenously, usually for about seven days (up to ten days if pulmonary embolism has occurred). The patient is also usually given the oral anticoagulant warfarin for about six weeks (three to six months if pulmonary embolism has occurred). These drugs do not dissolve an existing clot, but serve to prevent new clots from forming while the old ones are resolving. Newer drugs do dissolve clots but are still used only in special situations.

Prevention

Prevention of thrombophlebitis is a controversial subject. In hospitalized patients who are immobilized for long periods or who are about to undergo major surgery, doing leg exercises, wearing long support stockings or compression boots (soft plastic bags or sacks that are wrapped around the legs and rapidly inflated and deflated), and increasing activity as soon as feasible may be helpful. Heparin therapy has also been beneficial in preventing deep-vein thrombophlebitis in certain patients. For nonhospitalized patients who are susceptible to this condition, regularly exercising the legs, elevating the legs when lying down, and wearing support hose may be helpful. Heparin or warfarin may be prescribed.

Transient ischemic attacks

Transient ischemic attacks (TIAs) are neurologic deficits (such as

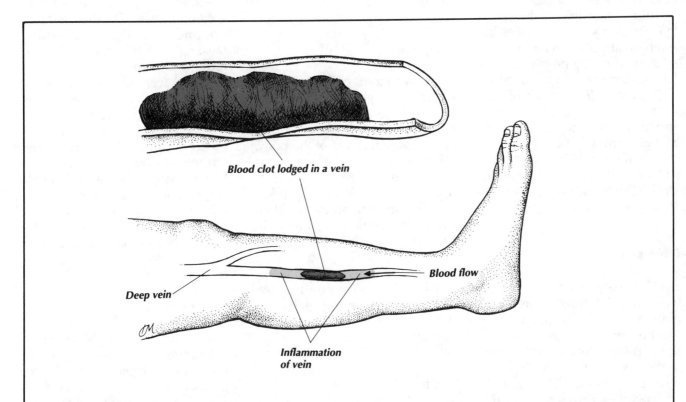

Blood clot lodged in a vein

Deep vein

Blood flow

Inflammation of vein

Thrombophlebitis (inflammation of a vein accompanied by the formation of a blood clot) often occurs in the deep veins of the legs. The condition is suspected if moving the foot forward or backward causes pain.

A transient ischemic attack is caused by an interruption in blood flow to an area of the brain. This could be the result of a blood clot that temporarily blocks an artery into the brain before breaking up and restoring blood flow.

loss of vision in one eye, inability to speak, paralysis, or weakness of one side of the body) of sudden onset that last for less than 24 hours. Although they are symptomatically similar to minor strokes, they do no discernible lasting damage to brain function.

The major importance of TIAs is their role as a predictor of stroke. When a person describes a "light stroke," it is often a TIA that is meant. If left untreated, TIAs can indeed lead to major strokes, with permanent damage to all parts affected.

Causes

TIAs are probably due to a temporary interruption in blood flow to an area of the brain. They can be caused by a narrowing in the carotid arteries (the arteries in the neck that supply the brain with oxygenated blood). This narrowing is usually due to the presence of atherosclerosis (clogging of the arteries). Blood vessel spasms and showers of tiny em-

boli (clots that travel through the bloodstream) are also possible causes.

Symptoms

The symptoms of TIAs are both varied and frightening to the victim. They can include weakness on one side of the face, numbness in various parts of the body, blindness in one eye, weakness in the arms or legs on one side, difficulty in speaking and understanding speech, and a prickling ("pins and needles") sensation in parts of the body. Vertigo (a sensation of spinning) combined with any of these or other symptoms can also be due to TIAs (this is rare). Fainting spells and light-headedness alone are usually not due to TIAs.

Diagnosis

The first step in diagnosis is a complete examination, including a history and physical, neuro-

logic, and eye examinations. Bruits (noises caused by narrowing in an artery) may be heard in a carotid artery. Detailed testing, commonly with angiography (also called arteriography) is performed to pinpoint the problem. In this procedure, a thin catheter is inserted into an artery in the arm or leg and advanced to the site to be studied; a special dye is then injected through the catheter to outline the area so that X rays may be taken. Prior to angiography, an ultrasonic examination (see pages 407-408) of the carotid arteries is usually done to determine if disease (narrowing) is present.

Treatment

Treatment of TIAs is aimed at preventing more TIAs and, hopefully, stroke. There are two basic methods of treatment: medical, with anticoagulant drugs; and surgical, with the opening and "cleaning out" of the obstructed arteries (endarterectomy). Anticoagulation is usually done with aspirin or heparin and warfarin. Which of these methods—medication or surgery—is more effective in preventing further TIAs or a stroke is dependent on many factors and is a subject of considerable controversy. TIAs can be an indication of serious problems and must be brought to the attention of a physician immediately.

Varicose veins

Varicose veins are swollen, stretched veins in the legs, close to the surface of the skin, caused by pooling of blood. Varicose veins alone are not too serious, but they may lead to a more serious condition, such as a skin ulcer, phlebitis (inflammation of a vein), or thrombosis (blood clot formation).

Causes

Blood from the legs must return to the heart uphill, against the force of gravity, so the veins in the legs have one-way valves to prevent blood from flowing back down toward the feet. When pressure on the veins stretches them or when the valves are injured in some way, the valves cannot close properly, and some blood travels back down. This blood accumulates in pools, which stretch the veins even more.

Varicose veins are caused by a number of factors that put excess pressure on the veins in the legs: prolonged standing; prolonged sitting, especially with the legs crossed; lack of exercise; confining clothes; obesity (which puts excess pressure on the legs and contributes to the inability of the muscles to push blood upward); heredity (a tendency toward

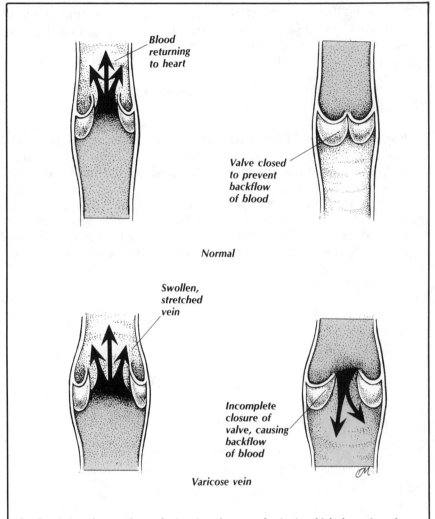

The drawing at the top shows the interior of a normal vein, in which the action of a valve prevents blood returning to the heart from flowing backward. In the drawing of a varicose vein, the valve has been weakened and cannot completely close, causing the blood to accumulate.

weak vein walls and valves seems to be inherited); and even height (tall people may be more susceptible because their blood needs to travel farther in its return trip to the heart).

Women are more susceptible to varicose veins than men, largely due to hormonal factors. Pregnancy accentuates this difference because special hormones released at this time tend to relax the walls of the veins. Also, varicose veins often appear during the last few months of pregnancy due to the increased

strain from the weight of the growing uterus. These veins may recede, however, after the birth.

Symptoms

Varicose veins are very noticeable since they form close to the skin. They appear as bulging, bluish, cordlike lines running down the legs. Symptoms that accompany varicose veins are feelings of achiness, heaviness, and fatigue in the legs, especially at the end of the day; itchy, scaly skin covering the affected areas; and, in advanced cases, swollen ankles, pain shooting down the leg, and leg cramps at night.

Diagnosis

Diagnosis can most often be made on the basis of physical examination because the affected superficial veins can be readily seen and palpated. If involvement of deeper veins is suspected, Doppler imaging (a technique used to detect obstructions by changes in the sounds made by flowing blood) may be performed.

Treatment

Varicose veins are usually treated by wearing elastic stockings, which act to aid the muscles pushing the blood upward. Very severe cases may require a surgical procedure called vein stripping, in which the afflicted veins are tied off and removed; other healthy veins in the area will take over the job of pushing blood toward the heart. A chemical can also be injected into the veins, closing them off and forcing the blood to find other channels to the heart.

Those with varicose veins may need to lose weight, exercise regularly, and stretch their legs or put their feet up whenever possible. Exercises to improve circulation in the legs may help relieve pressure.

Varicose veins tend to recur, particularly if adequate preventive measures are not taken.

THE DIGESTIVE SYSTEM

Digestion is the process by which the body converts food into basic substances that can be either absorbed in the bloodstream as nutrients or passed out of the body as waste. This process of breakdown and assimilation occurs within the digestive tract, a convoluted tube more than 30 feet long that is lined with a mucous membrane. The tract includes several hollow organs—the mouth, esophagus, stomach, small intestine, and large intestine (colon)—each of which has a specific function in digestion. The muscles of these organs move the food through the system, while mucus lubricates the tract and prevents irritation. The liver and pancreas are also critical organs in digestion. The gallbladder is involved in digestion as well.

Food first enters the digestive tract through the mouth. Movement of the jaws allows the teeth to cut and grind the food into smaller pieces, which are mixed with saliva (a secretion of the glands in the mouth). Saliva moistens food for easier swallowing and contains an enzyme (a special type of protein) that begins the chemical breakdown of starches.

From the mouth, food passes down the throat and into the esophagus, the muscular tube through which the food is conducted to the stomach. The stomach is a large pouch in the abdominal cavity where food is combined with acid- and enzyme-containing digestive juices secreted by glands within the stomach walls. The food becomes semifluid, which allows it to pass easily into the small intestine. The small intestine consists of three portions—the upper section, or duodenum; the middle section, or jejunum; and the lower section, or the ileum.

The digestive system includes the mouth, esophagus, stomach, small intestine, large intestine, liver, gallbladder, and pancreas—each of which plays a specific role in digestion.

In the duodenum, the first ten inches of the small intestine, digestive juices from the liver and pancreas continue the process of breaking down the food into its constituent nutrients, which can then be absorbed into the bloodstream in the remainder of the small intestine.

Aiding digestion is the liver, an accessory organ of digestion. The liver produces bile, which is necessary for absorption of fat in the small intestine. The liver also removes some wastes from the blood, produces and stores glucose (a form of sugar), and processes many drugs.

The gallbladder, located on the underside of the liver, is another organ that performs an indirect digestive function. The gallbladder stores the bile manufactured by the liver. As bile is needed, the gallbladder contracts and releases the fluid into the duodenum. If the gallbladder needs to be removed for medical reasons (such as in severe gallbladder disease), however, the liver can compensate for its role, and digestion is not hindered.

Other digestive juices required by the small intestine to digest and absorb food, particularly fats and starches, come from the pancreas, an organ located just behind the stomach. The pancreas also secretes insulin and other hormones into the blood. Insulin is the hormone responsible for aiding absorption and use of glucose.

Whatever substances are not assimilated into the bloodstream through the small intestine move into the large intestine. Within the large intestine, waste material is processed into stool (feces), and water and certain chemicals are absorbed into the bloodstream to preserve the body's fluid balance.

The fecal matter continues to move through the colon to the rectum (the lower part of the large intestine). Once in the rectum, waste is ready to be passed out of the body through the anus (the opening at the end of the digestive tract), thus completing the process of digestion.

Appendicitis

Appendicitis is an inflammation of the appendix, frequently caused by some type of hard material getting lodged at its tip.

The appendix is a small, wormlike pouch located at the juncture of the small and large intestines. Although it may have had a function at some point in evolutionary development, it serves no purpose now.

Causes

Despite its uselessness, the appendix can cause problems when it becomes inflamed. Inflammation occurs when the hollow, tubular structure becomes

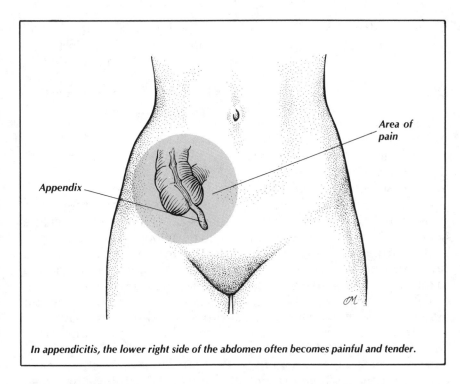

In appendicitis, the lower right side of the abdomen often becomes painful and tender.

clogged with masses of waste matter, intestinal worms, or other material that can prevent normal drainage. The blockage provides a fertile environment for bacteria to grow and multiply, causing infection and inflammation.

Symptoms

In the beginning, appendicitis may produce a dull or sharp pain in the navel area of the abdomen. Any movement, coughing, or sneezing can intensify the pain. In early stages, patients may also feel nauseated and may be unable to eat. Constipation can accompany appendicitis; however, about ten percent of patients have diarrhea instead. Adults may run a mild fever (up to 101°F), but children generally experience higher fevers. Occasionally, the pulse rate accelerates to about 100 beats per minute.

Within hours, the pain moves to the lower right side of the ab-

domen over the appendix and becomes continuous. Because the location of the appendix may vary from one individual to another, pain may emanate from the back, side, or pelvis—or even from the opposite side of the abdomen. The entire area around the appendix becomes extremely tender as abdominal muscles tighten.

As the fever rises and the pain grows more intense, chances of rupture also become greater. Rupture results when the appendix becomes so swollen and filled with pus that it bursts, spreading infection to surrounding organs. One serious complication of rupture is peritonitis (inflammation of the lining of the abdominal cavity).

Any fever with nausea and abdominal pain should be reported to a physician. More severe pain is an immediate medical emergency that must be evaluated and treated to prevent potential complications. Appendicitis can affect anyone, but the disease is more prevalent among persons between 10 and 30 years of age.

Diagnosis

When confirming appendicitis, the doctor checks for tenderness over the appendix. A blood test determines whether there is an elevated white blood cell count (in response to infection, the body produces extra white blood cells to help fight it). The doctor may perform more tests to rule out disorders sometimes mistaken for appendicitis, such as inflammation of the gallbladder, kidney stones, or a kidney infection. In women, a twisted ovarian cyst (a sac filled with fluid or semisolid material) or a ruptured ectopic pregnancy (one that develops outside the uterus) may produce symptoms similar to those of appendicitis.

Treatment

Although appendicitis cannot be prevented, prompt diagnosis can lead to effective treatment. Patients who suspect appendicitis should not eat, drink, or take drugs to relieve pain until a doctor has been consulted. Eating or drinking any substance, especially taking a laxative, will stimulate activity in the intestine, which may cause the appendix to rupture.

The most common treatment for acute appendicitis is surgery to remove the inflamed organ. To ensure against further infection, antibiotics may also be prescribed after surgery.

Bile

Bile is a fluid produced by the liver, stored in the gallbladder, and discharged into the small intestine, where it helps in the digestion of food, particularly fats. Bile is made up of water, salts, bile acids, cholesterol (a fatlike substance), and lecithin (a fatty acid).

Functions

Bile acts like a detergent to break down fat in the intestine into tiny globules that can be dissolved and suspended in water; the tiny globules can then pass through the walls of the small intestine into the bloodstream (to provide fuel for the body). The bile salts are also absorbed through the walls of the intestine but are returned to the liver to form new bile. The yellow-green or golden color of bile is due to the pigments bilirubin and biliverdin. Bilirubin is a yellow pigment derived from decomposed red blood cells. Biliverdin is a green pigment derived from conversion of bilirubin by a chemical reaction. These pigments are also responsible for some of the coloration of body wastes.

Bile is produced continuously in the liver and passes through ducts to be stored in the gallbladder until mealtime, when it is emptied into the duodenum. Digestive disturbances result if the flow of bile is stopped or reduced, either because of a liver disorder or because a duct has been blocked by inflammation or a gallstone (a solid mass of material—usually composed of calcium, cholesterol, bilirubin, or a combination thereof—formed in the gallbladder). Any of these conditions can also cause jaundice, in which the pigments bilirubin and biliverdin accumulate in the blood. Jaundice is a sign of trouble, not a disease in itself, and shows up as yellow staining of the skin, eyes, and body fluids.

Cholecystitis

Cholecystitis is an inflammation of the gallbladder. The gallbladder is a small, pear-shaped organ that stores the bile produced by the liver and releases it as needed to help digest foods—particularly fats—in the small intestine. Cholecystitis may be either acute (sudden and severe) or chronic (recurring but less severe).

Acute cholecystitis

In about 90 percent of cases, acute cholecystitis results when the outlet of the gallbladder or the duct leading from it is plugged by a gallstone. A gallstone is formed in the gallbladder from cholesterol (a fatty substance), calcium, bile pigments, or a combination of these substances. Unless the stone becomes dislodged, inflammation and pressure build up behind it. In severe cases, the swollen gallbladder may not receive enough blood, resulting in tissue death. The gallbladder may become gangrenous or perforated, causing bile to spill into the abdominal cavity. An abscess (a collection of pus within a cavity) usually forms, and bacteria may colonize the region. Occasionally, the resulting leakage of infected bile causes peritonitis (an inflammation of the lining of the abdominal cavity). However, not all gallbladder attacks progress to this extreme; they may subside only to recur later. Cholecystitis may also result from a blockage caused by enlargement of the veins in the common bile duct, which the gallbladder shares with the liver.

Acute cholecystitis often begins following a meal rich in fats, such as one containing fried foods, chocolate, or cream. The individual may awaken in the middle of the night with indigestion, gas, and a sharp pain in the upper right quarter of the abdomen, which is often hard and tender to the touch. Pain may also be felt in the middle of the abdomen and may spread to the tip of the right shoulder blade. The pain is crampy and severe. Vomiting is likely to occur and provides some relief. If fever is present, infection of the gallbladder or of the bile duct is likely. If jaundice (yellowing of the eyes and skin, caused by bile pigment in the blood) is present, then the symptoms are probably due to blockage of the common bile duct by a gallstone or tumor.

Nuclear medicine scanning confirms the diagnosis of cholecystitis. In this procedure, a radioactive material is administered, and its distribution in the affected area is recorded on X-ray film. X-ray examination and ultrasonography, a technique that uses sound waves to create images of internal structures, may also be used to confirm the diagnosis and to locate gallstones.

Treatment of an acute attack may include rest, intravenous feeding, painkilling drugs, and antibiotics. Because attacks are likely to recur, however, the usual solution is surgical removal of the gallbladder. This is often done immediately. If the patient has another illness, it should be brought under control before the operation is performed. Removal of the gallbladder does not hinder the digestive process, since the liver can compensate for the lost organ.

The mere presence of gallstones found incidentally during tests for other problems does not always mean that surgery is necessary, however. In many cases, gallstones can be present for life without ever causing acute cholecystitis.

Recently, a technique for removing the gallbladder without the standard incision—via a laparoscope—has been used. A laparoscope is a periscopelike instrument inserted through a puncture in the abdominal wall. After the laparoscope is inserted, a laser is used to free the gallbladder from its bed underneath the liver. The gallbladder is then removed through a puncture by suction. This procedure has shortened hospital stays and decreased complications from surgery. In addition, instead of having a large scar, the patient usually has only four small punctures. This procedure is not for everyone with gallbladder problems, however. Individuals who have had numerous abdominal surgeries are usually not candidates. Furthermore, if the attempted laparoscope surgery is unsuccessful, the standard incision may need to be made.

Other nonsurgical methods for removing gallstones, including drug and chemical therapy and lithotripsy (the use of shock waves to shatter the stones), have been tried with varying degrees of success on a select group of patients. The criteria for using these methods, however, is very strict; removal of the gallbladder is still the method of choice in most cases.

Chronic cholecystitis

Chronic cholecystitis is a continued inflammation of the gallbladder, with repeated attacks over time that are similar to, but milder than, those of acute cholecystitis. Gallstones are usually present; whether they develop before or after the emergence of the disease is unknown. The causes of chronic cholecystitis are not entirely understood, although occasionally bacterial infection is the reason. Diet, heredity, and hormones appear to be involved, and the disease is more likely to affect women.

The pains of chronic cholecystitis commonly appear over the pit of the stomach and in the upper right quarter of the abdomen. They may range in intensity from mild to unbearable. The pains are crampy and usually come on suddenly, but they may be separated by pain-free intervals of 15 minutes to an hour. The pains may disappear after 15 minutes or continue for several hours; the average attack lasts about an hour. Although the pains may appear together with nausea, gas, and belching and may occur after eating fatty foods, these indications may not be directly related to the disease.

Diagnosis is based on the symptoms and can be confirmed by the same studies used for diagnosis of acute cholecystitis—nuclear medicine scanning (see pages 406-407) and ultrasonography (see pages 407-408). The doctor must make a careful investigation of other possible causes of the symptoms, including peptic ulcer (which occurs in the stomach or in the beginning of the small intestine), inflammation of the pancreas, and bowel disease.

The ideal way to treat chronic cholecystitis is to remove the gallbladder, together with any gallstones in the duct leading from the liver to the duodenum (the first part of the small intestine). If it is not clear that the symptoms are caused by gall-bladder inflammation, or if the patient cannot withstand an operation, other methods are used. These include a low-fat diet (which lowers the need for bile), weight reduction, and use of medications. The use of medication, chemicals, or lithotripsy (the use of shock waves to shatter stones) to get rid of the stones has very strict criteria, and in most cases, removal of the gall-bladder is still the method of choice. (For more on gallstones, see pages 237-239.)

Cirrhosis

Cirrhosis is a disease in which cells throughout the liver are progressively destroyed. They are replaced by areas containing normal new cells but also by much scar tissue, which alters the structure of the organ. The flow of blood and lymph through the damaged liver is much less efficient, and eventually the liver fails.

Causes

Cirrhosis represents an attempt by the liver to rebuild itself and continue despite injury. The injury may be a sudden and massive infection, as in acute hepatitis, or it may occur in a less dramatic manner over a period of months or years, as in chronic active hepatitis or obstruction of the bile ducts within the liver. The process of obstruction starts with inflammation and progresses to scarring and then closure of the ducts. A similar condition is caused by obstruction of the external bile ducts by a stone, scar, inborn defect, or tumor. The damage is done over an even longer time, slowly and

steadily, by alcohol abuse, which is by far the most common cause of cirrhosis. Other causes include the following:
• Use of certain medications
• Inborn errors in physical or chemical processes
• Syphilis
• Passive liver congestion, due to inability of the heart to accept a normal flow of blood from the liver or to obstruction of one of the drainage systems of the liver

Symptoms

Frequently, cirrhosis is not suspected until it is well advanced, because it imitates many other diseases. Symptoms include general weakness, a vague feeling of being unwell, loss of appetite, loss of weight, and a loss of interest in sex. There may be a dull abdominal ache, nausea, constipation, or diarrhea. In a malnourished patient, the tongue may be inflamed. Many symptoms are the result of high blood pressure in the portal vein, which brings blood from the intestinal area to the liver. In cirrhosis, the liver cannot handle a normal flow of blood, so the pressure in the portal vein rises. One result is that fluid from the blood is lost into the abdominal cavity. The fluid may accumulate and press against the diaphragm (the muscular wall separating the abdominal and chest cavities) and interfere with breathing. Collateral blood vessels form to carry away the excess blood into the general circulation. There may be bleeding in the esophagus or stomach when these smaller collateral vessels burst under pressure. The patient may vomit blood. Serious, life-threatening hemorrhage (internal bleeding) may occur.

The liver may be enlarged and firm or, in advanced cases, shrunken. Other symptoms include an enlarged spleen, mottled redness of the mound at the base of the thumb, "spider veins" on the skin of the upper body, loss of hair from the chest and the pubic area, diminished size of the testes, and tingling sensations in the skin of the hands and feet.

Diagnosis

Proof of cirrhosis of the liver is furnished by liver biopsy. A hollow needle is inserted through the skin and into the liver itself to obtain a tissue sample for analysis. Examination of tissue from a diseased liver reveals destruction of cells and scarring. Other diagnostic procedures include nuclear medicine scanning, in which radioactive material is administered and its distribution to the liver is recorded on X-ray film. X-ray pictures are taken of the gallbladder and of bile ducts both inside the liver and leading from it. Important clues that may be found on blood and urine tests include the presence of high levels of bile pigments in the blood, a low red blood cell count (anemia), vitamin and mineral deficiencies, and protein in the urine.

Treatment

Treatment is aimed first at removing the cause of the original injury. For example, an alcoholic patient is told to stop drinking and is placed on a well-balanced diet. Often, thiamin (vitamin B_1) and folic acid supplements are also given. If a stone is obstructing an external bile duct and thus causing liver damage, it can be removed. Fluids and salt are usually restricted, to prevent fluid buildup in the body.

Good care includes getting plenty of rest and avoiding infection, which places stress on the liver. Avoidance of alcohol intake is paramount in the treatment of cirrhosis and most other liver diseases. All medications, including over-the-counter preparations, should be cleared by a physician.

Prevention

Many of the various causes of cirrhosis of the liver cannot be predicted and guarded against, but the major one can be. Drinking moderately or not at all is the best way to reduce the risk.

Colostomy

Colostomy is the creation of a stoma (opening) in the wall of the abdomen to which an opening in the colon is attached. Thereafter, the contents of the colon are eliminated through the stoma instead of through the rectum and anus (the normal opening to the outside of the body).

The opening may be permanent (as in some operations for cancer of the rectum, which eliminate the normal exit of the bowel), or it may be temporary (as in treatment of severe diverticular disease or Hirschsprung's disease).

Correction of Hirschsprung's disease

In Hirschsprung's disease, an inherited disorder of newborns, the last portion of the bowel lacks specialized nerves and cannot function normally. The

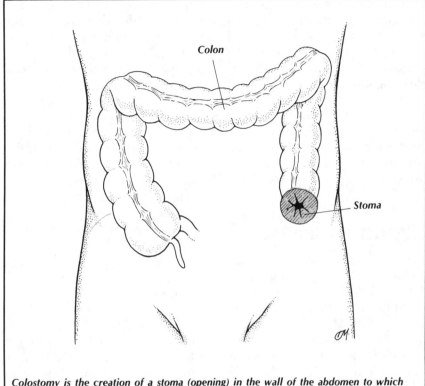

Colostomy is the creation of a stoma (opening) in the wall of the abdomen to which an opening in the colon is attached. The contents of the colon can then be eliminated through the stoma rather than through the rectum and anus.

healthy portion of the bowel above this segment is connected to a stoma. Elimination takes place via this route for several months until the baby is strong enough for a second surgical procedure, in which the defective portion of the bowel is removed and the healthy portion is connected to the anus, permitting normal bowel movements.

Permanent colostomy

Having a permanent colostomy does not prevent a person from leading a normal life. The patient is taught how to empty the colon once a day by using irrigations (enemas) and a special collecting device. By manipulating the diet, it becomes possible to anticipate bowel movements. At first, patients wear a pouch over the stoma to collect any leakage from the colon. An adhesive is used to form a tight seal around the opening of the pouch and the stoma, and a deodorant in the pouch controls odor. After a while, many patients with so-called dry colostomies need only wear a stoma cap or a small gauze patch over the stoma to absorb mucous secretions. Physical activities can be resumed, with or without a pouch, including swimming, other noncontact sports, and sexual relations. The only exceptions are heavy lifting, which could cause a hernia through the weakened abdominal muscles, and any activity that could injure the stoma or abdomen.

To avoid infection of the stoma and irritation of the skin around it, the patient needs to wash the surrounding skin area with mild soap and water each day and then rinse and dry it. Special adhesive materials that protect and soothe the skin have become available. These are applied after cleaning the skin.

Support and practical advice from those who have undergone the operation are available through local chapters and the national headquarters of the United Ostomy Association.

Crohn's disease

Crohn's disease (also known as regional enteritis and ileitis) is characterized by inflammation of a section or sections of any part of the digestive tract—most often, the ileum (the last third of the small intestine). The disease may begin as patches of tiny ulcers in the innermost lining of the intestine, with swelling of nearby tissues. The inflammation eventually extends through all layers of the intestine, which becomes thickened, hard, and brittle. Deepening ulcers, scarring, and swelling may obstruct the intestinal tract.

Causes

The cause is unknown. However, research indicates that infection, immune disorders, or an inherited defect may play a part. There is some evidence of an increased incidence of Crohn's disease in Jews; black persons are least likely to have the disease. The disease usually begins between age 15 and age 35, but can occur at any age.

Symptoms

Symptoms usually develop gradually, with spells of diarrhea (four to six stools a day, frequently bloody), low fever, weight loss, loss of appetite, general weakness, and steady or colicky pains in the abdomen, commonly on the right side. Milk, milk products, and coarse foods may make symptoms worse.

Occasionally an acute (sudden) case resembles appendicitis, with sharp pain in the lower right portion of the abdomen, cramping, nausea, fever, and diarrhea. There may be bloody stools. An acute case can resemble infectious diarrhea.

Diagnosis

While probing the abdomen and pelvis, the doctor may detect a tender mass of thickened or matted loops of intestine. The chronic form of the disease can occasionally be mistaken for other problems, such as irritable bowel syndrome. However, an X ray of the small intestine taken after administration of the contrast medium barium may reveal the characteristic pattern of narrowed portions of the bowel sharply differentiated from healthy portions. The doctor may use a proctosigmoidoscope (a lighted, hollow instrument) to inspect the lower intestinal lining for patchy areas of inflammation or to perform a biopsy (obtain a sample of tissue for microscopic examination).

Complications

Complications include abscesses (pus-filled cavities) and fistulas. Fistulas are abnormal connecting channels that originate from inflamed portions of the bowel and commonly extend into and around adjacent tissue. In the anorectal area, they may sometimes be seen as openings in the skin. They can also extend from one section of the bowel to another, from the bowel to the bladder or vagina, and from the bowel to the abdominal wall. Fistulas are often infected and discharge pus.

Perforation of the intestine can also occur, leading to peritonitis (inflammation of the lining of the abdominal cavity). This is marked by severe abdominal pain and rigidity of the abdomen, and is most often a surgical emergency. On occasion, a small perforation may become walled off, creating an abscess.

Malnutrition is a very common complication of Crohn's disease because areas of inflamed intestine cannot properly absorb nutrients. The risk of cancer of the colon and rectum is also increased. Arthritis, eye disorders, kidney stones, and certain skin disorders may also accompany this illness.

Treatment

At present, there is no cure for Crohn's disease. Surgery is sometimes necessary to remove an entire section of diseased bowel, drain an abscess, or eliminate a fistula. This relieves the condition for a time, but symptoms almost always recur, and another operation may be necessary. Treatment of the disease is directed at making the patient as comfortable and functional as possible by reducing the severity of his or her symptoms.

A diet rich in calories and vitamins with adequate protein is desirable, to compensate for the patient's poor absorption of nutrients from the intestines. Individuals with severely inflamed or obstructed bowels may be placed temporarily on intravenous feeding or a special diet. Patients with anemia may need supplements of vitamins and minerals (such as iron, folic acid, and vitamin B_{12}) and sometimes blood transfusions; those with severe diarrhea or dehydration may need intravenous fluids.

Cramps and diarrhea are frequently controlled by various medications that relax the bowel wall, while preparations such as psyllium may help to firm stools.

Antibiotics are used on a short-term basis to treat abscesses and infected fistulas. Sulfa-salicylate combination drugs may be used on a long-term basis to curb inflammation and prevent acute episodes, particularly in disease involving the large intestine. The steroid drug prednisone is a mainstay in treating flare-ups of symptoms. Newer salicylates, either in enema or oral form, are quite effective in relieving symptoms.

Diverticulitis is the inflammation of diverticula (small pouches that balloon out from the colon wall when the inner lining is forced through weak spots in the muscular lining). Inflammation often develops when a mass of hardened feces becomes trapped in a diverticulum, reducing the blood supply to the pouch wall and making it more susceptible to infection by bacteria in the colon.

Diverticulosis and diverticulitis

Diverticulosis is the occurrence of diverticula (little pouches) that form when the inner lining of the colon (large intestine) is forced, under pressure, through weak spots in the muscular outer layer of the colon. Diverticulosis may be present in about one third of persons over the age of 60 in the United States, and both its incidence and the frequency of complications increase with age. Diverticulitis is inflammation and/ or infection of the diverticula.

Causes

One theory about the cause of diverticulosis is that abnormal movement of the colon (possibly because of too little bulk in the diet) produces intense pressure, which forces the intestinal lining through weak spots in the muscular layer. Most people with simple diverticulosis have no symptoms. Occasionally, however, a pouch next to a blood vessel may ulcerate, causing it to bleed. If the vessel is an artery, severe bleeding can result, seen as bleeding from the anus. Shock and even death may result if the condition is not treated.

It has been estimated that about one-fifth to one-fourth of the persons who have diverticulosis will suffer from diverticulitis. Diverticulitis develops when a mass of hardened waste matter (called a fecalith) forms in a pouch and reduces the blood supply to the thin walls of the pouch (by means of pressure against the wall), making them more susceptible to infection by the bacteria of the colon. The inflammation that follows can lead to perforation, formation of an abscess (an enclosed sac of pus around the perforation), or peritonitis (infection of the lining of the abdominal cavity). Not infrequently, the inflamed section of bowel becomes attached to the urinary bladder or vagina, burrowing out from the colon to create a fistula (abnormal channel), which leaks infectious material into the other organ. Repeated inflammation can cause thickening of the wall of the colon, thus narrowing the colon and causing partial or total obstruction.

Symptoms

Symptoms of diverticulitis include intermittent crampy abdominal pains and tenderness, usually on the lower left side, but sometimes in other areas of the lower abdomen, in which case the pains may resemble those of appendicitis. Pain that worsens during urination may indicate that the inflamed colon has become attached to the bladder. Stool (feces) or air in the urine may indicate a colon-to-bladder fistula. Constipation alone or constipation alternating with diarrhea is common. Fever is usually present with acute attacks.

Diagnosis

The diagnosis of diverticulitis usually is made if there is a history of pain in the left lower section of the abdomen, accompanied by fever and a change in bowel habits. A physical examination may reveal a mass in that area, along with extreme tenderness. After the acute episode has subsided, the doctor may insert a proctosigmoidoscope (a lighted, tubelike instrument) through the anus and into the lower part of the colon to see if there is any evidence of cancer that might be causing the symptoms. X-ray studies with a contrast medium such as barium are usually done to further rule out cancer of the colon and to locate diverticula, obstructions, and fistulas.

Treatment

Treatment of severe diverticulitis begins with bed rest in a hospital and intravenous feeding; no food is given by mouth, to give the intestines a rest. Antibiotics are given if there is fever or other evidence of infection. If peritonitis develops, it may be necessary to operate. The inflamed section of the colon may simply be cut

out, and the remaining sections joined. More often, a temporary colostomy (a surgically created opening in the abdominal wall, which allows the colon to empty to the outside of the body) is necessary. Later, after all inflammation and infection have subsided, the redirected portion of the colon is reconnected to the remaining portion of the colon or to the rectum.

Prevention

A diet high in bulk appears to be a way to avoid diverticulosis. Persons who have diverticulosis should eat a relatively high-fiber diet. Supplements, such as psyllium, that increase bulk may be recommended to move the stool through the colon at a normal rate.

Food poisoning

The term "food poisoning" generally refers to an illness caused by the ingestion (taking into the body) of food that is either poisonous itself (such as certain kinds of wild mushrooms) or that has been contaminated, usually by bacteria or their toxic (poisonous) by-products.

The symptoms commonly associated with food poisoning—nausea, vomiting, and diarrhea—are unpleasant but not generally life threatening and usually subside within a relatively short period of time without treatment. However, for some groups—the very old, the very young, and the seriously ill—food poisoning can be extremely serious, and some forms, such as botulism and mushroom poisoning, are potentially fatal for anyone.

In general, bacterial food poisoning can be prevented by care-

ful observance of proper procedures in food processing and preparation, especially hand washing by food handlers, prompt refrigeration of food, and cleanliness in food preparation areas.

Botulism

The *Clostridium botulinum* bacterium produces a toxin which, when ingested, prevents the transmission of nerve impulses to muscle. Nausea, vomiting, and abdominal cramps are also common. The effects on the nervous system begin in the head, causing double or blurred vision and difficulty in swallowing, and then proceed downward as paralysis of the arms, the muscles that aid in breathing, and eventually the legs. These symptoms usually appear 4 to 36 hours after ingestion of the toxin, but can be delayed as long as eight days.

The foods most commonly implicated in botulism are home-canned preparations, and the best way to prevent botulism is to strictly follow established guidelines when canning foods at home. Contaminated foods sometimes have a foul odor, but this warning is not always present. Also, honey should not be given to infants because it has been reported as a source of fatal botulism in that age group.

With the availability of *Botulinum* antitoxin, fewer than ten percent of cases are now fatal. However, suspicion of botulism should still be considered a medical emergency.

Salmonellosis

The term salmonellosis refers to a number of diseases caused by *Salmonella* bacteria. One of those diseases is typhoid fever, which fortunately is now uncommon in the United States. A very common form of salmonellosis is *Salmonella* gastroenteritis.

The foods that most commonly harbor *Salmonella* bacteria are meat, poultry, milk, and eggs. *Salmonella* bacteria are frequently transmitted by contact with human or animal fecal material or by eating food contaminated with such material. The symptoms of *Salmonella* gastroenteritis include nausea, abdominal cramps, and diarrhea. In severe cases, mucus and blood are present in the stools. The symptoms usually appear 12 to 24 hours after ingestion of contaminated food. Most cases of *Salmonella* gastroenteritis occur in children during the summer and early fall. The illness is generally mild, usually lasting two to five days. However, salmonellosis can be fatal for very young infants, seriously ill patients, and the elderly.

Treatment of most *Salmonella* infections involves replacing the fluids lost because of diarrhea. If fluid loss is severe, hospitalization and intravenous fluid supplementation may be necessary. Use of antibiotics is reserved for patients with severe symptoms because, if used indiscriminately, such drugs can actually prolong the illness. Antidiarrheal medications can also prolong the illness and should be used only to control the most severe symptoms. Laboratory analysis of stool or blood samples may be necessary to establish the diagnosis and prescribe the appropriate treatment. Cultures of the stool should also be performed after the illness has passed to confirm that the bacteria are not still being shed, creating the potential for spread of infection.

Staphylococcal gastroenteritis

Gastroenteritis caused by the *Staphylococcus aureus* bacterium is a very common form of food poisoning. Foods cooked at low temperatures and then allowed to cool at room temperature for long periods of time are most often the source.

The symptoms—excessive salivation, nausea, diarrhea, abdominal cramps, and vomiting—usually occur within two to four hours after eating the contaminated food. The illness usually lasts less than 24 hours and requires no treatment in otherwise healthy individuals. Antibiotics and antidiarrheals can, in fact, prolong the illness. In elderly or ill persons, hospitalization and intravenous fluid replacement may be necessary. Symptoms of dehydration, such as dry mouth and light-headedness, merit prompt medical attention.

Other bacterial causes

Clostridium perfringens is a bacterium commonly found in raw meat and poultry. Its growth in foods is encouraged by slow cooking at low temperatures. Symptoms of infection—abdominal cramps, nausea, and diarrhea—usually appear about 8 to 12 hours after ingestion of contaminated food, but can be delayed as long as 24 hours. The illness generally lasts less than one day and requires no treatment other than getting plenty of fluids.

Infection with the *Vibrio parahaemolyticus* bacterium is most often associated with ingestion of raw or improperly refrigerated seafood. This illness usually occurs during the warmer months and is most common in the coastal regions of the United States. The primary symptom—severe, watery, occasionally blood-tinged diarrhea—generally occurs 12 to 24 hours after eating the contaminated food. The illness rarely lasts more than two days. In severe cases, antibiotics may be necessary.

Bacillus cereus infection is commonly associated with rice products, particularly fried rice and unrefrigerated boiled rice. The primary symptoms—nausea and vomiting—are usually mild.

Mushroom poisoning

It is all but impossible for anyone but the most highly trained expert to discriminate nontoxic mushrooms from the more than 50 species of toxic wild mushrooms. Therefore, all wild mushrooms should be avoided. The illness usually begins 6 to 24 hours after ingestion. Starting with severe abdominal cramps, nausea, vomiting, and diarrhea, the illness rapidly progresses to involve the liver, kidneys, and heart and can be fatal.

Gallstones

Gallstones are hardened masses that consist mainly of cholesterol (a fatlike substance found only in animal products), blood, bile (fluid produced in the liver and stored in the gallbladder, which is required for fat absorption in the small intestine), calcium, and other substances. The stones form in the gallbladder or in the bile duct leading from the gallbladder into the small intestine.

Causes

When bile contains excessive amounts of cholesterol, the un-

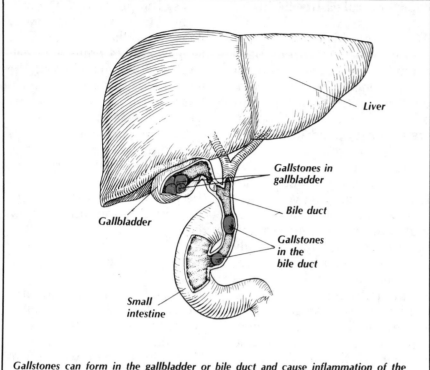

Gallstones can form in the gallbladder or bile duct and cause inflammation of the gallbladder or liver damage if they block the flow of bile from the gallbladder to the small intestine.

necessary cholesterol separates from the solution and forms stonelike masses. Unfortunately, since the body itself produces cholesterol, formation of these types of stones cannot always be prevented merely by controlling cholesterol intake in the diet.

Pregnancy, obesity, diabetes, liver disease, and certain forms of anemia can increase the risk of gallstones. Overweight people who frequently lose and gain large amounts of weight seem more susceptible to gallstones, as do women who have had two or more children. Although the reasons are unclear, twice as many women as men over age 40 develop gallstones.

Symptoms

By themselves, gallstones often produce no signs of disease.

About half the people with gallstones have no symptoms. Symptoms that do appear are usually chronic (long-term) in nature, including discomfort and pain in the upper abdomen, indigestion, nausea, and intolerance of fatty foods. Sometimes stones pass through the bile duct into the intestines to be excreted naturally.

However, symptoms can occur if the stones lodge in the bile duct. In an acute gallbladder attack, a sharp pain (often on the right side of the upper abdomen) may travel to the back and under the right shoulder blade. Frequently, the pain develops suddenly after a meal and leads to fever, chills, vomiting, and possibly jaundice (yellowing of the skin and whites of the eyes caused by the presence of excess bile pigment in the bloodstream). These symptoms occur when a stone that had been floating in

the gallbladder becomes trapped in the bile duct.

Complications

Serious complications of liver damage may develop if stones block the flow of bile.

When gallstones remain in the gallbladder, the organ may become inflamed. This condition, called chronic cholecystitis, may cause no symptoms. However, in most cases, repeated attacks of pain occur.

Diagnosis

Gallstones that cause no symptoms may be detected by an X-ray study of the gallbladder, called a cholecystogram. A cholecystogram is performed after the patient has swallowed a tablet containing dye that outlines the gallbladder and any stones that may be present. Nowadays, most physicians prefer to use ultrasound (see pages 407-408). Some studies using radioactive isotopes can be used to differentiate between acute and chronic cholecystitis.

Treatment

For acute gallbladder attacks due to gallstones with severe and prolonged symptoms, doctors generally recommend a cholecystectomy (surgical removal of the gallbladder). This treatment is one of the most common forms of abdominal surgery. Recently, a technique for removing the gallbladder without a standard incision—via a laparoscope—has also been used (see page 231). Other nonsurgical methods for removing gallstones, including drug and chemical therapy and lithotripsy (the use of shock waves to shatter the stones), have been tried with varying degrees of success on a select group of patients. The criteria for using these methods, however, is very strict; removal of the gallbladder is still the method of choice in most cases. Since the gallbladder is not necessary to maintain life, some doctors suggest removing a gallbladder containing stones even if they are not causing symptoms. However, unless there are extenuating circumstances, this is becoming a less common practice.

Gastroenteritis

Gastroenteritis is an inflammation of the lining of the stomach and the intestines.

Causes

Gastroenteritis can be caused by bacteria or viruses; by allergic reactions to certain foods or drinks; by infectious diseases, such as typhoid fever and influenza; by food poisoning; by overconsumption of alcohol; or by certain drugs.

Symptoms

Symptoms include headache, nausea, vomiting, diarrhea, and gas pains in the stomach and the intestines. Often, the individual will feel that gas is "caught" in certain portions of the intestine. On occasion, cramps may produce severe pain.

Diagnosis

The first task in treating gastroenteritis is to identify the cause or causes of the inflammation. Blood tests and cultures for viruses or bacteria may be done. If the problem is caused by an allergic reaction, the source of the reaction may sometimes be identified by allergy tests.

Treatment

Antibiotics can be used to treat bacterial infections. A variety of medicines (many of them nonprescription) can ease the effects of stomach cramps and gas pains. Diarrhea may necessitate replacement of lost fluids. Elderly or extremely ill persons may have to be hospitalized for intravenous replacement of fluids.

Prevention

Maintaining a clean kitchen, eating in restaurants where the kitchens are kept clean, washing fresh foods thoroughly, and cooking foods carefully are all safeguards against bacterial and viral infections. Identification of allergy-causing foods and moderation in alcohol consumption also help prevent gastroenteritis, if these are the causes of the problem.

Hemorrhoids

Hemorrhoids (often called piles) are enlarged veins inside or just outside the anal canal, which is the opening at the end of the large intestine. As veins swell, they cause severe inflammation and discomfort.

Causes

In some cases, hemorrhoids are the result of poor toilet habits. Habitual postponement of bowel movements can lead to loss of rectal function and undesirable straining during elimination. Straining puts increased pressure on veins and slows the flow of blood, thereby contributing to swelling and inflammation of veins. If bowel movements are postponed, the stools retained in the bowels may lose moisture. When feces becomes dry and hard, the added strain of constipation favors the development of hemorrhoids.

Another source of hemorrhoid irritation comes from pressure on the veins due to diseases of the liver or heart or from a tumor. Pregnancy may also contribute to the development of hemorrhoids because the enlarged uterus increases pressure on the veins. Moreover, prolonged pressure from pushing during labor and delivery can lead to hemorrhoids.

Diet plays a major role. A diet containing a high proportion of refined foods rather than foods with natural roughage increases the likelihood of constipation and, therefore, the likelihood of hemorrhoids.

Hemorrhoids seem to be more prevalent in some families. However, this tendency has been attributed to similar dietary and personal habits.

Symptoms

Hemorrhoids may take years to develop and almost always cause irritating symptoms. The first signs of hemorrhoids include itching and discomfort during and after bowel movements. Continued straining during elimination will eventually produce slight swelling of the lining of the anal canal. This swelling may not be noticed until hard stools scrape the anal lining and cause bleeding—an early clue that a hemorrhoid has developed.

With prolonged straining, a portion of the anal canal may jut out of the anus during a bowel movement. As long as the elastic connective tissue is still strong enough to pull the hemorrhoid back into the anal canal unassisted, the individual may not notice the growing problem. However, with persistent pressure, the protruding tissue may remain outside the anus after a bowel movement and need to be manually returned to the anal canal. Once outside the anal canal, the hemorrhoid creates a dull aching sensation or ulcerates and bleeds.

A more involved problem develops when the hemorrhoid is difficult or impossible to return within the anal canal, and permanent swelling at the anal opening interferes with elimination. The patient may then postpone bowel movements in an effort to avoid pain. This intensifies the problem because it leads to constipation.

Diagnosis

To diagnose a hemorrhoid, a physician inspects the anal canal, often with special instruments. An anoscope (a short, lighted, tubelike instrument) inserted into the anus can reveal hemorrhoids. The proctosigmoidoscope, a longer instrument that provides a view of the lower portion of the large intestine, may be used to rule out other causes of bleeding or pain.

Treatment

Painful hemorrhoids can be treated at home by taking warm

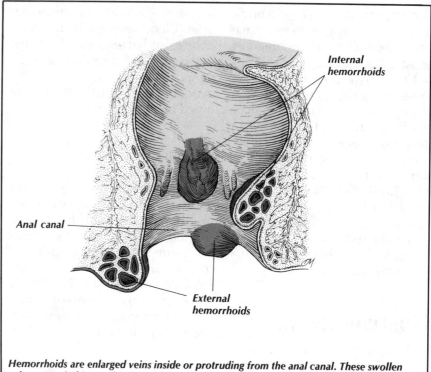

Hemorrhoids are enlarged veins inside or protruding from the anal canal. These swollen veins cause itching and pain, which may be accompanied by bleeding.

sitz baths (sitting in a tub of warm water). Over-the-counter preparations cannot cure hemorrhoids, but they can help relieve itching and swelling. Should symptoms worsen after application of any remedy, its use should be suspended and a doctor consulted. Chemicals in these preparations may produce an allergic reaction. Nonirritating laxatives may be useful in softening stools and easing bowel movements.

In the early stages of hemorrhoid development, adjustment of personal habits may prevent progression of the condition. A bowel movement should never be delayed once the urge is felt. During bowel movements, straining should be avoided. A diet including plenty of roughage—natural grains, fresh fruits, and vegetables—also softens stools. Fiber supplements are also quite helpful.

For severe cases of hemorrhoids, a doctor may recommend a surgical procedure called hemorrhoidectomy to remove dilated portions of the affected veins and to tie off the remaining parts of the vein. Newer procedures, such as cryosurgery and laser surgery, remove the hemorrhoid, but with less pain and fewer postoperative complications. Laser surgery uses an intensified beam of light to burn off the hemorrhoid. With cryosurgery, the hemorrhoid is frozen with an extremely cold probe. The frozen tissue dies, and the hemorrhoid falls off within several days. Physicians can perform cryosurgery in their offices in a matter of minutes. Frequently, the only postoperative complaint is a slight watery discharge from the anal canal for a few days.

Another technique used to eliminate hemorrhoids is rubberband ligation. With this procedure, which can be performed in the physician's office, the blood supply of the hemorrhoid is cut off by tying a rubber band around the swollen tissue. The hemorrhoid drops off within three to nine days. Unfortunately, as is the case with the nonsurgical procedures, this procedure is not suitable for all patients. It is often done only in the presence of internal hemorrhoids.

Recurrence of hemorrhoids after any type of treatment is not uncommon.

Hepatitis

Hepatitis is an inflammation of the liver, usually caused by a viral infection, which is characterized by jaundice (yellowing of the eyes and skin).

Causes and types

The disease is caused by several viruses, but the most common are those that cause hepatitis A (infectious hepatitis) and hepatitis B (serum hepatitis). The hepatitis A virus and the hepatitis B virus both attack cells in the liver.

Hepatitis A is transmitted from person to person via contaminated food or water or contact with the stools of an infected person. This disease may occur in epidemics where sanitation is poor and the water supply is contaminated. The incubation period (the time between exposure to the disease and the appearance of symptoms) is between 14 and 40 days. Sometimes, hepatitis A is so mild that symptoms never appear, but the infected person can still be a carrier and can transmit the disease to others.

In hepatitis B, the virus enters the bloodstream through contact with contaminated blood or other body fluids, such as semen, or with stool or through the use of contaminated hypodermic needles. Hepatitis B begins more gradually than does hepatitis A, so the disease may be present 40 to 180 days before the onset of symptoms. Because the virus can live in stool and almost all body fluids, including saliva, semen, and tears, hepatitis B can be transmitted by sexual contact or, rarely, by casual contact.

Recently, a hepatitis C virus has been characterized. The virus is presumed to be a major cause of what was previously known as "non-A, non-B hepatitis." Its incubation period is somewhere between that of A and B, and its mode of transmission is similar to B.

Hepatitis that is not due to any of the above may also result as a complication of infectious mononucleosis.

Symptoms

Early signs of hepatitis include general fatigue, joint and muscle pain, and loss of appetite. Nausea, vomiting, and diarrhea or constipation may follow, with a low-grade fever of 101°F or less. As the disease develops, the liver enlarges and becomes tender. Chills, weight loss, and distaste for smoking appear along with the characteristic jaundice. Jaundice results from an accumulation of yellow bile pigment in the blood, which turns the skin and whites of the eyes yellow.

In hepatitis A, the disappearance of jaundice generally signals the beginning of recovery. However, in hepatitis B or C, the virus may persist for years or even a lifetime.

Any sudden rise in fever, extreme drowsiness, or severe prolonged pain requires immediate medical attention to avoid permanent liver damage. Chronic (long-term) active hepatitis can lead to irreversible liver failure or cirrhosis (a condition in which normal cells of the liver are replaced by fibrous scar tissue that inhibits liver function).

Diagnosis

To determine the extent and severity of hepatitis, a physician analyzes blood and urine specimens from the patient. If the disease has progressed, the patient may have yellow skin and soreness in the upper abdomen over the liver.

More severe acute or chronic hepatitis may necessitate a liver biopsy—a diagnostic procedure in which a needle is inserted into the liver to obtain a sample of liver tissue. A local anesthetic is first injected into the upper abdomen to reduce discomfort from the test.

Treatment

There is no cure for viral hepatitis. Even treatment is limited, especially for individuals with acute hepatitis. Once the hepatitis virus attacks, recovery is usually up to the body's natural defense mechanisms.

To encourage the healing process, physicians advise patients to avoid strenuous activity. Bed rest is important during the acute phase of hepatitis. More serious cases may require hospitalization to ensure adequate nutrition. All hepatitis patients must avoid alcoholic beverages, because processing alcohol puts a tremendous strain on the liver. All drugs taken, including any over-the-counter (nonprescription) preparations, must first be okayed by the individual's physician since the liver is responsible for clearing most drugs from the body. Inflammation of the liver may lessen the liver's ability to do this and thus lead to increased levels of the drugs in the body, which can cause toxic effects.

Prevention

Persons exposed to hepatitis may prevent or minimize the severity of the disease by obtaining an injection of gamma globulin, a disease-fighting substance derived from blood. Gamma globulin usually defends against hepatitis A virus and may offer modest protection against hepatitis B virus.

A hepatitis B vaccine is now available. (A vaccine is a preparation of a disease-causing agent that stimulates the body to produce antibodies to fight the disease.) Hepatitis B vaccine is recommended for persons who are in direct contact with hepatitis carriers, for health-care workers, and for persons in certain other high-risk groups (for example, travelers to regions where hepatitis is prevalent and hemophiliacs who receive pooled blood products).

Hiatal hernia

A hernia is a protrusion of a body part through the structures that surround it. A hiatal hernia (also called a hiatus or diaphragmatic hernia) occurs when a portion of the stomach protrudes above the diaphragm (the muscular wall separating the chest and abdominal cavities) into the chest.

Normal

Sliding hiatal hernia

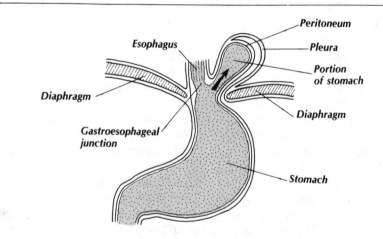

Paraesophageal hiatal hernia

A hiatal hernia occurs when a portion of the stomach protrudes through the hiatus (the tight muscular collar that normally prevents the stomach from pushing through the diaphragm into the chest). In a sliding hiatal hernia, the top part of the stomach and the gastroesophageal junction (the junction of the stomach and the esophagus) move upward through the hiatus. In a paraesophageal hiatal hernia, the gastroesophageal junction retains its normal position while a portion of the stomach and its peritoneal covering roll up through the hiatus.

Sliding hiatal hernia

Normally, the esophagus (the passageway from the throat to the stomach) passes through a tight muscular collar, called a hiatus, that prevents the stomach from squeezing up into the chest cavity. However, if the collar is too large or if it relaxes, a sliding hiatal hernia may occur. Pressure in the abdominal cavity (such as may be caused by obesity, pregnancy, tight clothing, bending or other changes in position, coughing, or straining) causes the top part of the stomach to herniate (slide through the opening) along with the gastroesophageal junction (the junction of the stomach and the esophagus). This condition is very common, especially in women and older persons. It is often without symptoms. Surgical treatment is recommended in only the most severe cases.

Until recently it was believed that the mere presence of a sliding hiatal hernia causes regurgitation (backward flow) of food and harsh stomach acid into the esophagus, which produces the burning sensation of heartburn. Current thinking, however, is that regurgitation and heartburn are the result of the functional ability of the esophageal sphincter.

Paraesophageal hiatal hernia

A relatively uncommon but quite dangerous type of hiatal hernia is the paraesophageal, or rolling, hiatal hernia. In this type, the gastroesophageal junction retains its normal position while a portion of the stomach and part of its peritoneum (covering membrane) rolls up through the opening in the diaphragm, alongside the junction. The danger is that the herniated section may be-

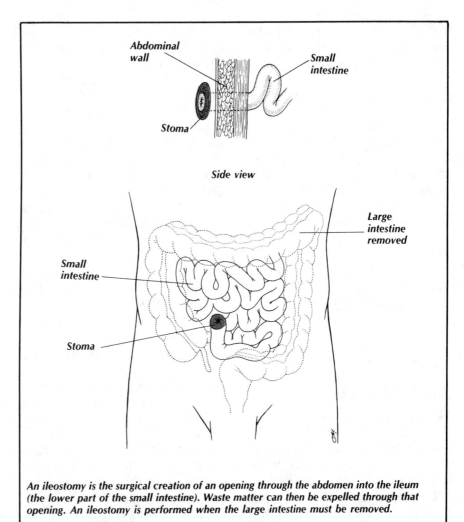

Side view

An ileostomy is the surgical creation of an opening through the abdomen into the ileum (the lower part of the small intestine). Waste matter can then be expelled through that opening. An ileostomy is performed when the large intestine must be removed.

come trapped in the chest with its blood supply choked off, thereby causing death of stomach tissue. Bleeding is also a common complication. Although dangerous, this condition may have no symptoms and is usually found accidentally on an X ray taken for another purpose. The only common symptom is a sense of fullness in the chest after eating.

Because of the potential complications of the paraesophageal hernia, many authorities recommend surgery, even in the absence of symptoms. Surgery for the paraesophageal hernia involves entering the abdomen and pushing the herniated portion of

the stomach back into its proper position while removing the sac of peritoneum around it. After this, the muscular collar of the diaphragm is tightened with stitches.

Ileostomy

An ileostomy is the surgical creation of an opening, or stoma, through the abdomen into the ileum (the lower part of the small intestine). An ileostomy is performed if the large intestine and rectum must be removed because of disease or abnormality. The opening into the small intestine then becomes an artificial anus through which waste material is expelled, since waste matter can no longer travel through the normal anus.

The waste matter that is discharged through the stoma is collected in a bag that the patient wears continuously. Because this waste does not pass through the large intestine, where water is absorbed from the waste, the material excreted through the stoma is watery.

Patients learn to care for their stomas in the hospital after the operation. Equipped with this knowledge, a patient can lead a normal life after an ileostomy.

Intestinal and gastric bypass surgery

Intestinal bypass surgery and gastric bypass surgery are methods of treating massive obesity. Because of their potential dangers, such methods are usually limited to persons who are at least 100 pounds over their ideal weight and who have failed to lose weight by other means, such as diet and exercise. These persons are at serious risk for diabetes, high blood pressure, heart disease, arthritis, and other disorders.

Various types of operations have been tried to detour digesting food around a long section of the small intestine, thus limiting the area of intestine that can absorb fats and carbohydrates from the food. One such operation is the jejunoileal bypass—named for the jejunum (the middle portion of the small intestine) and the ileum (the final portion of the small intestine). In this procedure, all but 18 inches of the 240 inches of the small intes-

tine is bypassed (the unused portion remains in the body and drains into the colon). The method is very effective in reducing weight—from 80 to 150 pounds in most patients—but frequently produces persistent diarrhea, severe liver disease, imbalances in body salts, kidney stones, bladder stones, mental disturbances, and joint inflammations. Because the mortality rate associated with those complications may be as high as five percent, many physicians believe that the intestinal bypass method should no longer be used. This surgery is now seldom performed since there are safer treatment methods.

Replacements for the intestinal bypass procedure, which are reported to have far fewer complications, are gastric bypass and gastric stapling. Both are designed to reduce the capacity of the stomach so that only a small amount of food can be eaten at one time. In the gastric bypass operation, the lower part of the stomach is cut off, and the remaining top part is connected to the upper portion of the small intestine. In the gastric stapling operation, stomach capacity is reduced by stapling off most of the fundus (the uppermost portion of the stomach).

Recently, a nonsurgical technique for reducing stomach capacity has been developed. A specially designed balloon is placed in the stomach and then inflated. Since the balloon takes up a significant portion of the volume of the stomach, there is less room for food. The patient feels full after eating a relatively small quantity of food. This technique has the advantage that it is readily reversible: the balloon can be removed relatively easily if problems arise or the patient reaches the desired weight.

The long-term results and side effects of gastric bypass, gastric stapling, and gastric balloon placement, when known, will determine whether these procedures are widely employed. Until then, it should be remembered that they are drastic measures that carry the risk of potentially serious complications.

Irritable bowel syndrome

Irritable bowel syndrome, also called spastic colon and mucous colitis, is a collection of symptoms caused by irritability and irregularity in the movement of both the small and large intestines. The syndrome is usually influenced by emotions. Feelings of nervousness, anxiety, guilt, depression, or anger may bring on or aggravate this very common disorder. Coffee, raw fruits and vegetables, hormones, drugs, and overuse of laxatives can promote it, as can an inability of the body to digest the natural sugar in milk.

Symptoms

Irritable bowel syndrome is not a disease, but a collection of symptoms that includes both constipation and diarrhea, often alternating and sometimes accompanied by abdominal cramps and straining during elimination. Stools may be loose or compacted and may include mucus, which is produced by the bowel lining in greater than usual amounts as a response to irritation. Gas, bloating, nausea, headache, and fatigue may accompany the other symptoms.

There are two main types of irritable bowel syndrome. The first type, spastic colon, is marked by cramps or a dull, aching pain in the abdomen, usually the lower part. The discomfort often begins at mealtime and may disappear after a bowel movement. The second type of irritable bowel syndrome is characterized by painless diarrhea, especially an urgent need for a bowel movement on awakening or during or right after a meal. Fecal incontinence (loss of voluntary bowel control) can occur.

Diagnosis

If a patient appears to have irritable bowel syndrome, the doctor will first want to rule out diseases with similar symptoms. The patient may be asked to bring in a stool specimen to be examined for traces of blood and microorganisms. The colon may be X-rayed following a barium enema. The doctor may examine the lower portion of the colon with a proctosigmoidoscope (a lighted tubelike instrument inserted through the anus) to check for serious disorders, such as ulcerative colitis.

Treatment

If no organic disease is found, the doctor will reassure the patient and discuss ways in which the symptoms can be relieved. There may be methods by which the patient can reduce the anxiety or depression that may be causing the syndrome. The doctor may prescribe a tranquilizer, sedative, antidepressant, or antispasmodic medication—but only on a short-term basis, so that the individual does not become dependent on the drug. Long walks, bike rides, or other exercise may help to relax the person while promoting better bowel action.

If constipation is a problem, the doctor will advise the patient to add bulk, such as whole bran, to the diet; to stop depending on laxatives; and to take pills that absorb water, add bulk, and help to stabilize the large intestine. If diarrhea is present, avoiding laxative foods, such as prunes, may help. Patients bothered by gas will be warned against foods such as cabbage and beans. Milk may be barred from the diet. Most people, with the general exception of those of northwestern European origin, lose some or all of the ability to digest lactose, the natural sugar in milk, by the time they are 20 years old. A test for this is an oral dose of lactose. If it results in diarrhea and bloating, it is a tip-off that the symptoms could have been caused by drinking milk.

If irritable bowel syndrome continues despite treatment, it is important to remember that it is not dangerous. However, to be safe, regular medical checkups should be scheduled, especially if the patient is over 40.

Jaundice

Jaundice is a yellowish discoloration of the skin, the whites of the eyes, the mucous membranes, and other tissues of the body, which is caused by the abnormal accumulation of the bile pigment bilirubin in the blood.

Bilirubin consists primarily of the hemoglobin of used red blood cells and is found in bile, a bitter, yellow-green fluid that aids in digestion by breaking down fat. Bile is secreted by the liver, stored in the gallbladder, and discharged into the small intestine when it is needed for digestion.

Causes

In many cases, jaundice occurs when bile is prevented from being discharged into the small intestine by an obstruction. The obstruction may be caused by gallstones, tumors, or parasites in the bile ducts. Jaundice may also be a sign of hepatitis, in which the inflamed or damaged liver cannot process the bilirubin it receives. Occasionally, jaundice appears if red blood cells are destroyed too rapidly and the liver cannot accommodate the excess pigment. Jaundice is also associated with many other diseases in which the functioning of the liver is disrupted, including various forms of cancer and certain viral and parasitic infections. More than 50 percent of full-term newborn infants and 80 percent of premature newborn infants show signs of jaundice by the third day after birth. In most of these cases, the condition is nothing to worry about and disappears in a week or so.

Symptoms

Usually when jaundice occurs, the liver has become enlarged and is functioning less than optimally. Bowel movements may be clay-colored, and urine can vary in hue from light yellow to brownish green. Jaundiced skin ranges in color from lemon yellow to olive green.

Diagnosis

Routine blood testing will determine the origin of some cases of jaundice, but usually it is necessary to examine the bile ducts using ultrasound, in which sound waves are used to create images of internal structures, and computed tomography, a special X-ray technique that provides cross-sectional pictures of an area. Endoscopic retrograde cholangiopancreatography (ERCP) is a technique whereby the pancreas and bile ducts are examined after direct injection of a contrast medium into a bile duct. This is accomplished by threading an endoscope (a flexible, lighted, tubelike instrument) through the mouth, down the esophagus, through the stomach, and into the duodenum. A small flexible tube is then inserted into the opening of the bile duct, and the contrast medium is infused. λ rays are immediately taken. Bile samples for testing can also be obtained in this manner. During this procedure, the patient is asleep but is not under general anesthesia. Usually the individual goes home the same day or the following day, depending on the underlying condition. Complications, such as perforation of an organ, pancreatitis (inflammation of the pancreas), or infection, can occur, but they are uncommon.

Treatment

Surgery may be necessary if an obstruction is present. Otherwise, treatment depends on the underlying condition that is causing the jaundice.

Occult blood

Occult blood is blood that is present in an amount so small that it is detectable only with a chemical test or microscopic examination. This term is generally used to refer to blood that is present in the stools that indicates bleeding somewhere along the gastrointestinal tract.

Symptoms

Often, the only symptom of occult bleeding is fatigue due to loss of oxygen-carrying red blood cells. A significant amount of blood can be passed in one stool with no visible indication.

Diagnosis

Occult bleeding is not always constant, so tests are typically performed on stool samples obtained on three separate occasions if a problem is suspected. The patient must not eat red meat for three days before the samples are obtained because even cooked blood from meat that has been eaten can cause a positive test result. Aspirin can also cause minute amounts of blood to appear in the stools and should not be taken for at least several days before starting to test for occult blood in the stools. Tests for occult blood are commonly done to screen for colon cancer and polyps. These tests are highly effective in early diagnosis of these conditions.

Pancreatitis

The pancreas has many functions. The endocrine portion of the pancreas secretes hormones directly into the bloodstream, such as the hormones insulin and glucagon, which are critical to the processing of glucose (the form of sugar used by the body for energy). The exocrine portion of the pancreas secretes digestive enzymes (proteins that promote chemical reactions), such as amylase, which aids in the breakdown of starches, and lipase, which aids in the breakdown of fats. Pancreatitis is an inflammation of the pancreas.

Causes

Pancreatitis commonly results from an obstruction of the pancreatic ducts, which convey enzymes to the small intestine. Why these blockages occur is often hard to determine; however, most cases of pancreatitis are related to gallbladder disease or alcoholism. Acute attacks are frequently associated with gallstones or alcoholic binges. If hereditary factors are involved, the disease may begin in childhood, as early as eight or ten years of age. Direct blows to the abdomen or injury during an operation may also lead to pancreatitis, sometimes a year or more later. Mumps and other viral infections; use of certain drugs, including steroids, thiazide diuretics, and oral contraceptives; and tumors have been associated with pancreatitis.

Symptoms

The disease is characterized by the sudden onset of steady, severe, piercing, upper abdominal pain (frequently radiating to the middle portion of the back) accompanied by nausea and persistent vomiting. Eating—or even the sight of food—may bring on the pain or make it worse. Vomiting provides no relief, a feature that distinguishes pancreatitis from some stomach or intestinal disorders. Fever, shock (circulatory collapse), jaundice (yellowing of the eyes and skin), dehydration (excessive fluid loss), bleeding, and infection may occur in severe attacks.

Diagnosis

The existence and degree of inflammation in the pancreas

may be hard to determine, not only because of the hidden position and dual purpose of the gland, but also because the symptoms are easily confused with those of other abdominal disorders. Blood and urine tests, as well as microscopic tissue examination, may be inconclusive, but can at least be helpful in excluding other abdominal disorders.

A special X-ray study, endoscopic retrograde cholangiopancreatography (ERCP), may be used to inspect the pancreatic ducts. The technique is performed by inserting an endoscope (a flexible, lighted, tube-like instrument) through the mouth and stomach into the duodenum. In the duodenum is the opening to the common bile and main pancreatic ducts. A special device is inserted through this opening, and X-ray contrast material is injected. Obstructions, tumors, and characteristic ductal patterns that are associated with chronic pancreatitis can be seen on the X-ray films that are obtained from this study.

Treatment

The patient is usually hospitalized for 3 to 14 days for a mild to severe acute attack. Correction of an underlying problem (for example, removal of stones) improves the chances for complete recovery.

Initial treatment is aimed at relieving the pain and reducing stomach secretions, which can stimulate the pancreas. To allow the pancreas to rest, eating and drinking are replaced by intravenous feeding, and stomach acids are suctioned out through a tube inserted through the nose. Antacids and antibodies are also frequently given.

During convalescence, a low-fat, high-protein diet should be followed, and antacids may be prescribed. If the disease is chronic, it may be necessary to use pancreatic extracts to supplement the insufficient quantities of enzymes secreted by the diseased pancreas. This helps to normalize digestion and thereby maintain adequate nutritional status.

After an acute episode of pancreatitis, tissue debris, blood, and pancreatic enzymes may form a pseudocyst (an internal space filled with a collection of material but not within a sac). Rupture or enlargement of a pseudocyst can be a very serious or even fatal event. If a pseudocyst does not clear up spontaneously, surgery is necessary to drain it.

Chronic pancreatitis is an indication of continued degenerative tissue damage, which may impair pancreatic function. In some cases of recurrence, surgical exploration might be considered to locate a previously unidentified blockage or to remove diseased tissue; however, surgery is unlikely to help the patient who continues to drink excessive amounts of alcohol. Recently, procedures to remove stones or otherwise relieve obstruction have been successfully performed through a gastroscope (see page 404), eliminating the need for surgery.

Periodontal disease

Periodontal disease (also known as periodontitis or, less accurately, as pyorrhea) is a progressive deterioration of the gums, bones, and other tissues around the teeth.

Causes

One theory is that the condition begins with an accumulation of bacteria and food particles within tissues surrounding the teeth. These bacteria emit toxins (poisons) that cause gum tissues to swell, bleed, and deteriorate.

Stages of periodontitis

Gingivitis (inflammation of the gums) is the first stage of periodontitis. The second stage results when the soft tissues become separated from the bone and teeth, leading to "pocket" formation. Pockets of bacteria and pus accumulate around the teeth, leading to weakening of the tissues holding the teeth in their sockets, as well as to destruction of the bone supporting the teeth. As the disease advances, teeth become loose and fall out. They may also move out of alignment with one another, causing problems with chewing.

Symptoms

In the early stage of periodontal disease, gums become sore, red, and slightly swollen. They may be sensitive to the touch and may bleed when brushed or flossed. The presence of pus in the gums around the teeth signals the beginning of the second stage. If pus remains in the gum tissue without draining, extreme pain and swelling can result.

Diagnosis

The diagnosis of periodontal disease is based on the presence of swollen gums and deposits of plaque around the teeth.

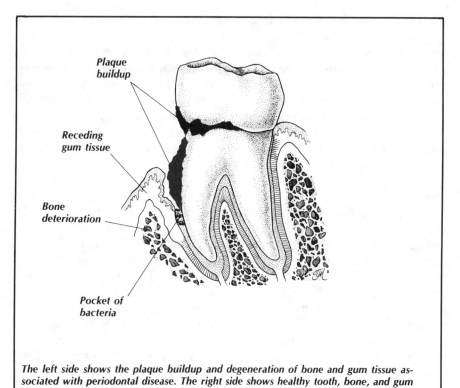

The left side shows the plaque buildup and degeneration of bone and gum tissue associated with periodontal disease. The right side shows healthy tooth, bone, and gum tissue.

Treatment and prevention

Once periodontal disease has been detected, continued care of the mouth at home can help prevent extension of disease and can reduce gum problems.

Oral hygiene to prevent gum disease is the same as treatment to prevent tooth decay. Ideally, the mouth should be cleaned after every meal. At the least, a thorough cleansing at bedtime is necessary. Dentists suggest brushing with a soft-bristled toothbrush. Gentle movements within the crevices dislodge decay-causing material, and firm strokes over the teeth remove plaque. Flossing is recommended to clear plaque from between teeth. After brushing and flossing, rinsing with mouthwash containing an antimicrobial agent (a substance that kills bacteria) can help eliminate bacterial growth, but mouthwash alone cannot prevent plaque formation.

For self-checking, a dental mirror provides a view of the teeth and gums in the back of the mouth. Disclosing wafers, which discolor plaque when chewed, reveal any invisible film that needs to be removed.

In advanced cases, a dentist may scrape the affected tissue pockets and apply antiseptics (germ-killers) every few months in an effort to kill the bacteria. Should this procedure fail to check the spread of the disease, surgery may be needed to remove deep pockets in the gums. Once the bacteria have been eliminated, good oral hygiene should control the disease.

Peritonitis

Peritonitis is a term used to describe an inflammation and/or infection of the peritoneum, the thin, double-layered membrane that lines the abdominal cavity and covers the abdominal organs.

Causes

The condition occurs when the peritoneum is invaded by bacteria or irritated by toxins (poisons), bile (a substance produced by the liver and stored in the gallbladder), blood, or urine. Because the peritoneum is well sealed, it can be infiltrated only when one of the hollow organs of the abdomen ruptures; when a solid organ is somehow damaged, causing it to leak; or when there is a penetrating injury from the outside. If the colon is perforated, feces, which contain bacteria and toxins, are discharged, causing bacterial peritonitis. Immediate treatment is necessary for this condition.

Symptoms

A main symptom of peritonitis is severe pain that intensifies with any movement and often forces the person to lie very still with the legs drawn up. The abdominal area becomes very tender and rigid; commonly there is vomiting, fever, and dehydration (excessive loss of body fluids). When the peritoneum is inflamed, fluid begins to leak out of the blood vessels into the peritoneum. If this condition is not corrected, it may lead to shock (failure of the circulatory system, marked by rapid, shallow breathing and a weak, rapid, irregular pulse). Swelling of the abdomen is a sign that the intestines have become paralyzed and bloated with air and/or a large amount of fluid is accumulating.

Treatment

These symptoms of peritonitis call for immediate medical care, including intravenous administration of antibiotics to fight infection. Intravenous fluids are also given to replace lost fluids. In addition, a tube is usually inserted through the nose and into the stomach to relieve bloating and remove pooled fluids. After the patient's condition has been stabilized, surgery is performed to remove or repair the cause of peritonitis. Chances for recovery are usually excellent.

Pyloric stenosis

Pyloric stenosis is a constriction (narrowing) of the passage between the stomach and the small intestine. The stomach has two openings—one at the top, where it joins with the esophagus (food tube), and one at the bottom, where it joins with the small intestine. The lower opening is called the pylorus.

Causes

Pyloric stenosis can be caused by many conditions, including cancer, spasm, a nearby ulcer in the part of the intestine directly below the pyloric opening, gastritis (inflammation of the stomach), and enlargement of the pyloric sphincter (the muscle that rings the pyloric opening and controls its movement).

Symptoms

In the case of congenital (present at birth) pyloric stenosis, ten days to three weeks after birth the infant will experience regurgitation ("spitting up" of part of

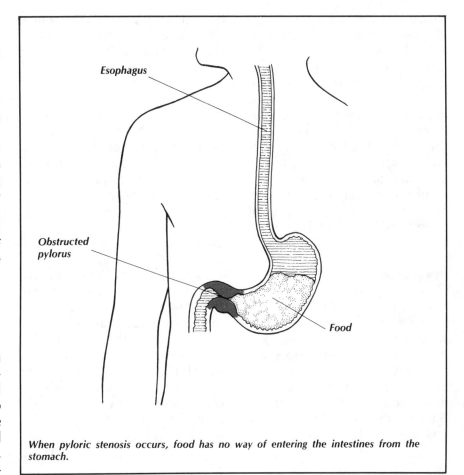

Esophagus

Obstructed pylorus

Food

When pyloric stenosis occurs, food has no way of entering the intestines from the stomach.

the stomach's contents), projectile vomiting (vomiting with great force), weight loss, and dehydration without appetite loss. Adults with pyloric stenosis experience discomfort in the upper and middle portions of the abdomen, pain, bloating of the abdominal area, nausea, vomiting, and weight loss.

Treatment

In mild cases of temporary pyloric stenosis, such as that due to an ulcer, the condition can be treated by offering only small meals or intravenous feeding, restoring normal fluid levels, and administering antacid drugs (drugs that block the production of stomach acid).

In severe cases, a pyloromyotomy (a lengthwise incision into the pyloric muscle) may be indicated. A portion of the pyloric sphincter may also be removed.

Tooth decay

Tooth decay (dental cavities, or caries) is the gradual process of destruction and mineral loss that affects the enamel (outer layer) and dentin (the bony second layer) of a portion of a tooth, causing it to become soft, discolored, and porous.

Causes

A combination of factors causes tooth decay. A substance

called plaque, made up of sugars, starches, bacteria, and proteins, builds up on dental surfaces, especially near the gums and in other hard-to-clean areas. The plaque prevents the saliva from performing its natural protective function. The bacteria in the plaque feed on the sugars and starches that cling to the teeth and produce acid as a byproduct of their metabolism. That acid is probably the agent of destruction of dental tissue.

Symptoms

When the cavity has progressed into the dentin or the surface of an exposed root, the tooth becomes sensitive to touch and rapid temperature changes. Sweet foods can cause pain as dissolved sugar enters the cavity. Bacteria may pass through tiny channels in the dentin and inflame the pulp, which contains blood vessels and nervous tissue, producing toothache.

Diagnosis

The cavity reveals itself to the dentist as a darkened area or as an area of softness when probed with a sharp instrument. It is also apparent on X ray.

Treatment

Cavities are treated by drilling out the decayed material and replacing it with a filling. In front teeth, where appearance is important, the filling may be of porcelain or a plastic resin (which is also used to fill pits and tiny cracks in the enamel). In other teeth, the filling is usually silver-colored or an alloy of gold, which is the most durable material. When a tooth is badly damaged, with involvement of the root, the dentist removes all decay, fills the cavity and root canal with dental cement, then grinds and tapers the outer surface and covers it with what is known as a gold crown. On teeth toward the front, the gold crown is overlaid with porcelain to provide a natural appearance.

Prevention

To prevent decay, teeth should be cleaned daily with a soft-bristled brush, preferably after each meal, to remove food particles and plaque. Equally important is the use of dental floss to remove debris between the teeth. Avoiding sweet, sticky foods, or at least rinsing or brushing shortly after eating them, may also help prevent decay. A child's teeth will be more resistant to decay if

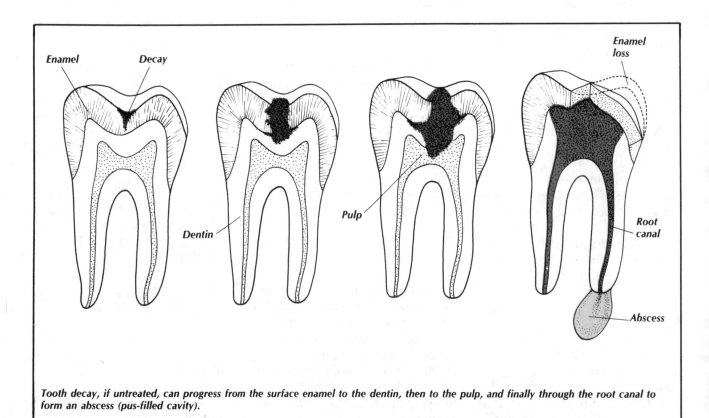

Tooth decay, if untreated, can progress from the surface enamel to the dentin, then to the pulp, and finally through the root canal to form an abscess (pus-filled cavity).

the child drinks water containing the proper amount of fluoride in the first 12 years of life, while the teeth are developing. If the water supply is not fluoridated, a vitamin supplement containing fluoride can be taken daily. Adults and children alike can benefit by using a fluoride-containing toothpaste or mouthwash.

Traveler's diarrhea

Of all the illnesses likely to afflict travelers to foreign countries, the most common is "traveler's diarrhea." This disorder, an intestinal infection caused by microorganisms to which the traveler is unaccustomed, is characterized by loose, watery stools, often accompanied by nausea and abdominal cramps.

Causes

The organism most commonly responsible is probably the *Escherichia coli* (*E. coli*) bacterium. This bacterium is a normal inhabitant of the intestines, but in some areas of the world it has evolved into a strain called enterotoxigenic *E. coli*, or ETEC, which can cause moderate to severe diarrhea. Other organisms that can cause traveler's diarrhea include *Campylobacter, Salmonella,* and *Shigella* bacteria; parasitic protozoa (one-celled organisms), such as *Entamoeba histolytica* (the cause of amoebic dysentery) and *Giardia lamblia*; and a number of viruses.

Symptoms

The major symptom of the illness is, of course, diarrhea, which can range in intensity from mild (three to four loose, watery stools per day) to severe (10 to 20 bloody stools per day). The severity of traveler's diarrhea is largely dependent on the type of organism that is causing the infection and the health status of the individual. Traveler's diarrhea caused by bacteria usually begins a few days after the beginning of the trip and may last for several days to a few weeks if not properly treated. *Campylobacter* and *Shigella* infections commonly are marked by severe, bloody diarrhea. The diarrhea caused by *Giardia* organisms is usually characterized by abundant stools (rarely blood-tinged) and can be associated with other symptoms, such as fever, weight loss, and weakness. Traveler's diarrhea caused by protozoa can be mild or very severe, with involvement of other organs, such as the liver.

Diagnosis

Knowledge of which foreign countries have been visited recently will help the doctor in making a preliminary diagnosis. Because it is very difficult to differentiate among the various infectious causes of diarrhea, laboratory studies, such as stool cultures and blood tests, are often needed. Parasitic diarrhea is especially difficult to diagnose; occasionally, multiple cultures are necessary, as well as proctosigmoidoscopy (visual examination of the rectum and lower portion of the large intestine with a special instrument).

Treatment

Prescription antidiarrheal medications are often sought by individuals about to leave on a trip so that they can treat themselves if they suffer some form of traveler's diarrhea. Physicians are justifiably reluctant to prescribe these medications routinely because in many forms of diarrheal illness, such drugs can actually cause complications and prolong the course of the disease. These medications should never be taken except on the advice of a physician.

Mild cases of traveler's diarrhea usually clear up without treatment in a few days. Diarrhea that lasts for more than several days or that is associated with persistent fever or with the presence of blood, pus, or mucus in the stools calls for immediate medical attention.

Prevention

Much has been written in recent years about prevention of traveler's diarrhea by taking medication before and during the trip. It must be remembered that all medications have potential side effects and that the indiscriminate use of antibiotics and antidiarrheal medications can be dangerous. Except in special circumstances (for example, a person with severe health problems, for whom an episode of severe diarrhea could be catastrophic), routine prophylaxis (preventive treatment) with antibiotics is not recommended.

Because there are no vaccines or universally effective prophylactic drugs to use against traveler's diarrhea, caution should be exercised when eating or drinking in many foreign countries. Avoid unboiled water (and ice made from unboiled water). Be careful of water that you use to brush your teeth, too. Do not assume that bottled water avail-

THE DIGESTIVE SYSTEM

able locally is safe. Lettuce and other fresh vegetables are common culprits. Fruit with intact skin is usually safe if you wash it with safe water and peel it yourself before eating. Beer, wine, and carbonated beverages are usually safe, but it must be remembered that the addition of alcoholic beverages to water does not kill infectious organisms. Food obtained from local street vendors should be avoided.

Ulcer

An ulcer is an erosion (open sore) on the surface of an organ or tissue. Ulcers most commonly erupt in the esophagus, stomach, and duodenum, in which case they are known as peptic ulcers.

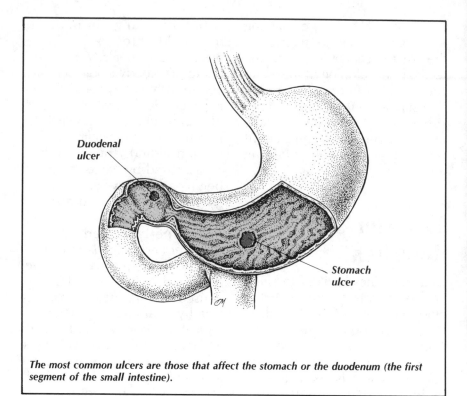

The most common ulcers are those that affect the stomach or the duodenum (the first segment of the small intestine).

Causes

Although the cause of peptic ulcers has not been fully established, scientists believe that the more common duodenal ulcers may result from the presence of excessive amounts of acid produced by the stomach. The stomach may increase acidic secretions after coffee, alcohol, and certain medications are consumed or after cigarettes are smoked. Therefore, these substances are thought to contribute to ulcers. Aspirin and aspirinlike compounds exert a direct damaging effect on the lining of the stomach.

The less common stomach ulcers may be due to an inherent weakness in the wall of the stomach. However, this weakness may result from the same environmental conditions that aggravate duodenal ulcers.

Emotional stress may play a role in ulcer development. However, physicians distinguish be-

tween stress as a factor by itself and certain ways of dealing with stress that may increase susceptibility to ulcers.

Heredity plays an important role in contributing to ulcers. Persons who have a family history of ulcers seem to have a greater likelihood of acquiring the condition, as do persons with type O blood. In addition, liver disease, rheumatoid arthritis, and emphysema may increase vulnerability to ulcers.

Symptoms

Ulcers can produce mild symptoms resembling heartburn or severe pain radiating throughout the upper portion of the body. The most common discomfort of ulcers is a burning sensation in the abdomen above the navel that may feel like hunger pangs. Pain comes about 30 to 120 minutes after eating or

in the middle of the night when the stomach is empty. At this time, the acidic stomach juices are more apt to irritate the unprotected nerve endings in the exposed ulcer. Usually, pain subsides after eating or drinking something or taking an antacid.

Some people experience nausea, vomiting, and constipation. Blood in the feces (discoloring them black), blood in the vomit, extreme weakness, fainting, and excessive thirst are all signs of internal bleeding, and may appear in more advanced cases.

While ulcers are not usually life threatening, they can cause serious damage if left untreated. Ulcers may erode nearby blood vessels and cause internal seepage of blood or hemorrhage (massive internal bleeding). A perforated ulcer may penetrate an adjoining organ, causing infection. In addition, scar tissue growing around the ulcer may lead to an obstruction or narrowing.

Diagnosis

Physicians diagnose peptic ulcers primarily on the basis of an X-ray examination after the patient has swallowed a special chalky substance called barium. The barium makes the digestive tract visible on X-ray film, allowing the doctor a view of any abnormalities.

A second diagnostic technique is called an upper GI endoscopy (also called gastroscopy). The doctor inserts an endoscope (a flexible, lighted, tubelike instrument) through the mouth and down the esophagus to directly view the lining of the esophagus, stomach, and duodenum. An endoscopic examination and a biopsy (removal of a tissue sample for analysis) are necessary to confirm that an apparent ulcer is not actually a cancerous growth.

Treatment

Treatment of ulcers involves relieving the irritation so that healing is able to progress naturally. Antacids counteract stomach acid and relieve symptoms, but they can cause complications. For example, sodium bicarbonate, a primary antacid ingredient, contains large amounts of sodium, which can aggravate kidney disease or high blood pressure.

For treatment of more problematic ulcers, a physician may prescribe other preparations to promote healing. Sucralfate coats the stomach, protecting it against gastric acid. Cimetidine, ranitidine, and other medications known as "H_2 blockers" inhibit gastric acid production and secretion.

Although recent studies have shown that a bland diet is not necessary for ulcer management, such a diet may be recommended until acute symptoms disappear. Thereafter, many doctors suggest avoiding only those foods known to cause stomach distress.

The effect of milk on ulcers is also questionable. Its neutralizing action on stomach acid is mild and temporary at best. Nevertheless, people who substitute milk for known irritants, such as alcohol and caffeine, are less likely to irritate their ulcers.

Most ulcers heal within two to six weeks after treatment begins. To prevent recurrence, patients should continue to refrain from use of cigarettes, caffeine, alcohol, and other substances that stimulate stomach acid production or irritate the digestive tract lining.

When drug therapy and diet cannot cure an ulcer, surgical repair may be necessary. Surgery is appropriate for repeated ulcers that recur or are life threatening, such as perforated ulcers. Sometimes, surgeons remove a portion of the stomach and parts of the vagus nerve (which controls digestive secretions) to reduce stomach acid production. Usually, ulcers do not reappear after surgery.

Recently, endoscopic cautery (burning of tissue through the endoscope), direct injection of medications, and laser surgery have been quite successful in stopping bleeding, reducing the size of tumors, and correcting strictures (narrowing due to scar formation). These procedures have spared many individuals a surgical procedure.

Ulcerative colitis

Ulcerative colitis is a chronic inflammatory disease of the large intestine characterized by bloody diarrhea and the development of erosions (open sores) on the lining of the colon.

Causes

Although there is a familial tendency to develop ulcerative colitis, the cause of the disorder is unknown. Any age group may be affected, but it tends to begin in persons between the ages of 15 and 40.

Among possible contributing factors are infection, immunologic derangement (a breakdown in the body's defense system), lack of protective elements in the bowel wall, nervous or psychological disturbances, and alterations in the connective tissue in the colon.

Symptoms

The first sign of ulcerative colitis is usually a series of attacks of bloody diarrhea. The attacks can vary in intensity and duration and are usually interspersed with periods of normal bowel movements. The onset of the attacks may be severe, with sudden violent diarrhea, high fever, symptoms of abdominal inflammation, and bacterial invasions. Often, an attack will be preceded by mild lower abdominal cramps and the appearance of small amounts of blood or mucus in the feces.

If ulceration is confined to the rectum and the terminal portion of the colon (ulcerative proctitis), the bowel movements may be normal or bloody, with discharges of mucus containing red and white blood cells between stools. If the disorder extends to other portions of the colon, however, stools become looser and more frequent (perhaps 10 to 20 per day), and the patient suffers severe cramps, watery stools, fever, anemia (due to blood loss), and loss of appetite.

Complications

If the condition persists in this severe form, hemorrhage (internal bleeding) is the most common complication. In toxic colitis, a serious complication, the colon loses muscular tone and dilates almost completely, resulting in perforations of the organ. The risk of colon cancer and cancer of the bile ducts is also increased in patients with ulcerative colitis. Arthritis, skin and eye disorders, and biliary tract disease are also associated with ulcerative colitis.

Diagnosis

Ulcerative colitis is diagnosed with the use of a stool examination and colonoscopy (in which a lighted, flexible, tubelike instrument is inserted through the anus and into the entire colon for a visual examination of the interior). X-ray studies with a barium enema are indicated, except in cases in which risk of perforation makes the barium enema procedure a potential danger for the patient.

Treatment

Mild cases of ulcerative colitis may sometimes be treated with

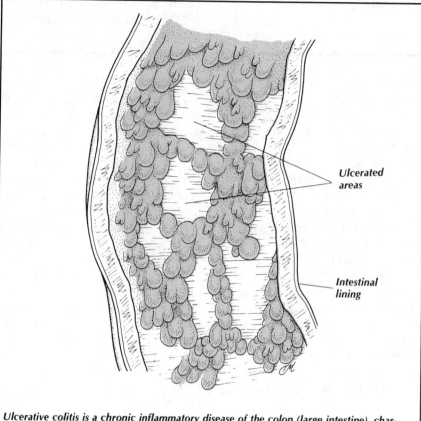

Ulcerated areas

Intestinal lining

Ulcerative colitis is a chronic inflammatory disease of the colon (large intestine), characterized by bloody diarrhea and the development of ulcerated areas in the intestinal lining.

adequate physical and mental relaxation (since the severity of the disease appears to be stress-related in some patients); a diet low in milk, milk products, nuts, kernels, and seeds; and antidiarrheal medication. More severe cases may respond to the drug sulfasalazine. Salicylate drugs (aspirinlike compounds), either in oral or enema form, and antibiotics have also been helpful. In cases that do not respond to salicylate or sulfasalazine therapy, hydrocortisone (a steroid hormone) may be given by enema, along with oral cortisone preparations. The only cure for ulcerative colitis is total colectomy (removal of the entire large intestine) sometimes with the rectum left in. Newer surgical techniques have, in many cases, eliminated the need for ileostomy (see pages 243-244). In ulcerative proctitis, surgery is usually not necessary to treat the condition, and individuals do not commonly progress to full-blown ulcerative colitis.

THE KIDNEYS AND
URINARY SYSTEM

The urinary system includes those organs of the body that produce and eliminate urine (a combination of water and waste products that passes out of the body as fluid). By controlling urine flow, the system maintains proper water balance throughout the body. Individual parts of the urinary system monitor the concentration of salts and other necessary nutrients.

Functions of urinary system organs

The organs most responsible for the control of the balance of chemicals and water in the blood are the two kidneys. The kidneys are bean-shaped structures located in back of the abdomen. Their chief functions are to filter wastes from the blood and to ensure reabsorption of essential chemicals back into the bloodstream. They also play a major role in blood pressure regulation, and they influence the production of red blood cells. In the kidneys, waste products combine with water and salts to form urine.

Urine passes from each kidney into the bladder through tubes called ureters. The bladder stores the urine prior to elimination from the body. A sphincter muscle around the exit from the bladder prevents urine from escaping. When the bladder is about half full, the body feels an urge to empty the organ. At this time, the muscle can be relaxed voluntarily to release the urine.

The urethra is a tube that conveys urine from the bladder to the exterior of the body. The female urethra is about an inch and a half long and is enclosed within the body. The male urethra passes through the penis and is approximately eight inches

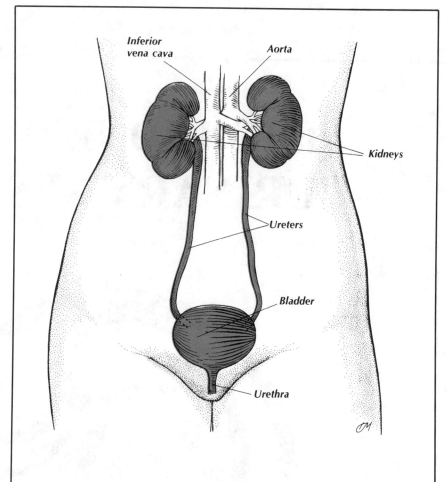

The role of the urinary system (the female urinary tract is shown here) is to cleanse the blood. Arterial blood is filtered through the kidneys and returned to the circulation. Waste products, plus excess water, are sent through the ureters to the bladder, to be excreted as urine.

long. For the male, the urethra serves the dual function of transporting urine and semen (the fluid from the male reproductive organs). Semen is released during sexual intercourse, at which time urine is blocked from leaving the bladder.

Disorders of the urinary system

Changes in urine and urinary habits that do not seem to have an obvious cause may be symptoms of disease.

Some symptoms that require medical attention are changes in

frequency, timing, and control of urination; changes in the quantity and color of urine; and the presence of pain accompanying urination. A doctor should be contacted immediately if any of the following symptoms is noted: extreme pain while urinating, blood in the urine, a noticeable increase or decrease in frequency of urination (a symptom of kidney failure), marked changes in the color of the urine, or cloudiness in the urine accompanied by pain or fever.

Changes in urine or urinary habits may be caused by a variety of disorders involving the kidneys, urinary tract, bladder, and prostate (a gland that surrounds the male urethra).

Increased frequency may be caused by inflammation of the kidneys, bladder, or urethra; diabetes mellitus; or an enlarged prostate gland.

A change in timing of urination, usually in the form of very frequent nighttime awakenings accompanied by the urge to urinate (called nocturia), is often coupled with painful urination, a poor stream, or difficulty in starting urination. These may be symptoms of an enlarged prostate gland or an inflammatory or infectious disease within the urinary tract, as well as tumors or other disorders that result in increased pressure on the bladder.

Difficulty in controlling, starting, and maintaining the flow of urine may also be symptoms of an inflammation of the prostate gland. Inability to hold back urine is a common problem of elderly people, as their control of the sphincter muscle of the bladder weakens. Also affected by this problem are women in the late stages of pregnancy, when the enlarged uterus continuously presses on the bladder.

Changes in the quantity of urine normally produced can also signal disease. Producing an excessive amount of urine (called polyuria) may be a symptom of kidney disease, diabetes, or glandular disorders. Decreased production of urine may indicate the presence of dehydration, internal hemorrhaging, or acute renal failure.

Slight changes in the color and clarity of the urine from day to day are normal, but strikingly obvious color changes and extreme cloudiness may signal infection, tumors, kidney stones, prostate problems, or other abnormalities in the urinary tract.

Pain while urinating, most commonly in the form of a burning sensation felt along the urethra, may be a sign of a lower urinary tract infection. Excruciating pain across the abdomen or the back may signal the presence of kidney stones.

Treatment of urinary problems usually involves treating the underlying cause of the change, which can range from a mild infection to a very serious disease. An accurate diagnosis by a physician is the first step to proper treatment of these disorders.

Cystitis

Cystitis is an inflammation of the urinary bladder; the term, however, is commonly used to mean bladder infection.

Causes

Cystitis is usually caused by bacteria that have invaded the urethra and entered the urinary bladder. Women are more susceptible than men because their urethras are shorter (approximately one and a half inches long, compared with about eight inches in men), thus presenting less distance for the bacteria to travel. Also, in women, the anus and the external openings of the urethra and the vagina (birth canal) are so close together that bacteria can easily migrate from one to another. Almost always the bacteria responsible are types that normally live harmlessly in the human intestine but that can cause infection if they invade the area around the opening of the urethra and enter the bladder.

Obstruction is also a common cause of urinary tract infection. When obstruction occurs, the bladder may not empty properly. The urine remaining in the bladder can then create a breeding ground for bacteria to multiply. Causes of obstruction include tumors, kidney stones, and an enlarged prostate gland.

The urethral lining may have a defect that allows bacteria to enter the urinary tract. For example, frequent intercourse may traumatize the urethra, disrupting its lining and making it more susceptible to infection.

Cystitis in men is uncommon. When it does occur, the usual cause is an infection that has spread from an inflamed prostate gland or that has developed in the bladder because of an enlarged prostate.

Urethritis, an infection or inflammation of the urethra, often sets the stage for the development of cystitis. Urethritis occurs in both men and women and is usually acquired through sexual intercourse with an infected individual. Gonorrhea and chlamydia are the two most common causes of urethritis.

Symptoms

The symptoms of cystitis include a painful sensation or burning on urination, a frequent and often urgent need to urinate (sometimes causing nighttime awakening), and, occasionally, low back pain. These symptoms, along with bloody urine, indicate hemorrhagic cystitis, which is relatively common in women. Although quite frightening, this is most often a minor, easily treatable condition when it occurs in women. However, repeated episodes or persistent bleeding, either visible or microscopic, requires further investigation. In men, however, bloody urine is not usually attributable to hem-

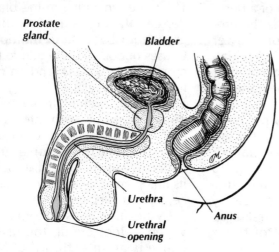

The male urethra is about eight inches long.

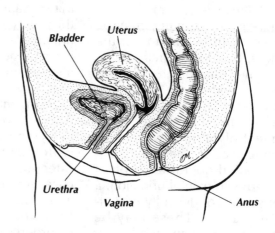

The female urethra is about an inch and a half long.

Cystitis is nearly ten times more common in women than in men. Because the female urethra is much shorter than the male urethra, infecting bacteria have a shorter distance to travel in women.

orrhagic cystitis and demands immediate investigation.

With the exception of visibly bloody urine, all of the symptoms mentioned can be present in urethritis, which is also commonly accompanied by a discharge. High fever, chills, and back pain (usually one-sided), with or without any other symptoms, usually indicate pyelonephritis (kidney infection), which demands the immediate attention of a doctor.

Diagnosis

The diagnosis rests on the urinalysis and urine culture results. The presence of moderate to large numbers of white blood cells, along with at least 100,000 colonies of any one type of bacterium, provides conclusive evidence of infection.

Not infrequently, it is difficult to determine which part of the urinary tract is infected, or if there is infection at all. In women, some white blood cells and bacteria are usually present at the opening of the urethra. Therefore, in order to keep the urine specimen free of these contaminants, a midstream specimen is usually requested. The first spurt of urine is thought to wash away the urethral contaminants, and the rest of the urine sample is then normally uncontaminated. For the vast majority of cases of simple cystitis, this procedure is adequate; however, if a question exists as to the validity of the specimen or if for some reason the specimen must be absolutely free of contaminants, a catheter (thin, flexible tube) may be inserted into the bladder through the urethra. In women, this is an easy procedure and eliminates vaginal and anal contaminants. If the catheterized specimen is free of pus and bacteria, the symptoms are the result of another condition—commonly vaginitis or urethritis. In a man, the procedure is somewhat more difficult and often not necessary. If prostatitis is the suspected cause of the infection, the physician can insert a gloved finger into the anus and feel the gland directly. A specimen of prostatic fluid is usually obtained (by massaging the gland at the time of examination) through the urethra for culture.

Appropriate treatment is dependent on correct identification of the site of infection of the urinary tract. The experience of the physician, the patient's history of signs and symptoms (such as discharge, back pain, or fever), and the findings obtained with more sophisticated diagnostic techniques are all important in making the correct diagnosis.

In difficult chronic cases of cystitis in both men and women, in which the cause of recurring infection may be an obstruction or a drainage problem, special X-ray studies are necessary; contrast material is placed in the bladder by means of a catheter, and X-ray pictures are taken of the bladder and the urethra during urination. With such studies, narrowing of a portion of the urethra, the presence of kidney stones, and incomplete emptying of the bladder (which promotes cystitis) may be detected. The bladder may also be examined through cystoscopy (examination by means of a flexible, lighted, tubelike instrument called a cystoscope, which is inserted through the urethra). Most often, these procedures are preceded by an intravenous pyelogram, in which contrast material injected through a vein is eliminated by the kidneys, providing an X-ray picture of the kidneys, ureters, and bladder.

Treatment

Treatment of first-time cystitis is usually by means of antibiotics taken by mouth. Occasionally, large single doses of drugs are used. Recurrences may be treated in the same way if they are due to a different organism. If the same organism is causing the trouble, the condition may require larger doses of medication or long-term treatment (for up to four to six weeks). If cystitis persists, daily doses of medications may be necessary for up to six months. It is important that dosage instructions be followed exactly, because a person is vulnerable to a new infection or reinfection if the entire course of recommended drug therapy is not completed.

Some individuals are prone to repeated episodes of cystitis or upper urinary tract infection. If there is an anatomic defect, such as a narrowed urethra, dilation (enlarging) of the urethra may be needed. If stones are present, they may have to be removed. If an infected prostate is the source of infection, antibiotics are usu-ally tried first; surgery is a last resort. If no obvious cause of recurrent cystitis is found, low doses of antibiotics may be prescribed for long periods of time (this is called prophylactic, or preventive, therapy).

Prevention

Women may be able to guard against recurrent cystitis by front-to-back wiping with toilet tissue and by cleansing with soap and water after each bowel movement. They should also try to urinate immediately after sexual intercourse to wash away infecting bacteria that might enter the urethra. Loose, absorbent underclothes allow evaporation and absorption of body fluids and thus help prevent infection. Both men and women should drink plenty of fluids and urinate frequently, completely emptying the bladder each time.

Dialysis

Dialysis is the removal of wastes and other undesirable substances from the blood by means of a special membrane that is selective in what it allows to cross. In the healthy body, this task is performed by the kidneys.

Hemodialysis

In a patient suffering from temporary or permanent kidney failure, cleansing of the blood can be done with an artificial kidney machine; this is known as hemodialysis. Two plastic tubes, one connected to an artery and one to a vein, are implanted in the patient's arm or leg. During dialysis, which can take three to five hours per treatment, blood from the artery tube enters the machine and comes into contact with a thin membrane. Wastes from the blood pass through the membrane into circulating fluid on the other side of the membrane. The blood cells themselves, along with other protein elements, cannot cross the membrane. The cleansed blood is then piped back into the patient through the vein tube.

Peritoneal dialysis

In peritoneal dialysis, the patient's own peritoneum (lining of the abdominal cavity) is used as the dialysis membrane. A sterile plastic catheter (tube) is passed into the abdominal cavity, and a solution of glucose (a form of sugar) and mineral salts is periodically injected into and withdrawn from the cavity. The fluid comes into contact with delicate blood vessels in the peritoneum. Because of the difference in concentration of certain chemical elements in the blood and the dialysis solution, wastes from the blood are forced through the membrane of the peritoneal wall. The dialysis liquid is periodically withdrawn and replaced with fresh solution.

Continuous ambulatory peritoneal dialysis

A new method called continuous ambulatory peritoneal dialysis has greatly lowered the cost of dialysis and made it more convenient. It can be done at home by the patient without the complex equipment and the skilled supervision that has made machine dialysis so expensive. A tube is surgically implanted in the patient, just below the navel. About every four to five hours and just before bedtime, the patient drains out the old fluid and empties a bag of fresh dialysis fluid into the abdominal cavity through a tube. The fluid remains in the cavity, soaking up wastes from the blood, while the patient sleeps or goes about his or her usual daily activities. The procedure takes only about 30 minutes each time and enables the patient to be independent and mobile.

Glomerulo-nephritis

Each kidney contains more than a million filtering units called nephrons, in which wastes are drawn from the blood to form urine. In each nephron is a network of capillaries (tiny blood vessels) called a glomerulus. Glomerulitis is an inflammation of the glomeruli (the plural of glomerulus), which interferes with the normal functioning of the kidney. First described in 1827 by the English physician Richard Bright, the condition used to be called Bright's disease, but doctors today are more likely to refer to it as glomerulonephritis (from *glomerulus*; *nephro*, referring to the kidney; and *itis*, meaning inflammation).

Causes

Glomerulonephritis can be caused by an infection in the kidneys, but most often it is due to an allergic or immune response to infections in other parts of the body. Although many different kinds of infections can lead to glomerulonephritis, including pneumonia, bacterial infection of the heart, syphilis, malaria, hepatitis, and measles,

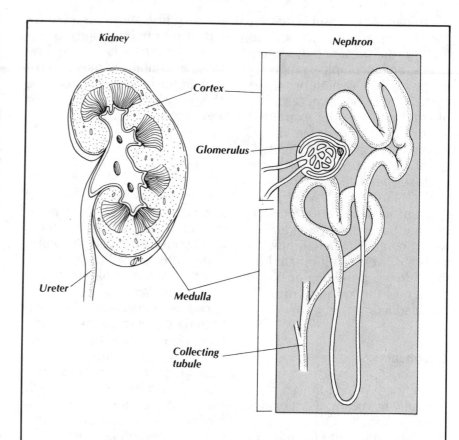

Each kidney contains more than a million filtering units called nephrons, in which wastes and excess water are drawn from the blood to form urine. In each nephron is a network of tiny blood vessels called a glomerulus. The glomeruli (plural of glomerulus) are located in the cortex (outer portion) of the kidney; their tubules lead into the medulla (central portion), from which the urine drains into the ureter.

the most common cause is infection of the throat, tonsils, or skin by certain types of *Streptococcus* bacteria. The immune response to the infection occurs as an inflammation of the capillaries in the glomeruli. The capillaries become congested and surrounded by blood cells and pus. Fluid builds up in surrounding tissues, sometimes causing the kidneys to enlarge. Protein, which should remain in the blood, is discharged into the urine through the diseased glomeruli, and there is edema (fluid buildup) in body tissues. These two signs—edema and the presence of albumin (a type of protein) in the urine—are the chief indicators of the disease.

If the disease continues to progress, the tiny arteries in the kidneys become thickened and scarred so that some can no longer carry blood. The parts of the kidneys that they serve shrink. The eventual result of this process over many years may be total kidney failure. The disease affects both kidneys.

Symptoms

Symptoms of glomerulonephritis usually begin one to three weeks after an initial infection, such as strep throat. The patient has headaches, a mild fever, a puffy face, pain in the area between the ribs and the hips, and decreased urine output. The urine may be bloody, smoky, or coffee-colored. Shortness of breath may occur, together with increased heartbeat and a rise in blood pressure. Detection of protein and red blood cells in the urine confirms the diagnosis. In extreme cases, bloating due to accumulation of fluids can cause the symptoms of heart failure, including rapid heartbeat, heart enlargement, and congestion of the lungs.

Treatment

Treatment consists of antibiotics, if strep are still present, and rest and symptomatic treatment until one to two weeks after tests of blood, blood pressure, and the urine indicate that the kidneys are back to normal. Sodium and protein may be restricted or even forbidden for a time. Fluids are restricted until the output of urine returns to normal. Heart failure is treated with restriction of salt and water and with use of oxygen and medications. Any infection is treated promptly with antibiotics. The overwhelming majority of patients with glomerulonephritis due to streptococcal infection recover fully.

Guarding against infection, injury, and fatigue can help prevent flare-ups of the disease. Intake of protein may have to be limited, depending on how well the kidneys are working. A return to normal activity is desirable, but strenuous exercise should be avoided, to prevent fatigue.

If the disease is still present after one to two years, it may be considered chronic. This occurs in 5 percent to 20 percent of patients. Typically, the damage to the kidneys continues to progress, but so slowly that the pa-

tient is without symptoms; the only evidence may be the presence of protein and red and white blood cells in the urine. A normal life may be possible for 20 or 30 years, until the kidneys can no longer function. At that time, replacement with a kidney transplant or dialysis is necessary.

There are also many other types of glomerulonephritis other than that due to strep; their treatment and prognosis vary significantly.

Incontinence

Urinary incontinence is the loss of voluntary bladder control. It occurs frequently in children and in older persons.

Causes

Most often, incontinence is caused by some underlying condition, such as obstruction, infection, or inflammation of any portion of the urinary tract. Successful treatment of the underlying cause clears up the problem of incontinence.

Stress incontinence is the leakage of urine on coughing, sneezing, straining, or laughing. This type of incontinence is common in women whose pelvic muscles have been weakened by childbirth.

Treatment

Although the first step in treating incontinence is to detect and correct any underlying problem, it is important to remember that many children do not establish complete bladder control before they are four or five years old. Children of any age may have

occasional accidents, especially if they are ill or exhausted.

Persons who have problems with incontinence can help themselves by going to the bathroom often and regularly, by arranging sleeping and living quarters near bathrooms, and by wearing clothes that can be removed quickly and easily. It may also help to keep a bedpan or urinal next to the bed and to drink only a small amount of water, if any, before going to bed.

Drugs are available to aid in controlling urination in certain conditions. Stress incontinence can usually be surgically corrected.

Kidney failure

Kidney failure occurs when certain abnormalities within the kidneys prevent them from functioning normally, leading to chemical imbalances and the buildup of toxic substances and fluid in the body. This may eventually lead to organ damage and possibly death.

Forms of kidney failure

There are two forms of kidney failure. In the acute form, there is a sudden malfunction of the kidneys, leading to a rapid buildup of toxins and fluid within the body, often within several hours. In the chronic form of kidney failure, there is a slow, progressive deterioration of kidney function, leading to a buildup of toxins and fluid, often occurring over several months or years.

Causes

Numerous conditions can cause kidney failure. High blood

pressure, kidney stones or other urinary tract blockage, adverse reactions to chemicals or drugs, serious injury, infectious disease, shock following surgery, heart attack, blood transfusion with incompatible blood, severe dehydration (excessive loss of body fluid), complications during pregnancy, immunologic disease, and congenital (existing from birth) kidney defects may all lead to kidney failure.

Symptoms

The most characteristic symptoms of kidney failure are a reduction in the volume of urine and edema (excessive accumulation of fluid in the tissues). As a result, the feet and hands and the area around the eyes may swell and become puffy. The urine may be bloody, wine-colored, or cloudy.

More generalized signs of kidney failure include drowsiness and fatigue, loss of appetite, diarrhea, nausea, dry skin, and difficulty in breathing. Delirium, coma, and death will eventually occur in untreated cases.

Diagnosis

Analysis of blood and urine samples is used to diagnose kidney failure. Urine tests may show that white blood cells, sugars, or protein have slipped through the normally efficient filtering system of the kidneys. Similarly, when the kidneys are not filtering waste materials from the blood, blood analysis will detect waste products remaining in the blood. X-ray studies, ultrasound scans (see pages 407-408) of the kidneys, or cystoscopy (see pages 404-405) may identify structural abnormalities or blockage.

Treatment

In the case of acute kidney failure, treatment begins with diagnosing and correcting the cause of the kidney damage and restoring normal kidney function as rapidly as possible. For example, shock may be treated with intravenous fluids, drugs, and, if necessary, blood transfusions; kidney stones may be removed.

Rest is essential as the kidneys recover. Limiting fluid intake, except in cases of unusual fluid loss from diarrhea or vomiting, may prevent congestive heart failure due to kidney overload. Physicians often recommend a low-protein diet due to the inability of the kidneys to process the waste products of protein metabolism.

Should these measures prove ineffective, the patient may be helped by dialysis. Dialysis is a process that cleans and filters toxic substances from the blood with an artificial kidney machine. Most dialysis patients receive treatment by traveling to the hospital three times a week. However, newer portable techniques allow more freedom for dialysis patients (see page 259).

In the case of chronic kidney failure, destruction of the kidney has progressed so much that treatment cannot bring kidney function back to normal. Treatment of these patients involves dialysis and a diet low in salt and protein. Dialysis will offer a chance to prolong life, but it is not a cure; only surgically replacing the damaged kidneys will cure the condition. In recent years, methods of matching kidney donors with recipients have improved, thereby limiting transplant rejection and serious complications. Today, transplants are a highly successful treatment for chronic kidney failure.

Kidney stones

Kidney stones are deposits of mineral or organic substances that form in the kidneys. When abnormally high levels of certain minerals, such as calcium, are in the urine, they may condense into hard masses, forming stones in the kidneys or urinary tract. The stones may be as small as a tiny pebble or as large as a walnut.

Causes

Increased levels of calcium in the urine may come from drinking large quantities of milk. Eating foods that are rich in vitamin D, which helps the body to absorb calcium, can also contribute to an overaccumulation of calcium in the body. In addition, fractured bones can release extra calcium, which may condense into stones in the kidneys.

Certain disorders encourage the buildup of mineral deposits in the kidneys. For example, gout is a joint disease that results from high blood levels of uric acid (a waste product that results from the breakdown of protein), which may crystallize into stones in the urine. Urinary infections that impede bladder function can also cause retention of urine, which then harbors higher concentrations of elements that can solidify into stones. In addition, overactive parathyroid glands (endocrine glands that regulate calcium absorption) permit increased mineral absorption into the body.

Middle-aged men and persons with gout or chronic urinary tract infections are more susceptible to the development of kidney stones. However, in many cases, it is not possible to pinpoint the cause of the kidney stones.

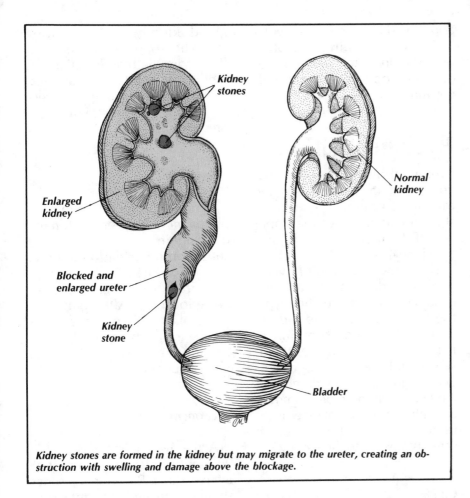

Kidney stones are formed in the kidney but may migrate to the ureter, creating an obstruction with swelling and damage above the blockage.

Symptoms

Kidney stones may be present for years and never produce any symptoms. Problems arise when a stone becomes so large that it obstructs or irritates a part of the kidney or causes problems as it passes out of the kidney. Symptoms include severe pain and tenderness over the affected kidney, frequent and painful urination, nausea, blood in the urine, fever, chills, and extreme exhaustion.

A more serious condition can develop if a stone becomes lodged in a ureter. It produces excruciating pain across the back, abdomen, and reproductive organs. If blockage occurs in the urethra, urine output decreases. The trapped urine may back up, distending and injuring the urinary tract. This situation requires immediate medical treatment.

Kidney stones that are too small to be noticed may still cause damage to delicate tissues in the urinary tract.

Diagnosis

To determine the type of kidney stone formation, a physician analyzes blood and urine samples taken from the patient. Analysis of stone fragments or the actual stone is critical in determining the exact chemical imbalance involved. An ultrasound (see pages 407-408) or X-ray study may reveal the location and nature of the stones.

Treatment

Treatment is aimed at keeping the patient well hydrated and as comfortable as possible until the stone is passed.

For kidney stones too large to pass, surgical removal may be necessary. A new, nonsurgical method of treating kidney stones called extracorporeal shock-wave lithotripsy is becoming more widely available. With this technique, tiny shock waves are pulsed into a water bath in which the anesthetized patient is placed. The shock waves are used to pulverize the stones so that they can pass out of the urinary tract. Removal of an impacted stone low in the urinary tract is frequently done through a cystoscope (a flexible, lighted, tubelike instrument). Once the cystoscope is in the bladder, a tiny guide wire attached to a basket is inserted into the ureter and withdrawn, hopefully with the stone inside.

Prevention

To prevent recurrence of kidney stones, patients need to drink a great deal of fluid to dilute their urine. Drinking large amounts of fluids, particularly at night, reduces urine concentration so that stones cannot form. Surplus water can also flush the system of any small stones. For individuals with excess calcium and/or uric acid and other minerals in their urine, medication and dietary therapy can be helpful in preventing recurrences.

Proteinuria

Excessive proteinuria (protein in the urine) can be a symptom of kidney problems.

Causes

Proteinuria can be caused by, among other conditions, kidney malfunction, heart disease, the consumption of certain foods, pregnancy, and overexertion from certain sports, such as jogging and marathon running.

Symptoms

Most cases of proteinuria in adults are discovered unexpectedly in a routine physical examination. Usually, the person will have experienced no symptoms and will be essentially healthy, with no evidence of kidney disease.

Treatment

Treatment of proteinuria depends on its cause and severity. In about half of the diagnosed cases, proteinuria ceases spontaneously within a year to several years. However, there are instances in which the patient continues to lose greater and greater amounts of protein in the urine. Eventually, high blood pressure and kidney failure may develop.

When proteinuria is constant, measurements of protein excretion should be made on a regular basis. Alteration in the protein level should be followed up with other appropriate testing of kidney function.

Pyelonephritis

Pyelonephritis is an inflammation of both the kidney tissue and the renal pelvis (the funnel-shaped expansion of the upper end of the ureter where it joins the kidney).

There are two types of pyelonephritis, descending and ascending. In the descending type, the bacteria reach the kidney through the bloodstream, infecting first the kidney tissues themselves and then moving downward to infect the renal pelvis of the kidney. In the more common ascending type, the bladder is infected first, and the infection spreads upward to the kidney.

Causes

Most cases of pyelonephritis are caused by bacterial infection. Conditions that increase the likelihood of such an infection include scars from previous infections, urinary tract infections, abnormal growth of the prostate gland, kidney stones, tumors, stagnation of urine due to backflow from the bladder, diabetes mellitus (a condition characterized by the presence of excess sugar in the bloodstream), and pregnancy.

Symptoms

Symptoms of acute pyelonephritis include fever, back pain, difficulty in urinating, a burning sensation on urination, mental confusion, nausea, vomiting, and, in extreme cases, loss of consciousness. Although some cases of chronic pyelonephritis can be traced to an initial attack, many patients have no signs of past or current infections.

Treatment

Acute pyelonephritis is treated with antibiotics given orally or intravenously. Recurrent episodes should be treated with an appropriate antibiotic. Chronic pyelonephritis requires careful management and frequent reevaluation. Patients are generally treated with an antibiotic even during periods when they feel no symptoms and usually receive long-term therapy after that.

THE ENDOCRINE SYSTEM

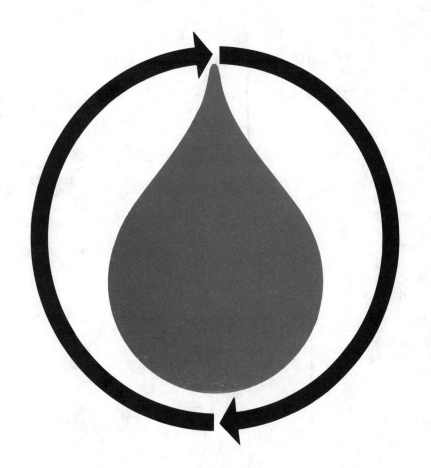

The endocrine system comprises a number of glands that produce hormones with a varied array of vital functions. Hormones are chemical substances that are secreted by organs or by cells of organs in one part of the body and are carried by the bloodstream to other organs or tissues, where they control or regulate the development or function of those structures.

Endocrine glands are also called ductless glands because they secrete hormones directly into the bloodstream. In contrast, exocrine glands release their secretions through ducts (for example, the sweat glands produce fluid that flows to the skin's surface through tiny tubelike sweat ducts).

Hormones can be considered chemical messengers. They are targeted at specific cells in the body, and their arrival in those cells causes specific activities to occur. One of the major tasks of hormones is to coordinate the activities of organ systems. For example, when a person has to run or do other physical exercise, the hormone epinephrine acts on the heart to increase its rate and force of contraction and on the blood vessels to increase blood flow to the muscles and decrease blood flow to the gastrointestinal tract (so that more blood will reach the muscles, where the need is temporarily greater). Hormones also help control the type and rate of body growth and metabolism, and they help the body maintain a consistent internal environment.

The endocrine system has a large influence on the way we feel and act. In turn, our energy and other needs in any given situation set the activity of the endocrine system. This feedback relationship is crucial in maintaining our general well-being.

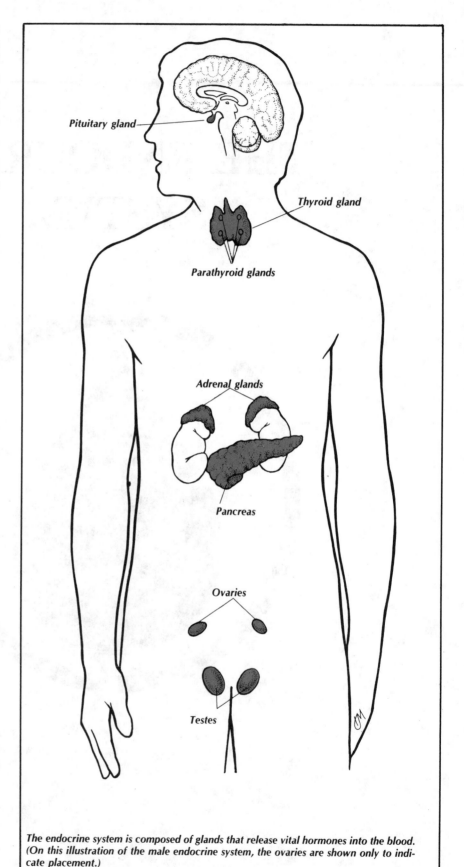

The endocrine system is composed of glands that release vital hormones into the blood. (On this illustration of the male endocrine system, the ovaries are shown only to indicate placement.)

Adrenal glands

The adrenal glands are critical to normal body functions, such as maintenance of fluid balance, reaction to stress, and reproduction. There are two adrenal glands, each of which lies above a kidney. The adrenal glands have two distinct parts: the cortex (outer layer), which secretes steroid hormones, and the medulla (inner part), which secretes epinephrine and norepinephrine. The more than 30 steroid hormones regulate a wide array of processes throughout the body. Epinephrine and norepinephrine are responsible for the changes in heart rate, blood pressure, and level of usable glucose (a form of sugar) that are necessary to cope with stress.

Pancreas

The pancreas is located in the rear center of the abdominal cavity, behind the stomach. Specialized cells in the pancreas produce two hormones, insulin and glucagon, needed to maintain stable blood sugar levels. Insulin helps cells utilize glucose for energy, reducing the amount of sugar in the bloodstream. To balance this action, the hormone glucagon stimulates the liver to release its stored sugar into the blood, raising the blood sugar levels.

The pancreas also functions in digestion. Nonendocrine cells in the pancreas produce special chemicals called enzymes, which are secreted directly into the small intestine through ducts. These enzymes help break down proteins, carbohydrates (sugars and starches), and fats in the small intestine.

This dual activity of the pancreas means that it functions as both an endocrine and an exocrine organ.

Pituitary gland

The pituitary gland is a small organ located just beneath the base of the brain, between the two frontal lobes and directly above a cavity called the sphenoid sinus. It is sometimes called the master gland because all other endocrine glands come under its control. Its job is to receive messages about the need for a particular hormone and to secrete either the hormone or substances that cause the manufacture and release of the hormone.

The anterior (front) lobe of the pituitary gland secretes somatotropin (also known as growth hormone), which affects the body's general growth; thyrotropic hormone (also known as thyroid-stimulating hormone), which acts on the thyroid gland to stimulate production of thyroid hormones; adrenocorticotropic hormone (ACTH), which stimulates the adrenal cortex; follicle-stimulating hormone and luteinizing hormone, which are necessary for maturation and release of egg and sperm cells; and prolactin, which acts on the mammary glands to promote the secretion of milk.

The posterior lobe of the pituitary gland secretes oxytocin, which stimulates smooth muscle tissue to contract and is of critical importance during childbirth, and vasopressin, which regulates kidney function with respect to water balance.

Sex glands

The primary responsibility for hormone production for the reproductive system lies with the testes (male sex glands) and ovaries (female sex glands).

The testes are two oval organs in the scrotum (the pouch of skin behind the penis). They produce sperm and sex hormones that govern the male secondary sex characteristics, such as facial hair growth.

The two ovaries are located in the pelvis. They secrete the hormones estrogen and progesterone, which govern ovulation (monthly release of an egg from an ovary) and the female secondary sex characteristics, such as breast development.

Thyroid and parathyroid glands

The thyroid gland is located at the front of the neck above the top of the breastbone. It consists of two main lobes on either side of the trachea (windpipe) that are connected by a narrow band of tissue called the isthmus. The hormones secreted by the thyroid influence the rate of metabolism (the chemical processes in the body having to do with energy production).

The four parathyroid glands are located on the back and side of each lobe of the thyroid gland. Their secretion, parathyroid hormone, controls calcium levels in the blood.

Addison's disease

Addison's disease is a condition that occurs when the adrenal cortex fails to produce enough of its hormones.

Causes

Formerly, the cause of this disease in most cases was tuberculosis or a fungal infection. However, in recent years, the disease is more likely to be idiopathic (of unknown cause). One theory is that most cases are due to autoimmune destruction of the adrenal cortex (that is, the body produces antibodies against its own tissues). Other known causes include partial destruction of the adrenal cortex by cancer, surgery, degeneration of the tissue, or deposition of a substance called amyloid. A similar condition, known as secondary adrenal insufficiency, is caused by failure of the pituitary gland to produce enough adrenocorticotropic hormone (ACTH), which stimulates the adrenal cortex to produce its hormones.

Symptoms

Early symptoms of Addison's disease are weakness, fatigue, and a tendency to become faint when rising suddenly from a bed or chair. Increased pigmentation of the skin, producing a "tan" all over the body, on exposed and unexposed areas alike, with even darker pigmentation on creases and bony pressure points, occurs in most cases. In certain places, the tan may be broken by completely white patches, known as vitiligo. Black freckles appear on the forehead, face, shoulders, and neck. There may be skin discoloration around the nipples, and the mucous membranes of the mouth may have dark-blue patches.

Symptoms that may appear later include weight loss, dehydration (excessive loss of body fluids), low blood pressure, and sometimes loss of appetite, nausea, vomiting, diarrhea, dizziness, and inability to keep warm.

The most alarming symptoms are those of a condition called adrenal crisis, which requires immediate attention and hospitalization. Signs of this are extreme weakness; severe pains in the lower back, abdomen, or legs; shock (collapse of the circulatory system); and renal shutdown (kidney failure). Such a crisis may be brought on by severe stress, such as infection, injury, or surgery, or by a loss of salt through perspiration during hot weather.

Diagnosis

One laboratory sign of Addison's disease is a high level of ACTH but a low level of cortisol (one of the adrenal gland hormones) in the blood. This indicates that the pituitary gland is working overtime, stimulating the adrenal cortex with ACTH to produce cortisol, but that the cortex is failing to produce it.

Treatment

The basic treatment for Addison's disease is to provide steroid hormones, principally cortisone, to replace those not being produced by the adrenal cortex. An additional steroid drug may be prescribed to promote retention of salt, and thereby water, in tissues and blood, so that the low blood pressure of severe Addison's disease can be avoided.

The outlook for patients receiving hormone treatment is excellent. Continued medical supervision is necessary to prevent emergencies caused by a sudden withdrawal of treatment or by an increased need for hormones because of infection, injury, surgery, pregnancy, or other stress on the body. It is important to avoid infection and to treat infection that develops as soon as possible. At all times, patients should carry a card or wear a bracelet describing the condition and the need for cortisone. It is also critical to take the medication exactly as prescribed and to be monitored by a physician who can increase or decrease the dosage as the need arises. With proper care, a person with Addison's disease can lead a nearly normal life.

Corticosteroids

Corticosteroids are hormones produced in the cortex of the adrenal glands in response to stimulation by adrenocorticotropic hormone (ACTH), which is secreted by the pituitary gland. There are more than 30 corticosteroids, which regulate essential processes throughout the body. They are divided into three groups: mineralocorticoids, glucocorticoids, and androgens (male sex hormones).

Natural forms

Mineralocorticoids are involved in maintaining salt and water balance in the body. Without these hormones, the tissues and blood would become depleted of salt and water; the resultant decrease in blood volume would cause a drop in blood pressure that could lead to shock (collapse of the circulatory system).

Glucocorticoids help regulate the body's use and reserves of sugars and proteins, among other complex metabolic processes. They also participate in the inflammatory response and the body's reaction to stress. The most important of these hormones is cortisol, which plays a major role in protein breakdown and formation, blood sugar control, and reduction of inflammation. Cortisol is also necessary to mount an effective response against severe stress due to disease or injury.

Androgens (which are also produced in the testes) stimulate the development of the male secondary sex characteristics, such as beard growth and increased muscle mass.

Drug forms

Pharmacologic preparations of both ACTH and corticosteroids are used to treat disease in the same way that the natural hormones would or as substitute or supplemental hormones for patients who have lost the ability to manufacture their own. The primary difference is that ACTH acts less directly and more generally than corticosteroid drugs. ACTH stimulates the adrenal glands to enlarge and secrete more of all the steroids that they produce, rather than any one specific hormone. Corticosteroid drugs can be administered to the part of the body that needs them most. For example, a dab of hydrocortisone cream will eliminate a rash, and a hydrocortisone injection will diminish the swelling of a painful knee joint, generally with little effect on the rest of the body. Sometimes, however, corticosteroids are considered for generalized use throughout the body. Corticosteroids have an advantage over ACTH in that they can be taken by mouth and may be given in doses that far exceed what the adrenal glands can naturally produce. ACTH must be injected because it would otherwise be destroyed by digestive enzymes; these enzymes, however, do not affect the corticosteroids.

Cushing's syndrome

Cushing's syndrome is a group of abnormalities resulting from an excess of the hormones produced by the cortex of the adrenal glands. The hormones produced in excess are chiefly cortisol, which has many complex functions; various hormones that regulate the body's use of sugars and proteins; male sex hormones; and a hormone that controls the distribution of fluids and salts in the body.

Causes

In most cases, Cushing's syndrome is caused by excess production of adrenocorticotropic hormone (ACTH), which is normally manufactured by the pituitary gland to stimulate production of hormones by the adrenal glands. This excess of ACTH can be caused by an ACTH-producing tumor in another organ, such as the lung or pancreas; by overmedication with ACTH or corticosteroid drugs; by tiny, nonmalignant ACTH-producing tumors on the pituitary gland; or by a tumor (usually nonmalignant) on the adrenal gland. The effect of too much ACTH, for whatever reason, is overgrowth of tissue in the adrenal cortex, resulting in overproduction of all its hormones. Since these hormones regulate essential processes throughout the body, excess production causes widespread disorders.

Symptoms

One of the most obvious signs of Cushing's syndrome is the moon-shaped face, caused by

excess fluid in the tissues. Because of deposition of excess fat, the trunk of the body is obese (although the arms and legs are thin), and there are fat pads over the shoulders and neck, producing a "buffalo hump." Purple "stretch marks" on the skin (usually of the abdomen), poor wound healing, easy bruising, muscle weakness, fractures in weakened bones, and emotional instability may also be part of the syndrome. Hairiness, acne, and decreased or absent menstruation may occur in women, due to the increase in male hormones. Diabetes and high blood pressure are also very common.

Diagnosis

Diagnosis of Cushing's syndrome requires measurement of adrenal cortex hormones in the blood and urine. In normal persons, cortisol levels in the blood are high on awakening but decrease during the day; in the person with Cushing's syndrome, cortisol levels are high all of the time. Various tests can determine whether the cause of the syndrome is a tumor of the pituitary gland (in which case the disorder is known as Cushing's disease) or a tumor on the adrenal gland or elsewhere. Tumors on the adrenal glands may be identified by X rays, ultrasound studies (see pages 407-408), and computed tomography (see page 407), or CT scans. CT scans and other special X rays of the head can also often locate tumors of the pituitary gland.

Treatment

Cushing's syndrome is treated by restoring a normal balance of hormones. This may involve surgery, radiation treatments, or drugs. Tumors on the adrenal glands are removed by surgery. If there is a tumor on just one adrenal gland, the other gland usually shrinks and ceases normal productivity. Hormone supplements are usually given before surgery and must be taken for weeks or months after surgery until the second gland recovers normal function. In a rapidly worsening case of Cushing's syndrome in which the cortex is greatly enlarged on both sides, one treatment is to remove both adrenal glands. This is usually a last-resort measure, however; more commonly, another method, such as chemotherapy (drug treatments), radiation treatments of the pituitary gland (to weaken it and lower its output of ACTH), or removal of any adenomas (nonmalignant growths) on the pituitary gland, is tried first. If other measures fail, the adrenal glands are removed, and the patient must take daily supplements of adrenal cortex hormones for the rest of his or her life.

If Cushing's syndrome is being caused by production of ACTH by a cancerous tumor in a part of the body other than the adrenal glands, the cancer is removed, if possible. However, in many cases it is inoperable, so drugs to suppress production of the adrenal glands are given.

Cushing's syndrome is a very serious, possibly fatal, disease unless it is detected and treated early. The outlook is best for those whose condition is caused by noncancerous growths and who receive early treatment.

Those who must take replacement hormones after treatment should carry a medical identification card and immediately tell their doctor about any infections, injuries, or stressful situations that might require an increase in hormone dosage. They should also report signs of underdosage, such as weakness, dizziness, or fatigue, as well as signs of overdosage, such as swollen tissues and rapid weight gain. Anyone whose adrenal glands have been removed must always take replacement hormones; stopping these medications for any length of time is fatal.

Diabetes mellitus

Diabetes mellitus, often called sugar diabetes, is a condition in which the body is unable to properly process carbohydrates (sugars and starches), which are the body's major source of energy.

Cause

Normally, digestion causes carbohydrates to release a form of sugar called glucose into the blood. As the blood glucose level rises, the pancreas is stimulated to secrete the hormone insulin. Insulin acts to reduce the sugar content in the blood by transporting glucose from the blood to body cells, where it is used for fuel, or to the liver, where it is stored until needed for fuel.

When the pancreas produces insufficient insulin or the body cannot use the insulin it manufactures, diabetes results. The glucose concentration in the blood increases because glucose circulates throughout the body

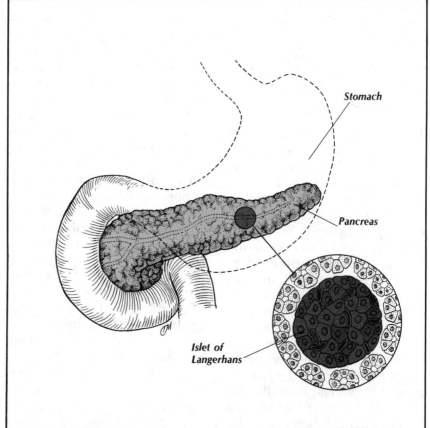

The islets of Langerhans in the pancreas secrete insulin, the hormone that helps the cells utilize sugar as fuel. One type of diabetes results from a defect in the islets of Langerhans, which causes decreased production of insulin.

without being absorbed. Eventually, the kidneys filter glucose from the blood, and urine carries the excess sugar from the body.

Types

There are two major forms of diabetes. Type I (or insulin-dependent) diabetes results from a defect of unknown origin in the islets of Langerhans (the areas in the pancreas where insulin is produced). This form of diabetes can develop in young children.

With Type II (or non-insulin-dependent) diabetes, either the pancreas functions inadequately or the body is unable to use insulin efficiently. Sometimes, a shortage of insulin-receptor cells (sites throughout the body where the interaction of glucose and insulin occurs) allows the insulin to be present in the bloodstream without working properly. Obesity often contributes to the problem because the presence of excess fat cells leads to increased resistance to insulin. Type II diabetes, which appears most often in adults over the age of 40, may evolve from a gradual slowing of insulin production within the pancreas. In addition, other disorders of the endocrine system may cause hormonal imbalances that disturb glucose regulation.

Research shows that people who have a family history of Type II diabetes may have a greater tendency to acquire the condition. Women are more likely to be affected, but for all adults, the risk of developing Type II diabetes doubles with every decade after the age of 40.

In some women, pregnancy triggers diabetes. The condition usually subsides after childbirth. However, women who show signs of diabetes during pregnancy and deliver babies weighing over ten pounds have a greater risk of diabetes later in life.

Complications

Although patients with diabetes can usually control the condition, untreated diabetes can lead to serious complications. Extremely high blood sugar levels place great strain on other organs. Diabetes may accelerate atherosclerosis (clogging of the arteries). Insufficient blood supply contributes to heart attack, stroke, kidney disease, eye disorders, impotence, gangrene (death of tissue due to inadequate blood circulation), and even death.

Symptoms

Symptoms of Type I diabetes are excessive thirst and urination, fatigue, altered vision, fainting, irritability, and slow healing of cuts and bruises. Weight loss may occur despite constant hunger and voracious eating.

The same symptoms may signal Type II diabetes, or no symptoms may appear at all. Physicians frequently detect this form when they perform routine examinations or tests for other problems.

Diagnosis

Doctors can diagnose diabetes by analyzing blood samples for elevated sugar concentrations. They may also test blood and urine for excess ketones, the chemical by-products of the breakdown of fat for energy. Since people with diabetes do not use glucose normally, their bodies burn fat for fuel, and as a result, ketones are eliminated in the urine.

Treatment

Both forms of diabetes mellitus require a treatment plan that maintains normal, steady blood glucose levels. Once blood sugar levels have been brought under control with insulin injections, diet, or medication, a person with diabetes can usually lead a nearly normal life.

Type I diabetes requires injections of insulin to maintain blood sugar levels evenly all day. If the blood glucose concentration rises, imbalance may be signalled by weakness, fatigue, and thirst. These symptoms mean that more insulin is needed. However, if blood glucose concentration falls too low, an insulin reaction sets in, causing dizziness, hunger, fatigue, headache, sweating, trembling, and (in severe cases) unconsciousness. A quick remedy for this problem is to give the person simple sugar, such as is found in orange juice and some kinds of candy. This should be done only if the person is conscious and alert, however; nothing should be given by mouth to an unconscious or semiconscious person, because of the risk of choking.

Ideally, a doctor can prevent these fluctuations of sugar levels by coordinating the type and timing of insulin injections with meal content and energy output. A special diet is important to balance daily insulin injections. Young children with diabetes, in particular, need sufficient calories to grow and develop normally. Insulin requirements for persons with Type I diabetes differ greatly. Some patients may maintain balanced blood sugar levels with one insulin injection taken before breakfast. Other patients may require several insulin injections per day. Insulin requirements may change as the patient grows older, undergoes surgery, becomes pregnant, or develops an unrelated illness.

Many people with Type II diabetes can regulate their condition with proper diet. Sometimes, oral antidiabetic drugs, which work by stimulating the pancreas to produce more insulin and/or stimulating insulin receptors, may be prescribed.

Special attention to diet is critical for diabetes control. Overweight individuals need to lose weight. Thereafter, emphasis is on eating balanced meals that will sustain the recommended weight. Fats need to be limited to reduce susceptibility to atherosclerosis, and the diet should be low in simple sugars. The diet should include plenty of fibrous roughage, such as is contained in fruits, vegetables, and whole grains; fiber in the diet has been shown to reduce or slow sugar absorption in the digestive tract. A doctor can provide a medically approved diet plan, with enough flexibility to allow the diabetic patient to share in regular family meals while meeting his or her special dietary needs.

With either type of diabetes, follow-up is important to plan diet, determine changes in insulin dosage (in Type I), and monitor blood for sugar levels. Testing urine for sugar has been shown to be inaccurate, and the availability of home blood glucose monitoring has all but replaced urine sugar testing for most diabetic patients. Urine ketone testing, however, is still important. It has been shown in recent years that meticulous control of blood glucose levels can delay or prevent many of the complications of diabetes mellitus. Therefore, strict adherence to the regimen prescribed by the physician is of major importance.

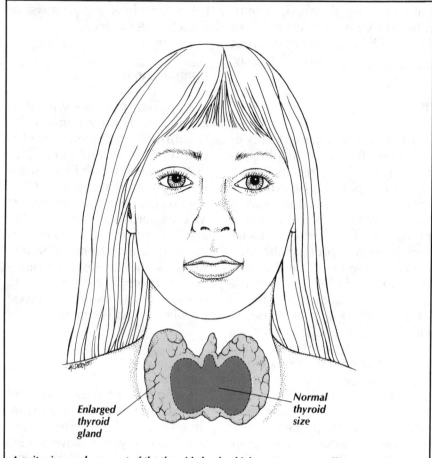

A goiter is an enlargement of the thyroid gland, which appears as a swelling at the front of the neck.

Enlarged thyroid gland

Normal thyroid size

Goiter

A goiter is an enlargement of the thyroid gland, which appears as a swelling at the front of the neck.

Causes

Goiter may be caused by a lack of dietary iodine, which is necessary for the production of thyroid hormone. In this case, the thyroid gland enlarges in an attempt to satisfy the body's demand for more hormone. The cells in the gland enlarge but do not increase in number.

At one time, goiter was common in areas where there is a lack of iodine in the soil and water. Since the ocean is the basic source of iodine, inland areas were the most deficient (in the United States, the Great Lakes region was such an area; in Europe, inland regions in the Alps were affected). In recent times, however, the use of iodized table salt has largely solved this problem.

Some forms of goiter are associated with an overactive thyroid gland, (one that produces more hormone than the body needs).

Symptoms

Often, the only symptom is the swelling in the neck. If the

thyroid is active, nervousness, weight loss, bulging eyes, rapid heartbeat, and high blood pressure may be noted. If the thyroid is underactive, sluggishness, weight gain, dry skin and hair, and fatigue may be present.

Diagnosis

The diagnosis is made primarily on the basis of the classic appearance and the dietary history of the patient. Blood tests to determine the concentration of thyroid hormones and a nuclear medicine study (see pages 406-407) of the thyroid may be performed to rule out more serious thyroid disorders.

Treatment

The chief objective of goiter treatment is reduction of the swelling. The first step is usually to suppress the overfunctioning of the thyroid gland. If the goiter is caused by simple iodine deficiency, small doses of iodine can be given. Sometimes, administering synthetic thyroid hormone, in an attempt to halt the increased efforts by the gland to produce the natural hormone, will reduce the enlargement. If treatment is started early enough, surgery to remove portions of the enlarged gland can be avoided. Surgery may be necessary if the size of the goiter interferes with normal breathing by pressing on the windpipe.

Hirsutism

Hirsutism is excessive hair growth or hair growth in areas that are not usually hairy. In general, this condition is due to a hormonal imbalance.

Causes

Some degree of hirsutism is present in about 30 percent of women, and it may be a symptom of some other disorder. Family and racial tendencies, however, account for a large percentage of cases of hirsutism in women. Many cases have no known cause. It is thought, though, that hirsute women may have hair follicles that are hypersensitive to normal female androgen levels. (Androgen is a male sex hormone, but it is normally present to a lesser extent in women as well.)

In some cases, hirsutism is only one sign of virilization (masculinization), which is characterized by acne, balding, and increased muscle mass, as well as by hirsutism. This condition may be due to overactive adrenal glands (which secrete some sex hormones), ovarian tumors, adrenal tumors, or use of steroid medications. However, the majority of hirsute women are not masculinized.

A common cause of hirsutism is polycystic ovaries; in this condition, the presence of numerous cysts on the ovaries leads to infrequent menstruation or absence of menstruation, absence of ovulation, obesity, and enlarged ovaries. Hirsutism is also seen in Cushing's syndrome, a condition that in women is characterized by excessive fat tissue in the face, neck, and trunk; absence of menstruation; convex (outward) curvature of the spine; high blood pressure; and muscular weakness. Mild hirsutism also appears in young girls with underactive thyroid glands. Absence of or damage to the pituitary gland, anorexia nervosa (self-inflicted starvation), and use of some drugs can also cause hirsutism.

Symptoms

The only symptom of hirsutism is excessive growth of hair in men or women or growth of hair in normally hairless areas in women (for example, on the face, neck, breasts, chest, and abdomen). The hair may be soft and fine or coarse, depending on many factors.

Diagnosis

Diagnosis is usually confirmed through visual examination and medical history.

Treatment

The treatment of hirsutism is based on removing the cause. For example, adrenal hyperplasia (an abnormal increase in the number of cells in the adrenal gland) can be suppressed by corticosteroid drugs. Patients with polycystic ovaries can be treated with low-dose estrogen birth control pills or with other drugs.

Removing the cause does not always diminish the hair growth, however, and hair removal may be desired for cosmetic reasons. The only safe, permanent local treatment is electrolysis (destruction of individual hair follicles with an electric current). Other measures, such as plucking, shaving, waxing, or using a depilatory chemical, will mask the problem temporarily.

Prevention

Other than prompt diagnosis and treatment of the primary cause or underlying disorder (provided there is one), there are no known preventive measures against hirsutism.

Hyperthyroidism

Hyperthyroidism is a general term that encompasses several different disorders with the common feature of excessive production of thyroid hormone. The two most common forms of hyperthyroidism are Graves' disease and toxic multinodular goiter.

Causes

The production of thyroid hormone is normally regulated by the pituitary gland, which secretes thyroid-stimulating hormone (TSH) when a need for thyroid hormone is present and decreases secretion of TSH when it senses an adequate supply of the hormone. Generally speaking, some malfunction occurs in hyperthyroidism, and the thyroid is no longer sensitive to this regulatory mechanism. Graves' disease is probably due to the presence of an abnormal chemical stimulator of thyroid hormone production. In toxic multinodular goiter, nodules (lumplike clusters) of thyroid tissue form, for reasons that have yet to be determined, and secrete abnormally large amounts of thyroid hormone, independent of the amount of hormone in the body.

Symptoms

Because thyroid hormone is involved in so many vital processes throughout the body, including maintenance of body temperature, conversion of food to energy, and regulation of growth and fertility, the effects of an excess of that hormone are many and varied. The symptoms common to all forms of hyperthyroidism include rapid heartbeat, weight loss despite increased appetite and food intake, generalized hyperactivity, tremors (shakiness), increased sweating, severe nervousness and emotional instability, alterations of menstruation and fertility, and muscle weakness.

In addition to these symptoms, patients with Graves' disease often have bulging eyes. Their skin is characteristically warm, moist, and velvety, and there may be areas of raised, thickened, sometimes itchy skin with the texture of orange peel on the legs and feet. The thyroid gland is frequently enlarged, smooth, and soft. This disease occurs most often in those in their 30s and 40s. It is more common in women than in men.

In toxic multinodular goiter, the thyroid gland is lumpy but not uniformly enlarged. This condition occurs most often in the middle-aged and elderly.

Diagnosis

The diagnosis of hyperthyroidism is made on the basis of the history and findings from a physical examination and various laboratory studies. Significant elevation of the level of thyroid hormone in the blood can be detected with special blood tests. The diagnosis can be further established through the use of nuclear medicine scans obtained after the injection of radioactive iodine, which becomes concentrated in the thyroid gland. The nuclear medicine study yields not only a picture of the gland, but also an estimate of the degree of hyperactivity.

Treatment

Specific treatment of hyperthyroidism depends on which condition is present. However, treatment of the hyperthyroid state in general has several common elements. The drug propranolol, a beta blocker, is commonly used to block the effects of the hormonal overstimulation that greatly contributes to the tremors, increased heart rate, and sweating. This drug, although it diminishes symptoms, does not get at the root problem of too much thyroid hormone. To decrease the amount of thyroid hormone being produced, an antithyroid drug, such as propylthiouracil, is used. Antithyroid drugs actually interfere with the production of thyroid hormone. However, this is only a temporary solution; when the drug is stopped, the excess production usually resumes. The definitive therapy for hyperthyroidism is the destruction or removal of most or all of the gland using radioactive iodine or surgery.

Graves's disease is usually first treated by blocking hormonal overstimulation with propranolol. Simultaneously, an antithyroid drug is started. This drug may be maintained for several years. If relapse occurs (which it frequently does) or if the level of thyroid hormone is not normalized, the question then is how to reduce the amount of thyroid tissue. Whether surgery or radioactive iodine is used depends on many complex factors. Both treatments frequently result in too little thyroid hormone in the blood, but this problem is easily remedied by supplementation with synthetic thyroid hormone.

The treatment of toxic multinodular goiter is less controversial than that for Grave's disease. In addition to a beta blocker and, frequently, an antithyroid drug, radioactive iodine is generally the therapy of choice.

Hypoglycemia

Hypoglycemia is the state of having an abnormally low blood glucose level. (Glucose is a sugar released into the blood as a result of digestion of carbohydrates.)

The two main forms of this condition are reactive hypoglycemia and fasting hypoglycemia. To understand how both forms occur, it is helpful to understand how glucose utilization is normally regulated.

During digestion, elevated blood glucose levels trigger the secretion of the hormone insulin from the pancreas. Insulin acts to reduce the sugar level in the blood by helping body cells absorb the glucose for fuel.

Reactive hypoglycemia

Reactive hypoglycemia is caused by oversecretion of insulin and consequent rapid lowering of blood glucose levels in response to ingestion of glucose. Reactive hypoglycemia is also known as postprandial (after meals) hypoglycemia because it occurs only in response to ingestion of food.

The specific causes of reactive hypoglycemia are unknown in most cases. However, certain persons—for example, those in the early stage of adult-onset diabetes mellitus and patients who have had part or most of the stomach removed surgically—are particularly susceptible to reactive hypoglycemia.

Fasting hypoglycemia

Fasting hypoglycemia is caused by insufficient production of glucose or overutilization of the glucose present in the blood.

Often, these two factors combine to severely depress the blood glucose level. An insulin-producing tumor on the pancreas can also cause fasting hypoglycemia. Because alcohol disturbs the normal mechanisms of sugar storage and release within the liver, heavy drinkers are at greater risk of developing the disorder. Fasting hypoglycemia can also occur in anyone who has not eaten for an unusually long interval, but this is a temporary situation. Chronic (long-term) hypoglycemia is uncommon.

Symptoms

The symptoms of both types of hypoglycemia include fatigue, nervousness, perspiration, dizziness, headache, hunger pangs, visual impairment, and accelerated heartbeat. The condition may also cause anxiety, difficulty in concentrating, confusion, and blackouts. If sugar deprivation continues unchecked, severe hypoglycemia may produce convulsions (short-term loss of consciousness, accompanied by jerking muscle movements) or deep coma (prolonged loss of consciousness).

True hypoglycemia is an uncommon condition. Since many of the symptoms of anxiety and hypoglycemia are alike, the two conditions are often confused with one another.

Diagnosis

To diagnose hypoglycemia, a doctor analyzes a blood sample to detect abnormally low sugar levels. Blood drawn during an attack of the condition allows the most accurate assessment, since symptoms can then be correlated with actual blood glucose levels.

Treatment

Treatment for hypoglycemia is often aimed at the underlying cause of the disease. For example, surgical removal of a pancreatic tumor or adjustment of a diabetic patient's insulin dosage may be necessary. In most cases of reactive hypoglycemia, however, there is no known cure for the tendency of the pancreas to overproduce insulin when it is not needed. The most effective treatment is to avoid all foods that generate attacks.

A good diet for a patient who is susceptible to episodes of hypoglycemia is one that is low enough in sugar and starches to moderate the reaction of the pancreas to sugar intake and rich enough in protein to help maintain gradual elevations of blood sugar. Eating several smaller meals a day, rather than three large meals, may help to keep blood sugar levels stable.

Hypothyroidism

Hypothyroidism is a disorder in which an underactive thyroid gland produces too little thyroid hormone.

Causes

Hypothyroidism can result from chronic (long-term) thyroid inflammation or a deficiency of thyroid-stimulating hormone, which is secreted by the pituitary gland. Autoimmune disorders (in which the immune system destroys the body's own tissues) are also a common cause of hypothyroidism. In addition, heredity may play a role in the development of the condition. Women seem more prone to thyroid disorders, and in some women, pregnancy triggers the hormonal imbalance. Hypothyroidism can also develop after suppression or partial removal of the thyroid gland as treatment for hyperthyroidism (a condition that results when an overactive thyroid gland produces too much thyroid hormone).

Symptoms

Because thyroid hormone influences every tissue in the body (for example, by participating in maintenance of body temperature, conversion of food to energy, and regulation of growth and fertility), the effects of having too little of the hormone are many and varied. People with hypothyroidism may be overweight, easily exhausted, and subject to recurrent infection. They may also experience menstrual disorders, be intolerant of cold, have dry skin and hair, exhibit puffiness of the hands and face, and suffer depression.

Diagnosis

The diagnosis of hypothyroidism is based on laboratory tests of the blood. Determination of levels of thyroid and pituitary hormones is fundamental. Cardiac enzymes and cholesterol may also be measured. A special nuclear medicine study, which is an X ray taken after the injection of a radioactive isotope, may be performed.

Chronic hypothyroidism may cause signs of reduced general body functioning. Anemia (deficiency of red blood cells) may result from diminished function of the bone marrow, where red blood cells are formed. Heart rate may decrease, and reflexes may become sluggish. An elec-

troencephalogram (see page 403) may reveal irregular patterns. Evaluation of growth patterns often provides the first clue to the diagnosis in children.

Treatment

Since hypothyroidism develops from a shortage of thyroid hormone, the most effective treatment is generally thyroid hormone supplementation. Supplements are either natural hormones extracted from the thyroid glands of animals or synthetic hormones. Both types control the problem, but the newer, synthetic forms are much more efficient and their effects are more easily regulated. Although treatment provides the necessary hormone control, hypothyroidism often continues throughout life, and the patient may require lifelong follow-up to monitor treatment.

Contrary to popular belief, the correction of hypothyroidism will not cause an obese person to lose a significant amount of weight.

Ketosis

Ketosis is an abnormal condition that occurs when the body burns fat instead of glucose (the form of sugar that is the body's chief source of energy) and, as a result, produces more of the chemical substances called ketones than is normal.

Causes

Ketones are the by-product of the chemical process that occurs in the cells when fat is broken down to produce energy. Under normal circumstances, ketones

are broken down into carbon dioxide and water by the liver and other organs. In ketosis, the body is producing more ketones than it can process. The buildup of ketones disrupts the chemical balance of the body; if left unchecked, it can be fatal.

Ketosis occurs most often in persons with insulin-dependent diabetes mellitus, a disorder in which the pancreas produces little or no insulin (a hormone secreted into the bloodstream to regulate glucose levels). This deficiency prevents the body from absorbing enough glucose and forces it to obtain its energy by burning fat. If ketosis is allowed to progress in a diabetic patient, a condition called diabetic ketoacidosis may occur. This is a life-threatening disorder that involves severe dehydration (excessive loss of body fluids) and coma.

Ketosis is also a consequence of starvation (and the self-induced starvation of excessive dieting), in which the body must rely on stores of fat for energy. Ketosis or ketoacidosis can also occur with heavy, long-term intake of alcohol.

Symptoms

The most common symptoms are a slightly sweet breath odor (similar to the smell of acetone or nail-polish remover), extreme dryness of the mucous membrane, weight loss, increased thirst and urination, weakness, abdominal pains, generalized aches, nausea and vomiting, and breathlessness.

Diagnosis

Ketosis is diagnosed by testing the glucose and ketone levels in blood or urine. The urine test is less accurate.

Treatment

In insulin-dependent diabetics, administration of insulin corrects diabetic ketoacidosis. Diabetics are especially susceptible to ketosis before their condition is diagnosed, while they are fighting an infection, or when they neglect their diet or medication. Treatment of ketosis caused by starvation consists of feeding the patient substances that contain sugar or administering glucose solution intravenously. Alcoholic ketoacidosis is treated the same as that caused by starvation, usually with vitamins added.

Pituitary disorders

Because of the vital role of the pituitary gland in regulating many body functions, disorders of this gland (often due to tumors) can result in disastrous abnormalities in growth and body maintenance.

Persons who have excessive secretion of growth hormone by the anterior lobe during the years in which the skeleton is growing

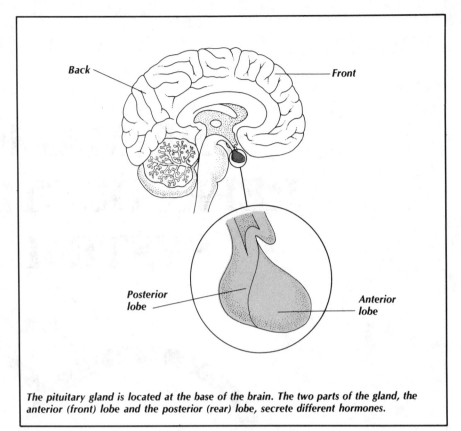

Back   Front

Posterior lobe   Anterior lobe

The pituitary gland is located at the base of the brain. The two parts of the gland, the anterior (front) lobe and the posterior (rear) lobe, secrete different hormones.

become giants; those who have deficient secretion at that time become dwarfs. If oversecretion occurs after a person has become an adult, a condition called acromegaly results, in which the victim's hands, feet, jaws, and facial bones grow disproportionately large.

A condition known as diabetes insipidus (which is related only symptomatically to the more common diabetes mellitus) is due to a malfunction of the posterior lobe of the pituitary gland. In this disorder, a deficiency of the pituitary hormone vasopressin results in abnormally high urinary output of water. Control can be regained with the use of synthetic vasopressin to inhibit excessive water release.

THE MALE REPRODUCTIVE SYSTEM

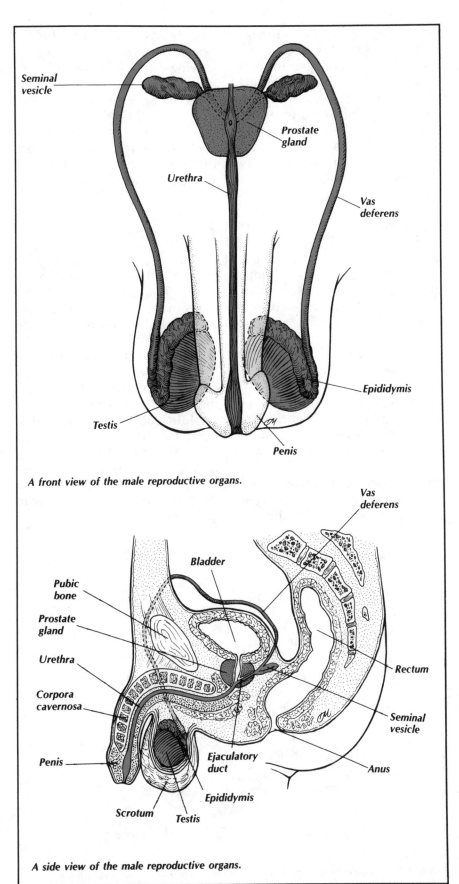

Seminal vesicle

Prostate gland

Urethra

Vas deferens

Epididymis

Testis

Penis

A front view of the male reproductive organs.

Vas deferens

Bladder

Pubic bone

Prostate gland

Urethra

Corpora cavernosa

Penis

Ejaculatory duct

Epididymis

Scrotum

Testis

Rectum

Seminal vesicle

Anus

A side view of the male reproductive organs.

The male reproductive system consists of those structures in the male body designed to create life. The system includes the two testes, a network of ducts, the seminal vesicles, the prostate gland, and the penis.

The testes are two oval glands located in the scrotum (the pouch of skin that hangs behind the penis). They produce the male sex hormone testosterone and sperm (male reproductive cells). Sex hormones control the secondary male sex characteristics (such as growth of the penis and of body hair, voice change, and increased muscle mass), which begin to appear at puberty.

The testes discharge sperm into the epididymis, the first structure in the duct system. Other passageways include the two vasa deferentia (the plural of vas deferens), the ejaculatory duct, and the urethra (the tube that connects the bladder to the outside of the body).

The epididymis runs along the top and side of each testis. Inside the epididymis are several ducts that conduct sperm from the testis into the vas deferens. The vas deferens loops up into the body before descending into a duct in the seminal vesicle. This duct joins the ejaculatory duct, which extends through the prostate gland and enters the upper segment of the urethra. At different times, the urethra functions as a passageway for urine and for sperm.

As sperm travel through the duct system, they combine with fluids from the seminal vesicles, the prostate gland, and the urethra to form semen. The two seminal vesicles, which lie near the underside of the urinary bladder, discharge a thick, sticky fluid. The prostate gland is a small, doughnut-shaped organ that completely surrounds the urethra. The prostate gland secretes an alkaline substance that makes up the major portion of seminal fluid. The sperm are protected from acid (present both in the male urethra and in the vagina) by the alkalinity of the prostatic secretions. Sperm are also capable of the greatest mobility when in a slightly alkaline medium. Proper prostate secretion is thus essential to effective sperm action.

The penis is the external organ that propels sperm into the female during sexual intercourse. During sexual excitement, the corpora cavernosa (large internal spaces within the penis) become filled with blood, making the penis rigid enough to enter the vagina (the entryway to the female reproductive tract). The semen, which is formed in the urethra, then travels out of the penis during ejaculation (sudden discharge of fluid).

Gynecomastia

Gynecomastia is excessive development of the breasts in a male. Breast enlargement is a normal, short-term occurrence in some newborn boys, whose breasts enlarge in response to female hormones they receive from their mother during pregnancy. The condition may also appear at puberty, when a boy's body is undergoing normal hormonal changes.

Causes

In most cases, gynecomastia is the result of too much estrogen (a female sex hormone) in the male's body. Breast enlargement at birth and at puberty usually occurs because the estrogen

level has not yet adjusted to normal (both females and males normally have estrogen in their bodies). Abnormal gynecomastia occurs when some condition, such as a tumor of one of the testes or an estrogen-secreting tumor of one of the adrenal glands, results in abnormally high levels of estrogen.

Symptoms

In addition to the obvious enlargement of the breasts, symptoms may include tenderness in the breasts and, in extreme cases, secretion of milk.

Treatment

Gynecomastia should always be brought to the attention of a doctor. It is especially important that tumors of the adrenal glands or testes be ruled out or treated. Such tumors are usually removed surgically. In severe or prolonged cases of gynecomastia, the excess breast tissue can be removed through plastic surgery, leaving little visible scarring. In most cases, patients can be reassured that the condition is both normal and temporary. Especially in need of such reassurance are teenage boys, who are often embarrassed and fearful that they are abnormal.

Hydrocele

A hydrocele is an abnormal collection of fluid around a testis, which is noticeable as a soft mass in the scrotum. The term hydrocele literally means a sac of water.

There is normally a double-layered covering around each testis. Within these two layers there is usually just enough fluid for lubrication. Occasionally, however, the amount of fluid is increased, causing the swelling around the testis. As a rule, hydroceles are harmless. They are relatively common, especially in older men.

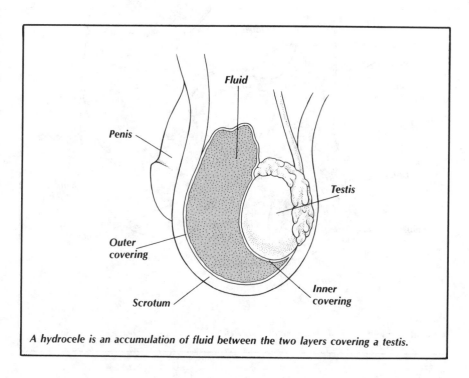

A hydrocele is an accumulation of fluid between the two layers covering a testis.

Causes

If the hydrocele is caused by an injury or inflammation in the scrotum, it is called a secondary hydrocele. If there is no apparent cause, it is called a primary hydrocele.

Symptoms

The most obvious symptom is the swelling. Although hydroceles are usually painless, pain may also be present.

Treatment

A small, painless hydrocele often requires no treatment. However, care must be taken not to dismiss something more serious as a hydrocele. Only a physician can make the diagnosis. Therefore, any scrotal mass merits immediate medical attention. The treatment for hydrocele is surgical removal of the fluid. The condition can recur.

Impotence

Impotence is the inability to achieve and maintain an erection of the penis, which is necessary to penetrate the vagina during sexual intercourse. The corpora cavernosa of the penis normally fill with blood during sexual excitement, which causes the penis to become rigid and erect. Impotence is a partial or total impairment of this function.

Types

There are two types of impotence: primary impotence, in which a man is never able to have an erection adequate for sexual intercourse; and secondary impotence, in which a man quite often fails to complete intercourse to the satisfaction of both partners. Secondary impotence is the more common type.

Many men experience temporary impotence at some point in their lives, but chronic (recurring) impotence can lower a man's self-esteem and put a strain on his marriage or social relationships.

Causes

Impotence can be caused by either physical or psychological problems. It may be brought on by job-related stress, fear of causing pregnancy, unresolved conflicts about sexuality, or fear of sex after a heart attack or major surgery. Drug and alcohol abuse are also among the leading causes of impotence.

Until recently, psychological problems were thought to be the only cause of impotence, but underlying physical factors are now also known to trigger the problem. These factors include the following: an imbalance in the hormonal system that causes a decrease in production of testosterone (the male hormone necessary for an erection); the use of certain drugs for the treatment of high blood pressure, particularly diuretics and beta blockers; diseases of the nervous system, such as multiple sclerosis; structural abnormalities of the penis; injury to the penis; and malfunctioning of the circulatory system, which can interfere with the blood flow to the penis.

Symptoms

The major symptom of impotence is inability to attain or maintain erection of the penis for sexual intercourse. This may be accompanied by a lack of interest in sex, but not necessarily infertility (the inability to father a child).

Diagnosis

Several tests can help to diagnose the cause of impotence. A blood test will show whether adequate levels of testosterone are present. With a blood pressure cuff specially designed to wrap around the penis and an ultrasound study (a technique that uses sound waves to create images of internal structures), blood vessel problems in the penis can often be detected. Another test registers the size of erections that naturally occur during sleep; if erections do not occur during sleep, a physical, rather than an emotional, cause is likely.

Treatment

If impotence has a physical basis, a number of treatments are available. Injections of testosterone and other hormones may relieve some problems. Surgery may be necessary to repair the arteries and veins that carry blood to and from the penis.

The use of penile implants is a successful new treatment for impotence, with several varieties now in use. One is a silicone rod that is implanted in the corpora cavernosa, resulting in a permanent partial erection. Another is a flexible silver wire surrounded by silicone, which allows manipulation of the penis to an erect position for intercourse. A third model consists of balloon-like cylinders implanted in the corpora cavernosa and connected to a container of fluid; with the use of a hand pump, the cylinders may be filled with the fluid, in much the same way that blood normally fills the penis during an erection.

Counseling by psychologists or trained sex therapists may be recommended for men whose impotence seems to stem from emotional problems. Counseling may also help those with physical disorders in learning to deal with their impotence.

Prevention

Avoiding the abuse of alcohol and drugs, as well as eliminating or coping with stress, should help to prevent at least some episodes of secondary impotence.

Prostatitis

Prostatitis is an infection or inflammation of the male sex gland called the prostate. It predominantly affects older men, usually in the form of chronic (recurring) flare-ups. Though not generally a serious disorder, prostatitis can be irritating and uncomfortable because it disrupts normal urination; in advanced stages, it can cause bladder or kidney damage.

Located just below the bladder, the prostate is a small, doughnut-shaped gland that surrounds the neck of the bladder and the urethra. As men get older, the prostate often becomes enlarged, which may constrict the urethra. This will eventually develop into a condition called prostatism, which causes disruption of normal urination, marked by prolonged effort or repeated attempts to start the flow, decreased force, and dribbling toward the end of the flow. Some urine is almost always left in the

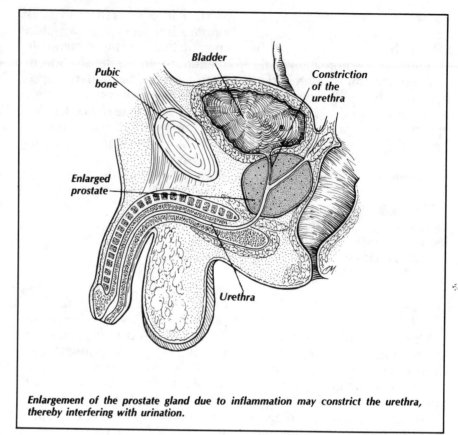

Enlargement of the prostate gland due to inflammation may constrict the urethra, thereby interfering with urination.

bladder, providing a fertile breeding ground for bacteria. Bladder infection is a common consequence of prostatism, which may in turn cause prostatitis. Advanced cases of prostatitis may cause a sudden, total blockage of urine flow, requiring emergency treatment before the backup of urine can cause bladder and kidney damage.

Causes

Sexually transmitted diseases and urinary tract infections are the most common underlying causes of prostatitis.

Symptoms

The most common symptoms are trouble in starting the urine flow, reduced force in urination,

dribbling at the end of urination, and increased frequency of urination. Prostatitis may be signaled by discomfort in the lower back and genital area, a burning sensation while urinating, fever, and chills.

Diagnosis

Prostatitis is diagnosed by an examination of the prostate to check its size, shape, and firmness. An infected prostate will be tender to the touch; when it is massaged by the doctor, pus cells will be forced out and will then appear in the urine. A culture of the urine specimen will be examined for bacteria, although very often no bacteria are identified in a case of chronic prostatitis. However, a urinalysis may show some evidence of infection, and if a trace of blood is present, the urine may be additionally tested for the presence of malignant cells.

Enlargement of the prostate can be diagnosed by means of a procedure called an intravenous pyelogram (IVP), in which dye is injected into a vein in the arm and allowed to travel through the bloodstream to the kidneys and urinary bladder and out through the penis. The dye may show enlargement or obstruction in the ureters. The patient will then be asked to urinate; if the IVP shows a large quantity of urine left in the bladder, a partial obstruction caused by an enlarged prostate can generally be diagnosed.

Treatment

Most prostate infections can be treated quite successfully with antibiotics. Chronic nonbacterial prostatitis, however, is not treated with antibiotics. Instead, drinking large quantities of water and taking hot baths are often recommended.

Enlargement of the prostate gland that causes symptoms is normally treated by surgical removal of the excess tissue through one of two procedures: transurethral surgery, in which the center of the prostate gland is scraped out by an instrument that has been inserted into the penis; or prostatectomy, a more complicated procedure requiring an incision in the lower abdomen or between the legs. There is little danger of impotence resulting from either of these surgical procedures, but they may lead to retrograde ejaculation, a condition in which the semen is passed back into the bladder to be expelled with the urine, rather than being released during intercourse (although this condition presents no health risk, it is a cause of male infertility).

Urethritis

Urethritis is an infection or inflammation of the urethra (the tube that runs through the penis and connects the bladder to the outside). It is the most common condition affecting the male reproductive system and may occur in men of all ages.

Causes

Two sexually transmitted diseases, gonorrhea and chlamydia, are the most common causes of urethritis in both men and women. Irritation may also be caused after sexual intercourse by chemicals contained in vaginal spermicides and douches. Once inside the urethra, these bacteria and chemicals will cause the urethra to become irritated and swollen.

Symptoms

The most common symptoms of urethritis are burning during urination and a creamy white or yellow discharge from the penis. Unlike a bladder infection, urethritis does not cause an increase in the frequency of urination.

Diagnosis

Urethritis is diagnosed by an examination of the penis to check for discharge. The doctor will then take specimens of the discharge for examination under a microscope and for bacterial culture.

Treatment

Infections of the urethra are treated with antibiotics. A person who has urethritis should abstain from sexual activity until a full course of antibiotics has been taken and until all tests indicate that the infection is no longer present. Every sexual partner of the infected person needs to be examined and, if necessary, treated.

Prevention

Urethritis can be prevented by avoiding sexual contact with someone who is infected with either gonorrhea or chlamydia. Using condoms also helps reduce the risk of contracting these infections. If urethritis is caused by irritation from vaginal spermicides or douches, these should be avoided or a condom should be used.

THE FEMALE REPRODUCTIVE SYSTEM

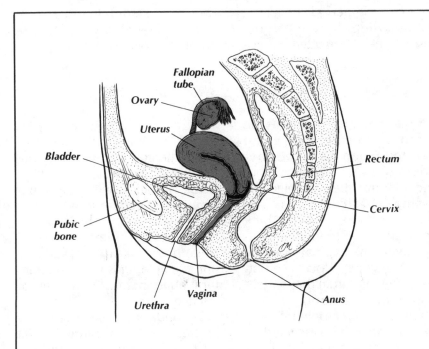

A side view of the female reproductive organs.

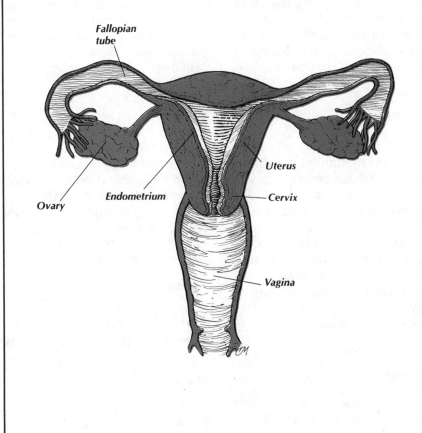

A front view of the female reproductive organs.

The female reproductive system consists of those structures within the female body that are designed to create and nourish new life. The system includes the ovaries, fallopian tubes, uterus, cervix, and vagina.

Although the breasts, or mammary glands, are actually a type of sweat gland, their function (supporting new life) is closely related to that of the reproductive system. For that reason, disorders affecting the breasts will also be covered in this chapter.

The reproductive process begins in the ovaries. The ovaries are small, egg-shaped glands located in the lower abdomen. These glands control the cyclic functions of the reproductive system—ovulation and menstruation. Ovulation is the monthly production and release of a mature egg (occasionally two or more eggs). This process and other reproductive functions are regulated by two hormones, estrogen and progesterone, which are secreted by the ovaries. Estrogen regulates the secondary sex traits of body hair growth, breast development, ovulation, and menstruation. Progesterone is responsible for preparing the uterus for pregnancy, as well as contributing to enlargement of the breasts during pregnancy and milk production after childbirth. The two hormones coordinate to control the menstrual cycle.

Once an egg has been released, it travels through the fallopian tubes, which extend from each ovary into the uterus. Their reproductive function is to contain the egg until fertilization (union of an egg and a sperm, or male sex cell) takes place and to provide a passageway leading the sperm to the egg and the fertilized egg to the uterus.

The uterus is a pear-shaped, hollow organ that is normally

about the size of a lemon. Its muscular walls are lined with rich, soft tissue called the endometrium. Each month, the lining adds layers in anticipation of receiving a fertilized egg. Should fertilization occur, the lining nourishes the fertilized egg in the uterus until birth. However, if the egg remains unfertilized, the uterus sheds the endometrium and the egg, which leave the body as menstrual discharge.

The cervix is a narrow structure with an inch-long canal connecting the lower end of the uterus to the upper portion of the vagina. This canal is the conduit for sperm on their way to fertilize an egg and for menstrual discharge and babies leaving the uterus.

The vagina, or birth canal, is a passageway leading from the cervix to the outside of the body. In the average adult woman, it measures four to five inches in length. Although the vaginal walls are normally close together, they separate to accommodate the infant during childbirth and the erect penis during sexual intercourse. The vagina continually produces secretions that lubricate and cleanse it.

Amenorrhea

Amenorrhea is the absence of menstruation. There are two categories of this disorder. Primary amenorrhea is the failure to begin menstruating by the age of 16. Secondary amenorrhea, the more common of the two conditions, is the absence of three or more periods in a row in a woman who has been menstruating for some time. Primary amenorrhea is specifically defined at the age of 16 and can go on indefinitely. Secondary amenorrhea is usually a temporary condition; the periods generally resume when the underlying cause has been corrected.

Causes

Primary amenorrhea may be caused by an endocrine gland disorder (such as hyperthyroidism or hypothyroidism); genetic abnormalities; damaged or missing ovaries, uterus, or vagina; or an excessively thick hymen (the membrane that usually covers the vaginal opening in virgins), which blocks the outflow of the menstrual discharge.

Secondary amenorrhea is caused most commonly by pregnancy. It can also be triggered by strenuous sports training, poor nutrition, drastic weight gain, jet lag, certain medications (including corticosteroids, tranquilizers, and birth control pills), major surgery or serious disease, emotional shock, or the loss of a large percentage of body fat.

Symptoms

Primary amenorrhea is commonly accompanied by abnormal or inhibited physical development; the young girl may fail to develop breasts or body hair, indicating that a genetic disorder may be preventing her from attaining sexual maturity. These girls are also usually short.

Secondary amenorrhea has no symptoms other than the absence of menstrual periods.

Diagnosis

Diagnostic evaluation of both types of amenorrhea will probably include a test to rule out pregnancy, tests to detect genetic or hormonal disorders, and X rays or ultrasound studies (see pages 407-408) to check the reproductive organs.

Treatment

Primary amenorrhea may be treated with an extensive hormone therapy program to stimulate physical development. If the cause is a thick hymen, a minor surgical procedure may be performed to open the hymen. Some cases of primary amenorrhea, however, are untreatable (for example, those due to structural abnormalities of the reproductive organs).

Secondary amenorrhea may be treated with a hormone that will trigger ovulation and reestablish the menstrual cycle. However, quite often this condition will reverse itself without treatment, especially if the cause is merely an interruption in the patient's normal routine, an emotional upset, or pregnancy.

Prevention

Maintaining good nutritional habits and a normal weight and avoiding overly strenuous sports can probably be beneficial in preventing secondary amenorrhea. No specific precautions can be taken, however, to prevent primary amenorrhea.

Cystocele

A cystocele is a protrusion into the vagina of a portion of the urinary bladder.

Cause

Cystocele is usually the result of damage to the wall of fibrous

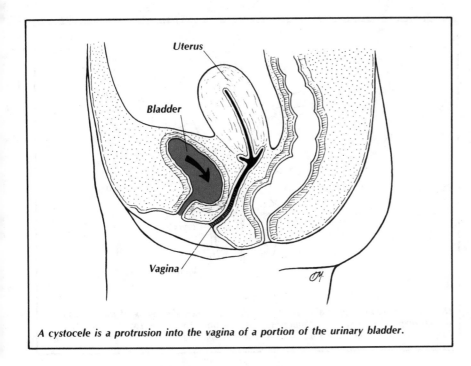

A cystocele is a protrusion into the vagina of a portion of the urinary bladder.

tissue that normally separates the vagina and the bladder. Such an injury often occurs during childbirth and may happen with the birth of a baby of any size. However, women who have never given birth may also develop a cystocele. A cystocele may not appear until menopause, when the damaged area is weakened further, permitting the rear and base portions of the bladder to protrude into the vagina. A portion of the rectum, the small intestine, or the urethra (the tube through which urine leaves the body) may also bulge into the vagina, or prolapse of the uterus (in which the uterus drops through the vagina and in very severe cases protrudes through the vaginal opening) may occur.

The protrusion of the bladder into the vagina creates a pool of stale urine in the bladder, which cannot be easily emptied and as a result, becomes a breeding ground for bacteria. Cystitis (inflammation of the bladder), signaled by painful and difficult urination, often results.

Symptoms

A woman with a cystocele may feel a fullness in the vagina and may find it difficult to empty her bladder completely. However, many women with a cystocele have no symptoms at all.

Diagnosis

Diagnosis is made by examining the inside of the vagina. If a bulge can be seen in front of the cervix, a cystocele is suspected. Also, if a catheter inserted into the bladder after urination can draw out more than two ounces of leftover urine, the diagnosis is even more likely. If a special X-ray study in which dye is injected into the bladder reveals a bulged-out section of the bladder, the diagnosis is confirmed.

Treatment

The preferred treatment for cystocele is surgery to repair the damaged wall and put the protruding section of bladder back in its original place. A pessary (a device inserted into the vagina to support the vagina and reduce the cystocele) may be used in women who cannot or do not wish to undergo surgery. A cystocele does not always require treatment. However, if frequent bouts of cystitis occur, some form of treatment will be necessary.

DES

Diethylstilbestrol (DES) is an artificial estrogen (female sex hormone) used to treat a variety of disorders. For nearly three decades, this drug was frequently prescribed to prevent miscarriage. In 1971, however, the Food and Drug Administration banned its use for this purpose because it had been found ineffective.

Use of DES has been linked to an increased incidence of adenocarcinoma (a rare cancer of the glandular cells of the reproductive organs) in the daughters of the several million women who took it to prevent miscarriage and other complications of pregnancy. Testicular cancer in male offspring has also been associated with maternal DES use. Persons exposed to DES before birth also have a higher than average incidence of benign (noncancerous) growths, structural changes involving the reproductive organs, and infertility problems. These abnormalities usually appear in the late teens to early 30s. Although the incidence of serious complications is small, physicians strongly advise that persons who were exposed to DES before·birth be routinely examined to detect any abnormalities.

Because of the potential problems, DES should not be taken by a woman who is pregnant or suspects that she is pregnant. DES may be used safely by non-pregnant women to treat a variety of disorders, including certain vaginal conditions and estrogen deficiency that may occur at menopause or after the surgical removal of the ovaries. Recently, DES has also been shown to be effective in some male patients in reducing the growth of advanced prostate cancer. Since DES is a hormone that may produce a variety of effects in the body, its use must always be supervised by a physician.

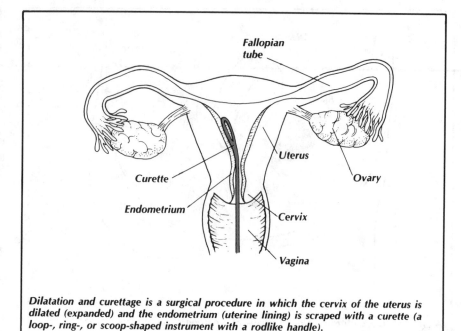

Dilatation and curettage is a surgical procedure in which the cervix of the uterus is dilated (expanded) and the endometrium (uterine lining) is scraped with a curette (a loop-, ring-, or scoop-shaped instrument with a rodlike handle).

Dilatation and curettage

Dilatation and curettage, also called a D&C, is a surgical procedure in which the cervix of the uterus is dilated (expanded) and the endometrial lining of the uterus is scraped with a curette (a loop-, ring-, or scoop-shaped instrument with a long, rodlike handle).

Purpose

This procedure is often used in the diagnosis of diseases of the uterus (such as cancer) and to halt excessive bleeding. It is also used to perform an abortion and may be employed after a miscarriage (involuntary expulsion of a fetus before it is able to live on its own) to remove any remains of tissue and thereby lower the risk of hemorrhage and infection.

Dilatation alone may be performed to enlarge the passageway out of the uterus. This might be done if a severely narrowed cervix is causing painful menstruation because of restricted flow of menstrual fluid. For treatment of this problem, multiple dilatations may be necessary since the cervix will often become narrow again after several months.

The procedure

Although a D&C is a relatively minor procedure, hospital admission is sometimes recommended. Because the large intestine should be empty before the procedure, an enema is often given; the urinary bladder should also be emptied.

The procedure is performed in an operating room under sterile conditions. Anesthesia may be general (the patient is put to sleep) or local. The patient rests on her back with her feet in stirrups. The surgeon inserts metal dilators of progressively larger sizes into the cervix until it is open enough to permit the insertion of the surgical instruments.

(An alternative method of cervical dilatation employs a small tube of dried seaweed that is left in the cervical canal for 8 to 12 hours. As the seaweed absorbs moisture from the cervical canal, it expands and enlarges the canal.)

A curette is used to remove endometrial tissue. Special forceps may also be used to remove tissue. When the operation is finished, an absorbent pad is placed over the entrance to the vagina. The pad is checked every 15 minutes for two hours, and excessive bleeding is reported to the physician.

Mild painkillers should be enough to control discomfort from the operation. If there is pain in the abdomen that cannot be relieved in this way or that is continuous or sharp, it should be reported immediately. Some difficulty in urinating is to be expected immediately after the procedure.

In most cases, the patient stays in bed for one to two hours following surgery. Most women return home several hours after the procedure or the next day. A return to many daily activities is possible immediately, and in a week all normal physical activities may be resumed. Sexual intercourse and use of tampons should not be attempted, however, until after the follow-up visit to the doctor (usually about two weeks after the procedure).

Risks

The principal risks of a D&C are hemorrhage, infection, and perforation (puncture) of the uterus. The latter is more likely during pregnancy, when the uterine walls are especially soft and thin.

Dysmenorrhea

Dysmenorrhea is the term for painful menstruation. It occurs most commonly in teenagers and in women who have never been pregnant.

There are two types of dysmenorrhea. Primary dysmenorrhea is a recurring condition, usually beginning shortly after the onset of menstruation in a young girl. Secondary dysmenorrhea develops later in life, after a woman has been menstruating for some time.

Dysmenorrhea is not a serious condition, but it can be annoying, uncomfortable, and even incapacitating. Since secondary dysmenorrhea usually indicates that another disorder is present, treatment should always be sought for this condition.

Causes

The cause of primary dysmenorrhea is thought to be the release of prostaglandins from the lining of the uterus shortly before the beginning of a menstrual period. (Prostaglandins are substances that, among other functions, stimulate uterine contractions.) The resulting contractions constrict blood vessels in the uterus, causing pain in the same way that a decrease in blood supply to the heart causes chest pain. The reason for this excessive production of prostaglandins is not known. Secondary dysmenorrhea is usually a result of another reproductive problem, such as fibroid tumors, a narrow cervix, or endometriosis (the displacement of tissue from the uterine lining to areas elsewhere in the body).

Symptoms

The major symptoms of dysmenorrhea are cramps and pain in the lower abdomen, possibly extending around to the back. Nausea, vomiting, diarrhea, headache, fatigue, and nervousness are mainly associated with primary dysmenorrhea. These symptoms usually appear at the beginning of, or slightly before, the menstrual period, and may last several hours or several days.

Diagnosis

Diagnostic evaluation will include a complete physical examination as well as medical and menstrual histories. If the symptoms have been present from the onset of menstruation at puberty, primary dysmenorrhea is usually the diagnosis. If the symptoms appeared suddenly in a woman who has been menstruating for some years, secondary dysmenorrhea can be assumed. In that case, further diagnostic evaluation of the reproductive organs will then be necessary to identify the underlying disorder. Ultrasound examinations (in which the echoes of sound waves are used to create images of internal structures) or X-ray studies often prove useful.

Treatment

Primary dysmenorrhea has been treated successfully with nonsteroidal anti-inflammatory drugs (such as ibuprofen, naproxen, meclofenamate, diflunisal, and mefenamic acid), which, when taken just before a period is to begin, act to suppress the release of prostaglandins and thereby reduce the intensity of the contractions that cause pain.

Secondary dysmenorrhea is treated by correcting the problem that is causing the painful menstration. For instance, if endometriosis is the underlying problem, it may be treated with hormone therapy or through surgery, thereby relieving the dysmenorrhea as well.

Home remedies often help to ease menstrual pain and relieve pressure. These include placing a hot-water bottle or heating pad on the abdomen, taking hot baths, and lying on the back with the knees bent. A woman who experienced dysmenorrhea before pregnancy may find that the problem is lessened after childbirth, possibly because of enlargement of the cervix or destruction of some nerve fibers in the uterus.

Dyspareunia

Dyspareunia is difficulty or pain for a woman during sexual intercourse.

Causes

Dyspareunia may be caused by a resistant hymen (the membrane that usually covers the opening to the vagina in virgins) or by inflammation of or injury to the vagina, the urethra (the tube that carries urine from the bladder to the outside), the vulva (the structures around the opening to the vagina), or the anus. It can be the result of formation of scar tissue around an episiotomy (a surgical cut to enlarge the opening of the vagina immediately before childbirth) or surgery to repair the vagina. Other physical causes of dyspareunia include tight muscles in the area around the vagina, an "hourglass" contraction of the vagina, a divided vagina, inflammation of the cervix, prolapsed (fallen) uterus, infection of the fallopian tubes, and endometriosis.

Inadequate lubrication of the vagina is a common cause of dyspareunia. This deficiency may be due to inadequate arousal of the woman before insertion of the penis or to menopause, which is accompanied by a decrease in vaginal secretions and thinning of the vaginal lining. Unconscious tightening of the vaginal muscles, called vaginismus, is another possible cause—perhaps the result of fear, unreadiness or unwillingness to perform the sex act, or other psychological reasons. Improperly fitted or improperly lubricated birth control devices (condoms or diaphragms) and an allergy to contraceptive spermicides are other causes.

Symptoms

Pain during or following sexual intercourse is the primary symptom.

Diagnosis

Diagnosis is made on the basis of both a physical and an emotional evaluation. In some cases, physical abnormalities can be detected during the physical examination. In other cases, careful inquiry into the patient's emotional state and sexual history may reveal factors that account for the discomfort.

Treatment

Treatment for dyspareunia is correction of any underlying disease, injury, or structural defect, if such a problem exists. For some couples, counseling by a psychiatrist or sex therapist is helpful in removing psychological barriers to sexual closeness that may result in dyspareunia.

Water-soluble lubricating jelly (not petroleum jelly), obtainable in any drugstore, provides a good vaginal lubricant. Estrogen creams can be used along with water-soluble jelly to restore lubrication to a dry vagina after menopause. Soothing creams and temporary avoidance of intercourse can relieve the soreness of dyspareunia.

Endometriosis

Endometriosis is a condition in which tissue from the endometrial lining of the uterus becomes detached and grows in the abdominal cavity outside the uterus. It occurs only in women of childbearing age, especially in women between the ages of 30 and 40.

Cause

During each menstrual cycle, the endometrium normally thickens and swells in preparation for

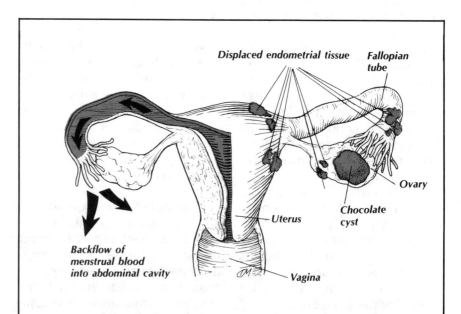

Endometriosis is a condition in which tissue from the endometrium (uterine lining) becomes detached and grows outside the uterus, usually elsewhere in the abdominal cavity. One possible cause may be backflow of menstrual blood through one of the fallopian tubes into the abdominal cavity. Blood-filled pockets called "chocolate cysts" sometimes form when scar tissue surrounds accumulations of blood and displaced endometrial tissue.

possible pregnancy. If no pregnancy occurs, portions of endometrial tissue break down and pass out of the uterus as part of the menstrual flow. When endometriosis develops, displaced endometrial tissue continues to swell and bleed each month in an abnormal location, but the blood has no outlet. The body responds to the presence of this accumulated blood by surrounding it with scar tissue, which builds up month after month, until blood-filled pockets, or cysts (often called "chocolate cysts"), are formed on the affected organs.

The exact cause of endometriosis is not known, but several conditions are thought to lead to its development: menstrual blood may flow backward through the fallopian tubes and into the abdominal cavity; the cervix or vagina may be blocked, so that the menstrual blood cannot flow out normally; or surgery or another condition may lead to the displacement of some tissue from the uterus.

Symptoms

The symptoms of endometriosis are pain immediately before, during, or immediately after the menstrual period; pain during intercourse; discomfort in the lower urinary tract or intestine; irregular or excessively heavy menstrual flow; bleeding from the rectum; blood in the urine; and infertility. Some women may experience all of these symptoms, while others may experience only one or two.

Diagnosis

Diagnostic evaluation begins with a complete medical and menstrual history. Pelvic examinations may be performed— once during menstruation and once between periods—to investigate the changes in the reproductive organs during the cycle. The doctor may also perform a laparoscopy, in which a small, lighted, tubelike instrument is inserted into the lower abdomen through a tiny incision, often allowing visualization of displaced tissues.

Treatment

Treatment of this disorder consists of halting the condition, reducing the pain, and restoring normal menstruation and fertility. The best way to halt endometriosis is to modify the body's natural hormonal secretions with drugs in order to stop menstruation and ovulation for some time, thus allowing the endometrial tissue to shrink. Naturally, the patient will be unable to become pregnant during this type of drug therapy, but since endometriosis often causes infertility, many patients are already unable to conceive.

Three types of drugs are usually used in this treatment. Birth control pills, as well as several other medications that modify female hormonal secretions, are sometimes prescribed in doses high enough to stop menstruation and ovulation. However, an excessive dosage often brings with it undesirable side effects, such as nausea, fluid retention, and blood clotting.

A synthetic hormone called danazol creates a condition similar to menopause, causing menstruation and ovulation to stop and the endometrial tissue to shrink almost immediately. Danazol does not have some of the side effects associated with other hormonal drugs. However,

it is relatively expensive and is not effective in all cases.

The newest form of treatment of endometriosis is a nasal spray that causes the brain to stop producing hormones that cause ovulation and menstruation. As with the use of danazol, the nasal spray causes endometrial tissue to shrink almost immediately. If drug therapy is unsuccessful, surgery may be necessary, involving either the removal of scar tissue and endometrial tissue or, in advanced cases, the removal of the uterus and ovaries, rendering the patient sterile. In certain cases, endometriosis may be destroyed by using very precise medical lasers. This form of therapy has been used to successfully dissolve areas of endometriosis while sparing surrounding normal tissue.

Fibrocystic disease of the breast

Fibrocystic disease is a condition in which benign (noncancerous) lumps form in the breast, either temporarily or for the duration of the childbearing years.

This condition is not dangerous in itself, but it has been found that women with certain forms of fibrocystic disease may be two to four times more likely to develop breast cancer than are other women. To complicate matters, the presence of these benign lumps makes it difficult to detect any new, possibly dangerous growths.

Cause

The exact cause of fibrocystic disease is not known. However, the tendency to develop it may be inherited. Also, it is seen more often in women who have never breast-fed a child; the reason for this is not known.

Symptoms

The most noticeable symptom of this disorder is the presence of the lumps, which may take the form of either solid masses or fluid-filled sacs called cysts. Large cystic lumps near the surface can be moved about freely, unlike cancerous lumps, which are usually firmly attached to surrounding tissue. Changes in hormonal secretions during the menstrual period tend to slightly increase the size of the lumps, which causes additional pain, but the size of the cysts decreases following the period. Other symptoms may include a slight discharge from the nipple, as well as persistently heavy and tender breasts, not only before and during menstruation (as is commonly seen in healthy breasts) but all the time.

Diagnosis

Diagnostic evaluation will begin with a physical examination. Mammography (a special X-ray study of the breasts) is often done to determine whether the lumps are fluid-filled cysts or solid masses. If they are found to be solid, a biopsy (the removal of a small piece of tissue for analysis) may be performed to detect the presence of cancerous cells.

Treatment

Fibrocystic disease often requires no treatment. In some cases, the lumps may disappear

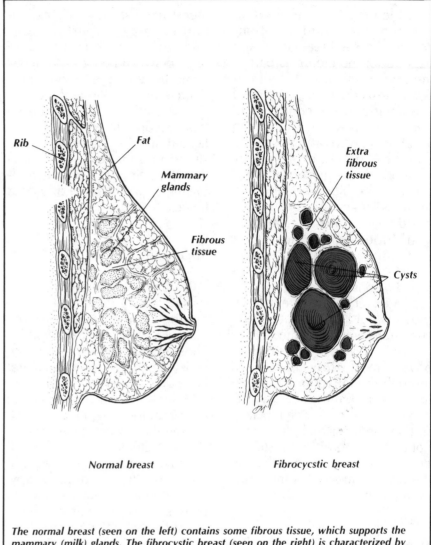

The normal breast (seen on the left) contains some fibrous tissue, which supports the mammary (milk) glands. The fibrocystic breast (seen on the right) is characterized by the presence of extra fibrous tissue and solid masses or fluid-filled sacs (cysts).

in a few months. However, cysts that are unusually large or particularly bothersome may be drained of their fluid by the insertion of a hollow needle in a procedure called aspiration. If there are many small lumps or if there is continuous development of new ones, other forms of treatment may be necessary to prevent the formation of cysts. Birth control pills may be prescribed, since they act to equalize the concentration of hormones in the body throughout the monthly cycle; however, birth control pills have also been found to cause cysts in some women. Large doses of vitamin E (taken under a doctor's supervision) have also reportedly been effective in treating this disorder.

Prevention

Relieving or preventing fibrocystic disease may be promoted by discontinuing or drastically limiting the intake of nicotine and a chemical called methylxanthine, found most commonly in coffee, tea, cola, chocolate, and some cold medications. It is thought that both nicotine and methylxanthine may promote the growth of fibrocystic tissue.

Because certain forms of this disorder carry a greater risk of breast cancer, women with fibrocystic disease should have a physical examination at least twice a year, report any new growths or enlargements of existing lumps, and perform self-examination of their breasts each month following the menstrual period.

Fibroid tumors

Fibroid tumors are solid, noncancerous growths composed of smooth muscle fibers and connective tissue that grow in the walls of the uterus or out from the uterus. Only rarely do they appear on the cervix. Occasionally they fill the entire uterus, push through the cervix, and appear in the vagina. These tumors usually grow slowly and vary in size and shape.

Fibroid tumors are thought to be the most common type of abdominal tumor, found in about 25 percent of all women over the age of 30 (more frequently in black women). Cancer rarely develops in fibroid tumors; however, they do sometimes cause problems. For example, the tumors tend to enlarge during pregnancy, which can cause complications as the fetus grows.

Causes

The cause of fibroid tumors is not known, but their growth seems to be related to the female hormone estrogen, since these tumors rarely appear before puberty and tend to recede by the

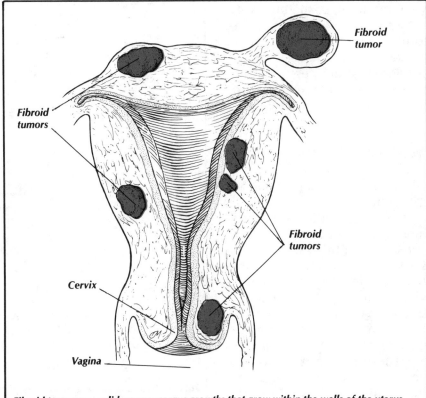

Fibroid tumors are solid, noncancerous growths that grow within the walls of the uterus or out from the uterine wall on a stalk.

menopause years. They most commonly appear in the middle to late reproductive years, when the estrogen level is at its peak.

Fibroid tumors may occur along with other disorders, such as endometriosis (the displacement of tissue from the uterine lining to areas elsewhere in the body) or pelvic inflammatory disease (an infection of the fallopian tubes).

Symptoms

Common symptoms of fibroid tumors are dysmenorrhea (pain during menstruation) and gushing or flooding of the menstrual flow. Occasionally, there is abdominal pain; however, pain is not usually a symptom unless a complication develops (for example, if the tumor becomes

twisted, cutting off its blood supply). If fibroid tumors become very large, they may press on surrounding organs, such as the intestines and bladder, which may result in constipation or frequent urination. If they extend into the uterus, heavy and prolonged menstrual periods may result. If the tumor is advanced, the abdomen may be noticeably enlarged. Sometimes, however, these tumors cause no symptoms at all and are simply discovered during a routine physical examination.

Diagnosis

Diagnostic evaluation begins with a physical examination and may include curettage (scraping the uterus walls) or endometrial biopsy (removal of some tissue from the lining of the uterus) to test for cancer. X rays and ultrasound (a technique that uses sound waves to create an image of internal structures) may also be used to establish the location, size, and nature of the tumor.

Treatment

Fibroid tumors may require no treatment at all, other than regular checkups with the doctor. Those that are causing complications may require one of two types of surgery: removal of the tumor (called a myomectomy), which is usually recommended for women in their early reproductive years whose symptoms are somewhat mild and who desire a future pregnancy, or removal of the uterus (called a hysterectomy), which is usually recommended for older women and for those who do not want to become pregnant, since this operation makes pregnancy impossible.

Hysterectomy

Hysterectomy is the surgical removal of the uterus, which causes the termination of menstruation and the inability to bear children.

A hysterectomy may be either total or partial. Total hysterectomy entails removal of the entire uterus, including the cervix. Partial hysterectomy, which is rarely done today, involves removal of only the body of the uterus but not the cervix (the narrow structure that connects the uterus to the vagina). Oophorectomy (removal of one or both ovaries) and salpingectomy (removal of one or both fallopian tubes) may be performed at the same time as hysterectomy (for

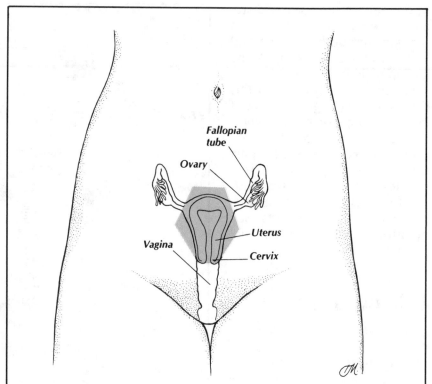

Total hysterectomy is the surgical removal of the uterus and the cervix. Oophorectomy (removal of the ovaries) and salpingectomy (removal of one or both of the fallopian tubes) is sometimes performed at the same time.

more information on oophorectomy, see page 299).

Removal of the uterus may be done through an abdominal incision (cut) or through the vagina. In the latter procedure, the top of the vagina is stitched together after the uterus has been removed; this technique requires no external incision and, therefore, leaves no external scar.

Hysterectomies are most commonly performed when the uterus is diseased. Symptomatic fibroid tumors, uterine prolapse (falling of the uterus out of its normal position), and cancer of the uterus are common reasons for a hysterectomy.

Contrary to common belief, a hysterectomy, in and of itself, does not interfere with, or diminish the pleasure of, sexual intercourse, nor does it cause weight gain.

Leukorrhea

Leukorrhea is an abnormal discharge from the vagina. All women have some normal discharge in the form of mucous secretions from the cervix and the vagina. This normal discharge helps to lubricate the vagina and, to some extent, prevent infection. This discharge is most noticeable at the time of ovulation (when an egg is released from the ovary), but it is generally present during the entire menstrual cycle.

Causes

Abnormal discharge is usually caused by an infection of the vagina by fungi, parasites, or bacteria. It may also be caused by an infection of the cervix, a tumor or other abnormal growth, the presence of foreign matter (such as a forgotten tampon) in the vagina, or an inflammation of the vagina caused by chemicals in douches or contraceptive creams or jellies.

Symptoms

An abnormal vaginal discharge usually is heavy, is accompanied by itching of the genital organs and anal area, and may have a disagreeable odor.

Diagnosis

To diagnose the cause of the discharge, the doctor will perform a pelvic examination and will often take a sample of the discharge for microscopic examination. Sometimes a culture of the discharge may also be performed so that the organism causing the problem can be identified.

Treatment

Once the cause of the abnormal discharge has been identified, specific steps are taken to treat it. If the discharge is caused by a bacterial infection, oral antibiotics or antibiotic vaginal creams may be prescribed. Specific oral drugs or vaginal preparations will be prescribed if the discharge is caused by a type of yeast or trichomonad (a single-celled parasite). In some cases, a biopsy of the cervix or vagina may be required if the doctor suspects that a tumor may be causing the discharge.

Douching with vinegar and water or other solutions available without a prescription generally will not cure the discharge, even

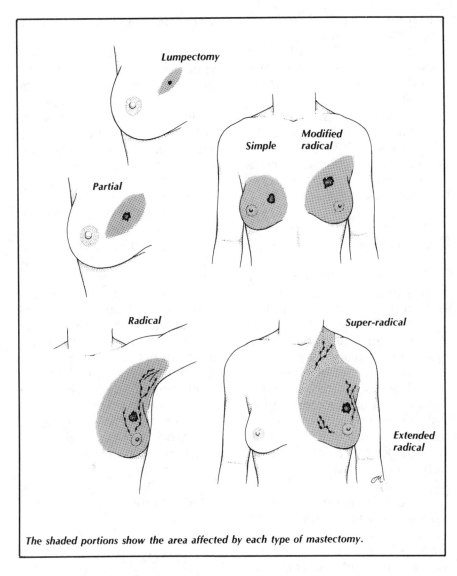

The shaded portions show the area affected by each type of mastectomy.

though symptoms may improve for a few days. A woman with an abnormal vaginal discharge should consult her doctor rather than attempt to treat herself.

Mastectomy

Mastectomy is the surgical removal of a breast or part of a breast, usually to treat cancer.

Types

There are several types of mastectomy, each characterized by which muscles, glands, and other tissues are removed.

- Lumpectomy—removal of the tumor along with some of the surrounding breast tissue
- Partial mastectomy—removal of the tumor along with as much as one half of the breast
- Simple mastectomy—removal of the entire breast
- Modified radical mastectomy—removal of the entire breast plus the armpit lymph nodes on the affected side
- Radical mastectomy—removal of the entire breast, the lymph nodes in the armpit, and the muscles below the breast

- Extended radical mastectomy—removal of the entire breast plus additional tissue in the chest, as well as the lymph nodes in the armpit and the chest muscles
- Super-radical mastectomy—removal of the same tissues and muscles as in the extended radical mastectomy, as well as some tissues and lymph nodes in the neck

Choice of type

The type of mastectomy to be performed is determined by a multitude of factors, including the location, size, and type of tumor. The age and general health of the patient are also extremely important. A biopsy (removal of a small tissue sample for microscopic examination) will be performed prior to mastectomy. In addition, other tests may be done to determine if the cancer has spread to other areas of the body.

There is some question about how extensive the surgery should be. In recent years, the modified radical mastectomy has become the most frequently chosen procedure. However, there are differences of opinion in medical circles, and a woman facing a mastectomy should thoroughly discuss all of the procedures and available options with her doctor.

Treatment

The operation is performed while the patient is under general anesthesia. Afterward the patient remains hospitalized for about a week and may begin radiation therapy or chemotherapy. Checkups every 6 to 12 months are recommended.

Early detection of breast cancer

One of the best measures a woman can take is establishing the habit of examining her breasts monthly. With this simple routine, a woman can often detect a cancerous lump before cancer cells can spread beyond the breast. The effectiveness of breast self-examination is shown by the high percentage of breast tumors that are discovered by patients themselves during a monthly breast self-examination. (For instructions on breast self-examination, see page 392).

Many experts recommend annual mammography (X-ray examination of the breasts) for women over the age of 40 and for younger women who are considered to be at high risk of developing breast cancer (those who have had breast cancer in the past or who have a mother or sister who has had the disease). A mammogram at the age of 35 is recommended for every woman to provide a baseline for later comparison.

Menopause

Menopause is the normal, natural stage in a woman's life when her menstruation and ovulation cycles stop, ending her reproductive years. Also called the climacteric, or the change of life, it occurs around age 50 but can start anywhere between the ages of 40 and 60.

Cause

Scientists do not fully understand what causes menopause. They believe it is triggered when the ovaries stop responding to the sex hormones that are secreted by the pituitary gland to control normal functioning of the ovaries. The subsequent decline in the production of the female hormone estrogen by the ovaries sets off the bodily changes.

Symptoms

During the years immediately preceding the onset of menopause, menstrual periods may become irregular and menstrual flow scanty.

Other physical symptoms may include hot flashes (a warm and flushed feeling over the face, neck, and chest that lasts a few minutes and recurs throughout the day), excessive perspiration, dryness in the vagina (which can lead to painful or difficult sexual intercourse), pounding heartbeat, joint pains, headaches, itching skin, increased facial hair, and decreased armpit and pubic hair.

Nonphysical symptoms may include depression, anxiety, irritability, apprehension, decreased ability to concentrate, lack of confidence, and insomnia.

The duration of symptoms may range from a few weeks to more than five years. Not every woman experiences the same changes, other than an end to menstruation; about 25 percent notice no other changes, 50 percent discern some physical or psychological symptoms, and the other 25 percent are troubled by very uncomfortable or distressing symptoms.

Diagnosis

It is important not to attribute all physical changes to menopause to the point of overlooking the symptoms of some disease. This is a good time to schedule an examination and discuss the bodily changes with a doctor. A woman should see a doctor immediately if she starts to bleed in between menstrual periods, bleeds excessively, or has another period six months or more after they had apparently stopped.

Treatment

The primary treatment for the physical symptoms of menopause is replacement of the female sex hormones (commonly estrogen or a combination of estrogen and progesterone in the form of an oral tablet). Estrogen in the form of a vaginal cream may be prescribed specifically to treat vaginal dryness. The lowest effective dose is administered (because of possible side effects). Any treatment merely lessens the discomfort of menopause, however; it cannot stop or slow down the process. Because of the many beneficial effects of hormone replacement therapy, most physicians now believe that it should continue for the remainder of the patient's life.

Estrogen is not usually given to women with severe circulatory or liver disorders and is carefully controlled when prescribed to those with diabetes, epilepsy, or heart or kidney disease. Progesterone is not prescribed for women with liver disease and is carefully controlled in those with asthma, epilepsy, or heart or kidney disease. The benefits and hazards should be discussed with a doctor; other medication is available to treat certain menopausal symptoms in women who cannot take hormones.

Treatment for the psychological or emotional symptoms may include tranquilizers, antidepressants, sleeping pills, or psychotherapy. During this time, it may also be difficult for a

woman to face the aging process and its physical ramifications—the end of the childbearing years and a sense of uselessness because of a possible decrease in family responsibilities. Some form of counseling may be helpful in such a situation.

Fertility and the need to practice birth control at this stage depend upon a woman's age at the time of her last period. In general, a woman under the age of 50 may still be able to conceive for up to 24 months after the date of her last period; over 50, conception may be possible for up to one year.

After menopause, a woman is more liable to suffer osteoporosis (a disease that makes bones porous and brittle). This can often be prevented or controlled with estrogen therapy and calcium supplementation under medical supervision. The risk of heart attack also increases after menopause, and it is currently believed that estrogen therapy helps to substantially decrease that risk.

Menorrhagia

Menorrhagia is a term referring to an abnormally long (more than seven days) or heavy menstrual flow, frequently accompanied by the passing of large blood clots.

The condition, which is especially common in women in their late 30s and 40s, seldom indicates the existence of a serious disorder. However, it may result in iron deficiency anemia because of excessive blood loss.

Causes

Menorrhagia is a common problem, often caused by a dis-

turbance in the hormones controlling the menstrual cycle. It can also be caused by fibroid tumors in the uterus, inflammation of the pelvic region, and hypothyroidism (underactivity of the thyroid gland).

Diagnosis

If abnormal menstrual flow continues or recurs or if there is any chance of pregnancy, a physician should be consulted. The physician may perform a number of tests (including a Pap test) to determine whether there is a serious underlying cause. Biopsy (removal of a small tissue sample for laboratory examination) of the cervix or the uterine lining may be performed to check for cancer or other abnormalities. The physician may also do a blood test to check for iron deficiency anemia.

Treatment

It is suggested that women who experience this disorder reduce the level of their activities during menstruation and be sure to get enough iron so that they will not become anemic.

Hormones (estrogen and progesterone) may also be used to control heavy bleeding if the underlying problem is a hormonal disturbance. Hysterectomy may be necessary in severe cases that do not respond to estrogen therapy and in cases of extensive fibroid tumors.

Menstruation

Menstruation is the monthly breakdown and discharge of portions of the endometrial tissue that lines the uterus.

THE FEMALE REPRODUCTIVE SYSTEM

The normal process

Endometrial tissue thickens during each menstrual cycle to prepare the uterus for possible pregnancy. Approximately midway through the cycle, ovulation occurs. Ovulation is the process by which an ovary produces and releases an egg. The fingerlike projections at the end of the nearby fallopian tube sweep the egg into the tube, where it begins inching toward the uterus. If the egg is fertilized by a sperm, the fertilized egg moves to the uterus and becomes implanted in the rich uterine lining, where it grows for the next nine months. If the egg does not become fertilized, the thickened endometrial tissue breaks down and passes, along with the unfertilized egg, out of the cervix, through the vagina, and out of the body as the menstrual discharge. This monthly cycle is controlled by the female hormones estrogen and progesterone, which are secreted by the ovaries.

Young women start menstruating and ovulating at puberty, which usually occurs between the ages of 9 and 14. Thereafter, they normally menstruate and ovulate once every month (except while pregnant) until they reach menopause.

Menstrual disorders

Menstruation may be accompanied by complications of varying degrees of seriousness. Most women will experience at least one such problem at some point in their reproductive lives. The most common problems are dysmenorrhea (painful menstruation), amenorrhea (the absence of one or more menstrual periods), and premenstrual syndrome (a complex of physical and emo-

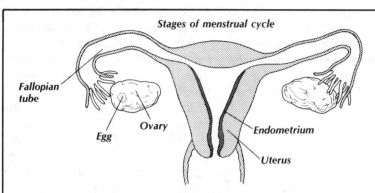

Stages of menstrual cycle

While the egg (shown greatly enlarged, for purposes of illustration) is still inside the ovary, the endometrium (uterine lining) is fairly thin.

When the egg is released and begins to move into the fallopian tube, the endometrium begins to thicken in preparation for a possible pregnancy.

The egg moves through the tube toward the uterus. This is the point at which conception may occur. The egg is met by the sperm cell in the fallopian tube, and the fertilized egg moves on to the uterus. During this time, the endometrium continues to grow.

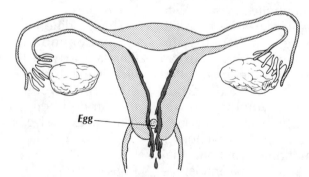

If conception does not occur, the endometrium ceases to grow and thicken. At this stage, the endometrium breaks down and is discharged, along with the unfertilized egg, from the uterus as the menstrual discharge.

tional symptoms that appear in the days before the period begins).

For many years, the symptoms of these disorders have been attributed to emotional factors. Research has shown, however, that most menstrual disorders are caused by very real physical changes in a woman's body, and many new methods of treatment have been developed.

Although the disorders themselves are generally not dangerous to a woman's health, they can be physically and emotionally incapacitating. Furthermore, they may be symptoms of disease in the reproductive organs. Therefore, to be on the safe side, medical evaluation and/or treatment for annoying symptoms accompanying menstruation should always be sought.

Oophorectomy

Oophorectomy is the surgical removal of an ovary. An oophorectomy is a major operation, usually performed through either a vertical or a horizontal incision in the abdominal area, but occasionally performed through an incision in the vagina.

Removal of one ovary is called a unilateral oophorectomy. A salpingectomy (removal of all or part of the nearby fallopian tube) is usually performed at the same time. Removal of both ovaries is called a bilateral oophorectomy. A bilateral oophorectomy ends a woman's ability to conceive children and brings on menopause (if it has not already occurred). A hysterectomy (removal of the uterus) is generally performed in conjunction with a bilateral oophorectomy because the uterus has no purpose without both ovaries and, if left, can later harbor tumors.

Purpose

Oophorectomy is used to correct a number of conditions in which the ovaries are the site of the trouble, including ovarian ectopic pregnancy (in which the embryo begins to develop in the ovary, rather than in the uterus) and benign (noncancerous) and malignant (cancerous) ovarian cysts and tumors. In women with recurrent cancer or endometriosis (the displacement of tissue from the uterine lining to areas elsewhere in the body), oophorectomy is performed to stop the production of hormones, which tend to aggravate the problem. Breast cancer, as well, may be dependent on hormones to grow; about one third of women with breast cancer show a decrease in breast cancer growth after removal of their ovaries.

Pros and cons

Some physicians recommend a bilateral oophorectomy when a hysterectomy must be performed. There are pros and cons when it comes to removing healthy ovaries. Arguments for their removal are that it reduces the risk of ovarian cancer; that a small number of women will develop painful cystic ovaries, which would necessitate a second operation; and that for a woman in her 40s, the ovaries will naturally stop functioning within a few years anyway. Arguments against routine oophorectomy are that it causes the premature onset of menopause, which brings with it a greater risk of osteoporosis (loss of bone mass) and heart attack; that the abrupt end of hormone production is less natural than the gradual tapering off of natural menopause, provoking severe

menopausal symptoms, such as hot flashes and vaginal shrinkage; and that estrogen, the hormone usually prescribed after the procedure, may increase the risk of cancer of the reproductive system.

If a woman is in her childbearing years, her doctor will make every effort to save healthy ovarian tissue. Because the ovaries are fed by an excellent blood supply, they heal quickly and even a small bit of preserved ovarian tissue will function, secrete hormones, and release eggs. The woman remains fertile and avoids early menopause.

In women past menopause, for whom fertility is no longer an issue and in whom the ovaries are no longer producing estrogen anyway, the ovaries and uterus are commonly removed even if only one ovary is abnormal.

Ovarian cysts

An ovarian cyst is an abnormal swelling or saclike growth on an ovary.

Ovarian cysts may be filled with liquid or may contain a semifluid substance. Most cysts are small, but they can vary in size from less than an inch in diameter to as large as 15 to 20 inches in diameter. Depending on their size, type, and location, they can cause severe pain and complications or no symptoms at all. They are common among women between the ages of 20 and 50 and can grow alone or in groups, on one ovary or both. Approximately 85 percent are benign (noncancerous).

Causes

The origin of most ovarian cysts is unknown. In some instances, they develop from an abnormal egg. Others originate as eggs in polycystic ovaries (ovaries in which the eggs are not released after they mature). Still others are related to abnormalities in the ovary. Women with endometriosis (the displacement of tissue from the uterine lining to elsewhere in the body) tend to develop growths on the ovaries. Dermoid cysts, which are most often found in women under the age of 30, arise from the ovarian cells that produce the eggs, and may contain fragments of hair, teeth, bone, and sweat and oil glands.

Complications

Cysts can rupture during sexual intercourse, a fall, childbirth, or surgery, or for no apparent reason. The resulting effect depends on how irritating the cystic fluid is to the surrounding tissues. The situation can be dangerous if the fluid is infected, cancerous, or extremely irritating. Also, in response to the injury caused by cystic fluid, surrounding tissues may produce adhesions (fibrous, scarlike material), which can further complicate the situation.

Symptoms

Symptoms of ovarian cysts vary with the type of growth. Some cause no symptoms and are discovered during a routine pelvic examination. Others cause firm, painless swelling in the lower abdomen; pain during sexual intercourse; frequent urination (if they press against the bladder); irregular vaginal bleeding; or pain, nausea, and fever (if the cysts rupture or grow on stalks that become twisted). Ex-

cessive and abnormal body hair growth and the development of acne may result from hormonal imbalances caused by polycystic ovaries.

Diagnosis

Ovarian cysts are diagnosed by pelvic examination, ultrasound (a technique that uses sound waves to create an image of internal structures), or laparoscopy (a surgical procedure in which a tubelike instrument is inserted through the abdominal wall to view the pelvic organs). The condition may be difficult to diagnose accurately because the symptoms can resemble those of acute appendicitis or other abdominal problems. In addition, it can be hard to determine if a cyst is malignant and if it is actually on the ovary rather than some other pelvic organ. Ovarian cysts that develop during pregnancy are also difficult to diagnose.

Treatment

Cysts that are small, are not creating any problems, or are likely to disappear on their own require no treatment. If treatment is necessary, cysts may be removed surgically. Removal involves either taking out the entire ovary (called an oophorectomy) or taking out only the cyst (called a cystectomy).

If the ovarian cyst is found to be cancerous, it is necessary to remove both ovaries, both fallopian tubes, and the uterus, since the cancer may have spread from the ovarian cyst to these other structures. This procedure is also performed if an ovarian cyst is found after menopause because these cysts are cancerous.

Ovulation

Ovulation is the process by which an ovary produces and releases an egg.

The egg develops within the ovary in a small, fluid-filled sac called a follicle. When the egg is mature, this sac ruptures, releasing the egg from the ovary. The fingerlike projections on the nearby fallopian tube sweep the egg into the tube, where it begins to inch toward the uterus. If the egg is fertilized by a sperm, the fertilized egg moves along the tube to the uterus and becomes implanted in the rich uterine lining, where it grows for the next nine months. If the egg does not become fertilized, the uterine lining breaks down and passes, along with the unfertilized egg, out of the cervix, through the vagina, and out of the body as the menstrual discharge.

Ovulation is regulated by a complex system of hormonal and chemical secretions from the ovaries, the hypothalamus (part of the brain), and the pituitary gland (the master gland, which controls most hormonal secretions). Ovulation and menstruation begin during puberty, which usually occurs between the ages of 9 and 14, and normally continue every month (except during pregnancy) until menopause occurs (around age 50).

One way to recognize when ovulation is happening is to take the body temperature with a basal thermometer (a special thermometer that will show even slight changes in body temperature) before rising in the morning. In most women, the body temperature rises slightly soon after ovulation occurs each month and does not return to normal until the menstrual flow begins. Another way is to count 14 days forward from the first

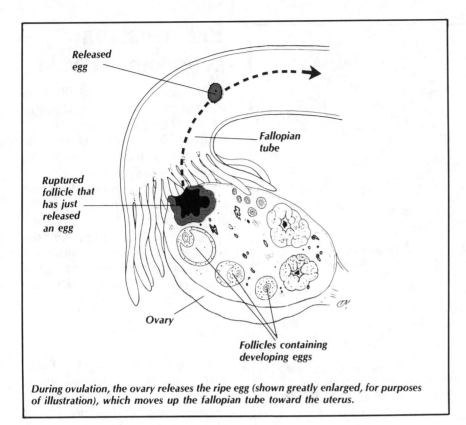

During ovulation, the ovary releases the ripe egg (shown greatly enlarged, for purposes of illustration), which moves up the fallopian tube toward the uterus.

day of the last menstrual period in an average 28-day cycle (count 15 days for a cycle that is normally 29 days long, 16 days for a cycle that is normally 30 days long, and so on). However, this method is less accurate than the thermometer method because the length of the menstrual cycle can vary from month to month. Some women feel cramps in the lower abdomen during ovulation.

A sperm that has been released into the vagina as long as two days before the release of a ripe egg can still fertilize it; and an egg, once released, is capable of being fertilized for about two days. Because of this variability, there is a period of four to ten days in each menstrual cycle during which a woman can become pregnant. (For more information on the role of ovulation in family planning, see pages 311-312.)

Pelvic inflammatory disease

Pelvic inflammatory disease (PID), or salpingitis, is an inflammation of one or both of the fallopian tubes. Although the term is widely used to refer to infections of other organs in the pelvic cavity, PID properly refers only to an inflammation of the fallopian tubes.

Causes

Pelvic inflammatory disease is usually caused by certain bacteria transmitted during sexual intercourse, the presence of an intrauterine device (IUD) that has become a source of infection, or certain vaginal infections. Two of the most common causes of PID are gonorrhea and chlamydia, both sexually transmitted diseases.

Under normal circumstances, the cervix prevents bacteria in the vagina from entering the uterus. However, a woman becomes more vulnerable to PID if the opening of her cervix has been dilated (enlarged) by recent surgery, childbirth, or miscarriage.

Symptoms

Symptoms include severe pain and tenderness in the lower abdomen, fever, a foul-smelling vaginal discharge, menstrual irregularities, pain during sexual intercourse, nausea, vomiting, fatigue, and pain during urination or defecation.

Diagnosis

It is important to seek medical attention as soon as symptoms occur, so that the infection can be treated before it worsens and spreads. The physician will perform a physical examination and take a sample of fluid from the cervix to identify the infecting organism.

Complications

If PID is not diagnosed and treated early, the infection can cause abscesses (pus-filled cavities) to form in the fallopian tubes or around the ovaries. The inflammation can also damage and irreversibly scar pelvic tissues. If the fallopian tubes are blocked, conception can become impossible. The infection can also result in septicemia (in which bacteria enter the bloodstream and are spread to other

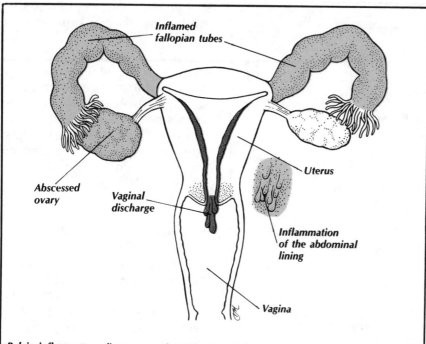

Pelvic inflammatory disease, or salpingitis, is an inflammation of one or both of the fallopian tubes, which can lead to an ovarian abscess, an inflammation of the abdominal lining, and blockage of the fallopian tubes. Vaginal discharge is a common sign of the condition.

Inflamed fallopian tubes

Abscessed ovary

Vaginal discharge

Uterus

Inflammation of the abdominal lining

Vagina

Premenstrual syndrome (PMS)

Premenstrual syndrome (PMS) is a term used to encompass the varying complex of physical and emotional symptoms experienced by some women during the week before their period begins. In the past, this and other menstrual problems were thought to be caused by emotional instability, but current research, while not yet offering conclusive findings, indicates there may be physical reasons.

Cause

Many researchers believe that PMS is caused by fluctuations in the production of female hormones during the menstrual cycle. Hormonal changes influence the amounts of salt and fluid retained in the body, especially during the week before the period begins. Neither the exact cause for this retention nor the reason for its effect on certain women is fully understood.

Symptoms

The symptoms appear from 5 to 14 days before menstruation and usually disappear as soon as the menstrual flow begins. In addition to nervousness and irritability, a bloated feeling that results from fluid retention often characterizes PMS. Other possible symptoms include depression, headache, fatigue, breast tenderness, and acne.

Diagnosis

The diagnosis is based on a physical examination and men-

parts of the body) and in peritonitis (inflammation of the membrane lining the pelvic and abdominal cavities).

Treatment

The doctor will prescribe antibiotics to fight the infection and aspirin or other painkillers for pain relief. The woman may be advised to rest in bed, abstain from sexual intercourse, and apply heat to the lower abdominal area. In some cases, the woman may have to enter the hospital to receive antibiotics intravenously. Laparoscopy (examination of the internal organs through a special tubelike instrument) or surgery to drain blocked tubes or abscessed tissue may be performed. Sometimes, the damage is too extensive, and the fallopian tubes, the uterus, and the ovaries have to be removed.

Prevention

When the cervix is dilated for any reason, a woman is more susceptible to pelvic inflammatory disease for the following several weeks. Since the cervix is dilated in childbirth, abortion, miscarriage, and the surgical procedure called dilatation and curettage (D&C), a woman can minimize her chances of contracting PID by taking special precautions after any of those events. Such precautions include avoiding sexual intercourse, tub baths, and the use of douches and tampons. She should check with her doctor before resuming any of these activities. Also, if a woman suspects that she may have gonorrhea or chlamydia, she should seek treatment for the infection immediately. The use of condoms during sexual intercourse will help prevent these infections.

strual history. The occurrence of any of the symptoms with some regularity before each period and their disappearance soon after menstrual flow begins are the key diagnostic clues.

Treatment

At present, there is no single or sure remedy for PMS. Depending on the symptoms present, various medications may be helpful. The edema is often treated by reducing salt intake or by taking diuretics, medications that help to eliminate excess fluid from the tissues. The avoidance of methylxanthines (chemicals contained in coffee, tea, cola, chocolate, and certain medications) will often help reduce headache and irritability. Tranquilizers and psychological counseling may be recommended for patients in whom PMS causes emotional distress. A balanced diet, moderate exercise, and adequate rest may also be beneficial. The use of hormones (for example, progesterone in the form of a vaginal suppository) is controversial but has significantly reduced PMS symptoms in some women.

Prevention

A reduction of salt intake may help to prevent the initial edema that often accompanies PMS. Self-treatment with diuretics without the advice of a physician is not recommended.

Prolapse of the uterus

Prolapse refers to a collapse, descent, or other change in the po-

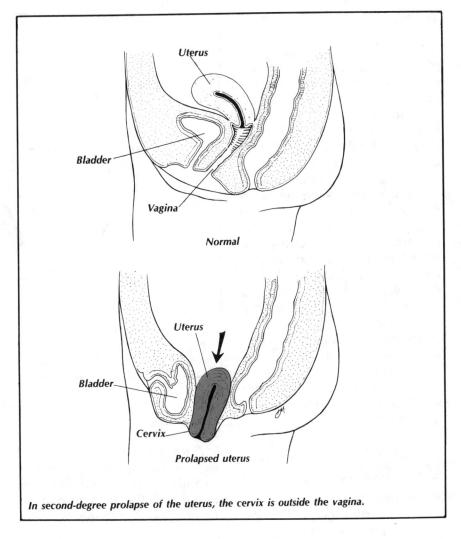

In second-degree prolapse of the uterus, the cervix is outside the vagina.

sition of an organ in relation to surrounding structures. Prolapse of the uterus may be one of three types, depending on severity:
- First-degree prolapse, in which the uterus sags downward so that the cervix is flush with the entrance to the vagina
- Second-degree prolapse, in which the cervix is outside the vagina
- Third-degree prolapse, in which the entire uterus is outside the vagina

Cause

Prolapse of the uterus occurs when the muscles and ligaments that normally hold the uterus in place become stretched or slack. This is most often due to a long or difficult childbirth or multiple childbirths.

Symptoms

There may be a feeling of heaviness in the vagina, backache, or inability to control urination.

Diagnosis

Prolapse of the uterus is apparent to the physician during a pelvic examination.

Treatment

It is especially important to treat prolapse of the uterus because it can make childbirth difficult and may damage other organs. In mild cases, exercises for the muscles of the pelvic floor may be helpful. If the prolapse is the result of injury or stress, surgical repair may be indicated, in which the uterus is returned to its proper place and sewn or stapled into position. If the prolapse is due to disease or swelling, the underlying disorder must first be controlled or eliminated before the uterus can be returned to its original position and secured there. In some cases, a pessary (a plastic ring or donut) may be inserted into the vagina to hold the uterus in its proper position. If childbearing is no longer desired, a hysterectomy may be performed.

Rectocele

Rectocele is a condition in which a part of the rectum (the terminal portion of the large intestine) protrudes into the vagina.

Cause

The usual cause of this condition is a weakening of the back wall of the vagina as a result of the stretching caused by childbirth.

Symptoms

A minimal protrusion may produce no symptoms or only a mild pressure sensation during bowel movements. More severe protrusion of the rectum may lead to chronic constipation and painful bowel movements.

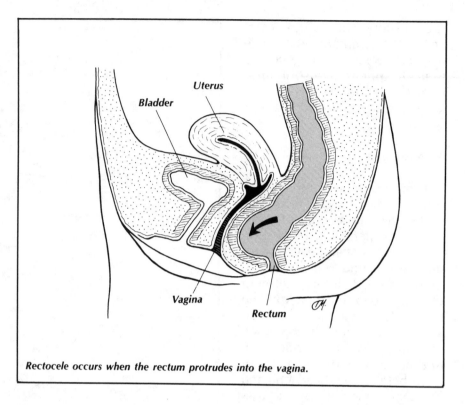

Rectocele occurs when the rectum protrudes into the vagina.

Diagnosis

A rectocele is easily identified by the doctor during a pelvic examination. On straining or coughing, the rectum may be found to bulge into the vagina.

Treatment

Rectocele is not dangerous and generally requires no treatment. If severe constipation or painful bowel movements develop, surgical repair is often curative. Mild symptoms may be relieved by avoiding straining and heavy lifting and by ensuring soft bowel movements with use of drugs and dietary therapy.

Toxic shock syndrome

Toxic shock syndrome (TSS) is a rare, sometimes fatal disease that develops very suddenly and progresses rapidly when a bacterial infection spreads through the bloodstream. The disorder was first defined in 1978, when its link to the use of tampons was suspected. Most of the reported cases have occurred in menstruating women under the age of 30 who use tampons. A significant number of these cases have been fatal.

Cause

Most researchers believe that TSS occurs when the *Staphylococcus aureus* bacterium enters the bloodstream and produces a toxin (poison) that causes leaks in blood vessel walls, allowing blood to seep into the tissues. This results in a sudden, very dangerous drop in blood pressure; shock; and sometimes death.

In serious cases, low blood pressure and weakening of the

cell membranes can leave the victim susceptible to further complications, such as heart and liver damage. Often, the body cannot produce enough antibodies (protective substances) to fight off the invasion of organisms through the weakened cell membranes, so TSS can easily recur.

Although the use of tampons is considered to be a definite risk factor for toxic shock syndrome, tampons do not actually cause the disease; rather, they promote the growth of bacteria that leads to the disorder. The tampons swell to fill the vagina and thereby inhibit the elimination of blood, creating a breeding ground for infection. Also, if tampons are left in the vagina for long periods of time, the chances for infection are increased. Tampon applicators, moreover, may scratch the walls of the vagina, allowing bacteria to enter.

Since about 25 percent of cases of toxic shock syndrome now occur in men and nonmenstruating women, it is clear that the bacteria can enter the body in ways other than through the vagina. In these cases, TSS often occurs when the body has been weakened by major surgery, severe burns, or boils or abscesses. Also, women who have recently given birth to a child are at a higher risk of contracting TSS because the vagina is more susceptible to the invasion of bacteria at this time.

Symptoms

The symptoms of TSS are high fever, vomiting, diarrhea, a rash that looks like sunburn, peeling of skin on the soles of the feet and the palms of the hands, blurred vision, and disorientation.

Diagnosis

The occurrence of the high fever, the characteristic rash, low blood pressure, and involvement of several organ systems strongly points to the diagnosis of TSS. Cultures of the blood and mucous membranes will be performed to search for evidence of infection by the *Staphylococcus aureus* bacterium.

Treatment

Emergency medical treatment should be sought immediately. This will necessitate hospitalization, during which the patient will be given therapy similar to that administered to poisoning victims. Fluids or whole-blood transfusions are given to raise blood pressure, an ice blanket is used to reduce fever, and antibiotics are administered to fight the infection.

Precautions

The best precaution is probably to discontinue or limit the use of tampons. Tampons can still be worn safely, but they should be changed every three to four hours and alternated with sanitary napkins as often as possible, especially before bed.

Vaginitis

Vaginitis is an inflammation of the vagina, usually marked by burning and itching of the external genital organs.

Causes

Vaginitis is most commonly caused by an imbalance of the microorganisms that are normally present in the vagina, resulting when some factor causes one of the strains to reproduce more quickly than the others. The microorganisms most often involved in vaginitis are the fungus *Candida albicans* (also called monilia), the bacterium *Hemophilus vaginalis*, and the protozoan (one-celled organism) *Trichomonas vaginalis*. Possible causes of overgrowth of microorganisms in the vagina include the use of birth control pills (oral contraceptives), which produce changes in the vaginal lining; the use of certain antibiotics, which may kill some types of bacteria but allow others to flourish; the presence of a warm, moist environment (such as may be created by wearing tight pants or panty hose, nylon underwear, or a wet bathing suit), which acts as a breeding ground for infection; and, particularly for infection by *Hemophilus vaginalis* or *Trichomonas vaginalis*, the introduction of an infectious microorganism through direct sexual contact with an infected individual. Vaginitis tends to occur more often in the summer, because excessive heat and moisture are known to promote the disease.

One variety of the disease, called noninfectious vaginitis, is not caused by overproduction of microorganisms, but rather by direct irritation of the vagina by some outside agent, such as the chemical irritation that arises from the excessive use of douches, feminine hygiene sprays, bubble baths, talcum powder, and scented or colored toilet paper.

Pregnant women and those who have diabetes or gonorrhea (a sexually transmitted disease) are at a higher risk of developing vaginitis than are other women.

Symptoms

Infection by *Candida albicans* causes severe itching of the external genital organs and pain during intercourse. Because of the thick, white vaginal discharge, which resembles cottage cheese in texture and has a "yeasty" odor, this condition is commonly known as a yeast infection. This is the type of vaginitis most frequently contracted by diabetic and pregnant women.

Infection by *Hemophilus vaginalis* causes a creamy white or grayish, foul-smelling discharge.

The presence of *Trichomonas vaginalis* is indicated by itching and burning, as well as by a greenish-white discharge and foul odor. These symptoms are likely to appear during or immediately following menstruation.

Noninfectious vaginitis is characterized only by irritation and dryness, usually with no discharge.

Diagnosis

Vaginitis is diagnosed by determining which microorganism is causing the infection. Microscopic examination of a sample, or "smear," of vaginal secretions is used to make the diagnosis.

Treatment

Treatment will vary according to the type of microorganism. Fungal infections are generally treated with an antifungal cream, which is applied directly to the vagina, or as a vaginal suppository (forms of which are now available without a doctor's prescription).

Bacterial infections are treated with antibiotics, administered either orally or as vaginal suppositories. Because bacterial infections can be transferred between sexual partners, both are usually treated with oral antibiotics.

An oral antibiotic called metronidazole is given to women with protozoan infections and to their partners. Because some studies have linked this drug to cancer and genetic damage in laboratory animals, it should not be taken during the first half of pregnancy.

Noninfectious vaginitis is usually treated by avoiding the irritants that may cause it, such as perfumed soaps, chemical sprays, and scented tissues, and by not wearing tight clothing.

Prevention

Some types of vaginitis can probably be prevented by using only nonscented, white toilet paper; wearing cotton underwear and loose-fitting pants; avoiding the overuse of douches, feminine hygiene sprays, and scented toiletries; and having any sexual partners use condoms.

PROBLEMS OF COUPLES

A couple can encounter health problems in three areas: contraception (birth control), infertility, and venereal (sexually transmitted) diseases. Decisions or problems in all three areas affect both partners.

Although sex is a topic that arouses considerable curiosity and interest, it unfortunately is also surrounded by many myths and misconceptions that can lead to needless anxiety. Fortunately, societal attitudes have been changing, and there is now more free and open discussion about subjects that used to be considered taboo.

The best approach to solving any problem includes two ingredients: an understanding by both persons of how the male and female reproductive systems work and a willingness to communicate openly and honestly.

Responsibility for these areas of health should not be shouldered by either the man or the woman alone. Both partners need to work together to weigh consequences, consider alternatives, and provide support.

Birth control

Couples who want to delay or prevent pregnancy can choose from several different kinds of contraceptives: physical devices (intrauterine devices); barrier methods (condoms, cervical caps, diaphragms); chemical methods (spermicides, sponges, pills, implants), a combination of barrier and chemical methods (diaphragm with a spermicide); permanent birth control (vasectomy for men and blocking of fallopian tubes for women); and abstinence from intercourse during the woman's fertile period.

Some birth control methods require a doctor's prescription; others can be purchased over the counter. Methods vary in effectiveness, convenience, and safety. It's a good idea for a couple to discuss with a doctor the advantages and disadvantages of the various methods of birth control, especially the side effects, ease of use, and reliability. Choose the birth control method that best suits your needs as a couple; a contraceptive method that works well for one couple may not appeal to another.

Infertility

About one of every five couples who want to conceive a child is unsuccessful at doing so. If pregnancy does not occur after a year of regular sexual intercourse without contraceptives, the couple may want to consult with an obstetrician/gynecologist or a urologist who specializes in infertility.

During the last ten years or so, medical science has made tremendous inroads into diagnosing and treating causes of infertility and has thus given new hope to childless couples. Improved testing procedures, new drugs that stimulate ovulation, new methods of fertilizing a woman's egg both inside and outside of the body, and surgical techniques that can correct female or male structural problems or sometimes reverse sterilization procedures have enabled many couples to become parents.

Sexually transmitted diseases

One of the risks of intimate sexual contact, especially for men and women who have more than one partner, is infection with a sexually transmitted disease (STD), or venereal disease (VD). Despite improved diagnosis and treatment for these diseases, their incidence has increased, probably because of the sexual freedom of the last 20 years, which has resulted in large part from more reliable birth control.

Sexually transmitted diseases are caused by organisms that thrive in the warm, moist environment of the reproductive system and are transmitted by sexual contact.

Gonorrhea is the most prevalent of the STDs, but herpes, syphilis, and chlamydia are common enough to be of concern to sexually active people. Although, with the exception of herpes, these diseases can be cured, the consequences of delaying treatment are too important to ignore. Permanent sterility can result.

STDs are particularly serious for pregnant women. The diseases can be transmitted to a baby passing through the birth canal and can critically affect the child.

A person who does become infected with any of these diseases must abstain from further sexual contact until the problem has been controlled. Any sexual partners need to be informed of the possibility of infection and must seek treatment, whether or not symptoms develop.

Birth control

Birth control, also called contraception, is the voluntary prevention of pregnancy. A variety of methods are available for preventing pregnancy. Couples who use no contraceptive method have an 80 to 90 percent chance of achieving pregnancy over a 12-month period, provided that they have no underlying infertility problem.

Condom

A condom is a thin rubber or synthetic sheath that the man fits over his erect penis just before sexual intercourse. A condom used alone is about 70 percent to 90 percent effective, depending on the care with which it is used. Several problems may occur with the use of the condom. For example, tiny holes or tears may develop in the sheath, causing leakage of sperm. Also, when the penis is withdrawn from the vagina as intercourse is completed, the condom sometimes breaks or partially unrolls inside the vagina, releasing its contents. However, a condom used regularly with a spermicide is approximately 95 percent effective in preventing pregnancy. Condoms have the great advantage of being readily available in any drugstore without a prescription. They also have the advantage of helping to prevent the spread of venereal disease and acquired immune deficiency syndrome (AIDS).

Diaphragm

The diaphragm is a molded rubber cap that the woman places inside the vagina to cover the cervix. The diaphragm blocks sperm from entering the uterus. It must be inserted for each act of intercourse and left in place for six hours afterward.

Diaphragms come in different sizes and must be fitted by a physician. Used alone, diaphragms occasionally fail, either because they were not inserted correctly or because they shifted during sexual intercourse. Used with spermicides, however, diaphragms are quite effective, with only about a three percent chance of pregnancy.

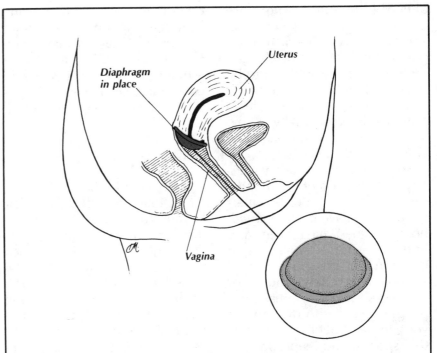

The diaphragm is a molded rubber cap that is placed inside the vagina to cover the cervix (the opening at the lower end of the uterus) before sexual intercourse. Ideally, the diaphragm blocks sperm from entering the uterus, but it should not be relied on as the sole means of contraception.

Cervical cap

The cervical cap is a molded rubber cap that fits over the outside of the cervix. While the diaphragm covers both the cervix and the back of the vagina, the smaller cervical cap fits only over the cervix. Like a diaphragm, the cervical cap blocks sperm from entering the uterus. It must be inserted for each act of intercourse and left in place for six to eight hours afterward. Cervical caps come in different sizes and must be fitted by a physician. Effectiveness in preventing pregnancy is similar to that of the diaphragm.

Spermicide

Spermicide is a chemical foam, cream, suppository, or jelly applied to the woman's vagina to kill sperm. Used alone, a spermicide is about 75 percent to 85 percent effective. Some disadvantages of a spermicide are that it must be applied before each individual act of sexual intercourse, it has chemical odors, and it may irritate the vagina. A chief advantage is that spermicides are readily available at drugstores without a prescription.

Contraceptive sponge

The contraceptive sponge is a disposable, spongelike device saturated with spermicide. A woman inserts the sponge into the vagina up against the cervix, where the device works by continuously releasing spermicide for up to 24 hours. Additional applications of spermicide are not necessary, even for multiple acts of intercourse. There are other advantages as well: the sponge is available without a prescription; unlike a diaphragm, the sponge does not have to be fitted; and the sponge can be inserted ahead of time, which allows greater spontaneity in sex. The sponge has been found to be about 85 percent effective.

Some side effects are associated with the use of the sponge. Cases of local irritation or allergic reaction have been reported; however, these have been mild and infrequent. There is also concern that the sponge could become a breeding ground for infection, especially if used improperly. You should consult your doctor about the contraceptive sponge and its proper use before trying this method of birth control.

IUD

The intrauterine device (IUD) is a small plastic device inserted into the woman's uterus by a physician. The IUD has a string attached to it that hangs into the cervix, so that the woman or her partner can check to be sure that the IUD is still in place. Most researchers believe that the IUD prevents pregnancy by causing changes in the uterine lining that disrupt the normal environment of an egg. For the woman who can use an IUD, the advantages are great, because she does not have to worry about contraception each day. The effectiveness rate is high, with only about a 5 percent chance of pregnancy.

However, there are several disadvantages to use of an IUD. Severe menstrual cramps and increased menstrual bleeding may follow the insertion of an IUD. Sometimes these side effects lessen after a month or two. In other cases, severe cramps and prolonged bleeding continue, and the physician may advise removal of the IUD. The IUD is thought to increase the risk of pelvic infection and ectopic (outside the uterus) pregnancy.

Sterilization

A woman may be sterilized by an operation that blocks the fallopian tubes (the structures through which eggs travel from the ovaries to the uterus). A man may be sterilized by a procedure called a vasectomy, in which each vas deferens (one of the two ducts through which the sperm travel from the testes to the urethra) is cut. These procedures may be reversed, but only by complicated surgery, which is not always successful. Doctors recommend sterilization only if a couple has decided, without reservation, that no future pregnancies are desired.

Oral contraceptives

Oral contraceptives, or birth control pills, are the most effective reversible method of contraception. A woman taking the pill has less than a one percent chance of getting pregnant.

The pill—which is available by prescription only—uses synthetic female hormones (estrogen and progestin) to override the natural hormonal regulation that results in the release of an egg. The pill signals the pituitary gland, which directs hormonal activity in the body, not to re-

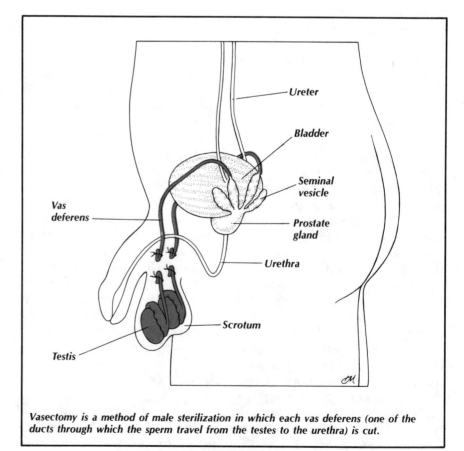

Vasectomy is a method of male sterilization in which each vas deferens (one of the ducts through which the sperm travel from the testes to the urethra) is cut.

lease the hormones that would normally stimulate the ovary to release an egg.

Each day you take one pill, at about the same time of day, removing it from a container that has the required number of pills for one cycle (usually 21). One to three days after you take the last pill for that cycle, your menstrual period begins. Menstrual periods may be lighter in flow, and cramps are reduced or absent.

If you forget to take one pill or more, menstrual bleeding may begin. In that case, you should continue taking the pills daily, but you should also use an additional contraceptive method, such as a condom, until after your next regular period.

Birth control pills are not recommended for women with a history of high blood pressure, blood-clotting problems, hepatitis, or cancer of the uterus or breast. A woman over age 35 who smokes heavily is advised to stop smoking if she wants to take the pill. Birth control pills should not be taken by a woman who suspects she may be pregnant. In addition, women with diabetes, epilepsy, heart disease, or thyroid disease may be advised not to take the birth control pill, depending on the nature and severity of the disease.

It is important for a woman taking birth control pills to report to her doctor if any of the following symptoms occur: blurred vision; severe chest pain; sudden shortness of breath; abdominal pain; unusual bleeding or bruising; breakthrough vaginal bleeding (spotting); changes in menstrual flow; pain in the calves; depression; difficult or painful urination; enlarged or tender breasts; hearing changes; increase or decrease in hair growth; migraine headaches;

numbness or tingling; rash; skin color changes; swelling of the feet, ankles, or lower legs; vaginal itching; weight changes; or yellowing of the eyes or skin.

Hormonal implants

The newest form of contraception is the hormonal implant. With this method, five small plastic rods containing the synthetic female hormone progestin are inserted with a needle under the skin of the upper arm or forearm. The hormone is gradually and slowly released from the plastic rods, thus preventing ovulation. This method is effective for about five years from the time the implants are inserted. The major advantage of this method is that the woman does not need to remember to take birth control pills or use a spermicidal agent or diaphragm before each sexual act. Disadvantages include the high cost of the implants, possible infection at the site of insertion, irregular menstruation, and the necessity for surgical incisions on the arm when the implants need to be removed. Hormonal implants are about as effective as oral contraceptives.

Natural family planning

Natural family planning is based on calculating when ovulation (release of an egg from one of the woman's ovaries each month) occurs. The couple then abstains from intercourse during the fertile period.

A man's sperm can live in a woman's body for about two days. The egg can live for about 24 hours after ovulation. A few days are added to this fertile period for safety's sake because it is so difficult to determine just

when ovulation occurs. All told, a couple needs to abstain from intercourse seven to ten days a month in order to have the greatest chance of preventing pregnancy.

There are three methods a woman can use to determine when she ovulates. The temperature method is one of the most reliable. Each morning on awakening and before getting out of bed, she takes her temperature with a special basal temperature thermometer (which measures temperatures only between 96°F and 100°F) and records it on graph paper. Near the middle of the menstrual cycle, the temperature may drop slightly (indicating that ovulation is about to occur) and then rise rapidly and continue to climb for the next three days. The temperature will not return to preovulation levels until the beginning of the menstrual period. The "safe" days to have sexual intercourse are from four days after the sudden rise in temperature until three or four days after the end of the period. It is important to become familiar with the menstrual cycle by recording temperature levels for several months before relying on this method of birth control.

The mucus method may also help determine the time of ovulation. Each morning the mucus from the vagina and cervix is examined. Cervical mucus undergoes changes as hormone levels vary during the course of the cycle. To detect these changes, the vaginal area is blotted each morning with a facial tissue and then the mucus is tested between the thumb and forefinger. After the menstrual period, there will be several days with no mucous discharge. This is followed by several days of a thick, sticky, yellow or white discharge. There will then be one or two days

No mucus for several days after period

Thick, sticky mucus for several days before ovulation

Slippery, stringy mucus indicates that ovulation is occurring

Thick, sticky mucus or no mucus after ovulation

Mucus from the cervix (neck of the uterus) undergoes changes as hormone levels vary during the menstrual cycle. The mucus can be tested between the thumb and the forefinger to detect the changes shown here.

at all. The fertile period begins with the thick, sticky, yellow or white discharge and continues until about three days after the phase when the mucus has the consistency of egg whites. Intercourse should be avoided during this time. In other words, the safe period is from three days after the slippery mucus stage to about three days after the end of the menstrual period. The use of certain medications (such as antihistamines), which alter mucus production throughout the body, will make determination of ovulation by this method difficult.

The calendar method is also an option. A record of menstrual cycles is kept for one year or more. The doctor will then use the record to work out the probable day of ovulation, based on the fact that the average woman menstruates 14 days after she ovulates. However, a woman may vary from that average, so this method is not precise.

Natural family planning does not require the use of mechanical aids or drugs. The effectiveness rate for this kind of birth control is up to about 80 percent, depending on the care with which the techniques are followed. However, even in women with regular cycles, such factors as illness, fatigue, stress, and use of certain drugs can delay ovulation or cause the techniques to become inaccurate, thereby throwing off all careful calculations.

Chlamydia

Chlamydia is a sexually transmitted bacteria that affects the reproductive organs in both males and females. Like other venereal diseases, chlamydia is a highly contagious illness spread primarily through direct sexual contact.

Complications

Left untreated, chlamydia infection can lead to prostatitis (inflammation of the prostate gland, where seminal fluid is produced) and epididymitis (inflammation of the ducts leading from the testes) in men and to pelvic inflammatory disease (an inflammation in the pelvic cavity affecting the fallopian tubes) and infertility in women. It can be transmitted from a mother to her baby during childbirth, resulting in ear infections and pneumonia in the newborn; it has also been linked to an increased risk of stillbirths and sudden infant death syndrome (SIDS).

Cause

Chlamydia is transmitted by direct sexual contact with an infected person. It displays symptoms similar to those of gonorrhea.

Symptoms

Sometimes no symptoms are evident. In other cases, there is a discharge from the penis or vagina, pain and burning during urination, and other symptoms similar to those of gonorrhea. In fact, chlamydia can occur with gonorrhea, so if symptoms persist after treatment for gonorrhea, they may be due to chlamydia.

Diagnosis

A physician can test for the presence of chlamydia infection by taking a sample of secretions from the penis or cervix. Results of this test can be obtained in as little as 30 minutes. Since gonorrhea can produce the same

when the mucus becomes transparent and very slippery, with the consistency of raw egg whites. The mucus will form a string between the thumb and forefinger. This is when ovulation occurs. After ovulation, the mucus again becomes thick and sticky, or there may be no mucus symptoms as a chlamydia infection, the doctor will usually test for both infections.

Treatment

Penicillin has no effect on chlamydia, so this disease is treated with another antibiotic, such as doxycycline, tetracycline, or erythromycin. This is why treatment of gonorrhea with penicillin will not affect a coexisting case of chlamydia.

A person who has chlamydia or any other sexually transmitted disease should abstain from sexual activity until all tests have indicated that the disease is no longer present. Every sexual partner of the infected person needs to be examined and, if necessary, treated.

Prevention

Chlamydia infection can be prevented by avoiding sexual contact with someone who has the disease. Because the chances of contracting chlamydia or any other sexually transmitted disease increase with the number of sexual partners a person has, limiting the number of partners is the first step toward prevention. Using condoms also helps to reduce the risk of contracting chlamydia.

Genital warts

Genital warts (known medically as condylomata acuminata) are viral growths that appear on the external genital organs. The condition is considered to be a sexually transmitted disease.

If left untreated, genital warts can grow quite large, causing discomfort during sexual inter-course, urination, and bowel movements. They are seen more frequently in uncircumcised men than in those who have been circumcised. Scientists now believe that some viruses that cause genital warts may, over a period of several years, lead to the development of certain genital tumors such as cancer of the cervix and cancer of the penis.

Pregnancy may make genital warts grow faster, but they usually shrink after the baby is born. They may even become large enough during pregnancy to block the birth canal, making a cesarean (through an incision in the walls of the uterus and abdomen) delivery necessary. The wart virus can be transmitted from a mother to her child during birth, sometimes causing the development of warts within the throat of the baby.

Cause

Genital warts are caused by direct sexual contact with an infected person. About 60 percent of all those exposed to genital warts will develop the condition. However, the warts will not appear until six weeks to eight months after the initial exposure.

Symptoms

The only symptom of genital warts is the warts themselves, which appear most frequently on the penis, vagina, vulva (the structure surrounding the vagina), and anus. They may also be found in the mouth or on the cervix. They are soft, moist, and pink, occurring alone or in clusters; cluster formations tend to resemble cauliflower in their uneven, puffy appearance. They are seldom painful, but they can be irritated by sexual intercourse; in fact, they often grow on the parts of the sex organs that receive the most friction during sexual intercourse.

Diagnosis

Genital warts can usually be diagnosed by a simple physical examination because their appearance is so distinctive. If there is any doubt, a sample of tissue from the wart can be tested to rule out other disorders, such as cancerous growths or the warts that often accompany syphilis (another sexually transmitted disease). Sometimes a magnifying instrument called a colposcope is used to detect small warts that are not visible to the naked eye.

Treatment

Small genital warts are treated with a drug called podophyllin, which is applied directly to the warts and then washed off several hours later. More than one application may be necessary. Because podophyllin is toxic in large quantities, very large or persistent warts are often removed by cryotherapy (a process in which liquid nitrogen is used to freeze the growths, which then fall off); by heat treatments, which dry out and destroy the warts; or by laser therapy, which literally vaporizes the growths.

A person who has genital warts or any other sexually transmitted disease should abstain from sexual activity until all tests have indicated that the disease is no longer present. As is the case with all other sexually transmitted diseases, every sexual partner of the infected person needs to be examined and, if necessary, treated.

Prevention

Genital warts can be prevented by avoiding sexual contact with someone who has the condition. Because the chances of contracting this disease increases with the number of sexual partners, limiting the number of partners is the first step in prevention. Using condoms also helps reduce risk.

Gonorrhea

Gonorrhea is one of the most frequently reported sexually transmitted diseases. It is a highly contagious bacterial infection, spread primarily through direct sexual contact.

Gonorrhea predominantly affects the penis in men, the vagina in women, and the throat and anus in both sexes. Left untreated, it can lead to a generalized blood infection, sterility (inability to conceive), arthritis, and heart trouble. In men it can also spread throughout the prostate gland and the ducts of the reproductive system, causing painful inflammation.

Gonorrhea can also lead to eye infections if the genital secretions come in contact with the eyes—for instance, if a person rubs his or her eyes after handling infected genital organs. Because the infant passes through the potentially infected birth canal during the birth process, every state requires that a few drops of silver nitrate or penicillin be placed in the eyes of all newborns to prevent infection and possible blindness.

Symptoms

In females, this disease may exist entirely without symptoms,

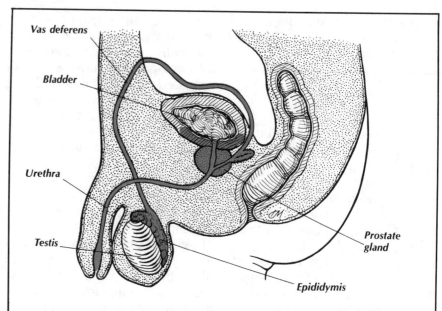

In males, untreated gonorrhea may involve the prostate gland, the male duct system (including the epididymis, which connects each testis to its vas deferens, and the vas deferens, which conducts the sperm cells to the urethra), the bladder, and the uretha.

but in many cases it is marked by a discharge from the vagina and urethra and by frequent, painful urination. Gonorrhea often leads to pelvic inflammatory disease (PID), which results when the infection extends to the fallopian tubes; the scar tissue that forms may block the tubes, often causing sterility. The symptoms of PID are lower abdominal pain, fever, chills, vaginal discharge, and vomiting.

The primary symptom of gonorrhea in men is a yellowish discharge from the penis that develops within two to ten days of exposure to the disease. The discharge is accompanied by painful and burning urination.

Gonorrhea of the anus is marked by an often bloody or mucus-filled discharge from the anus and pain during bowel movements. Gonorrhea of the throat may have no noticeable symptoms or may reveal itself only as a scratchy, sore throat or a severe, flame-red sore throat.

Diagnosis

Diagnosis is accomplished by taking a sample of the discharge, examining it under a microscope to identify the gonorrhea bacterium, and confirming the diagnosis by performing a culture (a technique in which the sample of the discharge is placed in a special substance that encourages the growth of bacteria).

Treatment

Gonorrhea is usually treated with penicillin or tetracycline, either injected or taken orally.

Men being treated for gonorrhea should avoid alcohol because recent studies have shown that drinking may increase the chances of developing an inflammation of the urethra (the canal leading from the urinary bladder through the penis).

While under treatment, the patient should abstain from sexual

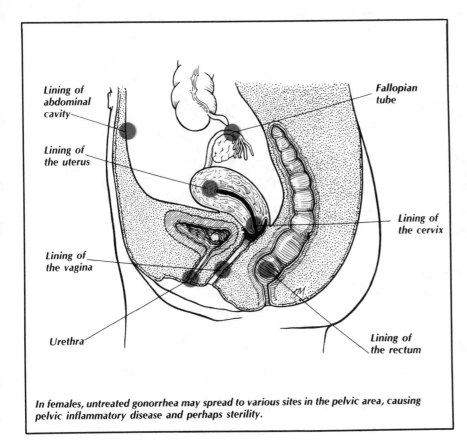

Lining of
abdominal
cavity

Lining of
the uterus

Lining of
the vagina

Urethra

Fallopian
tube

Lining of
the cervix

Lining of
the rectum

In females, untreated gonorrhea may spread to various sites in the pelvic area, causing pelvic inflammatory disease and perhaps sterility.

activity until further tests have confirmed that gonorrhea is no longer present. This testing is usually done two weeks after the beginning of treatment. If signs of the disease are still present, drug therapy can be reinstated with a different antibiotic.

A culture to detect a chlamydia infection is usually performed along with the culture to detect gonorrhea (since symptoms of the two infections are the same). If chlamydia is found, it will be treated with the antibiotic tetracycline.

Every sexual partner of the infected person should be examined and, if necessary, treated.

Prevention

Gonorrhea can be prevented by avoiding sexual contact with someone who has the disease.

Because the chance of contracting this and other venereal diseases increases with the number of sexual partners, limiting the number of partners is the first step in prevention. Using condoms helps to reduce the risk of contracting gonorrhea.

Herpes

Herpes is a sexually transmitted disease—a highly contagious illness spread primarily through direct sexual contact.

Herpes can be treated but not cured. Its symptoms appear briefly and then disappear; the disease lies dormant in nerve cells, but it may be reactivated by stress or illness. It is believed to be contagious only during active periods, when blisters are present. Persons taking drugs that suppress the body's immune sys-

tem (for instance, cancer or organ transplant patients) are at a higher risk of contracting herpes because their bodies are in a weakened state. There is also some evidence that links genital herpes with a higher rate of cancer of the cervix in women.

Herpes is spread primarily by direct sexual contact. It can also be transmitted to an infant during childbirth, causing brain damage or death. Therefore, if a woman shows signs of the active disease while in labor, the baby will be delivered by cesarean section (through an incision in the uterus and abdomen), rather than through the vagina, where the blisters may be present.

Cause

Herpes is caused by herpes simplex virus type 2, which is similar to the virus (herpes simplex virus type 1) that causes cold sores and fever blisters on the lips.

Symptoms

The predominant symptom of herpes is the outbreak of painful, itching blisters filled with fluid on and around the external sexual organs. Females may have a vaginal discharge. Symptoms vaguely similar to those of the flu may accompany these outbreaks, including fever and fatigue.

The blisters will disappear without treatment in about two to ten days, but the virus will remain, lying dormant among clusters of nerve cells until another outbreak is triggered by such factors as stress, a cold, fever, or menstruation. Many patients are able to anticipate an outbreak—they notice a warning sign, a tingling sensation called a pro-

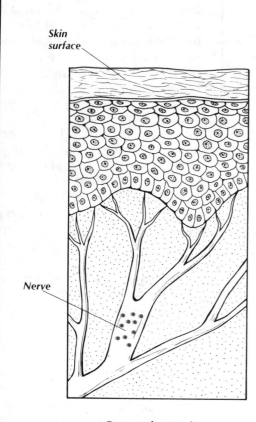

Skin surface

Nerve

Dormant herpes virus

Herpes blister

Active herpes virus

In its active stage, herpes simplex virus type 2 causes painful, itching blisters. The blisters eventually disappear, but the virus lies dormant within nerve cells until stress or illness reactivates it, triggering a new outbreak of active herpes blisters.

drome, of the approaching illness. Herpes is thought to be contagious only during actual outbreaks, so sexual activity should be avoided while blisters or other symptoms are present.

Diagnosis

Diagnosis of herpes is accomplished by microscopic examination and culture of the fluid contained in the blisters.

Treatment

Unlike other sexually transmitted diseases, herpes cannot be cured, because any medication that will attack the virus while it lies dormant in the nerve cells will also damage the nerve cells. However, there is treatment now available for acute outbreaks that involves the use of either the antiviral drug acyclovir or laser therapy, both of which will heal blisters, reduce pain, and, most important, kill large numbers of the herpes virus organisms. Acyclovir has also been found to reduce the reproduction of the virus in initial outbreaks, thus possibly lessening the number of subsequent outbreaks. It should be noted, however, that to be effective, therapy must be started immediately after the first sores appear. Every sexual partner of the infected person needs to be examined and, if necessary, treated.

Prevention

Herpes can be prevented by avoiding sexual contact with an infected person whose disease is in its active period. Because the chances of contracting this or any other sexually transmitted disease increase with the number of sexual partners a person has, limiting the number of partners is the first step toward prevention. Using condoms also helps to reduce the risk.

Infertility

Infertility is defined as a couple's failure to conceive a child after one year of regular sexual intercourse without birth control. In about 40 percent of all cases of infertility, the problem lies with the man; in 60 percent it lies with the woman or with both partners.

Infertility is not sterility. The term infertility implies that the condition can be treated and reversed—that it may be a temporary problem. The term sterility is applied to a permanent, irreversible inability to have children.

Recent research has shown that a woman's fertility drops off significantly between the ages of 31 and 35 and continues to decline thereafter until menopause, when it ceases. A man's fertility also declines after the age of 40, although men can remain fertile until old age.

Causes of male infertility

One of the major causes of male infertility is a low sperm count. It is measured by the number of active sperm present in a milliliter (there are approximately five milliliters in one teaspoon) of semen (the fluid ejected from the penis during intercourse). An average sperm count is 90 million or more sperm per milliliter. A count of at least 40 to 60 million is thought to be necessary for fertilization; when the count is less than 20 million, it is unlikely that the man can father a child (although, since only one sperm is needed to fertilize an egg, it is still possible).

A low sperm count can be caused by low levels of testosterone (the male sex hormone); by exposure to chemicals, pesticides, or radiation; by engaging in sexual intercourse too frequently, which depletes the sperm supply too quickly; and by heat (which slows sperm production) generated by wearing tight underwear or pants, sitting for long periods in hot cars or trucks, or working near ovens and kilns. Infertility can also result if sperm cannot propel themselves through the female reproductive tract to reach the egg, or if sperm are irregularly shaped (only sperm with oval-shaped heads can fertilize an egg).

In addition to problems with the sperm themselves, male infertility can be caused by any obstruction in the tubes that convey the sperm from the testes (the male sex organs where sperm are produced) to the penis. Infertility may also be caused by varicose veins in the scrotum (the pouch containing the testes), perhaps because the increased blood flow in these swollen veins brings extra heat to the area, or by a local infection or injury; the infertility problem will probably reverse itself when the condition is corrected. In addition, surgical removal of part of the prostate gland (one of the organs in which most of the fluid in semen is produced), as well as the use of certain drugs for high blood pressure, can lead to retrograde ejaculation (a disorder in which the semen is passed backward into the bladder, to exit with the urine, rather than out through the penis).

Causes of female infertility

A woman may be infertile because of a variety of conditions. It may be that she is not ovulating (releasing an egg each month); this is true in about 25 percent of all cases of female infertility. The fallopian tubes (through which the eggs travel on their way from the ovaries to the uterus) may be obstructed, often as a result of pelvic inflammatory disease (PID), which irritates the tubes and causes scar tissue to form. PID can develop as a reaction to an IUD (intrauterine device used for birth control), a sexually transmitted disease, or an infection of the lower reproductive tract. Endometriosis (the displacement of tissue from the uterine lining to elsewhere in the body) may also cause the formation of scar tissue that blocks the fallopian tubes. An imbalance of the female hormones estrogen and progesterone or of other hormones secreted from the pituitary or thyroid glands can interfere with the reproductive cycle. A "hostile" cervix (one that creates an environment that in some way prevents sperm from surviving) may also be the cause of the infertility.

Diagnosis

Diagnosis of the reason for the infertility problem will usually begin with physical examinations and complete medical and sexual histories of both partners.

A fresh sample of the man's semen will be examined under a microscope to determine the quantity and quality of the sperm. This will provide a sperm count and will also indicate whether the sperm are adequately mobile and whether the heads of the sperm are oval, both characteristics that are necessary for conception.

To determine whether ovulation is taking place in the female, the basal body temperature (the body temperature on awakening, before eating or drinking) will be taken every morning for several months. If the temperature rises by 0.6°F to 1.0°F for a few days in the middle of the menstrual cycle, ovulation is probably taking place. An endometrial biopsy, in which a sample of the lining of the uterus is obtained for examination, can also indicate whether ovulation is occurring and whether hormonal secretion is normal.

Obstruction of the fallopian tubes can be diagnosed by injecting a dye into the reproductive tract and then taking an X ray. Another test consists of injecting carbon dioxide gas into the fallopian tubes and waiting for the patient to feel pain in the upper part of the body, indicating that the gas is passing through the fallopian tubes and that there are no obstructions.

A hostile cervix can be identified by a microscopic examination of the mucus in the cervix shortly after sexual intercourse to determine the rate of sperm survival. Endometriosis is diagnosed by inserting into the abdomen a laparoscope (a small, lighted instrument), through which the doctor can actually see the uterus, fallopian tubes, ovaries, and any displaced endometrial tissue that may be causing the infertility.

Hormonal imbalances in both men and women can be diagnosed with blood tests.

Treatment

Treatment for a low sperm count caused by a testosterone deficiency is usually hormone therapy to increase testosterone levels. If the low sperm count is due to chemicals, radiation, or excess heat, exposure to these factors must be corrected or

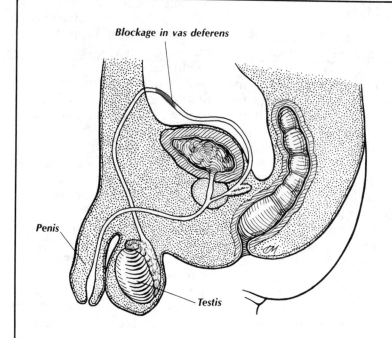

Male infertility can be caused by a blockage anywhere in the tubes that convey sperm from the testes to the penis.

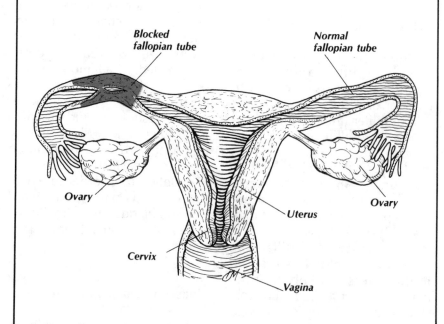

Female infertility can be caused by an obstruction in a fallopian tube, through which the egg passes from the ovary to the uterus.

avoided. If the sperm count is low for some unknown reason, there is often little more that can be done.

If male infertility is caused by varicose veins, surgery may be necessary. If an obstruction exists somewhere in the tubes leading to and through the penis, microsurgery to open the blockage may correct the problem.

Failure to ovulate is often treated with a fertility drug called clomiphene, which stimulates production of the hormone that regulates ovulation. About 60 percent of the patients who receive clomiphene become pregnant; the chances of multiple births are very low. A stronger drug, which is a combination of certain pituitary gland hormones, may also be prescribed, but it carries with it a greater risk of multiple births.

Obstructed fallopian tubes may require microsurgery in order to open the blockage, or a new procedure in which an egg is removed and replaced beyond the point of the obstruction, where it may be fertilized normally. A hostile cervix (one that creates an environment that in some way prevents sperm from surviving) can be treated with the female hormone estrogen, which stimulates the increased production of mucus, which is necessary to transport the sperm. Sometimes, sperm can be placed directly into the uterus, bypassing the cervix completely. Endometriosis can sometimes be treated by the surgical removal of displaced tissue and the scar tissue that has formed around it. Hormonal imbalances can be corrected with hormone therapy.

Test-tube, or *in vitro*, fertilization is a relatively new technique in which an egg is removed from the woman's ovary and then placed in a test tube or special sterile dish containing the man's sperm. Once the egg has been fertilized, it is placed into the woman's uterus, where it will continue to grow and develop into a baby. This technique is used primarily in women whose blocked fallopian tubes cannot be opened by surgery.

Another new technique used to treat infertility is called gamete intra fallopian transfer (GIFT). In this procedure, clomiphene or another fertility drug is given to the woman to stimulate ovulation. When an egg is produced by the ovary, it is removed via laparoscopy and immediately mixed with sperm from the man. This sperm-egg mixture is then transferred by laparoscopy into a fallopian tube, where fertilization may then take place normally. Fertilization occurs in the woman's body and not in a test tube. GIFT is a complicated and expensive procedure that should be used only by couples who have not been able to conceive using standard treatments for infertility.

Although recent advances in treating infertility have led to greater and greater success, about 15 percent of all female infertility problems and about 10 percent of all male fertility problems remain undiagnosed and therefore untreatable.

Artificial insemination

Artificial insemination is the introduction of semen (the fluid containing sperm) into a woman's vagina or uterus by means other than sexual intercourse (usually with a special syringe) at or before the time of ovulation in the hope of achieving fertilization. The semen may be from the woman's partner or from a donor.

Artificial insemination using semen from the partner is sometimes done when he has a low sperm count—that is, when there are not enough sperm per unit of fluid to be likely to fertilize an egg. To obtain enough sperm, several collections may be made over a period of days or weeks; the sperm obtained is frozen, pooled, and used in one insertion. Artificial insemination may also be used when one or the other partner cannot perform the sexual act in a normal manner, perhaps because of a physical condition or because of an emotional problem.

Artificial insemination using semen from a donor can be an alternative to adoption when the partner cannot father a child, whether because of low sperm count, absence of sperm, poor quality of sperm, or lack of motion by sperm or because of inability to perform sexual intercourse. It may also be considered when the partner carries a genetic defect that he does not want to transmit.

Syphilis

Syphilis is a serious, highly contagious disease spread primarily by direct sexual contact with an affected individual. Syphilis is caused by spiral-shaped bacteria called spirochetes.

Over time, syphilis can affect all parts of the body—the brain, bones, spinal cord, and heart, as well as the reproductive organs. If left untreated, blindness, brain damage, heart disease, and even death can result. Syphilis can also be passed from a mother to her unborn baby, causing congenital syphilis in the child. Congenital syphilis may eventually result in blindness and deafness, among other serious consequences in the newborn baby. Syphilis in a pregnant woman must be treated prior to the eighteenth week of the pregnancy in order to prevent passage of the disease to the fetus.

Stages and symptoms

Syphilis is a progressive disorder that passes through three stages: primary, secondary, and tertiary.

Primary syphilis is characterized by the appearance of a painless, open sore (called a chancre) 10 to 90 days after exposure to the disease. As a rule, there is usually only one sore, appearing most commonly on the genital organs, but also appearing at times on the rectum, cervix, lips, tongue, fingers, or anywhere that direct contact was made. The chancre first appears as a red bump, sometimes surrounded by a red ring that oozes clear fluid; it soon turns into a painless ulcer and disappears within several weeks without treatment. Although the chancre itself is gone, the disease is still active in the body.

Secondary syphilis usually appears within six weeks to six months of initial contact. Symptoms resembling those of the flu (fever, sore throat, headache, fatigue, aching joints, and enlarged lymph nodes) are common. Secondary syphilis is also characterized by extremely contagious, red or reddish-brown erosions that can be seen on the lining of the mouth, the penis, the external female sex organs, the anus, and warm, moist areas, such as the underarms; by growths resembling warts in the genital area (not to be confused with the more common nonsyphilitic genital warts; for more information on nonsyphilitic genital warts,

In its final stages, syphilis can seriously damage the brain, spinal cord, bones, heart, and reproductive organs.

see pages 313-314); and by a rash on the palms of the hands or the soles of the feet in the form of round, reddish spots that occur in patches and do not itch. These sores, growths, and rashes heal within three to six weeks without treatment, and the disease enters the third stage.

At the beginning of the third stage, all symptoms disappear and the disease becomes latent (present but not showing symptoms) for a time. The patient appears to be healthy, and the disease is probably no longer contagious (except in the case of pregnant women, who can still pass it on to their offspring). This latent stage can last indefinitely, but in about one third of patients the disease will most likely

progress, and the entire body may come under siege. The brain, bones, spinal cord, and heart may be affected, resulting in blindness, brain damage, heart disease, or even death.

Diagnosis

Syphilis is diagnosed on the basis of the patient's medical and sexual history and findings from the physical examination, blood tests, and microscopic examination of a sample taken from the sores or rash areas. Several blood tests may be necessary because the bacteria may not show up on blood tests during the first one to two weeks after exposure to the infection.

Treatment

Treatment consists of the administration of penicillin (or another antibiotic, if a penicillin allergy exists). Some cases of late syphilis are so advanced, however, that they cannot be treated.

A person who has syphilis or any other sexually transmitted disease should abstain from sexual activity until all tests have confirmed that the disease is no longer contagious. Every sexual partner needs to be tested and, if necessary, treated.

Prevention

Syphilis can be prevented by avoiding sexual contact with someone who has the disease. Because the chances of contracting this or any other sexually transmitted disease increase with the number of sexual partners a person has, limiting the number of partners is the first step toward prevention. Using condoms also helps to reduce the risk of contracting syphilis and other sexually transmitted diseases.

PREGNANCY AND CHILDBIRTH

This chapter considers the normal course of the childbearing process—from conception to childbirth—as well as common disorders that may arise during pregnancy.

CONCEPTION

Conception is the union of a sperm cell from the father with an egg from the mother to begin a new life.

Ovulation

During the course of her life, the average woman produces 350 to 400 eggs, or ova. The two organs in which the eggs are produced, known as ovaries, are located near the top and on either side of the uterus. Ducts known as fallopian tubes conduct the eggs toward the uterus. At the midpoint of the average 28-day menstrual cycle, an egg matures in one of the ovaries, is expelled from the ovary during the process called ovulation, and starts to travel through the nearby fallopian tube toward the uterus. The egg is propelled by the waving action of tiny hairlike structures, known as cilia, that line the tube. If the egg meets a sperm cell en route, conception may occur.

Fertilization

Sperm cells—which look like tadpoles through a microscope—originate in the man's testes. At the climax of sexual intercourse, an average of 300 million to 500 million sperm cells, contained in a teaspoonful of thick white fluid, spurt from the tip of the man's penis deep into the woman's vagina. Immediately

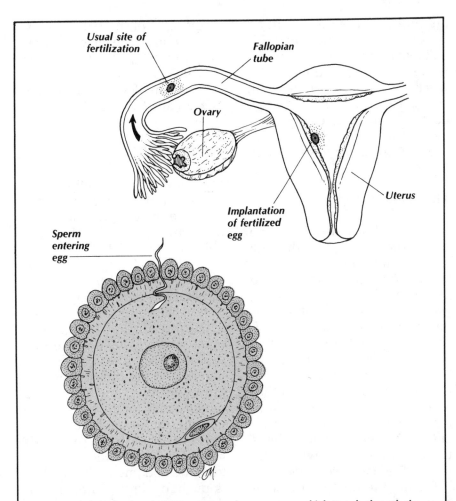

Once a month, one of a woman's ovaries releases an egg, which travels through the nearby fallopian tube toward the uterus. Conception occurs if a sperm unites with the egg. The fertilized egg then continues its progress toward the uterus, where it becomes implanted in the endometrial lining.

the sperm start swimming forward, propelled by their long, waving tails and aided by contractions of the muscles of the woman's vagina and uterus. The goal of the sperm is to swim through the cervix, into the uterus, and up one of the fallopian tubes to fertilize an egg.

Millions of sperm are killed by the acidic secretions of the vagina and the cervix or become trapped by mucus in the vagina. (During the middle of the woman's menstrual cycle, when the egg is moving along a fallopian tube, the secretions are thinner, less acidic, and less of a barrier; also, there are alkaline chemicals in the fluid accompanying the sperm, which act to neutralize the woman's acidic secretions.) The vast majority of sperm fail to pass through the uterus and up one of the fallopian tubes. During most of the woman's menstrual cycle, both tubes are empty and the sperm find nothing to fertilize. Only for a few days is an egg present in one of the tubes, and then it may be reached by only a few of the millions of sperm cells that began the journey. The sperm completely surround the egg, their tails waving furiously in an attempt to force their pointed heads into the female cell. Finally, one succeeds. The tail detaches, and the head moves toward the center of the egg. In seconds, a chemical change comes about in the egg that prevents the entry of any other sperm. Conception has occurred.

The fertilized egg

Unlike all other cells in the body, the sperm and the egg each contain only 23 chromosomes (chromosomes are the chemical "blueprints" that together determine all of the inherited characteristics of an individual; all of the other cells contain twice that number). In the first 12 hours after conception, the 23 chromosomes from the mother and the 23 chromosomes from the father join to form a new nucleus of 46 chromosomes. This is the basic unit from which the new individual will develop.

During the next four or five days, as the fertilized egg, or zygote, drifts down the fallopian tube and into the uterus, the original cell divides and subdivides into anywhere from 16 to 48 cells. In another two or three days, the growing cluster of cells becomes implanted in the nourishing, blood-rich lining of the mother's uterus, which soon forms the beginning of a placenta around the baby-to-be, called an embryo at this stage. (The placenta is the structure through which oxygen and nutrients pass from the mother to the fetus and through which carbon dioxide and other waste products pass from the fetus to the mother.) Within about 17 days after conception, the placenta begins blood circulation to the embryo. In the embryo, various cells are specializing to form dif-

ferent parts of the baby's body. By the end of the seventh week of pregnancy, all of the basic structures of the body have been formed. The developing embryo now is called a fetus until birth.

PREGNANCY

Pregnancy is the condition that exists in a woman between the time one of her eggs is fertilized by a sperm and the time her child is born.

Physical changes

During normal pregnancy, many changes take place in a woman's body. The abdomen expands, and the breasts enlarge, grow sensitive, and prepare to produce milk for the baby. Blood volume increases by up to 30 percent. Breathing proceeds more from the chest and less from the abdomen. The bladder is pushed higher into the abdomen because of the increased abdominal space taken up by the growing fetus. The amount of blood flowing through the kidneys increases by 25 percent to 40 percent because wastes must be eliminated from both the mother and fetus. There is a slight increase in the acidity of the saliva (this may be one of the causes of the nausea and vomiting that are so common). The nipples and external genitalia may darken, and brown spots or splotches may appear on the skin. A hormone called relaxin causes the ligaments (connective tissues that link bones together at joints) to begin to loosen during the tenth or twelfth week of pregnancy; this will be particularly important in the pelvic area because it will allow greater flexibility at the time of delivery.

Many of the glands increase in size as well.

Symptoms

Usually the first symptom noticed by a pregnant woman is a missed menstrual period. Nausea and vomiting ("morning sickness") are also common symptoms of pregnancy.

The nine months of pregnancy are usually thought of medically as three three-month periods, or trimesters. During the first trimester, the woman may experience nausea and vomiting, her breasts and nipples will become enlarged, and her waistline may expand. In the second trimester, the uterus expands, abdominal enlargement becomes more apparent, and the woman can feel the fetus move. Many women feel their best during this trimester. During the last three months, pregnancy tends to become a more cumbersome condition, and the woman may feel tired much of the time. The fetus often "drops" lower in the uterus in the last month.

Prenatal care

Many women wait until they have missed a second period before consulting their doctor. Once the doctor has confirmed the pregnancy, a program of prenatal (before birth) care will be prescribed for the mother-to-be. Prenatal care consists chiefly of making sure that nothing goes wrong with this completely normal and natural process—in other words, that there are no complications.

Good nutrition is especially important during pregnancy. The body's requirements for calcium and phosphorus, two essential

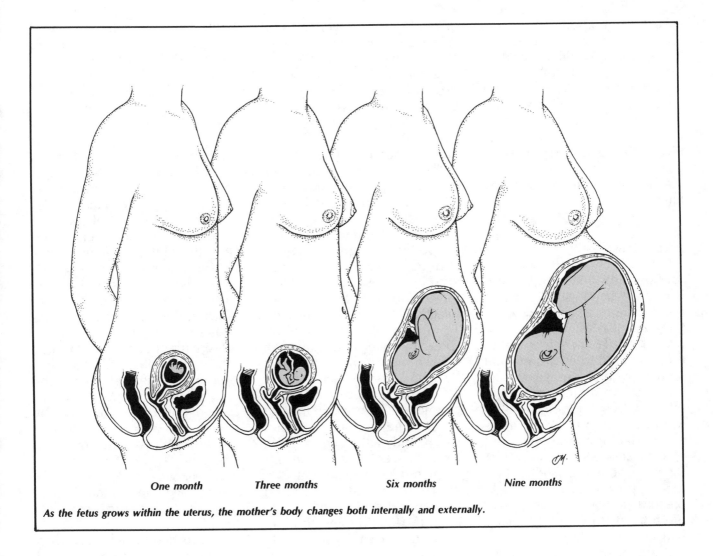

| One month | Three months | Six months | Nine months |

As the fetus grows within the uterus, the mother's body changes both internally and externally.

minerals in food, almost double, and there is an increase in the demand for iron and many other elements. Gradual caloric increases are not only allowed but advisable, provided that the additional food does not consist of empty calories, such as excess starches and sugars. Fresh fruits and vegetables and appropriate amounts of high-protein, low-fat foods are good choices. Generally, if the woman was consuming 2,000 calories before pregnancy with no weight gain, she should raise her intake to 2,200 to 2,400 calories in early pregnancy; she may be advised to increase that figure to 2,600 calories by the later stages.

If the baby's weight is included, most women should gain approximately 23 to 26 extra pounds by the ninth month. This additional weight puts more stress on the back and on the legs, sometimes resulting in such problems as swayback and varicose veins (swollen veins close to the skin surface) in the legs. These conditions can be eased by getting proper rest and exercise and by wearing special hosiery to alleviate or prevent varicose veins.

Once the initial period of nausea and vomiting is over (usually after two or three months), many women increase their caloric intake too much, sometimes in a

mistaken attempt to "make up for what the baby is taking." As a consequence, they experience a drastic gain in weight. At the other extreme are those mothers who cannot eat normally because nausea persists throughout pregnancy. In each of these cases, both the mother and the fetus may suffer. If any sudden weight gain or loss is experienced, the physician should be informed.

Due to either rapid weight gain or inadequate kidney function, some women experience significant swelling in the ankles and lower legs and, to a lesser extent, in the hands and fingers. Under no circumstances should nonprescription diuretics (drugs that increase urinary output) be taken for this condition. The doctor should be consulted.

Proper rest and exercise are important throughout pregnancy. In general, a woman can participate in most, if not all, of the activities and sports she was taking part in before her pregnancy. Her doctor can advise her about any limitations.

Precautions

Many substances and organisms have been found to affect the development and survival of the fetus. It is estimated that 20 percent of all birth defects are directly related to environmental factors such as drugs, viruses, and vitamin deficiencies. Another 60 percent are caused by the interaction of an environmental factor and an inherited predisposition. So it is important for every woman who is contemplating pregnancy or is already pregnant to beware of the possible hazards to which her baby may be vulnerable.

One of the most important aspects of prenatal care is safety in the use of medications and the ingestion of nonfood substances. A pregnant woman (or one who even suspects she is pregnant) should never take a medication without her doctor's recommendation or approval. This caution includes over-the-counter preparations—even aspirin—as well as prescription drugs. In addition, a woman should not smoke during pregnancy, and she should limit, if not eliminate, consumption of alcoholic beverages. Smoking has been linked to miscarriage (the expulsion of the fetus before it is capable of surviving on its own), low birth weight, and prematurity. Alcohol, too, has been

linked to miscarriage, and studies have shown that alcohol can affect the brain of the fetus. Products containing caffeine should probably also be limited. The best guideline to remember is that no drug or nonfood substance can be assumed to be harmless during pregnancy.

The fetus is also susceptible to infections that affect the mother-to-be, especially rubella (German measles) and certain sexually transmitted diseases, such as herpes. A pregnant woman should avoid immunizations with live viruses and postpone travel to foreign countries where infectious diseases are prevalent. Toxoplasmosis, an infection spread by eating or preparing uncooked meat or handling a cat's litter box, presents another risk. The parasite that causes toxoplasmosis is harbored in the bodies of some food animals (pigs, sheep, and cattle) and in the intestinal tracts of cats. A pregnant woman need not forgo meat or get rid of her cat. She should, however, be certain to cook meat thoroughly and to avoid emptying or cleaning the cat's litter box.

A woman's doctor will also advise against unnecessary X rays during pregnancy.

As the medical profession has learned more about inherited diseases, it has been able to offer genetic counseling to couples concerned about the possibility of having a child with an inherited disease or abnormality. A genetic counselor or specialist in genetic disorders can estimate the likelihood that a couple's offspring will be afflicted with a problem due to an inherited trait or to the age of the parents. For some genetic disorders, tests can determine whether one or both parents are carriers or can detect whether a defect is present in a

fetus. However, genetic counseling cannot guarantee the health of a child; it can only be a source of advice.

CHILDBIRTH

A normal pregnancy that has run its full course is called a "full-term pregnancy"—the baby is born after a full gestational (developmental) period of about 40 weeks. If the birth occurs earlier than the thirty-seventh week, it is considered premature.

There are three stages of normal labor and vaginal childbirth. During the first stage, contractions of the uterus open the cervix (the neck of the uterus). The plug of mucus that has been sealing off the uterus from the vagina for nine months is expelled. This is often followed by either a slow trickle or a sudden gush of amniotic fluid as the amniotic sac, in which the baby has been growing, breaks. At this point, the woman should notify her physician and go to the hospital.

The second stage begins when the cervix is completely dilated (opened). The contractions become much stronger, accompanied by an urge to bear down and push the baby along the birth canal. A doctor or midwife will instruct the woman to push down only during a contraction so that she conserves her energy and strength. After the baby has emerged, the umbilical cord, which connects the baby to the placenta, is tied and cut.

The baby, who usually gasps and cries on delivery, is immediately checked by the obstetrician or pediatrician. After being cleaned off, the baby may be given to the mother to hold.

Five or ten minutes later, the placenta, or afterbirth, is pushed out by more contractions of the uterus. After this third stage has been completed, the physician will stitch any tears or incisions that were made in the vagina and give the woman medication to stop excessive bleeding.

The entire birthing process can last anywhere from 5 to 24 hours; the average is about 12 hours. Childbirth usually takes longer if it is the woman's first delivery.

In about one out of six pregnancies, vaginal delivery is not possible or desirable, and a cesarean section must be performed. The baby is delivered through an incision in the mother's abdominal wall. (For more information on cesarean delivery, see the following section.)

More and more expectant fathers are taking active roles in the birthing process by attending prenatal classes and participating in the delivery. Most hospitals now welcome fathers into the delivery room so that they can witness the miracle of childbirth and can comfort and support the mother while she goes through labor.

Anesthesia

Although once the norm, general anesthesia is now rarely used during vaginal childbirth because, among other reasons, it slows uterine contractions and causes sluggishness and the possibility of respiratory problems in the baby. Other forms of anesthesia that are used during childbirth include pudendal block; paracervical block; and spinal, epidural, and caudal anesthesia.

In pudendal block, local anesthetic is injected through the wall of the vagina or through the skin of the buttock to reach the pudendal nerve. Blocking this nerve eliminates pain and feeling from the lower part of the vagina, the rear portion of the vulva (the external genitals), and the surrounding skin. It is often used when delivery is going well and the mother wants to push. Sometimes this type of anesthesia is used following a paracervical block, in which a local anesthetic is injected around the opening of the uterus.

Various types of spinal anesthesia are used in childbirth. In one method, a solution containing local anesthetic is injected between the fourth and fifth vertebrae of the lower back into the fluid-filled sac surrounding the spinal cord. The heavy solution mixes with the spinal fluid and settles downward, blocking off pain messages from below the waist for about an hour.

Epidural anesthesia has an effect similar to that of spinal anesthesia. The anesthetic is injected at the same place, but instead of being introduced into the spinal fluid in a single injection, it can be administered over a period of hours through a fine plastic tube with its tip resting against the tough dural membrane covering the spinal cord (the prefix *epi* means upon, hence the term epidural). The nerves are blocked where they enter the spinal cord, producing a numbing effect. Because the dural membrane is not punctured, the chance of complications, such as headache and infection, is reduced. Caudal anesthesia is the same as epidural except that the tube is introduced at the very tip of the spine (caudal comes from the Latin word meaning tail). Because both epidural and caudal anesthesia can slow labor if administered too soon, they are not given until the woman is in active labor.

Cesarean section

Cesarean section is a way of delivering a baby by cutting through the external walls of the mother's abdomen and uterus and removing the baby through these incisions. Cesarean section is performed when a vaginal delivery would cause injury to either the mother or the baby.

In the United States today, about 10 percent to 20 percent of births are by cesarean section. While cesarean delivery is still considered major surgery, the availability of antibiotics, improved anesthetic techniques, and blood transfusions has made cesareans much safer than in the past. Nevertheless, the indications for performing a cesarean section and the disadvantages of the procedure should be weighed carefully by the woman and her physician.

Types

There are two main types of cesarean section.

In the *classic cesarean,* an incision is made vertically on the skin of the abdomen, extending from the navel to the pubic bone. A vertical cut is also made directly down the center of the uterus in its thick upper section. This operation is generally used only if the baby is lying in an abnormal position or if the placenta is located in an abnormally low position in the cavity of the uterus.

The *lower-segment cesarean* is the more commonly performed procedure. The incision in the uterus is made in the lower, thinner section. This incision may be either a vertical cut down the middle or a curved, smile-shaped cut near the lower part of the abdomen.

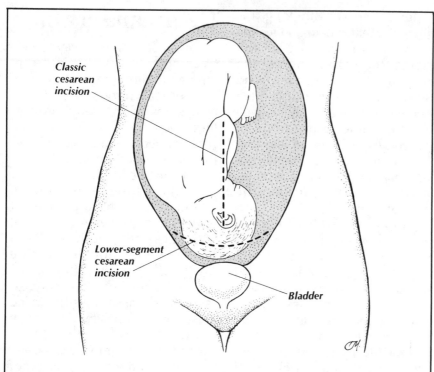

A cesarean section is a way of delivering a baby by cutting through the walls of the mother's abdomen and uterus and removing the baby through these incisions. The incision for the classic cesarean is a vertical cut down the center of the abdomen and uterus. One type of incision for the lower-segment cesarean is a curved cut near the lower part of the abdomen.

The classic cesarean produces more bleeding than the lower-segment cesarean. Also, the incision is more difficult to repair, and the uterus is more likely to rupture during a future pregnancy. For these reasons, the classic cesarean is seldom used today unless there are specific reasons.

Reasons

Some of the reasons for a cesarean section include:

- To save the baby's life when the umbilical cord (the fetus' supply line from the placenta) is being pinched off during the birth process, or any other time that the fetus is not getting enough blood and oxygen to survive. (These conditions may be indicated by abnormal heart rate patterns during fetal monitoring.)
- To prevent infection of the baby by a dangerous vaginal infection, such as herpes.
- To prevent injury to the baby that may result from a breech birth, during which a baby emerges through the vagina buttocks or feet first rather than head first. (Many obstetricians believe that cesarean delivery is necessary for all breech births in first-time mothers and all premature breech births.)
- To ease the birth or prevent injury when the baby is too large for a vaginal delivery.
- To deliver the baby if the mother fails to give birth after a long labor.
- To save the baby's life if problems with the placenta cause a decrease in the blood supply to the fetus.

- To facilitate delivery if immediate birth would allow more effective treatment of disease in the mother or the baby.
- To be safe if the mother has had a previous cesarean delivery. (The rule used to be that any woman who had one cesarean would have to have cesarean sections for all subsequent births; however, in recent years, many vaginal deliveries have been performed successfully on women who had previous lower-segment cesarean sections.)

Disadvantages

Risks of a cesarean section include possible infection, bleeding, and the formation of dangerous blood clots. There is a small chance that the uterus will rupture during a subsequent pregnancy, before or during birth. The cesarean may be inconvenient for the mother, requiring her to stay in the hospital for five to seven days instead of going home with her baby in three days or less. She may not be able to see the baby for a number of hours after delivery if she has undergone general anesthesia. Breast-feeding may be difficult if the mother is being given strong medications to relieve pain, which keep her asleep for long periods of time. There is pain from the abdominal incision, and the mother's activity is restricted once she arrives home. It takes up to six weeks for complete healing of the incision. The expense of the surgical procedure and the extra hospitalization is also a consideration. However, these disadvantages are relatively unimportant if they save the baby from permanent brain damage or save the life of the infant or the mother.

Ectopic pregnancy

An ectopic pregnancy is one in which the fertilized egg develops outside the uterus. Usually it occurs in one of the two fallopian tubes, through which the egg travels from the ovary to the uterus. (In that case, it is also known as a tubal pregnancy.) However, on rare occasions, the fertilized egg starts to develop in the ovary, on the cervix, or attached to the outside of a nearby organ in the abdominal cavity. (The ovary is not directly connected to the fallopian tube. There is a slight gap, which sometimes permits an egg to enter the abdominal cavity.)

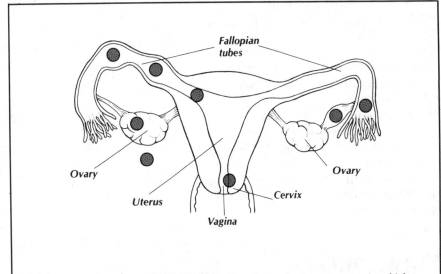

The circles indicate some of the possible sites of an ectopic pregnancy, in which a fertilized egg develops outside the uterus. The most common site is in one of the fallopian tubes, but development in an ovary, on the cervix, or attached to another organ in the abdominal cavity can also occur.

Causes

The usual cause of an ectopic pregnancy is an obstruction or narrowing of the fallopian tube that prevents the egg from passing through the tube to the uterus. The obstruction or narrowing is usually the result of inflammation or scarring from an infection, such as gonorrhea, but it may also develop after abdominal surgery or because of a growth, such as a pelvic tumor. Tubal infections can occur after miscarriage or childbirth or during the use of an intrauterine contraceptive device (IUD); if severe, blockage may result.

Complications

An ectopic pregnancy may be fatal unless it is promptly treated. The danger of a tubal pregnancy is that it will not be detected until the tube has ruptured (broken), causing massive bleeding. When a fertilized egg begins to develop in an area other than the uterus, such as the ovary or the cervix, nearby large blood vessels may be invaded, causing massive bleeding.

Symptoms

Symptoms of ectopic pregnancy usually begin two to four weeks after a woman misses her menstrual period. She may be bothered by sharp, continuous pains on one side of her lower abdomen and by slight bleeding from her vagina. When rapid bleeding occurs, which is usually not until after the sixth week of the pregnancy, she may experience sudden sharp pains in the lower abdomen, backache, low blood pressure, fainting, and shock (circulatory shock).

Diagnosis

The examining doctor may discover a tender swelling on one side of the pelvis. Movement of the uterus during a pelvic examination may cause pain. When ectopic pregnancy is suspected, the patient is hospitalized immediately. An ultrasound study (see pages 407-408) may reveal the outline of the expanding mass. In most cases, there is slow bleeding from the end of the fallopian tube into the abdominal cavity, which may be detected by inserting a hollow needle through the wall of the vagina beneath the cervix. The diagnosis is confirmed by inserting a laparoscope (a lighted tubelike instrument) through a small incision in the abdomen to inspect the area directly.

Treatment

Treatment for ectopic pregnancy is surgical removal of the embryo and surrounding tissues. When the condition occurs in a fallopian tube, the entire tube and sometimes the ovary must be removed. It is sometimes possible to reconstruct the tube.

A woman who has had one ectopic pregnancy has about a 15 percent chance of having a second one. This does not mean that she should not try to become pregnant again; however, when she does try, she should be especially watchful for symptoms of ectopic pregnancy, and when she suspects that conception has occurred, she should see her physician immediately so that the location of the embryo can be determined.

Episiotomy

An episiotomy is a surgical incision into the tissues surrounding the opening of the vagina during childbirth in order to make the delivery easier and to avoid extensive tearing of the tissues. The advantage of the procedure is that it substitutes a controlled surgical incision for excessive stretching and tearing of all the tissues. The incision itself is easier to repair later than a tear or break in the tissues would be.

Episiotomy is often performed in women who are having their first baby. With subsequent pregnancies, episiotomy may not be necessary, since the tissues surrounding the vagina have often been stretched sufficiently by the first delivery to allow an easy second delivery.

The most common type of episiotomy is an incision made with surgical scissors from the midpoint of the vaginal opening directly down toward the anus. An important risk with this type of incision is that during the birth, the opening might further extend into the anal sphincter (the ring of muscle surrounding the opening from the rectum) or the rectum itself; however, such a tear can be repaired relatively easily and will eventually heal itself. To

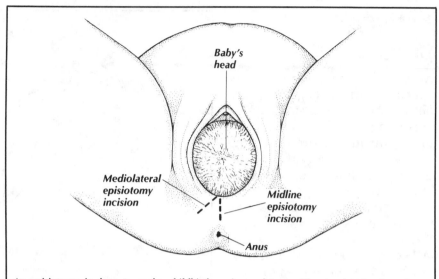

An episiotomy is done to make childbirth easier and to avoid extensive tearing of tissues. The most common type of episiotomy is a midline incision from the midpoint of the vaginal opening directly downward toward the anus. Some doctors, however, prefer an incision at an angle, called a mediolateral episiotomy.

avoid the risks of entering the rectum, some physicians prefer the mediolateral episiotomy, in which the incision is made at an angle, thus avoiding the rectum and anus.

Hyperemesis gravidarum

Hyperemesis gravidarum is a term that refers to excessive vomiting during pregnancy. This type of vomiting is more severe than that caused by ordinary morning sickness, which usually clears up on its own within a few months. In hyperemesis gravidarum, the vomiting leads to starvation, dehydration (excessive loss of water from the tissues), and a disruption of the chemical balance in the body.

Symptoms include loss of weight, dehydration, and, in very severe cases, jaundice (yellowing of the skin and the whites of the eyes). The condition is most often treated in the hospital through the use of antivomiting drugs and intravenous feeding to correct the possible malnutrition, dehydration, and chemical imbalance. A pregnant woman should not attempt to treat the vomiting with drugs without consulting her doctor.

Mastitis

Mastitis is an inflammation of the breast, most often caused by bacterial invasion and infection.

Causes

This condition occurs most frequently in nursing mothers and is caused by bacteria normally found on the skin and nipples. The bacteria enter the breast through the nipple and infect the milk glands and ducts. In many cases, the condition occurs on the third to fifth day after the birth of the baby because of the development of cracked nipples, through which bacteria enter.

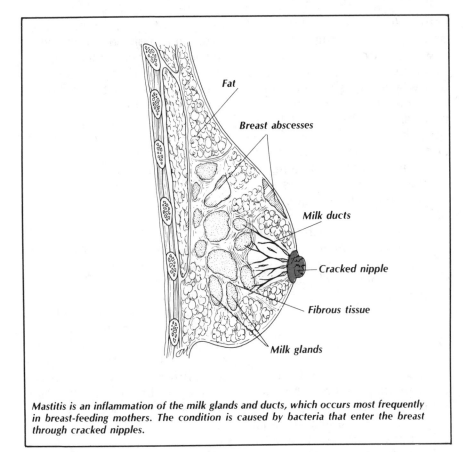

Fat

Breast abscesses

Milk ducts

Cracked nipple

Fibrous tissue

Milk glands

Mastitis is an inflammation of the milk glands and ducts, which occurs most frequently in breast-feeding mothers. The condition is caused by bacteria that enter the breast through cracked nipples.

Symptoms

Symptoms of mastitis include pain, swelling, redness, high fever, and a tender lump in the breast. Sometimes the lymph nodes in the armpit next to the affected breast may be tender and swollen. In cases of severe infection, there may be pus in the breast.

Diagnosis

The diagnosis of mastitis is generally made on the basis of the physical examination and the patient's medical history. If there is a severe infection, signaled by the appearance of pus coming from the nipple, a specimen of the pus may be examined under a microscope in order to identify the causative organism.

Treatment

Antibiotics are given to combat the infection. A nursing mother can continue nursing from the unaffected breast, but her physician may recommend that she discontinue nursing from the infected breast and expel the milk by hand to prevent painful breast swelling. Even though most antibiotics will enter the breast milk in small quantities, this will not harm the baby. When the infection clears, nursing from the previously infected breast can be resumed. If there is a great deal of pus, the pus may have to be drained.

Prevention

A woman who is breast-feeding a baby can reduce the risk of developing mastitis by keeping her nipples clean and dry between feedings and by wearing clothing that does not rub or irritate the nipples.

Miscarriage

A miscarriage (in medical terms, a spontaneous abortion) is the ending of a pregnancy due to the premature delivery of the fetus before the beginning of the twentieth week of pregnancy. At that point, the fetus is not developed enough to survive outside the uterus on its own. (After the twentieth week of pregnancy, a spontaneous abortion is considered a premature delivery or, if the fetus is dead at delivery, a stillbirth. A pregnancy that is ended artificially is commonly known as an abortion, although the medical term is termination of pregnancy.) Most miscarriages occur within the first 14 weeks of pregnancy.

It is impossible to know the number of miscarriages that occur during the first month of pregnancy before a woman realizes that she is pregnant; the only indication is a slightly late menstrual period with a heavier than normal flow. However, about 12 percent of known pregnancies end in miscarriage.

Types

There are several different types of miscarriages. A *threatened miscarriage* is experienced by about one of every five pregnant women when vaginal bleeding occurs during the first three months. Although such bleeding may indicate a spontaneous abortion, it is rarely more than a threat, and the pregnancy will continue normally. An *in-*

evitable miscarriage refers to a situation in which bleeding occurs, the cervix begins to dilate (open), but the uterine contents are not yet expelled. A *missed miscarriage* occurs when the fetus dies in the uterus but is not naturally expelled, and the woman has no bleeding or pain to signify that the pregnancy is not progressing; the physician usually diagnoses the condition when the uterus stops enlarging.

Causes

The reason that a miscarriage occurs is not always understood, but it is believed that a fetus is usually aborted because it is not developing normally. Several factors can contribute to a miscarriage, including abnormalities in the father's sperm; abnormalities in the egg; disease in the mother (for example, an infection, a glandular disorder, high blood pressure, kidney or heart disease, or diabetes); uterine abnormalities; the mother's poor nutrition or use of cigarettes, alcohol, or drugs; and exposure to environmental pollutants. Because the fetus is so well protected within the uterus, a fall or other trauma suffered by the mother is rarely, if ever, the cause of miscarriage.

The expulsion of the fetus resulting from an abnormality is thought to be a chance event, not due to a problem or defect in either parent. Of women who miscarry once, most (about 80 percent) have a successful subsequent pregnancy.

Symptoms

The symptoms of miscarriage are vaginal bleeding (from a few drops to a heavy flow) and cramps (either dull and constant or sharp and intermittent) in the lower abdomen or back. The bleeding can start suddenly or follow a brownish discharge. A solid clot of material or tissue may pass from the vagina. If possible, this should be saved for the doctor, who may be able to examine it and determine a reason for the expulsion. A miscarriage can be complete (the uterus expels all the tissue) or incomplete (tissue remains inside the uterus).

A pregnant woman who starts bleeding or experiences pain should contact her physician immediately.

Diagnosis

Depending on the type of miscarriage, diagnosis may be made on the basis of the medical history, physical examination, analysis of any discharge, blood and urine tests, or ultrasound studies (in which sound waves are used to visualize the fetus).

Treatment

There is no medical treatment to stop or avert an inevitable miscarriage. (The drug diethylstilbestrol, or DES, used to be prescribed to deter miscarriages until it was discovered that it had little effect and could cause fetal abnormalities.) The physician generally directs the woman with symptoms to rest in bed and abstain from sexual intercourse.

After an inevitable, incomplete, or missed miscarriage, any remaining fetal or placental tissue must be removed by a surgical procedure known as dilatation and curettage (D&C), in which the physician expands the cervix and gently scrapes out residual material from inside the uterus. Without this precaution, a woman is more susceptible to infections and heavy bleeding.

It is normal for a woman to feel depressed by the loss of the expected child, but it is usually safe for her to attempt to conceive soon afterward (six to eight weeks later) on the advice of her physician.

Prevention

More and more information is becoming available about the effect of drugs and nutritional and environmental factors on pregnancy. It is advisable for a woman, at the beginning of her pregnancy, to obtain adequate prenatal care and the most up-to-date information on the substances and practices that may contribute to a miscarriage.

Placenta previa

Placenta previa is an abnormal condition in which the fertilized egg, or zygote, travels to the lower portion of the uterus and attaches itself to a part of the uterine wall near or even over the uterine opening. As a result, the placenta (a temporary organ in the uterus, which develops during pregnancy to conduct nourishment and oxygen from the mother to the fetus) forms in such a way as to cover all or part of the uterine opening and thus interfere with normal delivery.

There are three types of placenta previa: partial, in which only a portion of the cervix is covered; complete, in which the cervix is completely covered; and low-lying (or marginal), in which the placenta does not cover the cervix, but is close enough to it to potentially interfere with normal delivery.

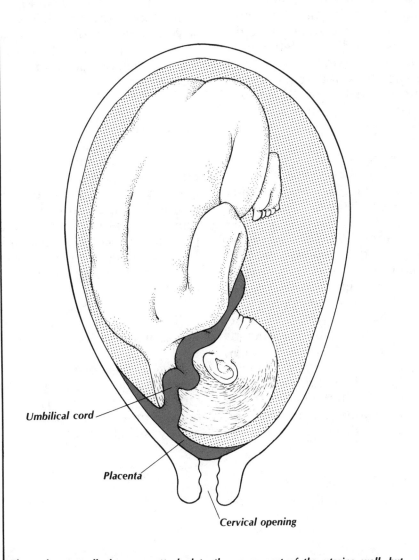

Umbilical cord

Placenta

Cervical opening

The embryo usually becomes attached to the upper part of the uterine wall, but sometimes implantation takes place in a lower location. As the placenta grows, it can partially or completely cover the cervical opening, thus interfering with a normal delivery.

Placenta previa occurs in one of every 100 to 500 pregnancies. It is more prevalent among women who have had two or more children than among those in their first pregnancy.

Cause

The cause of placenta previa is unknown. Some authorities believe that placental implantation cannot take place on the same part of the uterine wall more than once. If a woman has had several pregnancies, the lower part of the uterus may be the only place left on which the placenta can become implanted.

Symptoms

The major symptom of placenta previa is painless vaginal bleeding. Profuse bleeding may begin as early as the twenty-fourth week of pregnancy, with no apparent cause. The blood will be bright red, indicating that it is fresh. Bleeding occurs as the placenta separates from the wall of the uterus near the uterine opening. This bleeding occurs without any injury (from a fall, for example). In some cases, there is only spotting (light blood flow).

Diagnosis

Any vaginal bleeding during pregnancy is abnormal and should be reported to the doctor immediately. An ultrasound scan (in which sound waves are used to visualize internal structures) of the abdomen will then be performed. If placenta previa is present, it will be seen on an ultrasound scan.

Treatment

There are two types of treatment: delayed and active. The purpose of delayed treatment is to give the fetus time to mature. With active treatment, the fetus is delivered by cesarean section as soon as possible.

The degree of vaginal bleeding will usually dictate the type of treatment. If vaginal bleeding is slight, delayed treatment is generally chosen. If vaginal bleeding is heavy, a cesarean section will be performed immediately.

Bleeding from placenta previa may be extremely heavy, leading to severe blood loss by the mother. This bleeding stops only after the fetus and placenta have been delivered by cesarean section. Unless treatment is rapid, death of both the mother and fetus may occur.

Toxemia of pregnancy

Toxemia of pregnancy is a severe condition that sometimes occurs in the last stage of pregnancy and is marked by high blood pressure; swelling of the extremities, especially the hands, feet, and ankles; and the presence of protein in the urine. If it is allowed to worsen, convulsions and coma may develop.

The term *toxemia of pregnancy* is actually a misnomer; formerly it was thought that the condition was caused by toxic substances in the blood. It is more accurately called preeclampsia before the convulsive stage and eclampsia after.

Causes

The causes of toxemia of pregnancy are not clearly understood. It tends to be more common among mothers from lower socioeconomic groups. One theory is that dietary deficiencies may be at the root of some cases. Some types of toxemia may be the result of a deficiency of blood flow in the uterus.

Symptoms

Toxemia is divided into three progressively more serious stages, each with its own characteristic symptoms. *Mild preeclampsia* is marked by edema (swelling due to fluid retention), hypertension (high blood pressure), and the presence of protein in the urine. The symptoms of *severe preeclampsia* may include headache, dizziness, fever, drowsiness, tachycardia (abnormally rapid heart rhythm), tinnitus (ringing in the ears), double vision, nausea, vomiting, and scanty or absent urine production. In full-blown *eclampsia*, convulsions may be followed by severe hypotension (low blood pressure) and coma. The condition ultimately leads to death if not treated.

Treatment

Toxemia cannot be completely cured until the pregnancy is over. Until then, treatment includes stimulation of kidney function, control of high blood pressure and convulsions, and, in severe cases, early delivery of the infant to ensure the survival of the mother.

Prevention

There is no known preventive. The first line of defense is the monitoring of all bodily functions in order to spot symptoms as they begin to appear.

CARING FOR YOUR CHILD

Every parent knows the uneasy feeling that comes with the knowledge (or even the suspicion) that a child is sick. Part of the problem is that it can be very difficult to assess the seriousness of a childhood illness. How can you prepare yourself to make the best decisions about your child's health?

First, educate yourself. Carefully read this book so that you will know which symptoms to watch for and what to do about them. An informed parent is in the best possible position to deal with both the major and the minor crises of childhood.

Second, trust your instincts. As a parent, you know better than anyone else when your child is not acting or feeling right. Sometimes there are visible signs of illness, like diarrhea and a fever; at other times, a change in your child's behavior alerts you to a problem, even though there are no physical symptoms. If you feel that there is a problem or an emergency situation, act on it.

Third, ask questions. Don't worry that you will inconvenience the doctor or appear stupid if you are uncertain about a diagnosis or plan of treatment. It is the doctor's responsibility to make sure that you are fully informed about all matters that concern your child's health.

WHEN TO CALL A DOCTOR

Here are some rules of thumb about the need for medical attention for common ailments. Call your doctor if the following situations occur:

- *Fever* is higher than 101°F for more than 24 hours, or a child with a fever looks and acts extremely ill, is difficult to arouse, is incoherent, or is particularly irritable.
- *Common cold* lasts more than ten days or is accompanied by a fever higher than 101°F, a sore throat or puslike nasal discharge for longer than two days, or a persistent cough or wheezing.
- *Sore throat* is present for more than three days or is accompanied by a fever higher than 101°F.
- *Earache* lasts more than one hour, or a child with an earache looks very ill or has a temperature higher than 101°F.
- *Cough* is persistent or short, dry, and sharp or is accompanied by wheezing, difficulty in breathing, a fever of more than 101°F, or a cold that has lasted more than ten days.
- *Headaches* are frequent, and the child appears very ill or a headache wakens a child at night.
- *Stomachache* pain has been constant for more than two hours or is accompanied by bloody stools or recurrent vomiting of green or yellow material.
- *Vomiting* is accompanied by fever, lasts more than 12 hours, or produces green or yellow material more than twice, or a vomiting child appears very ill or is difficult to arouse.
- *Diarrhea* is bloody, lasts more than one day, or is accompanied by vomiting, fever of more than 101°F, or absence of urination for eight hours.

Illness in babies may be a little harder to detect. Call the doctor when an infant:
- Refuses to nurse or take liquids.
- Urinates very little.
- Vomits repeatedly.
- Becomes extremely fretful or lethargic.
- Becomes hoarse, has difficulty in breathing, or has a crowing cry, especially with a fever.
- Becomes fretful and pulls on his or her ear.
- Has a marked increase in bowel movements.
- Has blood or mucus in his or her stool.
- Displays noticeable protrusion of the fontanelle (soft spot on the head).

Call the doctor if an existing condition is not improving or if you do not know what to do about certain symptoms. Although parents need to use common sense in calling the doctor, it is always better to err on the side of being overcautious. A doctor can often give directions and reassure you over the telephone.

Respiratory disorders account for almost half of all childhood illnesses. Fortunately, they are easy to diagnose, and the availability of antibiotics makes many respiratory infections fairly simple to cure.

Although children are helpless in the sense that they cannot provide for themselves, they are remarkably tough when it comes to recovering from illness and overcoming physical disorders. This resilience sees them through a time of life when their undeveloped bodies make them vulnerable to mishaps and infections.

MEDICATIONS

Treating a sick child with medication is an example of how parent and doctor must work together in the interests of the child's health. The doctor is responsible for making an accurate diagnosis of the child's condition and prescribing the appropriate drug. It then becomes the parent's responsibility to make sure that the drug is administered correctly.

It has been estimated that in 10 percent to 30 percent of cases in which medication apparently failed to work, the cause of the failure was improper administration of the medication. Whenever a doctor prescribes a medication for your child, make sure that you understand completely how much to give, how to give it, how often to give it, and for how long.

How much medication to give

The quantity of medication the doctor prescribes for your child is determined by the child's weight and age. Thus, for a given medication, the dosage prescribed for a baby will be much different from that for an adolescent. Make sure that the child takes the complete dose—no more and no less. If the child vomits within 20 minutes of receiving a dose, you can assume that the medication was lost and can give another dose.

Do not use an ordinary kitchen teaspoon when measuring liquid medications; instead, use a specially marked measuring spoon for medication, which should be available from any pharmacy. If your child insists on taking medication from his or her "special" spoon, transfer the medication from the measuring spoon to the child's spoon after measuring.

When to give medication

Medications vary in the amount of time it takes for them to be absorbed by the body. Some medications need to be given at very precisely regulated intervals. Therefore, make sure you fully understand the instructions on the label. For example,

"four times a day" and "every six hours" do not mean the same thing; the former means that the child should have four doses at fairly equally spaced intervals within the waking hours, whereas the latter means that each dose should be given six hours after the previous one, even if the child must be awakened to do so.

How long to give medication is also important. A common mistake is to assume that because a child acts as if he or she is well, the child is well. The symptoms of an illness can subside long before the illness itself is over; in fact, the healing process may have barely begun. Stopping a child's medication too soon can cause a relapse and complications. For example, streptococcal infections require ten straight days of antibiotic treatment, and stopping too soon can allow disease-causing organisms to flourish again. Therefore, such instructions as "Give for ten full days," "Continue for two weeks," and "Give until finished" should be followed exactly.

How to give medication

Every parent needs to know how to give medication to a child, and every child needs to understand that taking medicine is an unpleasant but unavoidable fact of life. A young child, approached in a reassuring and matter-of-fact manner, will usually accept medication without any trouble.

Liquid medicine can be given directly from the spoon (after careful measurement). An alternative method is to use a nonglass medicine dropper to squirt the liquid slowly into the child's mouth. Be careful not to direct

the stream of liquid forcefully against the back of the throat and down the windpipe; instead, it should be released against the inside of the cheek.

If the medicine tastes unpleasant, you can give the child a sweet treat afterward. You may also be able to disguise the medicine in a little applesauce, ice cream, or juice. Be sure, however, to check with your pharmacist first, because some medications should not be diluted or taken with certain kinds of foods or beverages. Also, make sure that the child takes the entire portion.

Do not give pills or capsules to a child under the age of five; the child may choke. If the medication is not available in liquid form, you may be able to mash a tablet or empty the contents of a capsule and mix it with a small quantity of juice or food. Always check with your pharmacist or physician first, though, to be certain that the medication will be effective if given in this way, and always make sure that the child takes the whole dose. After the age of five or six, your child can probably swallow tablets or capsules whole. You can help the child learn how to do this by practicing when he or she needs a nonprescription remedy such as acetaminophen. Show the child how to put the pill on the back of the tongue and swallow it with a drink or with a spoonful of ice cream, applesauce, or jelly. You can also buy a special glass that delivers the pill into the mouth automatically with the first gulp of liquid. Whenever a child is taking a pill, watch to be sure that the medication goes down smoothly and that the child is in no danger of choking.

Don't encourage a child to take medication by saying that it is candy. Indeed, many cases of poisoning have occurred in children who took overdoses of medications that looked or tasted like candy. Indeed, many doctors discourage the use of children's vitamin pills that are sweet, brightly colored, or shaped like cartoon characters, believing that such products tend to blur the distinction in the child's mind between candy and drugs.

Apgar score

The Apgar score is a general evaluation of a baby's condition, made soon after birth, to determine immediately whether the newborn needs emergency care. The Apgar scoring system was devised by the late Virginia Apgar, M.D., and the letters of her last name are an acronym for the factors being scored.

Procedure

At one minute and five minutes after an infant's birth, a delivery room nurse, anesthesiologist, or pediatrician rates five factors, using a scale of 0 to 2:

A (Appearance)—A score of 2 is given if the skin is completely pink; 1 if it is pink except for the hands and feet, which are bluish; and 0 if the entire body is blue (indicating lack of oxygen).

P (Pulse)—A score of 2 is given for a pulse above 100; 1 for a rate of less than 100; 0 for no pulse.

G (Grimace, or reflex irritability)—A score of 2 is given if the baby cries vigorously when slapped lightly on the soles of the feet; 1, if the baby makes only a grimace or slight cry; 0, if there is no response.

A (Activity)—An active infant is given a score of 2; an infant who makes some movement of arms and legs, 1; a limp and motionless infant, 0.

R (Respiration)—Strong efforts to breathe, together with vigorous crying, score a 2; slow, irregular breathing, 1; no breathing at all, 0.

Scores

Most babies score between 7 and 10 when tested one minute after birth. They are breathing well, crying, pinkish in color, active, and need no emergency measures.

Those babies who score from 4 to 6 usually need help immediately. The throat is suctioned to remove thick mucus, small blood clots, or bits of swallowed membrane (from the amniotic sac that enclosed the baby before birth). Oxygen is sometimes given to assist breathing and restore color.

The baby with an Apgar score of less than 4 is limp, pale or bluish, and perhaps without a heartbeat, and is in grave danger. The throat is suctioned, and the baby is placed on a mechanical respirator until the baby can breathe on his or her own.

A second Apgar score is determined five minutes after birth and recorded on the baby's chart beside the first score. The second score is a good measure of the baby's adaptation to the world outside the womb.

Attention Deficit Disorder

Attention deficit disorder (ADD) is a nervous disorder that usually affects children. The condition is characterized by very high levels of physical activity, consistently impulsive and immature behavior, and an extremely short atten-

tion span. Because of these behavioral patterns, the condition is also known as minimal brain dysfunction and, in common usage, hyperactivity.

Although ADD does no physical damage to the body, it can trigger long-lasting social, emotional, and educational problems. Because affected children cannot sit still and concentrate for long periods, they may have trouble with schoolwork. They often appear to be immature, uncoordinated, and boisterous and may have trouble getting along with classmates, teachers, and parents; consequently, they often suffer from a poor self-image.

Causes

The cause of ADD is not known, but several theories have been proposed in recent years. None of these theories has been proved or disproved.

The condition may be the result of a nervous system malfunction or a deficiency of neurotransmitters (chemicals in the brain that transmit impulses between the nerves). According to one theory, based on the supposition that the brain has two systems for responding to situations—one that prompts immediate action and one that encourages hesitation and consideration—the neurotransmitters that control the hesitation response are malfunctioning in the child with ADD. In some cases, damage to a fetus during pregnancy or a complication of childbirth may have caused a neurologic defect.

Because the condition is four to five times more common in boys than in girls, some researchers believe that the tendency toward ADD may be inherited as a sex-linked hereditary trait. Support for a genetic basis for ADD comes from the finding that parents who had ADD as children tend to have children with ADD.

It has also been suggested that the additives, preservatives, and colorings found in processed foods may have a toxic or allergic effect on some children.

Symptoms

A variety of symptoms point to ADD. The child with ADD is overly active, fidgety, restless, overly talkative or boisterous, impulsive, and seemingly uncoordinated. In school, this child has a very short attention span and seems to forget facts quickly, disrupts the classroom, does schoolwork hastily and incorrectly, skips or adds words when reading, laughs too loud and hard, and prefers to play with younger children.

Diagnosis

There are no specific tests to diagnose ADD. These symptoms seem to be present in all children to some degree, and since ADD is rather vaguely defined, the symptoms displayed by an individual child should be carefully observed. The quantity, intensity, and duration of these symptoms may single out children with ADD from others who are merely bored with school or who are having other behavior problems. Care must be taken in diagnosis, since a real danger is that a child will be saddled with the label of hyperactivity not because he or she has an abnormally high energy level, but rather because his or her parents have a very low level of tolerance.

Treatment

Although controversial, drug therapy has proved successful in treating ADD. Several stimulant drugs appear to have a calming effect on children with ADD because they seem to affect the hesitation response. However, these drugs have been shown to have unpleasant side effects, such as stomach cramps, susceptibility to colds, nervous mannerisms, and stunted growth. Therefore, many children on this therapy are required by their doctors to take "drug holidays" to give their bodies a break.

Special diets that are designed in an attempt to eliminate all food additives have been prescribed, in keeping with the theory that additives cause ADD. The findings from studies on this treatment have been contradictory. However, many parents report dramatic changes in behavior after this treatment, although part of the change is most likely to be due to the extra attention paid to the child whose meals have to be specially prepared.

Parents can help to influence the child's actions by praising or rewarding good behavior and ignoring bad behavior.

Autism

Autism is a form of mental illness. The word *autism* comes from *auto,* Greek for self, and literally means self-absorption. The autistic child is wrapped up in his or her own inner thoughts, unable to communicate with or relate to others.

Causes

Although the cause of autism remains a mystery, several rea-sons for the disorder have been suggested. In some cases, an inborn mental defect may play a part, since many affected children do not smile or respond to affectionate cuddling. In other instances, severe mental or physical trauma during childhood may have contributed to the disorder. Gender may also be a factor; boys are four times as likely as girls to be autistic.

Symptoms

Autism is a collection of symptoms that appear in the first 30 months of life. The autistic child is very withdrawn, unaffectionate, and uninterested in people, including parents and siblings. The child behaves as if he or she were alone in the world. There is a speech and language disorder: the child may learn to speak late or not at all, and, if speech develops, it is odd and limited. Common characteristics are echolalia (repetition of the last phrase or word of everything another person says); a total resistance to change (even something so minor as rearrangement of furniture); and the repetition of some meaningless act, such as rocking, arm-flapping, or head-banging. Mental development is often uneven. Usually the child does best in learning nonverbal skills, and teaching methods that emphasize memorization and drill may be most useful. There are no established signs of nervous system defects, although half of all autistic children experience seizures before the teen years.

Diagnosis

In diagnosing autism, the doctor must distinguish it from childhood schizophrenia, a mental illness that may also cause a child to be silent and withdrawn but that usually strikes later than autism. The doctor must also make certain that deafness or severely impaired hearing is not present. The child is given neurologic and intelligence tests, to help determine the potential for training and education. A tranquilizer may be prescribed for emergency use to quiet violent outbursts.

Treatment

An autistic child may have to be cared for in an institution or a specialized school. Day-care programs for autistic children are available in some cities, and the trend is to train parents to care for their children at home. The method of treatment most often used by professionals, and taught to parents, is known as behavior therapy. The main goals are to limit self-destructive or meaningless actions, to promote language development, and to make the child more social. In behavior therapy, the professional or parent works to develop a close relationship with the child, so that the child will want to imitate the adult. The adult also uses direct action (such as rewards and praise) to promote speech, play with other children, self-care skills (such as dressing and washing), and helpfulness. With such methods, some autistic children of average or near-average intelligence are able to develop into normal adults.

Prevention

Unfortunately, because the cause is unknown, there are no preventive measures.

Cerebral palsy

Cerebral palsy (CP) is a general term to describe various disorders of muscle control caused by a period of lack of oxygen to the brain.

Cause

Cerebral palsy is caused by brain or nerve damage that usually occurs before or around the time of birth. The damage may result when brain tissue becomes starved for oxygen for any reason. It may result from separation and bleeding of the placenta (the organ that anchors the fetus to the wall of the uterus and provides nourishment) in late pregnancy or from disorders caused by diabetes in the mother. It is characteristic of cerebral palsy that the neurologic problems are not progressive.

Types

There are four major types of CP: spastic, athetoid, ataxic, and mixed. About 70 percent of cases of CP are the spastic type. Patients with spastic CP move stiffly and with great difficulty because their affected muscles are constantly tense and tight. One arm and one leg may be affected, or both arms or both legs. Affected extremities appear thin and wasted, are weak, and are likely to twist and jerk. Walking on the toes or with a scissorslike movement is typical. When all four limbs are affected, the mouth, tongue, and palate may also be affected, interfering with speech, eating, and drinking and causing constant drooling.

Athetoid, or dyskinetic, CP accounts for about 20 percent of cases. This disorder, which is caused by damage to the basal ganglia (a mass of nerve-cell bodies at the base of the brain), is characterized by continual slow, twisting movements of the fingers and hands during waking hours. Similar movements of the upper arms or legs and trunk may occur. There may also be sudden, jerky movements.

Ataxic CP results from damage to the cerebellum (a portion of the brain highly involved in muscular coordination) or the nerves leading from it. The characteristic signs of this type of CP are weakness, lack of balance and coordination, tremor, difficulty with fine or quick movements, and a clumsy way of walking, with feet wide apart.

Mixed CP occurs frequently. Often, spastic and athetoid types are combined. Ataxic and athetoid are mixed less often.

Symptoms

Possible signs of CP in a baby include twitching, convulsions, back-arching muscle spasms, partial paralysis of the face, and very late development of the ability to lift the head, sit, crawl, stand, walk, and talk. Any baby who may have suffered brain damage around the time of birth should be watched carefully for signs of CP (such a baby may have been born nearly lifeless or very small and premature, or may have suffered a severe infection soon after birth). Although it is difficult to diagnose any particular form of CP in the first two years of life, parents should report any suspicion promptly to their doctor.

After infancy, symptoms of cerebral palsy range from simple clumsiness or slight incoordination of muscles to multiple handicaps that prevent normal movement. Frequently, the brain damage that causes CP also causes mental retardation, epilepsy, hearing problems, visual defects, and learning and behavior disorders. However, some CP children are normal except for disordered muscle control.

Diagnosis

Early diagnosis and treatment of CP are essential if a child is to develop as fully as possible. An important part of the diagnostic evaluation is to discover if there is any other reason for the symptoms. A wide range of medical diagnostic studies and psychological tests will be performed.

Treatment

Treatment of a CP child may involve many different elements, such as speech therapy, physical therapy, special dental care, specially designed clothes, braces, corrective glasses, surgery, a hearing aid, special furniture, and special schooling. Occupational therapy can help the patient in self-care, including dressing and eating. About 25 percent of CP patients have convulsions, which usually can be controlled with drugs. Ideally, a physician will work with a team of specialists in a setting where treatments can be coordinated.

Because CP is a lifelong condition, parents need to learn as much as possible about caring for a CP child. The parents can learn how to continue therapy at home. Every effort must be made to help the child become self-reliant. Parents can often get valuable advice and support from other parents of CP children and from professionals at the local chapter of the United Cerebral

Palsy Association. Therapy for CP children and adults is provided at rehabilitation centers sponsored by the National Easter Seal Society and other agencies.

Prevention

Expectant mothers can guard against CP with good prenatal care emphasizing adequate diet, rest, exercise, frequent checkups, and avoidance of drugs and infections. During labor and birth, the doctor can keep track of the baby's heartbeat with use of a fetal monitor and, if necessary, operate quickly to save the baby from brain damage caused by oxygen starvation. Expectant mothers with difficult pregnancies should try to have their babies delivered at a hospital with a newborn intensive care unit, directed by a certified neonatologist (a physician who specializes in the care of newborn babies). In such a unit, premature and ill babies can be watched closely and cared for by specially trained nurses and doctors using the latest methods.

Child abuse

Child abuse encompasses all types of mistreatment—physical, emotional, and sexual—that can be inflicted on a child, particularly by a parent, guardian, or other family member. Closely related is child neglect, in which the parent or guardian chooses not to provide for the nutritional, emotional, physical, or health needs of a child.

Causes

The principal cause of child abuse is emotional inadequacy

of the parent or guardian. Most parents who abuse their children were themselves abused as children. They did not learn how to give or receive affection from their parents and thus find it hard to develop a good relationship with their own children. They often use the same harsh punishment methods—threats, ridicule, and physical violence—that were used on them as children, often because they do not know any other way of managing family problems.

Some parents who neglect their children are incompetent because of drug or alcohol abuse, medical or psychological disorders, or overwhelming socioeconomic problems. Parents who do not have a support system of close friends or relatives living nearby may feel isolated and overwhelmed by the constant demands of raising children. Others who may abuse their children are young parents with their first child, parents of ill or premature babies who are separated from them shortly after birth, and parents who did not want a child in the first place. Such parents need special attention and support in order to get their families off to a good start.

Symptoms

Physical symptoms of abuse (also known as the battered child syndrome) include old and new bruises; scars from cuts and burns; serious damage to the eyes, mouth, or internal organs; and X-ray evidence of bone fractures in various stages of healing. When parents cannot give reasonable explanations for the child's injuries, child abuse may be suspected.

Signs of emotional abuse are more difficult to detect. Babies who have been neglected emotionally may appear uninterested in people or even retarded. Another sign in babies is the condition known as failure to thrive, which is unexplained lack of growth even though no illness is present. Older children who are excessively well behaved and overly anxious to please adults, but who do not get along well with other children and are mistrustful may be victims of emotional abuse. At school, they may have trouble with teachers as well as with other children.

Sexual abuse by a parent or other relative is often difficult to detect. There may be no physical symptoms, although venereal disease in a child is grounds for suspicion. The child may be too fearful or too embarrassed to reveal the situation to anyone outside the family.

Outside intervention

When physicians, teachers, or other professionals suspect child abuse, they are required by law in most states to report it to a government social service agency or welfare department. However, punishment of the parents is not the goal of the law. Jailing a parent might injure the child as much as the original abuse if the parent is capable of being a good father or mother in the future. Removing the child from the family may be necessary to protect the youngster from future injury, but in most cases this is not done or the removal is only temporary.

The child may stay in the hospital for a few days while the case is studied and parents are interviewed. In many communities, a team made up of a social worker, a pediatrician, a psychiatrist, and other specialists talk to the child and the parents and develop a long-term treatment plan. This often involves periodic visits by a social worker to the home and psychological help for one or both parents. Practical help, such as day care for small children and household help by a trained homemaker, can ease the burdens on an overworked mother. If there is a local chapter of Parents Anonymous, an organization of parents who formerly abused their children, this may be another source of support.

Prevention

Parents who are afraid that they might abuse their children should talk frankly to their family doctor or a social worker. Joining a parent support group may be a helpful way to share child-care ideas and experiences.

If a baby is born ill or prematurely and must stay in the hospital after the mother comes home, the parents should visit the baby every day and stay as close as possible so that the baby will not be a stranger when he or she comes home.

Circumcision

Circumcision is the surgical removal of the foreskin, the retractable sleeve of skin covering the glans (the head of the penis). In some religions, the operation is performed as a religious ritual on the eighth day following birth. In hospitals, it is usually done on the day before a baby boy goes home. In any event, if it is to be done for nonmedical reasons, it should be done in infancy and not later, when it is a more serious operation and might harm the child psychologically.

During the five-minute operation, which is usually done without anesthesia, the foreskin is carefully cut away. Gauze coated with petroleum jelly is applied to the incision. In most cases, the incision heals rapidly, forming a dry scab that drops off after a few days. Although the incision should be kept clean (but not submerged in bathwater), no other special care is necessary. Other than a few drops of blood that might be produced if the diaper rubs against the cut, there is normally no bleeding.

Pros and cons

Routine circumcision for newborns is controversial. The decision should be made by the parents after consideration of both sides of the question.

The operation has become standard in American hospitals in recent decades as a cleanliness measure. In a young boy, the foreskin completely covers the head of the penis and cannot be pulled back very far. If the penis is not kept clean, urine and other substances can cause irritation of the glans and perhaps lead to infection between the foreskin and the glans. However, normal care can prevent this problem. There is some recent evidence that uncircumcised males have a higher rate of bladder and kidney infections, but further information is needed before any strong conclusions can be drawn. Even though the foreskin at first cannot be pulled back very far because of bands of tissue that bind it to the glans, it is necessary to wash only the part of the glans that can be uncovered comfortably at any one stage (the foreskin should never be forced back). The bands of tissue gradually dissolve, and by later childhood, the foreskin can be pulled back completely.

Some researchers believe that circumcision reduces the risk of cancer of the penis in the circumcised man and cancer of the cervix (the neck of the uterus) in his sexual partner and may help prevent venereal disease. However, there is insufficient evidence to support these views.

Very seldom is there a medical reason to perform a circumcision. It should never be done on the first day of life, or if the baby is ill or premature. Furthermore, it should be delayed indefinitely if there is any abnormality of the glans or penis, so that the foreskin can be used later as graft tissue to repair the defect. It should not be done if the mother was taking any medication that promotes bleeding, such as an anticoagulant or aspirin, during pregnancy or is taking such a medication while breast-feeding, nor should it be done if there is

any family history of hemophilia or other bleeding disorders.

Risks of circumcision include local infection, which may lead to significant hemorrhage and mutilation. Many medical authorities feel that there is no absolute medical reason for routine circumcision of the newborn. Adequate hygiene offers the same advantages as routine circumcision without the risks of the operation.

Parents, therefore, should consider all factors—cultural, religious, and medical—before making a decision about circumcision.

Cleft lip and cleft palate

Cleft lip and cleft palate, a defect in one of every 700 to 800 newborns, is characterized by a split running through all or part of the

upper structure of the mouth. A cleft lip (or harelip) may be only a small notch near the center of the upper lip, or it may extend into the nostril. A cleft in the palate can be as minor as a split in the uvula (the little projection of tissue that hangs down in the back of the throat), or it may divide the entire soft palate (the muscular tissue that covers the roof of the mouth). In its most severe form, a cleft splits not only the soft palate but the entire hard palate (the bony roof of the mouth) and upper jaw, joining with a cleft lip. The cleft may even divide the palate into three parts, resulting in a split on either side of the nose and leaving the middle section of the upper jaw and gum dangling.

Causes

The formation of a cleft lip occurs in the early stage of preg-

Palate

Normal palate   Cleft palate   Cleft palate with cleft lip on one side   Cleft palate with cleft lip on both sides

A cleft palate is a division of the tissues that form the roof of the mouth. This condition does not deform the outward appearance of the face, but makes feeding difficult for the child. The division may also extend through the entire palate and one side of the upper jaw, resulting in a cleft palate with cleft lip. In the most severe form, a cleft palate with a cleft lip on both sides, the palate is divided into three parts, resulting in a split on either side of the nose and leaving a middle section of upper jaw and gum dangling.

nancy, soon after the fourth week, when the baby's face starts to form. Bulges of tissue on either side of the face grow toward the midline to form the nostrils and lips. At about the seventh week they normally meet and join; if they do not, a cleft lip is the result.

A failure of development in the eighth week of pregnancy causes cleft palate. The palate is formed from two plates of tissue, which originally are on either side of the developing tongue. As the head and neck grow, the tongue moves downward and the tissue plates move into position and fuse into one—unless there is an error or weakness, which results in cleft palate.

The underlying causes of cleft lip and cleft palate are not fully understood. There is an inherited tendency toward the defects. More than one-fourth of children with cleft lip also have a relative with a cleft. If parents without cleft defects have one child with a cleft, they have a five percent risk of having a second child with a cleft; if they have two children with clefts, there is a 12 percent risk of a cleft in future children. Perhaps some difference in the uterus, such as poor blood supply to the fetus, combines with an inherited weakness to produce the error of development. Certain chemicals or medications, too many vitamins or not enough, and viruses have been suggested as possible causes of cleft defects.

Cleft lip and cleft palate are often associated with other birth defects. Of every six children who have a cleft lip, with or without cleft palate, one will have one or more other birth defects. Almost 50 percent of children with cleft palate also have another defect, such as joined fingers or toes, malformed ears,

spina bifida, heart disease, or clubfoot.

Treatment

Treatment of a patient with a cleft lip or a cleft palate (or both) requires the services of a specialized team that includes a pediatrician, an orthodontist (a dentist who specializes in the prevention or correction of misalignment of the teeth), a speech therapist, a plastic surgeon, a psychologist, an audiologist (a specialist in communication disorders), and an otolaryngologist (a physician who specializes in the treatment of disorders of the ears, nose, and throat). Treatment may take place at a specialized clinic or hospital center or may be coordinated by a pediatrician who consults experts as needed.

Before any treatment can begin, however, steps must be taken to permit the child to eat. A cleft lip prevents normal sucking, and a cleft palate allows milk to run out of the nose, often causing choking and vomiting. Special feeding devices are used, such as a nipple with an enlarged flange to cover the cleft or a regular nipple with enlarged holes. A small syringe with a short rubber tube, like one used to baste a turkey, may be used to feed a child with a cleft lip, although sometimes such a child can be breast-fed. A few days after birth, an orthodontist skilled in cleft palate repair may be able to fashion an appliance that provides a temporary roof for the mouth, enabling regular feeding. At the same time, the appliance prevents the mouth from being distorted before the palate can be closed.

Some surgeons correct a cleft lip in the first few days of the child's life because it will make

the baby more acceptable to his or her parents and make it easier to feed the baby by bottle. However, other surgeons delay the operation for two to eight months, so that surgery will not interfere with the growing bonds of affection between mother and baby (for one thing, the baby cannot breast-feed for six weeks after the operation) and to rule out other birth defects that might interfere with recovery.

Plastic surgery to correct cleft palate usually takes place in the second year of life. Some surgeons repair the soft palate first, when the child is between 6 and 18 months of age, and the hard palate much later—sometimes not until the age of five years. Although early surgery helps the child's emotional and speech development, some surgeons wait because they are concerned that early surgery may cause distortion of growth in the middle third of the face. While waiting, the child wears an appliance that acts as a roof over the mouth.

The problems created by cleft palate and cleft lip cannot be solved only by surgery. The services of an orthodontist are needed for youngsters with cleft palate, not only to make appliances but to straighten teeth that are poorly positioned. A speech therapist aids the child in developing speech, which is altered because of the missing or inadequate soft palate or artificial palate. A psychologist helps to treat emotional and social problems sometimes caused by being different in speech or appearance. An otolaryngologist should examine the child monthly for middle ear infections, which are common in young children with cleft palate. An audiologist helps those children who develop hearing loss because of middle ear infections. With proper care and encouragement and with modern plastic surgery, the average child with a cleft can make a good recovery.

Clubfoot

Clubfoot, or talipes, is a common birth defect in which one or both feet are fixed in an awkward, twisted position. The foot resists efforts to stretch or turn it back. In talipes equinovarus, the most frequent form, the foot points down and turns in while the front of the foot curls toward the heel. If not corrected, the condition worsens and interferes with walking. The person seems to walk on the ankle and the outside or inside edge of the foot.

Talipes equinovarus　　　　*Metatarsus varus*

The most common form of clubfoot is talipes equinovarus, in which the foot points down and turns in while the front of the foot curls toward the heel. Related to clubfoot is metatarsus varus ("pigeon toe"), in which the front of the foot turns inward.

Causes

The cause of clubfoot is unknown. However, there seems to be an inherited tendency for development to be arrested around the ninth week of pregnancy, when the fetus' feet are being formed. Clubfoot may begin as a muscle abnormality. The Achilles tendon is shortened, the ankle and its muscles are deformed, and the heel bone is shortened and flattened to some extent.

Treatment

Correction of clubfoot should begin as early as the first week after birth, when the bones, muscles, ligaments, and tendons are soft and pliable. The correction is usually done in stages. In talipes equinovarus, the first stage is to uncurl the front of the foot away from the heel. The next stage is to turn the foot so that the sole faces outward. The third stage is to put the foot in a cast

with the toes pointing up. This may require surgery to lengthen the Achilles tendon and to free the ankle joint.

Correction generally takes place in a series of small, painless, gradual adjustments. Typically, the doctor flexes and stretches the foot by hand and then fixes it in a cast in a partially corrected position. After a week or so the cast is removed, the foot is manipulated into a better position, and a new cast is applied. Sometimes, instead of making a new cast each time, the doctor places wedges inside the existing cast to adjust the foot. The entire casting process may take three months.

Once the correction has been made, it must be followed up with exercises, devices that hold the feet in place at night while the baby is sleeping, and orthopedic shoes. A night splint (corrective shoes with soles joined by a flat metal bar that keeps the feet in exactly the right position) is often used.

Because clubfoot sometimes recurs, periodic checkups are necessary until the child becomes an adult. However, in most cases, the correction is completely successful, and the individual can walk and run normally.

If early treatment has not succeeded, or if a child is not treated until the age of nine or ten years, more extensive surgery may be necessary. This is followed by several weeks with the foot in a cast. Satisfactory results are usually obtained. The foot is rather stiff, but this does not prevent the individual from engaging in the most active sports.

Related to true clubfoot is a condition called metatarsus varus, in which the front of the foot turns inward. Also known as apparent clubfoot and pigeon toe, this is a milder deformity that may not be diagnosed in the first several weeks. Unlike a true clubfoot, the apparent clubfoot can be moved easily into a correct position. It can usually be corrected by manipulation and exercise, without the need for casts or surgery.

Colic

Colic means different things to different people, but the universal characteristic is crying—not just short periods of fussiness that can be stopped by changing or feeding or cuddling—but long periods of crying with no apparent cause that defy all attempts to stop them.

Causes

It has long been assumed that colic arises from some gastrointestinal disorder. However, studies have shown no correlation between colic and poor weight gain or excessive vomiting, constipation, or diarrhea. Colicky babies are generally quite healthy, with no sign of nutritional problems. Nor does the problem appear to be hunger; the crying spells often begin after a feeding, not before one. It has been suggested that bottle-feeding is at fault, but breast-fed infants are just as likely to have colic. Lactose intolerance, food sensitivities, and allergies have also been suggested as causes.

Some babies with colic seem to have no such digestive symptoms—their crying seems to be related to general irritability, possibly because of immaturity of the nervous system or exceptional sensitivity to the environment. Other babies have a combination of the two types.

Symptoms

Colic most often begins when an infant is two to four weeks old. The baby will cry inconsolably for hours a day. These bouts of crying often occur as if on schedule (most often in the late afternoon or early evening). The colicky baby pulls his or her legs up, clenches his or her fists, screams, and turns red. The baby may nurse briefly but then stop to continue crying. The abdomen may be distended as if with gas, and the baby may even pass gas frequently. Generally, there are no other gastrointestinal symptoms; the bowel movements are normal, and the baby doesn't spit up any more than most babies. The baby's sleep pattern is often disrupted—he or she may wake frequently (every two hours or so), cry fretfully, take one to two ounces of formula or a few minutes at the mother's breast, fall into a fitful sleep, and then awaken to repeat the sequence.

Diagnosis

Before assuming that your baby has colic, check for other possible causes of crying, such as pain from an open diaper pin or discomfort from being overheated, constipated, hungry, or wet. See whether your baby responds promptly to talking and cuddling—a baby in pain can be distracted, but only temporarily. Also check for signs of illness: colic is not associated with fever, diarrhea, vomiting, cough, a runny nose, or reddened eyes.

Your pediatrician will want to rule out more serious causes of crying before assuming that your baby has colic. Signs of illness, such as sores in the mouth or gastrointestinal or urinary tract problems, will be sought. Although conclusive scientific evidence for a dietary basis for colic is lacking, your doctor may want to investigate the possibility that something in the baby's diet (or in the mother's diet if the baby is breast-fed) may be causing the condition.

Treatment

If the colic seems to be due, at least in part, to an accumulation of gas in the abdomen, do not overfeed the baby and be sure to burp him or her thoroughly after feedings. If you are bottle-feeding, check the nipple hole; if it is too large or too small, the baby may be swallowing too much air. A warm hot-water bottle on the abdomen may relieve some discomfort. The baby may be most comfortable lying on his or her stomach.

If the colic seems to be due to irritability, it might be helpful to restrict visitors and to keep the home environment as peaceful as possible. Some researchers believe that overly sensitive babies may be upset by an atmosphere charged with too much noise, too much activity, and too much emotional stress.

Your physician will probably not recommend any medical treatment for colic. Colic usually ends two or three months after it begins, with no physical or emotional consequences.

Congenital hypothyroidism

Congenital (present at birth) hypothyroidism is a condition that leads to defective physical and mental development because of a deficiency of thyroid hormone. If untreated, a person born with congenital hypothyroidism grows to a maximum height of three or four feet and has a large, flat, broad head; short forehead;

puffy, wide-set eyes; broad, short, upturned nose; thick lips; large tongue protruding from a drooling mouth; narrow chest; potbelly; swayback; rough skin; dry hair; and severe mental retardation.

Causes

Iodine is necessary for the body to produce thyroid hormone, and foods obtained from the ocean are the best sources of iodine. Before the widespread use of iodized salt, hypothyroidism was much more common in inland areas, where foods naturally contain little iodine.

Congenital hypothyroidism can result from a defect in the development of a child before birth. The thyroid gland may be missing or underdeveloped, possibly because of a severe deficiency of iodine in the mother's diet during pregnancy. In rare cases, congenital hypothyroidism is caused by an inherited absence of a body chemical needed to produce thyroid hormone.

When hypothyroidism first appears in children over the age of two years, it is usually due to an inflammation of the thyroid gland resulting from an immune disorder. It can also be caused by certain diseases of the pituitary gland or hypothalamus.

Symptoms

The first symptoms of untreated congenital hypothyroidism usually appear between the ages of three and six months or whenever the mother stops breast-feeding (breast milk contains tiny quantities of thyroid hormone). The baby is "too good," in the sense that he or she seldom cries (when the baby does cry, it is a strange, hoarse cry), sleeps more than normal, is inactive, and thus is easy to care for. This behavior is a result of the baby's lack of thyroid hormone, which regulates the rate of body processes, and increasing mental retardation. The baby's movements are slow and awkward, and the child has feeding difficulties, is constipated, and develops jaundice. The stomach protrudes, and a hernia may develop at the navel.

These symptoms are followed by the appearance of the characteristic facial features: the thick tongue, which interferes with breathing; the wide-set eyes; the turned-up nose; and the dull expression, indicating mental deficiency. The baby's heart beats slowly, resulting in poor circulation and cold skin. The hair is dry and dull. Teeth come in late and decay easily.

The child in whom symptoms of hypothyroidism first appear after the age of two is typically short and fat, with short legs and arms and a head that appears too large. Sexual development in an older child may be delayed.

Diagnosis

Early diagnosis is now much more common since all states began to require that every newborn be tested for thyroid hormone level.

Diagnosis of congenital hypothyroidism may require not only a blood test to determine thyroid hormone levels, but also a nuclear medicine study after the administration of radioactive iodine to evaluate thyroid function. Special X rays may be used to detect delayed skeletal development, and an electrocardio-gram (which measures the electrical impulses generated in the heart) may be done to reveal heartbeat patterns.

Treatment

Treatment for congenital hypothyroidism is lifelong replacement of thyroid hormone with a synthetic substitute, ideally starting at birth. Those who receive the hormone before the age of three months usually develop normally. Children born without a thyroid gland are more at risk than those whose thyroid gland works poorly; if not treated by three months of age, they will be mentally retarded even though their growth is corrected.

Prevention

Pregnant women can help prevent congenital hypothyroidism in their offspring by eating a well-balanced diet that includes iodine-rich foods, such as fish and seafood, and by using iodized salt. At birth, every child's blood should be tested for thyroid hormone level.

Croup

Croup is a condition marked by a hoarse, barking cough that sometimes follows a cold or fever in very young children, most commonly those under the age of two years. A croup attack may occur only once, or it may linger or reappear after it seems to have gone.

Causes

Croup is usually caused by a viral infection of the larynx

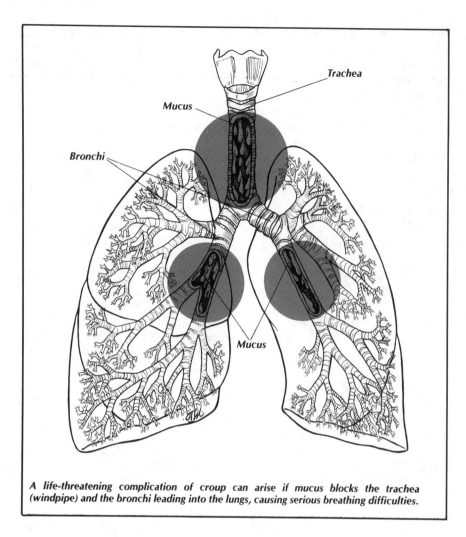

A life-threatening complication of croup can arise if mucus blocks the trachea (windpipe) and the bronchi leading into the lungs, causing serious breathing difficulties.

Diagnosis

The emphasis in diagnostic evaluation is on establishing that the difficulty in breathing is actually due to croup and not to epiglottitis, a life-threatening emergency condition in which the inflamed epiglottis (the lid-like structure covering the opening to the windpipe) rapidly becomes completely obstructed. Epiglottitis is usually caused by bacteria, most often *Hemophilus influenza*, and is associated with sudden onset of high fever (up to 104°F). This is an important diagnostic clue to help doctors differentiate between epiglottitis and viral croup.

Choking on a foreign object may also resemble croup, since both conditions share the symptom of frantic efforts to breathe. An X-ray examination may be performed to rule out this possibility.

Treatment

Croup can usually be treated at home. The first step is calming the child. The barking cough, especially when accompanied by difficulty in breathing, can frighten the child, and this fear can only aggravate the symptoms. Sometimes the child can be told to imagine a relaxing scene or can listen to a calming bedtime story; a relaxed child will respond much better to home remedies.

The goal of the treatment is to relieve the cough by reducing the inflammation and swelling in the larynx. This can be accomplished by breathing in moist air from a humidifier or vaporizer, by leaning over a pan of hot water with a towel draped over the head, or by sitting in a steamy bathroom with a hot

(voice box). The characteristic barking cough is produced when air forces its way through the child's swollen larynx. The air passageways in a child's throat are very narrow; when an infection causes swelling, little room is left for air to pass through, and breathing can be severely hampered. Also, the windpipe and the bronchi (the main breathing tubes that connect the windpipe and the lungs) may become blocked with mucus, further impairing breathing.

Symptoms

The identifying symptoms of croup are a deep, barking cough and breathing difficulties, especially when the child is inhaling. Sometimes a fever and hoarseness are also present. The child may gag while he or she is coughing, causing vomiting, which usually relieves the cough somewhat. The coughing attack often occurs in the evening and usually lasts less than an hour.

Symptoms that indicate a worsening condition include blue skin and lips, drooling, and extreme exhaustion. When the croaking sound continues while the child is inhaling, a condition called stridor has developed. If any of these symptoms occurs or if there are severe breathing difficulties, medical help should be obtained *immediately*.

shower running. Moist air reduces the swelling in the larynx and makes breathing easier. Of course, precautions should be taken to protect a young child from being scalded while taking part in these treatments, and the child should never be left alone.

Drinking extra fluids (not milk or orange juice) at room temperature is also recommended. Cough medicine will not help (and may even harm) a child with croup, nor is it advisable to put a spoon or any other object into the child's mouth in an attempt to aid the breathing. In a severe case, a physician may administer medications to control the inflammation in the throat; also, antibiotics can sometimes control the infections that are connected with croup.

Prevention

It is not known why some children develop croup after a cold or fever and others do not; therefore, there is really no way to prevent croup.

The fontanelles are the gaps between the bony plates of an infant's skull. The largest and most noticeable of these gaps is the "soft spot" on top of the head toward the front. The fontanelles permit the head to adapt without injury to being squeezed during birth. After birth, they allow room for the brain to grow. Shortly before adolescence, the bony plates meet and knit together.

Fontanelles

Fontanelles are the gaps between the bony plates of an infant's skull. The largest and most noticeable of these gaps is the "soft spot" on top of the head, toward the front. There is also a groove that runs like a center part toward the back of the head, where a much smaller soft spot is located. The fontanelles serve two purposes. During birth, they permit the head to adapt without injury to being squeezed as it passes through the birth canal. After birth, they permit the brain to grow. During the first two or three years of a child's life, the skull plates grow toward each other until they meet, covering the soft spots. However, the plates do not fully knit together until shortly before adolescence, when the brain stops growing.

The baby's soft spot is supported by a tough membrane and does not have to be treated more delicately than any other part of the head. It is normal for it to be slightly depressed, to tense up when the baby cries, and to pulsate in rhythm with the heartbeat. (The pulsation is not that of an artery directly beneath the soft spot. Instead, it is caused by changes in the pressure of the cerebrospinal fluid, which surrounds and protects the brain and spinal cord.)

Gilles de la Tourette's syndrome

Gilles de la Tourette's syndrome is a neuromuscular disorder marked by intense tics (twitchy, repetitive movements of certain muscles). It occurs most often in boys. Tourette's syndrome generally begins around the age of seven or eight years. At first, the tics are simple: facial twisting, blinking, grimacing, shoulder shrugging, or twitching. Later, however, the tics progress to vocal tics that are accompanied by psychological involvement.

349

Causes

The causes are unknown. It is still disputed whether the disorder is of physical or psychological origin.

Symptoms

The symptoms of Gilles de la Tourette's syndrome are at first limited to the muscles in the face, head, neck, and shoulders. Often, the first symptom is a characteristic breathing noise from the larynx (voice box), as if the patient were barking, wheezing, or gasping for air. As the tics spread to the shoulders and arms, there are shoulder shrugs and twitches, as well as twisting of the neck and arms. Vocal tics, such as grunting, snuffing, shouting, and barking sounds, then begin to develop. As the vocal symptoms worsen, the patient begins to exclaim in a loud voice words or phrases with obscene meanings or "swear words." Echolalia (repetition by the patient of words that have been said to him or her) is common. The patient will seem to fixate on a word or phrase and repeat it over and over with increasing speed. Often, too, the individual will spasmodically and automatically repeat or mimic the actions of those nearby.

The symptoms tend to come and go, especially as the patient approaches puberty and adulthood. Tics that are very violent during waking hours often stop during sleep. Some tics are intensified by emotional upheavals. The tics of Gilles de la Tourette's syndrome, unlike those of most neuromuscular disorders, are often suppressed in school or social settings and expressed more often when the patient is alone or with family members. In some cases, the tics can be controlled voluntarily. The excessive swearing, however, occurs only in the presence of others; some patients attempt to cover it up by coughing, thus developing another tic. Often symptoms decrease in adult life and disappear, only to return during a period of stress. Mental activity remains normal.

Diagnosis

Diagnosis is often difficult, since symptoms in the early stages often resemble common childhood tics seen in many young school-age children. Also, early- and middle-stage symptoms are difficult to distinguish from those of certain brain conditions. However, the syndrome can often be diagnosed with some assurance as the course of the illness unfolds.

Treatment

Gilles de la Tourette's syndrome can be treated with medications starting with small doses and increasing the dosage until the tics are controlled. Often a combination of drugs is used. Group psychotherapy can be helpful in some cases. In extreme cases, leukotomy (surgical interruption of white nerve fibers of the frontal lobe of the brain) is considered. There are no known preventive measures for Gilles de la Tourette's syndrome.

Hyaline membrane disease

Hyaline membrane disease (HMD) is a respiratory distress syndrome that occurs in premature infants who do not have fully functioning lungs. It is the leading cause of illness and death in premature infants.

Cause

The cause of HMD is the inability of the immature lungs to produce enough pulmonary surfactant, which is a chemical in the alveoli (the tiny air sacs in the lungs) that keeps them expanded. Without adequate surfactant, the alveoli tend to collapse when the infant exhales. As a result, the lungs do not expand completely, and the blood passing through them cannot obtain enough oxygen to sustain life.

Symptoms

The symptoms of HMD are easily observable. The skin is bluish due to lack of oxygenation of the blood, and there are other symptoms of oxygen deprivation—irregular heartbeat; rapid, labored, and shallow breathing; flaring of the nostrils; grunting when breathing out; and edema (swelling of tissues due to fluid accumulation).

Treatment

Treatment of HMD is aimed at maintaining adequate oxygen levels. Until the lungs can sufficiently oxygenate the blood, oxygen must be provided in such a way as to prevent damage to the infant. An oxygen face mask is often used to provide warmed, moisturized oxygen. In more severe cases, a ventilator is necessary to "breathe" for the infant.

Great strides in the treatment of HMD have been made in the

last few years. An artificial surfactant (a lubricant for the lungs), has been produced that, when administered via the baby's trachea (windpipe), markedly relieves the baby's respiratory distress.

Fluids, glucose (a form of sugar), and electrolytes (certain chemicals needed by the body) are provided intravenously.

Either the condition will clear up as the lungs develop and begin to produce their own natural surfactant or the infant will not survive.

Prevention

The best preventive measure is to guard against premature birth. Women should be carefully monitored during the last weeks of pregnancy for any signs of premature labor.

If the mother is diabetic, the fetal lungs may not be fully formed until the fortieth week of pregnancy, and HMD is possible until then.

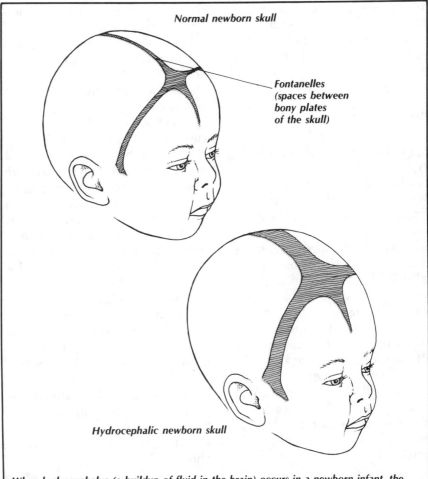

Normal newborn skull

Fontanelles (spaces between bony plates of the skull)

Hydrocephalic newborn skull

When hydrocephalus (a buildup of fluid in the brain) occurs in a newborn infant, the loosely connected bony plates of the skull spread apart to accommodate the swelling.

Hydrocephalus

Hydrocephalus (sometimes inaccurately referred to as "water on the brain") is an abnormal accumulation of cerebrospinal fluid within the cavities (hollow spaces) of the brain.

Normally, cerebrospinal fluid is secreted in the cavities of the brain and absorbed by a membrane that lines the cavities. If the membrane does not absorb the fluid or if the fluid is blocked, it builds up in the cavities. The fluid buildup causes the head to become enlarged and the brain to become compressed. This condition can lead to paralysis, blindness, mental retardation, inability to speak, and convulsions.

Cause

Hydrocephalus is usually the result of a brain infection or a malformation in the fetus prior to birth. Although the baby's head may not appear abnormally large at birth, it expands rapidly from month to month; if untreated, the child usually dies by the end of the second year. If the blockage of the cerebrospinal fluid is only partial, the child may live for a number of years or may even live a normal life span.

Although hydrocephalus is usually a congenital (present at birth) condition, it can occur later as a result of an infection or tumor.

Symptoms

When hydrocephalus occurs in an infant, the loosely connected bony skull plates pull apart to accommodate the swelling. As a result, the head becomes greatly enlarged. In addition to having an oversized head, the child with hydrocephalus may have an abnormally enlarged forehead and swollen or enlarged blood vessels in the scalp.

Diagnosis

Diagnosis is accomplished through the use of X rays and

computed tomography scanning (see page 407). If infection is suspected, samples of the blood and cerebrospinal fluid will be examined.

Treatment

Surgery can make it possible, in some cases, to bypass the blockage or obstruction, causing the fluid buildup to escape through other exits. Often, the insertion of a small tube connecting a brain cavity with the abdomen or a major blood vessel will allow the fluid to drain. As the child grows, the tube may become blocked, again allowing pressure to build in the brain. If this happens, the tube must be replaced or the blockage removed. When surgery is successful, the probability of mental retardation is greatly reduced, and the prospects of normal physical and intellectual development are increased.

Immunization

Immunization is the means of producing immunity, or resistance by the body, to a specific disease. (For information about how immunizations work, see pages 83-84.) Immunization can provide protection against measles, mumps, rubella (German measles), some types of meningitis, polio, pertussis (whooping cough), diphtheria, and tetanus, all of which can cripple or kill.

Every child should receive injections of the combined diphtheria-tetanus-pertussis (DTP) vaccine at 2, 4, 6, and 18 months of age. The child should also receive a dose of the oral polio vaccine (OPV) at 2, 4, and 18 months of age. At 15 months,

a child should receive the combined measles, mumps, and rubella (MMR) vaccine and a test for tuberculosis (TB). Booster shots of DTP vaccine and OPV should be given around the time of school entry (when the child is four to five years old). A diphtheria-tetanus toxoids (DT) booster shot should be given between 14 and 16 years of age. Doctors are also recommending that a relatively new vaccine against *Hemophilus influenzae* type B (HiB), the most common cause of bacterial meningitis in children, be given to infants. The recommended schedule for HiB vaccination depends upon the brand of vaccine used. For example, one brand of the vaccine should be given at 2, 4, and 12 months of age; another should be given at 2, 4, 6, and 15 months of age. The physician who performs the initial vaccination can tell you which schedule should be followed for your child.

Immunization and testing schedule

2 months	DTP, OPV, HiB*
4 months	DTP, OPV, HiB*
6 months	DTP, HiB*
12 months	HiB*
15 months	MMR, TB test, HiB*
18 months	DTP and OPV
4-5 years	DTP and OPV
11-12 years	Measles booster**
14-16 years	DT booster

* The schedule for HiB depends on the brand of vaccine. Injections should be given either at 2, 4, 6, and 15 months or at 2, 4, and 12 months. Check with your doctor.

** If there is a measles outbreak, anyone between the ages of 4 years and 21 years of age should receive a booster.

If the family does not have a family physician, immunizations can usually be obtained through the local public health department. If a child has an acute illness with fever, immunization should be delayed.

Nephrotic syndrome

Nephrotic syndrome is a kidney disorder in which the glomeruli (tiny clumps of blood vessels, which filter the blood to produce urine) do not work properly. The defective glomeruli allow proteins, most notably albumin, to escape from the bloodstream and seep into the urine, while letting fluid that should be eliminated as waste build up in the tissues.

Nephrotic syndrome most often affects children, particularly those between the ages of one and six years. Boys are more likely than girls to be affected.

Causes

Nephrotic syndrome is caused by other diseases that affect the kidneys. The syndrome in turn creates vulnerability to other infections, including peritonitis (inflammation of the lining of the abdominal cavity).

Symptoms

As a result of fluid accumulation, the body gradually swells (a condition called edema), becoming especially bloated around the face, abdomen, and ankles. The child may urinate very little (approximately one-fifth the normal amount).

To prevent complications, a doctor should be consulted as

soon as either less frequent urination or unusual swelling in the face, abdomen, or ankles is noted.

Diagnosis

If initial blood and urine tests point to nephrotic syndrome, the doctor will order more tests and possibly a kidney biopsy (removal of a tissue sample for microscopic examination).

Treatment

The condition can be controlled with proper medical care, usually in a hospital, where medication (diuretics to eliminate excess fluid from the tissues and steroids to control inflammation) and diet can be carefully supervised. Symptoms are likely to clear up after a few weeks, and the patient can finish recuperating at home, sometimes with no aftereffects.

Osteomyelitis

Osteomyelitis is inflammation of the bone and bone marrow, usually due to a bacterial infection. It is considered a childhood disease, occurring most often in boys between the ages of 5 and 14 years, but it also occurs in adults. Since the introduction of antibiotics, osteomyelitis has become rare in the United States, but it is still common in countries lacking good medical care and proper nutrition.

Causes

Along with essential oxygen and nutrients, blood may also carry bacteria and other organ-

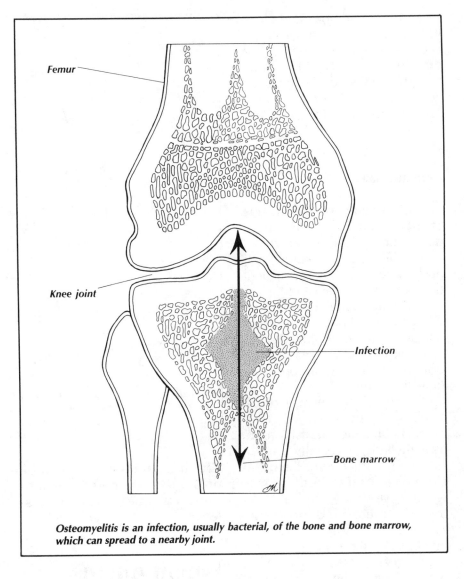

Osteomyelitis is an infection, usually bacterial, of the bone and bone marrow, which can spread to a nearby joint.

isms, which tend to settle in the capillaries (tiny blood vessels) of the long bones of the arms and legs. Infectious agents can also reach the bones directly from adjacent infected tissue or through an open wound or fracture. Osteomyelitis usually affects only one area of the bone or bone marrow, but it can attack more than one bone at a time.

Symptoms

Symptoms include pain and excruciating tenderness near a joint or at the affected area, fever

in the range of 102°F to 104°F, redness, and swelling.

Diagnosis

Although a physician can often diagnose osteomyelitis from the symptoms, X rays and blood tests confirm its presence.

Treatment

The child with osteomyelitis may be hospitalized and given antibiotics in liquid, tablet, or intravenous form. It may be necessary to drain any pus and clean the area in a minor surgical procedure and then immobilize the limb in a splint. The child is released from the hospital once the healing begins, but may have to take antibiotics for six more weeks.

Complications

Possible complications include septicemia (blood poisoning); destruction of the bone; spread of the infection to a nearby joint, possibly resulting in a permanent deformity; transference of the infection to the surface of the skin, where it erupts as an abscess; damage to the cartilage adjacent to the bone, which may retard bone growth; and suppurative (infectious) arthritis.

Chronic (long-term) osteomyelitis may be a delayed complication of acute (sudden-onset) osteomyelitis, especially if it results from a fracture or the presence of a foreign body in the wound, such as a bullet or a piece of metallic debris. The major sign of chronic osteomyelitis is a flare-up or reopening of an abscessed wound, with periodic pain and discharge of pus. X rays show irregular bone and pieces of dead bone. Treatment for chronic osteomyelitis may require several operations to remove all the dead bone and other tissue, completely drain the abscess, and repair the bone when possible. Large doses of antibiotics may be necessary.

Prevention

To prevent osteomyelitis, clean and disinfect all wounds thoroughly and, especially in children, apply a bandage to keep the area clean until it has healed.

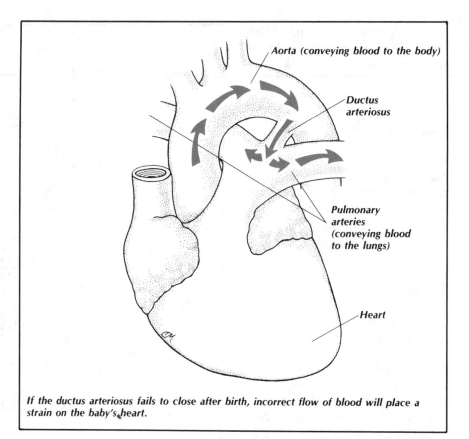

If the ductus arteriosus fails to close after birth, incorrect flow of blood will place a strain on the baby's heart.

Chronic osteomyelitis can be prevented by immediate antibiotic treatment of acute osteomyelitis.

Patent ductus arteriosus

Patent ductus arteriosus is a congenital (present at birth) heart disorder in which the ductus arteriosus, an extra blood vessel present in the fetus that allows the blood to pass from the pulmonary artery (which conveys blood from the heart to the lungs) to the aorta (the main blood vessel that conveys blood from the heart to the rest of the body) fails to close after birth. This condition is most common in premature babies.

During the nine months of growth and development in the uterus, the fetus is immersed in amniotic fluid, and the lungs are not used. The blood bypasses the lungs through the ductus arteriosus, and the fetus receives oxygen from the placenta.

If the ductus arteriosus remains open after birth, some blood is rerouted from the aorta back through the lungs. As a result, less oxygen-rich blood can be supplied to the tissues throughout the body, and the work of the left side of the heart (which pumps blood from the heart to the rest of the body) is increased.

Cause

In most babies, the duct begins to close before birth and is completely closed by the age of three months. The reasons for this normal closure (and for failure to close) are poorly understood.

Symptoms

Although obvious symptoms are rare, the affected infant may display shortness of breath or develop congestive heart failure.

Treatment

Patent ductus arteriosus can be treated with medication if diagnosed very early. Various prenatal (before birth) tests have become available in recent years for diagnosis if the condition is suspected. After birth, the condition can be corrected by tying off the duct in a relatively simple surgical procedure.

Phimosis

Phimosis is a constriction of the foreskin (the skin fold over the head of the penis), which prevents the foreskin from being drawn back over the glans (the head of the penis).

Causes

Phimosis is either congenital (present at birth) or acquired. The acquired form is usually due to an infection involving the penis that leaves adhesions (growths of tissue that adhere both to the inner aspect of the foreskin and to the glans itself). Phimosis also allows debris (dirt, dead cells, and normal fluid secretions) to accumulate between the foreskin and the glans, providing a breeding ground for bacteria to grow.

Symptoms

If infection becomes established, ulcers (open sores) may appear on the glans, and swelling of the lymph nodes in the groin may occur.

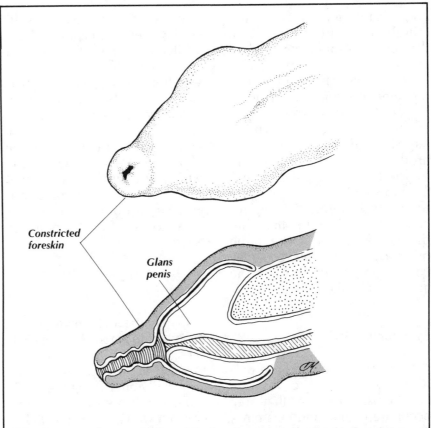

Phimosis occurs when constriction of the foreskin prevents the foreskin from being drawn back over the glans penis (the head of the penis).

Diagnosis

The condition will be apparent on physical examination of the child. If infection is present, cultures may be performed.

Treatment

The definitive treatment is circumcision (the surgical removal of the foreskin). If circumcision must be delayed, there must be careful attention to keeping the area clean and dry and free from infection until the procedure can be performed.

Pinworms

Pinworms (any of a variety of worms called oxyurids) are parasites that may infect the gastrointestinal tract and occasionally other sites, such as the female reproductive tract. These worms are tiny (about one-eighth to one-half inch in length).

Cause

The usual cause of the infection is eating food contaminated with fertilized oxyurid eggs. Contamination results from contact with infected feces. Eggs can also survive on clothes and bedding for two or three weeks.

After being ingested (taken into the body), the eggs hatch

and release their larvae (an immature form of the worm) into the upper portion of the small intestine. The larvae mature as they pass through the first part of the large intestine. After mating, the adult male worms die and the females migrate down the large intestine and lay their eggs around the anus. The eggs are transferred by the child's hands from the anus to the mouth, and the cycle continues. Pinworms can be transmitted to other children and adults in the same manner. Also, the hatched larvae can migrate back through the anus and into the bowel.

Symptoms

Many children who have pinworms do not have obvious symptoms. Symptoms that may occur are itching and inflammation around the anus. Worms can also cause irritation, inflammation, and obstruction in the appendix. In females, pinworms can work their way into the vagina and urethra and cause inflammation or infection in the reproductive system and bladder.

Diagnosis

Aside from noting the symptom of itching, diagnosis is made by identifying the eggs or worms through a microscope. The physician will usually place a piece of clear adhesive tape against the child's anus. The eggs will adhere to the tape, which is placed under a microscope for examination.

Treatment

Treatment of pinworms is not difficult. Usually one dose of the drug pyrantel pamoate is sufficient. Other medications are also available. In addition, all members of a family should be treated simultaneously, and their bedclothes, towels, and underwear should be laundered at the same time. Also, the eggs around the anus should be removed by cleaning the anal area thoroughly at the time of treatment. Reinfection is common, and when symptoms develop, another course of treatment is necessary.

Prevention

To help prevent pinworms, it is important to teach children clean eating habits, to encourage them to wash their hands frequently (especially after using the washroom), and to be alert to other children who may be infected (as evidenced by scratching around the anus).

Reye's syndrome

Reye's syndrome is a relatively rare condition in which encephalitis (inflammation of the brain) is associated with liver damage due to the collection of fatty deposits in that organ. It strikes children and adolescents (most commonly, children between the ages of 5 and 11 years), often while they are recovering from a viral infection, such as influenza or chicken pox. For some unknown reason, it occurs most often between December and March.

Reye's syndrome is a serious disease that requires *immediate* treatment. Brain damage, coma, or death can result if it is not diagnosed and treated quickly. It is fatal in about 25 percent of cases.

Cause

The exact cause of Reye's syndrome is not known, but since it almost always follows a viral infection, scientists suspect that the virus combines with an unknown substance in the body to produce a toxin (poison). There is some evidence that use of aspirin during a viral illness increases the risk of Reye's syndrome. Thus, physicians caution parents not to give aspirin products to their children during chicken pox or influenza infections.

Symptoms

The symptoms of Reye's syndrome are sudden vomiting, abnormal sleepiness or hyperactivity, and confusion. Convulsions and coma may occur as the disease progresses.

Diagnosis

Early diagnosis is crucial. Reye's syndrome is diagnosed by careful observation of the symptoms, testing of a sample of cerebrospinal fluid (the clear fluid of the central nervous system, which is produced in the brain), blood tests to determine the presence of liver damage, and tests of the blood sugar level, which is often low in young children with this disease.

Treatment

There is no known cure. Treatment consists in helping the child to weather the first few days of the illness, maintaining normal blood sugar levels and reducing pressure on the swollen brain. Usually, if the child survives for three or four days, the symptoms will subside and recovery will follow.

If the blood sugar level is low, a normal concentration is restored with the intravenous administration of glucose (a form of sugar). Increased pressure on the brain from the swelling is also reduced with medication.

Prevention

An association has been established between aspirin use during and immediately after viral infections (particularly chicken pox and influenza) and Reye's syndrome. It is therefore strongly recommended that aspirin not be given to a child or adolescent with such an infection. A doctor can suggest an aspirin substitute, such as acetaminophen, if needed for discomfort or fever.

Scoliosis

Scoliosis is curvature of the spine. There is usually a main curve in one direction and an upper curve or lower curve, or both, to compensate for it in the opposite direction.

Before the age of three years, boys are more likely to be affected, developing an upper curve to the left and a lower curve to the right. Between the ages of four and ten years, boys and girls are affected in equal numbers, and the direction of curvature varies. Most prevalent is the adolescent form, usually affecting girls between the age of ten and the time their skeletons mature. Most often, the upper spinal area curves to the right, with compensating curves to the left in the lower neck and in the small of the back.

Severe, untreated scoliosis can cause diminished lung capacity,

Severe scoliosis can be seen when viewing a child from the back, and even mild scoliosis can be noticed when the child bends at the waist. Bending forward rotates the chest, making one side of the back more prominent.

back pain, spinal arthritis, and disease of the cartilage disks between the vertebrae.

Causes

Scoliosis can result from unequal leg lengths, or it may be due to defective development of the vertebrae (the bones of the spine) while the fetus was growing in the uterus. Paralysis of the trunk muscles on one side of the body caused by polio, cerebral palsy, or muscular dystrophy; tilting of the pelvis due to hip disease; or deformities of the spine caused by rickets or rheumatism can also lead to scoliosis. Idiopathic scoliosis, the most common kind of the disorder, has no known cause.

Symptoms

Parents should be alert for the signs of scoliosis. At first the

child may appear to have an uneven hemline, unequal pant legs, or one hip higher than the other. To make a preliminary assessment, ask your child to stand up straight with his or her shirt off while you observe from the rear. Notice if one shoulder is higher than the other or if one shoulder blade sticks out. When the child's arms hang loosely at the sides, notice if one arm hangs farther away from the body than does the other. See if one hip appears higher or more prominent than the other. See if the child seems to tilt to one side. Finally, ask your child to bend forward, arms hanging in front and palms together at the level of the knees. A hump on the back at the ribs or near the waist may also be a sign of scoliosis.

Diagnosis

If you have any suspicions, report them to your child's doctor, who will give the child a similar checkup and, if necessary, take X rays or refer you to an orthopedic surgeon (bone specialist) to confirm the diagnosis.

Treatment

Treatment of scoliosis may involve only exercises if the curvature is mild. Sit-ups, exercises to stretch the spine, and breathing exercises may strengthen the muscles of the trunk enough to correct the situation. Frequent X rays and physical examinations may be needed to determine if the exercises are working.

More severe scoliosis may require the wearing of a special leather brace or a plastic pelvic girdle with one vertical brace in front and two in back, connected to a ring around the neck. In many cases, this must be worn 24 hours a day, except when the patient is bathing or exercising, until the child's skeleton has matured. It is adjustable for growth.

The use of specially designed electrical stimulation devices has met with some success.

The most severe scoliosis requires spinal-fusion surgery, in which certain vertebrae are fused together, with stabilization provided by metal rods, cable, or staples. Frequent checkups are needed after surgery.

Spina bifida

Spina bifida is a congenital (present at birth) defect of development, marked by defective closure of some of the vertebrae (the bones of the spine) that normally encase the spinal cord. If the meninges (the membranes that cover the brain and spinal cord) protrude as a sac through the gap in the spine, the condition is

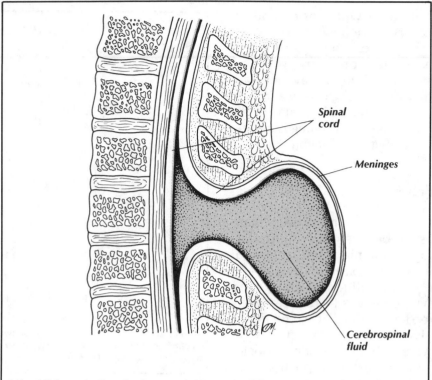

Spina bifida cystica is a developmental defect in which one or more of the vertebrae (bones of the spine) fail to completely encircle the spinal cord, allowing the meninges (membranes surrounding the spinal cord) to protrude as a sac through the opening.

known as spina bifida cystica; if not, it is called spina bifida occulta. The severity of the defect can range all the way from a form with few visible symptoms to a completely open spine.

Cause

The cause is unknown.

Description

Spina bifida commonly affects the chest and lower back regions of the spine and extends for three to six segments of the spinal column. If there is a sac, it may collapse while the child is still in the uterus, but it fills with cerebrospinal fluid soon after birth. If the sac is not covered with skin, it can rupture, perhaps leading to

meningitis (inflammation of the meninges).

Spina bifida can be accompanied by varying degrees of paralysis, depending on the extent of involvement of the spinal cord and its nerve roots. The paralysis can lead to orthopedic problems, such as clubfoot and dislocated hip, and may also affect the sphincters (closure muscles) of the bladder and rectum, resulting in genitourinary disorders. Abnormal curvature of the spine can hinder surgical closure. Hydrocephalus (accumulation of cerebrospinal fluid within the skull) also accompanies many cases of spina bifida.

Diagnosis

Diagnostic evaluation of the condition begins with X rays of the spine, skull, hips, and lower extremities. Urine tests are also necessary. The need for further tests depends on the extent of the defect. Such tests may include a computed tomography scan (see page 407) and an evaluation of the cerebrospinal fluid.

Treatment

Treatment requires an extensive evaluation of the child's condition by neurosurgeons, urologists, orthopedists, and pediatricians. In some cases, social service workers and psychiatrists will work with the parents. Closure of the defect ensures a better outcome. Long-term survival and quality of life depend on the type and extent of the spinal defect, other defects present, the infant's general health, and treatment resources. In addition to surgical closure of the spine, the infant may need other surgery to correct accompanying problems. The most common complications are loss of kidney function, clubfoot, dislocation of the hip joints, scoliosis (curvature of the spine), pressure sores, and muscle weakness and spasm.

Prevention

There is no known preventive for spina bifida. Prenatal (before birth) diagnosis through amniocentesis (for more information, see page 408) is growing progressively more accurate.

Strabismus

Strabismus is commonly referred to as "squint-eye" or "cross-eye." Technically, the term refers to a deviation of one eye from being parallel with the other.

When a light is shined into the eyes, the highlight should normally be on the same spot in each eye. The eyes shown above are properly aligned, while the eyes of a child with strabismus, shown below, are not parallel.

Causes

In most cases, strabismus is congenital (present at birth), although it can result from later injury to one eye or impaired vision because of disease. The cause of congenital strabismus is unknown, but the effect is generally paralysis or malfunction of the tiny muscles that control the movement of the eyes.

Symptoms

Symptoms include obviously crossed, wandering, or squinting eyes, although in some cases lack of parallelism of the eyes is so subtle that it can be detected only by special testing.

Diagnosis

Complete evaluation of the eyes is essential to rule out more serious eye or nervous disorders and to determine how best to correct the strabismus. Such an evaluation is usually performed by an ophthalmologist (a physician who specializes in eye disorders).

Treatment

If muscle imbalance alone is responsible, the strabismus can usually be treated easily with corrective glasses or contact lenses. Eye exercises are effective in many less severe cases. Surgical restoration of the muscle balance can be done in more extreme cases. Permanent visual loss can result if strabismus is not treated by the time the child is four to six years old.

Sudden infant death syndrome (SIDS)

Sudden infant death syndrome (also called crib death) is the unexplained and sudden death of a baby—often, the baby is perfectly well when put to bed but dies silently during sleep. In the United States, SIDS is second only to accidents as a cause of death in infants from two weeks to one year of age, causing 8,000 to 10,000 deaths per year. Most deaths from SIDS occur in the third or fourth month of life, with higher death rates for boys, children of teenage mothers, infants from poor families, and babies who were premature. Cigarette smoking by the mother during pregnancy appears to be one of the biggest risk factors for SIDS, as is use of drugs such as cocaine or heroin during pregnancy. There are more SIDS deaths in the winter than in the summer.

Cause

It once was thought that SIDS is caused by smothering in the bedding, but this is untrue. It is also not attributable to clogging of the airways by vomited food, to bottle feeding, or to any other cause that parents could prevent. Some investigators believe that a combination of conditions is necessary to trigger SIDS, including a narrowed and inflamed airway, temporary airway obstruction, chronic oxygen deficiency, and irregular breathing, leading to a spasm of the trachea (windpipe) and death. Research continues.

Counseling for parents

Parents who lose a child to SIDS are totally unprepared for the death and usually have overwhelming guilt feelings—that something they did or did not do caused the death of their child. An autopsy will usually prove

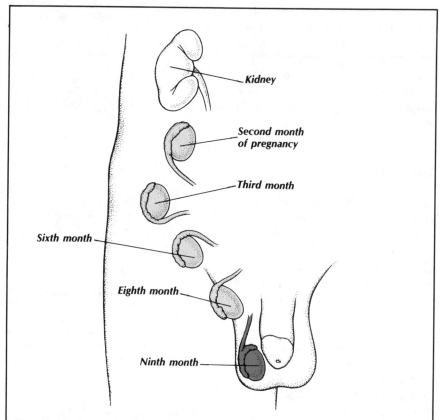

The testes (male sex glands) develop in the abdomen and gradually descend into the scrotum before birth. Occasionally, this progression does not occur, and the boy is born with undescended testes.

that the death was not the parents' fault. Doctors and nurses who take the time to discuss the death fully with the parents can be very helpful. So can another parent who has lost a child to SIDS. There are now many local chapters of the National Sudden Infant Death Syndrome Foundation and the International Council for Infant Survival, both of which can be valuable sources of counseling and information.

Undescended testes

Undescended testes is a condition in which one or both of the testes (male sex glands) do not descend into the scrotum (the sac between the legs that normally contains the testes), but remain in the abdomen, where they developed before birth. This condition is not uncommon.

If the testes do not descend, they often degenerate or atrophy (shrink), and thus do not secrete the male sex hormones that they ordinarily supply. This, in turn, can cause the elimination or suppression of the development during puberty of secondary male sex characteristics such as body hair, heavier musculature, deepening voice, and so forth. Damaged sperm, or insufficient production of them, can also result from undescended testes, especially if the situation is still present in adolescence or adulthood. If one testis is damaged but the other has descended and is normal, sexual development will be normal.

Causes

The causes of this condition are not clearly understood. It is conjectured that a membrane in the abdomen gets in the way of normal testicular positioning. If only one testis is undescended, the problem is most likely mechanical in nature; if both are involved, the underlying cause may well be hormonal.

Treatment

Treatment for this condition is controversial. In deciding on treatment, three important considerations must be kept in mind: the potential lack of fertility if the testes do not descend, the likelihood that they will descend without intervention, and the risk that the undescended testes will become cancerous. Hormone therapy is sometimes an effective treatment for undescended testes, but in many cases in which it has apparently been successful, some doctors think that the testes would probably have descended into the scrotum by themselves anyway. Surgery to bring the testes into the scrotum is usually successful if done before the age of five years. The physician can sometimes cause the testes to descend by manipulation of the tissues around them.

Prevention

There is no known means of preventing undescended testes.

EMOTIONAL AND
MENTAL ILLNESS

Emotional and mental problems vary greatly in degree. Today, many mentally healthy people turn to psychotherapy for help in coping with an emotional crisis, such as the loss of a loved one or a divorce. At the other extreme are people who are so disturbed that they cannot take care of their basic needs.

All of us experience emotional ups and downs throughout our lives and are prone to feelings of anxiety, fear, guilt, or depression from time to time. It is when these feelings seriously interfere with the ability to work or to deal with home or social life that a problem exists.

Warning signs

The borderline between "normal" and distorted actions and feelings is not scientifically exact. However, there are general warning signs of emotional or mental difficulties that indicate a need for professional help:
- Severe anxiety that is not attributable to reality
- Unreasonable fears of people, places, or events
- Prolonged depression or the inability to recover from a major crisis or loss
- Difficulty in getting along with others or in holding a job
- Self-destructive behavior, such as compulsive drinking, gambling, or drug use
- Sexual dysfunction, such as impotence, frigidity, promiscuity, or perversion
- Sleeping difficulties, insomnia, or recurring nightmares
- Feelings of hopelessness or confusion or suicidal thoughts
- Inability to make simple decisions, moodiness, or feeling out of control
- In children, failure at school, disruptive behavior at school and home, senseless destructiveness, delinquency, or frequent physical complaints

Since some medical disorders (for example, having a low blood sugar level or an overactive thyroid gland) can produce physical symptoms that resemble those of an emotional problem (such as shakiness, which may result from anxiety), the first step in seeking treatment is to have a thorough physical examination. In addition to ruling out a physical problem that may be causing symptoms, the doctor can make a referral to a competent therapist or mental health agency.

Types of professional help

There are several different kinds of professional therapists qualified to treat emotional and mental difficulties:
- Psychiatrists are doctors with a medical degree plus three or more years of training in psychiatry. Psychiatrists are the only therapists qualified to prescribe drugs. Like other medical specialists, they must be licensed by the state in which they practice and certified by their specialty board.
- Clinical or psychiatric social workers are professionals with a master's or doctoral degree in mental health plus two years of internship in a clinical setting. They may be certified by the state in which they practice and are listed in the *National Registry of Health Care Providers in Clinical Social Work.*
- Clinical psychologists are therapists with a doctoral degree in psychology and one year of supervised clinical training. Psychologists are licensed by the state in which they practice, certified by their specialty board, or listed in the *National Registry of Health Service Providers in Psychology.*
- Psychiatric nurses are nurses with a master's degree in psychiatry or mental health who are accredited by the American Nurses' Association Division on Psychiatric and Mental Health Nursing Practice.
- Psychoanalysts are psychiatrists or clinical psychologists with special psychoanalytic training. (However, a person with little or no training can use the title of psychoanalyst—be careful to check the person's credentials.) At present, psychoanalysts are licensed only in California, but others may be listed in the *National Registry of Psychoanalysts.*
- Pastoral counselors are members of the clergy with training or a degree in psychology or social work. They are certified by the American Association of Pastoral Counselors.

Finding help

One of the biggest keys to success in therapy is finding a qualified professional with whom the person seeking treatment feels comfortable. Before making an initial appointment, ask the therapist about his or her credentials. During the first appointment, ask for an explanation of the methods or forms of therapy the therapist uses, for an estimate of how long treatment may last and how much it will cost, and for an opinion on the results that can be expected.

The patient seeking treatment should ask himself or herself these questions: Do I feel comfortable talking to this therapist? Do I trust him or her? Do the proposed method of treatment and the expected results sound plausible? It may take more than one appointment or session with the therapist to answer these questions. If you have doubts, it is perfectly permissible to look around for another therapist. It is also possible that the therapist will feel unqualified to work successfully with you and will refer you to another professional.

Types of therapy

There are many kinds of therapy, but the most common are the following:

- Psychoanalysis—an intensive (four or five times a week for several years) program of sessions with a therapist with the aim of understanding and changing long-standing personality problems
- Individual psychotherapy—a series of one-on-one discussions with a therapist about problems, worries, emotional attitudes, and ways of coping with life
- Group therapy—a series of discussions with peers (under the guidance of a professional therapist), in which experiences are shared and criticism, praise, and support may be offered
- Family therapy—sessions in which family members work with a therapist to arrive at better ways of interacting with one another
- Behavior modification—use of special techniques to break old habits that cause problems and to learn new ways of dealing with people
- Drug therapy—use of medication to modify body chemistry, usually complemented by some form of "talk" therapy
- Relaxation training—use of special biofeedback techniques to increase awareness

and control of body processes so as to relieve physical conditions, such as tension headaches and high blood pressure

There is a lot of misinformation about the subject of emotional and mental illness, which is left over from the days when little was known about the workings of the mind and body. Some people still label those who have sought and received treatment for mental or emotional disorders as crazy, unpredictable, and dangerous. Such labels are not only unfair, but usually inaccurate; the number of persons with such problems who pose any threat at all to others is very small.

Fortunately for all of us, emotional and mental illness is gradually becoming better understood and accepted as a condition that can be treated and frequently cured. Even more important, emotional health is being recognized as a goal that should and can be attained.

Anorexia nervosa

Anorexia nervosa is an eating disorder that is most common in young women. Anorexics suppress the urge to eat and continue to lose weight to the point of malnutrition and starvation. This disorder can be fatal, because an anorexic can literally starve himself or herself to death.

The reasons for anorexic behavior are still unknown, but theories abound. One theory is that anorexics continue to starve themselves because they mistakenly believe that they are fat and need to diet. The result is not only an unattractively thin appearance but also abnormality of menstrual periods (which very frequently cease when a certain percentage of body fat has been

lost) and, most important, the destruction of healthy muscle and organ tissue, which the body uses as sources of energy when faced with starvation.

Those at risk

Ninety-five percent of all anorexics are female; most are teenagers from upper- or upper-middle-class homes. It is estimated that about one in 200 young women of this age and social class has anorexia nervosa.

Anorexia seems to be mostly a psychiatric disorder, since it often develops in young women with deep-seated problems, although the classic anorexic may not seem to be a "troubled" teenager. The young girl who has always been "perfect" and obedient and who has tried to fulfill all the wishes of her parents, teachers, and friends may become anorexic because of an unconscious need to have total control over at least one area of her life.

Impending adulthood and all that it entails may scare the anorexic into dieting away those characteristics that are symbolic of her developing maturity—larger breasts, fuller hips and thighs, and the monthly cycle of menstrual periods.

Our culture's obsession with thinness as the ideal in beauty can also trigger in an adolescent girl a desire to diet down to her "perfect" weight; often a casual remark that a girl is slightly overweight can lead to a case of anorexia in a susceptible person.

In addition, people with jobs or hobbies that require strict weight control, such as athletes, ballerinas, and fashion models, may find that simply watching their weight has become an obsession with dieting. In fact, the

A person with anorexia nervosa often has a distorted body image that makes her perceive herself as fat even when viewing her extremely thin body in a mirror.

few males who develop this disorder often do so in an attempt to qualify for an athletic team.

Symptoms

The most obvious symptom of anorexia nervosa is drastic weight loss to the point of extreme underweight, which can be accompanied by overly vigorous exercise that burns off the few calories that are consumed. Menstrual periods often stop completely, and a growth of fine, downy hair appears all over the body.

Anorexics cannot be convinced to eat by threats or reasoning. Many have a distorted body image that tells them they are fat even as they view their extremely thin bodies in a mirror. Despite the refusal to eat more than tiny amounts of particular foods, the anorexic may be obsessed with the idea of food and may prepare elaborate meals for others. The anorexic may also suffer from another eating disorder, bulimia, which is characterized by binge-eating, followed by self-induced vomiting and excessive use of laxatives and/or diuretics.

Diagnosis

Diagnostic evaluation of anorexia nervosa begins by ruling out the possibility that the extreme weight loss has been caused by a serious physical illness, such as cancer, an infectious disease, a disorder of the digestive organs, or inadequate absorption of vitamins and minerals. Anorexia can usually be diagnosed when the patient displays the classic symptoms before the age of 25 and has lost 25 percent of her body weight.

Treatment

Anorexia is sometimes treated with hospitalization and forced feeding, but anorexics can usually be treated on an outpatient basis by a medical doctor, psychiatrist, or specialist in eating disorders. The anorexic's distorted body image as well as her eating habits must be changed in order for her to conquer this disorder. Most important, the underlying psychological problems must be resolved. Often, this means psychological therapy for both the anorexic and her family.

Bulimia

Bulimia is abnormal and excessive eating, usually triggered by emotional factors. Victims of the disorder overeat far beyond the needs of their bodies. In extreme cases, they resemble alcoholics, employing food instead of drink as an escape from their problems. They may even go on food binges and eat themselves into a stupor. They often feel guilty after overeating and force themselves to vomit; overuse of laxatives to purge the food from their bodies is also common.

Causes

To a bulimic person, food provides a way to relieve stress. Some experts think that excessive eating is an unconscious attempt to recapture the feelings of security experienced in childhood when food was received from the mother. Psychiatrists have speculated that overeating may also represent a hunger for affection that was denied in early childhood, when the child's attention was focused on the mouth and eating. It may be a substitute for affection, attention, or sexual contact that the person is not receiving. It may be an outlet for hostile feelings, since food is being destroyed by the acts of biting and chewing. Another possibility is that the person may unconsciously seek to become more important and safer by becoming physically larger. Bulimia is sometimes found among mental patients, especially those who have regressed to infantile behavior.

Excessive eating may also result from hyperthyroidism (overactivity of the thyroid gland), a disorder in which great quantities of calories may be eaten without weight gain. In a very small percentage of cases, bulimia may be caused by damage to the appetite control center of the brain.

Treatment

Attempts to cure bulimia have not been very successful and have frequently caused the patient to become even more distressed. However, it is generally agreed that a logical first step is to help the patient discover the emotional causes of the disorder. This may require individual or family counseling by a psychiatrist or clinical psychologist, who also tries to help the patient gain confidence and become more sociable and self-reliant. New satisfactions are sought to replace those formerly found in overeating. Nutritional counseling by a registered dietician and a sensible exercise program may be recommended.

Delirium

Delirium is a confused mental state marked by disorganized or incoherent speech and hallucinations (imagined perceptions). Often, the person is unaware of time or place; is fearful, excited, and restless; and suffers from delusions. The heartbeat is rapid, the pupils are dilated (enlarged), and sweating is common.

Causes

Delirium can occur because of fever, disease, injury, poisoning, or mental disease. It may result from the sudden withdrawal of alcohol or another drug on which the individual has become dependent; from liver, kidney, or heart failure; or from deficiencies of certain B vitamins or thyroid hormone. It can also result from bruising or by pressure on brain tissue, caused by fluid, inflammation, hemorrhage, a tumor, or an abscess.

Symptoms

Delirium often develops rapidly and fluctuates in severity. The patient usually cannot remember what happened during the episode of delirium and does not recall past events well. Depending on its cause, delirium may last from hours to weeks.

Treatment

Treating the underlying disease or condition is the first step in treating delirium. In the meantime, the patient should be cared for patiently and sympathetically in a quiet, relaxed environment. Every effort should be made to answer questions, remove fears, and keep the patient in touch with reality.

Partial or complete recovery depends on the nature, severity, and treatability of the underlying cause.

Depression

Depression, the most common form of emotional disorder, is characterized by prolonged sadness, combined with other negative mood symptoms, such as indecisiveness, inability to concentrate, anxiety, apathy, loneliness, lowered self-esteem, self-blame, and loss of interest in others, in work, and in recreation.

Temporary depression

Deep sadness or depression is a normal reaction of an emotionally healthy person to discouraging life events such as loss, separation, death of a family member, and disappointment. It is probably a protective reaction, possibly enabling a person to withdraw from everyday concerns long enough to sort out his or her feelings and prepare for a new approach to life.

Temporary depression can also occur because of normal chemical changes in the body. Two examples are premenstrual depression and postpartum (after childbirth) depression—both of which are thought to be linked to female hormonal activity. In addition, alcohol and certain drugs, including oral contraceptives, reserpine (used to lower high blood pressure), and some sedatives, may cause depression as a side effect in some people. Certain infections (including influenza, viral hepatitis, infectious mononucleosis, and tuberculosis) can depress a person's mood, as can deficiency of vitamin B_{12}, overproduction or underproduction of hormones by the outer layer of the adrenal gland, and various diseases of the nervous system.

Temporary depression can be eased by the support of family and friends or simply by the passage of time and by steps the person takes to change his or her life situation. Medication is not usually necessary, nor is any other treatment. However, a visit to a physician can provide valuable reassurance that the depression is not abnormal.

Severe depression

Unlike temporary depression, which is sometimes called reactive depression because it is a reaction to a specific circumstance, severe depression does not always have an obvious cause. Even if there is an apparent cause, the reaction is out of proportion, and it may continue for weeks or months.

The causes of severe depression are unclear. Loss of a parent at an early age or growing up in a cold, critical, unstable, or unfriendly family setting may make a person susceptible to depression. There is also an inherited tendency to suffer certain forms of depression.

Symptoms

The symptoms of severe depression include crying spells, slowing of speech and thought processes, agitation, feelings of hopelessness and helplessness, withdrawal from usual activities, recurring thoughts of death and suicide, and irritability. (Some of these symptoms also occur in temporary depression, to a lesser degree.) Early awakening, insomnia, fatigue, loss of appetite, weight loss or gain, loss of sexual desire, and imagined pains are also common. Depressed patients with certain mental diseases may hear voices accusing them of unpardonable crimes, see visions of coffins or dead relatives, believe that others are watching or persecuting them, or suffer delusions that they are worthless, sinful, or ill with some incurable disease.

Sometimes periods of deep depression alternate with periods of elation, high hopes, grandiose ideas, and overactivity. This is known as manic-depressive disorder. When in the manic phase, the person is overwhelmingly confident and inexhaustible, racing from thought to thought. Eventually, however, the mood changes to bleakest despair.

Diagnosis

Diagnosis of severe depression can be complicated. Some depression is masked—the person is "smiling on the outside, crying on the inside" and may not even be aware of his or her depressed mental state. Instead, the depression is expressed in symptoms, such as headaches and backaches, that have no physical cause. In addition, the person may seem to have lost all emotion, including the ability to take pleasure in anything.

The physician needs to rule out physical causes of depression, such as nutritional deficiencies and the side effects of certain medications. Drug abuse and alcoholism may be involved (however, they may be the result, rather than the cause, of the depression). Schizophrenia and other mental disorders must be considered.

Treatment

With appropriate treatment, the symptoms of severe depression can often be reduced or eliminated. Hospitalization is not usually necessary, unless the patient is suicidal, in a stupor, agitated and out of touch with reality, or physically deteriorated as a result of the depression. Hospital treatment for the first three types of cases may involve treatment with antidepressant drugs or electroconvulsive therapy (for more on "electroconvulsive therapy," see page 368).

Most severe depression, however, can be managed with a combination of drugs and psychotherapy (counseling by a psychiatrist or psychologist, with office visits once or twice a week at the beginning of treatment and less often as improvement occurs). It is extremely important to find a professional who is not only knowledgeable but also reassuring and encouraging, and who is trusted by the patient. An extended course of psychotherapy is usually not called for unless there is a serious personality disorder. If depression is a result of a serious physical illness, individual reassurance and support groups may provide the most help.

Lithium carbonate is used to treat manic-depressive illness both in its extreme form and in its moderate form, known as cyclothymia. In the latter condition, the person alternates between brief periods (usually days) of gloom and elation.

Suicide is a major risk in depression and should be guarded against, especially when the person seems to be recovering from the depression but is still feeling "low," when anniversaries of landmarks in the person's life occur, and in the days preceding menstruation.

Electroconvulsive therapy

Electroconvulsive therapy (ECT) is a procedure in which an electric current is passed through the brain to create a convulsion of the central nervous system, like an epileptic seizure, after which the patient is often in a clearer state of mind. Also referred to as electroshock therapy and shock treatment, ECT is used chiefly in cases of severe depression and manic-depressive illness. Occasionally, it is employed to arouse a schizophrenic patient from catatonia (an unresponsive state).

Prior to treatment, the patient is examined and given appropriate tests, which may include an electroencephalogram (brain wave test) to detect brain injury that might be related to the patient's condition. Such an injury would rule out the use of ECT.

Usually, ECT is given early in the morning, because the patient must not have had anything to eat or drink for eight hours before treatment. The patient is put to sleep with an anesthetic given intravenously. Electrodes are placed on one or both sides of the head, and electric current is administered. The seizure that results lasts from 5 to 20 seconds. Recovery is rapid; after half an hour or an hour of drowsiness, most patients are alert and willing to talk. Some temporary memory loss is common, and headaches sometimes occur. However, the use of general anesthesia prevents the anxiety and spinal injuries that used to occur occasionally during ECT treatments. The incidence of serious complications of ECT has been reported to be less than one case in a thousand.

A usual course of ECT treatments is two or three times a week for three to four weeks. A faster method, in which the patient's heart rate is monitored with an electrocardiograph, employs repeated surges of electric current in one to three sessions.

Hyperventilation

Hyperventilation is abnormally rapid and deep breathing, as a result of which large quantities of air are drawn into the lungs and abnormally large amounts of carbon dioxide are expelled.

Causes

Although hyperventilation can result from a physical disorder that interferes with the exchange of oxygen and carbon dioxide in the lungs, most often hyperventilation is a physical response to stress, anxiety, and emotional upset. It begins slowly and builds up to the point at which symptoms appear and the person panics. The breathing then becomes even more rapid and difficult.

Symptoms

The diminished level of carbon dioxide in the blood can lead to buzzing in the ears; a tingling feeling in the fingers, toes, and lips; light-headedness; and fainting. It may also cause tightness in the chest and a feeling of suffocation. Episodes may last longer than half an hour, and they may recur several times in a 24-hour period.

Symptoms may be strikingly similar to those of heart disease and other serious illnesses. The individual experiencing these symptoms should, therefore, consult a doctor to rule out the existence of these conditions.

Treatment

The symptoms of hyperventilation can often be relieved by having the person breathe into a paper bag. In this way, the needed carbon dioxide that has been exhaled into the bag can be inhaled again; as a result, the level of carbon dioxide in the blood can be restored to normal, and the breathing rate is slowed.

Hypochondria

Hypochondria is persistent, exaggerated worry—usually based on self-diagnosis—about one's health, especially in the absence of any real illness. The condition reflects an often morbid concern over any unusual physical or mental sensation or feeling. For example, to the hypochondriac, a headache indicates a brain tumor; a cough has to mean tuberculosis; and a mole is sure to be cancerous. Despite normal test results and reassurances to the contrary, the person is convinced that he or she either has a serious illness or will have one very soon.

Symptoms

Frequently, the hypochondriac complains of pain or discomfort in the stomach, chest, head, or neck. Symptoms common among hypochondriacs include nausea, loss of appetite, vomiting, and belching. These symptoms become worse after the person has received expressions of sympathy and concern from family members or friends. The hypochondriac often makes repeated visits to the doctor or consults several doctors at the same time, without their knowledge, in order to obtain prescriptions for a variety of drugs.

Treatment

Hypochondria is very difficult to treat. It has been estimated that only a small percentage of persons afflicted with this disorder recover completely. Psychotherapy is sometimes useful; in many cases, however, a more helpful approach is to encourage the individual to divert the energy spent on worrying about health to more productive interests and activities.

Mania

Mania refers to an abnormal elevation of mood, characterized by wild excitement, overactivity, and lack of concentration. It is also marked by excessive irritability, hostility, and sometimes violence.

Mania is a component of the manic-depressive disorder, in which periods of mood elevation alternate with periods of depression, with periods of normalcy in between.

Symptoms

Persons in a manic state are likely to go on spending sprees; start, but not finish, new projects; become sexually promiscuous; exhibit restlessness and distractibility; and chatter rapidly and often incoherently. In addition to these symptoms, the judgment of a person in a manic state is often impaired. Because persons in the manic state think they are functioning at their very best, they tend to overextend themselves, becoming involved in many activities without considering the consequences.

Diagnosis

Mania must always be diagnosed by a doctor because apparently manic behavior may actually have a physical basis. Certain disease states can cause similar symptoms. Mood elevation can also be a side effect of some medications. Both possibilities must be ruled out (and treated, if necessary) before assuming that a purely psychiatric disorder is present.

Treatment

Mania and manic-depressive disorder are usually treated with medication and psychotherapy. The medication most commonly used is lithium carbonate. The chief value of lithium is in preventing manic episodes. However, it may take several weeks for the effects of the drug to become apparent. Tests to monitor the level of lithium in the blood are essential, since excessive amounts of lithium can cause serious side effects. It is not known exactly how lithium works to combat mania, although it has been shown that lithium affects chemical transmitters in the central nervous system (the brain and spinal cord).

Paranoia

Paranoia is a personality disorder characterized by delusions of grandeur and suspicions of persecution.

Causes

An internal conflict between the need for recognition and the compulsion to guard certain aspects of emotional life may be the root of paranoia. Unconscious sexual conflicts often play a role.

Symptoms

Paranoid persons display unreasonable distrust and constant unfounded suspicion that others are out to do them harm; interpret innocent comments as personal attacks; develop grandiose or exaggerated estimations of their own worth, yet feel that others do not recognize their value; believe they are the center of attention because everyone else openly criticizes them; and strenuously defend their fears with reason and logic. Paranoia differs from paranoid schizophrenia, a much more serious problem in which the individual not only has delusions of grandeur and a persecution complex, but also demonstrates deranged thought processes, hallucinations, and other signs of disturbed personality.

Diagnosis

Almost everyone exhibits short-lived symptoms that suggest paranoia at some time, usually from excessive worry over an embarrassment or from disappointment. It is only when paranoid behavior persists or worsens and impairs the person's ability to function that concern is warranted. Like the symptoms of many other mental disorders, paranoid symptoms can have an underlying physical cause, such as a brain disease or a drug side effect. Diagnosis should always be made by a physician, who will first rule out (or treat) purely physical causes and then recommend appropriate therapy.

Treatment

Paranoid persons can often be helped with psychotherapy and medication.

Phobia

A phobia is a psychological disorder characterized by persistent, abnormal, excessive, or unfounded dread of something that is often not inherently dangerous or considered threatening by most people. A phobic reaction resembles acute or chronic anxiety, but rather than being a generalized response, it is linked to specific environmental stimuli, such as being alone or in an open space, seeing a spider, or hearing thunder.

Phobias affect fewer than one percent of the total population. They seem to occur more often in some families and more often in women than in men.

Causes

Anxiety is a fearful reaction to the emergence of forbidden or unconscious drives. In most cases, the psychological mechanisms called projection and displacement focus anxiety on specific external objects, persons, or

situations, which then come to represent the original cause of the anxiety. In shifting attention to a secondary symbol, a patient learns to use avoidance of the object or situation (spiders, heights, open places, and so on) to prevent rearousal of the painful anxiety. The "choice" of the phobic object is often at random; it may be the first object, location, or situation at hand when the original anxiety first appeared.

Phobias usually begin in early adulthood and follow a long course of alternate improvement and worsening of symptoms. The longer a patient has phobic symptoms, the less likely he or she is to achieve a complete recovery.

Symptoms

The symptoms of a phobia depend on the phobic object. Often, the very thought or mention of the object induces anxiety in the patient. The more inescapable the exposure or contact becomes, the more anxiety mounts toward panic. As a result, the patient spends more and more time avoiding the phobic stimulus, and this avoidance often begins to restrict his or her daily activities (for example, he or she becomes unable to travel because of fear of flying).

Common phobias

Agoraphobia (a fear of open, public places, such as stores, malls, parks, theaters, and stadiums, or of crowds and crowded situations) is the most common phobia, accounting for about 60 percent of all cases. This abnormal fear of being in open places greatly restricts the life of the vic-

tim, who in extreme cases will not leave home, except perhaps if accompanied by a close friend or relative. The first sign of the condition may be a panic attack when out in public, with feelings of anxiety and a sense of approaching doom, restlessness, breathlessness, and rapid or irregular heartbeat. Thereafter, the person may stay at home to avoid another panic attack. Often, the agoraphobic person experiences the phobia selectively—he or she can face the phobic situation fairly well in the company of someone close or trusted.

Another common phobia, claustrophobia, is an intense and unrealistic fear of being confined in an enclosed space, such as an elevator or a small room. Commonly, the claustrophobic person becomes anxious at even the thought of being "trapped" in a small room or passageway. If the person unexpectedly has to face the phobia, as when caught in a stuck elevator, real panic may result. Unlike some phobias, such as a fear of mice, snakes, or spiders, which the average person seldom sees, claustrophobia can cripple one's vocational and social life, since enclosed spaces are part of the everyday environment.

Some childhood phobias, such as fear of the dark or of animals, disappear with age. But adults, too, experience phobias of specific objects or situations, such as arachnophobia (fear of spiders), ophidiophobia (fear of snakes), acrophobia (fear of heights), and monophobia (fear of being alone). If the objects are easily avoided, like spiders and snakes, there is usually no great problem. However, fear of flying due to acrophobia may cause great inconvenience for a person whose work or social life involves frequent air travel, and monophobia may handicap a worker whose job requires long periods of isolation.

The phobias of function, or social phobias, are those in which the presence of others causes the anxiety. Among them are erythrophobia (fear of blushing), haphephobia (fear of being touched), and phagophobia (fear of being seen eating, which makes the victim incapable of eating in the presence of others).

Treatment

A type of psychotherapy called insight therapy may be helpful in less severe cases; patients learn to recognize the real, underlying object of anxiety and come to see the phobic object as merely symbolic of that other fear. More extreme cases often respond better to behavioral therapy, in which the patient is deconditioned to the phobic stimulus by being required to confront it. At the same time, the patient is encouraged to try various relaxation techniques to combat anxiety. In the most severe cases, a psychiatrist may use a technique called flooding, by which the patient is forced to experience prolonged phobic anxiety with a constant exposure to the object.

Although drug therapy generally is less effective when used alone than when it is combined with psychotherapy, mild tranquilizers and antidepressants can often delay the onset of panic attacks or reduce their severity.

Psychosomatic illness

Psychosomatic illnesses are a broad category of disorders in which psychological or emotional factors cause or contribute to physical symptoms. Psychosomatic illnesses are often considered to be imaginary. This is unjustified, since the patient is not pretending to be ill, and his or her symptoms are no less real than if there were a purely physical basis for the complaint. (There is a psychiatric disorder called Munchausen's syndrome, in which a person knowingly pretends to be ill or intentionally injures himself or herself in order to become ill; however, this rare condition is quite different from psychosomatic illness).

Causes

It is known that psychological factors can contribute directly or indirectly to some physical disorders. For example, having a Type A personality (characterized by aggressiveness, competitiveness, preoccupation with deadlines and time constraints, and chronic impatience) has been associated with an increased risk of heart disease. In addition, there is evidence that stress can change the response of the body's immune system to disease.

Emotional stress may also be reflected in the appearance of physical symptoms, especially if a person has a hard time expressing emotions. In some families, having pain due to physical illness is accepted and elicits a caring response, whereas expressing unhappiness and anger is not tolerated. For someone in such a family, a physical symptom may be an unconscious expression of his or her emotional state.

It is also quite common for someone who is unhappy at home or at work to become preoccupied with everyday aches and pains. For that person, a genuine—albeit minor—illness may take on unwarranted importance because of the emotional state.

Symptoms

Almost any type of symptom may be psychosomatic. In fact, it has been estimated that one third of all complaints reported by patients to their doctors are at least partially psychosomatic. The most typical psychosomatic symptom is pain—for example, facial pain, headaches, generalized abdominal pain, and backache.

Diagnosis

It is important not to dismiss a person's seemingly psychosomatic illness as being "all in his or her head." A physician should always give serious consideration to a patient's complaints, even when it may seem obvious that those complaints are psychosomatic in nature. There have been cases in which symptoms with a purely physical basis have been disregarded because of a suspicion that they were psychosomatic. It should also be remembered that psychosomatic factors can sometimes set the stage for a serious physical disorder, and that psychosomatic symptoms, although they may be exaggerated, may nonetheless reflect an actual physical illness.

A physician who takes the time to learn about the patient's particular life circumstances can often discover the stresses that may be contributing to an illness, even though the patient himself or herself may be overlooking or denying the underlying emotional factors.

Treatment

If, after a thorough examination, no physical cause can be discovered for a disorder, the best treatment the doctor can offer may be to listen sympathetically and to show concern. Some patients may demand more dramatic treatment methods and may go from doctor to doctor until they find someone who will prescribe the treatment they want. It is important to avoid risky or expensive procedures and testing, as well as unnecessary medication. Helping the patient to recognize that certain symptoms are caused or worsened by stress and to learn how to deal effectively with that stress can often be helpful.

Schizophrenia

Schizophrenia is not a single mental disorder, but rather a group of mental disorders that are characterized by disturbances of thought processes, emotional response, and behavior. Among the characteristics common to most types of schizophrenia are extreme mental confusion, withdrawal from reality, delusions, hallucinations, extreme mood changes, and bizarre behavior.

Causes

Most cases of schizophrenia are due to a combination of inherited and environmental factors. A genetic predisposition appears to be an important factor in schizophrenia. It has been estimated that approximately 10 percent of relatives of schizophrenics are schizophrenic themselves. Schizophrenia is not inherited, however. Even if the genetic predisposition is present, the occurrence of the illness is often related to stressful life events and the individual's ways of coping with them.

Symptoms

Schizophrenia affects persons of all ages, although it commonly begins in late adolescence or early adult life. There is no specific personality type that can be singled out as predisposing to development of schizophrenia, but many schizophrenics show such traits as extreme sensitivity, shyness, lack of emotion, antisocial behavior, and paranoid attitudes early in life.

The onset may be sudden or gradual. Some or all of the following symptoms will be present:
- Mental disturbances—progressive confusion of thought and speech; disruption of logical reasoning
- Emotional disorders—absent or inappropriate emotional responses; extremes of depression, excitability, anxiety, and elation
- Hallucinations—distorted or imaginary perceptions involving any of the senses, such as hearing voices or seeing things that are not there
- Delusions—mistaken notions that one is being persecuted, that one is more powerful or important than one is (called delusions of grandeur), or that one's thoughts are being broadcast to others or are being controlled by some outside agency
- Movement disorders—extreme hyperactivity; stupor and immobility; adoption of strange positions, facial expressions, mannerisms, and abnormal activity patterns, such as rocking and pacing
- Violent behavior—such as threats of violence and assassination attempts against authority figures and persons in the public eye
- Withdrawal from reality and social contact

Diagnosis

The physician will obtain a personal and medical history from (or about) the patient and will conduct a physical examination to rule out the possibility that some medical condition or drug reaction may be causing the symptoms of schizophrenia.

Treatment

Chief treatment measures include drug therapy, psychotherapy, counseling, social support, and rehabilitation. For a first illness or acute relapse, hospitalization is usually indicated in order to stabilize the patient's condition. However, hospitalization for more than a few months may be inadvisable; if the patient is able to function outside an institution, leading some semblance of a normal life may be therapeutic.

Schizophrenia is not necessarily a chronic condition. About 30 percent of patients recover completely, and most of the rest show marked improvement with appropriate treatment, although impaired emotional response and motivation may persist.

Senility

Senility is the medical term applied to the gradual process of mental and physical deterioration that is sometimes associated with old age.

Causes

The causes of senility are many—arteriosclerosis (hardening of the arteries), other blood vessel diseases, heart diseases, and lung diseases (all of which may decrease the amount of oxygen available to the brain and other body tissues) and diseases of the liver, the kidneys, and other organs. Senility is not linked to a single disease, nor is it inevitable. However, the years take their toll, and chronic disorders hasten senility. Lifelong harmful habits are also a cause of early senility; alcohol, tobacco, and drug abuse are among the worst offenders.

Symptoms

Gradual loss of physical and mental vigor is the most common symptom of oncoming senility. A lack of interest in the surroundings or in activities once enjoyed is another symptom. Victims experience a loss of complex skills, such as the ability to do puzzles, math problems, or logic problems, or even to balance their checkbooks. If the onset of senility is relatively sudden, as it is with a condition called Alzheimer's disease, the victim will often be in a panic, as he or she feels the mental powers waning. Short-term memory is one of the first faculties to go, and many victims are painfully aware of their condition.

Physical senility is gradual, unless a chronic illness accelerates the process. The skin becomes dry and loses its resilience, the muscles lose their tone and become weak, the bones become brittle, and the organs gradually fail.

Diagnosis

Do not assume that a relative is suffering from senility simply on the basis of confusion and apparent loss of mental skills. Depression and a number of physical conditions can cause similar symptoms. Such symptoms may also be related to the use of certain medications (or combinations of medications). Always consult a physician so that such conditions can be ruled out (or, in some cases, treated).

Prevention

Although there is no way to stop the clock, there are many ways that one can continue leading a vigorous, active life. Getting regular exercise; avoiding toxic substances, such as tobacco, alcohol, drugs, and pollutants; and eating a balanced diet, with adequate amounts of vitamins and minerals, seem to have a positive effect at any age. Protection from debilitating disease and avoidance of injuries (such as broken bones) can also add years of activity to the lives of the elderly.

Mental senility can often be avoided simply by not "turning off" the mind on retirement. The mind begins to deteriorate quickly if it is not used, in much the same way that muscles shrink when they are not used.

HEREDITY AND INHERITED DISEASES

To understand how some disorders can be passed from one generation to another, one must first understand the role played by the genes in determining the form and function of each cell in the body.

The genes are the basic units that determine the hereditary (inborn) characteristics of an organism. Genes, which are composed of molecules of deoxyribonucleic acid (DNA), can be thought of as chemical instructions. Each gene, by virtue of the particular structure of its DNA molecule, contains the code for a specific trait, determining both what a cell is and how it works (as if a computer program not only told the computer what to do but helped to form the machine itself).

Within each cell, thousands of genes are linked in a specific order, like beads on a necklace, to form structures called chromosomes, which are, in effect, continuous strands of DNA. It has been estimated that each cell contains about five feet of coiled DNA strands and that each strand is made of about 100,000 genes.

The particular composition of the genes and their arrangement on the chromosomes are what constitute the genetic blueprint for each individual. Cells that develop into liver tissue, rather than blood cells or nerve fibers, for example, do so because that is what their genetic coding dictates. In this way, the cells of the body are programmed to create a person with a certain color of eyes and hair, as well as the hundreds of thousands of other characteristics that make each human being unique.

Sex cells

Each cell in the human body contains 46 chromosomes. The only exceptions are the sex cells—the ovum (egg) and the sperm—each of which contains only 23 chromosomes. When these sex cells unite in the fertilization of the ovum by a sperm, the result is a full complement of 46 chromosomes, with genes donated by both parents. Since each parent contributes only 23 chromosomes (half of the genetic coding that makes each parent a unique individual), the genetic makeup of their offspring is a blend of components of both parents' genetic material.

Dominant and recessive traits

The traits that genes give rise to may be either dominant or recessive. A recessive gene is one that produces a certain trait only

Chromosomes

Detail of chromosome structure

DNA strand

Protein coating

Genes are contained within the chromosomes of every cell in the body. Chromosomes are threadlike coils that contain the genetic code for the cell. Chromosomes are composed of DNA, which has a spiral, ladderlike structure. The composition and arrangement of the DNA determine the genetic code of the cell.

if its effects are not overridden by those of a dominant gene.

Eye color provides a relatively straightforward illustration of how inheritance of traits works. The gene for brown eyes is dominant; the gene for blue eyes is recessive. The child of a brown-eyed parent who has two brown-eye genes and a blue-eyed parent (who must have two blue-eye genes) will have brown eyes because the brown-eyed parent has only dominant brown-eye genes to contribute to the child's genetic makeup. However, if the brown-eyed parent has a dominant brown-eye gene and a recessive blue-eye gene, the child has a fifty-fifty chance of receiving a blue-eye gene from each parent and thereby having blue eyes. (Actually, inheritance does not always work with such textbook simplicity—sometimes the child of a brown-eyed parent and a blue-eyed parent will have green or hazel eyes.) The union of two blue-eyed persons, because it involves only recessive blue-eye genes, will always produce blue-eyed offspring. The offspring of two brown-eyed persons who each have a recessive blue-eye gene have a one-in-four chance of receiving a blue-eye gene from each parent and, as a result, having blue eyes. (This final combination illustrates how recessive genes can be present but unsuspected, allowing a trait to appear unexpectedly after skipping generations.)

Mutation

Genes are normally transmitted unchanged from one generation to the next. Sometimes, however, mutations occur—that is, the structure of the gene itself is changed, perhaps due to the effect of a toxic substance, an infection, or exposure to radiation. Offspring that receive a mutated gene will exhibit a characteristic that is not present in either of the parents.

The discovery of the structure of the DNA molecule opened a new era in medical research. Scientists in the new field of genetic engineering are exploring ways of artificially creating mutations in genes so that someday it may be possible to correct the errors in genetic coding that cause various disorders.

Genetic counseling

As the medical profession has learned more about inherited diseases, it has been able to offer genetic counseling to couples concerned about the possibility of having a child with an inherited disease or abnormality. A genetic counselor or specialist in genetic disorders can estimate the likelihood that a couple's offspring will be afflicted with a problem due to an inherited trait or to the age of the parents. For some genetic disorders, tests can determine whether one or both parents are carriers or can detect whether a defect is present in a fetus. However, genetic counseling cannot guarantee the health of a child; it can only be a source of advice.

Celiac disease

Celiac disease, or celiac sprue, is a chronic disorder of the small intestine caused by sensitivity to gluten, a protein found in wheat and rye and, to a lesser extent, in oats and barley. The disorder causes poor absorption by the intestine of fat, protein, carbohydrates, iron, water, and vitamins A, D, E, and K. Removal of gluten from the diet normally brings improvement.

Causes

The basic cause is probably an inherited defect found mostly in people of northwestern European ancestry. It affects one person in 300 in western Ireland, and approximately one in 5,000 in the United States. It is twice as likely to affect women as men.

One theory about celiac disease holds that the body reacts to gluten and its derivative gliadin as if they were viruses or bacteria. When food containing gluten reaches the portion of the small intestine called the jejunum, antibodies in the intestinal wall are stimulated. In the process, for some unknown reason, the intestinal villi (hairlike projections through which nutrients from the intestine are absorbed into the bloodstream) are destroyed. Destruction of the villi is almost total in the jejunum, less so in the rest of the small intestine. Poor absorption of food and water is the result. Another theory states that gluten and gliadin act directly on the intestinal wall as toxins (poisons). One or both of these theories may be correct.

Symptoms

Symptoms of celiac disease may begin in infancy when the child starts eating wheat cereal or other foods containing gluten. The child does not thrive, suffers painful bloating in the abdomen, and passes pale, foul-smelling, bulky stools. Failure to absorb enough iron produces anemia (deficiency of oxygen-carrying red blood cells). Poor absorption of protein may cause edema (swelling of body tissues). There is little fat on the body. Growth may be stunted, signs of vitamin deficiency appear, and softening of bones may produce bone deformities and fractures. Sometimes the symptoms disappear in adolescence and reappear in adulthood.

Adults with celiac disease have many of the same symptoms, including the bulky, foul-smelling stools; weight loss; vitamin deficiencies; edema; anemia; and bone pain. The disease can also cause strange sensations (burning, pricking, tickling, or tingling) in the hands and feet; dry skin; eczema; acne; cessation of menstruation; mood changes; and irritability. The disease may appear for the first time as late as age 60.

Diagnosis

The most definitive test for celiac disease is microscopic examination of a piece of tissue taken from the wall of the small intestine. The sample is taken with the aid of a flexible tube with a cutting instrument at the tip, which is inserted through the mouth into the intestine. The specimen from a celiac patient has almost no villi, and the surface is alternately flat and bumpy, with a disorganized network of blood vessels. Various blood tests taken after the patient has eaten specific substances reveal how well the intestine has absorbed these substances. In addition, blood tests may reveal low levels of protein, calcium, potassium, and sodium. Tests of stools reveal excess fat.

Treatment

The primary treatment of celiac disease is to remove all gluten from the diet, which is easier said than done. Hot dogs, ice cream, commercial soups and sauces, candy bars, and all kinds of baked goods can be sources of gluten (even small amounts of gluten must be avoided). Many doctors refer the patient to a dietitian for detailed lists of foods to avoid and for advice on following a healthful diet, which should be high in calories and protein and low in fat. Vitamin and mineral supplements are given as needed. In stubborn cases, a cortisone drug may be given, which will often result in improvement.

The outlook is good for most patients. Recovery is most dramatic in children. In severe cases, complete return to normal bowel function and normal absorption may take months or may never occur. For that reason, and to rule out other diseases of nutritional deficiency or poor absorption, it is best to see a doctor as soon as symptoms appear. This is one ailment that is almost completely treatable.

Cystic fibrosis

Cystic fibrosis is a serious hereditary disease characterized by abnormal secretions that affect many parts of the body, but primarily the lungs, pancreas, and digestive tract.

Cause

Cystic fibrosis is caused by an inherited defective gene. This defective gene is recessive, meaning that it must be inherited from both parents for the child to suffer from the disease. If the gene is received from only one parent, the child is a carrier but will not get the disease. About five percent of the white population in the United States are carriers; the incidence in the black and Oriental populations is much lower. Approximately one in every 400 marriages involves two carriers. A child of two carriers has a 25 percent chance of getting the disease, a 50 percent chance of being a carrier, and a 25 percent chance of being completely free of the defective gene.

The effect of the defective gene is to cause the exocrine glands to release abnormal mucus, sweat, and other secretions. (Exocrine glands are those that release their secretions through ducts, rather than directly into the bloodstream.) The most serious effects of cystic fibrosis occur when the mucous glands release thick, gummy mucus rather than the normal clear, free-flowing fluid. This thick mucus accumulates in the glands, causing swelling, forming cysts, and, most important, blocking various ducts throughout the body. One of the more serious complications of cystic fibrosis occurs when the mucus in the lungs, which normally sweeps bacteria and foreign particles from the lungs, becomes thick and sticky, accumulating in the airways and creating a breeding ground for infection, rather than preventing it. Consequent infections cause still more mucus to be produced, and the airways, already narrowed from the swelling, become even more clogged. Recurrent infections can lead to long-term breathing difficulties. Most deaths from cystic fibrosis are due to respiratory failure caused by obstruction of the airways and by persistent infections.

Also affected is the pancreas, the organ that normally secretes digestive enzymes through a series of ducts into the small

Heat exhaustion is another problem related to this disease, because of the large salt loss due to excessive sweating.

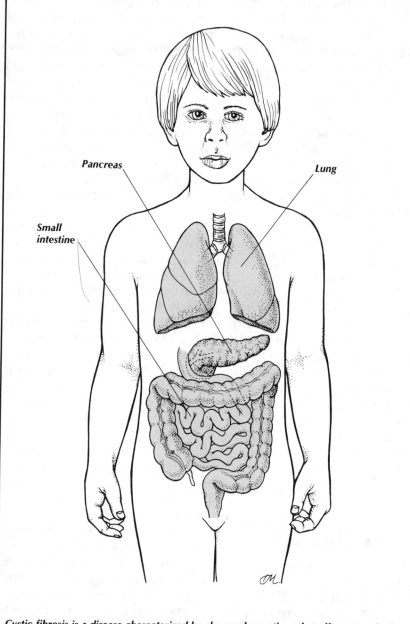

Cystic fibrosis is a disease characterized by abnormal secretions that affect many body parts, particularly the lungs, the pancreas, and the intestinal tract. In the lungs, thick mucus hampers breathing and promotes infection. Thickened secretions can obstruct the ducts in the pancreas and block the passage of pancreatic digestive enzymes into the small intestine.

Pancreas

Lung

Small intestine

Symptoms

The symptoms of cystic fibrosis may show up at birth or may not appear until adolescence. About ten percent of babies with cystic fibrosis are born with a mucous plug in their intestinal tract, which must be corrected surgically.

Because the pancreas is prevented from releasing the enzymes necessary to digest fat, digestive problems are common, and stools are large and foul-smelling. Typically, children afflicted with the disease eat well but gain weight slowly and show signs of malnutrition because the fat in their food is excreted from the body without being used. In addition, the patient usually has excessively salty sweat, a chronic cough accompanied by mucous discharge, and rapid and difficult breathing, and frequently experiences fatigue and muscle cramps from salt loss. Sinusitis (inflammation of the air-filled cavities in the facial bones), nasal polyps (growths in the nose), and a barrel-shaped chest from overinflated lungs may also develop.

Because many of these symptoms are also indications of less serious disorders, cystic fibrosis often remains undiagnosed or undetected for some time while the disease progresses.

Diagnosis

Diagnostic evaluation usually includes a physical examination, medical history, chest X ray, and a sweat test. (Most cystic fibrosis

intestine. These ducts become blocked by abnormally thickened mucus, preventing important enzymes from reaching the small intestine, where they are needed to digest fats.

Reproductive tract secretions are also thickened. In women, an overabundance of mucus in the cervix may block the passage of sperm, making it difficult to become pregnant. About 98 percent of male patients are sterile because the ducts through which the sperm normally travel are blocked by thickened mucus.

patients have excessively salty sweat, although the salt level does not indicate the severity of the condition.) Tests of the stool and digestive juices can show how well the pancreas is functioning.

Treatment

Although cystic fibrosis cannot be cured, its symptoms can be relieved to some extent. Dietary management is extremely important; patients are advised to reduce the fat in their diets, to eat nutritious foods with high amounts of essential minerals and vitamins, to take salt tablets, and to take pancreatic enzyme tablets to aid digestion of fats. The risk of respiratory infections can be reduced by means of antibiotics, aerosol mists, appropriate vaccinations, and postural drainage (in which the patient is positioned so that gravity can be used to help clear mucus from clogged lungs). Regular exercise may also be useful.

Prevention

There is no means of preventing cystic fibrosis today. Researchers continue to look for a reason why the defective gene causes mucus to become abnormal, as well as for a way to identify carriers of the gene. One new test measures certain chemicals present in the amniotic fluid (the liquid that surrounds a fetus in the womb), so that an unborn baby with the gene can be identified. Meanwhile, scientific advances in this area have at least helped those with the disease to live more comfortably. Until the 1960s, few patients lived beyond the age of 10, but today those with cystic fibrosis can live to age 25 or beyond because of medical advances in managing the condition.

Down's syndrome

Down's syndrome is a congenital (present at birth) disorder characterized by varying degrees of mental retardation and a variety of physical abnormalities.

Cause

Normally, each cell in the human body has 46 chromosomes; the cells in someone with Down's syndrome, however, have 47. In ways that are as yet unknown, the presence of the extra chromosome causes all of the unusual characteristics of Down's syndrome. In 95 percent of cases, the condition is called trisomy 21 (because the extra chromosome is attached to the twenty-first pair of chromosomes), and the mistake in genetic coding is one that apparently could happen to anyone. In five percent of cases, the syndrome is caused by a defect that is believed to run in families.

Symptoms

Down's syndrome is marked by a number of physical characteristics: somewhat slanted eyes in small sockets (which is why it used to be called mongolism); a small, short head, flattened in back and front; a nose flattened at the bridge; a thick tongue; short hands, feet, neck, trunk, arms, and legs; a single, rather than a double, crease across the top of the palm; flabby arms and legs with poor muscle tone; a wide gap between the first and second toes; and generally retarded physical development. A child with Down's syndrome may have a poorly functioning thyroid gland (which regulates metabolism, the rate at which the body uses energy) and pituitary gland (which regulates other glands, including those responsible for growth, maturation, and reproduction). About one third are born with heart defects, and both the skin and mucous membranes are especially susceptible to infection.

Education

Characteristically slower than other children to walk, talk, and learn, youngsters with Down's syndrome benefit from "early intervention" programs designed to help them develop their abilities as much as possible. Such programs are frequently available from the time the mother and baby leave the hospital after the birth. A number of organizations exist to promote such programs and assist parents in developing their child's potential. The degree of retardation that accompanies Down's syndrome ranges from mild to severe (the average IQ is about 50), and the extent to which an individual will be affected is not predictable at birth. Some children with Down's syndrome can attend special education classes in public schools; others can attend special schools for the mentally retarded. As adults, some may be able to live independently or semi-independently and work in the community. Depending on the degree of mental retardation that is present, other adults with Down's syndrome will require more supervised living arrangements and may be able to hold simple, routine jobs, perhaps in what is called a "sheltered workshop."

The normal human cell contains 23 pairs of chromosomes, one of which is a pair of sex chromosomes (either two X chromosomes or one X and one Y chromosome), for a total of 46 chromosomes. In Down's syndrome (also called trisomy 21), however, there are three number 21 chromosomes, rather than two; the presence of this extra chromosome is responsible for the collection of symptoms that characterize Down's syndrome.

Hemophilia

Hemophilia is a sex-linked hereditary bleeding disorder in which the clotting mechanism of the blood does not function properly. Blood normally contains several factors that enable clotting to occur. These are designated coagulation factors I through XIII. In the most common form of hemophilia—classic hemophilia, or hemophilia A—factor VIII is deficient. In this case, factors I through VII function adequately, but the clotting process is interrupted by a lack of sufficient amounts of factor VIII. Hemophilia B is the other common form of hemophilia, although it occurs significantly less often than hemophilia A. Hemophilia B is caused by a deficiency of factor IX. Hemophilia B is also known as Christmas disease.

Cause

Hemophilia is inherited as a sex-linked recessive trait—a woman can pass on the defective gene for the trait without being affected herself. The gene that causes the disorder appears on the X chromosome, which is the female sex chromosome. (Males have one X chromosome and one Y chromosome, while females have two X chromosomes.) If a woman has one defective X chromosome, the presence of her other, normal X chromosome ensures that she will not suffer from the disease herself. However, she can pass on her defective X chromosome to her sons, who will have the disease because they do not have a normal X chromosome to counteract the defect. If she passes the defective chromosome to her daughters, they, too,

Prevention

Prospective parents can reduce their chances of having a child with Down's syndrome by starting their families early. At age 20 a woman's risk of giving birth to a child with Down's syndrome is only one in 2,000 live births, but at age 35 the risk is one in 300, at age 40 it is one in 100, and at age 45 it is one in 40 live births. The age of the father also has some bearing on the risk, but not as much as the age of the mother. Diagnosis of Down's syndrome can be made between the sixteenth and eighteenth weeks of pregnancy through a procedure called amniocentesis. During an amniocentesis, the doctor will insert a needle through the mother's abdominal wall and into the uterus. A sample of the amniotic fluid (the amniotic fluid contains cells discarded from the fetus) is then drawn into a syringe, grown on a special culture plate, and analyzed to see if there are abnormal chromosomes present in the fetus. A newer technique used to check the chromosomes of the growing fetus is called chorionic villus biopsy. This procedure, performed during the eighth or ninth week of pregnancy, involves the removal of a small portion of the placenta by a small instrument inserted through the woman's cervix. Tissue that is obtained can be immediately evaluated for chromosome abnormalities.

will be carriers but will not have the disease. A male hemophiliac passes his defective X chromosome to his daughters, making them carriers. However, he passes on only his normal Y chromosome to his sons, who therefore will not have the disease (unless their mother is a carrier). Although the condition appears almost exclusively in males, a woman can be a hemophiliac if her mother is a carrier and her father is a hemophiliac (in such a case, she inherits two defective X chromosomes).

Symptoms

Although affected individuals are born with the disease, the onset of symptoms is variable. Milder cases may not be readily apparent. The symptoms of hemophilia usually appear during early childhood. When a cut in the skin occurs or an injury is suffered, the bleeding may be substantial and prolonged. In severe cases, spontaneous internal bleeding may occur without any obvious cause. Blood may appear in the urine due to internal bleeding. Pain is also a symptom when the bleeding occurs internally, between muscles and into joints. The course of the disease may result in irreversible damage to the joints, which, in turn, results in greater pain and in limitation of movement.

Diagnosis

If a child has any of the symptoms of hemophilia, or if there is a family history of hemophilia, a physician should be consulted. The physician will order laboratory tests to establish the diagnosis. The most common test for hemophilia is determination of the partial thromboplastin time (PTT), which indicates how long it takes for the blood to clot. Additional laboratory tests may be ordered in certain cases.

Treatment

Treatment of hemophilia has recently undergone dramatic changes. One important breakthrough has been the development of factor VIII replacement therapy. One factor VIII replacement, cryoprecipitate, is prepared from donated blood plasma (the fluid portion of blood, which contains more factor VIII than whole blood does). The plasma of an individual donor is quickly frozen by a special process and then slowly thawed, so that the portion rich in factor VIII can be separated out. This portion can then be prepared later for intravenous administration. Cryoprecipitate has the disadvantage of having to be stored and prepared in a hospital. Also, since cryoprecipitate is produced from the plasma of a single donor, the amount of factor VIII present in a given preparation is variable.

Treatment of hemophilia A has been further advanced by the development of a process of rapid freezing and dehydration (removal of water) of plasma, called lyophilization. Freeze-dried concentrates are prepared and packaged so that they can be readily dissolved by a simple mixing procedure. (This process is similar in concept to the preparation and use of freeze-dried coffee.) This concentrate, which quickly stops bleeding, is particularly efficient for home use in comparison with cryoprecipitate.

There is a drawback, however, to the use of freeze-dried concentrate. Whereas the cryoprecipitate is prepared from the blood plasma of a single donor, the concentrate is prepared from the plasma of thousands of donors. The recipient of concentrate is therefore placed at increased risk of infection compared with a recipient of cryoprecipitate. Hepatitis (a serious infection of the liver), for example, may be transmitted in blood products, and the virus that causes acquired immune deficiency syndrome (AIDS) is carried in bodily fluids. Both of these diseases have developed in a number of hemophilia patients who were treated with concentrate. (New blood-testing procedures have now reduced this risk.) Scientists are therefore continuing to investigate the relative risks and benefits of concentrate and cryoprecipitate for treatment of hemophilia A.

Treatment of hemophilia B involves the use of fresh or stored plasma. Concentrate is also available for hemophilia B and is known as prothrombin complex concentrate.

Prevention

There is no preventive for hemophilia. Genetic testing can now identify carriers of hemophilia with considerable accuracy, however, allowing affected individuals to decide whether they wish to risk transmitting the disorder to their offspring.

Huntington's chorea

Huntington's chorea is an inherited degenerative nerve disorder that seldom becomes apparent before early middle age. It is characterized by disorganized body movements (the word *chorea* comes from a Greek word meaning dance) and mental deterioration. It is thought that Huntington's chorea is the result of a disturbance in the part of the brain that automatically regulates voluntary movements.

Cause

The condition is transmitted as a dominant genetic trait from a parent who has the disease. There is about a 50 percent chance of a child's inheriting the disease from an affected parent. Since the symptoms of Huntington's chorea usually do not appear until the victim is between 30 and 50 years of age, a person with a family history of Huntington's chorea lives through the years of adolescence and early adulthood in dread of reaching the middle years, when the symptoms may begin. Even more tragic, a person who is unaware of a family history of Huntington's chorea may have children before discovering that he or she has the disease.

Symptoms

The first symptoms of mental deterioration are usually personality changes—obstinacy, moodiness, lack of interest in surroundings, and inappropriate behavior may be displayed. It should be noted, however, that all of these symptoms can also be due to psychological or other disorders that have nothing to do with Huntington's chorea.

These symptoms are accompanied by irregular, jerky movements that begin in the arms, the neck, and the face. They may start as "fidgeting" and gradually develop into facial grimaces,

halting speech, irregular movements of the torso, and muscle contractions in the neck that cause the head to be held to one side.

In advanced cases, a wide stance will be adopted in an attempt to maintain balance. The gait will become prancing, as control of the legs deteriorates. As the disease progresses, the victims usually become paranoid, walking ability is lost altogether, swallowing becomes difficult, and dementia (loss of intellectual capabilities) increases.

Treatment

No treatment has yet been found to control the symptoms or halt the disease. However, the body movements may be controlled somewhat by drugs, most notably haloperidol and chlorpromazine. There is no known treatment for the mental degeneration that accompanies the physical symptoms.

Prevention

There is no preventive for Huntington's chorea, other than advising affected patients not to have children.

Muscular dystrophy

Muscular dystrophy is the general term for a group of rare diseases in which the body's muscles weaken and waste away. Muscular dystrophy almost always strikes in childhood and is usually inherited. Duchenne muscular dystrophy, which is usually inherited through the

mother, is the most common form of the disease.

The disease is progressive; that is, it becomes gradually worse once it takes hold. In severe forms of muscular dystrophy, the child must use a wheelchair to get around by the age of 11 or 12. Scoliosis (curvature of the spine) may also result from the disease. Severe cases may be fatal, often when the patient is a young adult. Pneumonia is sometimes a fatal complication because of weakening of the muscles involved in breathing.

Muscular dystrophy is sometimes confused with multiple sclerosis, which is a disease of the nervous system that can ultimately result in spasticity and paralysis. There is no deterioration of the nervous system in muscular dystrophy.

Symptoms

Symptoms of muscular dystrophy vary. Muscles usually begin to weaken first in the hips, legs, and shoulders. A child of four or five who waddles from side to side, who has difficulty standing up properly, or who falls frequently should be examined by a physician. The child may also have difficulty in standing up straight or raising an arm high above the head.

Parents should not be overly concerned about the natural awkwardness that occasionally overtakes the older toddler. However, a child near five years of age who consistently has problems with muscular coordination should be checked.

Diagnosis

The diagnosis of Duchenne muscular dystrophy is rarely

made before the age of three. It is most commonly seen in boys; girls are rarely affected.

The physician may want to obtain a muscle biopsy specimen (a small tissue sample) to confirm a diagnosis of muscular dystrophy. The biopsy may be done on an outpatient basis in a hospital or in a physician's office.

Treatment

There is no treatment for the disease, but an exercise program designed by a physical therapist may be helpful. The patient's diet should be regulated so that he or she does not become over-weight; excess weight taxes the child's weakening muscles and hastens the course of the disease.

Prevention

Because muscular dystrophy is an inherited disease, women in the family of an affected child should be tested to see if they are carriers (they can pass on the disease to their children). Such women should receive genetic counseling regarding any pregnancy.

Phenylketonuria

Phenylketonuria (PKU) is a congenital (present at birth) disorder characterized by the presence of increased amounts of certain amino acids in the blood and urine. (Amino acids are the chemical building blocks of protein.) The condition is caused by the inability to convert phenyl-alanine (an amino acid essential for optimal growth in infants and for maintenance of nitrogen balance in adults) into tyrosine (another amino acid). Excess phenyl-

alanine is normally eliminated from the body by conversion to tyrosine. In PKU, this mechanism does not work, permitting an accumulation of phenylalanine. The result is mental retardation in infants or young children if the disorder is untreated.

Cause

Phenylketonuria is hereditary and is found in most population groups, although it is very rare in Jewish and black children. The incidence in the United States is about one in every 16,000 live births.

Diagnosis

Early diagnosis of phenylketonuria is essential because symptoms are usually not obvious in a newborn infant. Therefore, screening tests are now mandatory for all babies born in the United States and Canada. Sometimes, infants with PKU will have nervous system disorders, very light coloring of the skin and hair, eczema (a skin disorder), and a musty odor. Older children may be extremely hyperactive. The light coloring is often an early clue to the disease; the infant's skin, hair, and even eyes will be lighter than those of other members of the family.

Treatment

Treatment of this disorder within the first few days after birth is essential if mental retardation is to be prevented. Treatment consists of limiting the child's phenylalanine intake so that the essential amino acid requirement is satisfied without

any excess. This can be done by feeding the infant special formulas that contain little or no phenylalanine. Milk is a protein food that is rich in phenylalanine; therefore, it must be avoided. When it is time to introduce solid foods, natural foods that are low in protein, such as fruits, vegetables, and certain cereals, are permitted.

If PKU is not diagnosed in the first few days of life, extreme hyperactivity, seizures, and mental retardation usually occur. Some physicians think that treatment and special diet must be continued throughout the child's life; others believe it can be ended when brain development is virtually complete (around age five).

It is important to remember that, although untreated PKU can lead to retardation and other problems, early diagnosis and treatment can enable the child to develop normally and to lead a normal life.

Sickle cell anemia

Sickle cell anemia is an inherited blood disorder, occurring almost exclusively in black persons, in which the normally round red blood cells are transformed into crescentic, or sickle-shaped, cells that are less able to transport needed oxygen. The disease is chronic and is marked by fatigue, breathing difficulty on exertion, swollen joints, attacks of extreme illness, complications from other diseases, and shortened life. In the past, half of all victims of sickle cell anemia died by the age of 20 and few survived past the age of 40. With new technology and new forms of treatment, the outlook is much better, but sickle cell anemia remains a chronic debilitating disease.

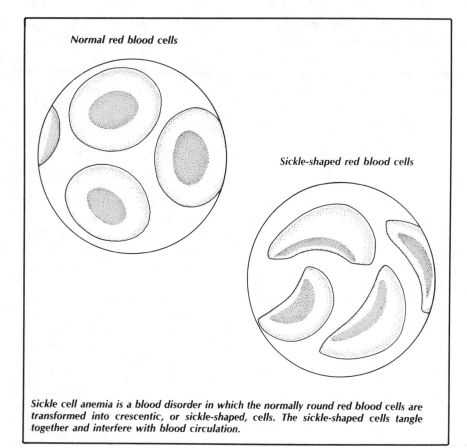

Normal red blood cells

Sickle-shaped red blood cells

Sickle cell anemia is a blood disorder in which the normally round red blood cells are transformed into crescentic, or sickle-shaped, cells. The sickle-shaped cells tangle together and interfere with blood circulation.

Cause

The deformation of the red blood cells occurs because of the presence of defective hemoglobin (the iron-protein compound in the red blood cells that carries oxygen). It occurs when part or all of the body is not getting enough oxygen. Because of their hooked shapes, the blood cells tend to tangle together and pile up, temporarily clogging tiny blood vessels and slowing circulation. Tissue formerly nourished by the clogged blood vessels becomes starved for oxygen and may die. The anemia (deficiency of red blood cells) that results from the accelerated breakdown of defective red blood cells not only weakens the body, but increases oxygen deficiency, which results in more "sickling" of the cells.

The disease occurs in about one of every 330 black persons in the United States. About one in ten black persons in America is a carrier of the defective gene for sickle cell anemia but has no symptoms and is not affected by the disease. However, if two carriers conceive a child together, the risk that their child will be afflicted by the disease is one in four. The risk that the child will also be a carrier is one in two. Both the carrier state and the active state of the disease can be established by a blood test.

Symptoms

In half the victims, symptoms begin between the ages of six months and two years. Among the first signs is unusual swelling of the fingers and toes. The bones of the hands and feet thicken, and clumping of sickle cells may affect the bone marrow, where new blood cells are produced. Youngsters are especially subject to "sickle cell crises," marked by severe pain in the abdomen, joints, bones, and muscles due to lack of oxygen. These crises may last from four days to several weeks, and commonly occur eight to ten times a year before the age of ten. They occur much less often in later years. Signs of a sickle cell crisis include pale lips, tongue, and palms; lack of energy; sleepiness and difficulty in awakening; irritability; pain; and a temperature of 104°F (or one over 100°F lasting for at least two days).

Thickening of the heart muscle; enlargement of the heart, liver, and spleen in children; heart murmurs; and gallstones are common. The heartbeat is usually rapid. Children with the disease are usually small for their age. Those who survive to adulthood may have narrow shoulders and hips, a barrel chest, a curved spine, long arms and legs, and an elongated skull.

Treatment

At present, there is no cure. Treatment includes giving painkillers, making the patient as comfortable as possible, and treating problems as they occur. These problems include severe anemia, which may require a blood transfusion, and frequent infections, which occur because the immune system is impaired.

Prevention

Avoiding cold, fatigue, and other stress may help to reduce the number of sickle cell crises.

Screening programs are available for those who wish to know whether they carry the gene for sickle cell anemia. Those who have the gene can obtain genetic counseling. There is no risk of disease in offspring if only one parent is a carrier, but each child will have a one in two chance of being a carrier.

Tay-Sachs disease

Tay-Sachs disease is a hereditary metabolic disorder that chiefly afflicts infants of eastern European Jewish descent. This disease is fatal, usually by the age of four years. It is marked by retarded development, loss of vision, and paralysis.

Cause

The disease is caused by a deficiency of a certain digestive enzyme (a substance that causes chemical changes without being altered itself). This deficiency results in the accumulation of fatty acids in the brain.

Symptoms

The symptoms of Tay-Sachs disease in an infant are most often noted after four to six months of normal development. A previously well infant begins to lose motor coordination skills that had been attained and to exhibit loss of interest in his or her surroundings. As the condition becomes more advanced, seizures occur, and the head becomes considerably enlarged.

Diagnosis

The physician may notice poor muscle tone and an exaggerated startle response to sound. A distinctive cherry-red spot may be seen in the retina of the eye. The diagnosis is confirmed with special blood tests.

Diagnosis of the disorder may be made before birth by amniocentesis, a procedure in which a small amount of amniotic fluid (the fluid in the sac surrounding the fetus in the uterus) is removed for laboratory examination.

Treatment

There is no known treatment for Tay-Sachs disease, other than supportive care.

Prevention

There is a blood test available that will help identify carriers of the defective gene. (A carrier has the defective gene but does not have the disease.) This test is especially recommended for all Jews of reproductive age. If two carriers have children, each child conceived has a one in four chance of having the disease. It is, therefore, a good idea for carriers to seek genetic counseling before starting their families.

CANCER

Cancer is the term used to describe a broad group of diseases in which certain body cells grow out of control.

RISK FACTORS

Who is most likely to develop cancer? This question is very difficult, if not impossible, to answer. There are, however, certain risk factors that increase the possibility that you may develop cancer in your lifetime. Among these are age (as a rule, the older you are, the higher your risk), family history (for example, if your mother or sister had breast cancer, your risk of developing it is increased), and environmental and other factors.

The rapid increase in cancer rates during this century has been blamed largely on the environment. Polluted air and water, food additives and colorings, and changes in diet from "natural" to "processed" foods all have been implicated as possible causes. Cigarette smoking has been shown conclusively to be a cause of lung and other related cancers. If you wish to reduce your risk of getting cancer, think about changing those factors that are within your control, such as diet and tobacco use.

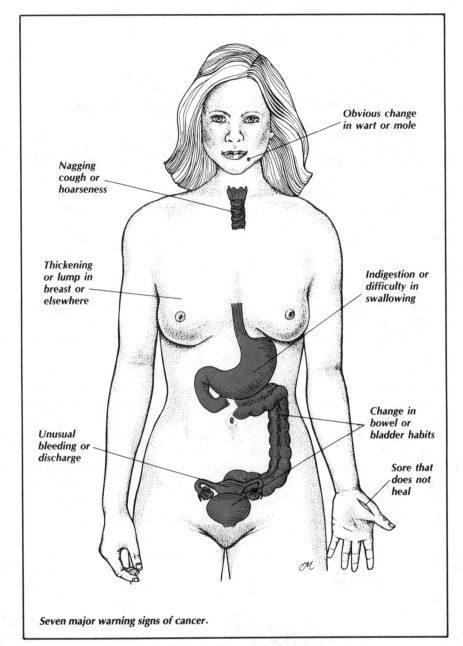

Seven major warning signs of cancer.

WARNING SIGNS

Often a patient is the first to suspect cancer. This is why it is important to learn some of cancer's most common warning signs:
- Change in bowel or bladder habits
- A sore that does not heal
- Unusual bleeding or discharge
- Thickening or lump in the breast or elsewhere
- Indigestion or difficulty in swallowing
- Obvious change in a wart or a mole
- A nagging cough or hoarseness

The chances of cure are greatest if the cancer is discovered at an early stage. If you are a woman, you should learn how to perform the breast self-examination to detect suspicious lumps as early as possible. If you are a man, many physicians recommend self-examination for testicular cancer.

CAUSES AND TYPES

Unlike normal cells, which grow and reproduce in the orderly manner dictated by their genetic coding in their chromosomes, cancer cells grow at an uncontrolled rate—taking over, causing the death of, or replacing normal cells. As the disease progresses, cancer cells often travel through the circulatory system to start growth in other parts of the

387

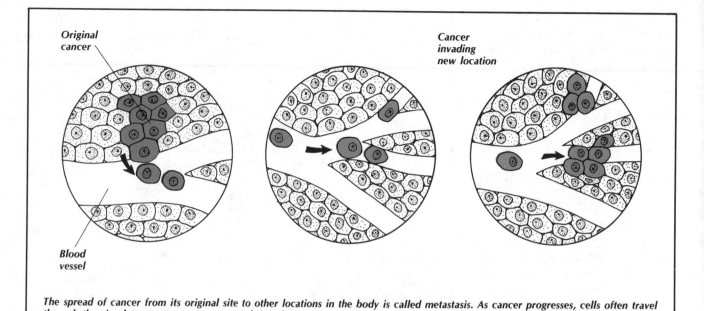

The spread of cancer from its original site to other locations in the body is called metastasis. As cancer progresses, cells often travel through the circulatory system to start growth in other parts of the body.

body; this process is called metastasis.

A tumor is an abnormal tissue growth. A tumor may be either malignant (cancerous) or benign (noncancerous). A benign tumor commonly grows within a capsule and does not invade surrounding tissue or spread throughout the body. Malignant tissues may grow out of control; quite often, they spread.

More than 200 types of cancer have been identified. There are three basic categories of cancer: carcinoma (cancer of the epithelial cells, which line organs and secrete mucus, among other functions), sarcoma (cancer of connective tissue, such as bone, fat, and muscle), and fluid cancers (for example, leukemia). Some cancers may fall into more than one category.

DIAGNOSIS

If you suspect you may have cancer, *do not delay* in seeing a

A tumor may be either benign (noncancerous) or malignant (cancerous). A benign tumor commonly grows within a self-produced capsule and does not invade surrounding tissue or spread itself throughout the body (metastasize). A malignant tumor may grow out of control and metastasize.

physician. Following a physical examination, if the doctor suspects abnormal growth, he or she may order a series of tests, including special X-ray examinations (for example, computed tomography or CT scans, in which successive X rays at slightly different levels are used to create a three-dimensional image of a structure), nuclear medicine scans (in which radioactive substances are used in the imaging process), ultrasound scanning (a technique that uses sound waves to create images of internal structures), cytologic tests (microscopic examination of cells), and various laboratory evaluations. The doctor may also order a biopsy (removal of a small tissue sample for microscopic examination) to determine the cell type of the suspected growth and to determine whether it is benign or malignant.

Your physician may also refer you to a specialist with expertise in treating the type of cancer that you have. This may be an oncologist (cancer specialist), a cancer surgeon, a radiation oncologist (radiologist who uses radiation to treat cancer), or a hematologist (specialist in blood diseases). These physicians are specially trained to deal with the diagnosis and treatment of cancer.

WHERE TO SEEK MEDICAL HELP

There are many places to get cancer treatment. Most cancers can be effectively treated at a well-equipped and well-staffed community hospital. There are, however, a number of large cancer centers throughout the country where specialized treatment programs (called protocols) are available. Often, diagnosis and treatment are initiated at a spe-cial center and then continued in the community by an oncologist or a family physician. If you need information or referrals, cancer hotlines and the American Cancer Society are valuable resources. They or your personal physician should be able to assist you in getting a second opinion, if you want one.

TREATMENT

There are many ways of treating cancer. Many treatment protocols have been developed that are effective in certain types of disease. Cancer therapy often includes surgery to remove the cancer, to clear obstructions of vital passageways caused by the cancer, or to cut nerves sending pain messages to the brain; chemotherapy (use of powerful drugs to kill cancer cells); radiation therapy (use of radioactive materials in the form of energy beams or radioactive implants to destroy cancer cells); and immunotherapy (use of naturally occurring substances to increase the activity of the body's immune system). Combinations of therapies are often used.

Surgery

Surgery is the most commonly used method of dealing with cancers that develop into tumors. If cancer is contained in one area, surgery can sometimes completely eliminate it. New surgical techniques are continually expanding the range of tumors that can be safely removed. Furthermore, if the surgeon is able to remove only a part of the tumor, the reduced tumor can often be successfully controlled with chemotherapy or radiation therapy.

More precise surgical techniques mean that surgery today is often less disfiguring than in the past. In addition, new developments in skin grafting make it possible to begin reconstructive work on patients—for instance, those with cancer of the head and neck—simultaneously with the cancer surgery.

Sometimes surgery is performed on a patient even though it is known that surgery will not cure the cancer. The removal of a tumor may simply make the patient more comfortable. In other cases, nerve pathways to the pain center in the brain may be cut. Certain noncancerous growths may be removed because they may develop into cancer or because they are exerting pressure on an adjacent anatomic structure (which may lead to functional problems).

Chemotherapy

Chemotherapy (the treatment of cancer with drugs) has gradually become much more widely used. Many kinds of cancer can be effectively treated with chemotherapy alone. Anticancer drugs are also often used as an adjuvant (supplement) to primary treatment, such as surgery. Once surgery has reduced a cancerous growth, chemotherapy can often eliminate it. Chemotherapy has proved effective against some forms of cancer that formerly were almost always fatal, in particular, Hodgkin's disease (cancer of the lymph system), acute lymphocytic leukemia (a blood disease predominantly of children), and cancer of the testes (male sex glands).

Most cancer drugs attack any rapidly reproducing cells in the body, whether they are cancerous or not, producing some of the side effects of chemotherapy. Destruction of normal cells that reproduce frequently, such as those in the digestive tract, the hair follicles, and the bone marrow, can lead to nausea, hair loss, and lowered red blood cell count.

Usually, several drugs are administered in combination. If the cancer does not respond, or if resistance to a medication develops, another combination of drugs may be tried.

Radiation therapy

Radiation destroys the ability of cells to divide. Cancer cells are far more susceptible to radiation than normal cells, although not all cancers respond to radiation. Like surgery, radiation therapy is usually a localized treatment, directed at a particular cancer site. Radiation treatment may also involve implanting a radioactive object directly into a tumor, destroying it from within. Radiation can be used before surgery to reduce a tumor to operable size, and frequently a patient receives radiation after surgery to destroy any cancer cells that might remain near the cancer site. Some tumors can be treated by radiation alone.

Radiation therapy is continually being refined. Drugs have been discovered that make cancer cells more sensitive to radiation. Different forms of radiation are being tested on resistant cancers. In addition, radiation today can be directed more precisely, and in stronger forms, with little harm to surrounding tissue. However, there are still side effects, including loss of appetite, nausea, and temporary hair loss. It is not certain how dangerous it is to be treated with radiation, which is itself carcinogenic (ca-

pable of causing cancer); however, it is generally considered that a cancer in the body is far more threatening than the future effects of radiation therapy.

Immunotherapy

The goal of immunotherapy is to enable the patient's body to produce substances that resist the growth of cancer. The basis of immunotherapy is the theory that cancer develops when, for some reason, the body fails to destroy abnormal cells. Immunotherapy for the treatment of cancer is still in the experimental stage.

Unorthodox treatments

Sometimes, in desperation, a patient or his or her family will seek unorthodox methods of treatment, such as various forms of dietary therapy and the use of drugs of unproved value.

One such unorthodox treatment is the use of laetrile, an extract of apricot pits that some have proclaimed is a cure for cancer. This substance has been banned in the United States because it has been shown to be of no value against cancer in laboratory animals and has yet to be adequately tested in humans. Furthermore, laetrile has been shown to be poisonous.

The medical community is actively researching all known methods of treating cancer and carefully evaluating those that look most promising. Many treatments are slow, and often have severe side effects. Many quack cures offer—but do not deliver—rapid cure with fewer side effects. The harm done by quack practitioners is that they prevent a patient from seeking effective

treatment until it is too late for any treatment to be of use. The best advice is to trust a physician to treat cancer and not waste time, money, and hope on an unproved "cure."

PROGNOSTIC FACTORS

If you do develop cancer, a number of prognostic factors (factors that predict length of survival) are important. Most important are the stage and the type of the disease. The earlier the stage of the disease (that is, the earlier in its course it is diagnosed) the better the prognosis will be. The type of tumor is also important, since the various types may respond differently to treatment. Furthermore, more than one type of cancer can occur within a specific organ. For example, all lung cancers do not involve the same kind of cell. Your age and overall physical condition are also important in determining your ability to win the fight against cancer.

Cancer should no longer be considered the dreaded scourge that it was 20 years ago. It is not always fatal and is, in many instances, curable. The keys to living today should be to avoid carcinogens (substances that cause cancer such as tobacco and asbestos), to consult your physician regularly (and discuss possible risk factors), and to perform regularly the important self-examination procedures that your doctor suggests. Early detection is extremely important.

Bladder cancer

This is the most common cancer of the urinary tract. It occurs most often between the ages of 50 and 70 and is the fourth leading cause of cancer death among men. Four times as many men as women are afflicted.

Bladder cancer has been connected with exposure to a number of carcinogens. This may be because the urinary tract comes into contact with so many foreign substances due to its excretory function. For many years it has been known that those who work with aniline dyes have a high incidence of cancer of the bladder. Bladder cancer is also associated with exposure to tar from tobacco smoke and with schistosomiasis (infestation with a tropical parasite).

Blood in the urine is usually the first symptom of bladder cancer. In addition, urination may be difficult, painful, and frequent. The appearance of blood in the urine may be intermittent, and if this symptom disappears, a doctor is sometimes not consulted. However, anyone with blood in the urine should consult a doctor, since in the early stages, this disease may be curable, and treatment is far more difficult later. If your doctor considers that the symptoms suggest bladder cancer, a cystoscopic examination may be ordered. With the patient under local or general anesthesia, a lighted tubelike instrument called a cystoscope is passed into the urinary tract through the urethra (the passageway from the bladder to the outside), so that the interior of the bladder can be examined. This instrument can also be used to obtain a biopsy specimen (a small sample of tissue for laboratory analysis) of a suspicious growth.

Treatment of bladder cancer depends on how far advanced the disease is. A small tumor can sometimes be completely removed with a cystoscope. More advanced cases are treated with surgery or radiation or a combination of the two. In certain cancers, chemotherapeutic agents are instilled directly into the bladder.

Bone cancer

This rare form of cancer is most common in those between the ages of five and 20. Predisposing factors include bone diseases, bone fractures, and exposure to radiation.

Bone cancer usually develops first in the arms or legs. Pain, swelling, and brittleness of the bone may be its symptoms. It is often far advanced by the time it is discovered. The first tool in diagnosis is the X ray, which may show whether the bone is cancerous and whether the disease has spread. If cancer is suspected, an orthopedic surgeon generally performs a biopsy. Bone cancer is usually treated with a combination of surgery, radiation, and chemotherapy.

Brain cancer

Any tumor in the brain, whether cancerous or not, is very dangerous. Because the brain occupies an enclosed space within the skull, even a small tumor that weighs only a fifth of a pound can cause crowding sufficient to bring on death. Brain cancer is most often the result of metastasis from other cancer sites, particularly the breast, lung, and skin.

Symptoms of brain cancer are of two kinds. Increased pressure in the skull can cause seizures, headaches, nausea, forgetfulness, and personality changes. However, symptoms may also arise in the part of the body controlled by the affected area in the brain.

For instance, coordination, vision, or strength of limbs may be affected.

In the past, brain tumors did not respond well to treatment, largely because diagnosis could not be made until late in the development of the disease. Recently, however, diagnostic techniques have improved. The computed tomography (CT) scanner produces a three-dimensional image of the brain that can show the size and location of a tumor and can be used to monitor the progress of treatment. A new technique, magnetic resonance imaging, is also being used.

Surgery is the primary treatment for brain cancer. It is often not used, however, when cancer is present in multiple areas or when the tumor originated in another organ. Surgery in the brain is a delicate procedure; often, a tumor deep in the brain cannot be totally removed without risking impairment of body function. However, new techniques in brain surgery—sometimes with the use of a microscope—permit treatment of tumors once considered inoperable. Radiation therapy and chemotherapy are often used after surgery, although the sensitivity of brain tissue demands that these be administered cautiously. Steroid drugs may be given to reduce the dangerous swelling that a tumor can produce.

Breast cancer

About one woman in 13 will develop breast cancer at some time in her life. It is the leading cause of cancer death in women and the leading cause of all deaths in women between the ages of 40 and 44. The high-risk group includes women over 35, women who have never had children or who had a child for the first time after the age of 30, women who began menstruation early, and women who experienced late menopause. Breast cancer also occurs more frequently in chemical workers, women with a family history of the disease, and women who have already had breast cancer.

Self-examination of the breasts can often lead to early detection. All women should perform these examinations monthly at the end of the menstrual period. About 90 percent of all breast tumors are discovered by self-examination. The recommended technique for breast self-examination is shown in the illustration on this page.

If a lump is discovered in a breast, the doctor will probably order an X-ray examination of the breast, known as a mammogram. The doctor may also take a biopsy specimen from the lump to test for the presence of cancer. If cancer is identified, surgery will probably be performed. Women with breast cancer often dread surgery because of the disfigurement that can result; however, surgery for a breast tumor is often less extensive today than in the past. At one time, all breast cancer patients received a radical mastectomy (removal of the breast, underlying chest muscles, and lymph nodes in the armpit). Now it is known that in many cases the removal of the breast, or even the tumor alone, may be equally effective. In addition, there are techniques for reconstruction of the breast after surgery and for rehabilitation of muscle tone in an arm that has been weakened by surgery. In some cases, radiation therapy and chemotherapy will be used after surgery to destroy remaining cancer cells.

In the shower, examine each breast with the opposite hand while keeping the other hand overhead. Having wet, soapy skin may make it easier to feel lumps.

Lie in bed with a pillow under one shoulder to elevate and flatten the breast. Examine each breast with the opposite hand, first with the arm on the same side as the breast under the head and then with that arm at the side.

Stand in front of a mirror, with hands resting on hips. Examine breasts for swelling, dimpling, bulges, and changes in skin.

Make rotary motions with the fat pads, not the tips, of the fingers, moving in concentric circles inward toward the nipple. Feel for knots, lumps, or indentations. Be sure to include the armpit area.

Standing in front of a mirror with arms extended overhead, examine breasts for changes. This position highlights bulges and indentations, which may indicate a lump.

Squeeze nipples gently to inspect for discharge. Report any suspicious findings to your doctor.

Cervical cancer

The cervix is the lower part of the uterus (womb), which extends into the vagina. Cancer of the cervix is the second most common cancer among American women. The death rate from this disease has decreased 50 percent over the last 50 years, largely as a result of early diagnosis. Early cervical cancer has no symptoms but can be detected by means of a Pap smear (Pap is short for Papanicolaou, the name of the doctor who developed the test). A Pap smear is performed routinely in a doctor's office by scraping the surface of the cervix. The collected material is tested for indications of cancer. Today, two out of three cases of cervical cancer are detected with this test before they display symptoms.

Cervical cancer has a higher incidence among black women and poor women. This cancer also occurs more frequently among women who were sexually active early with many partners and among those with genital herpes.

If a Pap smear indicates the possibility of cervical cancer, a biopsy of the affected area will probably be performed. Treatment depends on how far the disease has advanced; early forms are almost always curable by surgery. If a patient still hopes to bear children, and the cancer is in an early stage, this surgery can sometimes be put off until after children have been born. However, this is possible only if the disease does not seem to be progressing, and the cancer must be monitored carefully during this phase. The uterus should be removed eventually. More advanced forms of the disease are treated with radiation as well as surgery.

Colon cancer

Every year, many Americans die of cancer of the colon and rectum. About half of all cases of cancer of the colon can be cured by surgery, and early detection can greatly improve this percentage. A simple test for occult (not visible to the naked eye) blood in the stool can indicate whether further tests should be made for the presence of this type of cancer. Everyone who is over 40 or who has chronic digestive problems should have this test regularly. Cure is twice as likely if the disease is discovered before symptoms occur.

Symptoms of cancer of the colon include a change in bowel movements, bleeding from the rectum, pencil-thin stools, and abdominal discomfort not eased by bowel movement. If you have any of these symptoms, your doctor will probably perform a rectal exam, inserting a finger into the rectum to search for unusual growths. If further examination is necessary, the doctor may introduce a proctosigmoidoscope (a lighted, tubelike instrument) into the colon through the anus. This instrument permits examination of the inside of the colon and can also be used to obtain a biopsy specimen of a suspicious growth. Sometimes, a noncancerous growth called a polyp is removed with a similar instrument, because such a growth may become cancerous.

Surgery is the usual treatment for cancer of the colon. If the cancer is near or in the rectum, the surgeon may remove all of the rectum and create an artificial rectum, or colostomy, in the lower abdominal wall. A colostomy is covered with a bag to collect waste material. It is important to note that colostomy is not automatically done for any colon cancer. The type of operation performed is dictated by the size and location of the tumor along with other factors.

Leukemia

This is a disease that originates in the bone marrow, the site of blood cell production. The term *leukemia,* which is derived from Greek words that mean literally "white blood," refers to the fact that this disease is characterized by the presence of excessive numbers of white blood cells, especially immature and poorly functioning forms of these cells.

The symptoms of leukemia result from the impairment of normal blood cell functions. The primary role of white blood cells is fighting infection. Since many of the white blood cells present are immature, they function poorly and infections are common. Other blood cell types normally present in bone marrow (red blood cells, which carry oxygen, and platelets, which are needed for blood clotting) may be crowded out by the cancerous leukemic cells. As a result, symptoms of deficiency of these cell types are often evident in leukemia patients. Symptoms include poor blood clotting ability (due to a shortage of platelets) and tiredness resulting from anemia (due to decreased numbers of red blood cells). Other symptoms are easy bruising, bleeding gums, blood in the stools, fever, and frequent infections. The spleen and lymph nodes are usually enlarged.

A diagnosis of leukemia should be made by a cancer specialist. The doctor will probably insert a needle into the hipbone to withdraw a sample of the bone marrow which will be tested for the presence of cancer.

Leukemia is often treated first with intensive chemotherapy to kill the cancer cells. The patient may appear to become even more ill during treatment because of the side effects of the cancer-fighting drugs. After this initial treatment phase, radiation and additional drugs may be administered. Bone marrow transplants are now often used.

Leukemia is the most common form of cancer in children. In recent years, the outlook has improved dramatically for children with this disease. Twenty years ago, nearly all children who suffered from leukemia died. Today, the life spans of many have increased; some live normal life spans.

Liver cancer

Liver cancer usually results from the spread of cancer cells from another site in the body. However, cancer that originates in the liver can sometimes be traced to environmental carcinogens. It is known that anyone who has worked with vinyl chloride, a chemical used in plastics manufacture, has a higher risk of this disease. It also appears that cirrhosis of the liver (a disease in which normal liver cells are replaced by fibrous tissue) may cause an individual to be more susceptible to cancer of the liver.

Symptoms of liver cancer are difficult to identify. They may resemble the signs of a peptic ulcer—aching or burning pain in the upper abdomen, nausea, and vomiting. A swollen or hardened liver often indicates to the doctor the need for further testing.

If this form of cancer is diagnosed early and is confined to the liver, it can be treated surgically, but most often the prognosis is not good.

Lung cancer

Cigarette smoking is generally accepted as the major cause of lung cancer. Lung cancer is the leading cause of cancer death in men, and in recent years the incidence of lung cancer in women has been growing, probably as a result of the increase in the number of women who smoke. The incidence of lung cancer is also increasing among nonsmokers, possibly due to improved diagnostic techniques (many lung tumors were once diagnosed as tuberculosis) and to environmental pollution.

If you smoke and are over 45, or if you have a family history of lung cancer, you should be on the lookout for symptoms, since the early signs—a persistent cough or lingering respiratory discomfort—can be very mild. Later, coughing will increase, as will chest pain and shortness of breath, and blood may be found in the sputum (the material coughed up from the lungs).

A cancerous tumor in the lung is usually removed surgically. It is sometimes necessary to remove an entire lobe of the lung. Because lung cancers are usually not detected until they are well advanced, surgery alone may not be able to eliminate them, and radiation and chemotherapy may be used in combination with or in place of surgery.

In recent years, the deadliest form of lung cancer, small-cell carcinoma (also called oat-cell carcinoma), has yielded to a new drug therapy that has produced temporary remission (absence of symptoms) in some patients.

Lymphoma

This cancer attacks the lymphatic system, particularly the lymph nodes and the spleen. These organs manufacture lymphocytes (cells that protect the body against infection).

The first symptom of lymphoma is usually a swollen spleen or swollen lymph nodes in the neck, armpit, or groin. Fever and sweating are later symptoms. If these symptoms persist, a doctor should be consulted. If the doctor suspects cancer, a biopsy of the enlarged organ will probably be ordered.

There are two major forms of lymphoma: Hodgkin's disease and nonHodgkin's lymphoma. In recent years, there have been dramatic strides in the treatment of Hodgkin's disease. In the early stages, radiation alone can be very effective. Later in the course of the disease, more extensive radiation or a combination of radiation and chemotherapy may be required. Treatment of non-Hodgkin's lymphoma is much the same as that of Hodgkin's lymphoma. In the past, this form of lymphoma was usually discovered too late for treatment, but recent advances have made long periods of remission possible in many cases.

Ovarian cancer

This is the most dangerous form of cancer of the female reproductive organs, because it is so difficult to diagnose in its early stages. Women over 50 have a higher incidence of the disease, as do childless women and those with a family history of ovarian cancer.

Symptoms may include pelvic discomfort, constipation, abdominal swelling, and irregular menstruation. Diagnosis is often not possible without an exploratory operation known as a laparotomy, in which a surgical incision is made in the abdominal wall. Laparoscopy, during which a lighted tubelike instrument is inserted through a small incision in the abdominal wall for direct examination of the female organs and sometimes for treatment, has become a very useful tool in ovarian cancer. Sometimes, removing only one ovary is sufficient, but usually it is necessary to remove both ovaries and the uterus. Radiation therapy and chemotherapy may then be administered, if necessary.

Prostate cancer

After lung cancer, this is the most common cancer among men. Black Americans have a higher incidence of prostate cancer than any other group in the world. In general, it is more common in men over 55. Cancer of the prostate (the male sex gland that lies at the base of the bladder) can develop very slowly, often producing no symptoms until the disease is far advanced. Sometimes a routine examination discloses a lump in the prostate, which proves to be cancerous in about 50 percent of cases. Prostate examinations should be included in medical checkups of all men over 40.

When symptoms occur, they are usually the result of enlargement of the prostate, which causes difficult urination or blood in the urine. Prostate cancer often spreads to the bone, and patients may complain of bone pain before they show any other symptoms.

In cases in which prostate cancer is discovered before it has begun to spread, the cancer can frequently be cured by surgery or radiation. When the disease has spread, usually only its symptoms are treated as they occur.

Often a patient can live a long time with this form of treatment.

Skin cancer

About 300,000 cases of skin cancer are discovered every year. Its incidence increases every year, particularly among women, perhaps because people currently are getting more exposure to sunlight. The ultraviolet rays of the sun are a major cause of skin cancer. Fair-skinned people have less melanin (a protective substance in the skin) than dark-skinned people do and are therefore more susceptible to the effects of these rays. Skin cancer can also result from prolonged exposure to certain chemicals, such as arsenic compounds. Burn scars and skin diseases sometimes develop into cancer.

Symptoms of skin cancer are a change in the surface of the skin, a wound that does not heal, or a sudden major change in a wart, mole, or birthmark. Any such suspicious signs should be examined by a doctor.

Most skin cancers are highly treatable. Some can be removed in a doctor's office or an outpatient clinic. But since some forms of skin cancer can spread throughout the body, it is important that they be treated early. The most dangerous skin cancer, malignant melanoma, can metastasize through the lymph and vascular (blood vessel) systems. Melanomas can develop from moles.

Skin cancer is an unusual form of cancer in that it can be prevented easily. Fair-skinned people and anyone with a family history of skin cancer should avoid exposure to the sun. Additionally, everyone who spends time in the sun should apply a protective sunscreen to exposed

portions of the body. It is important that children, whose skin is more sensitive, be protected against the sun. The use of certain drugs, such as barbiturates, antibiotics, and birth control pills, can increase the sensitivity of the skin.

Stomach cancer

The incidence of stomach cancer has decreased by 50 percent in the last 25 years. A change in diet may account for this. Stomach cancer is more common in men than in women and usually occurs between the ages of 50 and 70. The high-risk group includes those with a history of pernicious anemia or alcoholism and those who choose a diet rich in smoked, pickled, or salted foods.

The symptoms of stomach cancer are similar to those of peptic ulcer (heartburn and abdominal discomfort), which makes diagnosis more difficult. It may not be until the disease is well advanced that the identifying symptoms of bloody stools or vomit appear. A special X-ray study may be obtained after the patient swallows barium (a contrast substance that coats the lining of the stomach), which allows visualization of irregularities in the stomach (such as the presence of a tumor) on X-ray films. If a tumor is identified, a flexible, lighted, tubelike instrument called an endoscope may be inserted down the throat into the stomach to examine the tumor more closely and perhaps obtain a biopsy specimen of it.

Surgery is the most effective treatment of this disease, but only about ten percent of victims survive more than five years after diagnosis. Surgery is most useful when the tumor has not begun to spread. It is sometimes necessary to remove all or part of the stomach. After such surgery, the patient will require a modified diet.

Uterine cancer

This disease is most common in women over the age of 50. Especially susceptible to cancer of the uterus are women who have never given birth, those who are obese or diabetic, and those who suffer from high blood pressure. Women who have taken the female hormone estrogen are probably at higher risk than those who have not taken it.

Vaginal bleeding after menopause is the most common symptom of uterine cancer. If a Pap smear shows no abnormalities, a minor surgical procedure known as dilatation and curettage (D&C) may be performed. This involves scraping the interior walls of the uterus in order to examine the tissue for the presence of cancer. If cancer is identified, a hysterectomy (surgical removal of the uterus) is usually performed. (Often, the ovaries are removed as well.) Cancer of the uterus is harder to detect than that of the cervix; it is often discovered too late for successful treatment.

Vaginal cancer

Once confined to women over 50 years of age, vaginal cancer has begun to appear in women between the ages of 17 and 20. The mothers of most of these young women took artificial estrogens, particularly diethylstilbestrol (DES), during pregnancy to prevent miscarriage. A woman whose mother took artificial estrogens during pregnancy should have a Pap smear twice a year. Symptoms of vaginal cancer include vaginal pain and bleeding. The disease is usually treated with radiation and surgery.

FACTS ABOUT MEDICAL TESTS

The basis of medical evaluation is a complete medical history and physical examination. Common health problems are primarily detected and diagnosed by means of the history and physical examination. Nevertheless, your doctor will also use a variety of diagnostic aids and tests to rule out a disease, to confirm a diagnosis, or to detect a disorder that is not apparent. Modern technology now enables medical professionals to inspect the structure of a cell, to see the inside of an organ, and to examine a detailed cross-sectional picture of the body. These tests provide essential information to aid your doctor in the diagnosis of illness and the selection of appropriate treatment.

This section is a guide to some of the more common medical tests and how they are performed.

Common tests

BLOOD TESTS

Although some blood tests can be done on a sample from a finger prick, most tests require a larger sample. The complete blood cell count (the most common of the blood tests) and blood chemistry screening tests are usually based on blood samples drawn by venipuncture (puncture of a vein by a hypodermic needle). The procedure is quick and relatively painless. The doctor who orders the blood tests will most often submit all the test orders together, so that more than one venipuncture is not needed.

Although some patients fear that a great volume of blood is being drawn in venipuncture, the usual laboratory tests do not or-

dinarily require more than 10 to 20 milliliters (two to four teaspoons). The total amount of blood circulating in the body of the average person is at least six quarts at any given time and is constantly being replenished. Therefore, fears about unusual blood loss from such testing are groundless. Also, with the use of disposable, single-use needles, the concern about transmission of disease is unfounded.

Complete blood cell count

A complete blood cell count (CBC) determines the number and types of blood cells in the blood. The CBC includes:

- Hematocrit—to measure how much of the blood is made up of red blood cells alone
- Hemoglobin test—to measure the amount of hemoglobin (the blood substance that carries oxygen to the body tissues) present in a given volume of red blood cells
- White blood cell count—to find out how many white blood cells are in the blood
- Differential count—to learn how many of the various types of white blood cells are present in the blood
- Platelet count—to determine the number of platelets (the blood elements that aid in clotting the blood) that are present

Blood chemistry tests

Besides the complete blood cell count, there are other blood tests that together constitute what is known as a blood chemistry panel. These tests, which analyze many components and chemicals in the blood, can be done from a single sample of blood within minutes, using an

automated blood chemistry machine.

Blood chemistry studies are performed routinely as screening tests for the detection of certain disorders, such as diabetes and kidney disease. They are also used as diagnostic tests when specific diseases, such as hepatitis, are suspected. Blood chemistry profiles are frequently used to determine the overall function of an organ, especially the liver (the usual profiles contain three or four indicators of liver function). These tests may not pinpoint a specific disease of the liver; instead, they provide a general indication of whether the liver is functioning normally and whether specific diagnostic tests need to be performed. Many illnesses affect more than one organ; furthermore, failure in one organ may cause problems in another. It is here that blood chemistry profiles have great utility; using one sample, they give information about the function of several organs (particularly the liver and kidneys).

The following list briefly explains the purpose of some of the more common blood chemistry tests:

- Blood glucose—to aid in diagnosing diabetes mellitus (glucose is a form of sugar)
- Blood urea nitrogen (BUN)—to assess kidney function
- Creatinine—to assess kidney function
- Electrolytes—to check body fluid and salt balance (salts include sodium, potassium, and chloride)
- Uric acid—to aid in diagnosing gout
- Cholesterol or triglycerides—to measure the levels of fat present in the blood
- Bilirubin—to assess liver function, to evaluate jaundice, and to help diagnose anemia

- Albumin—to assess general nutritional status and to get a general idea of liver function (albumin is a type of protein produced by the liver)

URINALYSIS

A routine urinalysis is a microscopic examination and chemical analysis of the urine. If red blood cells or white blood cells can be seen under the microscope, bleeding or an infection is present somewhere along the urinary tract. Other microscopic elements, such as casts (formations of protein with or without cellular elements, which usually indicate disease in the kidneys) and crystals (of uric acid or calcium, for example) may also be seen. A chemical analysis can determine the presence of sugar, protein, or other substances that may indicate kidney or bladder diseases, as well as disorders that are unrelated to the urinary tract, such as diabetes mellitus and starvation. There is no risk involved in this test.

The patient is given a clean container and told to urinate directly into it. When a urine culture is indicated, a "midstream" specimen is usually requested, that is, a specimen obtained after the urinary tract opening has been properly cleansed and the initial spurt of urine has been passed. If you are to collect the specimen at home, you should also be provided with a clean container with a cap. If not, you should use a clean plastic or glass container. A container that has held food, perfume, chemicals, or cosmetics should not be used. Such containers may be difficult to empty and may still contain traces of the original contents, which would invalidate the test results.

CHEST X RAY

The most common standard X-ray examination is the chest X ray, usually used to check for signs of lung diseases and abnormalities. Because the heart, parts of the aorta (the large artery that carries blood from the heart to much of the body), the ribs, the upper spine, the shoulders, the upper arm bones, and the collarbones are also seen, diseases other than those that affect the lungs, such as congestive heart failure (enlargement of the heart accompanied by fluid buildup in the lungs and their blood vessels), may be diagnosed and followed up with chest X rays.

The patient undresses from the waist up. The usual chest X ray is taken in two positions: with the patient standing sideways and with either the chest or back resting against the cassette containing the X-ray film. The patient must be correctly positioned and must remain motionless if good X-ray pictures are to be obtained. The test is painless. The actual time of exposure to radiation is quite short; however, if the test is overused, there may be a minimal risk of long-term effects of radiation exposure. Routine X rays should be avoided by pregnant women; if such an examination is necessary, a lead shield can be used to protect the developing baby.

ELECTROCARDIOGRAM

An electrocardiogram (ECG) is a visual record of the heart's electrical impulses, which control the rate and rhythm of beating and reflect many alterations in the heart muscle. This test, along with the history and physical examination, is used to diagnose a number of heart disorders, including previous and new myocardial infarctions (heart attacks), some congenital (present at birth) abnormalities of the heart, pericarditis (inflammation of the sac surrounding the heart), and abnormal thickness of the muscle (such as is seen in long-term high blood pressure). There is no risk to this test, and it is totally painless.

Electrodes (small metal disks that are sensitive to the heart's impulses) are taped onto the body at various points on the chest, arms, and legs. The electrode cables are connected to the electrocardiograph, a machine that produces a visual record of the impulses. The ECG tracing for a normal heart consists of regularly occurring wave patterns, whereas that for an abnormal heart will show alterations in the rhythm or appearance of the wave patterns.

STOOL BLOOD TEST

This test is used to detect tiny quantities of occult (hidden) blood in the stool (feces) that are not visible without a microscope. The presence of occult blood may signal bowel disease or bleeding somewhere along the digestive tract.

The test is usually done by the patient at home and mailed to a laboratory. The patient places a small sample of stool on specially coated paper that will reveal any blood when treated with a special developer. The test may have to be done several times, since the bleeding may be intermittent. The patient will be instructed to eat no red meat for at least three days before taking the stool specimen (the blood from meat, including cooked meat, may cause a falsely positive result on the test) and to take no aspirin-containing medications (aspirin may cause bleeding from the stomach).

This test is painless and has no risk. It is an excellent method of screening for colon cancer.

THROAT CULTURE

This common procedure is used to determine the type of microorganisms causing infection in the throat. A sample of bacteria is obtained by rolling a cotton-tipped applicator around the swollen area. The test is painless but may cause gagging.

The cell samples are placed in a culture medium (a special mixture of chemicals and nutrients designed to support growth of bacteria), so that growth of microorganisms can be detected and measured. Special procedures are used to identify the specific types of bacteria. It usually takes from 24 to 48 hours to get definitive results.

Recently, "instant" throat cultures specifically for the detection of streptococcal infection have become available. The results are known within 15 minutes and are generally reliable.

Special diagnostic tests

ALLERGY TESTS

Tests to determine the existence of various allergies are as numerous and complex as the substances (called allergens) that cause the allergic responses. One of the most common allergy tests is the skin test. This procedure can be either a scratch skin test or an intracutaneous skin test. In the scratch test, suspected allergens are applied in small amounts to individual, tiny scratches on the skin, often several at a time and in a prescribed order. In the intracutaneous skin test, small quantities of the suspected allergens are injected into or under the skin. After a short period of time (about half an hour), the doctor notes which substances have caused a reaction. In both of these tests, a swollen, reddish bump at the site of the application is a positive reaction to that allergen. The skin scratches and injections can be uncomfortable while the procedures are being performed. In addition, there is the risk that an extremely sensitive individual may have an allergic reaction.

There is also a blood test to help identify allergens. The test, called a radioallergosorbent test (RAST), measures specific antibodies in the blood. Antibodies are substances formed by the immune system in response to foreign invaders, such as allergens. The test can be used for those people who should not have skin tests—persons with extremely sensitive skin, very young children, and persons suspected of being extremely sensitive to an injected allergen. However, the RAST may not be as sensitive as skin tests and is more expensive.

In the case of food allergies, diagnosis is often difficult. One method of identifying allergens is to have samples of suspected allergy-causing foods eaten in small quantities at times when there is nothing in the digestive system. Symptoms, if any, are noted. Adequate time is required between food samples so that each sample can clear the system before the next food is given. Someone with a history of severe reactions should not be tested in this fashion. Skin testing may be useful.

BIOPSY

A biopsy is the removal of a small sample of tissue for examination under a microscope. This procedure is done to establish a precise diagnosis of abnormalities, including cancer. The tissue may be obtained by cutting, by aspirating (suctioning) with a needle, or by other methods, depending on the part of the body from which the sample is to be removed. For example, endoscopic biopsy is removal of tissue by instruments attached to or passed through an endoscope (a flexible, lighted tubelike device) into a hollow organ, such as the colon.

The procedure varies with the type of biopsy to be performed. Some biopsies require hospitalization, especially if surgery is necessary to obtain a specimen from an internal organ. Other procedures, such as biopsy of small skin growths and needle aspiration of a breast lump, can be done in a doctor's office or an outpatient clinic. Many biopsies are done with some type of anesthesia, and there may be discomfort if a biopsy involves cutting or an invasive technique (one involving the insertion of an instrument or other device into the body). Also, there is some risk, which varies with the procedure being performed. The risks of outpatient biopsies are usually minimal, but complications, such as excessive bleeding, can occur.

CARDIAC STRESS TEST

The cardiac stress test, also often called the treadmill test, is done basically to determine the reaction of the cardiovascular system (the heart and blood vessels) to physical exercise. Devices other than a treadmill, such as a bicycle, can also be used, depending on the situation. A stress test is done for many reasons—among them, to determine whether the cause of chest pain is a heart abnormality, to detect the presence of coronary artery disease, and to follow the progress of a patient in cardiac rehabilitation.

At the lab, the patient will put on exercise clothes and running shoes and will be questioned about his or her recent medical history and exercise habits.

For the test, electrodes for continuous electrocardiographic recording are attached so that the tester (usually a cardiologist) can monitor the heart rate and the response of the heart to graded exercise. A blood pressure cuff is attached to one arm.

The patient then starts walking on the treadmill at a low work load. The work load (determined by the speed and incline of the treadmill) is gradually increased, usually at three-minute intervals, until the patient: (1) attains about 90 percent of the predicted maximum heart rate for his or her age (obtained from standardized tables); (2) experiences symptoms or electrocardiographic changes consistent with heart disease; or (3) cannot continue the test for some reason (for example, leg cramps or shortness of breath).

The time it takes to reach the target heart rate is related to the degree of cardiovascular fitness, but is not necessarily related to the presence or absence of heart disease. That is, an individual who attains his or her peak heart rate at only six minutes is less fit than someone who can exercise for 12 minutes on the treadmill before attaining peak heart rate. However, either individual may have changes or symptoms indicating heart disease.

At the individual's maximum performance level, the closer he or she comes to the predicted maximum heart rate, the more meaningful the test. For example, a negative ECG (indicating that there is no heart disease) would have greater diagnostic significance if it was obtained at a particular patient's age-predicted maximum heart rate of 180 beats per minute than if the patient had had to stop the test at a rate of 130 beats because of a leg cramp, fatigue, or some other noncardiovascular reason.

Stress tests may cause discomfort because of fatigue, tired muscles, and so forth. The main risk is bringing about a cardiac event, such as arrhythmia (abnormal heart rhythm) or a heart attack.

CONTRAST EXAMINATIONS

Contrast media, known popularly as dyes, are materials that, when introduced into the body, alter radiopacity (the capacity to be "seen" on an X-ray examination of one part of the body in comparison with surrounding parts). The contrast materials are opaque, that is, they stop the passage of X rays, and are essential to visualize certain internal body organs, such as the stomach and intestines, which normally are not seen on X-ray examinations. When the contrast medium is introduced into the body, the radiologist performing the test often uses fluoroscopy (the projection of X rays through the body onto a special screen) to observe the working of the internal body organs and then takes still X-ray films of the area being examined. Commonly performed contrast examinations include the upper gastrointestinal tract examination (upper GI series), the lower gastrointestinal series (barium enema), the intravenous pyelogram (IVP, or kidney study), the gallbladder series, and the coronary angiogram (visualization of the heart and its blood vessels).

Barium is an inert (not active) substance that is either swallowed or introduced via enema. It coats the gastrointestinal tract and allows visualization of its anatomy. Ulcers, tumors, and other abnormalities are found in this manner. True allergic reactions to barium probably do not exist.

The contrast medium (dye) used for IVP, angiography, computed tomography scanning, and some other X-ray studies is usually injected directly into a vein. This substance is not inert and can cause severe reactions, such as hives, swelling, and rash. Less severe reactions include hot flashes, nausea, vomiting, and diarrhea. Kidney failure can also occur with this type of contrast if the individual has preexisting kidney disease or certain other illnesses. Prior to receiving these dyes, the patient should provide the physician with a careful medical history.

Upper GI series

The upper GI series is a contrast examination of the esophagus, stomach, and duodenum (first part of the small intestine). This X-ray study is used to detect ulcers, cancer, and other abnormalities. The contrast medium used is barium sulfate, which is introduced by having the patient drink it after fasting overnight. The patient's stomach must be empty to accommodate the barium meal and also to avoid having food particles confuse the results. The radiologist observes the filling of the stomach on the fluoroscope as the patient drinks. The time required for the exam is about 30 minutes. In some instances, the doctor will order what is known as a small bowel follow-through, a series of X rays taken to follow the movement of the barium through the small intestine. In this procedure, many films are taken at specified time intervals. This study may take hours. Patients can expect very light-colored stools after the test because of the presence of the barium sulfate. As with any X-ray examination, there may be a risk of effects from radiation exposure, but modern equipment and techniques have minimized this.

Lower GI series

The lower GI series, or barium enema, is a contrast examination of the colon (large intestine), which is useful in detecting tumors, polyps (abnormal outgrowths of tissue from the bowel's inner surface), and other problems. For this examination, the colon must be cleared of all fecal matter. This is usually accomplished by taking a liquid diet for 24 to 48 hours, accompanied by laxatives and enemas. Nothing is then allowed by mouth until the examination has been completed. The time for the examination itself is usually about 30 minutes. The patient is given an enema consisting of a barium solution (which makes the colon opaque) introduced into the large intestine through a tube inserted into the anus; the solution must be retained until all the films have been obtained. When looking for polyps or when a detailed view of the lining of the colon is required, air is put into the colon to form a double contrast with the barium.

This procedure is referred to as an "air-contrast barium enema" and is rapidly becoming more common than the plain lower GI series.

At the time of the examination, the radiologist observes the colon fluoroscopically as it fills with barium. X-ray films are made before, during, and after emptying of the barium-coated colon. Afterward, the patient is usually given a cleansing enema or a mild laxative to rid the colon of barium.

Although rare, obstruction of the colon by impacted (hardened) barium or perforation of the colon by the enema tube may occur. As with any X-ray study, there is the usual minimal risk from radiation exposure.

Intravenous pyelogram (IVP)

This test is used to evaluate the size and functioning of the kidneys and the urinary tract, as well as the presence of obstructions. In men, an enlarged prostate gland may also be noted. The test is done by injecting contrast material into a vein in the arm. The contrast material is then eliminated through the kidneys and urinary tract. X-ray films are made at specified time intervals to observe the rate of excretion, the concentration of the contrast medium inside the kidneys, and the outlines of the ureters (tubes from the kidneys to the bladder) and the bladder. Since fecal matter and gas in the intestinal tract obscure the observation of urinary tract structures, the lower bowel needs to be cleared for this examination. As with any X-ray study, there is a minimal risk from the effects of radiation exposure.

Patients with diabetes mellitus, kidney disease, or a history of previous reactions to X-ray contrast materials may be at risk of kidney damage or serious allergic reactions. These patients should inform the radiologist of such risk factors, because precautions can be taken to minimize the chance of complications.

Gallbladder series

A gallbladder series, or oral cholecystogram, is performed to test gallbladder function and to detect gallstones. The oral cholecystogram allows correct diagnosis of gallbladder disease (including both poor function and gallstones) about 96 percent of the time.

For this examination, it is helpful to clear the intestinal tract of fecal matter and gas to allow for adequate viewing of the gallbladder. This is done by giving a special diet for the 24 hours before the examination and by administering enemas. Avoidance of cream, butter, and other fatty foods (fats stimulate the gallbladder, which must be at rest in order to concentrate the contrast material well) is also necessary.

Contrast medium in tablet form is given to the patient after dinner the day before the X-ray study begins. Usually, nothing is then given by mouth until the examination has been completed. If the gallbladder does not show up on the X-ray film (does not concentrate the contrast material), the dose of contrast is repeated the next day, and another film is taken. If the gallbladder still is not visible, this indicates that the gallbladder is diseased (assuming that the gastrointestinal tract and liver are processing the contrast material normally). In some X-ray departments, after the films of the contrast-filled gallbladder have been made, the patient is given a fatty meal to stimulate the gallbladder to empty, and another film is then obtained to evaluate this function. The time required for the actual examination is about one hour, excluding the time for the fatty meal.

There may be side effects, such as nausea, vomiting, and diarrhea. As with any X-ray study, there is a minimal risk from radiation exposure. There is also a risk (although uncommon) of an allergic reaction to the contrast material. Patients with diabetes and kidney disease should inform the radiologist so that precautions can be taken. With the advent of ultrasound and nuclear isotope visualization, this test is becoming uncommon.

Angiography

Angiography (also called arteriography) is visualization of blood vessels (the heart is often included in this term), usually by introduction of a contrast medium (dye) via a tube, called a catheter, that is inserted directly into a blood vessel.

Coronary angiography is required before heart surgery and for diagnosis of some heart diseases. In this procedure, the cardiologist introduces a catheter into the body, usually through a puncture in an artery in the groin or arm, and threads it through the vascular system until it reaches the heart. Through this catheter, an opaque contrast medium is injected, allowing moving pictures of the heart to be obtained. With this procedure, the cardiologist and the cardiovascular surgeon obtain crucial information, such as the location of defects in the walls and valves of the heart, the loca-

tion and degree of narrowing of the coronary arteries (the arteries that supply blood to the heart muscle itself), and even the different pressures in the chambers (which reflect the overall functioning of the heart).

Nowadays, this procedure is commonly performed and carries a very low risk in the hands of experienced physicians. After the procedure, there is sometimes bleeding at the catheter introduction site, as well as mild discomfort there. During contrast injection, many patients complain of a "hot flash" or nausea. As with any X-ray study, there is a minimal risk of radiation exposure. Also, patients with diabetes, kidney disease, or a history of reaction to contrast media may be at risk from the contrast medium. Precautions can be taken to prevent complications if the physician performing the procedure is informed of these problems before the test. Other possible risks should be discussed with the doctor.

ELECTROENCEPHALOGRAM

An electroencephalogram, or EEG, is a visual record of electrical impulses discharged by brain cells. The EEG is used to detect abnormalities in the brain. The test is painless and without risk.

Electrodes (small metal disks) are placed at specified points on the surface of the head (in special circumstances, disks may be inserted through the nose into the throat, which may be uncomfortable) and then attached to the electroencephalograph, which is a machine that produces a visual tracing of the brain's electrical waves. If, for instance, the brain has been damaged or the patient has epilepsy, the waves produced by the elec-

trical discharges form characteristic patterns. Tracings are taken when the patient is awake and calm; when he or she has been asked to hyperventilate (breathe rapidly) and has been stimulated with a flashing light, which may evoke changes characteristic of epileptic grand mal seizures; and when the patient is asleep. An EEG usually takes about one hour to complete.

Careful pretest preparation of the patient is essential for accurate results. On the day of the test, no coffee, tea, cola drinks, or other stimulants are permitted. Alcohol, which as a depressant would affect the accuracy of the EEG, must also be avoided. The physician ordering the test must be informed of any medications the patient is taking, as these can have profound effects on the EEG. After shampooing, no hair preparations should be used until after the tracing has been made. If sleep recording is planned, it is helpful if no naps are taken on the day of the test.

ENDOSCOPY

Endoscopy is a method of directly viewing the inside of hollow organs by inserting an endoscope (a flexible, lighted tubelike instrument) into the organ. Five common endoscopic examinations are described here (in order, from the most frequently performed to the least frequently performed).

Proctosigmoidoscopy

This is an examination of the rectum and colon for detection of cancers and other ailments of the lower 12 inches of the large intestine. In addition to cancer, the examination can reveal hemorrhoids (swollen veins), infected areas, anal fistulas (abnormal passageways), rectal polyps (abnormal growths), and abnormal narrowing of the intestine, among other problems.

The examination is frequently recommended as part of a complete checkup. It is a must for anyone with rectal bleeding or a change in bowel habits. The examination usually takes place on a tilting-top table with the patient in the knee-chest position (resting on the knees and chest, with the face turned to the side) or lying in a head-down position. After a manual examination (insertion of the physician's gloved finger into the anus), the doctor inserts a lubricated anoscope (an instrument that enlarges the anus and lower rectum to allow close inspection). Then a proctosigmoidoscope (a lighted, hollow instrument, also known as a proctoscope or sigmoidoscope) is inserted through the anal canal into the large intestine. Formerly, such scopes were rigid, but these have largely been replaced by flexible ones. The advantages of the flexible devices are that they cause less discomfort and generally allow more accurate visualization of a greater length of intestine than was allowed by the traditional proctoscope.

Patients are advised to prepare for this examination by eating a light diet for 24 to 48 hours before the test and by emptying the lower intestinal tract with one or two enemas. If a barium X ray of the colon is to follow the proctosigmoidoscopy, more detailed preparation, involving laxatives and a number of enemas, is undertaken.

There are few risks to a routine screening. Perforation of the colon is possible, but quite rare. There may be some discomfort or cramping during the examina-

tion, but there should be no actual pain.

Gastroscopy (Esophago-gastro-duodenoscopy, or EGD)

Gastroscopy is an examination of the interior of the esophagus, stomach, and duodenum (the first part of the small intestine). The test is performed to detect and examine ulcers or tumors and to determine the cause of gastrointestinal bleeding or any other known or suspected abnormalities. The response of an ulcer to treatment can also be followed up endoscopically rather than by X-ray studies. During this procedure, biopsy specimens (tissue samples) can be collected, and stomach contents can be examined.

Recently, techniques utilizing lasers, chemical injections, and electrocautery (use of a heated needle to destroy tissue) have been developed for use through an endoscope. With these instruments, treatment as well as diagnosis can be accomplished.

The patient can have no solid food for the evening meal the night before the test is done. Water cannot be taken within eight hours before the test. Smoking is prohibited on the day of the test until the examination has been completed, since smoking stimulates secretion of digestive juices by the stomach. Any other stimulation, such as that triggered by alcohol, caffeine, or colas, should also be avoided.

In the procedure, the throat is first anesthetized with a spray or a gargle (or both). The patient is then given a sedative to induce relaxation. A gastroscope (a flexible, lighted, tubelike instrument) is then passed down the throat, through the esophagus, and into the stomach and duodenum.

There is little risk involved. The patient may gag and experience a temporary sore throat afterward. On very rare occasions, the gastroscope may injure or perforate an organ, or the patient may vomit and inhale the contents of the stomach.

Colonoscopy

This procedure is similar to proctosigmoidoscopy, but the entire colon (large intestine) is examined. The instrument used is a long, flexible, lighted, tubelike device. Usually, colonoscopy is performed to detect or remove polyps (small abnormal growths), to do a biopsy of tumors or suspicious areas, to look for sites of occult (hidden) or obvious bleeding, and to detect inflammatory bowel disease. The patient is asked to stay on a liquid diet for about 48 hours before the procedure. Laxatives and enemas are also given to cleanse the colon thoroughly. During the test, mild sedatives are given.

Some discomfort and cramping are common, but actual pain should not occur. The main risks are perforation and bleeding from the site of biopsy or growth removal; both are uncommon.

Cystoscopy

Cystoscopy is the direct viewing of the interior of the urinary bladder and the urethra (the passageway from the bladder to the outside of the body). A flexible, lighted, tubelike instrument called a cystoscope is passed through the urethra into the bladder. The bladder and urethra are examined for cancer, polyps, and other abnormalities. If indicated, biopsy specimens can be collected for later examination.

Men generally enter the hospital for the procedure, and are usually given a sedative before the test and a spinal or general anesthetic during the procedure. Women frequently need only local anesthesia and often have the procedure done on an outpatient basis. There is little risk involved in diagnostic cystoscopy, although there may be a slight chance of damage to the lining of the urethra, of perforation of the bladder, and of temporary retention of urine after the test is completed.

Part of the prostate gland is viewed during this procedure in men, and an overgrown prostate gland can be "shaved down" through the cystoscope. This is referred to as a transurethral resection of the prostate and is considered a surgical procedure. Some bladder cancers can be burned off via electrocautery (use of a heated needle to destroy tissue) through a cystoscope, thus eliminating the need for a surgical procedure.

Bronchoscopy

Bronchoscopy is the direct examination of the trachea (windpipe), larynx (voice box), and bronchi (the breathing tubes through which air travels from the trachea into the lungs). This examination can pinpoint the cause of an unexplained persistent cough, wheeze, or pneumonia. It is also used to investigate an unexplained abnormality on a chest X ray or to diagnose a lung tumor. Bronchoscopy may also be used to obtain a tissue sample or to remove a small obstruction, such as a foreign body.

A lighted tube, either flexible or rigid, is inserted from the mouth or nose through the trachea into the bronchi. Some bronchoscopes are small enough in diameter to offer a view of even the smallest structures in the bronchial tree. A sedative and an anesthetic are used; the anesthetic may be in the form of a spray for the mouth and nose or a lubricating jelly to protect and anesthetize the tissues of the nose and throat. The patient fasts for at least eight hours prior to the test.

Patients with a history of heart disease and those over age 50 are frequently monitored with an electrocardiograph. There is a minor risk of damage to the teeth, throat, and bronchial structures, but damage to the respiratory tract is very rare. Bleeding from biopsy sites and areas of growth removal also occurs, but uncommonly. This procedure is almost always done in a hospital setting on an outpatient basis.

LUMBAR PUNCTURE

The lumbar puncture (also called a spinal tap) is a procedure used to withdraw a small amount of cerebrospinal fluid from an area (the subarachnoid space) surrounding the spinal cord. The cerebrospinal fluid is then examined microscopically and analyzed chemically to detect conditions that may exist in the central nervous system. These conditions include bleeding, infections, and other abnormalities of the brain and spinal cord. Often the appearance of the fluid, which is normally crystal clear, will suggest a preliminary diagnosis of a problem; if, for example, the fluid is cloudy, it may indicate the presence of an infection.

The patient usually lies on his or her side with the knees drawn up sufficiently to bow the back. After administration of a local anesthetic, the subarachnoid space (where the cerebrospinal fluid circulates) is entered with a special needle inserted through the skin and soft tissues and between two of the lower lumbar vertebrae (bones of the spinal column). The pressure of the cerebrospinal fluid in the central nervous system is measured with a manometer (an instrument for measuring the pressure of liquids and gases). Some fluid is then collected in a series of small, sterile test tubes for subsequent laboratory analysis.

Although patients are sometimes apprehensive about the lumbar puncture procedure, it is usually not painful. Headache after the tap is not uncommon. Lying flat for an hour or so after the tap appears to decrease the incidence of headache. Furthermore, if a headache should develop, lying flat seems to ease the pain.

There is a slight risk of nerve damage from the needle, but this is extremely rare. The site of the puncture is below the end of the spinal cord, so the cord itself cannot be injured in any way. Special precautions are necessary if the pressure in the central nervous system is elevated due to swelling of the brain or the presence of a tumor. Computed tomography or magnetic resonance imaging may be used to evaluate the brain before a spinal tap is performed. Although any procedure that invades the body carries a risk of infection, the incidence of infections following lumbar punctures is quite low.

MAGNETIC RESONANCE IMAGING

Magnetic resonance imaging (MRI), sometimes referred to as nuclear magnetic resonance

(NMR), is one of the newest and most versatile imaging techniques currently available. With it, physicians are able to distinguish the fine details of internal body structures.

The main component of an MRI facility is a massive cylindrical magnet, which weighs as much as one hundred tons. The patient is positioned at the center of the magnet, and a radio signal is transmitted through the patient's body while a powerful magnetic field is simultaneously generated around him or her.

The magnetic field generated by such a huge magnet is extremely powerful—powerful enough to temporarily modify the position of the protons (charged particles in the center of each atom) in the patient's body. Under the influence of the magnet, these protons line up parallel to the magnetic field, in much the same way that a compass needle points toward the North Pole. The radio signal causes the protons to move out of alignment. When the radio signals are stopped, the protons once again align with the magnetic field, releasing energy in the process. This energy can be detected as tiny alterations in the magnetic field. The information can then be transmitted to a computer for analysis. The images generated by the computer are very thin cross-sectional "slices" through the body, which can show details unobtainable by any other means.

Physical effects from undergoing an MRI procedure are rare, but may include headache, nausea, and a warm, tingling sensation. No health risks from either the radio waves or the magnetic field have yet been reported. Any metal object present in the body should be reported to the physician prior to this procedure. Indi-

viduals who are claustrophobic may experience anxiety during this test due to the close quarters imposed by the machine. Mild sedation is commonly used and is quite effective in easing or preventing anxiety.

PHOTON ABSORPTIOMETRY

Due to increasing awareness of the risks associated with osteoporosis (a disease in which the bones become thinner and more easily breakable), a reliable means of determining the presence and degree of this disorder has been sought. Photon absorptiometry (also known as densitometry), a technique for measuring bone density, is being used increasingly for this purpose. Although this procedure is probably not harmful, its usefulness as a screening procedure is not yet fully known.

PULMONARY FUNCTION TESTING

Pulmonary function testing (PFT) is a procedure for assessing how well the lungs are working. The results of this group of tests may reveal the existence of various diseases of the lungs, including asthma and emphysema. Diseases that cause restriction of lung movement can be diagnosed and differentiated from those that cause airway obstruction. Pulmonary function tests are also used to obtain baseline values when monitoring the course of a disease and the effects of therapy.

Routine PFT is done with a spirometer—long tubes resembling vacuum-cleaner hoses are connected to a device that measures the volume of air breathed in and out over a period of time

and then displays that information on a graph. The patient breathes into the spirometer according to instructions given during the test. The amount of air inhaled and exhaled and the rate of inhalation and exhalation are measured; sometimes, specific exhaled gases are also measured. Some pulmonary function tests also require a blood sample from an artery to determine if the arterial blood (freshly oxygenated in the lungs) has adequate oxygen and a normal concentration of carbon dioxide.

The test is painless and without risk, with the possible exceptions of discomfort during, and complications after, an arterial puncture for the blood sample.

NUCLEAR MEDICINE (OR RADIOISOTOPE) SCANNING

Radioactive isotopes, or radioisotopes, are used primarily as a diagnostic tool to detect tumors, blood clots, and malfunctioning of organs in the body.

A radioisotope is a form of a chemical element in which the nucleus of each atom is unstable because it does not contain the usual number of neutrons. (The nucleus is the central portion of an atom, which is the smallest particle of an element.) Because the nucleus is unstable, it disintegrates and gives off electrically charged particles and energy (ionizing radiation).

Certain elements are concentrated in, or are used by, particular organs. For example, iodine, when given by mouth or injected, will travel to and be concentrated by the thyroid gland. Radioactive iodine, when administered to a patient, will also travel to the thyroid gland, where, because of its special properties, it will show up on X-ray films. A machine called a scanner is placed near the patient. It detects the radiation emitted by the radioactive isotope as it travels to the organ being studied. The scanner converts the radiation into flashes of light that form an image on X-ray film or that are projected onto a special screen.

Using this technique, a physician can determine the position, shape, and size of an organ or the presence of a tumor. By looking at the rate at which the radioisotope is absorbed and eliminated, the doctor can also evaluate how the organ is functioning.

Radioisotopes are used mainly to study organs, such as the thyroid gland, brain, liver, gallbladder, spleen, and kidneys, which do not show up well on ordinary X-ray images. The most recent advance in radioisotope diagnosis has allowed doctors to observe the heart muscle. Although the procedure is still quite costly, it appears promising for victims of heart attack and other abnormalities. This type of imaging, when coupled with a cardiac stress test, is excellent for detecting and localizing areas of heart muscle that are not getting enough oxygen. Some of the other conditions that can be detected by using radioisotopes are tumors, blood clots, injuries, bone marrow disease, red blood cell irregularities, cirrhosis of the liver (a condition in which the tissues of the liver are scarred and otherwise damaged), hepatitis (inflammation of the liver), nonabsorption of vitamin B_{12}, and certain anemias.

There is no danger of radiation poisoning with this study. Because very small amounts of radiation can be detected and measured, only a minute amount of a radioisotope is required.

TOMOGRAPHY

Tomography is a type of X-ray examination in which the shadows in front of and behind the part of the body being studied are blurred out on the X-ray picture. Successive exposures are made at different depths within the structure of the body part under study and from different angles. The effect is the same as that achieved when a microscope is adjusted back and forth and up and down while looking at a piece of tissue—it is possible to get a picture of a structure at different levels, each one pinpointed and sharply focused.

The combination of the tomographic X-ray technique and expanded computer capabilities led to the development of a highly sophisticated form of diagnostic imaging called computed tomography (also known as computerized axial tomography, CAT scanning, and CT scanning). With this special procedure, X rays are not used to create images directly on film. Instead, the X rays are detected by a scanner as they leave the body, and that information is analyzed by a computer to construct a cross-sectional "map" of the body part under study.

The most widely known use of the CT scan has been in the detection of brain disorders. However, in recent years, use of the technique has been extended to other parts of the body, so that, for example, cross-sectional images of organs in the abdomen, such as the liver and pancreas, can now be produced. These scans are quite sensitive and have greatly aided in the early detection of tumors. One of the breakthroughs that has made this possible is the development of equipment that can complete a scan in five seconds or less.

Brain scanning does not require such speed, since the head can easily be immobilized. The abdominal area, however, is in constant movement, because of the action of the stomach, the intestines, and the diaphragm. Consequently, the scan must be made fast enough to provide a clear image, in the same way that a fast shutter speed on an ordinary camera can "stop" the motion of the subject.

The test is painless and there is minimal risk from radiation exposure. Also, intravenous X-ray contrast medium is sometimes used to enhance the picture. Persons with kidney disease or diabetes mellitus may be at risk of kidney damage when contrast medium is used, and persons with a sensitivity to such dyes may suffer serious allergic reactions. These individuals should tell their radiologist of such risk factors so that adequate precautions can be taken to minimize the chance of complications. Oral contrast agents, similar to barium, are also routinely used. CT scanning is relatively expensive and therefore not done as a screening procedure.

ULTRASONOGRAPHY

Ultrasonography (often called ultrasound) is a method of visualizing the structures of the body by recording the reflections of high-frequency sound waves off those structures. The procedure is painless and uses no radiation. Ultrasound, the sound range used in this diagnostic procedure, is a vibration beyond the range of human hearing.

The instrument used in ultrasonography is called a transducer. The transducer, placed over the area to be examined, directs ultrasonic waves at the tissue. The sounds returning from the internal structure are processed by machines that produce a multidimensional, detailed image of the structure. Formerly, only still pictures could be obtained; now, however, moving pictures in "real time" are possible—for example, in pregnancy, the fetus' movements and beating heart can actually be visualized.

Sonography does not involve the use of contrast medium or invasive procedures (for example, sonography does not involve the use of injections, catheterization, and incisions). There is no known risk involved in sonography, although the long-term effects of sound waves have not been determined.

Tests for Women

AMNIOCENTESIS

Amniocentesis is performed during pregnancy. A hollow needle is inserted through the abdominal and uterine walls into the amniotic sac surrounding the fetus in order to withdraw some amniotic fluid for testing. The analysis of amniotic fluid is useful in determining the condition of the fetus, since the amniotic fluid contains discarded fetal cells. Examination of these cells for chromosomal and chemical makeup can detect a large number of genetic defects and hereditary disorders. Testing certain chemicals in the fluid itself is done to determine fetal lung maturity and to detect certain fetal abnormalities, such as spina bifida. The fetal cells will also indicate the sex of the baby, which is important if a sex-linked hereditary disorder, such as hemophilia (a blood-clotting disease that oc-

curs almost exclusively in males), is suspected. However, amniocentesis is never performed simply to satisfy curiosity about the sex of a baby.

The test is performed most often in women who are over the age of 35 or who have a family history of certain hereditary disorders. The incidence of chromosome abnormalities of the fetus increases rapidly after a woman reaches the age of 35. As each year passes, the chances of such abnormalities increase.

The procedure is relatively painless, since a local anesthetic is used around the injection site. The test is usually done during the sixteenth to eighteenth week of pregnancy (before this time the test results are inconclusive). The final results are not available for three to four weeks; therefore, the waiting period can be the most difficult part of the test. However, approximately 95 percent of amniocentesis results are normal.

There is some risk to this test, which is why it is not routinely used. There is a risk of miscarriage, as well as a chance of striking the placenta or the fetus. However, this risk is minimized by the use of ultrasonography to reveal the position of both the fetus and the placenta before the needle is inserted. In addition, as with any invasive technique (that is, one that involves an incision, an injection, or the insertion of something into the body), there is a chance of infection. A patient experiencing pain, fever, or discharge from the puncture site or from the vagina should notify her doctor immediately.

MAMMOGRAPHY

Mammography is a simple, generally painless examination of

the breasts by means of a special X-ray machine that is designed to be used for soft tissues. This procedure is especially valuable for the detection of early breast cancers before they can be felt manually by the woman or her doctor. Mammography can frequently differentiate between malignant (cancerous) and nonmalignant (noncancerous) lumps and can provide information about fibrocystic breast disease.

Many medical experts recommend that a mammogram of the normal breasts be made when a woman is around the age of 35. This baseline study can then be used for comparison with subsequent mammograms to detect changes in the breasts. After the first mammogram, it is recommended that the test be repeated every one to two years, depending on individual risk factors, such as a family history of breast cancer. Most doctors suggest a mammogram every year for women past the age of 50, regardless of risk factors. However, a mammogram should not replace monthly breast self-examinations (see page 392) and regular breast examinations by a doctor; rather, the mammogram should be done in conjunction with these manual examinations.

Other related techniques for breast examination are xerography and thermography. Xerography is a form of mammography that records the image using a photoelectric process rather than standard X-ray film. Thermography is a diagnostic technique that uses no X rays and thus can be repeated as often as desired. Thermography records differences in temperature among various parts of the breast. The basic premise of thermography is that rapidly growing cancer cells give off more heat than normal cells do. Thermography, however, is not as accurate as mammography and should be used only to augment information obtained from a physical examination and a mammogram.

There is some question about the risk of radiation exposure in mammography, especially for those women who receive a yearly mammogram. The radiation dosage has been reduced in modern testing, and many physicians feel that the benefits of early detection outweigh any risks. However, because of these risks, most doctors are conservative about the use of mammography. A woman should discuss the benefits and risks of this procedure with a doctor who knows her medical history. As a general rule, mammography should not be performed on a pregnant woman.

PAP TEST

The Pap test is a standard part of the gynecological examination for women. (Pap is an abbreviation of Papanicolaou, the name of the physician who developed the test.) Analysis of the specimen obtained is used to detect early cell changes that might indicate cancer or other abnormalities of the cervix (the neck of the uterus).

The Pap test involves scraping some cells from the surface of the area where the cervix opens into the vagina. The scraping is done with a small plastic spatula. The scrapings are smeared onto a glass slide for microscopic examination. The test is relatively painless, and there is virtually no risk.

The test results are categorized into five groups: Class I—no abnormal cells; Class II—atypical cells, usually caused by inflammation or infection; Class III—cells suspected of being cancerous; and Classes IV and V—cancer cells present. In some laboratories, a modification of this classification is used so that the report states that the smear is negative, doubtful, unsatisfactory, or positive.

A woman should have her first Pap test at about 18 years of age. The test should be repeated every one to two years. Women over age 40 should have an annual Pap test. Any woman with a history of cervical or uterine cancer or of abnormal Pap test results should have the test done every six months.

PELVIC EXAMINATION

The pelvic examination is a manual and visual inspection of the female reproductive tract. It is done to detect disorders in the reproductive organs, including the vagina, cervix, uterus, and ovaries. A pelvic examination can also reveal pregnancy.

The patient lies on an examination table and places her heels in metal holders resembling the stirrups on a horse's saddle. The doctor inserts into the vagina a speculum, a special instrument that expands the vagina to permit visual examination of the vagina and cervix. A specimen for a Pap test may be obtained. After removing the speculum, the doctor inserts two gloved fingers into the vagina while simultaneously pressing lightly on the patient's abdomen; this procedure enables the doctor to detect abnormalities in the uterus and ovaries. Sometimes, the doctor also inserts a finger into the rectum while pressing on the abdomen; this, too, enables the doctor to feel the uterus and ovaries.

A pelvic examination takes only a few minutes, is relatively painless, and entails virtually no risk.

PRESCRIPTION DRUGS

Introduction

The right drug for the right patient in the right dose by the right route at the right time. This rule sums up the decisions made when your doctor gives you a prescription. You've helped make those decisions by giving a complete medical history: You've informed your doctor of any previous allergic reactions you've suffered to drugs, foods, or dyes; of any other drugs you may be taking; of any chronic health problems you may have; and whether you are pregnant or breast-feeding an infant. Once you leave your doctor's office, prescription in hand, you have still more to do as a responsible patient.

You must know how to administer the medication you will be taking. You must understand and comply with your dosage schedule. You must know what to do should side effects occur. You must recognize the signals that indicate the need to call your doctor. All too often, patients leave their doctors' offices without a full understanding of the drug therapy they're about to start, with the result that they do not comply fully with their doctors' prescriptions. They may stop taking the medication too soon because it doesn't seem to work, or because they feel better, or because it causes bothersome side effects. They may take the drug improperly or at the wrong time or too often. They may continue drinking alcohol or taking other drugs, perhaps not even realizing that such products as cold pills, oral contraceptives (birth control pills), aspirin, and vitamins can affect the action of the newly prescribed drug. The end result may be that they do not get better; perhaps they will even get worse or suffer a dangerous overdose.

PRESCRIPTION DRUGS provides the information that you need to take medications safely. Along with general information on reading a prescription and buying, storing, and using drugs, it provides an introduction to the action of drugs—how drugs work to stop infection, to lower blood pressure, or to relieve pain. It provides detailed information on hundreds of the most commonly prescribed drugs and several over-the-counter (nonprescription) products, including how to alleviate certain side effects, whether you should take the drug on an empty stomach or with meals, whether the drug is likely to affect your ability to drive a car, and whether you can substitute a generic drug for a prescribed brand-name medication. You will discover which side effects are common to some medications and which are danger signals that require immediate attention from your physician.

Of course, this book is not a substitute for consulting your doctor and pharmacist. Those people should be your primary reference sources on the use of drugs. But to ensure that you receive the best health care possible, you, too, must be informed and knowledgeable about the drugs you use.

Filling Your Prescription

While you're having your prescription filled, you should make sure you understand what the drug is used for, your dosage schedule, how to store the medication properly, what kinds of precautions to take to prevent or reduce side effects, whether you should restrict your diet or drinking habits while taking the drug, which side effects are expected or unavoidable, and which side effects signal a need for a doctor's attention. Your first step in filling your prescription is reading what your doctor has written.

READING YOUR PRESCRIPTION

Prescriptions are not mysterious—they contain no secret messages. Many of the symbols and phrases doctors use on prescriptions are abbreviated Latin or Greek words; they are holdovers from the days when doctors actually wrote in Latin. For example, "gtt" comes from the Latin word *guttae,* which means drops, and "bid" is a shortened version of *bis in die,* which is Latin for twice a day.

You do not have to be a doctor, nurse, or pharmacist to read a prescription. You can (and should) learn how to read one yourself—after all, the prescription describes the drug you will be taking. You should understand what your doctor has written on the prescription blank to be sure that the label on the drug container you receive from your pharmacist coincides with your prescription.

The accompanying chart lists the most common prescription symbols and abbreviations. Use it as a guide to read the sample prescriptions that follow.

Common Abbreviations and Symbols Used in Writing Prescriptions

Abbreviation	Meaning	Derivation and Notes
aa	of each	*ana* (Greek)
ac	before meals	*ante cibum* (Latin)
AD	right ear	*auris dextra* (Latin)
AL	left ear	*auris laeva* (Latin)
AM	morning	*ante meridiem* (Latin)
AS	left ear	*auris sinistra* (Latin)
au	both ears	*auris* (Latin)
bid	twice a day	*bis in die* (Latin)
C	100	—
c̄	with	*cum* (Latin)
cap	capsule	—
cc or cm³	cubic centimeter	30 cc equals one ounce
disp	dispense	
dtd#	give this number	*dentur tales doses* (Latin)
ea	each	—
ext	for external use	—

Abbreviation	Meaning	Derivation and Notes
gtt	drops	*guttae* (Latin)
gt	drop	*gutta* (Latin)
h	hour	*hora* (Latin)
hs	at bedtime	*hora somni* (Latin)
M ft	make	*misce fiat* (Latin)
mitt#	give this number	*mitte* (Latin)
ml	milliliter	30 ml equals one ounce (1 ml=1 cc)
O	pint	*octarius* (Latin)
OD	right eye	*oculus dexter* (Latin)
OL	left eye	*oculus laevus* (Latin)
OS	left eye	*oculus sinister* (Latin)
OU	each eye	*oculus uterque* (Latin)
pc	after meals	*post cibum* (Latin)
PM	evening	*post meridiem* (Latin)
po	by mouth	*per os* (Latin)
prn	as needed	*pro re nata* (Latin)
q̄	every	*quaqua* (Latin)
qd	once a day; every day	*quaqua die* (Latin)
qid	four times a day	*quater in die* (Latin)
qod	every other day	
s̄	without	*sine* (Latin)
sig	label as follows	*signa* (Latin)
sl	under the tongue	*sub lingua* (Latin)
SOB	shortness of breath	—
sol	solution	—
ss	half unit	*semis* (Latin)
stat	at once; first dose	*statim* (Latin)
susp	suspension	—
tab	tablet	—
tid	three times a day	*ter in die* (Latin)
top	apply topically	
ung or ungt	ointment	*unguentum* (Latin)
UT	under the tongue	
ut dict or UD	as directed	*ut dictum* (Latin)
x	times	—

The first sample prescription is for a medication called Fiorinal. The prescription tells the pharmacist to give you 24 capsules (#24), and it tells you to take one capsule (cap i) every four hours (q̄ 4h) as needed (prn) for pain.

The prescription indicates that you may receive five re-fills (5x), that the label on the drug container should state the name of the drug (yes), and that the pharmacist may

---

John D. Jones MD
Anytown, U.S.A.

DEA# 123456789   PHONE# 123-4567

NAME *Your Name*   AGE __47__
ADDRESS *Anytown, U.S.A.*   DATE __5/10/92__

℞ Fiorinal
   #24
   Sig: caps i q̄ 4 h prn pain

REFILLS __5x__   DISPENSE AS WRITTEN
LABEL __yes__   *John D. Jones M.D.*
                        SUBSTITUTION

---

substitute (substitution) a less expensive equivalent product.

Look at the second prescription. It shows that you will receive 100 (dtd C) tablets of Lanoxin, 0.125 mg. You will take three tablets at once (iii stat), then two (ii) to-

---

John D. Jones MD
Anytown, U.S.A.

DEA# 123456789   PHONE# 123-4567

NAME *Your Name*   AGE __55__
ADDRESS *Anytown, U.S.A.*   DATE __5/23/92__

℞ Lanoxin 0.125
   dtd C
   Sig: iii stat, ii tomorrow AM,
   then i q̄ AM c̄ OJ
                        John D. Jones, M.D.
                        DISPENSE AS WRITTEN

REFILLS __prn__
LABEL __✓__   SUBSTITUTION

---

morrow morning (AM), and one (i) every (q̄) morning (AM) thereafter with (c̄) orange juice (OJ). You will re-ceive the specific brand noted (dispense as written), you may receive refills as needed (prn), and the name of the drug will be on the package (✓).

Do remember to check the label on the drug container. If the information on the label is not the same as on the prescription, question your pharmacist. Make sure you are receiving the right medication and the correct in-structions for taking it.

TALKING TO YOUR PHARMACIST

Once you have read the prescription, its directions may seem clear enough, but will they seem clear when you get home? For example, the prescription for the Fiorinal states that you should take one capsule every four hours as needed. How many capsules can you take each day—four, six, more? The phrase "as needed" is not clear, and unless you understand what it means, you don't know how much medication you can take per day. What if your prescription instructs you to take "one tablet four times a day?" What does four times a day mean? For some an-tibiotics, it may mean one tablet every six hours around the clock. For other medications, it may mean one tablet in the morning, one at noon, one in the early evening, and one at bedtime. For still others, it may mean one tablet every hour for the first four hours after you get up in the morning. Don't leave the pharmacy with unanswered questions; ask your pharmacist for an explanation of any confusing terms on your prescription.

Your pharmacist is a valuable resource in your health care. He or she should have a record of ALL the pre-scription drugs you receive, in order to detect any pos-sible life-threatening drug interactions. It is, therefore, a good idea to purchase your medications through one pharmacy—choose one that maintains careful records.

The pharmacist will be able to tell you if your therapy may be affected by smoking tobacco, eating certain foods, or drinking alcohol, and if the drugs you are taking can cause drowsiness or nausea. He or she can tell you what to expect from the medication and about how long you will have to take it. Of course, people's treatments vary tremendously, but you should ask whether you will have to take medication for five to ten days (for example, to treat a mild respiratory infection) or for a few months (for example, to treat a kidney infection).

You should discuss with your pharmacist the possible side effects of your medication and ask for a description of symptoms. The pharmacist can tell you which side ef-fects require prompt attention from your physician. For example, one of the major side effects of the drug phenylbutazone is the development of a blood disorder. Since a sore throat can be one of the early symptoms of a blood disorder, your pharmacist may instruct you to con-sult your physician if this symptom occurs.

Your pharmacist can also explain how to take your medicine. You need to know whether to take the drug before or after a meal or along with it. The timing of doses of a drug can make a big difference, and the effective-ness of each drug depends on following the directions for its use. Your pharmacist can tell you what is meant by the phrases "as needed," "as directed," and "take with fluid." For example, you may take water, but not milk, with some drugs. With other drugs, you should drink milk. Your pharmacist can also tell you how many refills you may have and whether you may need them.

OVER-THE-COUNTER DRUGS

Drugs that can be purchased without a prescription are referred to as over-the-counter (OTC) drugs. They are sold in a wide variety of settings, such as drugstores, gro-cery stores, and hotel lobbies. There are no legal re-quirements or limitations on who may buy or sell them.

Products sold OTC contain amounts of active ingredi-ents considered to be safe for self-treatment by consumers when labeling instructions are followed.

Many people visit a doctor for ailments that can be treated effectively by taking nonprescription drugs.

Actually, prescriptions are sometimes written for such drugs. Your pharmacist will be able to recommend appropriate use of OTC medications and preparations.

If your pharmacist recommends that you not take certain OTC drugs, follow the advice. OTC drugs may affect the way your body reacts to the prescription drugs you are taking. For instance, people taking tetracycline should avoid taking antacids or iron-containing products at the same time; their use should be separated by at least two hours. Antacids and iron interfere with the body's absorption of tetracycline, thereby decreasing its effectiveness. Be sure you know what you are taking. If you are unsure of the type or contents of your medications, ask your doctor or pharmacist.

GENERIC DRUGS

One way your pharmacist can help you save money is by dispensing generic drugs. "Generic" means not protected by trademark registration. The generic name of a drug is usually a shortened form of its chemical name. Any manufacturer can use the generic name when marketing a drug.

Usually, a manufacturer uses a trade name (or brand name) as well as a generic name for a drug. A trade name is registered, and only the manufacturer who holds the trademark can use the trade name when marketing a drug. For example, only Lederle Laboratories can call their tetracycline product Achromycin V, and only the Upjohn Company can use the trade name Panmycin for tetracycline. Most trade names are easy to remember, are capitalized in print, and usually include the registered symbol (®) after them. You should know the generic name and the trade name of every drug you are taking.

Many people think that drugs with trade names are made by large manufacturers and generic drugs are made by small manufacturers. But, in fact, a manufacturer may market large quantities of a drug under a brand name and may also sell the base chemical to several other companies, some of which sell the drug generically and some of which sell it under their own brand names. For example, the antibiotic ampicillin is the base for over 200 different products. However, all ampicillin is produced by only a few dozen drug companies.

Generic drugs are generally priced lower than their trademarked equivalents, largely because they are not as widely advertised. However, not every drug is available generically, and not every generic is significantly less expensive than its trademarked equivalent. Nevertheless, consumers may be able to save as much as 40 percent by purchasing a generic product. For example, 100 tablets of Inderal (40 mg) may cost $22 to $25. One hundred tablets of the generic equivalent product may cost about $18—a savings of $4 to $7.

For certain drugs, however, it's inadvisable to "shop around" for a generic equivalent. Although the Food and Drug Admin-istration has stated that there is no evidence to suspect serious differences between trade-name drugs and generic drugs, differences have been shown to exist between brands of certain drugs. The tablets or capsules from different manufacturers may not dissolve in the stomach at the same rate or to the same extent, because of variations in the way they are made or the fillers (nonac-

tive ingredients) that are used. This is especially true for the various generic digoxin and phenytoin products. It is, therefore, important to discuss with your doctor or pharmacist the advantages or disadvantages of any particular generic product.

All states have some form of substitution law that allows pharmacists to fill prescriptions with the least expensive equivalent product. However, your doctor can authorize the use of a specific brand of medication by signing on the appropriate line or otherwise noting this on the prescription form (see the sample prescriptions on page 9). You should be aware that certain patients can sometimes respond in different ways to various equivalent products, and your doctor may have good reasons for being specific. Discuss this with your doctor.

HOW MUCH TO BUY

On a prescription, your doctor specifies exactly how many tablets or capsules or how much liquid medication you will receive. But if you must take a drug for a long time, or if you are very sensitive to drugs, you may want to purchase a different quantity.

The amount of medication to buy depends on several factors. The most obvious is how much money you have or, for those who have a comprehensive insurance program, how much the insurance company will pay for each purchase. These factors may help you decide how much medication to buy, but you must also consider the kind of medication you will be taking (for example, how long it can be stored).

Medications to treat heart disease, high blood pressure, diabetes, or a thyroid condition may be purchased in large quantity. Patients with such chronic conditions take medication for prolonged periods. Chances are, they will pay less per tablet or capsule by purchasing large quantities of drugs. Generally, the price per dose decreases with the amount of the drug purchased. In other words, a drug that usually costs six cents per tablet may cost four or five cents per tablet if you buy 100 at a time.

Many doctors prescribe only a month's supply of drugs, even those drugs that will be taken for a long time. If you wish to buy more, check with your pharmacist. It is also important to make sure that you have enough medication on hand to cover vacation travel and long holidays. Serious side effects could occur if you miss even a few doses of such drugs as propranolol, prednisone, or clonidine.

If you have been plagued by annoying side effects or have had allergic reactions to some drugs, you may want to ask your pharmacist to dispense only enough medication on initial prescriptions for a few days or a week, so that you can determine how your body reacts to the drug. Pharmacists cannot take back prescription drugs once they have left the pharmacy. You may have to pay more per dose if the pharmacist gives you a small quantity of the prescription, but at least you will not be paying for a supply of medication your body cannot take. Be sure you can get the remainder of the prescribed amount of the drug if no serious or intolerable side effects occur. With some drugs, after you have received part of the intended amount, you cannot receive the remainder without obtaining another prescription.

STORING YOUR DRUGS

Before you leave the pharmacy, find out how you should store your medication. If drugs are stored in containers that do not protect them from heat or moisture, they may lose potency.

All medications should be kept in their original containers. Different medications should NOT be mixed in one container, in order to prevent confusion about which drug is being taken. In addition, some drugs may lose their potency when stored with other medications. Never remove the label from the prescription vial. It contains your prescription number (for refills), the name of the medication, and directions for proper use.

You can safely store most prescription drugs at room temperature and out of direct sunlight. Even those drugs dispensed in colored bottles or containers that reflect light should be kept out of direct sunlight.

Some drugs require storage in the refrigerator; other medications should not be refrigerated. For example, some liquid cough suppressants thicken as they become cold and will not pour from the bottle. Some people keep nitroglycerin tablets in the refrigerator because they believe the drug will be more stable when kept cold. Nitroglycerin, however, should not be stored in the refrigerator.

Even if the label on your medication states "keep refrigerated," this does NOT mean you can keep the drug in the freezer. If frozen and thawed, coated tablets may crack, and some liquids may separate into layers that can't be remixed.

Many people keep prescription drugs and other medications in the bathroom medicine cabinet, but this is one of the WORST places to keep drugs. Small children can easily climb onto the sink and reach drugs stored above it. Also, the temperature and humidity changes in the bathroom may adversely affect the stability of prescription and nonprescription drugs.

It is required by law that all prescription medications for oral use be dispensed in childproof containers. If you find the container difficult to open AND if there are no small children in your home, you can request that your pharmacist dispense your medication in a nonchildproof container.

Definitions Used to Describe Storage Temperatures

Excessive Cold	Any temperature under 36°F (2°C)
Refrigerated	Any cold place where the temperature is between 36° and 46°F (2°–8°C)
Cool	Any temperature between 46° and 59°F (8°–15°C)
Room temperature	Temperature usually between 59° and 86°F (15°–30°C)
Excessive heat	Any temperature above 104°F (40°C)

KEEP ALL MEDICATIONS AWAY FROM CHILDREN, and do not keep unused prescription drugs. Flush leftover medication down the toilet or pour it down the sink, and wash and destroy the empty container. Regularly clean out your medicine cabinet and discard all drugs you are no longer using and drugs that have expired (the expiration date is often listed on the prescription label). These drugs can be dangerous to your children, and you might be tempted to take them in the future if you develop similar symptoms. Similar symptoms may not be due to the same disease, however, and you may complicate your condition by taking the wrong medication.

If a child accidentally swallows medication or receives too much of a prescribed medication, IMMEDIATELY CALL YOUR LOCAL POISON CONTROL CENTER, A NEARBY EMERGENCY ROOM, OR YOUR DOCTOR for instructions and recommendations. These phone numbers should be written down in a readily accessible place. (For safety's sake, it is wise to keep a list of these and other important telephone numbers, such as those for the police and fire departments, at each and every telephone in your home.) You should also keep a bottle of syrup of ipecac (available without a prescription at your local drugstore) for each child under five years of age in your home (in case the poison control center or emergency room personnel or your doctor recommends that you induce vomiting in the child). Do not, however, use the syrup of ipecac unless instructed to do so by a health professional.

Administering Medication Correctly

You must use medicine correctly to obtain its full benefit. If you administer drugs improperly, you may not receive their full therapeutic effects. Furthermore, improper administration can be dangerous. Some drugs may become toxic if used incorrectly.

Before administering medications to children or elderly patients, ask your doctor for instructions. Children and older patients can be more sensitive to dosage amounts and side effects of medications.

LIQUIDS

Liquid medications are used in several different ways. Some are intended to be used externally on the skin; some are placed into the eye, ear, nose, or throat; still others may be taken internally. Before taking or using any liquid medication, look at the label to see if there are specific directions.

A suspension is a liquid product that contains particles that settle to the bottom of the container. It must be shaken before you use the medicine. If you don't shake it well each time, you may not get the correct amount of the active ingredient—as the amount of liquid remaining in the bottle becomes smaller, the drug becomes more concentrated. You will be getting more of the active ingredient with each dose. It may even reach toxic levels.

When opening the bottle, point it away from you. Some liquid medications build up pressure inside the bottle; the liquid could spurt out and stain your clothing. If the medication is for application to the skin, pour a small quantity onto a cotton pad or a piece of gauze. Do not use a large piece of cotton or gauze, since it will absorb the liquid and much will be wasted. Don't pour the medication into your cupped hand; you may spill some of it. If you're using it on only a small area, you can spread the medication with your finger or a cotton-tipped applicator. Never dip cotton-tipped applicators or pieces of cotton or gauze into the bottle, since this might contaminate the rest of the medication.

Liquid medications that are to be swallowed must be measured accurately. When your doctor prescribes one teaspoonful of medication, he or she is thinking of a 5-milliliter (ml) medical spoon. The teaspoons you have at home can hold anywhere from 2 to 10 ml of liquid. If you use one of these to measure your medication, you may get too little or too much drug with each dose. Ask your pharmacist for a medical teaspoon or one of the other plastic devices for accurately measuring liquid medications. Most of these cost only a few cents and are well worth their cost in ensuring accurate dosage. In addition, while many children balk at medication taken from a teaspoon, they often enjoy taking it from a "special" spoon.

CAPSULES, TABLETS, AND ORAL POWDERS

Many people find it hard to swallow a tablet or capsule. If tablets or capsules tend to catch in your throat, rinse your mouth with water, or at least wet your mouth, before attempting to take a tablet or capsule. Place the tablet or capsule on the back of your tongue, take a drink, and swallow. If it is too large, or still "sticks" in your throat, empty the capsule or crush the tablet into a spoon and mix it with applesauce, soup, or even chocolate syrup. But BE SURE TO CHECK WITH YOUR PHARMACIST BEFORE YOU DO SO. Some tablets and capsules should not be crushed or opened and must be swallowed whole—your pharmacist can tell you which ones they are.

If you have trouble swallowing a tablet or capsule and do not wish to mix the medication with food, ask your doctor to prescribe a liquid drug preparation or a chewable tablet instead, if one is available.

Occasionally, medications come in oral powder form (for example, cholestyramine and colestipol). Such medications should be carefully mixed with liquids, then swallowed. These medications should NOT be swallowed dry.

SUBLINGUAL TABLETS

Some drugs, such as nitroglycerin, are prepared as tablets that must be placed under the tongue. Such medications are more rapidly or more completely absorbed into the bloodstream from the lining of the mouth than they are from the stomach and intestinal tract.

To take a sublingual tablet properly, place the tablet under your tongue, close your mouth, and hold the saliva in your mouth and under your tongue as long as you can before swallowing (to allow the tablet to dissolve). If you have a bitter taste in your mouth after five minutes, the drug has not been completely absorbed. Wait at least five more minutes before drinking water. Drinking too soon may wash the medication into the stomach before it has been absorbed thoroughly. Do not smoke, eat, or chew gum while the medication is dissolving.

BUCCAL TABLETS

Some drugs, such as nitroglycerin, are prepared as tablets that must be placed under the lip or in the cheek. These products are designed to release a dose of the drug over a period of time.

To take a buccal tablet properly, place the tablet between the upper lip and gum (above the front teeth) or between the cheek and gum. If you eat or drink during the three to five hours that it takes for the tablet to dissolve, place the tablet between the upper lip and gum. Do not go to sleep with a tablet in your mouth because it could slip down your throat and cause choking. Do not use chewing tobacco when a tablet is in place.

EYE DROPS AND EYE OINTMENTS

Before administering eye drops or ointments, wash your hands. Then lie down or sit down, and tilt your head back. Using your thumb and forefinger, gently and carefully pull your lower eyelid down to form a pouch. Hold the dropper close to your eyelid without touching it. Drop the prescribed amount of medicine into this pouch and slowly close your eyes. Try not to blink. Keep your eyes closed, and place one finger at the corner of the eye next to your nose for a minute or two, applying slight pressure (this is done to prevent loss of medication through the duct that drains fluid from the surface of the eye into the nose and throat). Then wipe away any excess with a clean tissue. Do not wash or wipe the dropper before replacing it in the bottle—you might accidentally contaminate the rest of the medication. Close the bottle tightly to keep out moisture.

To administer an eye ointment, squeeze a line of ointment in the prescribed amount into the pouch formed as for administering eye drops (avoid touching the tube to your eyelid), and close your eye. Roll your eye a few times to spread the ointment.

Be sure the drops or ointments you use are intended for use in the eye (all products manufactured for use in the eye must be sterilized to prevent eye infections). Also, check the expiration date on the label or container of the medication. Don't use a drug product after the specified date, and never use any eye product that has changed color. If you find that the medication contains particles that weren't there when you bought it, don't use it.

EAR DROPS

Ear drops must be administered so that they fill the ear canal. To administer ear drops properly, tilt your head to one side, turning the affected ear upward. Grasp the earlobe and gently pull it upward and back to straighten the ear canal. When administering ear drops to a child, GENTLY pull the child's earlobe downward and back. Fill the dropper and place the prescribed number of drops (usually a dropperful) into the ear, but be careful to avoid touching the sides or edge of the ear canal. The dropper can easily become contaminated by contact with the ear canal.

Keep the ear tilted upward for five to ten seconds while continuing to hold the earlobe. Your doctor may want you to gently insert a small wad of clean cotton into the ear to ensure that the drops do not escape. Do not wash or wipe the dropper after use; replace it in the bottle and tightly close the bottle to keep out moisture.

Before administering the medication, you may warm the bottle of ear drops by rolling the bottle back and forth between your hands to bring the solution to body temperature. DO NOT place the bottle in boiling water. The ear drops may become so hot that they will cause pain when placed in the ear. Also, boiling water can loosen or peel off the label and might even destroy the medication.

NOSE DROPS AND SPRAYS

Before using nose drops or sprays, gently blow your nose if you can. To administer nose drops, fill the dropper, tilt your head back, and place the prescribed number of drops into your nose. To prevent contamination of the rest of the medicine do not touch the dropper to the nasal membranes. Keep your head tilted for five to ten seconds, and sniff gently two or three times.

Do not tilt your head back when using a nasal spray. Insert the sprayer into the nose, but try to avoid touching the inner nasal membranes. Sniff and squeeze the sprayer at the same time. Do not release your grip on the sprayer until you have withdrawn it from your nose (to prevent nasal mucus and bacteria from entering the plastic bottle and contaminating its contents). After you have sprayed the prescribed number of times in one or both nostrils, gently sniff two or three times.

Unless your doctor has told you otherwise, you should not use nose drops or sprays for more than two or three days at a time. If they have been prescribed for a longer period, do not administer nose drops or sprays from the same container for more than one week. Bacteria from your nose can easily enter the container and contaminate the solution. If you must take medication for more than a week, purchase a new container. NEVER allow anyone else to use your nose drops or spray.

RECTAL SUPPOSITORIES

Rectal suppositories are used to deliver various types of medication. They may be used as laxatives, sleeping aids, or tranquilizers or as preparations that are used to relieve the itching, swelling, and pain of hemorrhoids. Regardless of the reason for their use, all rectal suppositories are inserted in the same way.

In extremely hot weather, a suppository may become too soft to handle properly. If this happens, place the suppository in the refrigerator, in a glass of cool water, or under running cold water until it becomes firm. A few minutes is usually sufficient. Before inserting a suppository, remove any aluminum wrappings. Rubber finger coverings or disposable rubber gloves may be worn when inserting a suppository, but they are not necessary unless your fingernails are extremely long and sharp.

To insert a suppository, lie on your left side with your right knee bent. Push the suppository, pointed end first, into the rectum as far as is comfortable. You may feel like defecating, but lie still for a few minutes and try not to have a bowel movement for at least an hour. If you cannot insert a suppository, or if the process is painful, you can coat the suppository with a thin layer of petroleum jelly or mineral oil to make insertion easier.

Manufacturers of many suppositories that are used in the treatment of hemorrhoids suggest that the suppositories be stored in the refrigerator. Ask your pharmacist if the suppositories you have purchased should be stored in the refrigerator.

VAGINAL OINTMENTS AND CREAMS

Most vaginal products are packaged with complete instructions for use. If a woman is not sure how to administer vaginal medication, she should ask her pharmacist.

Before using any vaginal ointment or cream, read the directions. They will probably tell you to attach the applicator to the top of the tube and to squeeze the tube from the bottom until the applicator is completely filled. Then lie on your back with your knees drawn up. Hold the applicator horizontally or pointed slightly downward, and insert it into the vagina as far as it will go comfortably. Press the plunger down to empty the cream or ointment into the vagina. Withdraw the plunger and wash it in warm, soapy water. Rinse it thoroughly and allow it to dry completely. When the plunger is dry, return it to its original package.

VAGINAL TABLETS AND SUPPOSITORIES

Most packages of vaginal tablets or suppositories include complete directions for use, but you may wish to review these general instructions.

Remove any foil wrapping. Place the tablet or suppository in the applicator that is provided. Lie on your back with your knees drawn up. Hold the applicator horizontally or tilted slightly downward, and insert it into the vagina as far as it will comfortably go. Depress the plunger slowly to release the tablet or suppository into the vagina. Withdraw the applicator and wash it in warm, soapy water. Rinse it and let it dry completely. When the applicator is dry, return it to its package.

Unless your doctor has told you otherwise, do not douche two to three weeks before or after you use vaginal tablets or suppositories. Be sure to ask your doctor for specific recommendations on douching.

THROAT LOZENGES AND DISCS

Both lozenges and discs contain medication that is released in the mouth to soothe a sore throat, to reduce coughing, or to treat laryngitis. Neither should be chewed; they should be allowed to dissolve in the mouth. After the lozenge or disc has dissolved, try not to swallow or drink any fluids for a while.

THROAT SPRAYS

To administer a throat spray, open your mouth wide and spray the medication as far back as possible. Try not to swallow—hold the spray in your mouth as long as you can, and do not drink any fluids for several minutes. Swallowing a throat spray is not harmful, but if you find that your throat spray upsets your stomach, don't swallow it; simply spit the throat spray out.

TOPICAL OINTMENTS AND CREAMS

Most topical (used on the skin) ointments and creams exert only local effects—that is, they affect only the area on which they are applied. Most creams and ointments are expensive (especially steroid products, such as betamethasone valerate, fluocinolone, fluocinonide, hydrocortisone, and triamcinolone) and should be applied to the skin as thinly as possible. A thin layer is as effective as (but less costly than) a thick layer. Furthermore, some steroid-containing creams and ointments can cause toxic side effects if applied too heavily.

Before applying the medication, moisten the skin by immersing it in water or by dabbing the area with a clean, wet cloth. Blot the skin almost dry and apply the medication as directed. Gently massage it into the skin until the cream or ointment disappears. You should feel no greasiness after applying a cream. After an ointment is applied, the skin will feel slightly greasy.

If your doctor has not indicated whether you should receive a cream or an ointment, ask your pharmacist for the one you prefer. Creams are greaseless and do not stain your clothing. Creams are best to use on the scalp or other hairy areas of the body. However, if your skin is dry, ask for an ointment. Ointments help keep skin soft for a longer period.

If your doctor tells you to place a wrap on top of the skin after the cream or ointment has been applied, you may use a wrap of transparent plastic film like that used for wrapping food. A wrap holds the medication close to the skin and helps to keep the skin moist so that the drug can be absorbed. To use a wrap correctly, apply the cream or ointment as directed, then wrap the area with a layer of transparent plastic film. Follow your doctor's directions EXACTLY, and keep the wrap in place only as long as you are told to do so. If you keep a wrap on the skin too long, too much of the drug may be absorbed, which may lead to increased side effects. Do not use a wrap without your doctor's approval, and never use one on an oozing lesion.

AEROSOL SPRAYS

Many topical (applied to the skin) items are packaged as pressurized aerosol sprays. These sprays usually cost more than the cream or ointment form of the same medication. They are especially useful on very tender or hairy areas of the body, where it is difficult to apply a cream or ointment. Aerosols can provide a cooling effect on burns or rashes.

Before using an aerosol, shake the can to evenly disperse the particles of medication. Hold the container upright four to six inches from the skin. Press the nozzle for a few seconds, then release.

Never use an aerosol around the face or eyes. If your doctor tells you to use the spray on a part of your face, apply it to your hand and then rub it into the area. If you get it into your eyes or on a mucous membrane, it can be very painful; it may even damage the eyes.

Aerosol sprays may feel cold when they are applied. If this sensation bothers you, ask your pharmacist or doctor whether another form of the same product is available.

TRANSDERMAL PATCHES

Transdermal patches allow controlled, continuous release of medication. They are convenient and easy to use. For best results, apply the patch to a hairless or clean-shaven area of skin, avoiding scars and wounds. Choose a site (such as the chest or upper arm) that is not subject to excessive movement. It is all right to bathe or shower with a patch in place. In the event that the patch becomes dislodged, discard and replace it. Replace a patch by applying a new unit in another spot. By doing this, you allow for uninterrupted drug therapy and minimal skin irritation.

If redness or irritation develops at the application site, consult your physician. Some people are sensitive to the materials used to make the patches.

Coping with Side Effects

Drugs have certain desirable effects—that's why they are taken. The desirable effects of a drug are known as the drug's activity or therapeutic effects. Drugs, however, have undesirable effects as well. Undesirable effects are called side effects, adverse reactions, or, in some cases, lethal effects. An adverse reaction is any undesirable effect of a drug. It can range from minor to toxic or lethal.

Even if you experience minor side effects, it is very important that you take your medication exactly as it was prescribed. You should take the full dose at the appropriate times throughout the day for the length of time prescribed by your doctor. Taking a lesser amount of medication to avoid side effects or because your condition appears to be improving is NOT appropriate. A smaller dose may not provide any benefit whatsoever; that is, half of the dose may not provide half of the therapeutic effects.

Some side effects are expected and unavoidable, but others may surprise the doctor as well as the patient. Unexpected reactions may be due to a person's individual response to the drug.

Side effects generally fall into one of two major groups—those that are obvious and those that cannot be detected without laboratory testing. Discussion between you and your doctor about your medication should not be restricted to the most easily recognized side effects; other, less obvious side effects may also be harmful.

If you know a particular side effect is expected from a particular drug, you can relax a little. Most expected side effects are temporary and need not cause alarm. You'll merely experience discomfort or inconvenience for a short time. For example, you may become drowsy after taking an antihistamine or develop a stuffy nose after taking reserpine or certain other drugs that lower blood pressure. Of course, if you find minor side effects especially bothersome, you should discuss them with your doctor, who may be able to prescribe another drug or at least assure you that the benefits of the drug far outweigh its side effects. Sometimes, side effects can be minimized or eliminated by changing your dosage schedule or taking the drug with meals. Be sure, however, to consult your doctor or pharmacist.

Many side effects, however, signal a serious, perhaps dangerous, problem. If these side effects appear, you should consult your doctor immediately. The following discussion should help you determine whether your side effects require attention.

Obvious Side Effects

Some side effects are obvious to the patient; others can be discerned only through laboratory testing. We have divided our discussion according to the body parts affected by the side effects.

Ears

Although a few drugs may cause loss of hearing if taken in large quantities, hearing loss is uncommon. Drugs that are used to treat problems of the ear may cause dizziness, and many drugs produce tinnitus (a sensation of ringing, buzzing, thumping, or hollowness in the ears). Discuss with your doctor any persistent problem with your hearing or your ears.

Eyes

Blurred vision is a common side effect of many drugs. Medications such as digoxin may cause you to see a halo around a lighted object (a television screen or a traffic light), and other drugs may cause night blindness. Chlordiazepoxide and clidinium combination makes it difficult to judge distance accurately while driving and also makes the eyes sensitive to sunlight. While the effects on the eyes caused by digoxin are danger signs of toxicity, the effects caused by chlordiazepoxide and clidinium combination are to be expected. In any case, if any eye-related problems occur while you are taking medication, contact your physician.

Gastrointestinal System

The gastrointestinal system includes the mouth, esophagus, stomach, small and large intestines, and rectum. A side effect that affects the gastrointestinal system can be expected from almost any drug. Many drugs produce dry mouth, mouth sores, difficulty in swallowing, heartburn, nausea, vomiting, diarrhea, constipation, loss of appetite, or abnormal cramping. Other drugs cause bloating and gas, and some cause rectal itching.

Diarrhea can be expected after taking many drugs. Diarrhea caused by most drugs is temporary and self-limiting; that is, it should stop within three days. During this time, do not take any diarrhea remedy; drink liquids to replace the fluid you are losing. If the diarrhea lasts more than three days or is accompanied by fever, call your doctor.

Diarrhea sometimes signals a problem. For example, some antibiotics can cause severe diarrhea. When diarrhea is severe, the intestine may become ulcerated and begin to bleed. If you have severe diarrhea (diarrhea that lasts for several days, or stools that contain blood, pus, or mucus) while taking antibiotics, contact your doctor.

As a side effect of drug use, constipation is less serious and more common than diarrhea. It occurs when a drug slows down the activity of the bowel. Medications such as chlorpromazine and amitriptyline slow bowel activity. Constipation also occurs when drugs cause moisture to be absorbed from the bowel, resulting in a more solid stool. It may also occur if a drug acts on the nervous system to decrease nerve impulses to the intestine—an effect produced, for example, by methyldopa. Constipation produced by a drug can last several days. You may help relieve it by drinking eight to ten glasses of water a day, including more fiber in your diet, and getting plenty of exercise (unless your doctor directs you to do otherwise). Do not take laxatives unless your doctor directs you to do so. If constipation continues for more than three days, call your doctor.

Circulatory System

Drugs may speed up or slow down the heartbeat. If a drug slows the heartbeat, you may feel drowsy and tired or even dizzy. If a drug accelerates the heartbeat, you probably will experience palpitations (thumping in the chest). You may feel as though your heart is skipping a beat occasionally. For most people, none of these symptoms indicates a serious problem. However, if they occur frequently, consult your doctor, who may adjust your drug dosage or prescribe other medication.

Some drugs can cause edema (fluid retention), in which fluid from the blood collects outside the blood vessels. Ordinarily, edema is not a serious condition. But if you are steadily gaining weight or have gained more than three pounds within a week, be sure to talk to your doctor.

Drugs may increase or decrease blood pressure. When blood pressure decreases, you may feel drowsy or tired; you may become dizzy, or even faint, especially when you rise suddenly from a sitting or reclining position. If a drug makes you dizzy or light-headed, sit or lie down for a while. To avoid light-headedness when you stand, contract and relax the muscles of your legs for a few moments before rising. Push one foot against the floor while raising the other foot slightly, alternating feet so that you are "pumping" your legs in a pedaling motion. Get up slowly, and be careful on stairs. When blood pressure increases, you may feel dizzy, have a headache or blurred vision, hear a ringing or buzzing in your ears, or experience frequent nosebleeds. If these symptoms occur, call your doctor.

Nervous System

Drugs that act on the nervous system may cause drowsiness or stimulation. If a drug causes drowsiness, you may become dizzy or your coordination may become impaired. If a drug causes stimulation, you may become nervous or have insomnia or tremors. Neither drowsiness nor stimulation is cause for concern for most people. When you are drowsy, however, you should be careful around machinery and should avoid driving. Some drugs cause throbbing headaches, and others produce tingling in the fingers or toes. If these symptoms don't disappear in a few days to a week, call your doctor.

Respiratory System

Side effects common to the respiratory system include stuffy nose, dry throat, shortness of breath, and slowed breathing. A stuffy nose and dry throat usually disappear several days after starting a medication. If these side effects are bothersome, you may use nose drops (consult your doctor first) or throat lozenges, or you may gargle with warm salt water to relieve them. Shortness of breath is a characteristic side effect of some drugs (for example, propranolol). If shortness of breath occurs frequently, check with your doctor. It may be a sign of a serious side effect, or you may simply be overexercising.

Skin

Skin reactions include rash, swelling, itching, and sweating. Itching, swelling, and rash frequently indicate a drug allergy. You should NOT continue to take a drug if you develop an allergy to it, but be sure to consult your doctor before you stop taking the drug.

Some drugs increase sweating; others decrease it. Drugs that decrease sweating may cause problems during exercise or hot weather when your body needs to sweat to reduce body temperature.

If you have a minor skin reaction not diagnosed as an allergy, ask your pharmacist for a soothing cream. Your pharmacist may also suggest that you take frequent baths or dust the sensitive area with a suitable powder.

Another type of skin reaction is photosensitivity (also called phototoxicity or sun toxicity)—that is, unusual sensitivity to the sun. Tetracyclines can cause photosensitivity. If, while taking such a drug, you are exposed to the sun for even a brief period of time (10 or 15 minutes), you may experience a severe sunburn. You do not have to stay indoors while taking these drugs, but you should be fully clothed while outside, and you should not remain in the sun too long. Furthermore, you should use a protective sunscreen while in the sun—ask your pharmacist to help you choose one. Since medications may remain in your bloodstream after you stop taking them, you should continue to follow these precautions for two days after treatment with these drugs has been completed.

Subtle Side Effects

Some side effects are difficult to detect. You may not notice any symptoms at all, or you may notice only slight ones. Therefore, your doctor may want you to have periodic blood tests or eye examinations to ensure that no subtle damage is occurring while you are on certain medications.

Kidneys

If one of the side effects of a drug is to reduce the kidneys' ability to remove chemicals and other substances from the blood, these substances begin to accumulate in body tissues. Over a period of time, this accumulation may cause vague symptoms, such as swelling, fluid retention, nausea, headache, or weakness. Obvious symptoms, especially pain, are rare.

Liver

Drug-induced liver damage may result in fat accumulation within the liver. Since the liver is responsible for converting many drugs and body chemicals into compounds that can be eliminated by other organs of the body (kidneys, lungs, gastrointestinal tract), drug-induced liver damage can result in a buildup of these substances. Because liver damage may be quite advanced before it produces any symptoms, periodic blood tests of liver function are recommended during therapy with certain drugs.

Blood

A great many drugs affect the blood and the circulatory system but do not produce noticeable symptoms for some time. Some drugs decrease the number of red blood cells—the cells responsible for carrying oxygen and nutrients throughout the body. If you have too few red blood cells, you become anemic; you appear pale and feel tired, weak, dizzy, and perhaps hungry. Other drugs decrease the number of white blood cells—the cells responsible for combating infection. Having too few white blood cells increases susceptibility to infection and may prolong illness. If a sore throat or a fever begins after you start taking a drug and continues for a few days, you may have an infection and too few white blood cells to fight it. Call your doctor.

DRUG USE DURING PREGNANCY AND BREAST-FEEDING

Before taking ANY medication, it is very important to tell your doctor if you are pregnant (or planning to become pregnant) or are breast-feeding an infant. For most drugs, complete information on safety during pregnancy and while breast-feeding is lacking. This is not due to negligence or lack of concern on the part of regulatory agencies, but to the fact that it would be unethical to conduct drug experiments on pregnant and nursing women. With this in mind, you should discuss with your doctor the risks versus the benefits of taking any medications during pregnancy or while nursing an infant.

MANAGEMENT OF SIDE EFFECTS

Consult the drug profiles to determine whether the side effects you are experiencing are minor (relatively common and usually not serious) or major (symptoms that you should consult your doctor about). If your side effects are minor, you may be able to compensate for them (see the following table for suggestions). However, consult your doctor if you find minor side effects persistent or particularly bothersome.

If you experience any major side effects, contact your doctor immediately. Your dosage may need adjustment, or you may have developed a sensitivity to the drug. Your doctor may want you to switch to an alternative medication to treat your disorder. Never stop taking a prescribed medication unless you first discuss it with your doctor.

Common Minor Side Effects

Side Effect	Management
Constipation	Increase the amount of fiber in your diet; drink plenty of fluids*; exercise*
Decreased sweating	Avoid working or exercising in the sun or under warm conditions
Diarrhea	Drink lots of water to replace lost fluids; if diarrhea lasts longer than three days, call your doctor
Dizziness	Avoid operating machinery or driving a car
Drowsiness	Avoid operating machinery or driving a car
Dry mouth	Suck on candy or ice chips, or chew sugarless gum
Dry nose and throat	Use a humidifier or vaporizer
Fluid retention (mild)	Avoid adding salt to foods; keep legs raised, if possible
Headache	Remain quiet; take aspirin* or acetaminophen*
Insomnia	Take the last dose of the drug earlier in the day*; drink a glass of warm milk at bedtime;ask your doctor about an exercise program
Itching	Take frequent baths or showers, or use wet soaks
Nasal congestion	If necessary, use nose drops*
Palpitations (mild)	Rest often; avoid tension; do not drink coffee, tea, or cola; stop smoking
Upset stomach	Take the drug with milk or food*

*Consult your doctor first

How Drugs Work

Prescription drugs fall into a number of groups according to the conditions for which they are prescribed. In the following pages, we will provide you with a better understanding of the types of medications that are prescribed for different medical conditions. We'll describe the intended actions of drugs and the therapeutic effects you can expect from various types of medications.

CARDIOVASCULAR DRUGS

Antianginals

Since the heart is a muscle that must work continuously, it requires a constant supply of nutrients and oxygen. The chest pain known as angina can occur when there is an insufficient supply of blood, and consequently of oxygen, to the heart. There are several types of antianginal drugs. These drugs include vasodilators (nitroglycerin, isosorbide dinitrate), calcium channel blockers (diltiazem, nifedipine, verapamil), and beta blockers (acebutolol, atenolol, labetalol, metoprolol, nadolol, pindolol, propranolol, timolol). All of these drugs act by increasing the amount of oxygen that reaches the heart muscle.

Antiarrhythmics

If the heart does not beat rhythmically or smoothly (a condition called arrhythmia), its rate of contraction must be regulated. Antiarrhythmic drugs (disopyramide, mexiletine, procainamide, propranolol, tocainide, quinidine) prevent or alleviate cardiac arrhythmias by altering nerve impulses within the heart.

Antihypertensives

Briefly, high blood pressure is a condition in which the pressure of the blood against the walls of the blood vessels is higher than what is considered normal. High blood pressure, or hypertension, which can eventually cause damage to the brain, eyes, heart, or kidneys, is controllable. If a medication for high blood pressure has been prescribed, it is very important that you continue to take it regularly, even if you don't notice any symptoms of hypertension. If hypertension is controlled, other damage can be prevented. Drugs that counteract or reduce high blood pressure can prolong a hypertensive patient's life.

Several different drug actions produce an antihypertensive effect. Some drugs block nerve impulses that cause arteries to constrict; others slow the heart rate and decrease its force of contraction; still others reduce the amount of a certain hormone (aldosterone) in the blood that causes blood pressure to rise. The effect of any of these is to reduce blood pressure. The mainstay of antihypertensive therapy is often a diuretic, a drug that reduces body fluids. Examples of additional antihypertensive drugs include clonidine, hydralazine, methyldopa, prazosin, and reserpine.

Diuretics

Diuretic drugs, such as chlorothiazide, chlorthalidone, furosemide, hydrochlorothiazide, and spironolactone, promote the loss of water and salt from the body (this is why they are sometimes called "water pills"). This loss of water and salt results in lowering of blood pressure. They also lower blood pressure by increasing the diameter of blood vessels. Because many antihypertensive drugs cause the body to retain salt and water, they are often used concurrently with diuretics. Most diuretics act directly on the kidneys, but there are different types of diuretics, each with different actions. Thus, therapy for high blood pressure can be individualized for each patient's needs.

Thiazide diuretics, such as chlorothiazide, chlorthalidone, and hydrochlorothiazide are the most commonly prescribed water pills available today. They are generally well tolerated and can be taken once or twice a day. Since patients do not develop a tolerance to their antihypertensive effect, they can be taken for prolonged periods. However, a major drawback to thiazide diuretics is that they often deplete the body of potassium. This depletion can be compensated for with a potassium supplement. Potassium-rich foods and liquids, such as bananas, apricots, and orange juice, can also be used to help correct the potassium deficiency. Salt substitutes are another source of potassium. Your doctor will direct you as to which source of potassium, if any, is appropriate for you to use.

Loop diuretics, such as furosemide, act more vigorously than thiazide diuretics. (The term "loop" refers to the structures in the kidneys on which these medications act.) Loop diuretics promote more water loss but also deplete more potassium.

To remove excess water from the body but retain its store of potassium, manufacturers developed potassium-sparing diuretics. Drugs such as spironolactone, triamterene, and amiloride are effective in treating potassium loss, heart failure, and hypertension. Potassium-sparing diuretics are combined with thiazide diuretics in medications such as spironolactone and hydrochlorothiazide combination, triamterene and hydrochlorothiazide combination, and amiloride and hydrochlorothiazide combination. Such combinations enhance the antihypertensive effect and reduce the loss of potassium. They are now among the most commonly used antihypertensive agents.

Cardiac Glycosides

Cardiac glycosides include drugs that are derived from digitalis (for example, digoxin and digitoxin). This type of drug slows the rate of the heart but increases its force of contraction. Cardiac glycosides, therefore, act as both heart depressants and stimulants and may be used to regulate irregular heart rhythm or to increase the volume of blood pumped by the heart in heart failure.

Anticoagulants

Drugs that prevent blood clotting are called anticoagulants (blood thinners). Anticoagulants fall into two categories.

The first category contains only one drug, heparin. Heparin must be given by injection, so its use is generally restricted to hospitalized patients.

The second category includes oral anticoagulants, principally derivatives of the drug warfarin. Warfarin may be used in the treatment of conditions such as stroke, heart disease, and abnormal blood clotting. It is also used to prevent the movement of a clot, which could cause serious problems. It acts by preventing the liver from manufacturing the proteins responsible for blood clot formation.

Persons taking warfarin must avoid using many other drugs (including aspirin), because their interaction with the anticoagulant could cause internal bleeding. Patients taking warfarin should check with their pharmacist or physician before using any other medications, including over-the-counter products for coughs or colds. In addition, they must have their blood checked frequently by their physician to ensure that the drug is maintaining the correct degree of blood thinning.

Antihyperlipidemics

Drugs used to treat atherosclerosis (arteriosclerosis, or hardening of the arteries) act to reduce the serum (the liquified portion of blood) levels of cholesterol and triglycerides (fats), which form plaques (deposits) on the walls of arteries. Some antihyperlipidemics, such as cholestyramine and colestipol, bind to bile acids in the gastrointestinal tract, thereby decreasing the body's production of cholesterol. Clofibrate and probucol also decrease the body's production of cholesterol. Use of such drugs is generally recommended only after diet and lifestyle changes have failed to lower blood lipids to desirable levels. Even then, diet therapy should be continued.

Vasodilators

Vasodilating drugs cause the blood vessels to dilate (widen). Some of the antihypertensive agents, such as hydralazine and prazosin, lower blood pressure by dilating the arteries or veins. Other vasodilators are used in the treatment of stroke and diseases characterized by poor circulation. Ergoloid mesylates, for example, are used to reduce the symptoms of senility by increasing blood flow to the brain.

Beta Blockers

Beta-blocking drugs block the response of the heart and blood vessels to nerve stimulation, thereby slowing the heart rate and reducing high blood pressure. They are used in the treatment of a wide range of diseases including angina, hypertension, migraine headaches, and arrhythmias. Propranolol and metoprolol are two examples of beta blockers.

Calcium Channel Blockers

Calcium channel blockers (diltiazem, nifedipine, verapamil) are used for the prevention of angina (chest pain). Verapamil is also useful in correcting certain arrhythmias (heartbeat irregularities) and lowering blood pressure. This group of drugs is thought to prevent angina and arrhythmias by blocking or slowing calcium flow into muscle cells, which results in vasodilation (widening of the blood vessels) and greater oxygen delivery to the heart muscle.

DRUGS FOR THE EARS

For an ear infection, a physician usually prescribes an antibiotic and a steroid, or a medication that contains a combination of these. The antibiotic attacks the infecting bacteria, and the steroid reduces the inflammation and pain. Often, a local anesthetic, such as benzocaine or lidocaine, may also be prescribed to relieve pain.

DRUGS FOR THE EYES

Almost all drugs that are used to treat eye problems can be used to treat disorders of other parts of the body as well.

Glaucoma is one of the major disorders of the eye, especially in people over 40 years of age, and results in increased pressure within the eyeball. Although glaucoma is sometimes treated surgically, pressure in the eye can usually be reduced, and blindness prevented, through use of eye drops. Two drugs frequently prescribed as eye drops are epinephrine and pilocarpine.

Pilocarpine is a cholinergic drug. Cholinergic drugs act by stimulating parasympathetic nerve endings. Stimulation of these nerve endings alters the activity of many organs throughout the body. For example, a cholinergic drug can cause the heart rate to decrease, intestinal activity to increase, and the bronchioles within the lungs to constrict. When used in the eyes, pilocarpine causes constriction of the pupils and increases the flow of aqueous humor (fluid) out of the eye, thereby reducing the pressure.

Epinephrine is a newer name for the body chemical called adrenaline. Epinephrine is secreted in the body when one must flee from danger, resist attack, or combat stress. Epinephrine has adrenergic properties, such as increasing the amount of sugar in the blood, accelerating the heartbeat, and dilating the pupils. The mechanism by which epinephrine lowers pressure within the eye is not completely understood, but it appears to involve both a decrease in the production of aqueous humor and an increase in the outflow of this fluid from the eye.

Antibiotics are used to treat bacterial eye infections. Steroids can also be used to treat noninfectious eye inflammations, as long as these medications are not used for too long a period of time. Pharmacists carefully monitor requests for eye drop refills, particularly for drops that contain steroids, and may refuse to refill such medication until you have revisited your doctor because these products can cause further eye problems with long-term use.

GASTROINTESTINAL DRUGS

Antinauseants

Antinauseants reduce the urge to vomit. One of the most effective antinauseants is the phenothiazine derivative prochlorperazine. This medication acts on the vomiting center in the brain. It is often administered rectally and usually alleviates nausea and vomiting within a few minutes to an hour. Antihistamines are also commonly used to prevent nausea and vomiting, especially when those symptoms are due to motion sickness. This type of medication may also work at the vomiting center in the brain.

Anticholinergics

Anticholinergic drugs—for example, dicyclomine—slow the action of the bowel and reduce the amount of stomach acid. Because these drugs slow the action of the bowel by relaxing the muscles and relieving spasms, they are said to have an antispasmodic action.

Antiulcer Medications

Antiulcer medications are prescribed to relieve symptoms and promote healing of peptic ulcers. The antisecretory ulcer medications cimetidine, famotidine, and ranitidine work by suppressing the production of excess stomach acid. Another antiulcer drug, sucralfate, works by forming a chemical barrier over an exposed ulcer (like a bandage) thereby protecting the ulcer from stomach acid. These drugs provide sustained relief from ulcer pain and promote healing.

Antidiarrheals

Diarrhea may be caused by many conditions, including influenza and ulcerative colitis, and can sometimes occur as a side effect of drug therapy. Narcotics and anticholinergics slow the action of the bowel and can thereby help alleviate diarrhea. A medication such as diphenoxylate and atropine contains both a narcotic and an anticholinergic.

HORMONES

A hormone is a substance produced and secreted by a gland. Hormones stimulate and regulate body functions. Hormone drugs are given to mimic the effects of naturally produced hormones.

Hormone drugs are prescribed to treat various conditions. Most often, they are used to replace naturally occuring hormones that are not being produced in amounts sufficient to regulate specific body functions. This category of medication also includes oral contraceptives and certain types of drugs that are used to combat inflammatory reactions.

Thyroid Drugs

Thyroid hormone was one of the first hormone drugs to be produced synthetically. Originally, thyroid preparations were made by drying and pulverizing the thyroid glands of animals and then forming them into tablets. Such preparations are still used today in the treatment of patients who have reduced levels of thyroid hormone production. However, a synthetic thyroid hormone (levothyroxine) is also available.

Antidiabetic Drugs

Insulin, which is secreted by the pancreas, regulates the level of glucose (a form of sugar) in the blood, as well as the metabolism of carbohydrates and fats. Insulin's counterpart, glucagon, stimulates the liver to release stored glucose. Both insulin and glucagon must be present in the right amounts to maintain the proper blood sugar levels.

Treatment of diabetes mellitus (the condition in which the body is unable to produce and/or utilize insulin) may involve an adjustment of diet and/or the administration of insulin or oral antidiabetic drugs. Glucagon is given only in emergencies (for example, insulin shock, when blood sugar levels must be raised quickly).

Oral antidiabetic medications induce the pancreas to secrete more insulin by acting on small groups of cells within the pancreas that make and store insulin. Oral antidiabetic medications are prescribed for diabetic patients who are unable to regulate their blood sugar levels through diet modification alone. These medications cannot be used by patients who have insulin-dependent (juvenile-onset, or Type I) diabetes; their blood sugar levels can be controlled only with injections of insulin.

Steroids

The pituitary gland secretes adrenocorticotropic hormone (ACTH), which directs the adrenal glands to produce adrenocorticosteroids (for example, cortisone). Oral steroid preparations (for example, prednisone) may be used to treat inflammatory diseases such as arthritis or to treat poison ivy, hay fever, or insect bites. How these drugs relieve inflammation is currently unknown.

Steroids may also be applied to the skin to treat certain inflammatory skin conditions. Triamcinolone and the combination of fluocinonide, hydrocortisone, and iodochlorhydroxyquin are examples of steroid hormone creams or ointments.

Sex Hormones

Although the adrenal glands secrete small amounts of sex hormones, these hormones are produced mainly by the sex glands. Estrogens are the female hormones responsible for secondary sex characteristics such as development of the breasts and maintenance of the lining of the uterus. Testosterone (androgen) is the corresponding male hormone. It is responsible for secondary sex characteristics such as a beard, a deepened voice, and the maturation of external genitalia. Progesterone is also produced in females—it prepares the uterus for pregnancy.

Testosterone reduces elimination of protein from the body, thereby producing an increase in muscle size. Athletes sometimes take drugs called anabolic steroids (chemicals similar to testosterone) for this effect, but such use of these drugs is dangerous. Anabolic steroids can adversely affect the heart, nervous system, and kidneys.

Most oral contraceptives (birth control pills) combine estrogen and progesterone, but some contain only progesterone. The estrogen in birth control pills prevents egg production. Progesterone aids in preventing ovulation, alters the lining of the uterus, and thickens cervical mucus—processes that help to prevent conception and implantation. Oral contraceptives have many side effects, so their use should be discussed with a physician.

Conjugated estrogens are used as replacement therapy to treat symptoms of menopause in women whose bodies are no longer producing sufficient amounts of estrogen. Medroxypro-gesterone is used to treat uterine bleeding and menstrual problems. It prevents uterine bleeding by inducing and maintaining a lining in the uterus that resembles the lining produced during pregnancy. In addition, it suppresses the release of the pituitary gland hormone that initiates ovulation.

ANTI-INFECTIVES

Antibiotics

Antibiotics are used to treat a wide variety of bacterial infections. They are usually derived from molds or are produced synthetically. Antibiotics inhibit the growth of bacteria by interfering with their production of certain biochemicals necessary to sustain life or by interfering with their ability to use nutrients. The body's defenses then have a much easier time eliminating the infection.

When used properly, antibiotics are usually effective. To adequately treat an infection, antibiotics must be taken regularly for a specific period of time. If you do not take an antibiotic for the prescribed period, microorganisms resistant to the antibiotic are given the opportunity to continue growing, and your infection could recur. Aminoglycosides, cephalosporins, erythromycins, penicillins (including ampicillin and amoxicillin), and tetracyclines are some examples of antibiotics.

Antibiotics do not counteract viruses, such as those causing the common cold, so their use in cold therapy is inappropriate.

Antivirals

Antiviral drugs are used to combat viral infections. An antiviral drug called acyclovir is being used in the management of herpes. Acyclovir reduces the reproduction of the herpes virus in initial outbreaks, lessens the number of recurring outbreaks, and speeds the healing of herpes blisters. However, this antiviral drug does not cure herpes.

Vaccines

Vaccines were used long before antibiotics became available. A vaccine contains weakened or dead disease-causing microorganisms or parts of such organisms, which activate the body's immune system to produce a natural defense against a particular disease (such as polio or measles). A vaccine may be used to alleviate or treat an infectious disease, but most commonly it is used to prevent a specific disease.

Other Anti-infectives

Drugs called anthelmintics are used to treat worm infestations. Fungal infections are treated with antifungals (such as nystatin)—drugs that destroy and prevent the growth of fungi.

A pediculicide is a drug used to treat a person infested with lice, and a scabicide is a preparation used to treat a person with scabies.

ANTINEOPLASTICS

Antineoplastic drugs are used in the treatment of cancer. Most of the drugs in this category prevent the growth of rapidly dividing cells, such as cancer cells. Antineoplastics are, without exception, extremely toxic and can cause serious side effects. But for many cancer victims, the benefits derived from chemotherapy with antineoplastic drugs far outweigh the risks involved.

TOPICAL DRUGS

Drugs are often applied topically (locally to the skin) to treat skin disorders with minimal systemic (throughout the body) side effects. Antibiotic creams or ointments are used to treat skin infections, and adrenocorticosteroids are used to treat inflammatory skin conditions. Another common dermatologic (skin) problem is acne. Acne can be—and often is—treated with over-the-counter drugs, but it sometimes requires prescription medication. Antibiotics such as tetracycline, erythromycin, or clindamycin are used orally or applied topically to slow the growth of the bacteria that play a role in the formation of acne pustules. Keratolytics (agents that soften the skin and cause the outer cells to slough off) are also sometimes prescribed.

Some drugs applied to the skin do have effects within the body. For example, nitroglycerin is absorbed into the bloodstream from ointment or patches placed on the skin. The absorbed nitroglycerin dilates blood vessels and prevents anginal pain. Clonidine, scopolamine, and estrogen are available as transdermal patches, also.

CENTRAL NERVOUS SYSTEM DRUGS

Sedatives

Medications used in the treatment of anxiety or insomnia selectively reduce activity in the central nervous system (brain and spinal cord). Drugs that have a calming effect include barbiturates, chlordiazepoxide, clorazepate, diazepam, doxepin, hydroxyzine, meprobamate, and oxazepam. Drugs to induce sleep in insomniacs include butabarbital, flurazepam, temazepam, and triazolam.

Tranquilizers

Major tranquilizers or antipsychotic agents are usually prescribed for patients with psychoses (certain types of mental disorders). These drugs calm certain areas of the brain but permit the rest of the brain to function normally. They act as a screen that allows transmission of some nerve impulses but restricts others. The drugs most frequently used are phenothiazines, such as chlorpromazine and thioridazine. Haloperidol, a butyrophenone, has the same effect as chlorpromazine.

Antidepressants

Tricyclic antidepressants (such as amitriptyline), tetracyclic antidepressants (such as maprotiline), and monoamine oxidase (MAO) inhibitors (such as phenelzine) are used to combat depression. Antidepressants are also used in the preventive treatment of migraine headaches, although the manner in which they help these headaches is not clearly understood.

Antidepressants may produce serious side effects, and they can interact with other drugs. MAO inhibitors can also interact with certain foods, resulting in dangerous increases in blood pressure. Therefore, they should be used very carefully.

Amphetamines

Amphetamines or adrenergic drugs are commonly used as anorectics (drugs used to reduce the appetite). These drugs temporarily quiet the part of the brain that causes hunger, but they also keep a person awake, speed up the heart, and raise blood pressure. After two to three weeks, these medications begin to lose their effectiveness as appetite suppressants.

Amphetamines stimulate most people, but they have the opposite effect on hyperkinetic children. Hyperkinesis (the condition of being highly overactive) is difficult to diagnose or define and requires a specialist to treat. When hyperkinetic children take amphetamines or the adrenergic drug methylphenidate, their activity slows down. Most likely, amphetamines quiet these youngsters by selectively stimulating parts of the brain that ordinarily provide control of activity.

Anticonvulsants

Drugs such as phenytoin and phenobarbital are used to control seizures and other symptoms of epilepsy. They selectively reduce excessive stimulation in the brain.

Antiparkinsonism Agents

Parkinson's disease is a progressive disorder that is due to a chemical imbalance in the brain. Victims of Parkinson's disease have uncontrollable tremors, develop a characteristic stoop, and eventually become unable to walk. Drugs such as benztropine, trihexyphenidyl, levodopa, and bromocriptine are used to correct the chemical imbalance, thereby relieving the symptoms of the disease. Benztropine and trihexyphenidyl are also used to relieve tremors caused by other medications.

Analgesics

Pain is not a disease but a symptom. Drugs used to relieve pain are called analgesics. These drugs form a rather diverse group. We do not fully understand how most analgesics work. Whether they all act on the brain is not known. Analgesics fall into two categories; they may be either narcotic or nonnarcotic.

Narcotics are derived from the opium poppy. They act on the brain to cause deep analgesia and often drowsiness. Some narcotics relieve coughing spasms and are used in many cough syrups. Narcotics relieve pain and give the patient a feeling of well-being. They are also addictive. Manufacturers have attempted to produce nonaddictive synthetic narcotic derivatives but have not yet been successful.

Many nonnarcotic pain relievers are commonly used. Salicylates are the most commonly used pain relievers in the United States today. The most widely used salicylate is aspirin. While aspirin ordinarily does not require a prescription, many doctors may prescribe it to treat such diseases as arthritis.

The aspirin substitute acetaminophen may be used in place of aspirin to relieve pain. It does not, however, reduce inflammation (such as that caused by arthritis).

A number of analgesics contain codeine or other narcotics combined with nonnarcotic analgesics (such as aspirin or acetaminophen). These analgesics are not as potent as pure narcotics but are frequently as effective.

Because these medications contain narcotics, they have potential for abuse and must be used with caution.

Anti-inflammatory Drugs

Inflammation is the body's response to injury. It causes swelling, pain, fever, redness, and itching. Aspirin is one of the most effective anti-inflammatory drugs. Other drugs, called nonsteroidal anti-inflammatory drugs (for example, fenoprofen, ibuprofen, indomethacin, naproxen, and tolmetin), relieve inflammation and may be more effective than aspirin in certain individuals. Steroids are also used to treat inflammatory diseases.

When sore muscles tense, they cause pain, inflammation, and spasm. Skeletal muscle relaxants (for example, orphenadrine, aspirin, and caffeine combination; meprobamate and aspirin combination; and chlorzoxazone and acetaminophen combination) can relieve these symptoms. Skeletal muscle relaxants are often given in combination with an anti-inflammatory drug such as aspirin. Some doctors, however, believe that aspirin and rest are better for alleviating the pain and inflammation of muscle strain than are skeletal muscle relaxants.

RESPIRATORY DRUGS

Antitussives

Antitussives control coughs. There are numerous over-the-counter (nonprescription) antitussives available—most of them contain dextromethorphan. Codeine is a narcotic antitussive that is an ingredient in many prescription cough medications. These cough syrups must be absorbed into the blood and must circulate and act on the brain before they relieve a cough.

Expectorants

Expectorants are used to change a nonproductive cough to a productive one (one that brings up phlegm). Expectorants are supposed to increase the amount of mucus produced. However, drinking water or using a vaporizer or humidifier is probably more effective in increasing mucus production. Popular expectorant ingredients include ammonium chloride, guaifenesin, potassium guaiacolsulfonate, and terpin hydrate.

Decongestants

Decongestants constrict blood vessels in the nose and sinuses to open up air passages. They are available as oral preparations, nose drops, and nose sprays. Oral decongestants are slow-acting but do not interfere with production of mucus or movement of the cilia (special hairlike structures) of the respiratory tract. They can, however, increase blood pressure, so they should be used cautiously by patients with high blood pressure. Topical decongestants (nose drops or spray) provide almost immediate relief. They do not increase blood pressure as much as oral decongestants, but they do slow the movement of the cilia.

People who use these products may also develop a tolerance for them. Tolerance can be described as a need for ever-increasing dosages to achieve a beneficial effect. The additional disadvantage of developing tolerance is that the risk of side effects increases as the dosage increases. Topical decongestants should not be used for more than a few days at a time.

Bronchodilators

Bronchodilators (agents that open airways in the lungs) and agents that relax smooth-muscle tissue (such as that found in the lungs) are used to improve breathing. Theophylline and aminophylline are oral bronchodilators commonly used to relieve the symptoms of asthma and pulmonary emphysema. Albuterol and metaproterenol are inhalant bronchodilators, which act directly on the muscles of the bronchi (breathing tubes).

Antihistamines

Histamine is a body chemical that, when released in the body, typically causes swelling and itching. Antihistamines counteract these symptoms of allergy by blocking the effects of histamine. For mild respiratory allergies, such as hay fever, antihistamines can be used. Diphenhydramine and other antihistamines are relatively slow-acting. Severe allergic reactions sometimes require the use of epinephrine (which is not an antihistamine); in its injectable form, it is very fast-acting.

Some types of antihistamines are also used to prevent or treat the symptoms of motion sickness. Diphenhydramine and meclizine are examples of drugs used specifically for this purpose.

VITAMINS AND MINERALS

Vitamins and minerals are chemical substances that are vital to the maintenance of normal body function. Most people obtain enough vitamins and minerals in their diet, but some people have vitamin deficiencies. Serious nutritional deficiencies lead to diseases such as pellagra and beriberi, which must be treated by a physician. People who have an inadequate or restricted diet, people who have certain disorders or debilitating illnesses, and women who are pregnant or breast-feeding are among those who may benefit from taking supplemental vitamins and minerals. However, even these people should consult a doctor to see if a true vitamin deficiency exists.

Drug Profiles

On the following pages are drug profiles for the most commonly prescribed drugs, as well as a few selected over-the-counter medications. These profiles are arranged alphabetically according to the generic name.

A drug profile summarizes the most important information about a particular drug. By studying a drug profile, you will learn what to expect from your medication, when to be concerned about possible side effects, which drugs interact with the drug you are taking, and how to take the drug to achieve its maximum benefit. Each profile includes the following information:

generic name

The drugs profiled in this book are listed by generic names. You should know both the generic and the trade names of ALL of the medications you are taking. If you don't know the contents of your medication, check with your pharmacist.

BRAND NAMES (Manufacturers)
The most common trade names of each generic product are listed, along with the manufacturers' names. Not every available trade name is included, but as many as possible have been listed. "Various manufacturers" is listed for some of the generic names—this indicates that there are generic products available.

TYPE OF DRUG
The chemical or pharmacologic class or pharmacological effect is listed for each generic drug.

INGREDIENTS
The components of each drug product are itemized. Many drugs contain several active chemical components; all are included under this category.

DOSAGE FORMS
The most common forms (for example, tablets, capsules, liquid, suppositories) of each profiled drug are listed, as well as the drug's alcohol content, if any. Strengths or concentrations are also provided.

STORAGE
Storage requirements for each of the dosage forms listed are discussed. These directions should be followed carefully, in order to ensure the potency of your medications.

USES
It is important that you understand why you are taking each of your medications. This section includes the most important and most common clinical uses for each drug profiled. Your doctor may prescribe a drug for a reason that does not appear on this list. The exclusion does not

mean that your doctor has made an error. However, if the use for which you are taking a drug does not appear in this category and if you have any questions about why the drug was prescribed, consult your doctor. A description of how the drug is thought to work is also provided in this section.

TREATMENT
Instructions are provided on how to take each profiled medication in order to obtain its maximum benefit. Information can be found on whether the drug can be taken with food; how to apply the ointment, cream, ear drops, or eye drops; how to insert suppositories; and recommendations for what to do if you miss a dose of your medication.

SIDE EFFECTS
Minor. The most common and least serious reactions to a drug are listed in this section. Most of these side effects, if they occur, disappear in a day or two. Do not expect to experience these side effects; but if they occur and are particularly annoying, do not hesitate to seek medical advice.

Suggestions for preventing or relieving some of these side effects are also provided.

Major. Major side effects are less common than minor side effects, and you will probably never experience them. However, should any of the reactions listed in this section occur, you should call your doctor. These reactions indicate that something may be going wrong with your drug therapy. You may have developed an allergy to the drug, or some other problem could have occurred. If you experience a major side effect, it may be necessary to adjust your dosage or to substitute a different medication in your treatment. It is important to discuss this with your doctor.

New side effects are being reported daily. If you experience a reaction that is bothersome or severe, consult your doctor immediately, even if the side effect is not listed.

INTERACTIONS
This section lists the medications (both prescription and over-the-counter drugs) and foods that can interact with the profiled drug. Certain drugs are safe when used alone but may cause serious reactions when taken in combination with other drugs or chemicals or with certain foods. A description of how the profiled drug interacts with other drugs or foods and what to expect if the two are taken together is also provided. Not all possible drug combinations have been tested. It is, therefore, important that your pharmacist and health care providers be aware of ALL the drugs you are taking (both prescription and over-the-counter).

WARNINGS
This section lists the precautions necessary for safe use of the profiled drug. It provides information on drugs that should be avoided if you have had a previous allergic reaction or severe drug reaction, as well as information on the conditions or disease states that require close monitoring while this drug is being taken.

In this section you will find out whether the profiled drug is likely to affect your driving ability, whether you are likely to become tolerant to its effects, if it is dangerous to stop taking the drug abruptly, and if you should discuss with your doctor stopping the drug before having surgery or any other medical or dental procedure.

Certain individuals are allergic to the color additive FD&C Yellow No. 5 (tartrazine). This section provides information on the tartrazine content of the various dosage forms.

Other information included in this category might concern supplemental therapy—for example, drinking extra fluids while treating a urinary tract infection or wearing cotton panties while treating a vaginal infection.

A discussion of the known risks of treatment with this drug during pregnancy or while breast-feeding an infant is provided. It should be kept in mind that for the majority of drugs available, the risks to a fetus or nursing infant are not known. Experiments are not usually conducted on pregnant women and infants (for ethical reasons). You should, therefore dis-cuss the risks and benefits of any particular drug therapy with your doctor if you are pregnant, are planning to become pregnant, or are nursing an infant.

Accurbron—see theophylline

Accutane—see isotretinoin

acebutolol

BRAND NAME (Manufacturer)
Sectral (Wyeth-Ayerst)
TYPE OF DRUG
Beta-adrenergic blocking agent
INGREDIENT
acebutolol
DOSAGE FORM
Capsules (200 mg and 400 mg)
STORAGE
Acebutolol should be stored at room temperature in a tightly closed container.

USES
Acebutolol is used to treat high blood pressure or irregular heartbeat. Acebutolol belongs to a group of medicines known as beta-adrenergic blocking agents or, more commonly, beta blockers. These drugs work by controlling impulses along certain nerve pathways, thereby decreasing the workload on the heart and helping to regulate the heartbeat.

TREATMENT
Acebutolol can be taken either on an empty stomach or with food or milk (as directed by your doctor). In order to become accustomed to taking this medication, try to take it at the same time(s) each day.

If you miss a dose of this medication, take the missed dose as soon as possible, unless it is almost time for your next dose. In that case, do not take the missed dose at all; just wait until the next scheduled dose. Do not double the next dose of the medication.

It is important to remember that acebutolol does not cure high blood pressure, but it will help to control the condition as long as you continue to take it.

SIDE EFFECTS
Minor. Abdominal pain, anxiety, constipation, diarrhea, dizziness, dry eyes, fatigue, gas, headache, heartburn, nausea, runny nose, sleeping problems, or vomiting. These side effects should disappear as your body adjusts to the drug.

If you are extra-sensitive to the cold, be sure to dress warmly during cold weather.

Plain, nonmedicated eye drops (artificial tears) may help to relieve eye dryness.

To relieve constipation, increase the amount of fiber in your diet (bran, fresh fruits and vegetables, salads, and whole-grain breads) unless your doctor directs you to do otherwise.

If you feel dizzy, sit or lie down for a while; get up slowly from a sitting or reclining position, and be careful on stairs.

Major. Tell your doctor about any side effects that are persistent or particularly bothersome. IT IS ESPECIALLY IMPORTANT TO TELL YOUR DOCTOR about chest pain; cold fingers or feet (due to decreased blood circulation to skin, fingers, and toes); confusion; cough; depression; fluid accumulation; hair loss; impotence; itching; muscle, joint or back pain; numbness; rash; shortness of breath; sore throat; swelling of the feet; unusual bleeding or bruising; urination problems; visual disturbances or eye pain; or wheezing.

INTERACTIONS
Acebutolol may interact with other types of medications:
1. Indomethacin, other nonsteroidal anti-inflammatory agents, aspirin, or other salicylates may decrease the blood-pressure-lowering effects of beta blockers.
2. Concurrent use of beta blockers and calcium channel blockers (diltiazem, nifedipine, and verapamil) or disopyramide can lead to heart failure or very low blood pressure.
3. Side effects may also be increased if beta blockers are taken with digoxin, epinephrine, phenylephrine, phenylpropanolamine, phenothiazine tranquilizers, reserpine, clonidine, prazosin, or monoamine oxidase (MAO) inhibitors. At least 14 days should separate the use of a beta blocker and the use of an MAO inhibitor.
4. Beta blockers may antagonize (work against) the effects of theophylline, aminophylline, albuterol, isoproterenol, metaproterenol, and terbutaline.
5. Beta blockers can also interact with insulin or oral antidiabetic agents—raising or lowering blood sugar levels or masking the symptoms of low blood sugar.
6. The action of beta blockers may be increased if they are used with chlorpromazine, cimetidine, furosemide, hydralazine, or oral contraceptives (birth control pills), which could have a negative effect.
7. Alcohol, barbiturates, and rifampin can decrease blood concentrations of this drug, which can result in a decrease of effectiveness.

Before starting acebutolol, BE SURE TO TELL YOUR DOCTOR about any medications you are already taking, especially any of the medications listed above.

WARNINGS

• Before starting this medication, it is important to tell your doctor about any unusual or allergic reactions you have had to any medications, especially to acebutolol or any other beta blocker (atenolol, betaxolol, carteolol, esmolol, labetalol, metoprolol, nadolol, penbutolol, pindolol, propranolol, timolol).
• Tell your doctor if you now have or if you have ever had asthma, bronchitis, diabetes mellitus, heart block, heart failure, kidney disease, liver disease, peripheral vascular disease (poor circulation in the fingers or toes), severe bradycardia (slowed heart rate), or thyroid disease.
• You may want to check your pulse while taking this medication. If your pulse is much slower than your usual rate (or if it is less than 50 beats per minute), check with your doctor. A pulse rate that is too slow may cause circulation problems.
• This medicine may affect your body's response to exercise. Ask your doctor what an appropriate amount of exercise would be for you, taking into account your medical condition.
• It is important that you do not stop taking this medicine without first checking with your doctor. Some conditions may become worse when the medicine is stopped suddenly, and the danger of a heart attack is increased in some patients. Your doctor may want you to gradually reduce the amount of medicine you take before stopping completely. Make sure that you have enough medicine on hand to last through vacations, holidays, and weekends.
• Before having surgery or any other medical or dental treatment, tell your physician or dentist that you are taking this medicine. Often, this medication will be discontinued 48 hours prior to any major surgery.
• While taking this medicine, do not use any over-the-counter allergy, asthma, cough, cold, sinus, or diet preparation without first checking with your pharmacist or doctor. The combination of these drugs with a beta blocker can result in high blood pressure.
• Be sure to tell your doctor if you are pregnant. Although acebutolol appears to be safe in animals, studies in pregnant women have not been conducted. Also, tell your doctor if you are breast-feeding an infant. Small amounts of acebutolol may pass into human breast milk.

acetaminophen and codeine combination

BRAND NAMES (Manufacturers)
acetaminophen with codeine (various manufacturers)
Aceta with Codeine (Century)
Capital with Codeine (Carnrick)
Phenaphen-650 with Codeine (Robins)
Phenaphen with Codeine (Robins)
Tylenol with Codeine (McNeil)
Ty-tabs (Major)

TYPE OF DRUG
Analgesic combination
INGREDIENTS
acetaminophen and codeine
DOSAGE FORMS
Tablets (300 mg acetaminophen with 7.5 mg, 15 mg, 30 mg, or 60 mg codeine; 325 mg acetaminophen with 30 mg or 60 mg codeine; 650 mg acetaminophen with 30 mg codeine)
Capsules (325 mg acetaminophen with 15 mg, 30 mg, or 60 mg codeine)
Oral elixir (120 mg acetaminophen and 12 mg codeine per 5-ml spoonful, with 7% alcohol)
On the label of the vial of tablets or capsules, the name of this drug is followed by a number that refers to the amount of codeine present (#1 has 7.5 mg codeine, #2 has 15 mg codeine, #3 has 30 mg codeine, and #4 has 60 mg codeine).
STORAGE
This medication should be stored at room temperature. It should never be frozen.

USES
Acetaminophen and codeine combination is used to relieve mild to severe pain (formulations of this medication with higher codeine contents are used to relieve more severe pain). Codeine is a narcotic analgesic that acts upon on the central nervous system (brain and spinal cord) to relieve pain.

TREATMENT
In order to avoid stomach upset, you can take this medication with food or milk.

This medication works most effectively if you take it at the onset of pain, rather than waiting until the pain becomes intense.

Measure the dose of the liquid form of this medication carefully with a specially designed 5-ml measuring spoon. An ordinary kitchen teaspoon is not accurate enough for measuring the dosage.

If you are taking this medication on a regular schedule and you miss a dose, take the missed dose as soon as possible, unless it is almost time for the next dose. In that case, don't take the missed dose at all; just return to your regular dosing schedule. Do not double the next dose.

SIDE EFFECTS
Minor. Constipation, dizziness, drowsiness, dry mouth, false sense of well-being, flushing, light-headedness, loss of appetite, nausea, painful or difficult urination, or sweating. These side effects should disappear as your body adjusts to the medication.

If you are constipated, increase the amount of fiber in your diet (fresh fruits and vegetables, salads, bran, and whole-grain breads), exercise, and drink more water (unless your doctor directs you to do otherwise).

To reduce mouth dryness, chew sugarless gum or suck on ice chips or hard candy.

If you feel dizzy or light-headed, sit or lie down for a while; get up slowly from a sitting or reclining position, and be careful on stairs.

Major. Tell your doctor about any side effects that are persistent or particularly bothersome. IT IS ESPECIALLY IMPORTANT TO TELL YOUR DOCTOR about anxiety, difficulty in breathing, excitation, fatigue, palpitations, rash, restlessness, sore throat and fever, tremors, unusual bleeding or bruising, weakness, or yellowing of the eyes or skin.

INTERACTIONS

This medication interacts with several other types of drugs:

1. Concurrent use with other central nervous system depressants (such as alcohol, antihistamines, barbiturates, benzodiazepine tranquilizers, muscle relaxants, and phenothi-azine tranquilizers) or with tricyclic antidepressants can cause extreme drowsiness.

2. A monoamine oxidase (MAO) inhibitor taken within 14 days of this medication can lead to unpredictable and severe side effects.

3. Long-term use and high doses of the acetaminophen portion of this medication can increase the effects of oral anticoagulants (blood thinners, such as warfarin); this combination may lead to bleeding complications.

4. Anticonvulsants (antiseizure medications), barbiturates, and alcohol can increase the liver toxicity caused by large doses of the acetaminophen portion of this medication.

BE SURE TO TELL YOUR DOCTOR about any medications you are currently taking, especially any listed above.

WARNINGS

• Tell your doctor about unusual or allergic reactions you have had to any medications, especially to acetaminophen, codeine, or other narcotic analgesics (such as hydrocodone, hydromorphone, meperidine, methadone, morphine, oxycodone, and propoxyphene).

• Tell your doctor if you now have or if you have ever had an acute abdominal condition, asthma, a blood disorder, brain disease, colitis, epilepsy, gallstones or gallbladder disease, head injuries, heart disease, kidney disease, liver disease, lung disease, mental illness, prostate disease, thyroid disease, or urethral strictures.

• If this drug makes you dizzy or drowsy, do not take part in any activity that requires alertness, such as driving a car or operating potentially dangerous equipment.

• Before having surgery or any other medical or dental treatment, be sure to tell your doctor or dentist that you are taking this medication.

• Because this product contains codeine, it has the potential for abuse and must be used with caution. Usually, it should not be taken on a regular schedule for longer than ten days at a time. Tolerance develops quickly; do not increase the dosage or stop taking the drug abruptly unless you first consult your doctor. If you have been taking large amounts of this medication for long periods, you may experience a withdrawal reaction (diarrhea, excessive yawning, gooseflesh, irritability, muscle aches, nausea, runny nose, shivering, sleep disorders, stomach cramps, sweating, trembling, vomiting, or weakness). Your doctor may, therefore, want to reduce the dosage gradually.

• Because this product contains acetaminophen, additional drugs that contain acetaminophen should not be taken without your doctor's approval. Be sure to check the labels on over-the-counter pain, sinus, allergy, asthma, diet, cough, and cold products before you use them in order to see if they contain acetaminophen.

• Be sure to tell your doctor if you are pregnant. The effects of this medication during pregnancy have not been thoroughly studied in humans. Codeine used regularly in large doses during pregnancy can result in addiction of the fetus, leading to withdrawal symptoms (diarrhea, excessive crying, excessive yawning, irritability, fever, sneezing, tremors, or vomiting) at birth. Also, tell your doctor if you are breast-feeding an infant. Small amounts of this drug may pass into breast milk and cause drowsiness in the nursing infant.

acetaminophen and hydrocodone combination

BRAND NAMES (Manufacturers)

Amacodone (Trimen)
Bancap HC (Forest)
Co-Gesic (Central)
Damacet-P (Mason)
Dolacet (Hauck)
Duradyne DHC (Forest)
Hydrogesic (Edwards)
Hy-Phen (Ascher)
Lortab 5 (Russ)*
T-Gesic (T.E. Williams)
Vicodin (Knoll)
Zydone (DuPont)
*Available in different strengths

TYPE OF DRUG

Analgesic combination

INGREDIENTS

acetaminophen and hydrocodone

DOSAGE FORMS

Tablets (500 mg acetaminophen with 2.5 mg, 5 mg, or 7.5 mg hydrocodone; 650 mg acetaminophen with 7.5 mg hydrocodone; 750 mg acetaminophen with 7.5 mg hydrocodone)

Capsules (500 mg acetaminophen with 5 mg hydrocodone)

Liquid (120 mg acetaminophen with 2.5 mg hydrocodone per 5-ml spoonful, with 7% alcohol)

STORAGE

Acetaminophen and hydrocodone combination tablets, capsules, and liquid should be stored at room temperature in tightly closed, light-resistant containers.

USES

This medication is used to relieve moderate to severe pain. Hydrocodone is a narcotic analgesic that acts on the central nervous system (brain and spinal cord) to relieve pain.

TREATMENT

To avoid stomach upset, take this drug with food or milk.

Each dose of the oral liquid form of this medication should be measured carefully with a specially designed 5-

ml measuring spoon, not with an ordinary kitchen tea-spoon.

This medication works most effectively if you take it at the onset of pain, rather than waiting until it becomes intense.

If you are taking this medication on a regular schedule and you miss a dose, take the missed dose as soon as possible, unless it is almost time for your next dose. In that case, don't take the missed dose at all; just return to your regular dosing schedule. Do not double the next dose.

SIDE EFFECTS

Minor. Constipation, dizziness, dry mouth, false sense of well-being, flushing, light-headedness, loss of appetite, nausea, painful or difficult urination, or sweating. These side effects should disappear as your body adjusts to the medication.

If you are constipated, increase the amount of fiber in your diet (fresh fruits and vegetables, salads, bran, and whole-grain breads), exercise, and drink more water (unless your doctor directs you to do otherwise).

To reduce mouth dryness, chew sugarless gum or suck on ice chips or hard candy.

If you feel dizzy, sit or lie down for a while; get up from a sitting or reclining position slowly, and be careful on stairs.

Major. Tell your doctor about any side effects that are persistent or particularly bothersome. IT IS ESPECIALLY IMPORTANT TO TELL YOUR DOCTOR about anxiety, difficulty in breathing, excitation, fatigue, palpitations, rash, restlessness, sore throat and fever, tremors, unusual bleeding or bruising, weakness, or yellowing of the eyes or skin.

INTERACTIONS

This medication interacts with several other types of drugs:
1. Concurrent use of this medication with other central nervous system depressants (such as alcohol, antihistamines, barbiturates, benzodiazepine tranquilizers, muscle relaxants, and phenothiazine tranquilizers) or with tricyclic antidepressants can cause extreme drowsiness.
2. A monoamine oxidase (MAO) inhibitor taken within 14 days of this drug can lead to severe side effects.
3. Long-term use and high doses of the acetaminophen portion of this medication can increase the effects of oral anticoagulants (blood thinners, such as warfarin); this combination may lead to bleeding complications.
4. Anticonvulsants (antiseizure medications), barbiturates, and alcohol can increase the liver toxicity caused by large doses of the acetaminophen portion of this medication.

TELL YOUR DOCTOR about any medications you are currently taking, especially any of those listed above.

WARNINGS

• Tell your doctor about unusual or allergic reactions you have had to any medications, especially to acetaminophen, hydrocodone, or other narcotic analgesics (such as codeine, hydromorphone, meperidine, methadone, morphine, oxycodone, and propoxyphene).
• Tell your doctor if you now have or if you have ever had acute abdominal conditions, asthma, blood disor-

ders, brain disease, colitis, epilepsy, gallstones or gallbladder disease, a head injury, heart disease, kidney disease, liver disease, lung disease, mental illness, prostate disease, thyroid disease, or urethral strictures.
• If this drug makes you dizzy or drowsy, do not take part in any activity that requires you to remain alert, such as driving an automobile or operating potentially dangerous equipment.
• Before having surgery or any other medical or dental treatment, be sure to tell your doctor or dentist that you are taking this medication.
• Because this product contains hydrocodone, it has the potential for abuse and must be used with caution. Usually, it should not be taken on a regular schedule for longer than ten days at a time. Tolerance develops quickly; do not increase the dosage or stop taking the drug abruptly unless you first consult your doctor. If you have been taking large amounts of this medication for long periods, you may experience a withdrawal reaction (diarrhea, excessive yawning, gooseflesh, irritability, muscle aches, nausea, runny nose, shivering, sleep disorders, stomach cramps, sweating, trembling, vomiting, or weakness). Your doctor may, therefore, want to reduce the dosage gradually.
• Because this product contains acetaminophen, additional medications that contain acetaminophen should not be taken without your doctor's approval. Check the labels on over-the-counter (nonprescription) pain, sinus, allergy, asthma, diet, cough, and cold products to see if they contain acetaminophen.
• Be sure to tell your doctor if you are pregnant. The effects of this medication during pregnancy have not been thoroughly studied in humans. Regular use of hydrocodone in large doses during pregnancy can result in addiction of the fetus, leading to withdrawal symptoms (diarrhea, excessive crying, excessive yawning, fever, irritability, sneezing, tremors, or vomiting) at birth. Also, tell your doctor if you are breast-feeding an infant. Small amounts of this medication may pass into breast milk and cause excessive drowsiness in the nursing infant.

acetaminophen and oxycodone combination

BRAND NAMES (Manufacturers)
oxycodone hydrochloride with acetaminophen
   (various manufacturers)
Percocet (DuPont)
Tylox (McNeil-CPC)
TYPE OF DRUG
Analgesic combination
INGREDIENTS
acetaminophen and oxycodone
DOSAGE FORM
Tablets (325 mg acetaminophen with 5 mg oxycodone;
   500 mg acetaminophen with 5 mg oxycodone)
STORAGE
Acetaminophen and oxycodone tablets should be stored at room temperature in a tightly closed container.

USES

Acetaminophen and oxycodone combination is used to relieve moderate to severe pain. Oxycodone is a narcotic analgesic that acts on the central nervous system (brain and spinal cord) to relieve pain.

TREATMENT

In order to avoid stomach upset, you can take this medication with food or milk.

This medication works most effectively if you take it at the onset of pain, rather than waiting until the pain becomes intense.

If you are taking this medication on a regular schedule and you miss a dose, take the missed dose as soon as possible, unless it is almost time for your next dose. In that case, don't take the missed dose at all; just return to your regular dosing schedule. Do not double the next dose.

SIDE EFFECTS

Minor. Constipation, dizziness, drowsiness, dry mouth, false sense of well-being, flushing, light-headedness, loss of appetite, nausea, painful or difficult urination, or sweating. These side effects should disappear as your body adjusts to the medication.

If you are constipated, increase the amount of fiber in your diet (fresh fruits and vegetables, salads, bran, and whole-grain breads), exercise, and drink more water (unless your doctor directs you to do otherwise).

To reduce mouth dryness, chew sugarless gum or suck on ice chips or hard candy.

If you feel dizzy or light-headed, sit or lie down for a while; get up from a sitting or reclining position slowly, and be careful on stairs.

Major. Tell your doctor about any side effects that are persistent or particularly bothersome. IT IS ESPECIALLY IMPORTANT TO TELL YOUR DOCTOR about anxiety, difficulty in breathing, excitation, fatigue, palpitations, rash, restlessness, sore throat and fever, tremors, unusual bleeding or bruising, weakness, or yellowing of the eyes or skin.

INTERACTIONS

This medication interacts with several other types of drugs:
1. Concurrent use of this medication with other central nervous system depressants (such as alcohol, antihistamines, barbiturates, benzodiazepine tranquilizers, muscle relaxants, and phenothiazine tranquilizers) or with tricyclic antidepressants can cause extreme drowsiness.
2. A monoamine oxidase (MAO) inhibitor taken within 14 days of this medication can lead to unpredictable and severe side effects.
3. Long-term use and high doses of the acetaminophen portion of this medication can increase the effects of oral anticoagulants (blood thinners, such as warfarin); this combination may lead to bleeding complications.
4. Anticonvulsants (antiseizure medications), barbiturates, and alcohol can increase the liver toxicity caused by large doses of the acetaminophen portion of this medication.

BE SURE TO TELL YOUR DOCTOR about any medications you are currently taking, especially any listed above.

WARNINGS

• Tell your doctor about unusual or allergic reactions you have had to any medications, especially to acetaminophen, oxycodone, or other narcotic analgesics (such as codeine, hydrocodone, hydromorphone, meperidine, methadone, morphine, and propoxyphene).
• Tell your doctor if you now have or if you have ever had an acute abdominal condition, asthma, blood disorders, brain disease, colitis, epilepsy, gallstones or gallbladder disease, head injuries, heart disease, kidney disease, liver disease, lung disease, mental illness, prostate disease, thyroid disease, or urethral strictures.
• If this drug makes you dizzy or drowsy, do not take part in any activity that requires alertness, such as driving a car or operating potentially dangerous equipment.
• Before having surgery or any other medical or dental treatment, be sure to tell your doctor or dentist that you are taking this medication.
• Because this product contains oxycodone, it has the potential for abuse and must be used with caution. Usually, it should not be taken on a regular schedule for longer than ten days at a time. Tolerance develops quickly; do not increase the dosage or stop taking the drug abruptly unless you first consult your doctor. If you have been taking large amounts of this medication for long periods, you may experience a withdrawal reaction (muscle aches, diarrhea, gooseflesh, runny nose, nausea, vomiting, shivering, trembling, stomach cramps, sleep disorders, irritability, weakness, excessive yawning, or sweating). Your doctor may, therefore, want to reduce the dosage gradually.
• Because this product contains acetaminophen, additional medications that contain acetaminophen should not be taken without your doctor's approval. Check the labels on over-the-counter (nonprescription) pain, sinus, allergy, asthma, diet, cough, and cold products to see if they contain acetaminophen.
• Be sure to tell your doctor if you are pregnant. The effects of this medication during pregnancy have not been thoroughly studied in humans. Oxycodone, used regularly in large doses during pregnancy, can result in addiction of the fetus, leading to withdrawal symptoms (irritability, excessive crying, tremors, fever, vomiting, diarrhea, sneezing, or excessive yawning) at birth. Also, tell your doctor if you are breast-feeding an infant. Small amounts of this medication may pass into breast milk and cause excessive drowsiness in the nursing infant.

acetaminophen and propoxyphene combination

BRAND NAMES (Manufacturers)
Darvocet-N 50 (Lilly)
Darvocet-N 100 (Lilly)
Dolene AP-65 (Lederle)
Genagesic (Goldline)
Propacet 100 (Lemmon)
propoxyphene hydrochloride with acetaminophen
  (various manufacturers)

propoxyphene napsylate with acetaminophen (various manufacturers)
Wygesic (Wyeth)

TYPE OF DRUG
Analgesic combination

INGREDIENTS
acetaminophen and propoxyphene

DOSAGE FORMS
Tablets (325 mg acetaminophen with 50 mg propoxyphene napsylate; 650 mg acetaminophen with 100 mg propoxyphene napsylate; 650 mg acetaminophen with 6 mg propoxyphene hydrochloride)
Capsules (650 mg acetaminophen with 65 mg propoxyphene hydrochloride)

STORAGE
Acetaminophen and propoxyphene combination tablets and capsules should be stored at room temperature in tightly closed containers.

USES
This medication is used to relieve moderate to severe pain. Propoxyphene is a narcotic analgesic that acts on the central nervous system (brain and spinal cord) to relieve pain.

TREATMENT
In order to avoid stomach upset, you can take this medication with food or milk.

This medication works best if you take it at the onset of pain, rather than waiting until the pain becomes intense.

If you are taking this acetaminophen and propoxyphene combination on a regular schedule and you miss a dose, take the missed dose as soon as possible, unless you are nearing the time for the next dose. In that case, do not take the missed dose at all; just return to your regular dosing schedule. It is importsnt that you do not double the next dose.

SIDE EFFECTS
Minor. Constipation, dizziness, drowsiness, dry mouth, false sense of well-being, flushing, light-headedness, loss of appetite, nausea, painful or difficult urination, or sweating. These side effects should disappear as your body adjusts to the drug.

If you are constipated, increase the amount of fiber in your diet (fresh fruits and vegetables, salads, bran, and whole-grain breads), exercise, and drink more water (unless your doctor directs you to do otherwise).

To reduce excessive mouth dryness, you may want to chew sugarless gum or you may want to suck on ice chips or hard candy.

If you feel dizzy or light-headed, sit or lie down for a while; get up from a sitting or lying position slowly, and be careful on stairs.

Major. Tell your doctor about any side effects that are persistent or particularly bothersome. IT IS ESPECIALLY IMPORTANT TO TELL YOUR DOCTOR about anxiety, difficulty in breathing, excitation, fatigue, palpitations, rash, restlessness, sore throat and fever, tremors, unusual bleeding or bruising, weakness, or yellowing of the eyes or skin.

INTERACTIONS
This medication interacts with several other types of drugs:

1. Concurrent use of acetaminophen and propoxyphene combination with other central nervous system depressants (such as alcohol, antihistamines, barbiturates, benzodiazepine tranquilizers, muscle relaxants, and phenothiazine tranquilizers) or with tricyclic antidepressants can possibly cause extreme drowsiness.

2. A monoamine oxidase (MAO) inhibitor taken within 14 days of this medication can lead to unpredictable and severe side effects.

3. Long-term use and high doses of acetaminophen can increase the effects of oral anticoagulants (blood thinners, such as warfarin), which may lead to bleeding complications.

4. Anticonvulsants (antiseizure medication), barbiturates, and alcohol can increase the liver toxicity caused by large doses of the acetaminophen portion of this medication.

5. The propoxyphene portion of this medication decreases the elimination of carbamazepine from the body, which can lead to an increase in side effects.

Before starting to take this medication, BE SURE TO TELL YOUR DOCTOR about any medications you are currently taking, especially any of those listed above.

WARNINGS
• Tell your doctor about unusual or allergic reactions you have had to any medications, especially to acetaminophen, propoxyphene, or other narcotic analgesics (such as codeine, hydrocodone, hydromorphone, meperidine, methadone, morphine, and oxycodone).

• Tell your doctor if you now have or if you have ever had an acute abdominal condition, asthma, blood disorders, brain disease, colitis, epilepsy, gallstones or gallbladder disease, head injuries, heart disease, kidney disease, liver disease, lung disease, mental illness, prostate disease, thyroid disease, or urethral strictures.

• If this drug makes you dizzy or drowsy, do not take part in any activity that requires alertness, such as driving a car.

• Before having surgery or any other medical or dental treatment, be sure to tell your doctor or dentist that you are taking this medication.

• Because this product contains propoxyphene, it has the potential for abuse and must be used with caution. Usually, it should not be taken on a regular schedule for longer than ten days at a time. Tolerance develops quickly; do not increase the dosage or stop taking the drug abruptly unless you first consult your doctor. If you have been taking large amounts of this medication for long periods, you may experience a withdrawal reaction (muscle aches, diarrhea, gooseflesh, runny nose, nausea, vomiting, shivering, trembling, stomach cramps, sleep disorders, irritability, weakness, excessive yawning, or sweating). Your doctor may, therefore, want to reduce the dosage gradually to prevent or minimize this response.

• Because this product contains acetaminophen, additional medications that contain acetaminophen should not be taken without your doctor's approval. Check the labels on over-the-counter (nonprescription) pain, sinus, allergy, asthma, diet, cough, and cold products to see if they contain acetaminophen.

• Be sure to tell your doctor if you are pregnant. The effects of this medication during pregnancy have not been thoroughly studied in humans. Propoxyphene used regularly in large doses during pregnancy can result in addiction of the fetus, leading to withdrawal symptoms (irritability, excessive crying, tremors, fever, vomiting, diarrhea, sneezing, or excessive yawning) at birth. Also, tell your doctor if you are breast-feeding an infant. Small amounts of this medication may pass into breast milk and cause excessive drowsiness in the nursing infant.

acetaminophen with codeine—see acetaminophen and codeine combination

Aceta with Codeine—see acetaminophen and codeine combination

acetazolamide

BRAND NAMES (Manufacturers)
acetazolamide (various manufacturers)
AK-Zol (Akorn)
Dazamide (Major)
Diamox (Lederle)
Diamox Sequels (Lederle)
TYPE OF DRUG
Carbonic anhydrase inhibitor
INGREDIENT
acetazolamide
DOSAGE FORMS
Tablets (125 mg and 250 mg)
Sustained-release capsules (500 mg)
STORAGE
Acetazolamide tablets and capsules should be stored at room temperature in tightly closed containers.

USES
This medication is used to treat glaucoma, epilepsy, and edema (fluid retention) and to prevent or treat the symptoms of mountain sickness.

TREATMENT
In order to avoid stomach irritation, you can take acetazolamide with food or with a full glass of water or milk (unless your doctor directs you to do otherwise).

The sustained-release form of this medication should be swallowed whole. Chewing, crushing, or breaking these capsules destroys their sustained-release activity and possibly increases the side effects.

If you miss a dose of this medication, take the missed dose as soon as possible, unless it is almost time for the next dose. In that case, do not take the missed dose; just return to your regular dosing schedule. Do not double the next dose.

SIDE EFFECTS
Minor. Confusion, drowsiness, increased urination, loss of appetite, or a tingling feeling. These side effects should disappear as your body adjusts to the medication.
Major. Tell your doctor about any side effects that are persistent or particularly bothersome. IT IS ESPECIALLY

IMPORTANT TO TELL YOUR DOCTOR about back pain; bloody or black, tarry stools; blurred vision; convulsions; difficult or painful urination; fever; rash; unusual bleeding or bruising; or yellowing of the eyes or skin.

INTERACTIONS
Acetazolamide interacts with other types of medications:
1. Acetazolamide can decrease the excretion through the kidneys of amphetamines, ephedrine, flecainide, mexiletine, pseudoephedrine, tocainide, and quinidine, which can lead to an increased risk of side effects with these medications. Acetazolamide can also increase the side effects (to the bones) of phenobarbital, phenytoin, and primidone.
2. Dosage adjustments of insulin or oral antidiabetic medications may be necessary when this medication is started.
3. The therapeutic benefits of methenamine, methotrexate, lithium, or large doses of aspirin may be decreased by acetazolamide.

Before starting to take acetazolamide tablets or capsules, BE SURE TO TELL YOUR DOCTOR about any medications that you are currently taking, especially any of the medications that are listed above.

WARNINGS
• Tell your doctor about unusual or allergic reactions you have had to any medications, especially to acetazolamide, methazolamide, sulfonamide antibiotics, diuretics (water pills), oral antidiabetics, dapsone, sulfone, or sulfoxone.
• Before starting to take this medication, be sure to tell your doctor if you now have or if you have ever had acidosis, Addison's disease (underactive adrenal gland), chronic lung disease, diabetes mellitus, electrolyte disorders, gout, kidney disease, or liver disease.
• If this drug makes you dizzy or drowsy, avoid taking part in any activity that requires alertness, such as driving a car or operating potentially dangerous equipment.
• Although several generic versions of this drug are available, you should not switch from one brand to another without your doctor's or pharmacist's approval. Not all of these products are equivalent.
• Tolerance to this drug can develop quickly. Check with your doctor if you feel this drug is losing effectiveness.
• Be sure to tell your doctor if you are pregnant. Although this drug appears to be safe in humans, birth defects have been reported in the offspring of animals that received large doses during pregnancy. Also, tell your doctor if you are breast-feeding an infant. It is not known whether acetazolamide passes into breast milk.

acetohexamide

BRAND NAMES (Manufacturers)
acetohexamide (various manufacturers)
Dymelor (Lilly)
TYPE OF DRUG
Oral antidiabetic
INGREDIENT
acetohexamide

DOSAGE FORM
Tablets (250 mg and 500 mg)
STORAGE
This medication should be stored at room temperature in a tightly closed container.

USES
Acetohexamide is used for the treatment of diabetes mellitus (sugar diabetes) that appears in adulthood and cannot be managed by control of diet alone. This type of diabetes is known as non-insulin-dependent diabetes (sometimes called maturity-onset or Type II diabetes). Acetohexamide lowers blood sugar by increasing the release of insulin from the pancreas.

TREATMENT
In order for this medication to work correctly, it must be taken as directed by your doctor. It is best to take this medicine at the same time each day in order to maintain a constant blood sugar level. It is important, therefore, to try not to miss any doses of this medication. If you do miss a dose, take it as soon as possible, unless it is almost time for the next dose. In that case, do not take the missed dose at all; just return to your regular dosing schedule. Do not double the next dose. Tell your doctor if you feel any side effects from missing a dose of this drug.

Diabetics who are taking oral antidiabetic medication may need to be switched to insulin if they develop diabetic coma, have a severe infection, are scheduled for major surgery, or become pregnant.

SIDE EFFECTS
Minor. Diarrhea, headache, heartburn, loss of appetite, nausea, vomiting, or stomach pain or discomfort. These side effects usually disappear during treatment, as your body adjusts to the medication.

Acetohexamide may increase your sensitivity to sunlight. It is, therefore, important to use caution during exposure to the sun. You may want to wear protective clothing and sunglasses. Use an effective sunscreen, and avoid exposure to sunlamps.

Major. If any of the side effects you experience are persistent or particularly bothersome, it is important to notify your doctor. IT IS ESPECIALLY IMPORTANT TO TELL YOUR DOCTOR about dark urine, fatigue, itching of the skin, light-colored stools, rash, sore throat and fever, unusual bleeding or bruising, or yellowing of the eyes or skin.

INTERACTIONS
Acetohexamide interacts with a number of other types of medications:

1. When combined with acetohexamide, chloramphenicol, fenfluramine, guanethidine, insulin, miconazole, monoamine oxidase (MAO) inhibitors, oxyphenbutazone, oxytetracycline, phenylbutazone, probenecid, aspirin or other salicylates, sulfinpyrazone, and sulfonamide antibiotics can lower blood sugar levels—sometimes to dangerously low levels.

2. When combined with acetohexamide, thyroid hormones, dextrothyroxine, epinephrine, phenytoin, thiazide diuretics (water pills), and cortisone-like medications (such as dexamethasone, hydrocortisone, and prednisone) can actually increase blood sugar levels.

3. Rifampin can decrease the blood concentrations of acetohexamide, which can lead to a decrease in its effectiveness.

4. Oral antidiabetic medications can increase the effects of warfarin, which can lead to bleeding complications.

5. Beta-blocking medications (such as acebutolol, atenolol, labetalol, metoprolol, nadolol, pindolol, propranolol, and timolol) combined with acetohexamide can result in either high or low blood sugar levels. Beta blockers can also mask the symptoms of low blood sugar, which can be dangerous.

BE SURE TO TELL YOUR DOCTOR about any medications you are currently taking, especially any of those listed above.

WARNINGS
• It is important to tell your doctor if you have ever had an unusual or allergic reaction to this medicine or to any other medications, particularly acetazolamide, sulfonamide antibiotics, diuretics (water pills), and other oral antidiabetics.

• It is also important to tell your doctor if you now have or have ever had kidney disease, liver disease, severe infection, or thyroid disease.

• Follow the special diet that your doctor gave you. This is an important part of controlling your blood sugar and is necessary in order for this medicine to work properly.

• Avoid drinking alcoholic beverages while taking this medication (unless otherwise directed by your doctor). Some patients who take this medicine suffer nausea, vomiting, dizziness, stomach pain, pounding headache, sweating, and redness of the face and skin when they drink alcohol. Also, large amounts of alcohol can lower blood sugar to dangerously low levels.

• Be sure to tell your doctor or dentist that you are taking this medicine before having surgery or any other medical or dental treatment.

• Test for sugar in your urine as directed by your doctor. It is a convenient way to determine whether your diabetes is being controlled by this medicine.

• Eat or drink something containing sugar right away if you experience any symptoms of low blood sugar (anxiety, chills, cold sweats, cool or pale skin, drowsiness, excessive hunger, headache, nausea, nervousness, rapid heartbeat, shakiness, unusual tiredness, weakness). It is important that your family and friends know how to recognize the symptoms of low blood sugar and know what to do if they should observe any of these symptoms occuring in you.

Even if the symptoms of low blood sugar are corrected by eating or drinking sugar, it is important to contact your doctor as soon as possible after experiencing them. The blood-sugar-lowering effects of this medicine can last for hours, and the symptoms of low blood sugar may return during this period. Good sources of sugar are orange juice, corn syrup, honey, sugar cubes, and ordinary table sugar. You are at greatest risk of developing low blood sugar if you skip or delay meals, if you exercise more than usual, if you cannot eat because you are experiencing nausea or vomiting, or if you drink large amounts of alcoholic beverages.

• Be sure to tell your doctor if you are pregnant. Studies in animals have shown that this type of medicine can cause birth defects. Studies have not been conducted in humans, however. It is also important to tell your doctor if you are breast-feeding an infant. Small amounts of acetohexamide may pass into your breast milk.

Aches-N-Pain—see ibuprofen

Achromycin V—see tetracycline

Actagen-C Cough Syrup—see pseudoephedrine, triprolidine, and codeine combination

Acticort 100—see hydrocortisone (topical)

Actifed with Codeine—see pseudoephedrine, triprolidine, and codeine combination

acyclovir (topical)

BRAND NAME (Manufacturer)
Zovirax (Burroughs Wellcome)
TYPE OF DRUG
Antiviral
INGREDIENT
acyclovir
DOSAGE FORM
Ointment (5%)
STORAGE
Acyclovir ointment should be stored in a cool, dry place.

USES
Acyclovir is used to treat genital herpes and herpes infections of the skin. Acyclovir prevents the growth and multiplication of the Herpes virus. This drug does not cure a herpes infection, but may relieve the pain associated with the viral infection and may shorten its duration.

TREATMENT
Apply acyclovir as soon as possible after the symptoms of a herpes infection appear. Wash the infected area with soap and water, and allow it to dry. To avoid spreading the infection, use a rubber glove or a finger cot to apply the ointment. Apply enough acyclovir to cover the entire area of the infection.

Complete the full course of therapy (usually about ten days), even if your symptoms disappear sooner.

If you miss a dose of this medication, apply the missed dose as soon as possible. However, if you do not remember until it is almost time for the next dose, do not apply the missed dose at all; just return to your regular dosing schedule. Do not use a double dose of the medication at the next application.

SIDE EFFECTS
Minor. You may experience temporary pain, burning, stinging, itching, or rash when this medication is applied.

This sensation should disappear as your body adjusts to the medication.
Major. Tell your doctor about any side effects that are persistent or particularly bothersome.

INTERACTIONS
Acyclovir should not interact with other medications if it is used according to directions.

WARNINGS
• Be sure to tell your doctor about unusual or allergic reactions you have had to any medications.
• Acyclovir ointment is intended for use on the skin only; it should not be used in or around the eyes.
• Try to avoid sexual activity while you have signs or symptoms of genital herpes; this medication does not prevent the transmission of herpes to other individuals, nor does it prevent recurrences.
• This medication has been prescribed for your current infection only. A subsequent infection, or one that someone else has, may require a different medication. Do not use your medication to treat other infections, unless your doctor directs you to do so.
• Be sure to tell your doctor if you are pregnant. Although this drug appears to be safe in animals, studies in humans during pregnancy have not been conducted. Also, tell your doctor if you are breast-feeding an infant. It is not known whether acyclovir passes into breast milk.

Adalat—see nifedipine

Adapin—see doxepin

Adipex-P—see phentermine

Adphen—see phendimetrazine

Adipost—see phendimetrazine

Adsorbocarpine—see pilocarpine (ophthalmic)

Advil—see ibuprofen

Aerolate—see theophylline

Aeroseb-HC—see hydrocortisone (topical)

Akarpine—see pilocarpine (ophthalmic)

AK-Ramycin—see doxycycline

AK-Ratabs—see doxycycline

AK-Spore—see neomycin, polymyxin B, and bacitracin or gramicidin combination (ophthalmic)

AK-Spore H.C. Otic—see hydrocortisone, polymyxin B, and neomycin combination (otic)

AK-Sulf—see sodium sulfacetamide (ophthalmic)

AK-Sulf Forte—see sodium sulfacetamide (ophthalmic)

AK-Trol—see dexamethasone, neomycin, and polymyxin B combination (ophthalmic)

AK-Zol—see acetazolamide

Ala-Cort—see hydrocortisone (topical)

Ala-Quin—see hydrocortisone and iodochlorhydroxyquin combination (topical)

Ala-Scalp—see hydrocortisone (topical)

Alatone—see spironolactone

Alazide—see spironolactone and hydrochlorothiazide combination

Alazine—see hydralazine

albuterol

BRAND NAMES (Manufacturers)
Albuterol Sulfate (Copley)
Proventil (Schering)
Ventolin (Glaxo)
TYPE OF DRUG
Bronchodilator
INGREDIENT
albuterol
DOSAGE FORMS
Tablets (2 mg and 4 mg)
Inhalation aerosol (each spray delivers 90 mcg)
Inhalation solution (0.5%)
Oral syrup (2 mg per 5-ml spoonful)
STORAGE
Albuterol tablets and oral syrup should be stored at room temperature in a tightly closed, light-resistant container. The inhalation aerosol should be stored away from excessive heat—the contents are pressurized and can explode if heated.

USES
Albuterol is used to relieve wheezing and shortness of breath caused by lung diseases such as asthma, bronchitis, and emphysema. This drug acts directly on the muscles of the bronchi (breathing tubes) to relieve bronchospasms (muscle contractions of the bronchi), which allows air to move more freely to and from the lungs.

TREATMENT
To lessen stomach upset, take albuterol tablets and oral syrup with food (unless your doctor directs you to do otherwise).

Each dose of oral syrup should be measured carefully with a 5-ml measuring spoon designed for that purpose. Ordinary kitchen teaspoons are not accurate enough.

The inhalation aerosol form of this medication is usually packaged with an instruction sheet. Read the directions carefully before using this medication. You may wish to consult your doctor or pharmacist about the proper administration of this drug. The container should be shaken well just before each use. The contents tend to settle on the bottom, so it is necessary to shake the bottle in order to distribute the ingredients evenly and equalize the doses. If more than one inhalation is necessary, wait at least one full minute between doses, in order to receive the full benefit of the first dose.

If you miss a dose of this medication and remember within an hour, take the missed dose immediately; then follow your regular dosing schedule for the next dose. If you miss the dose by more than an hour, just wait until the next scheduled dose. Do not double the dose.

SIDE EFFECTS
Minor. Anxiety, dizziness, flushing, headache, insomnia, irritability, loss of appetite, muscle cramps, nausea, nervousness, restlessness, sweating, tremors, vomiting, weakness, or dryness or irritation of the mouth or throat (from the inhalation aerosol). These side effects should disappear as your body adjusts to the medication.

To help prevent dryness or irritation of the mouth or throat, rinse your mouth with water after each dose of the inhalation aerosol.

In order to avoid difficulty in falling asleep, check with your doctor to see if you can take the last dose of this medication several hours before bedtime each day.

If you feel dizzy, sit or lie down for a while; get up from a sitting or reclining position slowly, and be careful on stairs.
Major. Tell your doctor about any side effects that are persistent or particularly bothersome. IT IS ESPECIALLY IMPORTANT TO TELL YOUR DOCTOR about chest pain, difficult or painful urination, itching, palpitations, or rash.

INTERACTIONS
Albuterol interacts with several other types of drugs:
1. The beta blockers (acebutolol, atenolol, labetalol, metoprolol, nadolol, pindolol, propranolol, timolol) antagonize (act against) this medication, decreasing its effectiveness.
2. Monoamine oxidase (MAO) inhibitors, tricyclic antidepressants, antihistamines, levothyroxine, and over-the-counter (nonprescription) cough, cold, asthma, allergy, diet, and sinus medications may increase the side effects of this medication.
3. There may be a change in the dosage requirements of insulin or oral antidiabetic medications when albuterol is started.
4. The blood-pressure-lowering effects of guanethidine may be decreased by this medication.
5. The use of albuterol with other bronchodilator drugs (either oral or inhalant drugs) can have additive side effects. Discuss this with your doctor.

BE SURE TO TELL YOUR DOCTOR about any medications you are taking, especially any listed above.

WARNINGS
• Tell your doctor about unusual or allergic reactions you have had to medications, especially to albuterol or any related drug (metaproterenol, terbutaline, amphetamines, ephedrine, epinephrine, isoproterenol, norepinephrine, phenylephrine, phenylpropanolamine, pseudoephedrine).

• Tell your doctor if you now have or if you have ever had diabetes mellitus, an enlarged prostate gland, epilepsy, glaucoma, heart disease, high blood pressure, or thyroid disease.

• This medication can cause dizziness. Your ability to perform tasks that require alertness, such as driving a car or operating potentially dangerous equipment, may be decreased. Appropriate caution should, therefore, be taken.

• Before having surgery or any other medical or dental treatment, be sure to tell the doctor or dentist that you are taking this medication.

• Do not exceed the recommended dosage of this medication; excessive use may lead to an increase in side effects or a loss of effectiveness.

• Avoid contact of the aerosol inhalation with your eyes.

• Do not puncture, break, or burn the aerosol container. The contents are under pressure and may explode.

• Contact your doctor if you do not respond to the usual dose of this medication. It may be a sign of worsening asthma, which may require additional therapy.

• Be sure to tell your doctor if you are pregnant. The effects of this medication during pregnancy have not been thoroughly studied in humans, but it has caused side effects in the offspring of animals that received large doses during pregnancy. Also, tell your doctor if you are breast-feeding an infant. It is not known if albuterol passes into breast milk.

Albuterol Sulfate—see albuterol

Aldactazide—see spironolactone and hydrochlorothiazide combination

Aldactone—see spironolactone

Aldomet—see methyldopa

Aldoril—see methyldopa and hydrochlorothiazide combination

Allerest 12-Hour—see phenylpropanolamine and chlorpheniramine combination

Allerfrin with Codeine—see pseudoephedrine, triprolidine, and codeine combination

Allergen—see antipyrine, benzocaine, oxyquinoline, and glycerin combination

AllerMax—see diphenhydramine

allopurinol

BRAND NAMES (Manufacturers)
allopurinol (various manufacturers)
Lopurin (Boots)
Zurinol (Major)
Zyloprim (Burroughs Wellcome)
TYPE OF DRUG
Antigout

INGREDIENT
allopurinol
DOSAGE FORM
Tablets (100 mg and 300 mg)
STORAGE
Allopurinol tablets should be stored at room temperature in a tightly closed container.

USES
This medication is used to treat chronic gout and to lower blood uric acid levels. Allopurinol blocks the body's production of uric acid. Allopurinol should not be used to treat acute gout attacks.

TREATMENT
In order to avoid stomach irritation, you can take allopurinol with food or with a full glass of water or milk. It may take one to three weeks before the full effects of this medication are observed.

Drink at least ten to 12 glasses (eight ounces each) of fluids per day while taking this medication in order to prevent the formation of kidney stones.

If you miss a dose of this medication, take the missed dose as soon as possible, unless it is almost time for the next dose. In that case, do not take the missed dose at all; just return to your regular dosing schedule. Do not double the next dose.

SIDE EFFECTS
Minor. Diarrhea, drowsiness, nausea, stomach upset, or vomiting. These side effects should disappear as your body adjusts to the medication.
Major. Tell your doctor about any side effects that are persistent or particularly bothersome that may be the result of this medication. IT IS ESPECIALLY IMPORTANT TO TELL YOUR DOCTOR about blurred vision, chills, difficult or painful urination, fatigue, fever, loss of hair, muscle aches, numbness or tingling sensations, paleness, rash, sore throat, unusual bleeding or bruising, or yellowing of the eyes or skin.

INTERACTIONS
Allopurinol interacts with several other types of drugs:
1. Alcohol, diuretics (water pills), and pyrazinamide can increase blood uric acid levels, thus decreasing the effectiveness of allopurinol.
2. Allopurinol can increase the body's store of iron salts, which can lead to iron toxicity.
3. When combined with allopurinol, ampicillin can increase the chance of skin rash; thiazide diuretics and captopril can increase the chance of allergic reactions; and cyclophosphamide can increase the chance of blood disorders. Allopurinol can also increase the blood levels and side effects of mercaptopurine, azathioprine, oral anticoagulants (blood thinners, such as warfarin), and theophylline.
4. Vitamin C can make the urine acidic, which can increase the risk of kidney stone formation with allopurinol.

Before starting to take allopurinol, BE SURE TO TELL YOUR DOCTOR about any medications you are currently taking, especially any of those listed above.

WARNINGS

• Tell your doctor about unusual or allergic reactions you have had to any medications, especially to allopurinol.

• Tell your doctor if you now have or if you have ever had blood disorders, kidney disease, or liver disease. Also, tell your doctor if you have a relative with idiopathic hemochromatosis (a disorder of iron metabolism).

• This drug may cause dizziness or drowsiness. Do not take part in any activity that requires alertness, such as driving a car or operating potentially dangerous equipment.

• Be sure to tell your doctor if you are pregnant. Although this drug appears to be safe in animals, studies in pregnant women have not been conducted. Also, tell your doctor if you are breast-feeding an infant. It is not known whether allopurinol passes into breast milk.

Alphatrex—see betamethasone dipropionate (topical)

alprazolam

BRAND NAME (Manufacturer)
Xanax (Upjohn)
TYPE OF DRUG
Benzodiazepine sedative/hypnotic
INGREDIENT
alprazolam
DOSAGE FORM
Tablets (0.25 mg, 0.5 mg, 1 mg, and 2 mg)
STORAGE
This medication should be stored at room temperature in a tightly closed, light-resistant container.

USES

Alprazolam is prescribed to treat symptoms of anxiety and anxiety associated with depression. It may work by acting as a depressant of the central nervous system. This drug is currently used by many people to relieve nervousness. It is effective for this purpose for short periods, but it is important to try to remove the cause of the anxiety as well.

TREATMENT

This drug should be taken exactly as directed by your doctor. It can be taken with food or a full glass of water if stomach upset occurs. Do not take this drug with antacids, as they may retard its absorption from the gastrointestinal tract.

If you are taking this medication regularly and you miss a dose, take the missed dose immediately if you remember within an hour of the scheduled dose. If more than an hour has passed, skip the dose you missed and wait for the next scheduled dose. Do not double the dose.

SIDE EFFECTS

Minor. Bitter taste in mouth, constipation, diarrhea, dizziness, drowsiness (after a night's sleep), dry mouth, excessive salivation, fatigue, flushing, headache, heartburn, loss of appetite, nausea, nervousness, sweating, or vom-

iting. As you adjust to the drug, these effects should disappear.

To relieve constipation, increase the amount of fiber in your diet (fresh fruits and vegetables, salads, bran, and whole-grain breads), exercise, and drink more water (unless your doctor directs you to do otherwise).

Dry mouth can be relieved by chewing sugarless gum or by sucking on ice chips.

If you feel dizzy, sit or lie down for a while; get up slowly from a sitting or reclining position, and be careful on stairs.

Major. Tell your doctor about any side effects that are persistent or particularly bothersome. IT IS ESPECIALLY IMPORTANT TO TELL YOUR DOCTOR about blurred or double vision, chest pain, severe depression, difficulty in urinating, fainting, falling, fever, hallucinations, joint pain, mouth sores, nightmares, palpitations, rash, shortness of breath, slurred speech, sore throat, uncoordinated movements, unusual excitement, unusual tiredness, or yellowing of the eyes or skin.

INTERACTIONS

Alprazolam interacts with several other types of drugs:

1. To prevent oversedation, this drug should not be taken with alcohol, other sedative drugs, central nervous system depressants (such as antihistamines, barbiturates, muscle relaxants, pain medications, narcotics, medicines for seizures, and phenothiazine tranquilizers), or antidepressant medications.

2. This medication may decrease the effectiveness of carbamazepine, levodopa, and oral anticoagulants (blood thinners) and may increase the side effects of phenytoin.

3. Disulfiram, oral contraceptives (birth control pills), isoniazid, and cimetidine can increase the blood levels of alprazolam, which can lead to toxic effects.

4. Concurrent use of rifampin may decrease the effectiveness of alprazolam.

Before starting to take alprazolam, BE SURE TO TELL YOUR DOCTOR about any medications you are currently taking, especially any of those listed above.

WARNINGS

• Tell your doctor about unusual or allergic reactions you have had to any medications, especially to alprazolam or other benzodiazepine tranquilizers (such as chlordiazepoxide, clorazepate, diazepam, flurazepam, halazepam, lorazepam, oxazepam, prazepam, temazepam, or triazolam).

• Tell your doctor if you now have or if you have ever had liver disease, kidney disease, epilepsy, lung disease, myasthenia gravis, narrow-angle glaucoma, porphyria, mental depression, mental illness, or sleep apnea.

• This medicine can cause drowsiness. Avoid tasks that require mental alertness, such as driving a car or using potentially dangerous equipment.

• This medication has the potential for abuse and must be used with caution. Tolerance may develop quickly; do not increase the dosage of the drug without first consulting your doctor. It is also important not to stop this drug suddenly if you have been taking it in large amounts or if you have used it for several weeks. Your doctor may want to reduce the dosage gradually.

• This is a safe drug when used properly. When it is combined with other sedative drugs or alcohol, however, serious side effects can develop.

• Be sure to tell your doctor if you are pregnant. This medicine may increase the chance of birth defects if it is taken during the first three months of pregnancy. In addition, too much use of this medicine during the last six months of pregnancy may result in addiction of the fetus—leading to withdrawal side effects in the newborn. Also, use of this medicine during the last weeks of pregnancy may cause drowsiness, slowed heartbeat, and breathing difficulties in the infant. Also, tell your doctor if you are breast-feeding an infant. This medicine can pass into breast milk and cause excessive drowsiness, slowed heartbeat, and breathing difficulties in nursing infants.

Alupent—see metaproterenol

Amacodone—see acetaminophen and hydrocodone combination

amantadine

BRAND NAMES (Manufacturers)
amantadine hydrochloride (various manufacturers)
Symadine (Reid-Rowell)
Symmetrel (DuPont)
TYPE OF DRUG
Antiparkinsonism agent and antiviral
INGREDIENT
amantadine
DOSAGE FORMS
Capsules (100 mg)
Oral syrup (50 mg per 5-ml spoonful)
STORAGE
Amantadine should be stored at room temperature (never frozen) in a tightly closed container. This medication should never be frozen.

USES
Amantadine is used to treat the symptoms of Parkinson's disease and to prevent or treat respiratory tract infections caused by influenza A virus. It is thought to relieve the symptoms of Parkinson's by increasing the levels of dopamine, an important chemical in the brain, which is lacking in these patients. Amantadine is also an antiviral agent that slows the growth of the influenza virus.

TREATMENT
Amantadine can be taken on an empty stomach or with food or milk.

Each dose of the oral syrup should be measured carefully with a specially designed 5-ml measuring spoon. If you are taking amantadine to treat a viral infection, you should start taking it as soon as possible after exposure to the infection. Continue to take this medication for the entire time prescribed by your doctor (usually seven to 14 days), even if the symptoms of infection disappear before the end of that period. If you stop taking the drug too soon, the virus is given a chance to continue growing and the infection could recur.

Amantadine works best when the level of medicine in your bloodstream is kept constant. Therefore, take the doses at evenly spaced intervals day and night. For example, if you are to take two doses a day, the doses should be spaced 12 hours apart.

If you are taking amantadine to treat Parkinson's disease, you should know that the full effects of this medication may not become apparent for several weeks.

If you miss a dose of this medication, take the missed dose as soon as possible, unless it is almost time for the next dose. In that case, don't take the missed dose at all; just return to your regular dosing schedule. Do not double the next dose.

SIDE EFFECTS
Minor. Constipation, dizziness, dry mouth, fatigue, headache, insomnia, loss of appetite, nausea, or vomiting. These side effects should gradually disappear.

To relieve constipation, increase the amount of fiber in your diet (fresh fruits and vegetables, salads, bran, and whole-grain breads), exercise, and drink more water (unless your doctor directs you to do otherwise).

If you feel dizzy, sit or lie down for a while; get up slowly from a sitting or reclining position, and be careful on stairs.

To relieve mouth dryness, chew sugarless gum or suck on ice chips or hard candy.
Major. Tell your doctor about any side effects that are persistent or particularly bothersome. IT IS ESPECIALLY IMPORTANT TO TELL YOUR DOCTOR about anxiety, confusion, convulsions, depression, difficulty urinating, fluid retention, hallucinations, purplish-red spots on the skin, shortness of breath, skin rash, slurred speech, or visual disturbances.

INTERACTIONS
Amantadine interacts with several other types of drugs:
1. Concurrent use of amantadine and alcohol can lead to dizziness, fainting, and confusion.
2. Phenothiazine tranquilizers and tricyclic antidepressants in combination with amantadine can lead to confusion, hallucinations, and nightmares.

BE SURE TO TELL YOUR DOCTOR about any medications you are currently taking, especially any of those listed above.

WARNINGS
• Tell your doctor about unusual or allergic reactions you have had to any medications, especially to amantadine.

• Before starting to take amantadine, tell your doctor if you now have or if you have ever had epilepsy, heart or blood vessel disease, kidney disease, liver disease, mental disorders, or stomach ulcers.

• If this drug makes you dizzy, avoid taking part in any activity that requires alertness, such as driving a car or operating potentially dangerous equipment.

• If you are taking amantadine to treat Parkinson's disease, do not stop taking the medication unless you first consult your doctor. Stopping the drug abruptly may lead to a worsening of the disease. Your doctor may, therefore, want to reduce your dosage gradually to prevent this from occurring. In addition, tolerance to the benefits of amantadine can develop in several months. If you notice a loss of effectiveness, CONTACT YOUR DOCTOR.

• Be sure to tell your doctor if you are pregnant. Although amantadine appears to be safe in humans, birth defects have been reported in the offspring of animals that received large doses during pregnancy. Also, tell your doctor if you are breast-feeding an infant. Small amounts of amantadine pass into breast milk and can cause side effects in the nursing infant.

amantadine hydrochloride—see amantadine

Amaril D Spantab—see phenylpropanolamine, phenylephrine, chlorpheniramine, and phenyltoloxamine combination

Amen—see medroxyprogesterone

---

amiloride

BRAND NAMES (Manufacturers)
amiloride (various manufacturers)
Midamor (Merck Sharp & Dohme)
TYPE OF DRUG
Diuretic and antihypertensive
INGREDIENT
amiloride
DOSAGE FORM
Tablets (5 mg)
STORAGE
Amiloride should be stored at room temperature in a tightly closed container.

USES
Amiloride is often prescribed to treat high blood pressure. It is also used to reduce fluid accumulation in the body caused by chronic conditions such as heart failure, cirrhosis of the liver, kidney disease, and the long-term use of some medications. Amiloride reduces fluid accumulation in your body by increasing the elimination of salt and water through the kidneys. It may also be used in conjunction with other diuretics to prevent potassium loss.

TREATMENT
To decrease stomach irritation, you can take amiloride with a glass of milk or with a meal (unless your doctor directs you to do otherwise). Try to take it at the same time every day. Avoid taking a dose after 6:00 P.M.; otherwise, you may have to get up during the night to urinate.

If you miss a dose of this drug, take the missed dose as soon as possible, unless it is almost time for the next one. In that case, do not take the missed dose at all; just wait until the next scheduled dose.

This medication does not cure high blood pressure, but it will help to control the condition as long as you continue to take it.

SIDE EFFECTS
Minor. Constipation, diarrhea, dizziness, dry mouth, gas, headache, heartburn, loss of appetite, nasal congestion, nausea, sleeping problems, stomach upset, or vomiting. These side effects should disappear in time.

To relieve constipation, increase the amount of fiber in your diet (fresh fruits and vegetables, salads, bran, and whole-grain breads) and exercise more (unless your doctor directs you to do otherwise).

Dry mouth can be relieved by sucking on ice chips or a piece of hard candy or by chewing sugarless gum.

To avoid dizziness or light-headedness when you stand, contract and relax the muscles of your legs for a few moments before rising from a sitting position. Do this by alternately pushing one foot against the floor while raising the other foot slightly.

Major. Tell your doctor about any side effects that are persistent or particularly bothersome. IT IS ESPECIALLY IMPORTANT TO TELL YOUR DOCTOR about anxiety; black, tarry stools; chest pain; confusion; cough; extreme tiredness or weakness; hair loss; impotence; itching; joint pain; mental depression; muscle aches; muscle cramps; nervousness; palpitations; rash; ringing in the ears; shakiness; shortness of breath; tingling in the fingers, lips, or toes; visual disturbances; or yellowing of the eyes or skin.

INTERACTIONS
Amiloride interacts with several other types of medications and certain foods:
1. Concurrent use of this medication with spironolactone, triamterene, potassium salts, low-salt milk, salt substitutes, captopril, enalapril, lisinopril, or laxatives may cause serious side effects from hyperkalemia (high levels of potassium in the blood). Check with your physician before using any of these medications or products.
2. Amiloride may increase the side effects of lithium and digoxin.
3. Amiloride may decrease the effectiveness of oral anticoagulants and antigout medications.

Before starting to take amiloride, BE SURE TO TELL YOUR DOCTOR about any medications.

WARNINGS
• Be sure to tell your doctor if you have ever had unusual or allergic reactions to medications, especially to amiloride or any other diuretic.
• Tell your doctor if you now have or if you have ever had kidney disease or urination problems, hyperkalemia, diabetes mellitus, liver disease, or acidosis.
• Amiloride can cause hyperkalemia (high levels of potassium in the blood). Signs of hyperkalemia include palpitations (rapid or irregular heartbeat); confusion; numbness or tingling in your hands, feet, or lips; anxiety; or unusual tiredness or weakness. In order to avoid this problem, do not alter your diet and do not use salt substitutes unless you first consult your doctor.
• While taking this medication, limit your intake of alcoholic beverages in order to prevent dizziness and light-headedness.
• Do not take any over-the-counter (nonprescription) medication for weight control or for cough, cold, allergy,

asthma, or sinus problems, unless you first check with your doctor.

• To prevent severe water loss (dehydration) while taking this medication, check with your doctor if you have any illness that causes severe or continuous nausea, vomiting, or diarrhea.

• Be sure to tell your doctor if you are pregnant. This drug crosses the placenta. Although this drug appears to be safe in animals, studies in humans have not been conducted. Also, tell your doctor if you are breast-feeding an infant. Small amounts of this drug pass into breast milk.

amiloride and hydrochlorothiazide combination

BRAND NAMES (Manufacturers)
amiloride with hydrochlorothiazide (various manufacturers)
Moduretic (Merck Sharp & Dohme)
TYPE OF DRUG
Diuretic and antihypertensive
INGREDIENTS
amiloride and hydrochlorothiazide
DOSAGE FORM
Tablets (5 mg amiloride and 50 mg hydrochlorothiazide)
STORAGE
Amiloride and hydrochlorothiazide combination should be stored at room temperature in a tightly closed container.

USES
Amiloride and hydrochlorothiazide combination is prescribed to treat high blood pressure. It is also used to reduce fluid accumulation in the body caused by conditions such as heart failure, cirrhosis of the liver, and kidney disease, and by the long-term use of some medications. This medication reduces fluid accumulation by increasing the elimination of salt and water through the kidneys. Amiloride is combined with hydrochlorothiazide to prevent potassium loss from the body.

TREATMENT
To avoid stomach upset, you can take this medication with food or with a full glass of milk or water (unless your doctor directs you to do otherwise). Try to take it at the same time every day. Avoid taking a dose after 6:00 P.M.; otherwise, you may have to get up during the night to urinate.

If you miss a dose of this medication, take the missed dose as soon as possible, unless it is almost time for the next one. In that case, do not take the missed dose at all; just wait until the next scheduled dose. Do not double the dose.

This medication does not cure high blood pressure, but it will help to control the condition as long as you take it.

SIDE EFFECTS
Minor. Constipation, cramps, diarrhea, dizziness, drowsiness, headache, heartburn, loss of appetite, restlessness, or upset stomach. As your body adjusts to this medication, these side effects should disappear.

This medication can cause increased sensitivity to sunlight. Avoid prolonged exposure to sunlight and sunlamps, wear protective clothing, and use an effective sunscreen.

To relieve constipation, increase the amount of fiber in your diet (fresh fruits and vegetables, salads, bran, and whole-grain breads) and exercise more (unless your doctor directs you to do otherwise).

To avoid dizziness or light-headedness when you stand, contract and relax the muscles of your legs for a few moments before rising. Do this by alternately pushing one foot against the floor while raising the other foot slightly, so that you are "pumping" your legs in a pedaling motion.
Major. Tell your doctor about any side effects that are persistent or particularly bothersome. IT IS ESPECIALLY IMPORTANT TO TELL YOUR DOCTOR about anxiety; blurred vision; bruising; confusion; difficulty in breathing; dry mouth; excessive thirst; excessive weakness or tiredness; fever; impotence; itching; joint pain; mood changes; muscle spasms; nausea; nervousness; palpitations; skin rash; sore throat; tingling in your fingers, lips, or toes; unusual bleeding; vomiting; or yellowing of the eyes or skin.

INTERACTIONS
Amiloride and hydrochlorothiazide combination interacts with several other types of medications and certain foods:
1. Concurrent use with triamterene, spironolactone, potassium salts, low-salt milk, salt substitutes, captopril, enalapril, or laxatives can cause serious side effects from hyperkalemia (high levels of potassium in the blood).
2. This drug may decrease the effectiveness of oral anticoagulants, antigout medications, insulin, oral antidiabetic medicines, and methenamine.
3. Indomethacin may decrease the blood-pressure-lowering effects of this drug, which can be dangerous.
4. Fenfluramine may increase the blood-pressure-lowering effects of this drug, which can be dangerous.
5. Cholestyramine and colestipol can decrease the absorption of amiloride and hydrochlorothiazide from the gastrointestinal tract. Therefore, this drug should be taken one hour before or four hours after a dose of cholestyramine or colestipol.
6. The side effects of amphotericin B, calcium, cortisone and cortisone-like steroids (such as hydrocortisone, prednisone, and prednisolone), digoxin, digitalis, lithium, quinidine, sulfonamide antibiotics, and vitamin D may be increased when these drugs are taken concurrently with amiloride and hydrochlorothiazide.

TELL YOUR DOCTOR about any medications you are currently taking, especially any of those listed above.

WARNINGS
• Tell your doctor about unusual or allergic reactions you have had to any medications, especially to amiloride,

hydrochlorothiazide, or any other diuretic or to any sulfa drug, including acetazolamide, oral antidiabetic medications, or sulfonamide antibiotics.

• Tell your doctor if you now have or if you have ever had kidney disease or problems with urination, diabetes mellitus, gout, liver disease, asthma, pancreatic disease, systemic lupus erythematosus, acidosis, or hyperkalemia.

• This drug can occasionally cause potassium loss from the body. Signs of potassium loss include dry mouth, thirst, weakness, muscle pain or cramps, nausea, and vomiting. If you experience any of these symptoms, be sure to call your doctor.

• Amiloride can cause hyperkalemia (high levels of potassium in the blood). Signs of hyperkalemia include palpitations (rapid or irregular heartbeat); confusion; numbness or tingling in the hands, feet, or lips; anxiety; and unusual tiredness or weakness. In order to avoid this problem, do not alter your diet and do not use salt substitutes unless your doctor tells you to do so.

• While taking this medication, limit your intake of alcoholic beverages in order to prevent dizziness.

• Do not take any over-the-counter (nonprescription) medication for weight control or for cough, cold, asthma, allergy, or sinus problems unless you first check with your doctor.

• To prevent dehydration while taking this medication, check with your doctor if you have any illness that causes severe or continuous nausea, vomiting, or diarrhea.

• This drug can raise the blood sugar level in diabetic patients. Therefore, blood sugar levels should be monitored carefully with blood or urine tests when this drug is being taken.

• A doctor does not usually prescribe this drug or other "fixed-dose" products as the first choice in the treatment of high blood pressure. Usually the patient first receives each ingredient singly. If the response is adequate to the fixed dose contained in this product, it can then be substituted. The advantage of a combination product is increased convenience and (often) decreased cost.

• Be sure to tell your doctor if you are pregnant. Hydrochlorothiazide crosses the placenta and may cause adverse effects in the developing fetus. Also, tell your doctor if you are breast-feeding an infant. Small amounts of this drug pass into breast milk.

amiloride with hydrochlorothiazide—see amiloride and hydrochlorothiazide combination

aminophylline

BRAND NAMES (Manufacturers)
aminophylline (various manufacturers)
Amoline (Major)
Phyllocontin (Purdue Frederick)
Somophyllin (Fisons)
Somophyllin-DF (Fisons)
Truphylline (G & W)
TYPE OF DRUG
Bronchodilator

INGREDIENT
aminophylline (theophylline as the ethylenediamine salt)
DOSAGE FORMS
Tablets (100 mg and 200 mg)
Controlled-release tablets (225 mg)
Oral liquid (105 mg per 5-ml spoonful)
Suppositories (250 mg and 500 mg)
Rectal solution (300 mg per 5 ml)
STORAGE
Aminophylline tablets, liquid, and rectal solution should be stored at room temperature in tightly closed containers. This medication should never be frozen. The suppositories should be stored in a cool place. They can be refrigerated if they become too soft.

USES
Aminophylline is used to treat breathing problems (wheezing and shortness of breath) caused by asthma, bronchitis, or emphysema. It relaxes the smooth muscles of the bronchial airways (breathing tubes), thus opening the passages to the lungs and allowing air to move in and out more easily.

TREATMENT
Aminophylline should be taken on an empty stomach, 30 to 60 minutes before a meal or two hours after a meal. If this medication causes stomach irritation, however, you can take it with food or with a full glass of water or milk (unless your doctor directs you to do otherwise).

Aminophylline works best when the level of the medication in your bloodstream is kept constant. It is best, therefore, to take it at evenly spaced intervals day and night. For example, if you are to take four doses a day, the doses should be spaced six hours apart.

The controlled-release tablets should be swallowed whole (if the tablet is scored for breaking, you can break it along these lines). Chewing, crushing, or crumbling the tablets destroys their sustained-release activity and possibly increases the side effects.

Doses of the oral liquid should be measured carefully with a 5-ml measuring spoon or a cup specially designed for that purpose. Ordinary kitchen spoons are not accurate enough.

To use the suppository form of this medication, remove the foil wrapper and moisten the suppository with water (if it is too soft to insert, refrigerate it for half an hour or run cold water over it before removing the wrapper). Lie on your left side with your right knee bent. Push the suppository into the rectum, pointed end first. Lie still for a few minutes. Try to avoid having a bowel movement for at least an hour after inserting the suppository. Aminophylline suppositories can be irritating to rectal tissue. Therefore, they should not be used for prolonged periods.

Aminophylline rectal solution is packaged with detailed patient instructions. Be sure to read the instructions before using this medication. If crystals appear in the solution, redissolve the crystals by partially immersing the bottle in warm water. The syringe should be washed after each application. To prevent rectal irritation, do not use this solution continuously for longer than 24 to 36 hours.

Try not to miss any doses of this medication. If you do miss a dose, take the missed dose as soon as possible, unless it is almost time for the next dose. In that case, do not take the missed dose at all; just return to your regular dosing schedule. Do not double the next dose of this medication unless your doctor has directed you to do so.

SIDE EFFECTS

Minor. Diarrhea, dizziness, feeling faint, flushing, headache, heartburn, increased urination, insomnia, irritability, loss of appetite, nausea, nervousness, stomach pain, or vomiting. These side effects should disappear as your body adjusts to the medication.

If you feel dizzy or light-headed, sit or lie down for a while; get up slowly from a sitting or reclining position, and be careful on stairs.

Major. Tell your doctor about any side effects that are persistent or particularly bothersome. IT IS ESPECIALLY IMPORTANT TO TELL YOUR DOCTOR about black, tarry stools; confusion; convulsions; difficulty in breathing; muscle twitches; palpitations; rash; severe abdominal pain; or unusual weakness.

INTERACTIONS

Aminophylline interacts with several other types of medications:

1. It can increase the effects (increased urination) of furosemide.

2. Reserpine in combination with aminophylline can cause a rapid heart rate.

3. Beta blockers (acebutolol, atenolol, labetalol, metoprolol, nadolol, pindolol, propranolol, and timolol) can decrease the effectiveness of aminophylline.

4. Aminophylline can increase the side effects of the following products: over-the-counter (nonprescription) sinus, cough, cold, asthma, allergy, and diet preparations; digoxin; and oral anticoagulants (blood thinners, such as warfarin).

5. Aminophylline can decrease the effectiveness of phenytoin and lithium.

6. Phenobarbital, carbamazepine, and rifampin can increase the elimination of aminophylline from the body, thus decreasing its effectiveness.

7. Cimetidine, erythromycin, troleandomycin, oral contraceptives (birth control pills), allopurinol, and thiabendazole can decrease the elimination of aminophylline from the body, thus increasing its side effects.

8. Antidiarrheal medications prevent the absorption of aminophylline. Therefore, at least one hour should separate doses of these two types of medications.

Before starting to take aminophylline, BE SURE TO TELL YOUR DOCTOR about any of the medications you are currently taking, especially any of those listed above.

WARNINGS

• Tell your doctor about any unusual or allergic reactions you have had to medications, especially to aminophylline, theophylline, caffeine, dyphylline, oxtriphylline, or theobromine.

• Tell your doctor if you now have or if you have ever had an enlarged prostate gland, fibrocystic breast disease, heart disease, kidney disease, low or high blood pressure, liver disease, stomach ulcers, or thyroid disease.

• Cigarette or marijuana smoking may affect the action of this drug. Be sure to tell your doctor if you smoke. Also, do not suddenly stop smoking without informing your doctor.

• High fever, diarrhea, the flu, and influenza vaccinations can affect the action of this drug. You should tell your doctor about episodes of high fever or prolonged diarrhea. Before having any vaccinations, especially those to prevent the flu, tell your doctor that you are taking this medication.

• Avoid drinking large amounts of caffeine-containing beverages (coffee, cocoa, tea, and cola drinks) and avoid eating large amounts of chocolate. These products may increase the side effects of aminophylline.

• Do not change your diet without first consulting your doctor. Eating charbroiled foods or a high-protein, low-carbohydrate diet can affect the action of this drug.

• Before having surgery or other medical or dental treatment, tell your doctor or dentist you are taking this drug.

• Before taking any over-the-counter (nonprescription) asthma, allergy, cough, cold, sinus, or diet products, ask your doctor or pharmacist. These products may add to the side effects of aminophylline.

• Be sure to tell your doctor if you are pregnant. Although aminophylline appears to be safe during pregnancy, studies in humans have not been conducted. Birth defects have been observed in the offspring of animals that received large doses of this drug during pregnancy. Also, tell your doctor if you are breast-feeding an infant. Small amounts of aminophylline pass into breast milk and may cause irritability, fretfulness, or insomnia in nursing infants.

Amitril—see amitriptyline

---

amitriptyline

BRAND NAMES (Manufacturers)
Amitril (Park Davis)
amitriptyline hydrochloride (various manufacturers)
Elavil (Stuart)
Endep (Roche)
Enovil (Hauck)
TYPE OF DRUG
Tricyclic antidepressant
INGREDIENT
amitriptyline
DOSAGE FORM
Tablets (10 mg, 25 mg, 50 mg, 75 mg, 100 mg, and 150 mg)
STORAGE
Store at room temperature in a tightly closed container.

USES
Amitriptyline is used to relieve the symptoms of mental depression. This medication belongs to a group of drugs referred to as the tricyclic antidepressants. These medicines are thought to relieve depression by increasing the

concentration of certain chemicals necessary for nerve transmission in the brain.

TREATMENT

This medication should be taken exactly as your doctor prescribes. It can be taken with water or with food to lessen the chance of stomach irritation, unless your doctor tells you to do otherwise.

The effects of therapy with this medication may not become apparent for two or three weeks.

If you miss a dose of this medication, take the missed dose as soon as possible, and then return to your regular dosing schedule. However, if the dose you missed was a once-a-day bedtime dose, do not take that dose in the morning; check with your doctor instead. If the dose is taken in the morning, it may cause some unwanted side effects. Never double the dose.

SIDE EFFECTS

Minor. Constipation, cramps, diarrhea, dizziness, drowsiness, dry mouth, fatigue, heartburn, loss of appetite, nausea, peculiar tastes in the mouth, restlessness, sweating, vomiting, weakness, or weight gain or loss. As your body adjusts to the medication, these side effects should disappear.

This medication may cause increased sensitivity to sunlight. You should, therefore, avoid prolonged exposure to sunlight and sunlamps. Wear protective clothing and use an effective sunscreen.

Amitriptyline may cause your urine to turn blue-green; this effect is harmless.

Dry mouth can be relieved by chewing sugarless gum or by sucking on ice chips or hard candy.

To relieve constipation, increase the amount of fiber in your diet (fresh fruits and vegetables, salads, bran, and whole-grain breads), exercise, and drink more water (unless your doctor directs you to do otherwise).

To avoid dizziness when you stand, contract and relax the muscles of your legs for a few moments before rising. Do this by alternately pushing one foot against the floor while raising the other foot slightly, so that you are "pumping" your legs in a pedaling motion.

Major. Tell your doctor about any side effects that are persistent or particularly bothersome. IT IS ESPECIALLY IMPORTANT TO TELL YOUR DOCTOR about agitation, anxiety, blurred vision, chest pain, confusion, convulsions, difficulty in urinating, enlarged or painful breasts (in both sexes), fainting, fever, fluid retention, hair loss, hallucinations, headaches, impotence, mood changes, mouth sores, nervousness, nightmares, numbness in the fingers or toes, palpitations, ringing in the ears, seizures, skin rash, sleep disorders, sore throat, tremors, uncoordinated movements or balance problems, unusual bleeding or bruising, or yellowing of the eyes or skin.

INTERACTIONS

Amitriptyline interacts with a number of other types of medications:

1. Extreme drowsiness can occur when this medicine is taken with central nervous system depressants (such as alcohol, antihistamines, barbiturates, benzodiazepine tranquilizers, muscle relaxants, narcotics, pain medica-tions, phenothiazine tranquilizers, and sleeping medications) or with other antidepressants.

2. Amitriptyline may decrease the effectiveness of anti-seizure medications and may block the blood-pressure-lowering effects of clonidine and guanethidine.

3. Oral contraceptives (birth control pills) or estrogen-containing drugs can increase the side effects and reduce the effectiveness of the tricyclic antidepressants (including amitriptyline).

4. Cimetidine can decrease the elimination of amitriptyline from the body, thus increasing the possibility of side effects.

5. Tricyclic antidepressants may increase the side effects of thyroid medication and of over-the-counter (nonprescription) cough, cold, allergy, asthma, sinus, and weight-control medications.

6. The concurrent use of tricyclic antidepressants and monoamine oxidase (MAO) inhibitors should be avoided because the combination may result in fever, convulsions, or high blood pressure. At least 14 days should separate the use of amitriptyline and the use of an MAO inhibitor.

Before starting to take amitriptyline, BE SURE TO TELL YOUR DOCTOR about any medications you are currently taking, especially any of those listed above.

WARNINGS

• Tell your doctor if you have had unusual or allergic reactions to medications, especially to amitriptyline or any of the other tricyclic antidepressants (imipramine, doxepin, trimipramine, amoxapine, protriptyline, desipramine, maprotiline, nortriptyline).

• Tell your doctor if you have a history of alcoholism, or if you have ever had asthma, diabetes, high blood pressure, liver or kidney disease, heart disease, a heart attack, circulatory disease, stomach problems, intestinal problems, difficulty in urinating, enlarged prostate gland, epilepsy, glaucoma, thyroid disease, mental illness, or electroshock therapy.

• If this drug makes you dizzy or drowsy, do not take part in any activity that requires alertness, such as driving a car or operating potentially dangerous equipment.

• Before having surgery or other medical or dental treatment, tell your doctor or dentist you are taking this drug.

• Do not stop taking this drug suddenly. Abruptly stopping it can cause nausea, headache, stomach upset, fatigue, or a worsening of your condition. Your doctor may want to reduce the dosage gradually.

• The effects of this medication may last as long as seven days after you have stopped taking it, so continue to observe all precautions during that period.

• Be sure to tell your doctor if you are pregnant. Studies have not been done in humans; however, studies in animals have shown that this type of medication can cause side effects to the fetus when given to the mother in large doses during pregnancy. Also, tell your doctor if you are breast-feeding an infant. Small amounts of this drug can pass into breast milk and may cause unwanted side effects, such as irritability or sleeping problems, in nursing infants.

amitriptyline hydrochloride—see amitriptyline

Amodopa—see methyldopa

Amoline—see aminophylline

amoxapine

BRAND NAME (Manufacturer)
Asendin (Lederle)
TYPE OF DRUG
Tricyclic antidepressant
INGREDIENT
amoxapine
DOSAGE FORM
Tablets (25 mg, 50 mg, 100 mg, and 150 mg)
STORAGE
This medication should be stored at room temperature in a tightly closed container.

USES
Amoxapine is used to relieve the symptoms of mental depression. This medication belongs to a group of drugs referred to as the tricyclic antidepressants. These medicines are thought to relieve depression by increasing the concentration of certain chemicals necessary for nerve transmission in the brain.

TREATMENT
This medication should be taken exactly as your doctor prescribes. It can be taken with water or with food to lessen the chance of stomach irritation, unless your doctor tells you to do otherwise.

If you miss a dose of this medication, take the missed dose as soon as possible, then return to your regular dosing schedule. However, if the dose you missed was a once-a-day bedtime dose, do not take that dose in the morning; check with your doctor instead. If the dose is taken in the morning, it may cause some unwanted side effects. Never double the dose.

SIDE EFFECTS
Minor. Constipation, cramps, diarrhea, dizziness, drowsiness, dry mouth, fatigue, heartburn, loss of appetite, nausea, peculiar tastes in the mouth, restlessness, sweating, vomiting, weakness, or weight gain or loss. As your body adjusts to the medication, these side effects should disappear.

This medication may cause increased sensitivity to sunlight. Avoid prolonged exposure to sunlight and sunlamps. Wear protective clothing, and use an effective sunscreen.

Dry mouth can be relieved by chewing sugarless gum or by sucking on ice chips or hard candy.

To relieve constipation, increase the amount of fiber (bran, salads, fresh vegetables and fruits, and whole-grain breads) in your diet, exercise, and drink more water (unless your doctor directs you to do otherwise).

To avoid dizziness or light-headedness when you stand, contract and relax the muscles of your legs for a few moments before rising. Do this by alternately pushing one foot against the floor while raising the other foot slightly, so that you are "pumping" your legs in a pedaling motion.

Major. Tell your doctor about any side effects that are persistent or particularly bothersome. IT IS ESPECIALLY IMPORTANT TO TELL YOUR DOCTOR about agitation, anxiety, blurred vision, chest pains, confusion, convulsions, difficulty in urinating, enlarged or painful breasts (in both sexes), fainting, fever, fluid retention, hair loss, hallucinations, headaches, impotence, mood changes, mouth sores, nervousness, nightmares, numbness in the fingers or toes, palpitations, ringing in the ears, seizures, skin rash, sleep disorders, sore throat, tremors, uncoordinated movements or balance problems, unusual bleeding, or yellowing of the eyes or skin.

INTERACTIONS
Amoxapine interacts with a number of other types of drugs:
1. Extreme drowsiness can occur when this medicine is taken with central nervous system depressants, including alcohol, antihistamines, barbiturates, benzodiazepine tranquilizers, muscle relaxants, narcotics, pain medications, phenothiazine tranquilizers, and sleeping medications, or with other antidepressants.
2. Amoxapine may decrease the effectiveness of antiseizure medications and may block the blood-pressure-lowering effects of clonidine and guanethidine.
3. Birth control pills or estrogen-containing drugs can increase the side effects and reduce the effectiveness of the tricyclic antidepressants (including amoxapine).
4. Cimetidine can decrease the elimination of amoxapine from the body, increasing the possibility of side effects.
5. Tricyclic antidepressants may increase the side effects of thyroid medication and over-the-counter (nonprescription) cough, cold, allergy, asthma, sinus, and diet medications.
6. The concurrent use of tricyclic antidepressants and monoamine oxidase (MAO) inhibitors should be avoided, because the combination may result in fever, convulsions, or high blood pressure. At least 14 days should separate the use of amoxapine and the use of an MAO inhibitor.

BE SURE TO TELL YOUR DOCTOR about any medications you are currently taking, especially any of those listed above.

WARNINGS
• Tell your doctor if you have had unusual or allergic reactions to medications, especially to amoxapine or any of the other tricyclic antidepressants (amitriptyline, imipramine, doxepin, trimipramine, protriptyline, desipramine, maprotiline, nortriptyline).
• Tell your doctor if you have a history of alcoholism, or if you now have or ever had asthma, high blood pressure, liver or kidney disease, heart disease, a heart attack, circulatory disease, stomach problems, intestinal problems, difficulty in urinating, enlarged prostate gland, epilepsy, glaucoma, thyroid disease, mental illness, or electroshock therapy.
• If this drug makes you dizzy or drowsy, do not take part in any activity that requires alertness, such as driving a car or operating potentially dangerous equipment.

• Before having surgery or other medical or dental treatment, tell your doctor or dentist you are taking this drug.
• Do not stop taking this drug suddenly. Abruptly stopping it can cause nausea, headache, stomach upset, fatigue, or a worsening of your condition. Your doctor may want to reduce the dosage gradually.
• The effects of this medication may last as long as seven days after you have stopped taking it, so continue to observe all precautions during that period.
• Be sure to tell your doctor if you are pregnant. Studies have not been done in humans; however, studies in animals have shown that this type of medication can cause side effects to the fetus when large doses are given to the mother during pregnancy. Also, tell your doctor if you are breast-feeding an infant. Small amounts of this drug can pass into breast milk and may cause unwanted effects, such as irritability or sleeping problems, in nursing infants.

amoxicillin

BRAND NAMES (Manufacturers)
amoxicillin (various manufacturers)
Amoxil (Beecham)
Polymox (Bristol)
Trimox (Squibb)
Utimox (Parke-Davis)
Wymox (Wyeth)
TYPE OF DRUG
Antibiotic
INGREDIENT
amoxicillin
DOSAGE FORMS
Capsules (250 mg and 500 mg)
Chewable tablets (125 mg and 250 mg)
Oral suspension (125 mg and 250 mg per 5-ml spoonful)
Oral suspension drops (50 mg per ml)
STORAGE
Amoxicillin tablets and capsules should be stored at room temperature in tightly closed containers. The oral suspension should be stored in the refrigerator in a tightly closed container. Any unused portion of the suspension should be discarded after 14 days because the drug loses its potency after that time. This medication should never be frozen.

USES
Amoxicillin antibiotic is used to treat a wide variety of bacterial infections, including infections in the middle ear, skin, upper and lower respiratory tracts, and urinary tract. Amoxicillin acts by severely injuring the cell walls of the infecting bacteria, thereby preventing them from growing and multiplying.

Amoxicillin kills susceptible bacteria but is not effective against viruses, parasites, or fungi.

TREATMENT
Amoxicillin can be taken either on an empty stomach or with food or milk (in order to prevent stomach upset).

The suspension form of this medication should be shaken well just before measuring each dose. The contents tend to settle on the bottom of the bottle, so it is necessary to shake the container to distribute the ingredients evenly and equalize the doses. Each dose should then be measured carefully with a specially designed 5-ml measuring spoon or the 1-ml dropper provided, as directed by your doctor or pharmacist. An ordinary kitchen teaspoon is not accurate enough.

It is important to continue to take this medication for the entire time prescribed by your doctor (usually seven to 14 days), even if the symptoms of infection disappear before the end of that period. If you stop taking the drug too soon, resistant bacteria are given the chance to continue growing, and the infection could recur.

Amoxicillin works best when the level of medicine in your bloodstream is kept constant. It is best, therefore, to take the doses at evenly spaced intervals day and night. For example, if you are to take three doses a day, the doses should be spaced eight hours apart.

If you miss a dose of this drug, take the missed dose immediately. However, if you don't remember to take the missed dose until it is almost time for your next dose, take it; space the next dose about halfway through the regular interval between doses; then return to your regular schedule. Do not skip any doses.

SIDE EFFECTS
Minor. Diarrhea, heartburn, nausea, or vomiting. These side effects should disappear as your body adjusts to the drug.
Major. Tell your doctor about any side effects that are persistent or particularly bothersome. IT IS ESPECIALLY IMPORTANT TO TELL YOUR DOCTOR about bloating, chills, cough, darkened tongue, difficulty in breathing, fever, irritation of the mouth, muscle aches, rash, rectal or vaginal itching, severe or bloody diarrhea, or sore throat. Also, if your symptoms of infection seem to be getting worse rather than improving, you should contact your doctor.

INTERACTIONS
Amoxicillin interacts with other types of medications:
1. Probenecid can increase the blood concentration of this medication.
2. Amoxicillin may decrease the effectiveness of oral contraceptives (birth control pills), and pregnancy could result. You should, therefore, use a different or additional form of birth control while taking this medication. Discuss this with your doctor.
3. The concurrent use of amoxicillin and allopurinol can increase the risk of developing a rash.

BE SURE TO TELL YOUR DOCTOR about any medications you are currently taking.

WARNINGS
• Tell your doctor about unusual or allergic reactions you have had to any medications, especially to amoxicillin, ampicillin, or penicillin or to cephalosporin antibiotics, penicillamine, or griseofulvin.
• Tell your doctor if you now have or if you have ever had kidney disease, asthma, or allergies.

Tablet/Capsule Identification Guide

On the following pages, you will find color photos of hundreds of the most commonly prescribed drugs in tablet and capsule form. These photos will help you identify your prescription medications and will enable you to make certain that the prescription your doctor wrote refers to the same medication you received from your pharmacist. If you note any discrepancy, call your pharmacist immediately.

HOW TO USE THIS SECTION

Prescription drugs are displayed in alphabetical order by brand name. Included are one or more dosage forms of the particular medication. The generic name is listed below the brand name of each prescription medication. A generic name is generally a shortened form of the chemical name of the drug or, in the case of a combination medication, a list of its active ingredients. This is the name under which you will be able to read more about your medication in the Drug Profiles section of this book. For example, if you have been prescribed

the antibiotic Amoxil, you will find a detailed discussion of this medication under its generic name, amoxicillin. If you have been prescribed Darvon Compound-65, you will find your medication discussed in detail within the ``aspirin, caffeine, and propoxyphene combination'' profile.

For drugs that have only one active ingredient, the amount of that ingredient is listed. For example, in the sample photo for Amoxil on the following page, the quantity of amoxicillin in the capsule is indicated. Some medications however, are, composed of more than one active ingredient. For such medications, the quantities of each ingredient are listed in the order in which they appear in the generic name. For example, Darvon Compound-65 contains 389 mg of aspirin, 32.4 mg of caffeine, and 65 mg of propoxyphene. Note that the number 65 appears in the drug's brand name, thus indicating the drug's narcotic content. Other combination drugs containing a narcotic often use the terms No. 1, No. 2, No. 3, or No. 4 to designate the narcotic content. (This is described in more detail within the appropriate drug profiles.)

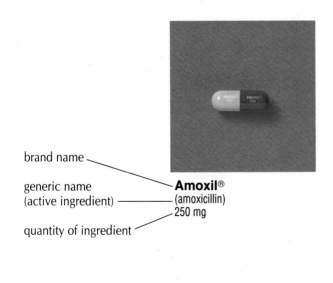

brand name

generic name
(active ingredient)

quantity of ingredient

Amoxil®
(amoxicillin)
250 mg

Darvon®———————— brand name

Compound-65 †—
(asprin, caffeine, and   narcotic content
propoxyphene combination)
389 + 32.4 + 65 mg   generic name
(active ingredients)

quantity of ingredient

† Drug contains multiple ingredients; ingredients and quantities are listed respectively.

Accutane®
(isotretinoin)
10 mg

Aldoril®†
(methyldopa and hydrochlorothiazide combination)
250 + 15 mg

Aldoril®†
(methyldopa and hydrochlorothiazide combination)
250 + 25 mg

Aldoril®†
(methyldopa and hydrochlorothiazide combination)
500 + 30 mg

Aldoril®†
(methyldopa and hydrochlorothiazide combination)
500 + 50 mg

Amoxil®
(amoxicillin)
250 mg

Amoxil®
(amoxicillin)
500 mg

Anaprox®
(naproxen sodium)
275 mg

Anaprox® DS
(naproxen sodium)
550 mg

Antivert®
(meclizine)
12.5 mg

Antivert®/25
(meclizine)
25 mg

Armour® Thyroid
(thyroid hormone)
60 mg

Asendin®
(amoxapine)
50 mg

Asendin®
(amoxapine)
100 mg

Atarax®
(hydroxyzine)
10 mg

Atarax®
(hydroxyzine)
25 mg

† Drug contains multiple ingredients; ingredients and quantities are listed respectively.

Ativan®
(lorazepam)
0.5 mg

Ativan®
(lorazepam)
1 mg

Ativan®
(lorazepam)
2 mg

Atromid-S®
(clofibrate)
500 mg

Augmentin®†
(amoxicillin and clavulanic acid
combination)
500 + 125 mg

Bactrim™†
(sulfamethoxazole and trimethoprim combination)
400 + 80 mg

Benadryl®
(diphenhydramine)
25 mg

Benadryl® Kapseals®
(diphenhydramine)
50 mg

Bentyl®
(dicyclomine)
10 mg

Bentyl®
(dicyclomine)
20 mg

Blocadren®
(timolol)
10 mg

Blocadren®
(timolol)
20 mg

Capoten®
(captopril)
25 mg

Carafate®
(sucralfate)
1 g

Cardizem®
(diltiazem)
30 mg

Catapres®
(clonidine)
0.1 mg

† Drug contains multiple ingredients; ingredients and quantities are listed respectively.

Catapres®
(clonidine)
0.2 mg

Catapres®
(clonidine)
0.3 mg

Ceclor®
(cefaclor)
250 mg

Ceclor®
(cefaclor)
500 mg

Cleocin HCl®
(clindamycin)
150 mg

Clinoril®
(sulindac)
150 mg

Cogentin®
(benztropine)
0.5 mg

Cogentin®
(benztropine)
1 mg

Cogentin®
(benztropine)
2 mg

Compazine® **Spansule**®
(prochlorperazine)
10 mg

Compazine® **Spansule**®
(prochlorperazine)
15 mg

Corgard®
(nadolol)
40 mg

Coumadin®
(warfarin)
5 mg

Cytomel®
(liothyronine)
25 mcg

Cytomel®
(liothyronine)
50 mcg

Dalmane®
(flurazepam)
15 mg

† *Drug contains multiple ingredients; ingredients and quantities are listed respectively.*

Dalmane®
(flurazepam)
30 mg

Darvocet-N® **50†**
(acetaminophen and propoxyphene
combination)
325 + 50 mg

Darvon® **Compound-65†**
(aspirin, caffeine, and
propoxyphene combination)
389 + 32.4 + 65 mg

Decadron®
(dexamethasone)
0.5 mg

Decadron®
(dexamethasone)
0.75 mg

Deconamine® **SR†**
(pseudoephedrine and chlorpheniramine combination)
120 + 8 mg

Desyrel®
(trazodone)
50 mg

Dexedrine® **Spansule**®
(dextroamphetamine)
15 mg

Diabinese®
(chlorpropamide)
250 mg

Dilantin® **Kapseals**®
(phenytoin)
100 mg

Dimetapp Extentabs®**†**
(phenylpropanolamine and
brompheniramine combination)
75 + 12 mg

Diulo®
(metolazone)
2.5 mg

Diulo®
(metolazone)
5 mg

Dolobid®
(diflunisal)
250 mg

Dolobid®
(diflunisal)
500 mg

Donnatal®**†**
(atropine, scopolamine,
hyoscyamine, and phenobarbital
combination)
0.0194 + 0.0065 + 0.1037 + 16.2

† Drug contains multiple ingredients; ingredients and quantities are listed respectively.

Duricef®
(cefadroxil)
500 mg

Duricef®
(cefadroxil)
1 g

Dyazide®†
(triamterene and hydrochlorothiazide combination)
50 + 25 mg

Dymelor®
(acetohexamide)
250 mg

Elavil®
(amitriptyline)
10 mg

**Empirin® with Codeine
No. 2†**
(aspirin and codeine combination)
325 + 15 mg

E-Mycin®
(erythromycin)
333 mg

Endep®
(amitriptyline)
150 mg

Entex® LA†
(phenylpropanolamine and guaifenesin combination)
75 + 400 mg

Eryc®
(erythromycin)
250 mg

**Erythrocin® Stearate
Filmtab®**
(erythromycin)
250 mg

Esidrix®
(hydrochlorothiazide)
25 mg

Esidrix®
(hydrochlorothiazide)
50 mg

Eskalith®
(lithium)
300 mg

Estinyl®
(ethinyl estradiol)
0.05 mg

Fastin®
(phentermine)
30 mg

† Drug contains multiple ingredients; ingredients and quantities are listed respectively.

Feldene®
(piroxicam)
10 mg

Fiorinal® **with Codeine
No. 3†**
(aspirin, caffeine, butalbital, and
codeine combination)
325 + 40 + 50 + 30 mg

Flexeril®
(cyclobenzaprine)
10 mg

Gantanol®
(sulfamethoxazole)
500 mg

Gantrisin®
(sulfisoxazole)
500 mg

Geocillin®
(carbenicillin)
382 mg

Halcion®
(triazolam)
0.125 mg

Halcion®
(triazolam)
0.25 mg

Haldol®
(haloperidol)
10 mg

Hydergine®
(ergoloid mesylates)
1 mg

HydroDIURIL®
(hydrochlorothiazide)
100 mg

Hygroton®
(chlorthalidone)
100 mg

Ilosone® **Pulvules**
(erythromycin)
250 mg

Imodium®
(loperamide)
2 mg

Inderal®
(propranolol)
10 mg

Inderal®
(propranolol)
20 mg

† Drug contains multiple ingredients; ingredients and quantities are listed respectively.

Inderal®
(propranolol)
40 mg

Inderal®
(propranolol)
80 mg

Inderal® **LA**
(propranolol)
80 mg

Inderal® **LA**
(propranolol)
120 mg

Inderide®†
(propranolol and hydrochlorothiazide combination)
40 + 25 mg

Indocin®
(indomethacin)
25 mg

Indocin®
(indomethacin)
50 mg

Indocin® **SR**
(indomethacin)
75 mg

Ionamin®
(phentermine)
15 mg

Isordil®
(isosorbide dinitrate)
5 mg

Keflex®
(cephalexin)
250 mg

Keflex®
(cephalexin)
500 mg

K-Tab®
(potassium chloride)
750 mg

Lanoxin®
(digoxin)
0.125 mg

Lanoxin®
(digoxin)
0.25 mg

Lasix®
(furosemide)
40 mg

† Drug contains multiple ingredients; ingredients and quantities are listed respectively.

Librax®†
(chlordiazepoxide and clidinium combination)
5 + 2.5 mg

Lithobid®
(lithium)
300 mg

Lomotil®†
(diphenoxylate and atropine combination)
2.5 + 0.025 mg

Lopid®
(gemfibrozil)
300 mg

Lopressor®
(metoprolol)
50 mg

Lopressor®
(metoprolol)
100 mg

Loxitane®
(loxapine)
25 mg

Ludiomil®
(maprotiline)
25 mg

Ludiomil®
(maprotiline)
50 mg

Macrodantin®
(nitrofurantoin)
50 mg

Maxzide®†
(triamterene and hydrochlorothiazide combination)
75 + 50 mg

Mevacor®
(lovastatin)
20 mg

Micro-K Extencaps®
(potassium chloride)
600 mg (8 mEq)

Minipress®
(prazosin)
1 mg

Minocin®
(minocycline)
50 mg

Minocin®
(minocycline)
100 mg

† Drug contains multiple ingredients; ingredients and quantities are listed respectively.

Minocin®
(minocycline)
50 mg

Minocin®
(minocycline)
100 mg

Moduretic®†
(amiloride and hydrochlorothiazide
combination)
5 + 50 mg

Motrin®
(ibuprofen)
300 mg

Motrin®
(ibuprofen)
400 mg

Motrin®
(ibuprofen)
600 mg

Naldecon®†
(phenylpropanolamine, phenylephrine, chlorpheniramine, and
phenyltoloxamine combination)
40 + 10 + 5 + 15 mg

Nalfon®
(fenoprofen)
300 mg

Nalfon®
(fenoprofen)
600 mg

Nalfon® 200
(fenoprofen)
200 mg

Naprosyn®
(naproxen)
250 mg

Naprosyn®
(naproxen)
375 mg

Naprosyn®
(naproxen)
500 mg

Norgesic®†
(orphenadrine, aspirin, and caffeine combination)
25 + 385 + 30 mg

Norgesic® Forte†
(orphenadrine, aspirin, and caffeine combination)
50 + 770 + 60 mg

Norpace®
(disopyramide)
100 mg

† Drug contains multiple ingredients; ingredients and quantities are listed respectively.

Omnipen®
(ampicillin)
250 mg

Omnipen®
(ampicillin)
500 mg

Optimine®
(azatadine)
1 mg

Pamelor®
(nortriptyline)
25 mg

Parlodel® SnapTabs™
(bromocriptine)
2.5 mg

Pen-Vee® K
(penicillin VK)
250 mg

Percocet®†
(acetaminophen and oxycodone combination)
325 + 5 mg

Percodan®†
(aspirin, oxycodone hydrochloride, and oxycodone terephthalate combination)
325 + 4.5 + 0.38 mg

Phenaphen® with Codeine No. 3†
(acetaminophen and codeine combination)
325 + 30 mg

Phenergan®
(promethazine)
50 mg

Polaramine® Repetabs®
(dexchlorpheniramine)
6 mg

Premarin®
(estrogens, conjugated)
0.3 mg

Premarin®
(estrogens, conjugated)
0.625 mg

Premarin®
(estrogens, conjugated)
0.9 mg

Premarin®
(estrogens, conjugated)
1.25 mg

Premarin®
(estrogens, conjugated)
2.5 mg

† Drug contains multiple ingredients; ingredients and quantities are listed respectively.

Prilosec™
(omeprazole)
20 mg

Pro-Banthine®
(propantheline)
15 mg

Procardia®
(nifedipine)
10 mg

Proventil®
(albuterol)
2 mg

Proventil®
(albuterol)
4 mg

Provera®
(medroxyprogesterone)
2.5 mg

Provera®
(medroxyprogesterone)
10 mg

Pyridium®
(phenazopyridine)
100 mg

Reglan®
(metoclopramide)
10 mg

Restoril®
(temazepam)
15 mg

Ritalin®
(methylphenidate)
5 mg

Rondec®†
(pseudoephedrine and carbinoxamine combination)
60 + 4 mg

Rufen®
(ibuprofen)
400 mg

Rufen®
(ibuprofen)
600 mg

Seldane®
(terfenadine)
60 mg

Serax®
(oxazepam)
15 mg

† Drug contains multiple ingredients; ingredients and quantities are listed respectively.

Sinequan®
(doxepin)
10 mg

Slow-K®
(potassium chloride)
600 mg (8 mEq)

Stelazine®
(trifluoperazine)
2 mg

Sumycin®
(tetracycline)
250 mg

Symmetrel®
(amantadine)
100 mg

Synthroid®
(levothyroxine)
0.025 mg

Synthroid®
(levothyroxine)
0.05 mg

Synthroid®
(levothyroxine)
0.1 mg

Synthroid®
(levothyroxine)
0.15

Synthroid®
(levothyroxine)
0.2 mg

Synthroid®
(levothyroxine)
0.3 mg

Tagamet®
(cimetidine)
200 mg

Tagamet®
(cimetidine)
300 mg

Talwin® Nx†
(pentazocine and naloxone combination)
50 + 0.5 mg

Tegopen®
(cloxacillin)
250 mg

Tegretol® Chewable
(carbamazepine)
100 mg

† Drug contains multiple ingredients; ingredients and quantities are listed respectively.

Tenormin®
(atenolol)
50 mg

Tenormin®
(atenolol)
100 mg

Tenuate®
(diethylpropion)
25 mg

Theo-Dur®
(theophylline)
200 mg

Theo-Dur®
(theophylline)
300 mg

Tigan®
(trimethobenzamide)
250 mg

Tofranil-PM®
(imipramine)
100 mg

Tolectin® DS
(tolmetin)
400 mg

Tranxene®-SD
(clorazepate)
11.25 mg

Tranxene®-SD™
(clorazepate)
22.5 mg

Tranxene® T-Tab™
(clorazepate)
3.75 mg

Tranxene® T-Tab™
(clorazepate)
7.5 mg

Tranxene® T-Tab™
(clorazepate)
15 mg

Triavil®†
(perphenazine and amitriptyline
combination)
2 + 10 mg

Triavil®†
(perphenazine and amitriptyline
combination)
2 + 25 mg

Triavil®†
(perphenazine and amitriptyline
combination)
4 + 10 mg

† Drug contains multiple ingredients; ingredients and quantities are listed respectively.

Triavil®†
(perphenazine and amitriptyline combination)
4 + 25 mg

Trimox®
(amoxicillin)
500 mg

Trinalin® Repetabs®†
(pseudoephedrine and azatadine combination)
120 + 1 mg

Tylenol® No. 1†
(acetaminophen and codeine combination)
300 + 7.5 mg

Tylenol® No. 2†
(acetaminophen and codeine combination)
300 + 15 mg

Tylenol® No. 3†
(acetaminophen and codeine combination)
300 + 30 mg

Tylenol® No. 4†
(acetaminophen and codeine combination)
300 + 60 mg

Tylox®†
(acetaminophen and oxycodone combination)
500 + 5 mg

Ultracef®
(cefadroxil)
500 mg

Urecholine®
(bethanechol)
10 mg

Urex®
(methenamine)
1,000 mg

Valium®
(diazepam)
5 mg

Valium®
(diazepam)
10 mg

Valrelease®
(diazepam)
15 mg

Velosef®
(cephradine)
250 mg

Velosef®
(cephradine)
500 mg

† Drug contains multiple ingredients; ingredients and quantities are listed respectively.

Ventolin®
(albuterol)
2 mg

Ventolin®
(albuterol)
4 mg

Vibramycin® Hyclate
(doxycycline)
100 mg

Vibra-Tabs®
(doxycycline)
100 mg

Vicodin®†
(acetaminophen and hydrocodone combination)
500 + 5 mg

Vistaril®
(hydroxyzine)
50 mg

Wellbutrin®
(bupropion)
100 mg

Wymox®
(amoxicillin)
250 mg

Wymox®
(amoxicillin)
500 mg

Xanax®
(alprazolam)
0.25 mg

Xanax®
(alprazolam)
0.5 mg

Xanax®
(alprazolam)
1 mg

Zantac® 150 Tablets
(ranitidine)
150 mg

Zarontin® Capsules
(ethosuximide)
250 mg

Zyloprim®
(allopurinol)
100 mg

Zyloprim®
(allopurinol)
300 mg

† Drug contains multiple ingredients; ingredients and quantities are listed respectively.

• This medication has been prescribed for your current infection only. Another infection later on, or one that someone else has, may require a different medicine. You should not give your medicine to other people or use it for other infections, unless your doctor specifically directs you to do so.

• Diabetics taking amoxicillin should know that this drug may cause a false-positive sugar reaction with a Clinitest urine glucose test. To avoid this problem while taking amoxicillin, you should switch to Clinistix or Tes-Tape to test your urine for sugar.

• Be sure to tell your doctor if you are pregnant. Although amoxicillin appears to be safe during pregnancy, extensive studies in humans have not been conducted. Also, tell your doctor if you are breast-feeding an infant. Small amounts of this medication pass into breast milk and may temporarily alter the bacterial balance in the intestinal tract of the nursing infant, resulting in diarrhea.

amoxicillin and clavulanic acid combination

BRAND NAME (Manufacturer)
Augmentin (SK-Beecham)
TYPE OF DRUG
Antibiotic
INGREDIENTS
amoxicillin and clavulanic acid
DOSAGE FORMS
Tablets (500 mg amoxicillin and 125 mg clavulanic acid; 250 mg amoxicillin and 125 mg clavulanic acid)
Chewable tablets (125 mg amoxicillin and 31.25 mg clavulanic acid; 250 mg amoxicillin and 62.5 mg clavulanic acid)
Oral suspension (125 mg amoxicillin and 31.25 mg clavulanic acid per 5-ml spoonful; 250 mg amoxicillin and 62.5 mg clavulanic acid per 5-ml spoonful)
STORAGE
Amoxicillin and clavulanic acid tablets should be stored at room temperature in a tightly closed container. The oral suspension should be stored in the refrigerator in a tightly closed container. Any unused portion of the suspension should be discarded after ten days because the drug loses its potency after that time. This drug should never be frozen.

USES

Amoxicillin and clavulanic acid combination is used to treat a wide variety of bacterial infections, including infections of the middle ear, skin, sinuses, lower respiratory tract, and urinary tract. Amoxicillin is an antibiotic that acts by severely injuring the cell membranes of infecting bacteria, thereby preventing them from growing and multiplying. Clavulanic acid has no antibacterial activity. It acts to prevent the breakdown of amoxicillin in the body.

Amoxicillin and clavulanic acid combination kills susceptible bacteria, but it is not effective against viruses, parasites, or fungi.

TREATMENT

Amoxicillin and clavulanic acid combination can be taken either on an empty stomach or with food or milk in order to prevent stomach upset.

The suspension form of this medication should be shaken well just before measuring each dose. The contents tend to settle on the bottom of the bottle, so it is necessary to shake the container to distribute the ingredients evenly and to equalize the doses. Each dose should then be measured carefully with a specially designed 5-ml measuring spoon. An ordinary kitchen teaspoon is not accurate enough.

It is important to continue to take this medication for the entire time prescribed by your doctor (usually seven to ten days), even if the symptoms of infection disappear before the end of that period. If you stop taking the drug too soon, resistant bacteria are given the chance to continue growing, and the infection could recur.

Amoxicillin and clavulanic acid combination works best when the level of medicine in your bloodstream is kept constant. It is best, therefore, to take the doses of this medication at evenly spaced intervals throughout the day and night. For example, if you are to take three doses a day, the doses should be spaced eight hours apart.

If you miss a dose of amoxicillin and clavulanic acid combination, take the missed dose of this medication immediately. However, if you do not remember to take the missed dose until it is almost time for your next dose, take the missed dose; space the next dose about halfway through the regular interval between doses; and then return to your regular schedule. Try not to skip any doses of this medication.

SIDE EFFECTS

Minor. Abdominal discomfort, bloating, diarrhea, gas, headache, heartburn, nausea, or vomiting. These side effects should disappear as your body adjusts to this medication.

Major. Tell your doctor about any side effects that are persistent or particularly bothersome. IT IS ESPECIALLY IMPORTANT TO TELL YOUR DOCTOR about bloody or prolonged diarrhea, chills, cough, darkened tongue, difficulty in breathing, fever, irritation of the mouth, itching, muscle aches, rash, rectal or vaginal itching, sore throat, or unusual bleeding or bruising. Also, if your symptoms of infection seem to be getting worse rather than improving, you should contact your doctor.

INTERACTIONS

Amoxicillin and clavulanic acid can interact with several other types of medications:

1. Probenecid can increase the blood concentration of amoxicillin.

2. Amoxicillin may decrease the effectiveness of oral contraceptives (birth control pills), and pregnancy could result. You should, therefore, use a different or additional form of birth control while taking this medication. Discuss this with your doctor.

3. Amoxicillin and clavulanic acid can increase the risk of side effects with disulfiram (Antabuse).

4. The risk of skin rash is increased when amoxicillin and allopurinol are taken concurrently.

Before starting this medication, BE SURE TO TELL YOUR DOCTOR about all of the medications you are currently taking.

WARNINGS

• Tell your doctor about unusual or allergic reactions you have had to any medications, especially to penicillin, amoxicillin, ampicillin, cephalosporin antibiotics, penicillamine, griseofulvin, or clavulanic acid.

• Tell your doctor if you now have or if you have ever had allergies, asthma, kidney disease, or mononucleosis.

• This medication has been prescribed for your current infection only. A subsequent infection, or one that someone else has, may require a different medication. You should not give your medicine to other people for their use or use it to treat other infections, unless your doctor specifically directs you to do so.

• Diabetics taking amoxicillin should know that this drug may cause a false-positive sugar reaction with a Clinitest urine glucose test. To avoid this problem while taking amoxicillin, you should switch to Clinistix or Tes-Tape to test your urine for sugar.

• Be sure to tell your doctor if you are pregnant. Although amoxicillin and clavulanic acid combination appears to be safe during pregnancy, studies in humans have not been conducted. Also, tell your doctor if you are breast-feeding an infant. Small amounts of this medication pass into breast milk and may cause diarrhea in the nursing infant.

Amoxil—see amoxicillin

---

amphetamine

BRAND NAME (Manufacturer)
Amphetamine Sulfate (Lannett)
TYPE OF DRUG
Amphetamine
INGREDIENT
amphetamine
DOSAGE FORM
Tablets (5 mg and 10 mg)
STORAGE
Store at room temperature in a tightly closed container.

USES

This medication is a central nervous system stimulant that increases mental alertness and decreases fatigue. It is used to treat narcolepsy (a disorder involving uncontrollable desires to sleep or actual sleep attacks that occur in a rapid and unpredictable manner) and abnormal behavioral syndrome in children (hyperkinetic syndrome or attention deficit disorder). The way this medication acts to control abnormal behavioral syndrome in children is not clearly understood.

Amphetamine is also used as an appetite suppressant during the first few weeks of dieting (while you are trying to establish new eating habits). It is thought to relieve hunger by altering nerve impulses to the appetite control center in the brain. Its effectiveness as an appetite suppressant lasts only for short periods (three to 12 weeks), however.

TREATMENT

In order to avoid stomach upset, you can take amphetamine with food or with a full glass of milk or water (unless your doctor directs you to do otherwise).

If this medication is being used to treat narcolepsy or abnormal behavioral syndrome in children, the first dose each day should be taken soon after awakening. Subsequent doses should be spaced at four- to six-hour intervals.

If this medication has been prescribed as a diet aid, it should be taken one hour before each meal.

In order to avoid difficulty in falling asleep, the last dose of this medication each day should be taken four to six hours before bedtime.

If you miss a dose of this medication, take the missed dose as soon as possible, unless it is almost time for your next dose. In that case, don't take the missed dose at all, just return to your regular dosing schedule. Do not double the next dose.

SIDE EFFECTS

Minor. Abdominal cramps, constipation, diarrhea, dizziness, dry mouth, false sense of well-being, insomnia, irritability, loss of appetite, nausea, overstimulation, restlessness, unpleasant taste in the mouth, or vomiting. These side effects should disappear as your body adjusts to the medication.

In order to prevent constipation while taking this medication, increase the amount of fiber in your diet (bran, fresh fruits and vegetables, salads, wholegrain cereals and breads), drink more water, and exercise more (unless your doctor directs you to do otherwise).

Dry mouth can be relieved by sucking on ice chips or a piece of hard candy or by chewing sugarless gum.

If you feel dizzy, sit or lie down for a while; get up from a sitting or lying position slowly, and be careful on stairs.

Major. Tell your doctor about any side effects that are persistent or particularly bothersome. IT IS ESPECIALLY IMPORTANT TO TELL YOUR DOCTOR about blurred vision, confusion, fatigue, headaches, impotence, mental depression, palpitations, rash, sweating, tightness in the chest, tremors, uncoordinated movements, or unusual bleeding or bruising.

INTERACTIONS

Amphetamine interacts with several other types of medications:

1. The concurrent use of amphetamine and a monoamine oxidase (MAO) inhibitor (isocarboxazid, pargyline, phenelzine, tranylcypromine) should be avoided, since the combination may result in convulsions, high blood pressure, or high fever. At least 14 days should separate the use of amphetamine and the use of an MAO inhibitor.
2. Barbiturate medications, phenothiazine tranquilizers (especially chlorpromazine), and tricyclic antidepressants can antagonize (act against) this medication.

3. Amphetamine can decrease the blood-pressure-lowering effects of antihypertensive medications (especially guanethidine) and may alter insulin and oral antidiabetic medication dosage requirements in diabetic patients.

4. The side effects of other central nervous system stimulants, such as caffeine, over-the-counter (nonprescription) appetite suppressants, and cough, cold, allergy, asthma, or sinus preparations, may be increased by amphetamine.

5. Acetazolamide and sodium bicarbonate can decrease the elimination and prolong the duration of action of the amphetamines.

BE SURE TO TELL YOUR DOCTOR about any medications you are currently taking.

WARNINGS

•Tell your doctor about unusual or allergic reactions you have had to any medications, especially to amphetamine or other central nervous system stimulants (albuterol, dextroamphetamine, ephedrine, epinephrine, isoproterenol, metaproterenol, norepinephrine, phenylephrine, phenyl-pro-panolamine, pseudoephedrine, terbutaline).

•Tell your doctor if you have a history of drug abuse, or if you have ever had problems with agitation, diabetes mellitus, glaucoma, heart or blood vessel disease, high blood pressure, or thyroid disease.

•Amphetamine can mask the symptoms of extreme fatigue and can cause dizziness. Your ability to perform hazardous tasks, such as driving a car or operating potentially dangerous machinery, may be decreased. Appropriate caution should, therefore, be taken.

•Before having surgery or any other medical or dental treatment, be sure to tell your doctor or dentist that you are taking this medication.

•Amphetamine may be habit-forming when taken for long periods of time (both physical and psychological dependence can occur). Therefore, you should not increase the dose of this medication or take it for longer than 12 weeks unless you first consult your doctor. It is also important that you not stop taking this medication abruptly-fatigue, sleep disorders, mental depression, nausea, vomiting, stomach cramps, or pain can occur. Your doctor may, therefore, want to decrease the dose gradually in order to prevent these side effects.

•Be sure to tell your doctor if you are pregnant. Although studies have not been done in humans, some of the amphetamines have caused heart, brain, and biliary tract abnormalities in the fetuses of animals who received large doses of these drugs during pregnancy. Also, tell your doctor if you are breast-feeding an infant. Small amounts of this drug pass into breast milk.

Amphetamine Sulfate—see amphetamine

---

ampicillin

BRAND NAMES (Manufacturers)
ampicillin (various manufacturers)
D-Amp (Dunhall)
Omnipen (Wyeth-Ayerst)
Polycillin (Apothecon)
Principen (Apothecon)
Totacillin (SK-Beecham)

TYPE OF DRUG
Antibiotic

INGREDIENT
ampicillin

DOSAGE FORMS
Capsules (250 mg and 500 mg)
Oral suspension (125 mg and 250 mg per 5-ml spoonful)
Oral suspension drops (100 mg per ml)

STORAGE
Ampicillin capsules should be stored at room temperature; ampicillin liquid suspension and drops should be refrigerated but should never be frozen. Do not keep any of these medications beyond the expiration date written on the container. All containers should be closed tightly to keep out moisture.

USES

Ampicillin is used to treat a wide variety of bacterial infections, including middle ear infections in children and infections of the respiratory, urinary, and gastrointestinal tracts. This type of antibiotic acts by severely injuring the cell walls of the infecting bacteria, thereby preventing them from growing and multiplying. Ampicillin kills susceptible bacteria but is not effective against viruses, parasites, or fungi.

TREATMENT

It is best to take ampicillin on an empty stomach (one hour before or two hours after a meal) with a full glass of water (not juice or soda pop). Always follow your doctor's directions.

If you have been prescribed the liquid suspension form of this drug, be sure to shake the bottle well before taking this medication. The contents tend to settle on the bottom of the bottle, so it is necessary to shake the container to distribute the ingredients evenly and equalize the doses. Be sure to use specially marked droppers or spoons to accurately measure the correct amount of liquid. Household teaspoons vary in size and may not give you the correct dosage.

Ampicillin works best when the level of medicine in your bloodstream is kept constant. It is, therefore, best to take the doses at evenly spaced intervals day and night. For example, if you are to take four doses a day, the doses should be spaced six hours apart.

If you miss a dose, take it as soon as possible. If it is already time for the next dose, take it; space the next two doses at half the normal time interval (for example, if you were supposed to take one tablet every six hours, take your next two doses every three hours); then resume your normal dosing schedule.

Please remember that it is very important that you continue to take this medication for the entire duration prescribed to you by your doctor (usually ten days), even if the symptoms are no longer apparent before the end of that period. If you stop taking this medication too soon, resistant bacteria are given a chance to continue growing, and the infection could recur.

SIDE EFFECTS

Minor. Diarrhea, nausea, or vomiting. These side effects should disappear as your body adjusts to the medication. **Major.** Tell your doctor about any side effects that are persistent or particularly bothersome. IT IS ESPECIALLY IMPORTANT TO TELL YOUR DOCTOR about darkened tongue, difficulty in breathing, fever, joint pain, mouth sores, rash, rectal or vaginal itching, severe or bloody diarrhea, or sore throat. Also, if your symptoms of infection seem to be getting worse rather than improving, you should contact your doctor.

INTERACTIONS

This drug interacts with other types of medications:
1. Ampicillin interacts with allopurinol, chloramphenicol, erythromycin, paromomycin, tetracycline, and troleandomycin.
2. Ampicillin may decrease the effectiveness of oral contraceptives (birth control pills), and pregnancy could result. You should, therefore, use a different or additional form of birth control while taking ampicillin.

BE SURE TO TELL YOUR DOCTOR about any medications you are taking, especially any of those listed above.

WARNINGS

• Tell your doctor about unusual or allergic reactions you have had to any medications, especially to penicillin, ampicillin, amoxicillin, cephalosporin antibiotics, penicillamine, or griseofulvin.
• Tell your doctor if you have or have ever had liver or kidney disease, asthma, hay fever, or other allergies.
• This medication has been prescribed for your current infection only. Another infection later on, or one that someone else has, may require a different medicine. Do not give your medicine to other people or use it for other infections, unless your doctor directs you to do so.
• Diabetics taking ampicillin should know that this drug may cause a false-positive sugar reaction with a Clinitest urine glucose test. To avoid this problem while taking ampicillin, you should switch to Clinistix or Tes-Tape to test your urine for sugar.
• Be sure to tell your doctor if you are pregnant. Although ampicillin appears to be safe during pregnancy, extensive studies in humans have not been conducted. Also, tell your doctor if you are breast-feeding an infant. Small amounts of this medication pass into breast milk and may temporarily alter the bacterial balance in the intestinal tract of the nursing infant, resulting in diarrhea.

Anamine T.D.—see pseudoephedrine and chlorpheniramine combination

Anaprox—see naproxen

Anaprox DS—see naproxen

Android—see methyltestosterone

Anorex—see phendimetrazine

Ansaid—see flurbiprofen

Anspor—see cephradine

Antabuse—see disulfiram

---

antipyrine, benzocaine, oxyquinoline, and glycerin combination

BRAND NAMES (Manufacturers)
Allergen (Goldline)
Auralgan (Ayerst)
Auromid (Vangard)
Auroto Otic (Barre)
Earocol (Mallard)
Oto (Vortech)
TYPE OF DRUG
Otic analgesic and anesthetic
INGREDIENTS
antipyrine, benzocaine, oxyquinoline, and glycerin
DOSAGE FORM
Otic solution (5.4% antipyrine, 1.4% benzocaine, oxyquinoline in glycerin)
STORAGE
This medication should be stored at room temperature in a tightly closed container. If the solution changes color or consistency, do not use it any longer. Never add water to the solution; it may lose its effectiveness.

USES

Antipyrine, benzocaine, oxyquinoline, and glycerin combination is used to relieve congestion, pain, and inflammation caused by an ear infection. It can also be used to help remove excess wax from the ear. Antipyrine is an analgesic (pain-reliever); benzocaine is a local anesthetic (deadens the nerve endings); and glycerin provides a drying effect.

TREATMENT

For accuracy, and in order to avoid contamination, another person should administer the ear drops if possible.

If you want to warm the ear drops before administration, roll the bottle back and forth between your hands. It is very important that you DO NOT place the bottle in boiling water.

To administer, tilt the head to one side with the affected ear turned upward. Grasp the earlobe and gently pull it upward and back to straighten the ear canal. (If administering ear drops to a child, gently pull the earlobe downward and back.) Fill the dropper and place the prescribed number of drops into the ear. Do not to touch the dropper to the ear canal. Keep the ear tilted upward for about five minutes. Your doctor may want you to put a piece of cotton soaked with the drug into your ear to keep the drug from leaking out. DO NOT wash or wipe the dropper after use.

If you miss a dose, use the drops as soon as possible, unless it is almost time for the next dose. In that case, do not use the missed dose; return to your regular schedule.

SIDE EFFECTS
Minor. Burning or itching immediately upon application. The burning or itching should last for only a few minutes.
Major. Be sure to tell your doctor about any severe or persistent burning or itching.

INTERACTIONS
This medication should not interact with other medications as long as it is used according to directions.

WARNINGS
• Tell your doctor about any unusual or allergic reactions you have had to medications, especially to antipyrine, benzocaine, or any local anesthetic or to oxyquinoline or glycerin.
• Before taking this medication, it is very important to tell your doctor if you have ever had a perforated eardrum or ear discharge.
• Be sure to tell your doctor if you are pregnant. The effects of antipyrine, benzocaine, oxyquinoline, and glycerin during pregnancy have not been studied. Also, tell your doctor if you are breast-feeding an infant. It is not known if this drug passes into human breast milk.

Antivert—see meclizine

Antivert/25—see meclizine

Antivert/50—see meclizine

Antrizine—see meclizine

Anturane—see sulfinpyrazone

Anumed HC—see hydrocortisone, benzyl benzoate, bismuth resorcin compound, bismuth subgallate, zinc oxide, and Peruvian balsam combination (topical)

Anusol HC—see hydrocortisone, benzyl benzoate, bismuth resorcin compound, bismuth subgallate, zinc oxide, and Peruvian balsam combination (topical)

Anxanil—see hydroxyzine

Apresoline—see hydralazine

Aquachloral Supprettes—see chloral hydrate

Aquaphyllin—see theophylline

Aquatensen—see methyclothiazide

Aristocort (systemic)—see triamcinolone (topical)

Aristocort (topical)—see triamcinolone (topical)

Aristocort A—see triamcinolone (systemic)

Armour Thyroid—see thyroid hormone

Artane—see trihexyphenidyl

Artane Sequels—see trihexyphenidyl

A.S.A. Enseals—see aspirin

Asbron G—see theophylline and guaifenesin combination

Asendin—see amoxapine

Asmalix—see theophylline

aspirin

BRAND NAMES (Manufacturers)
A.S.A. Enseals* (Lilly)
aspirin* (various manufacturers)
Bayer* (Glenbrook)
Bayer Children's* (Glenbrook)
Easprin (Parke-Davis)
Ecotrin* (SK-Beecham)
Empirin* (Burroughs Wellcome)
Measurin* (Winthrop Pharmaceuticals)
ZORprin (Boots)
*Available over-the-counter (without a prescription)
TYPE OF DRUG
Analgesic and anti-inflammatory
INGREDIENT
aspirin
DOSAGE FORMS
Tablets (65 mg, 81 mg, 325 mg, and 500 mg)
Chewable tablets (81 mg)
Enteric-coated tablets (325 mg, 500 mg, 650 mg, and 975 mg)
Sustained-release tablets (650 mg and 800 mg)
Caplets (325 mg and 500 mg)
Suppositories (60 mg, 120 mg, 130 mg, 195 mg, 200 mg, 300 mg, 325 mg, 600 mg, 650 mg, and 1.2 g)
STORAGE
Store at room temperature in a tightly closed container. Moisture causes aspirin to decompose. Discard the medicine if it has a vinegary odor.

USES
Aspirin is used to treat mild to moderate pain, fever, and inflammatory conditions, such as rheumatic fever, rheumatoid arthritis, and osteoarthritis. Because it prevents the formation of blood clots, aspirin has also been shown to be effective in reducing the risk of transient ischemic attacks (small strokes) and to have a protective effect against heart attacks in men with angina (chest pain).

Aspirin is a useful medication that is utilized in the treatment of a wide variety of diseases. Because it is so common and so readily available, you may not think of it as "real medicine." This is a common misconception; aspirin certainly is "real medicine." If your doctor prescribes or recommends aspirin for your condition, it is for a good reason. FOLLOW YOUR DOCTOR'S DIRECTIONS CAREFULLY!

TREATMENT

To avoid stomach irritation, you should take aspirin with food or with a full glass of water or milk.

Chewable aspirin tablets may be chewed, dissolved in fluid, or swallowed whole.

Swallow the sustained-release or enteric-coated tablets whole. Crushing, chewing, or breaking these tablets destroys their sustained-release activity and increases side effects.

To use the suppository, remove the foil wrapper and moisten the suppository with water (if it is too soft to insert, refrigerate the suppository for half an hour or run cold water over it before you remove the wrapper). Lie on your left side with your right knee bent. Push the suppository into the rectum, pointed end first. Lie still for a few minutes. Avoid having a bowel movement for at least an hour to give the drug time to be absorbed.

If you are using aspirin to treat an inflammatory condition, it may take two or three weeks until the full benefits are observed.

If you are taking aspirin on a regular schedule and you miss a dose, take the missed dose as soon as possible, unless it is almost time for the next dose. In that case, do not take the missed dose at all; just return to your regular dosing schedule. Do not double the next dose.

SIDE EFFECTS

Minor. Heartburn, nausea, or vomiting. These side effects should disappear as your body adjusts to the medication.

Major. Tell your doctor about any side effects that are persistent or particularly bothersome. IT IS ESPECIALLY IMPORTANT TO TELL YOUR DOCTOR about any loss of hearing or ringing in the ears; bloody or black, tarry stools; confusion; difficult or painful urination; difficulty in breathing; dizziness; severe stomach pain; skin rash; or unusual weakness.

INTERACTIONS

Aspirin interacts with a number of other types of medications:

1. Aspirin can increase the effects of anticoagulants (blood thinners), such as warfarin, leading to bleeding complications.

2. The antigout effects of probenecid and sulfinpyrazone may be blocked by aspirin.

3. Aspirin can increase the gastrointestinal side effects of nonsteroidal anti-inflammatory drugs, alcohol, phenylbutazone, and adrenocorticosteroids (cortisone-like medicines).

4. Ammonium chloride, methionine, and furosemide can increase the side effects of aspirin.

5. Acetazolamide, methazolamide, antacids, and phenobarbital can decrease the effectiveness of aspirin.

6. Aspirin can increase the side effects of methotrexate, penicillin, thyroid hormone, phenytoin, sulfinpyrazone, naproxen, valproic acid, insulin, and oral antidiabetic medications.

7. Aspirin can decrease the effects of spironolactone.

Before starting to take aspirin, BE SURE TO TELL YOUR DOCTOR about any medications you are currently taking, especially any of those listed above.

WARNINGS

• Tell your doctor about unusual or allergic reactions you have had to any medications, especially to aspirin, methyl salicylate (oil of wintergreen), tartrazine, diclofenac, diflunisal, flurbiprofen, fenoprofen, ibuprofen, indomethacin, ketoprofen, meclofenamate, mefenamic acid, naproxen, piroxicam, sulindac, or tolmetin.

• Before starting to take aspirin, be sure to tell your doctor if you now have or if you have ever had asthma, bleeding disorders, congestive heart failure, diabetes, glucose-6-phosphate dehydrogenase (G6PD) deficiency, gout, hemophilia, high blood pressure, kidney disease, liver disease, nasal polyps, peptic ulcers, or thyroid disease.

• Before having surgery or any other medical or dental treatment, be sure to tell your doctor or dentist that you are taking aspirin. Aspirin is usually discontinued five to seven days before surgery, in order to prevent bleeding complications.

• The use of aspirin in children (about 16 years of age or less) with the flu or chicken pox has been associated with a rare, life-threatening condition called Reye's syndrome. Aspirin should, therefore, not be given to children with signs of an infection.

• Large doses of aspirin (greater than eight 325-mg tablets per day) can cause erroneous urine glucose test results. Diabetics should, therefore, check with their doctor before changing insulin doses while taking this medication.

• Additional medications that contain aspirin should not be taken without your doctor's approval. Be sure to check the labels on over-the-counter (nonprescription) pain, sinus, allergy, asthma, cough, and cold preparations to see if they contain aspirin.

• Be sure to tell your doctor if you are pregnant. Aspirin has been shown to cause birth defects in the offspring of animals that received large doses during pregnancy. Large doses of aspirin given to a pregnant woman close to term can prolong labor and cause bleeding complications in the mother and heart problems in the infant. Also, tell your doctor if you are breast-feeding an infant. Small amounts of aspirin pass into breast milk.

aspirin and codeine combination

BRAND NAME (Manufacturer)
aspirin with codeine (various manufacturers)
Empirin with Codeine (Burroughs Wellcome)
TYPE OF DRUG
Analgesic combination
INGREDIENTS
aspirin and codeine
DOSAGE FORM
Tablets (325 mg aspirin with 15 mg, 30 mg, or 60 mg of codeine)

Note that on the label of the vial of tablets, the name of this drug is followed by a number. This number refers to the amount of codeine: #2 contains $\frac{1}{4}$ grain (15 mg) codeine, #3 has $\frac{1}{2}$ grain (30 mg) codeine, and #4 contains 1 grain (60 mg) codeine.

STORAGE

Aspirin and codeine combination tablets should be stored at room temperature in a tightly closed container. Care should be taken to prevent moisture from entering the container, as it will cause the aspirin in this product to decompose. Discard the medicine if it has a vinegary odor.

USES

This medication is used to relieve tension headaches and mild to severe pain. Codeine is a narcotic analgesic that acts on the central nervous system to relieve pain.

TREATMENT

In order to avoid stomach upset, you can take this medication with food or milk.

This medication works best if you take it at the onset of pain, rather than when the pain becomes intense.

If you are taking this medication on a regular schedule and you miss a dose, take the missed dose as soon as possible, unless it is almost time for your next dose. In that case, don't take the missed dose at all; just return to your regular dosing schedule. Do not double the next dose.

SIDE EFFECTS

Minor. Constipation, dizziness, drowsiness, dry mouth, false sense of well-being, flushing, indigestion, light-headedness, loss of appetite, nausea, sweating, and vomiting. These side effects should disappear as your body adjusts to the medication.

If you are constipated, increase the amount of fiber in your diet (fresh fruits and vegetables, salads, bran, and whole-grain breads), drink more water, and exercise (unless your doctor directs you to do otherwise).

Chew sugarless gum or suck on ice chips or a piece of hard candy to reduce mouth dryness.

If you feel dizzy or light-headed, sit or lie down for a while; get up from a sitting or lying position slowly, and be careful on stairs.

Major. Tell your doctor about any side effects that are persistent or particularly bothersome. IT IS ESPECIALLY IMPORTANT TO TELL YOUR DOCTOR about severe abdominal pain; bloody or black, tarry stools; chest tightness; difficult or painful urination; difficulty in breathing; fatigue; itching; palpitations; rash; ringing in the ears; tremors; or yellowing of the eyes or skin.

INTERACTIONS

This medication interacts with several other types of drugs:

1. Concurrent use of it with other central nervous system depressants (such as alcohol, antihistamines, barbiturates, benzodiazepine tranquilizers, muscle relaxants, and phenothiazine tranquilizers) or with tricyclic antidepressants can cause extreme drowsiness.

2. The concurrent use of aspirin and codeine combination and monoamine oxidase (MAO) inhibitors should be avoided. At least 14 days should separate the use of aspirin and codeine combination and the use of an MAO inhibitor.

3. Alcohol and anti-inflammatory medication can increase the gastrointestinal side effects of this medication.

4. The side effects of anticoagulants (blood thinners, such as warfarin), oral antidiabetic agents, phenytoin, and methotrexate may be increased by the aspirin in this product.

5. Large doses of antacids increase the elimination of the aspirin portion of this medication from the body and decrease its effectiveness.

6. Aspirin may decrease the antigout effects of probenecid and sulfinpyrazone.

BE SURE TO TELL YOUR DOCTOR about any medications you are currently taking, especially any listed above.

WARNINGS

• Tell your doctor about unusual or allergic reactions you have had to medications, especially to aspirin, methyl salicylate (oil of wintergreen), diclofenac, diflunisal, flurbiprofen, fenoprofen, ibuprofen, indomethacin, ketoprofen, meclofenamate, mefenamic acid, naproxen, piroxicam, sulindac, and tolmetin or to codeine or other narcotic analgesics (such as hydrocodone, hydromorphone, meperidine, methadone, morphine, oxycodone, and propoxyphene).

• Tell your doctor if you now have or if you have ever had abdominal disease, Addison's disease, bleeding or blood disorders, brain disease, colitis, epilepsy, gallstones or gallbladder disease, head injuries, heart disease, hemophilia, kidney disease, liver disease, lung disease, peptic ulcers, porphyria, enlarged prostate gland, or thyroid disease.

• If this drug makes you dizzy or drowsy, do not take part in any activity that requires alertness, such as driving a car or operating potentially dangerous equipment.

• Before having surgery or any other medical or dental treatment, be sure to tell your doctor or dentist that you are taking this medication. Aspirin-containing medication is usually discontinued five to seven days before surgery, to prevent bleeding complications.

• The use of aspirin in children (about 16 years of age or less) in an attempt to treat the flu or chicken pox has been associated with a rare, life-threatening condition called Reye's syndrome. Aspirin-containing products should, therefore, not be given to children with signs of infection.

• Because this drug contains codeine, it has the potential for abuse and must be used with caution. Usually, it should not be taken on a regular schedule for longer than ten days at a time. Tolerance develops quickly; do not increase the dosage or stop taking the drug abruptly, unless you first consult your doctor. If you have been taking large amounts of this medication for long periods, you may experience a withdrawal reaction (muscle aches, diarrhea, gooseflesh, runny nose, nausea, vomiting, shivering, trembling, stomach cramps, sleep disorders, irritability, weakness, excessive yawning, or sweating). Your doctor may, therefore, want to reduce the dosage gradually.

• Because this product contains aspirin, additional medications that contain aspirin should not be taken without your doctor's approval. Check the labels on over-the-counter (nonprescription) pain, sinus, allergy, asthma, cough, and cold products to see if they contain aspirin.

• Diabetic patients should be aware that large doses of aspirin (more than eight 325-mg tablets per day) may interfere with urine sugar testing. Diabetics should, therefore, check with their doctor before changing their insulin dose.

• Be sure to tell your doctor if you are pregnant. The effects of this medication during pregnancy have not been thoroughly studied in humans. Codeine, used regularly in large doses during pregnancy, may result in addiction of the fetus, leading to withdrawal symptoms (irritability, excessive crying, tremors, fever, vomiting, diarrhea, sneezing, or excessive yawning) at birth. Large amounts of aspirin taken close to the end of pregnancy may prolong labor and cause bleeding problems in the mother and heart problems in the newborn infant. Also, tell your doctor if you are breast-feeding an infant. Small amounts of this medication may pass into breast milk and cause excessive drowsiness in the nursing infant.

aspirin and meprobamate combination—see meprobamate and aspirin combination

aspirin and oxycodone combination

BRAND NAMES (Manufacturers)
Codoxy (Halsey)
oxycodone hydrochloride, oxycodone terephthalate, and aspirin (various manufacturers)
Percodan (DuPont)
Percodan-Demi (DuPont)
TYPE OF DRUG
Analgesic combination
INGREDIENTS
aspirin and oxycodone
DOSAGE FORM
Tablets (325 mg aspirin with 2.25 mg oxycodone hydrochloride and 0.19 mg oxycodone terephthalate; 325 mg aspirin with 4.5 mg oxycodone hydrochloride and 0.38 mg oxycodone terephthalate)
STORAGE
Store at room temperature in a tightly closed container. Moisture causes the aspirin in this product to decompose. Discard the medicine if it has a vinegary odor.

USES
This combination medication is used to relieve moderate to severe pain. Oxycodone is a narcotic analgesic that acts on the central nervous system to relieve pain.

TREATMENT
In order to avoid stomach upset, you can take this medication with food or milk.

This medication works most effectively if you take it at the onset of pain, rather than waiting until the pain becomes intense.

If you are taking this medication on a regular schedule and you miss a dose, take the missed dose as soon as possible, unless it is almost time for your next dose. In that case, don't take the missed dose at all; just return to your regular dosing schedule. Do not double the next dose.

SIDE EFFECTS
Minor. Constipation, dizziness, drowsiness, dry mouth, false sense of well-being, flushing, indigestion, lightheadedness, loss of appetite, nausea, sweating, or vomiting. These side effects should disappear as your body adjusts to the medication.

If you are constipated, increase the amount of fiber in your diet (fresh fruits and vegetables, salads, bran, and whole-grain breads), drink more water, and exercise (unless your doctor directs you to do otherwise).

Chew sugarless gum or suck on ice chips or a piece of hard candy to reduce mouth dryness.

If you feel dizzy, light-headed, or nauseated, sit or lie down for a while; get up from a sitting or lying position slowly, and be careful on stairs.

Major. Tell your doctor about any side effects that are persistent or particularly bothersome. IT IS ESPECIALLY IMPORTANT TO TELL YOUR DOCTOR about bloody or black, tarry stools; chest tightness; difficult or painful urination; difficulty in breathing; fatigue; itching; palpitations; rash; ringing in the ears; severe abdominal pain; tremors; or yellowing of the eyes or skin.

INTERACTIONS
This medication interacts with several other types of drugs:
1. Concurrent use of this medication with other central nervous system depressants (such as alcohol, antihistamines, barbiturates, benzodiazepine tranquilizers, muscle relaxants, and phenothiazine tranquilizers) or with tricyclic antidepressants can cause extreme drowsiness.
2. The concurrent use of aspirin and oxycodone combination and monoamine oxidase (MAO) inhibitors should be avoided. At least 14 days should separate the use of this drug and the use of an MAO inhibitor.
3. Alcohol and anti-inflammatory medications can increase the gastrointestinal side effects of this medication.
4. The side effects of anticoagulants (blood thinners, such as warfarin), oral antidiabetic agents, phenytoin, and methotrexate may be increased by the aspirin in this product.
5. Large doses of antacids increase the elimination of the aspirin portion of this medication from the body and decrease its effectiveness.
6. The aspirin portion of this medication may decrease the antigout effects of probenecid and sulfinpyrazone.

BE SURE TO TELL YOUR DOCTOR about any medications you are currently taking, especially any listed above.

WARNINGS
• Tell your doctor about unusual or allergic reactions you have had to medications, especially to aspirin, methyl

salicylate (oil of wintergreen), diclofenac, diflunisal, flurbiprofen, fenoprofen, ibuprofen, indomethacin, ketoprofen, meclofenamate, mefenamic acid, naproxen, piroxicam, sulindac, or tolmetin or to oxycodone or other narcotic analgesics (such as codeine, hydrocodone, hydromorphone, meperidine, methadone, morphine, or propoxyphene).

• Tell your doctor if you now have or if you have ever had abdominal disease, Addison's disease, bleeding or blood disorders, brain disease, colitis, epilepsy, gallstones or gallbladder disease, head injuries, heart disease, hemophilia, kidney disease, liver disease, lung disease, peptic ulcers, porphyria, enlarged prostate gland, or thyroid disease.

• If this drug makes you dizzy or drowsy, do not take part in any activity that requires alertness, such as driving a car or operating potentially dangerous equipment.

• Before having surgery or any other medical or dental treatment, tell your doctor or dentist that you are taking this drug. Aspirin-containing medications are usually stopped five to seven days before surgery, in order to prevent complications.

• The use of aspirin in children (about 16 years of age or less) with the flu or chicken pox has been associated with a rare, life-threatening condition called Reye's syndrome. Aspirin-containing products should, therefore, not be given to children who have any signs of infection.

• Because this drug contains oxycodone, it has the potential for abuse and must be used with caution. Usually, it should not be taken on a regular schedule for longer than ten days at a time. Tolerance develops quickly; do not increase the dosage or stop taking the drug abruptly, unless you first consult your doctor.

• If you have been taking large amounts of this medication for long periods, you may experience a withdrawal reaction (muscle aches, diarrhea, gooseflesh, runny nose, nausea, vomiting, shivering, trembling, stomach cramps, sleep disorders, irritability, weakness, excessive yawning, or sweating). Your doctor may, therefore, want to reduce the dosage gradually to prevent or minimize this response.

• Because this product contains aspirin, additional medications that contain aspirin should not be taken without your doctor's approval. Check the labels on over-the-counter (nonprescription) pain, sinus, allergy, asthma, cough, and cold products to see if they contain aspirin.

• Diabetic patients should be aware that large doses of aspirin (more than eight 325-mg tablets per day) may interfere with urine sugar testing. Diabetics should, therefore, check with their doctor before changing their insulin dose.

• Be sure to tell your doctor if you are pregnant. The effects of this medication during pregnancy have not been thoroughly studied in humans. Oxycodone, used regularly in large doses during pregnancy, may result in addiction of the fetus, leading to withdrawal symptoms (irritability, excessive crying, tremors, fever, vomiting, diarrhea, sneezing, or excessive yawning) at birth. Large amounts of aspirin taken close to the end of pregnancy may prolong labor and cause bleeding problems in the mother and heart problems in the newborn infant. Also, tell your doctor if you are breast-feeding an infant. Small amounts of this medication may pass into breast milk and cause excessive drowsiness in the nursing infant.

aspirin, caffeine, and butalbital combination

BRAND NAMES (Manufacturers)
B-A-C (Mayrand)
butalbital with aspirin and caffeine (various manufacturers)
Fiorgen PF (Goldline)
Fiorinal (Sandoz)
Isollyl Improved (Rugby)
Lanorinal (Lannett)
Marnal (Vortech)
TYPE OF DRUG
Analgesic combination and sedative
INGREDIENTS
aspirin, caffeine, and butalbital
DOSAGE FORMS
Tablets (325 mg aspirin, 40 mg caffeine, and 50 mg butalbital; 650 mg aspirin, 40 mg caffeine, and 50 mg butalbital) Capsules (325 mg aspirin, 40 mg caffeine, and 50 mg butalbital)
STORAGE
Aspirin, caffeine, and butalbital combination tablets and capsules should be stored at room temperature in tightly closed containers. Moisture causes the aspirin in this product to decompose. Discard the medicine if it has a vinegary odor.

USES
This combination medication is used to relieve tension headaches and mild to moderate pain. Butalbital belongs to a group of drugs known as barbiturates. The barbiturates act on the central nervous system (brain and spinal cord) to produce relaxation. Caffeine is a central nervous system stimulant. It constricts blood vessels in the head, which may help to relieve headaches.

TREATMENT
To avoid stomach upset, take this drug with food or milk.

This drug works most effectively if you take it at the onset of pain, rather than waiting until the pain is intense.

If you are taking this medication on a regular schedule and you miss a dose, take the missed dose as soon as possible, unless it is almost time for your next dose. In that case, don't take the missed dose at all; just return to your regular dosing schedule. Do not double the next dose.

SIDE EFFECTS
Minor. Dizziness, drowsiness, gas, loss of appetite, nausea, nervousness, sleeping disorders, or vomiting. These side effects should disappear as your body adjusts to the medication.

If you feel dizzy or light-headed, sit or lie down for a while; get up from a sitting or lying position slowly.

Major. Tell your doctor about any side effects that are persistent or particularly bothersome. IT IS ESPECIALLY IMPORTANT TO TELL YOUR DOCTOR about bloody or black, tarry stools; chest tightness; confusion; difficult or painful urination; light-headedness; loss of coordination; palpitations; rash; ringing in the ears; shortness of breath; severe abdominal pain; sore throat and fever; or yellowing of the eyes or skin.

INTERACTIONS
This medication interacts with several other types of drugs:
1. Concurrent use of this medication with other central nervous system depressants (such as alcohol, antihistamines, barbiturates, benzodiazepine tranquilizers, muscle relaxants, and phenothiazine tranquilizers) or with tricyclic antidepressants can cause extreme drowsiness.
2. Alcohol and anti-inflammatory medications can increase the gastrointestinal side effects of this medication.
3. The side effects of anticoagulants (blood thinners, such as warfarin), oral antidiabetic agents, phenytoin, and methotrexate may be increased by the aspirin in this product.
4. Large doses of antacids increase the elimination of the aspirin portion of this medication from the body and decrease its effectiveness.
5. Aspirin may decrease the antigout effects of probenecid and sulfinpyrazone.
6. Butalbital can increase the elimination from the body of oral contraceptives (birth control pills), carbamazepine, adrenocorticosteroids (cortisone-like drugs), digoxin, doxycycline, tricyclic antidepressants, griseofulvin, metronidazole, theophylline, aminophylline, and quinidine, thereby decreasing the effectiveness of these medications.
7. The side effects of cyclophosphamide may be increased by butalbital.

BE SURE TO TELL YOUR DOCTOR about any medications you are currently taking, especially any of those listed above.

WARNINGS
• Tell your doctor about unusual or allergic reactions you have had to medications, especially to aspirin, methyl salicylate (oil of wintergreen), diclofenac, diflunisal, flurbiprofen, fenoprofen, ibuprofen, indomethacin, ketoprofen, meclofenamate, mefenamic acid, naproxen, piroxicam, sulindac, or tolmetin; to caffeine; or to butalbital or other barbiturates (such as phenobarbital, pentobarbital, or secobarbital).
• Tell your doctor if you now have or if you have ever had bleeding problems, blood disorders, diabetes mellitus, heart disease, hemophilia, hyperactivity, kidney disease, liver disease, mental depression, peptic ulcers, or thyroid disease.
• If this drug makes you dizzy or drowsy, do not take part in any activity that requires alertness, such as driving a car or operating potentially dangerous equipment.
• Before having surgery or any other medical or dental treatment, be sure to tell your doctor or dentist that you are taking this medication. Aspirin-containing medication is usually discontinued five to seven days before surgery to prevent bleeding complications.

• The use of aspirin in children (about 16 years of age or less) in an attempt to treat the symptoms of the flu or chicken pox has been associated with a rare, life-threatening condition called Reye's syndrome. Therefore, it is very important that aspirin-containing products should, not be given to children with the signs of these infections.
• Because this drug contains butalbital, it has the potential for abuse and must be used with caution. Tolerance develops quickly; do not increase the dosage or stop taking the drug abruptly, unless you first consult your doctor. If you have been taking large amounts of this medication for long periods, you may experience a withdrawal reaction (muscle aches, diarrhea, convulsions, sleep disorders, nervousness, irritability, or weakness). Your doctor may, therefore, want to reduce the dosage gradually.
• Because this product contains aspirin, additional medications that contain aspirin should not be taken without your physician's approval. Check the labels on over-the-counter (nonprescription) pain, sinus, allergy, asthma, cough, and cold products to see if they contain aspirin.
• You should not take more than six tablets or capsules of this drug in one day, unless your doctor specifically directs you to do so.
• Diabetic patients should be aware that large doses of aspirin (more than eight 325-mg tablets or capsules per day) may interfere with urine sugar testing. Diabetics should, therefore, check with their doctor before changing their insulin dose.
• Be sure to tell your doctor if you are pregnant. The effects of this medication during pregnancy have not been thoroughly studied in humans. Butalbital, used regularly in large doses during pregnancy, may result in addiction of the fetus, leading to withdrawal symptoms (irritability, excessive crying, tremors, fever, vomiting, diarrhea, sneezing, or excessive yawning) at birth. Large amounts of aspirin taken close to the end of pregnancy may prolong labor and cause bleeding problems in the mother and heart problems in the newborn infant. Also, tell your doctor if you are breast-feeding an infant. Small amounts of this medication may pass into breast milk and cause excessive drowsiness in the nursing infant.

aspirin, caffeine, and dihydrocodeine combination

BRAND NAME (Manufacturer)
Synalgos-DC (Ives)
TYPE OF DRUG
Analgesic combination
INGREDIENTS
aspirin, caffeine, and dihydrocodeine
DOSAGE FORM
Capsules (356.4 mg aspirin, 30 mg caffeine, and 16 mg dihydrocodeine)
STORAGE
This medication should be stored at room temperature in a tightly closed container. Moisture causes the aspirin in this product to decompose.

USES

Aspirin, caffeine, and dihydrocodeine combination is used to relieve mild to moderate pain. Dihydrocodeine is a narcotic analgesic that acts on the central nervous system (brain and spinal cord) to relieve pain. Caffeine is a central nervous system stimulant. It constricts the blood vessels in the head, which may help to relieve headaches.

TREATMENT

In order to avoid stomach upset, you can take this medication with food or milk.

This medication works most effectively if you take it at the onset of pain, rather than waiting until the pain becomes intense.

If you are taking this drug on a schedule and you miss a dose, take the missed dose as soon as possible, unless it is almost time for your next dose. In that case, don't take the missed dose at all; just return to your regular dosing schedule. Do not double the next dose.

SIDE EFFECTS

Minor. Constipation, dizziness, drowsiness, dry mouth, false sense of well-being, headache, indigestion, loss of appetite, nausea, nervousness, restlessness, sleep disorders, sweating, or vomiting. These side effects should disappear as your body adjusts to the medication.

If you are constipated, increase the amount of fiber in your diet (fresh fruits and vegetables, salads, bran, and whole-grain breads), drink more water, and exercise (unless your doctor directs you to do otherwise).

Chew sugarless gum or suck on ice chips or a piece of hard candy to reduce mouth dryness.

If you feel dizzy or light-headed, sit or lie down for a while; get up from a sitting or lying position slowly.

Major. Tell your doctor about any side effects that are persistent or particularly bothersome. IT IS ESPECIALLY IMPORTANT TO TELL YOUR DOCTOR about black, tarry stools; blurred vision; chest tightness; difficult or painful urination; difficulty in breathing; fainting; itching; light-headedness; loss of coordination; palpitations; ringing in the ears; severe abdominal pain; skin rash; sore throat and fever; or unusual bleeding or bruising.

INTERACTIONS

This medication interacts with several other types of drugs:
1. Concurrent use of this medication with other central nervous system depressants (such as alcohol, antihistamines, barbiturates, benzodiazepine tranquilizers, muscle relaxants, and phenothiazine tranquilizers) or with tricyclic antidepressants can cause extreme drowsiness.
2. Concurrent use of this drug and monoamine oxidase (MAO) inhibitors should be avoided. At least 14 days should separate the use of aspirin, caffeine, and dihydrocodeine combination and the use of an MAO inhibitor.
3. Alcohol and anti-inflammatory medication can increase the gastrointestinal side effects of this medication.
4. The aspirin in this product may increase the side effects of anticoagulants (blood thinners, such as warfarin), oral antidiabetic agents, phenytoin, and methotrexate.
5. Large doses of antacids increase the elimination of the aspirin portion of this medication from the body and decrease its effectiveness.

6. The aspirin portion of this medication may decrease the antigout effects of probenecid and sulfinpyrazone.

BE SURE TO TELL YOUR DOCTOR about any medications that you are currently taking, especially any of the medications that are listed above.

WARNINGS

• Tell your doctor about unusual or allergic reactions you have had to medications, especially to aspirin, methyl salicylate (oil of wintergreen), diclofenac, diflunisal, flurbiprofen, fenoprofen, ibuprofen, indomethacin, ketoprofen, meclofenamate, mefenamic acid, naproxen, piroxicam, sulindac, or tolmetin; to dihydrocodeine or other narcotic analgesics (such as codeine, hydrocodone, hydromorphone, meperidine, methadone, morphine, oxycodone, and propoxyphene); or to caffeine.

• Tell your doctor if you now have or if you have ever had abdominal disease, Addison's disease, bleeding or blood disorders, brain disease, colitis, epilepsy, gallstones or gallbladder disease, head injuries, heart disease, hemophilia, kidney disease, liver disease, lung disease, peptic ulcers, prostate disease, or thyroid disease.

• If this drug makes you dizzy or drowsy, do not take part in any activity that requires alertness, such as driving a car or operating potentially dangerous equipment.

• Before having surgery or any other medical or dental treatment, be sure to tell your doctor or dentist that you are taking this medication. Aspirin-containing medication is usually discontinued five to seven days before surgery, to prevent bleeding complications.

• The use of aspirin in children (about 16 years of age or less) in an attempt to treat the symptoms of the flu or chicken pox has been associated with a rare, life-threatening condition called Reye's syndrome. Therefore, it is very important that aspirin-containing products should, not be given to children with the signs of these infections.

• Because this drug contains dihydrocodeine, it has the potential for abuse and must be used with caution. Usually, it should not be taken on a regular schedule for longer than ten days at a time. Tolerance develops quickly; do not increase the dosage or stop taking the drug abruptly, unless you first consult your doctor. If you have been taking large amounts of this medication for long periods, you may experience a withdrawal reaction (muscle aches, diarrhea, gooseflesh, runny nose, nausea, vomiting, shivering, trembling, stomach cramps, sleep disorders, irritability, weakness, excessive yawning, or sweating). Your doctor may, therefore, want to reduce the dosage gradually.

• Because this product contains aspirin, additional medications that contain aspirin should not be taken without your doctor's approval. Check the labels on over-the-counter (nonprescription) pain, sinus, allergy, asthma, cough, and cold products to see if they contain aspirin.

• Diabetics should be aware that large doses of aspirin (more than eight 325-mg tablets of aspirin per day) may interfere with urine sugar testing and should, therefore, check with their doctor before changing their insulin dose.

• Be sure to tell your doctor if you are pregnant. The effects of this medication during pregnancy have not been thoroughly studied in humans. Dihydrocodeine, used regularly in large doses during pregnancy, may result in addiction of the fetus, leading to withdrawal symptoms (irritability, excessive crying, tremors, fever, vomiting, diarrhea, sneezing, or excessive yawning) at birth. Large amounts of aspirin taken close to the end of pregnancy may prolong labor and cause bleeding problems in the mother and heart problems in the newborn infant. Also, tell your doctor if you are breast-feeding an infant. Small amounts of this medication may pass into breast milk and cause excessive drowsiness in the nursing infant.

aspirin, caffeine, and propoxyphene combination

BRAND NAMES (Manufacturers)
Darvon Compound (Lilly)
Dolene Compound-65 (Lederle)
Doxaphene Compound (Major)
propoxyphene hydrochloride compound
   (various manufacturers)
TYPE OF DRUG
Analgesic combination
INGREDIENTS
aspirin, caffeine, and propoxyphene
DOSAGE FORM
Capsules (389 mg aspirin, 32. 4 mg caffeine, and 32 mg propoxyphene; 389 mg aspirin, 32. 4 mg caffeine, and 65 mg propoxyphene)
STORAGE
Aspirin, caffeine, and propoxyphene capsules should be stored at room temperature in a tightly closed container. Moisture causes the aspirin to decompose. Discard the medicine if it has a vinegary odor.

USES
Aspirin, caffeine, and propoxyphene combination is used to relieve mild to moderate pain. Propoxyphene is a narcotic analgesic that acts on the central nervous system (brain and spinal cord) to relieve pain. Caffeine is a central nervous system stimulant. It constricts blood vessels in the head, which may help to relieve headaches.

TREATMENT
In order to avoid stomach upset, you can take this medication with food or milk.

This medication works most effectively if you take it at the onset of pain, rather than waiting until the pain becomes intense.

If you are taking this medication on a regular schedule and you miss a dose, take the missed dose as soon as possible, unless it is almost time for your next dose. In that case, don't take the missed dose at all; just return to your regular dosing schedule. Do not double the next dose.

SIDE EFFECTS
Minor. Constipation, dizziness, drowsiness, dry mouth, false sense of well-being, flushing, indigestion, loss of appetite, nausea, sweating, or vomiting. These side effects should disappear as your body adjusts to the medication.

If you are constipated, increase the amount of fiber in your diet (fresh fruits and vegetables, salads, bran, and whole-grain breads), drink more water, and exercise (unless your doctor directs you to do otherwise).

If you feel dizzy or light-headed, sit or lie down for a while; get up from a sitting or lying position slowly, and be careful on stairs.

Major. Tell your doctor about any side effects that are persistent or particularly bothersome. IT IS ESPECIALLY IMPORTANT TO TELL YOUR DOCTOR about severe abdominal pain; bloody or black, tarry stools; chest tightness; difficult or painful urination; difficulty in breathing; fatigue; itching; lightheadedness; palpitations; rash; ringing in the ears; tremors; or yellowing of the eyes or skin.

INTERACTIONS
This medication interacts with several other types of drugs:
1. Concurrent use of this medication with other central nervous system depressants (such as alcohol, antihistamines, barbiturates, benzodiazepine tranquilizers, muscle relaxants, or phenothiazine tranquilizers) or with tricyclic antidepressants can cause extreme drowsiness.
2. Concurrent use of this medication and monoamine oxidase (MAO) inhibitors should be avoided. At least 14 days should separate the use of aspirin, caffeine, and propoxy-phene combination and the use of an MAO inhibitor.
3. Alcohol and anti-inflammatory medication can increase the gastrointestinal side effects of this medication.
4. The aspirin in this product may increase the side effects of anticoagulants (blood thinners, such as warfarin), oral antidiabetic agents, phenytoin, and methotrexate.
5. Large doses of antacids increase the elimination of the aspirin portion of this medication from the body and decrease its effectiveness.
6. The aspirin portion of this medication may decrease the antigout effects of probenecid and sulfinpyrazone.
7. The propoxyphene portion of this medication can decrease the elimination of carbamazepine from the body, which can lead to an increase in side effects.

BE SURE TO TELL YOUR DOCTOR about any medications you are currently taking.

WARNINGS
• Tell your doctor about unusual or allergic reactions you have had to medications, especially to aspirin, methyl salicylate (oil of wintergreen), diclofenac, diflunisal, flurbiprofen, fenoprofen, ibuprofen, indomethacin, ketoprofen, meclofenamate, mefenamic acid, naproxen, piroxicam, sulindac, or tolmetin; to propoxyphene or other narcotic analgesics (such as codeine, hydrocodone, hydromorphone, meperidine, methadone, morphine, and oxycodone); or to caffeine.
• Tell your doctor if you now have or if you have ever had abdominal disease, Addison's disease, bleeding or blood disorders, brain disease, colitis, epilepsy, gallstones or gallbladder disease, head injuries, heart disease, hemophilia, kidney disease, liver disease, lung disease, peptic ulcer, prostate disease, or thyroid disease.

• If this drug makes you dizzy or drowsy, do not take part in any activity that requires alertness, such as driving a car or operating potentially dangerous equipment.

• Before having any surgery or other medical or dental treatment, be sure to tell your doctor or dentist that you are taking this medication. Aspirin-containing medication is usually discontinued five to seven days before surgery, to prevent bleeding complications.

• The use of aspirin in children (about 16 years of age or less) with the flu or chicken pox has been associated with a rare, life-threatening condition called Reye's syndrome. Aspirin-containing products should, therefore, not be given to children with signs of infection.

• Because this drug contains propoxyphene, it has the potential for abuse and must be used with caution. Usually, it should not be taken on a regular schedule for longer than ten days at a time. Tolerance develops quickly; do not increase the dosage or stop taking the drug abruptly, unless you first consult your doctor. If you have been taking large amounts of this medication for long periods, you may experience a withdrawal reaction (muscle aches, diarrhea, gooseflesh, runny nose, nausea, vomiting, shivering, trembling, stomach cramps, sleep disorders, irritability, weakness, excessive yawning, or sweating). Your doctor may, therefore, want to reduce the dosage gradually.

• Because this product contains aspirin, additional medications that contain aspirin should not be taken without your doctor's approval. Check the labels on over-the-counter (nonprescription) pain, sinus, allergy, asthma, cough, and cold products to see if they contain aspirin.

• You should not take more than six capsules of this drug in one day, unless your doctor specifically directs you to take more than six.

• Diabetics should be aware that large doses of aspirin (more than eight 325-mg tablets of aspirin per day) may interfere with urine sugar testing. Diabetics should, therefore, check with their doctor before changing their insulin dose.

• Be sure to tell your doctor if you are pregnant. The effects of this medication during pregnancy have not been thoroughly studied in humans. Propoxyphene, used regularly in large doses during pregnancy, may result in addiction of the fetus, leading to withdrawal symptoms (irritability, excessive crying, tremors, fever, vomiting, diarrhea, sneezing, or excessive yawning) at birth. Large amounts of aspirin taken close to the end of pregnancy may prolong labor and cause bleeding problems in the mother and heart problems in the newborn infant. Also, tell your doctor if you are breast-feeding an infant. Small amounts of this medication may pass into breast milk and cause excessive drowsiness in the nursing infant.

aspirin, caffeine, butalbital, and codeine combination

BRAND NAMES (Manufacturers)
B-A-C #3 (Mayrand)
Fiorinal with Codeine (Sandoz)

TYPE OF DRUG
Analgesic combination and sedative

INGREDIENTS
aspirin, caffeine, butalbital, and codeine

DOSAGE FORMS
Tablets (325 mg aspirin, 40 mg caffeine, 50 mg butalbital, and 30 mg codeine)
Capsules (325 mg aspirin, 40 mg caffeine, 50 mg butalbital, and 7.5 mg, 15 mg, or 30 mg codeine)
Note that on the label of the vial of tablets or capsules the name of this drug is followed by a number. This number refers to the amount of codeine present (#1 contains 7.5 mg codeine, #2 has 15 mg codeine, and #3 contains 30 mg codeine).

STORAGE
Aspirin, caffeine, butalbital, and codeine combination tablets and capsules should be stored at room temperature in tightly closed containers. Moisture causes the aspirin in this product to decompose. Discard the medicine if it has a vinegary odor.

USES
This combination medication is used to relieve tension headaches and mild to moderate pain. Codeine is a narcotic analgesic that acts on the central nervous system (brain and spinal cord) to relieve pain. Butalbital belongs to a group of drugs known as barbiturates. The barbiturates act on the central nervous system to produce relaxation. Caffeine is a central nervous system stimulant. It constricts blood vessels in the head, which may help to relieve headaches.

TREATMENT
In order to avoid stomach upset, you can take this medication with food or milk.

This medication works most effectively if you take it at the onset of pain, rather than waiting until the pain becomes intense.

If you are taking this medication on a regular schedule and you miss a dose, take the missed dose as soon as possible, unless it is almost time for your next dose. In that case, don't take the missed dose at all; just return to your regular dosing schedule. Do not double the next dose.

SIDE EFFECTS
Minor. Constipation, dizziness, drowsiness, flushing, headache, indigestion, loss of appetite, nausea, nervousness, sleep disorders, sweating, tiredness, or vomiting. These side effects should disappear as your body adjusts to the medication.

If you feel dizzy or light-headed, sit or lie down for a while; get up from a sitting or lying position slowly, and be careful on stairs.

If you are constipated, increase the amount of fiber in your diet (fresh fruits and vegetables, salads, bran, and whole-grain breads), drink more water, and exercise (unless your doctor directs you to do otherwise).

Major. Tell your doctor about any side effects that are persistent or particularly bothersome. IT IS ESPECIALLY IMPORTANT TO TELL YOUR DOCTOR about bloody or black, tarry stools; blurred vision; chest tightness; confusion; difficult or painful urination; loss of coordination; palpitations; rash; ringing in the ears; shortness of breath; severe abdominal pain; sore throat and fever; or yellowing of the eyes or skin.

INTERACTIONS

This combination medication interacts with several other types of drugs:

1. Concurrent use of this medication with other central nervous system depressants (such as alcohol, antihistamines, barbiturates, benzodiazepine tranquilizers, muscle relaxants, or phenothiazine tranquilizers) or with tricyclic antidepressants can cause extreme drowsiness.

2. Alcohol and anti-inflammatory medications can increase the gastrointestinal side effects of this medication.

3. The side effects of anticoagulants (blood thinners, such as warfarin), oral antidiabetic agents, phenytoin, and methotrexate may be increased by the aspirin content.

4. Large doses of antacids increase the elimination of the aspirin portion of this medication from the body and decrease its effectiveness.

5. Aspirin may decrease the antigout effects of probenecid and sulfinpyrazone.

6. Butalbital can increase the elimination from the body of oral contraceptives (birth control pills), carbamazepine, adrenocorticosteroids (cortisone-like drugs), digoxin, doxycycline, tricyclic antidepressants, griseofulvin, metronidazole, theophylline, aminophylline, and quinidine, thereby decreasing the effectiveness of these medications.

7. The side effects of cyclophosphamide may be increased by butalbital.

8. This medication may interact with monoamine oxidase (MAO) inhibitors.

BE SURE TO TELL YOUR DOCTOR about any medications you are currently taking, especially any of those listed above.

WARNINGS

• Tell your doctor about unusual or allergic reactions you have had to medications, especially to aspirin, methyl salicylate (oil of wintergreen), diclofenac, diflunisal, flurbiprofen, fenoprofen, ibuprofen, indomethacin, ketoprofen, meclofenamate, mefenamic acid, naproxen, piroxicam, sulindac, or tolmetin; to codeine or other narcotic analgesics (such as hydrocodone, hydromorphone, meperidine, methadone, morphine, oxycodone, and

propoxyphene); to caffeine; or to butalbital or other barbiturates (such as phenobarbital, pentobarbital, and secobarbital).

• Tell your doctor if you now have or if you have ever had abdominal disease, Addison's disease, bleeding or blood disorders, brain disease, colitis, epilepsy, gallstones or gallbladder disease, head injuries, heart disease, hemophilia, kidney disease, liver disease, lung disease, peptic ulcers, porphyria, prostate disease, or thyroid disease.

• If this drug makes you dizzy or drowsy, do not take part in any activity that requires alertness, such as driving a car or operating potentially dangerous equipment.

• Before having surgery or any other medical or dental treatment, be sure to tell your doctor or dentist that you are taking this medication. Aspirin-containing medication is usually discontinued five to seven days before surgery, to prevent bleeding complications.

• The use of aspirin in children (about 16 years of age or less) with the flu or chicken pox has been associated with a rare, life-threatening condition called Reye's syndrome. Aspirin-containing products should, therefore, not be given to children with signs of infection.

• Because this drug contains codeine and butalbital, it has the potential for abuse and must be used with caution. Usually, it should not be taken on a regular schedule for longer than ten days at a time. Tolerance develops quickly; do not increase the dosage or stop taking the drug abruptly, unless you first consult your doctor. If you have been taking large amounts of this medication for long periods, you may experience a withdrawal reaction (muscle aches, diarrhea, gooseflesh, runny nose, nausea, vomiting, shivering, trembling, stomach cramps, sleep disorders, irritability, weakness, excessive yawning, or sweating). Your doctor may, therefore, want to reduce the dosage gradually.

• Because this product contains aspirin, additional medications that contain aspirin should not be taken without your doctor's approval. Check the labels on over-the-counter (nonprescription) pain, sinus, allergy, asthma, cough, and cold products to see if they contain aspirin.

• You should not take more than six tablets or capsules of this drug in one day, unless your doctor specifically directs you to do so.

• Diabetic patients should be aware that large doses of aspirin (more than eight 325-mg tablets or capsules per day) may interfere with urine sugar testing. Diabetics should, therefore, check with their doctor before changing their insulin dose.

• Be sure to tell your doctor if you are pregnant. The effects of this medication during pregnancy have not been thoroughly studied in humans. Codeine and butalbital, used regularly in large doses during pregnancy, may result in addiction of the fetus, leading to withdrawal symptoms (irritability, excessive crying, tremors, fever, vomiting, diarrhea, sneezing, or excessive yawning) at birth. Large amounts of aspirin taken close to the end of pregnancy may prolong labor and cause bleeding problems in the mother and heart problems in the newborn infant. Also, tell your doctor if you are breast-feeding an infant. Small amounts of this medication may pass into breast milk and cause excessive drowsiness in the nursing infant.

aspirin with codeine—see aspirin and codeine combination

---

astemizole

BRAND NAME (Manufacturer)
Hismanal (Janssen)
TYPE OF DRUG
Antihistamine
INGREDIENT
astemizole

DOSAGE FORM
Tablets (10 mg)
STORAGE
Store this medication in a tightly closed container in a cool, dry place, away from heat or direct light, and out of the reach of children.

USES
Astemizole is indicated for the treatment of the allergic symptoms of conditions such as hay fever or hives. It belongs to a group of drugs known as antihistamines, which act by blocking the action of histamine, a chemical that is released by the body during an allergic reaction. It may be useful in patients unable to tolerate side effects, such as sedation, that other antihistamines may produce.

TREATMENT
Astemizole should be taken only as needed, and the prescribed dose should not be exceeded.

Because food significantly impairs the absorption of this medication, the drug should be taken on an empty stomach, at least two hours after a meal. No additional food should be taken for at least an hour after a dose is taken.

It may take up to two days for astemizole to achieve its full therapeutic effect.

SIDE EFFECTS
Minor. Abdominal pain, diarrhea, drowsiness, dry mouth, gas, headache, increased appetite, nervousness, increased sensitivity to sunlight, or weight gain.

To relieve mouth dryness, chew sugarless gum or suck on ice chips or hard candy.
Major. Tell your doctor about any side effects that are persistent or particularly bothersome. It is ESPECIALLY IMPORTANT TO TELL YOUR DOCTOR about symptoms of a hypersensitivity reaction such as shortness of breath or rash.

INTERACTIONS
Although clinical studies with astemizole have not shown significant interactions with central nervous system depressants, such as alcohol or diazepam, it is important to be aware of the possibility of interactions. BE SURE TO TELL YOUR DOCTOR about all medications you are taking before starting astemizole.

WARNINGS
• Tell your doctor about unusual or allergic reactions you have had to any medication, especially to astemizole.
• Although astemizole is a less-sedating antihistamine, some patients may be more sensitive to its effects. Until you are familiar with how astemizole affects you, be especially cautious in performing tasks that require alertness.
• Tell your physician of any known liver ailments. Patients with diseases of the liver may not eliminate astemizole as rapidly as those with normal liver function.
• Be sure to tell your doctor if you are pregnant or plan to become pregnant. The safety of astemizole in pregnant women has not been established. In animal studies in which administered doses of astemizole exceeded dosage levels used in humans, an increased incidence of low birth weight and risk of infant death was noted. Since breakdown products of the drug may remain in the body for up to four months after use, this fact should be taken into consideration if pregnancy is being planned.
• Because babies are more sensitive to the side effects of antihistamines, such as excitement or irritability, astemizole is not recommended in nursing mothers until its effects upon infants are more fully established.

Atarax—see hydroxyzine

atenolol

BRAND NAMES (Manufacturers)
atenolol (various manufacturers)
Tenormin (ICI Pharma)
TYPE OF DRUG
Beta-adrenergic blocking agent
INGREDIENT
atenolol
DOSAGE FORM
Tablets (25 mg, 50 mg, and 100 mg)
STORAGE
Atenolol should be stored at room temperature in a tightly closed, light-resistant container.

USES
Atenolol is used to treat high blood pressure and angina (chest pain). It belongs to a group of medicines known as beta-adrenergic blocking agents or, more commonly, beta blockers. These drugs work by controlling impulses along certain nerve pathways. The result is a decreased workload for the heart.

TREATMENT
Atenolol can be taken with a glass of water, with meals, immediately following meals, or on an empty stomach, depending on your doctor's instructions. Try to take the medication at the same time(s) each day.

Try not to miss any doses of this medication. If you do miss a dose, take the missed dose as soon as possible. However, if the next scheduled dose is within eight hours (if you are taking this medicine only once a day) or within four hours (if you are taking this medicine more than once a day), do not take the missed dose at all; just return to your regular dosing schedule. Do not double the next dose.

It is important to remember that atenolol does not cure high blood pressure, but it will help to control the condition as long as you continue to take it.

SIDE EFFECTS
Minor. Anxiety; constipation; decreased sexual ability; diarrhea; difficulty in sleeping; drowsiness; dryness of the eyes, mouth, and skin; headache; nausea; nervousness; stomach discomfort; tiredness; or weakness. These side effects should disappear as your body adjusts to the medicine.

If you are extra-sensitive to the cold, be sure to dress warmly during cold weather.

To relieve constipation, increase the amount of fiber in your diet (fresh fruits and vegetables, salads, bran, and whole-grain breads), and drink more water (unless your doctor directs you to do otherwise).

Plain, nonmedicated eye drops (artificial tears) may help to relieve eye dryness.

Sucking on ice chips or chewing sugarless gum helps relieve mouth or throat dryness.

Major. Tell your doctor about any side effects that are persistent or particularly bothersome. IT IS ESPECIALLY IMPORTANT TO TELL YOUR DOCTOR about breathing difficulty or wheezing; cold hands or feet (due to decreased blood circulation to skin, fingers, and toes); confusion; dizziness; fever and sore throat; hair loss; hallucinations; light-headedness; mental depression; nightmares; reduced alertness; skin rash; swelling of the ankles, feet, or lower legs; or unusual bleeding or bruising.

INTERACTIONS
Atenolol interacts with a number of other medications:

1. Indomethacin has been shown to decrease the blood-pressure-lowering effects of the beta blockers. This may also happen with aspirin or other salicylates.

2. Concurrent use of beta blockers and calcium channel blockers (diltiazem, nifedipine, and verapamil) or disopyramide can lead to heart failure or very low blood pressure.

3. Cimetidine and oral contraceptives (birth control pills) can increase the side effects of beta blockers.

4. Side effects may also be increased when beta blockers are taken with clonidine, digoxin, epinephrine, phenylephrine, phenylpropanolamine, phenothiazine tranquilizers, prazosin, or monoamine oxidase (MAO) inhibitors. At least 14 days should separate the use of a beta blocker and the use of an MAO inhibitor.

5. Alcohol, barbiturates, and rifampin can decrease the effectiveness of atenolol.

6. Beta blockers may antagonize (work against) the effects of theophylline, aminophylline, albuterol, isoproterenol, metaproterenol, and terbutaline.

7. Beta blockers can also interact with insulin or oral antidiabetic agents—raising or lowering blood sugar levels or masking the symptoms of low blood sugar.

8. The action of beta blockers may be increased if they are used with chlorpromazine, furosemide, or hydralazine, which may have a negative effect.

9. In patients who have congestive heart failure treated with digitalis glycosides (for example, digoxin or digitoxin), caution should be used as both betaxolol and digitalis products may slow heart conduction.

BE SURE TO TELL YOUR DOCTOR about any medications you are currently taking, especially any of those listed above.

WARNINGS
• Before starting to take this medication, it is important to tell your doctor if you have ever had unusual or allergic reactions to any beta blocker (acebutolol, atenolol, betaxolol, carteolol, esmolol, labetalol, metoprolol, nadolol, penbutolol, pindolol, propranolol, and timolol).

• Tell your doctor if you now have or if you have ever had allergies, asthma, hay fever, eczema, slow heartbeat, bronchitis, diabetes mellitus, emphysema, heart or blood vessel disease, kidney disease, liver disease, thyroid disease, or poor circulation in the fingers or toes.

• In diabetics, atenolol may block some of the warning signs of low blood sugar (hypoglycemia), such as rapid pulse rate, but not others, such as dizziness or sweating.

• You may want to check your pulse while taking this medication. If your pulse is much slower than your usual rate (or if it is less than 50 beats per minute), check with your doctor. A pulse rate that is too slow may cause circulation problems.

• Atenolol may affect your body's response to exercise. Make sure you discuss with your doctor a safe amount of exercise for your medical condition.

• It is important that you do not stop taking this medicine without first checking with your doctor. Some conditions may become worse when the medicine is stopped suddenly, and the danger of a heart attack is increased in some patients. Your doctor may want you to gradually reduce the amount of medicine you take before stopping completely. Make sure that you have enough medicine on hand to last through vacations, and holidays.

• Before having surgery or any other medical or dental treatment, tell the physician or dentist that you are taking this medicine. Often, this medication will be discontinued 48 hours prior to any major surgery.

• This medicine can cause dizziness, drowsiness, light-headedness, or decreased alertness. Therefore, exercise caution while driving a car or using any potentially dangerous equipment.

• While taking this medicine, do not use any over-the-counter (nonprescription) asthma, allergy, cough, cold, sinus, or diet preparations unless you first check with your pharmacist or doctor. Some of these medicines can cause high blood pressure when taken at the same time as a beta blocker.

• Be sure to tell your doctor if you are pregnant. Animal studies have shown that some beta blockers can cause problems in pregnancy when used at very high doses. Adequate studies have not been done in humans, but there has been some association between beta blockers used during pregnancy and low birth weight, as well as breathing problems and slow heart rate in the newborn infants. However, other reports have shown no effects on newborn infants. Also, tell your doctor if you are breast-feeding an infant. Small amounts of atenolol may pass into breast milk.

atenolol and chlorthalidone combination

BRAND NAME (Manufacturer)
Tenoretic (ICI Pharma)
TYPE OF DRUG
Beta-adrenergic blocking agent and diuretic
INGREDIENTS
atenolol and chlorthalidone

DOSAGE FORM
Tablets (50 mg atenolol and 25 mg chlorthalidone;
 100 mg atenolol and 25 mg chlorthalidone)
STORAGE
Atenolol and chlorthalidone combination tablets should
be stored at room temperature in a tightly closed, light-resistant container. The tablets should be protected from
moisture during storage.

USES
Atenolol and chlorthalidone combination is prescribed
to treat high blood pressure. Chlorthalidone is a diuretic,
which reduces fluid accumulation in the body by increasing the elimination of salt and water through the
kidneys. Atenolol belongs to a group of medicines known
as beta-adrenergic blocking agents or, more commonly,
beta blockers. They work by controlling impulses along
certain nerve pathways, thereby decreasing the workload
on the heart and lowering blood pressure.

TREATMENT
This medication can be taken with a glass of water, with
meals, immediately following meals, or on an empty
stomach, depending on your doctor's instructions.

Try to take the medication at the same times(s) each
day. Avoid taking a dose after 6:00 P.M.; otherwise, you
may have to get up during the night to urinate.

If you miss a dose of this medication, take the missed
dose as soon as possible, unless it is almost time for your
next dose. In that case, do not take the missed dose at all;
just wait until the next scheduled dose. Do not double
the dose.

Atenolol and chlorthalidone combination does not cure
high blood pressure, but it will help to control the condition as long as you continue to take it.

SIDE EFFECTS
Minor. Anxiety, constipation, cramps, decreased sexual
ability, diarrhea, difficulty in sleeping, dizziness, drowsiness, dryness of the eyes and skin, gas, headache, heartburn, loss of appetite, nervousness, restlessness, stomach
discomfort, sweating, or tiredness. These side effects
should disappear as your body adjusts to the medication.

Chlorthalidone can cause increased sensitivity to sunlight. It is important, therefore, to avoid prolonged exposure to sunlight and sunlamps. Wear protective clothing
and sunglasses, and use an effective sunscreen.

If you become extra-sensitive to the cold, be sure to
dress warmly during cold weather.

Plain, nonmedicated eye drops (artificial tears) may
help to relieve eye dryness.

To relieve constipation, increase the amount of fiber
in your diet (fresh fruits and vegetables, salads, bran, and
whole-grain breads) unless your doctor directs you to do
otherwise.

Sucking on ice chips or chewing sugarless gum helps to
relieve mouth and throat dryness.

To avoid dizziness or light-headedness when you stand
that may be a result of taking atenolol and chorthalidone
combination, contract and relax the muscles of your legs
for a few moments before rising. Do this by alternately
pushing one foot against the floor while raising the other
foot slightly, so that you are "pumping" your legs in a
pedaling motion. This will increase the blood flow
through your body.

Major. Tell your doctor about any side effects that are
persistent or particularly bothersome. IT IS ESPECIALLY
IMPORTANT TO TELL YOUR DOCTOR about blurred
vision, cold hands and feet, confusion, depression, difficulty in breathing, dry mouth, excessive thirst, excessive
weakness, fever, hair loss, hallucinations, itching, joint
pain, mood changes, muscle pain or spasms, nausea,
nightmares, numbness or tingling in the fingers or toes,
palpitations, rapid weight gain (three to five pounds within
a week), reduced alertness, ringing in the ears, skin rash,
sore throat, swelling, unusual bleeding or bruising, vomiting, or yellowing of the eyes or skin.

INTERACTIONS
Atenolol and chlorthalidone combination can interact
with other types of medications:

1. Indomethacin, aspirin, and other salicylates may decrease the blood-pressure-lowering effects of beta blockers.

2. Concurrent use of atenolol and calcium channel blockers (diltiazem, nifedipine, verapamil) or disopyramide
can lead to heart failure or very low blood pressure.

3. Cimetidine can increase blood levels of atenolol, resulting in greater side effects. Side effects may also be increased when atenolol is taken with clonidine, digoxin,
epinephrine, phenylephrine, phenylpropanolamine, phenothiazine tranquilizers, prazosin, reserpine, oral contraceptives (birth control pills), or monoamine oxidase
(MAO) inhibitors. At least 14 days should separate the
use of atenolol and the use of an MAO inhibitor.

4. Atenolol can antagonize (act against) the effects of
theophylline, aminophylline, albuterol, isoproterenol,
metaproterenol, and terbutaline.

5. Alcohol, barbiturates, and rifampin can decrease blood
levels of beta blockers, resulting in decreased effectiveness.

6. The action of beta blockers may be increased if they
are used with chlorpromazine, furosemide, or hydralazine,
which may have a negative effect.

7. Atenolol and chlorthalidone can interact with insulin
and oral antidiabetic agents—raising or lowering blood
sugar levels and masking the symptoms of low blood
sugar.

8. Chlorthalidone can decrease the effectiveness of oral
anticoagulants (blood thinners, such as warfarin), antigout
medications, and methenamine.

9. Fenfluramine may increase the blood-pressure-lowering effects of this drug, which can be dangerous.

10. Cholestyramine and colestipol can decrease the absorption of chlorthalidone from the gastrointestinal tract.
Chlorthalidone should, therefore, be taken one hour before or four hours after a dose of cholestyramine or
colestipol (if you have also been prescribed one of these
medications).

11. Chlorthalidone may increase the side effects of amphotericin B, calcium supplements, cortisone-like steroids
(such as cortisone, dexamethasone, hydrocortisone, prednisone, and prednisolone), digoxin, digitalis, lithium,
quinidine, sulfonamide antibiotics, and vitamin D.

BE SURE TO TELL YOUR DOCTOR about all of the medications you are currently taking, especially any of the ones listed above.

WARNINGS

• Tell your doctor about unusual or allergic reactions you have had to medications, especially to atenolol or any other beta blocker (acebutolol, betaxolol, carteolol, esmolol, labetalol, metoprolol, nadolol, penbutolol, pindolol, propranolol, and timolol), to chlorthalidone or other diuretics (such as bendroflumethiazide, benzthiazide, chlorothiazide, cyclothiazide, hydrochlorothiazide, hydroflumethiazide, methyclothiazide, metolozone, polythiazide, quinethazone, trichlormethiazide, and furosemide), or to any sulfa drug, including oral antidiabetic medications and sulfonamide antibiotics.

• Tell your doctor if you now have or if you have ever had asthma, diabetes mellitus, heart disease, gout, kidney disease or problems with urination, liver disease, lung disease, pancreatitis, poor circulation in the fingers or toes, systemic lupus erythematosus, or thyroid disease.

• Chlorthalidone can cause potassium loss. Signs of potassium loss include dry mouth, thirst, weakness, muscle pain or cramps, nausea, and vomiting. If you experience any of these symptoms, call your doctor. To help prevent this problem, your doctor may have blood tests performed periodically to monitor your potassium levels. To help avoid potassium loss, take this medication with a glass of fresh or frozen orange juice or cranberry juice, or eat a banana every day. The use of a salt substitute also helps to prevent potassium loss. Do not change your diet, until you discuss it with your doctor. Too much potassium may also be dangerous.

• While taking this medication, limit your intake of alcohol in order to prevent dizziness and light-headedness.

• Do not take any over-the-counter (nonprescription) medications for weight control or for allergy, asthma, cough, cold, or sinus problems unless you first check with your doctor.

• To prevent severe water loss (dehydration) while taking this medication, check with your doctor if you have any illness that causes severe or continuous nausea, vomiting, or diarrhea.

• This medication can raise blood sugar levels in diabetic patients. Blood sugar should be monitored carefully with blood or urine tests when this medication is being taken.

• You may want to check your pulse while taking this medication. If your pulse is much slower than your usual rate (or if it is less than 50 beats per minute), check with your doctor; a pulse rate that slow may cause circulation problems.

• Atenolol can affect your body's response to exercise. Make sure that you ask your doctor what an appropriate amount of exercise would be for you, taking into account your medical condition.

• Before having surgery or any other medical or dental treatment, tell your doctor or dentist that you are taking this medicine. Often, this medication will be discontinued 48 hours prior to any major surgery.

• This medication can cause dizziness, drowsiness, light-headedness, or decreased alertness. Therefore, exercise caution whenever driving a car or operating potentially dangerous equipment.

• A doctor does not usually prescribe a "fixed-dose" drug like this as the first choice in the treatment of high blood pressure. Usually the patient first receives each ingredient singly. If there is an adequate response to the fixed dose contained in this product, it can then be substituted. The advantage of a combination product is increased convenience and (often) decreased cost.

• It is important that you do not stop taking this medicine unless you first check with your doctor. Some conditions worsen when this medicine is stopped suddenly, and the danger of a heart attack is increased in some patients. Your doctor may, therefore, want you to gradually reduce the amount of medicine you take before stopping completely. Make sure that you have enough medicine on hand to last through vacations, holidays, and weekends.

• Be sure to tell your doctor if you are pregnant. Animal studies have shown that some beta blockers can cause problems in pregnancy when used at very high doses. Studies have not been conducted in humans, but there has been some association between use of beta blockers during pregnancy and low birth weight, as well as breathing problems and slow heart rate in newborn infants. However, other reports have shown no effects on newborn infants. Also, tell your doctor if you are breast-feeding an infant. Although problems in humans have not been reported, small amounts of this medication may pass into breast milk, so caution is warranted.

Ativan—see lorazepam

Atromid-S—see clofibrate

---

atropine, scopolamine, hyoscyamine, and phenobarbital combination

BRAND NAMES (Manufacturers)
Barophen (various manufacturers)
belladonna alkaloids with phenobarbital (various manufacturers)
Donnamor (H.L. Moore)
Donna-Sed (Vortech)
Donnatal (Robins)
Hyosophen (Rugby)
Kinesed (Stuart)
Malatal (Mallard)
Relaxadon (Geneva Generics)
Spasmolin (various manufacturers)
Spasmophen (Lannett)
Spasquid (Geneva Generics)
Susano (Halsey)

TYPE OF DRUG
Anticholinergic and sedative

INGREDIENTS
atropine, scopolamine, hyoscyamine, and phenobarbital

DOSAGE FORMS
Tablets (0.0194 mg atropine, 0.0065 mg scopolamine, 0.1037 mg hyoscyamine, and 16.2 mg phenobarbital)
Capsules (0.0194 mg atropine, 0.0065 mg scopolamine, 0.1037 mg hyoscyamine, and 16.2 mg phenobarbital)
Oral elixir (0.0194 mg atropine, 0.0065 mg scopolamine, 0.1037 mg hyoscyamine, and 16.2 mg phenobarbital, with 23% alcohol)

STORAGE
The medication should be stored at room temperature (never frozen) in a tightly closed, light-resistant container.

USES
Atropine, scopolamine, hyoscyamine, and phenobarbital combination is used to treat stomach and intestinal disorders, motion sickness, lack of bladder control, and premenstrual tension.

Atropine, scopolamine, and hyoscyamine belong to a group of drugs known as belladonna alkaloids or anticholinergic agents. These drugs block certain nerve pathways, thereby slowing the gastrointestinal tract and decreasing urination. Phenobarbital is a sedative that acts directly on the brain to slow the activity of the nervous system.

TREATMENT
Take this medication 30 minutes to one hour before meals (unless your doctor says otherwise). To reduce stomach upset, take it with food or with a glass of water or milk.

At least one hour should separate doses of this medication combination and either antacids or antidiarrheal medications—they may prevent gastrointestinal absorption of this drug.

Measure the liquid form of this medication carefully with a specially designed 5-ml measuring spoon. An ordinary kitchen teaspoon is not accurate enough.

If you miss a dose, don't take the missed dose; just return to your regular dosing schedule. Don't double the next dose.

SIDE EFFECTS
Minor. Confusion; constipation; decreased sexual desire; dizziness; drowsiness; dry mouth, nose, and throat; headache; insomnia; loss of taste; muscle pain; nausea; nervousness; reduced sweating; sensitivity of eyes to sunlight; vomiting; or weakness. These side effects should disappear as your body adjusts to the medication.

If you are constipated, increase the amount of fiber in your diet (fresh fruits and vegetables, salads, bran, and whole-grain breads), exercise, and drink more water (unless your doctor directs you to do otherwise).

Chew sugarless gum or suck on ice chips or a piece of hard candy to reduce mouth dryness.

Wear sunglasses if your eyes become sensitive to light.

To avoid dizziness or light-headedness when you stand, contract and relax the muscles of your legs for a few moments before rising. Do this by pushing one foot against the floor while raising the other foot slightly, alternating feet so that you are "pumping" your legs in a pedaling motion.

Major. Tell your doctor about any side effects that are persistent or particularly bothersome. IT IS ESPECIALLY IMPORTANT TO TELL YOUR DOCTOR about blurred vision, difficulty in breathing, difficulty in urinating, hallucinations, hot and dry skin, palpitations, rash, slurred speech, sore throat, or yellowing of the eyes or skin.

INTERACTIONS
Atropine, scopolamine, hyoscyamine, and phenobarbital combination interacts with several other types of drugs:
1. This medication can cause extreme drowsiness when combined with central nervous system depressants (such as alcohol, antihistamines, barbiturates, benzodiazepine tranquilizers, muscle relaxants, narcotics, and pain medications) or with tricyclic antidepressants.
2. Amantadine, antihistamines, haloperidol, monoamine oxidase (MAO) inhibitors, phenothiazine tranquilizers, procainamide, quinidine, and tricyclic antidepressants can increase the side effects of the belladonna alkaloids. At least 14 days should separate the use of this drug and the use of an MAO inhibitor.
3. The phenobarbital content in this drug can decrease the effectiveness of oral anticoagulants (blood thinners, such as warfarin), cortisone-like medications, digoxin, griseofulvin, doxycycline, metronidazole, phenytoin, and tricyclic antidepressants.

WARNINGS
• Tell your doctor about unusual or allergic reactions you have had to any medications, especially to atropine, scopolamine, hyoscyamine, phenobarbital, or to other barbiturates (such as butalbital, primidone, pentobarbital, and secobarbital).
• Tell your doctor if you now have or if you have ever had glaucoma, heart disease, hiatal hernia, high blood pressure, internal bleeding, kidney disease, liver disease, lung disease, myasthenia gravis, porphyria, enlarged prostate gland, obstructed bladder, obstructed intestine, ulcerative colitis, or thyroid disease.
• If this medication makes you dizzy or drowsy or blurs your vision, do not take part in any activity that requires alertness, such as driving a car or operating potentially dangerous equipment. Be careful on stairs, and avoid getting up from a lying or sitting position suddenly.
• This medication can decrease sweating and heat release from the body. Avoid strenuous exercise in hot weather, and avoid taking hot baths, showers, and saunas.
• Before having surgery or any other medical or dental treatment, tell the doctor or dentist that you are taking this drug.
• Be sure to tell your doctor if you are pregnant. This medication crosses the placenta. Phenobarbital given to the mother close to term can cause breathing problems and bleeding complications in the newborn infant. Also, tell your doctor if you are breast-feeding an infant. Small amounts of this medication pass into breast milk and may cause excessive drowsiness or irritability in the nursing infant.

Augmentin—see amoxicillin and clavulanic acid combination

Auralgan—see antipyrene, benzocaine, oxyquinoline, and glycerin combination

auranofin

BRAND NAME (Manufacturer)
Ridaura (Smith Kline & French)
TYPE OF DRUG
Antirheumatic
INGREDIENT
auranofin
DOSAGE FORM
Capsules (3 mg)
STORAGE
Auranofin should be stored at room temperature in a tightly closed container.

USES

Auranofin is a gold compound used to treat active rheumatoid arthritis. It is unclear how auranofin works to relieve the symptoms of rheumatoid arthritis.

TREATMENT

Auranofin can be taken either on an empty stomach or with food or milk (as directed by your doctor). It can be taken along with other antirheumatic medications.

The full effects of auranofin for the control of arthritis symptoms may not become apparent for several months. It is important to continue taking this medication until your doctor instructs you to do otherwise.

Auranofin is generally reserved for arthritis patients who have not responded to or did not tolerate other medications. It should be used in conjunction with, not in place of, a total treatment program, which can include diet, exercise, rest, and heat treatments.

If you miss a dose of this drug, take the missed dose as soon as possible, unless it is almost time for the next dose. In that case, don't take the missed dose at all; just wait until the next scheduled dose.

SIDE EFFECTS

Minor. Abdominal cramps, constipation, diarrhea, gas, heartburn, loss of appetite, nausea, or vomiting. As your body adjusts to auranofin, these effects should disappear.

To relieve constipation, increase the amount of fiber in your diet (fresh fruits and vegetables, salads, bran, and whole-grain breads), exercise, and drink more water (unless your doctor directs you to do otherwise).
Major. Tell your doctor about any side effects that are persistent or particularly bothersome. IT IS ESPECIALLY IMPORTANT TO TELL YOUR DOCTOR about black or tarry stools, blood in the urine, fever, gingivitis (inflammation of the gums), hair loss, itching, metallic taste, mouth sores, persistent diarrhea, rash, shortness of breath, sore throat, tingling or pain in the fingers or toes, tongue sores, unusual bleeding or bruising, or yellowing of the skin or eyes.

INTERACTIONS

Auranofin can increase the blood concentration of phenytoin, which can increase the risk of side effects.

Before taking auranofin, BE SURE TO TELL YOUR DOCTOR about any medications that you are currently taking. It is especially important to tell your doctor if you are taking phenytoin.

WARNINGS

• Tell your doctor about any unusual or allergic reactions you have had to any medications, especially to auranofin or injectable gold compounds (aurothioglucose or gold sodium thioglucose).
• Before taking auranofin, be sure to tell your doctor if you now have or if you have ever had blood disorders, bone marrow disease, heart disease, inflammatory bowel disease (ulcerative colitis or Crohn's disease), kidney disease, liver disease, or rash.
• Regular blood and urine tests should be performed to assess possible side effects of auranofin. It is important for you to keep all your scheduled appointments.
• Tell your doctor if you are pregnant. Complete studies in pregnant women have not yet been performed. However, birth defects have occurred in the offspring of pregnant animals that have been given large doses of auranofin. Also, tell your doctor if you are breast-feeding an infant. It is not yet known if auranofin passes into human breast milk, but it has been shown that this drug passes into the milk of animals.

Auromid—see antipyrine, benzocaine, oxyquinoline, and glycerin combination

Auroto Otic—see antipyrine, benzocaine, oxyquinoline, and glycerin combination

Aventyl—see nortriptyline

Azaline—see sulfasalazine

azatadine

BRAND NAME (Manufacturer)
Optimine (Schering)
TYPE OF DRUG
Antihistamine
INGREDIENT
azatadine
DOSAGE FORM
Tablets (1 mg)
STORAGE
Store at room temperature in a tightly closed container.

USES

This medication belongs to a group of drugs known as antihistamines (antihistamines block the action of histamine, a chemical released by the body during an allergic reaction). It is, therefore, used to treat or prevent symptoms of allergy.

TREATMENT

To avoid stomach upset, you can take azatadine with food or with a full glass of milk or water (unless your doctor directs you to do otherwise).

If you miss a dose of this drug, take the missed dose as soon as possible, unless it is almost time for your next dose. In that case, don't take the missed dose at all; just return to your regular dosing schedule.

SIDE EFFECTS

Minor. Confusion; constipation; diarrhea; difficult or painful urination; dizziness; dry mouth, throat, or nose; headache; irritability; loss of appetite; nausea; restlessness; ringing or buzzing in the ears; stomach upset; or unusual increase in sweating. These side effects should disappear as your body adjusts to the medication.

This medication can cause increased sensitivity to sunlight. Avoid prolonged exposure to sunlight and sunlamps. Wear protective clothing and use an effective sunscreen.

If you are constipated, increase the amount of fiber in your diet (fresh fruits and vegetables, salads, bran, and whole-grain breads), exercise, and drink more water (unless your doctor tells you not to do so).

Chew sugarless gum or suck on ice chips or a piece of hard candy to reduce mouth dryness.

If you feel dizzy or light-headed, sit or lie down for a while; get up from a sitting or lying position slowly, and be careful on stairs.

Major. Be sure to tell your doctor about any side effects that are persistent or particularly bothersome. IT IS ESPECIALLY IMPORTANT TO TELL YOUR DOCTOR about the following effects: blurred vision, change in menstruation, clumsiness, feeling faint, fever, flushing of the face, hallucinations, palpitations, rash, sleeping disorders, seizures, shortness of breath, sore throat, tightness in the chest, unusual bleeding or bruising, or unusual tiredness.

INTERACTIONS

Azatadine interacts with other types of medications:

1. Concurrent use of it with other central nervous system depressants (such as alcohol, barbiturates, benzodiazepine tranquilizers, muscle relaxants, narcotics, pain medications, and phenothiazine tranquilizers) or with tricyclic antidepressants can cause extreme drowsiness.

2. Monoamine oxidase (MAO) inhibitors (isocarboxazid, pargyline, phenelzine, and tranylcypromine) can increase the side effects of this medication. At least 14 days should separate use of this drug and use of an MAO inhibitor.

3. Azatadine can also decrease the activity of oral anticoagulants (blood thinners, such as warfarin).

BE SURE TO TELL YOUR DOCTOR about any medications you are currently taking, especially any listed above.

WARNINGS

• Tell your doctor about unusual or allergic reactions you have had to medications, especially to azatadine or any other antihistamine (brompheniramine, carbinoxamine, chlorpheniramine, clemastine, cyproheptadine, dexchlorpheniramine, dimenhydrinate, dimethindene, diphenhydramine, diphenylpyraline, doxylamine, hydroxyzine, promethazine, pyrilamine, trimeprazine, tripelennamine, and triprolidine).

• Tell your doctor if you now have or if you have ever had asthma, blood vessel disease, glaucoma, high blood pressure, kidney disease, peptic ulcers, enlarged prostate gland, or thyroid disease.

• Azatadine can cause drowsiness or dizziness. Your ability to perform tasks that require alertness, such as driving a car or operating potentially dangerous equipment, may be decreased. Appropriate caution should, therefore, be taken.

• Be sure to tell your doctor if you are pregnant. The effects of this medication during pregnancy have not been thoroughly studied in humans. Also, tell your doctor if you are breast-feeding an infant. Small amounts of azatadine pass into breast milk and may cause unusual excitement or irritability in nursing infants.

azathioprine

BRAND NAME (Manufacturer)
Imuran (Burroughs Wellcome)
TYPE OF DRUG
Immunosuppressant
INGREDIENT
azathioprine
DOSAGE FORM
Tablets (50 mg)
STORAGE
Azathioprine should be stored at room temperature in a tightly closed, light-resistant container.

USES

This medication is used to prevent rejection of kidney transplants and to control the symptoms of severe rheumatoid arthritis. It is not clear exactly how azathioprine works, but it is known to act on the body's immune system.

TREATMENT

In order to prevent nausea and vomiting, you can take azathioprine with food or after a meal (unless your doctor directs you to do otherwise).

Try not to miss any doses of this medication. If you do miss a dose, take the missed dose as soon as possible, unless it is almost time for the next scheduled dose. In that case, do not take the missed dose at all; just return to your regular dosing schedule. Do not double the next dose. If you miss more than one dose, CHECK WITH YOUR DOCTOR.

SIDE EFFECTS

Minor. Diarrhea, nausea, or vomiting. These side effects should disappear over time and as your body adjusts to the medication.

Major. Tell your doctor about any side effects that are persistent or particularly bothersome. IT IS ESPECIALLY IMPORTANT TO TELL YOUR DOCTOR about darkened urine, fever, hair loss, joint pains, mouth sores, muscle aches, skin rash, sore throat, unusual bleeding or bruising, or yellowing of the eyes or skin.

INTERACTIONS

BE SURE TO TELL YOUR DOCTOR if you are already taking allopurinol. This medication can possibly increase the blood levels of azathioprine, which can lead to serious side effects.

WARNINGS

• Be sure to tell your doctor about any unusual or allergic reactions that you have had to any medications, especially to those you may have experienced after taking azathioprine.

• Before starting to take this medication, be sure to tell your doctor if you now have or if you have ever had gout, kidney disease, liver disease, pancreatitis, or recurrent infections.

• Azathioprine is potent medicine. Your doctor will want to monitor your therapy carefully with blood tests, so that you take the least amount of the drug possible.

• Do not stop taking this medication unless you first check with your doctor. Stopping therapy with this drug abruptly may lead to a worsening of your condition. Your doctor may, therefore, want to start you on another drug before therapy with azathioprine is stopped.

• There is a chance that azathioprine may cause unwanted effects months or years later. These delayed effects may include certain types of cancer. Be sure to discuss these possible effects with your doctor.

• Azathioprine can increase your susceptibility to infections. It is, therefore, important to contact your doctor at the first sign of infection. Your dose of azathioprine may need to be adjusted.

• Be sure to tell your doctor if you are pregnant. Birth defects have been reported in the offspring of animals that received large doses of azathioprine during pregnancy. This drug also has the potential for producing birth defects in human offspring. Use of this drug is not recommended during pregnancy. There is a possibility that birth defects may occur in the offspring if either the male or female is using this drug at the time of conception. Use of birth control is recommended while taking this drug. Also, tell your doctor if you are breast-feeding an infant. It is not known whether azathioprine passes into breast milk.

azithromycin

BRAND NAME (Manufacturer)
Zithromax (Pfizer)
TYPE OF DRUG
Antibiotic
INGREDIENT
azithromycin
DOSAGE FORM
Capsules (250 mg)
STORAGE
This product should be stored at room temperature in a closed, light-resistant container.

USES

Azithromycin is used to treat a wide variety of bacterial infections, including those of the upper and lower respiratory tracts and skin and certain sexually transmitted diseases. This medicine acts by preventing bacteria from manufacturing protein and thereby preventing their growth. Azithromycin kills certain bacteria but is not effective against viruses, parasites, or fungi.

TREATMENT

It is best to take azithromycin on an empty stomach (one hour before and two hours after a meal). Azithromycin works best when the level of medicine in your bloodstream is kept constant. Therefore, it is best to take the doses at the same time every day.

If you miss a dose, take it immediately. However, if you don't remember to take your scheduled dose until the next day, skip the missed dose and go back to your regular dosing schedule. Do not double the next dose.

It is important to continue to take this medicine for the entire time period prescribed by the doctor (usually five days), even if the symptoms disappear before the end of that period. If you stop taking this drug too soon, resistant bacteria (bacteria that will not be killed by the antibiotic) are given a chance to continue to grow and infection could recur.

SIDE EFFECTS

Minor. Diarrhea, nausea, vomiting, headache, dizziness, abdominal pain. These effects should disappear as your body adjusts to the medication.

This medication can cause increased sensitivity to sunlight. It is important to avoid prolonged exposure to sunlight and sunlamps. Wear protective clothing and use an effective sunscreen.

If you feel dizzy or light-headed, sit or lie down for a while; get up slowly from a sitting or reclining position, and be careful on stairs.

Major. Tell your doctor about any side effects that are persistent or particularly bothersome. IT IS ESPECIALLY IMPORTANT TO TELL YOUR DOCTOR about fever, palpitations, rash, shortness of breath, swelling of the face or neck, sore throat, rectal or vaginal itching, unusual bruising or bleeding, or yellowing of the eyes or skin. Also, if your symptoms of infection seem to be getting worse rather than improving, you should contact your doctor.

INTERACTIONS

Azithromycin interacts with several medications:
1. Azithromycin potentially can increase blood levels of aminophylline, theophylline, carbamazepine, cyclosporin, phenytoin, digoxin, triazolam, phenobarbital, ergotamine, dihydroergotamine, or oral anticoagulants (blood thinners, such as warfarin); this may lead to serious side effects.
2. Antacids containing aluminum and magnesium will decrease the efficacy of azithromycin. Take antacids one hour before, or two hours after your dose of azithromycin.

BE SURE TO TELL YOUR DOCTOR about any medications you are currently taking, especially any listed above.

WARNINGS

• Tell your doctor about any unusual reactions you have to any medications, especially to azithromycin, erythromycin, or clarithromycin.

• Tell you doctor if you have or ever had kidney disease, liver disease, or heart disease.

• This medication has been prescribed for your current infection only. Another infection later on, or one that someone else has, may require a different medicine. You should not give your medication to other people or use it for other infections, unless your doctor specifically directs you to do so.

• Before having surgery or any other medical or dental treatment, be sure to tell your doctor or dentist you are taking azithromycin.

• Be sure to tell your doctor if you are pregnant. The effects of this medicine during pregnancy have not been thoroughly studied in humans. Also, tell your doctor if you are breast-feeding an infant. It is not known if azithromycin passes into breast milk.

Azo Gantanol—see sulfamethoxazole and phenazopyridine combination

Azo Gantrisin—see sulfisoxazole and phenazopyridine combination

Azo-Standard—see phenazopyridine

Azo-Sulfisoxazole—see sulfisoxazole and phenazopyridine combination

AZT—see zidovudine

Azulfidine—see sulfasalazine

Azulfidine EN-tabs—see sulfasalazine

B-A-C—see aspirin, caffeine, and butalbital combination

B-A-C #3—see aspirin, caffeine, butalbital, and codeine combination

---

baclofen

BRAND NAME (Manufacturer)
Lioresal (Geigy)
TYPE OF DRUG
Muscle relaxant
INGREDIENT
baclofen
DOSAGE FORM
Tablets (10 mg and 20 mg)
STORAGE
Baclofen should be stored at room temperature in a tightly closed container.

USES

This medication is used to relieve muscle spasms. It is unclear exactly how baclofen works to relieve spasticity, but it is known that the drug acts on the central nervous system (brain and spinal cord).

TREATMENT

Baclofen can be taken either on an empty stomach or with food or a full glass of milk or water.

If you miss a dose of this medication and remember within an hour, take the missed dose immediately. If more than an hour has passed, do not take the missed dose at all; just return to your regular dosing schedule. Do not double the next dose.

SIDE EFFECTS

Minor. Abdominal pain, constipation, diarrhea, dizziness, drowsiness, dry mouth, fatigue, headache, insomnia, loss of appetite, nasal congestion, vomiting, or weight gain. These side effects should disappear as your body adjusts to the medication.

To relieve constipation, increase the amount of fiber in your diet (fresh fruits and vegetables, salads, bran, and whole-grain breads), exercise, and drink more water (unless your doctor directs you to do otherwise).

If you feel dizzy, sit or lie down for a while; get up slowly from a sitting or lying position, and be careful on stairs.

To relieve mouth dryness, chew sugarless gum or suck on ice chips or a piece of hard candy.

Major. Tell your doctor about any side effects that are persistent or particularly bothersome. IT IS ESPECIALLY IMPORTANT TO TELL YOUR DOCTOR about chest pain, confusion, convulsions, depression, fainting, false sense of well-being, hallucinations, muscle pain, palpitations, ringing in the ears, slurred speech, tremors, or visual disturbances.

INTERACTIONS

Concurrent use of baclofen with other central nervous system depressants (such as alcohol, antihistamines, barbiturates, benzodiazepine tranquilizers, muscle relaxants, narcotics, pain medications, phenothiazine tranquilizers, and sleeping medicines) or with tricyclic antidepressants can lead to extreme drowsiness.

BE SURE TO TELL YOUR DOCTOR about any medications you are currently taking, especially any listed above.

WARNINGS

• Be sure to tell your doctor about any unusual or allergic reactions you have had to any drugs, especially to baclofen.

• Before starting to take baclofen, be sure to tell your doctor if you now have or if you have ever had diabetes mellitus, epilepsy, kidney disease, mental disorders, or a stroke.

• If this drug makes you dizzy or drowsy, avoid taking part in any activity that requires alertness, such as driving a car.

• Do not stop taking this medication unless you have first checked with your doctor. Stopping therapy with this medication abruptly can lead to hallucinations, nervousness, convulsions, and mood changes. Your doctor may, therefore, want to reduce your dosage of this medication gradually.

• Be sure to tell your doctor if you are pregnant. Although baclofen appears to be safe in humans, birth defects have been reported in the offspring of animals that received large doses of this drug during pregnancy. Also, tell your doctor if you are breast-feeding an infant. It is not known whether baclofen passes into breast milk.

Bactine Hydrocortisone—see hydrocortisone (topical)

Bactocill—see oxacillin

Bactrim—see sulfamethoxazole and trimethoprim combination

Bactrim DS—see sulfamethoxazole and trimethoprim combination

Bancap HC—see acetaminophen and hydrocodone combination

Banex-LA—see phenylpropanolamine and guaifenesin combination

Barbita—see phenobarbital

Baridium—see phenazopyridine

Barophen—see atropine, scopolamine, hyoscyamine, and phenobarbital combination

Bayer—see aspirin

Bayer Children's—see aspirin

Beepen-VK—see penicillin VK

Belix—see diphenhydramine

belladonna alkaloids with phenobarbital—see atropine, scopolamine, hyoscyamine, and phenobarbital combination

Benadryl—see diphenhydramine

Benadryl Kapseals—see diphenhydramine

Benemid—see probenecid

Bentyl—see dicyclomine

Benylin Cough Syrup—see diphenhydramine

bendroflumethiazide

BRAND NAME (Manufacturer)
Naturetin (Princeton)
TYPE OF DRUG
Diuretic and antihypertensive
INGREDIENT
bendroflumethiazide
DOSAGE FORM
Tablets (5 mg and 10 mg)
STORAGE
This medication should be stored at room temperature in a tightly closed container.

USES
Bendroflumethiazide is prescribed to treat high blood pressure. It is also used to reduce fluid accumulation in the body caused by conditions such as heart failure, cirrhosis of the liver, kidney disease, and the long-term use of some medications. This medication reduces fluid accumulation by increasing the elimination of salt and water through the kidneys.

TREATMENT
To decrease stomach irritation, you can take this medication with a glass of milk or with a meal (unless your doctor directs you to do otherwise). Try to take it at the same time every day. Avoid taking a dose after 6:00 P.M.; otherwise, you may have to get up during the night to urinate.

If you miss a dose of this medication, take the missed dose as soon as possible, unless it is almost time for the next dose. In that case, do not take the missed dose at all; just wait until the next scheduled dose. Do not double the dose.

This medication does not cure high blood pressure, but it will help to control the condition as long as you continue to take it.

SIDE EFFECTS
Minor. Constipation, cramps, diarrhea, dizziness, drowsiness, headache, heartburn, loss of appetite, restlessness, or upset stomach. As your body adjusts to the medication, these side effects should disappear.

This medication can cause increased sensitivity to sunlight. It is, therefore, important to avoid prolonged exposure to sunlight and sunlamps. Wear protective clothing and use an effective sunscreen.

To relieve constipation, increase the amount of fiber in your diet (fresh fruits and vegetables, salads, bran, and whole-grain breads) and exercise more (unless your doctor directs you to do otherwise).

To avoid dizziness or light-headedness when you stand, contract and relax the muscles of your legs for a few moments before rising. Do this by pushing one foot against the floor while raising the other foot slightly, alternating feet so that you are "pumping" your legs in a pedaling motion.

Major. Tell your doctor about any side effects that are persistent or particularly bothersome. IT IS ESPECIALLY IMPORTANT TO TELL YOUR DOCTOR about blurred vision, confusion, difficulty in breathing, dry mouth, excessive thirst, excessive weakness, fever, itching, joint pain, mood changes, muscle pain or spasms, nausea, palpitations, skin rash, sore throat, tingling in the fingers or toes, unusual bleeding or bruising, vomiting, or yellowing of the eyes or skin.

INTERACTIONS
This drug interacts with several other drugs:
1. It may decrease the effectiveness of oral anticoagulants, antigout medications, insulin, oral antidiabetic medicines, and methenamine.
2. Fenfluramine can increase the blood-pressure-lowering effects of bendroflumethiazide (which can be dangerous).
3. Indomethacin can decrease the blood-pressure-lowering effects of bendroflumethiazide, thereby counteracting the desired effects.

4. Cholestyramine and colestipol decrease the absorption of this medication from the gastrointestinal tract. Bendroflumethiazide should, therefore, be taken one hour before or four hours after a dose of cholestyramine or colestipol (if you have also been prescribed one of these medications).

5. The side effects of amphotericin B, calcium, cortisone-like steroids (such as cortisone, dexamethasone, hydrocortisone, prednisone, and prednisolone), digoxin, digitalis, lithium, quinidine, sulfonamide antibiotics, and vitamin D may be increased by bendroflumethiazide.

BE SURE TO TELL YOUR DOCTOR about any medications you are currently taking, especially any of those listed above.

WARNINGS

•Tell your doctor about unusual or allergic reactions you have had to any medications, especially to diuretics or any other sulfa drugs, including oral antidiabetic medications or sulfonamide antibiotics.

•Before you start taking bendroflumethiazide, tell your doctor if you now have or if you have ever had kidney disease or problems with urination, diabetes mellitus, gout, liver disease, asthma, pancreatic disease, or systemic lupus erythematosus.

•Bendroflumethiazide can cause potassium loss. Signs of potassium loss include dry mouth, thirst, weakness, muscle pain or cramps, nausea, and vomiting. If you experience any of these symptoms, call your doctor. To help avoid potassium loss, take this drug with a glass of fresh or frozen orange juice or cranberry juice, or eat a banana every day. The use of a salt substitute also helps to prevent potassium loss. Do not change your diet or use a salt substitute, however, before discussing it with your doctor. Too much potassium can also be dangerous. Your doctor may want you to have blood tests performed periodically in order to monitor your potassium levels.

•Limit your intake of alcoholic beverages while taking this medication, in order to prevent dizziness and light-headedness.

•If you have high blood pressure, do not take any over-the-counter (nonprescription) medications for weight control or for allergy, asthma, cough, cold, or sinus problems unless your doctor directs you to do so.

•To prevent dehydration (severe water loss) while taking this medication, check with your doctor if you have any illness that causes severe or continuous nausea, vomiting, or diarrhea.

•This medication can raise blood sugar in diabetic patients. Therefore, blood sugar levels should be carefully monitored by blood or urine tests when this medication is being taken.

•This product contains the color additive FD&C Yellow No. 5 (tartrazine), which can cause allergic-type reactions (rash, fainting, difficulty in breathing) in certain susceptible individuals.

•Be sure to tell your doctor if you are pregnant. Bendroflumethiazide can cross the placenta and may cause adverse effects in the developing fetus. Also, tell your doctor if you are breast-feeding an infant. Although problems in humans have not been reported, small amounts of this drug can pass into breast milk, so caution is warranted.

benzthiazide

BRAND NAMES (Manufacturers)
benzthiazide (various manufacturers)
Exna (Robins)
Hydrex (Trimen)
TYPE OF DRUG
Diuretic and antihypertensive
INGREDIENT
benzthiazide
DOSAGE FORM
Tablets (50 mg)
STORAGE
This medication should be stored at room temperature in a tightly closed container.

USES

Benzthiazide is prescribed to treat high blood pressure. It is also used to reduce fluid accumulation in the body caused by conditions such as heart failure, cirrhosis of the liver, kidney disease, and the long-term use of some medications. This medication reduces fluid accumulation by increasing the elimination of sodium and water through the kidneys.

TREATMENT

To decrease stomach irritation, you can take this medication with a glass of milk or with a meal (unless your doctor directs you to do otherwise). Try to take it at the same time every day. Avoid taking a dose after 6:00 P.M.; otherwise, you may have to get up during the night to urinate.

If you miss a dose of this medication, take the missed dose as soon as possible, unless it is almost time for the next dose. In that case, do not take the missed dose at all; just wait until the next scheduled dose. Do not double the next dose.

This medication does not cure high blood pressure, but it will help to control the condition as long as you continue to take it.

SIDE EFFECTS

Minor. Constipation, cramps, diarrhea, dizziness, drowsiness, headache, heartburn, loss of appetite, restlessness, or upset stomach. These side effects should disappear as your body adjusts to the medication.

This medication can cause increased sensitivity to sunlight. It is, therefore, important to avoid prolonged exposure to sunlight and sunlamps. Wear protective clothing, and use an effective sunscreen.

To relieve constipation, increase the amount of fiber in your diet (fresh fruits and vegetables, salads, bran, and whole-grain cereals and breads) and exercise (unless your doctor directs you to do otherwise).

To avoid dizziness or light-headedness when you stand, contract and relax the muscles of your legs for a few moments before rising. Do this by pushing one foot against the floor while raising the other foot slightly, alternating feet so that you are "pumping" your legs in a pedaling motion.

Major. Tell your doctor about any side effects that are persistent or particularly bothersome. IT IS ESPECIALLY IMPORTANT TO TELL YOUR DOCTOR about blurred vision, confusion, difficulty in breathing, dry mouth, excessive thirst, excessive weakness, fever, itching, joint pain, mood changes, muscle pain or spasms, nausea, palpitations, skin rash, sore throat, tingling in the fingers or toes, unusual bleeding or bruising, vomiting, or yellowing of the eyes or skin.

INTERACTIONS

Benzthiazide interacts with several other types of medications:

1. It may decrease the effectiveness of oral anticoagulants, antigout medications, insulin, oral antidiabetic medicines, and methenamine.

2. Fenfluramine can increase the blood-pressure-lowering effects of benzthiazide, which can be dangerous.

3. Indomethacin can decrease the blood-pressure-lowering effects of benzthiazide, thereby counteracting the desired effects.

4. Cholestyramine and colestipol decrease the absorption of this medication from the gastrointestinal tract. Benzthiazide should, therefore, be taken one hour before or four hours after a dose of cholestyramine or colestipol (if you have also been prescribed one of these medications).

5. The side effects of amphotericin B, calcium, cortisone-like steroids (such as cortisone, dexamethasone, hydrocortisone, prednisone, and prednisolone), digoxin, digitalis, lithium, quinidine, sulfonamide antibiotics, and vitamin D may be increased by benzthiazide.

BE SURE TO TELL YOUR DOCTOR about any medications you are currently taking, especially any of those listed above.

WARNINGS

• Tell your doctor about unusual or allergic reactions you have had to any medications, especially to diuretics or any other sulfa drugs, including oral antidiabetic medications or sulfonamide antibiotics.

• Before you start taking benzthiazide, tell your doctor if you now have or if you have ever had kidney disease or problems with urination, diabetes mellitus, gout, liver disease, asthma, pancreatic disease, or systemic lupus erythematosus.

• Benzthiazide can cause potassium loss. Signs of potassium loss include dry mouth, thirst, weakness, muscle pain or cramps, nausea, and vomiting. If you experience any of these symptoms, call your doctor. To help avoid potassium loss, take this drug with a glass of fresh or frozen orange juice or cranberry juice, or eat a banana every day. The use of a salt substitute also helps to prevent potassium loss. Do not change your diet or take a salt substitute, however, before discussing it with your doctor. Too much potassium can also be dangerous. Your doctor may want to have blood tests performed periodically in order to monitor your potassium levels.

• Limit your intake of alcoholic beverages while taking this medication, in order to prevent dizziness and light-headedness.

If you have high blood pressure, do not take any over-the-counter (nonprescription) medications for weight control or for allergy, asthma, cough, cold, or sinus problems unless your doctor directs you to do so.

• To prevent dehydration (severe water loss) while taking this medication, check with your doctor if you have any illness that causes severe or continuous nausea, vomiting, or diarrhea.

• This medication can raise blood sugar in diabetic patients. Therefore, blood sugar levels should be carefully monitored by blood or urine tests when this medication is being taken.

Some of these products contain the color additive FD&C Yellow No. 5 (tartrazine), which can cause allergic-type reactions (wheezing, rash, fainting, difficulty in breathing) in certain susceptible individuals.

• Be sure to tell your doctor if you are pregnant. Benzthiazide can cross the placenta and may cause adverse effects in the developing fetus. Also, tell your doctor if you are breast-feeding an infant. Although problems in humans have not been reported, small amounts of this drug can pass into breast milk, so caution is warranted.

benztropine

BRAND NAMES (Manufacturers)
benztropine (various manufacturers)
Cogentin (Merck Sharp & Dohme)
TYPE OF DRUG
Anticholinergic and antiparkinsonism agent
INGREDIENT
benztropine
DOSAGE FORM
Tablets (0.5 mg, 1 mg, and 2 mg)
STORAGE
Benztropine tablets should be stored at room temperature in a tightly closed container.

USES

Benztropine is used to treat the symptoms of Parkinson's disease or to control the side effects of phenothiazine tranquilizers. It is not understood how this medication works, but it may act by balancing certain chemicals in the brain.

TREATMENT

In order to reduce stomach irritation, you can take benztropine tablets with food or just after a meal.

Antacids and antidiarrheal medicines prevent the absorption of this medication, so at least one hour should separate doses of benztropine and one of these medicines.

If you miss a dose of this medication, take the missed dose as soon as possible, unless it is within two hours of your next dose. In that case, don't take the missed dose at all; just return to your regular dosing schedule. Do not double the next dose.

SIDE EFFECTS

Minor. Bloating; blurred vision; constipation; dizziness; drowsiness; dry mouth, throat, and nose; false sense of well-being; headache; increased sensitivity of the eyes to light; muscle cramps; nausea; nervousness; reduced sweating; or weakness. These side effects should disappear as your body adjusts to the medication.

If you are constipated, increase the amount of fiber in your diet (fresh fruits and vegetables, salads, bran, and whole-grain breads), exercise, and drink more water (unless your doctor directs you to do otherwise).

Chew sugarless gum or suck on ice chips or a piece of hard candy to reduce mouth dryness.

Wear sunglasses if your eyes become sensitive to light.

To avoid dizziness and light-headedness when you stand, contract and relax the muscles of your legs for a few moments before rising. Do this by pushing one foot against the floor while raising the other foot slightly, alternating feet.

Major. Tell your doctor about any side effects that are persistent or particularly bothersome. IT IS ESPECIALLY IMPORTANT TO TELL YOUR DOCTOR about depression, difficulty sleeping, difficulty in urinating, hallucinations, involuntary muscle movements, loss of balance, memory loss, mood changes, numbness of the fingers, palpitations, or unusual excitement.

Some side effects may occur for a short time after discontinuing this drug. Consult your doctor if they become bothersome.

INTERACTIONS

Benztropine can interact with several other types of medications:

1. It can cause extreme drowsiness when combined with alcohol or other central nervous system depressants (such as antihistamines, barbiturates, benzodiazepine tranquilizers, muscle relaxants, narcotics, and pain medications) or with tricyclic antidepressants.

2. Amantadine, antihistamines, haloperidol, monoamine oxidase (MAO) inhibitors, phenothiazine tranquilizers, procainamide, quinidine, and tricyclic antidepressants can increase the side effects of benztropine. At least 14 days should separate the use of this drug and the use of an MAO inhibitor.

Before starting to take this medication, BE SURE TO TELL YOUR DOCTOR about any medications you are currently taking, especially any of those listed above.

WARNINGS

• Be sure to tell your doctor about unusual or allergic reactions you have had to any medications, especially to benz-tropine.

• Tell your doctor if you now have or if you have ever had achalasia, glaucoma, heart disease, high blood pressure, kidney disease, liver disease, myasthenia gravis, blockage of the intestinal tract or urinary tract, enlarged prostate gland, stomach ulcers, or thyroid disease.

• If this drug makes you dizzy or drowsy, be sure to avoid any activity that requires alertness, such as driving a car or operating potentially dangerous equipment. Be careful on stairs, and avoid getting up suddenly from a lying or sitting position.

• This medication can decrease sweating and heat release from the body. You should, therefore, avoid getting overheated by strenuous exercise in hot weather and should avoid taking hot baths, showers, and saunas.

• Elderly patients are more sensitive to the effects of benztropine. Contact your doctor if confusion, disorientation, agitation, or hallucinations occur.

• Be sure to tell your doctor if you are pregnant. Extensive studies of the use of benztropine during pregnancy have not been conducted. Also, tell your doctor if you are breast-feeding an infant. Small amounts of this medication may pass into breast milk.

betamethasone (systemic)

BRAND NAME (Manufacturer)
Celestone (Schering)
TYPE OF DRUG
Adrenocorticosteroid hormone
INGREDIENT
betamethasone
DOSAGE FORMS
Tablets (0.6 mg)
Oral syrup (0.6 mg per 5-ml spoonful, with less than 1% alcohol)
STORAGE
Betamethasone should be stored at room temperature in a tightly closed container. Carefully dispose of any outdated medication or any medication that is no longer necessary.

USES

Your adrenal glands naturally produce certain cortisone-like chemicals. These chemicals are involved in various regulatory processes in the body (such as those involving fluid balance, temperature, and reaction to inflammation). Betamethasone belongs to a group of drugs known as adrenocorticosteroids (or cortisone-like medications). It is used to treat a variety of disorders, including endocrine and rheumatic disorders; asthma; blood diseases; certain cancers; eye disorders; gastrointestinal disturbances, such as ulcerative colitis; respiratory diseases; and inflammations such as arthritis, dermatitis, and poison ivy. How this drug acts to relieve these disorders is not completely understood.

TREATMENT

In order to prevent stomach irritation, you can take betamethasone with food or milk.

The oral syrup form of this medication should be measured carefully with a specially designed 5-ml measuring spoon. An ordinary kitchen teaspoon is not accurate enough.

If you are taking only one dose of this medication each day, try to take it before 9:00 A.M. This will mimic the body's normal production of this type of chemical.

It is important to try not to miss any doses of betamethasone. However, if you do miss a dose of this medication, follow these guidelines:

1. If you are taking it more than once a day, take the missed dose as soon as possible, and return to your regular schedule. If it is already time for the next dose, double the dose.

2. If you are taking this medication once a day, take the dose you missed as soon as possible, unless you don't remember until the next day. In that case, do not take the missed dose at all; just follow your regular schedule. Do not double the next dose.

3. If you are taking this drug every other day, take it as soon as you remember. If you missed the scheduled time by a whole day, take it when you remember; then skip a day before you take the next dose. Do not double the dose.

If you miss more than one dose of betamethasone, CONTACT YOUR DOCTOR.

SIDE EFFECTS

Minor. Dizziness, false sense of well-being, increased appetite, increased susceptibility to infections, increased sweating, indigestion, menstrual irregularities, muscle weakness, nausea, reddening of the skin on the face, restlessness, sleep disorders, or weight gain. These effects should disappear as you adjust to the medication.

Major. Tell your doctor about any side effects that are persistent or particularly bothersome. IT IS ESPECIALLY IMPORTANT TO TELL YOUR DOCTOR about abdominal enlargement; acne or other skin problems; back or rib pain; bloody or black, tarry stools; blurred vision; convulsions; fever and sore throat; glaucoma; growth impairment (in children); headaches; impaired healing of wounds; increased thirst and urination; menstrual irregularities; mental depression; mood changes; muscle wasting; nightmares; peptic ulcers; puffiness of the face; rapid weight gain (three to five pounds within a week); rash; shortness of breath; thinning of the skin; unusual bleeding or bruising; or unusual weakness.

INTERACTIONS

Betamethasone interacts with several other types of drugs:
1. Alcohol, aspirin, and anti-inflammatory medications (diflunisal, ibuprofen, indomethacin, ketoprofen, mefenamic acid, meclofenamate, naproxen, piroxicam, sulindac, tolmetin) aggravate the stomach problems that are common with use of this medication.

2. The dosage of oral anticoagulants (blood thinners, such as warfarin), oral antidiabetic drugs, or insulin may need to be altered when this medication is started or stopped.

3. The loss of potassium caused by betamethasone can lead to serious side effects in individuals taking digoxin. Thiazide diuretics (water pills) can increase the potassium loss caused by betamethasone.

4. Phenobarbital, phenytoin, rifampin, and ephedrine can increase the elimination of betamethasone from the body, thereby decreasing its effectiveness.

5. Oral contraceptives (birth control pills) and estrogen-containing drugs may decrease the elimination of this drug from the body, which can lead to an increase in side effects.

6. Betamethasone can increase the elimination of aspirin and isoniazid, thereby decreasing the effectiveness of these two medications.

7. Cholestyramine and colestipol can chemically bind this medication in the stomach and gastrointestinal tract and prevent its absorption.

BE SURE TO TELL YOUR DOCTOR about any medications you are currently taking, especially any listed above.

WARNINGS

•Tell your doctor about unusual or allergic reactions you have had to any medications, especially to betamethasone or other adrenocorticosteroids (such as cortisone, dexamethasone, hydrocortisone, methylprednisolone, paramethasone, prednisolone, prednisone, and triamcinolone).

•Be sure to tell your doctor if you now have or if you have ever had bone disease, diabetes mellitus, emotional instability, glaucoma, fungal infections, heart disease, high blood pressure, high cholesterol levels, myasthenia gravis, peptic ulcers, osteoporosis, thyroid disease, tuberculosis, ulcerative colitis, kidney disease, or liver disease.

•To help avoid potassium loss while using this drug, take your dose with a glass of fresh or frozen orange juice, or eat a banana each day. The use of a salt substitute also helps to prevent potassium loss. Discuss this with your doctor.

•If you are using this medication for longer than a week, you may need to receive higher dosages if you are subjected to stress, such as serious infections, injury, or surgery. Discuss this with your doctor.

•If you have been taking this drug for more than a week, do not stop taking it suddenly. If it is stopped suddenly, you may experience abdominal or back pain, dizziness, fainting, fever, muscle or joint pain, nausea, vomiting, shortness of breath, or extreme weakness. Your doctor may, therefore, want to reduce the dosage gradually. Never increase the dose or take the drug for longer than the prescribed time, unless you first consult your doctor.

•While you are taking this drug, you should not be vaccinated or immunized. This medication decreases the effectiveness of vaccines and can lead to overwhelming infection if a live-virus vaccine is administered.

•Before having skin tests, surgery, or any other medical or dental treatment, be sure to tell your doctor or dentist that you are taking betamethasone.

•Because this drug can cause glaucoma and cataracts with long-term use, your doctor may want you to have your eyes examined by an ophthalmologist periodically during treatment.

If you are taking this medication for prolonged periods, you should wear or carry an identification card or notice stating that you are taking an adrenocorticosteroid.

•This medication can raise blood sugar levels in diabetic patients. Blood sugar should, therefore, be monitored carefully with blood tests when this medication is being taken. If you notice a change in your blood sugar levels, contact your doctor.

•Be sure to tell your doctor if you are pregnant. This type of drug crosses the placenta. Although studies in humans have not been conducted, birth defects have been observed in the offspring of animals that were given large doses of this drug during pregnancy. Also, tell your doctor if you are breast-feeding an infant. Small amounts of this type of drug pass into breast milk and may cause growth suppression or a decrease in natural adrenocorticosteroid production in the nursing infant.

betamethasone dipropionate (topical)

BRAND NAMES (Manufacturers)
Alphatrex (Savage)
betamethasone dipropionate (various manufacturers)
Diprolene (Schering)
Diprosone (Schering)
Maxivate (Westwood)
TYPE OF DRUG
Adrenocorticosteroid hormone
INGREDIENT
betamethasone
DOSAGE FORMS
Ointment (0.05%)
Cream (0.05%)
Lotion (0.05%)
Aerosol (0.1%)
STORAGE
Betamethasone dipropionate ointment, cream, and lotion should be stored at room temperature in tightly closed containers. This medication should never be frozen.

The aerosol form of this medication is packaged under pressure. It should not be stored near heat or an open flame or in direct sunlight, and the container should never be punctured.

USES
Your adrenal glands naturally produce certain cortisone-like chemicals. These chemicals are involved in various regulatory processes in the body (such as those involving fluid balance, temperature, and reaction to inflammation). Betamethasone dipropionate belongs to a group of drugs known as adrenocorticosteroids (or cortisone-like medications). It is used to relieve the skin inflammation (redness, swelling, itching, and discomfort) associated with conditions such as dermatitis, eczema, and poison ivy. How betamethasone dipropionate acts to relieve these disorders is not completely understood.

TREATMENT
Before applying this medication, wash your hands. Then, unless your doctor gives you different instructions, gently wash the area of the skin where the medication is to be applied. With a clean towel, pat the area almost dry; it should be slightly damp when you put the medicine on.

If you are using the lotion form of this medication, shake it well before pouring it out. The contents tend to settle on the bottom of the bottle, so it is necessary to shake the container to distribute the ingredients evenly and equalize the doses.

Apply a small amount of the medication to the affected area in a thin layer. Do not bandage the area unless your

doctor tells you to do so. If you are to apply an occlusive dressing (like kitchen plastic wrap), be sure you understand the instructions. Wash your hands again after application.

Shake the aerosol spray form of this medication in order to disperse the medication evenly. Hold the can upright, six to eight inches from the area to be sprayed, and spray the area for one to three seconds. DO NOT SMOKE while you are using the aerosol spray; the contents are under pressure and may explode when exposed to heat or flames.

Avoid applying this medication to areas with cuts or open wounds.

If you miss a dose of this medication, apply the dose as soon as possible, unless it is almost time for the next application. In that case, do not apply the missed dose; just return to your regular schedule. Do not put twice as much of the medication on your skin at the next application.

SIDE EFFECTS
Minor. Acne, burning sensation, itching, skin dryness, or rash.

If the affected area is extremely dry or scaling, the skin may be moistened before applying the medication by soaking in water or by applying water with a clean cloth. The ointment form is probably better for dry skin.

A mild, temporary stinging sensation may occur after this medication is applied. If this persists, contact your doctor.

Major. Tell your doctor about any side effects that are persistent or particularly bothersome. IT IS ESPECIALLY IMPORTANT TO TELL YOUR DOCTOR about blistering, increased hair growth, irritation of the affected area, loss of skin color, secondary infection in the area being treated, or thinning of the skin with easy bruising.

INTERACTIONS
This medication should not interact with any other medications as long as it is used according to directions.

WARNINGS
• Tell your doctor about unusual or allergic reactions you have had to any medications, especially to betamethasone dipropionate or any other adrenocorticosteroid (such as amcinonide, clocortolone, cortisone, desonide, desoximetasone, dexamethasone, diflorasone, flumethasone, fluocinolone, fluocinonide, fluorometholone, flurandrenolide, halcinonide, hydrocortisone, methylprednisolone, prednisolone, prednisone, and triamcinolone).
• Tell your doctor if you now have or if you have ever had blood vessel disease, chicken pox, diabetes mellitus, fungal infection, peptic ulcer, shingles, tuberculosis, tuberculosis of the skin, vaccinia, or any other type of infection, especially at the site currently being treated.
• If irritation develops while using this drug, immediately discontinue its use and notify your doctor.
• This product is not for use in the eyes or on mucous membranes; contact may result in side effects.
• Do not use this product with an occlusive wrap unless your doctor directs you to do so. Systemic absorption of

this drug is increased if extensive areas of the body are treated, particularly if occlusive bandages are used. If it is necessary for you to use this drug under a wrap, follow your doctor's instructions exactly; do not leave the wrap in place longer than specified.

• If you are using this medication on a child's diaper area, do not put tight-fitting diapers or plastic pants on the child. This may lead to increased systemic absorption of the drug and a possible increase in side effects.

• Elderly patients and younger children have naturally thinner skin, and, therefore, betamethasone dipropionate is more likely to be absorbed. Be sure to report any adverse effects to your doctor.

• In order to avoid freezing skin tissue when using the aerosol form of betamethasone dipropionate, make sure that you do not spray for more than three seconds, and hold the container at least six inches from the skin.

• When using the aerosol form of this medication on the face, cover your eyes and do not inhale the spray.

• Use this medication only for your current condition. Do not use it for another problem later or give it to other people to use.

• Tell your doctor if you are pregnant. If large amounts of this drug are applied for prolonged periods, some of it may cross the placenta. Although studies in humans have not been conducted, birth defects have been observed in the offspring of animals that were given large oral doses of this type of drug during pregnancy. Also, tell your doctor if you are breast-feeding an infant. If absorbed through the skin small amounts of the drug may pass into breast milk and may cause growth suppression or a decrease in natural adrenocorticosteroid production in the nursing infant.

betamethasone dipropionate and clotrimazole combination (topical)

BRAND NAME (Manufacturer)
Lotrisone (Schering)
TYPE OF DRUG
Adrenocorticosteroid hormone and antifungal
INGREDIENTS
betamethasone dipropionate and clotrimazole
DOSAGE FORM
Topical cream (0.05% betamethasone dipropionate and 1% clotrimazole)
STORAGE
This medication should be stored at room temperature (never frozen) in a tightly closed container. Discard any outdated or unneeded medication.

USES
Betamethasone dipropionate and clotrimazole combination is used to treat fungal infections of the skin. Clotrimazole is an antifungal agent that prevents the growth and multiplication of a wide range of fungi and yeast, including *Candida*. Betamethasone dipropionate

belongs to a group of drugs known as adrenocorticosteroids (or cortisone-like medications). Your adrenal glands naturally produce certain cortisone-like chemicals. These chemicals are involved in various regulatory processes in the body. Betamethasone dipropionate is added to this combination to relieve skin inflammation (redness, swelling, itching, and discomfort).

TREATMENT
Before applying betamethasone dipropionate and clotrimazole combination, you should wash your hands. Then, unless your doctor tells you to do otherwise, cleanse the affected area with soap and water. Pat the skin with a clean towel until it is almost dry. Gently massage a small amount of the cream over the entire area that is affected and the skin immediately surrounding this area. Avoid applying the medication to areas with cuts or open wounds. Don't bandage or cover the area after applying the medication, unless your doctor instructs you to do so. Wash your hands again after application.

Improvement in your condition may not become apparent for as long as a week after you begin treatment with this drug. However, you should be sure to complete the full course of medication. If you stop using this drug too soon, resistant fungi are given a chance to continue growing, and the infection could recur. If your condition has not improved after four weeks, CONTACT YOUR DOCTOR. Clotrimazole may not be effective against the organism causing your infection.

If you miss a dose of this drug, apply the dose as soon as possible, unless it is almost time for the next application. In that case, do not apply the missed dose; just return to your regular schedule. Do not put twice as much of the drug on your skin at the next application.

SIDE EFFECTS
Minor. Acne and burning sensation. You may also experience some burning, itching, redness, or stinging when this drug is applied to the skin. These side effects should disappear as your body adjusts to this medication.
Major. Tell your doctor about any side effects that are persistent or particularly bothersome. IT IS ESPECIALLY IMPORTANT TO TELL YOUR DOCTOR about blistering, increased hair growth, irritation, loss of skin color, peeling of the skin, swelling, or thinning of the skin with easy bruising.

INTERACTIONS
Betamethasone dipropionate and clotrimazole combination should not interact with other medications as long as it is used according to directions.

WARNINGS
• Tell your doctor about unusual or allergic reactions you have had to any medications, especially to betamethasone dipropionate or other adrenocorticosteroids (amcinonide, clocortolone, cortisone, desonide, desoximetasone, dexamethasone, diflorasone, flumethasone, fluocinolone, fluocinonide, fluorometholone, flurandrenolide, halcinonide, hydrocortisone, methylprednisolone, prednisolone, prednisone, and triamcinolone) or to clotrimazole.

• Tell your doctor if you now have or if you have ever had blood vessel disease, chicken pox, diabetes mellitus, fungal infection, peptic ulcers, pulmonary tuberculosis, shingles, tuberculosis of the skin, vaccinia, or any other type of infection, especially at the site being treated.

• If irritation develops while using this drug, immediately discontinue its use and notify your doctor.

• This product is not for use in the eyes or on mucous membranes; contact may result in side effects.

• Do not use this product with an occlusive wrap unless your doctor directs you to do so. Systemic absorption of this drug is increased if extensive areas of the body are treated, particularly if occlusive bandages are used. If it is necessary for you to use this drug under a wrap, follow your doctor's instructions exactly; do not leave the wrap in place longer than specified.

• If you are using this medication on a child's diaper area, do not put tight-fitting diapers or plastic pants on the child. This may lead to increased systemic absorption of the drug and a possible increase in side effects.

• Elderly patients and younger children have naturally thinner skin, and, therefore, the drug is more likely to be absorbed. Report any adverse effects to your doctor.

• This medication has been prescribed for your current infection only. A subsequent infection, or one that someone else has, may require a different medication. Therefore, you should not give your medicine to other people or use it for other infections, unless directed to do so by your doctor.

• In order to avoid reinfection, keep the affected area clean and dry, wear freshly laundered clothing, and avoid wearing tight-fitting clothes.

• Be sure to tell your doctor if you are pregnant. If large amounts of this drug are applied for prolonged periods, some of it will be absorbed and may cross the placenta. Although studies in humans have not been conducted, birth defects have been observed in the offspring of animals that were given large oral doses of adrenocorticosteroids during pregnancy. Also, tell your doctor if you are breast-feeding an infant. Small amounts of this type of drug may pass into breast milk and cause growth suppression or a decrease in adrenocorticosteroid production in the nursing infant.

betamethasone valerate (topical)

BRAND NAMES (Manufacturers)
betamethasone valerate (various manufacturers)
Betatrex (Savage)
Beta-Val (Lemmon)
Valisone (Schering)
Valisone Reduced Strength (Schering)
TYPE OF DRUG
Adrenocorticosteroid hormone
INGREDIENT
betamethasone
DOSAGE FORMS
Cream (0.01% and 0.1%)

Ointment (0.1%)
Lotion (0.1%)
STORAGE
This medication should be stored at room temperature (never frozen) in a tightly closed container.

USES
Your adrenal glands naturally produce certain cortisone-like chemicals. These chemicals are involved in various regulatory processes in the body (such as those involving fluid balance, temperature, and reaction to inflammation). Betamethasone valerate belongs to a group of drugs known as adrenocorticosteroids (or cortisone-like medications). It is used to relieve the skin inflammation (redness, swelling, itching, and discomfort) associated with conditions such as dermatitis, eczema, and poison ivy. How this drug acts to relieve these disorders is not completely understood.

TREATMENT
Before applying this medication, wash your hands. Then, unless your doctor gives you different instructions, gently wash the area of the skin where the medication is to be applied. With a clean towel, pat the area almost dry; it should be slightly damp when you put the medicine on.

If you are using the lotion form of this drug, shake it well before pouring out the medicine to distribute the ingredients evenly and equalize the doses.

Apply a small amount of the medication to the affected area in a thin layer. Avoid applying medication to cuts or open wounds. Do not bandage the area unless your doctor tells you to do so. If you are to apply an occlusive dressing (like kitchen plastic wrap), be sure you understand the instructions. Wash your hands again after application.

If you miss a dose of this medication, apply the dose as soon as possible, unless it is almost time for the next application. In that case, do not apply the missed dose; just return to your regular dosing schedule. Do not put twice as much on your skin at the next application.

SIDE EFFECTS
Minor. Acne, burning sensation, itching, rash, or skin dryness.

If the affected area is extremely dry or scaling, the skin may be moistened before applying the medication by soaking in water or by applying water with a clean cloth. The ointment form is probably better for dry skin.

A mild, temporary stinging sensation may occur after this medication is applied. If this persists, contact your doctor.

Major. Tell your doctor about any side effects that are persistent or particularly bothersome. IT IS ESPECIALLY IMPORTANT TO TELL YOUR DOCTOR about blistering, increased hair growth, irritation of the affected area, loss of skin color, secondary infection of the area being treated, or thinning of the skin with easy bruising.

INTERACTIONS
This medication should not interact with any other medications as long as it is used according to directions.

WARNINGS

• Tell your doctor about unusual or allergic reactions you have had to any medications, especially to betamethasone valerate or other adrenocorticosteroids (such as amcinonide, clocortolone, cortisone, desonide, desoximetasone, dexamethasone, diflorasone, flumethasone, fluocinolone, fluocinonide, fluorometholone, flurandrenolide, halcinonide, hydrocortisone, methylprednisolone, prednisolone, prednisone, and triamcinolone).
• Tell your doctor if you now have or if you have ever had blood vessel disease, chicken pox, diabetes mellitus, fungal infection, peptic ulcers, shingles, tuberculosis, tuberculosis of the skin, vaccinia, or any other type of infection, especially at the site currently being treated.
• If irritation develops while using this drug, immediately discontinue its use and notify your doctor.
• This product is not for use in the eyes or on mucous membranes; contact may result in side effects.
• Use this drug only for your current condition. Do not use it for another problem or give it to others to use.
• Do not use this product with an occlusive wrap unless your doctor directs you to do so. Systemic absorption of this drug is increased if extensive areas of the body are treated, particularly if occlusive bandages are used. If it is necessary for you to use this drug under a wrap, follow your doctor's instructions exactly.
• If you are using this medication on a child's diaper area, do not put tight-fitting diapers or plastic pants on the child. This may lead to increased systemic absorption of the drug and a possible increase in side effects.
• Elderly patients and younger children have naturally thinner skin, and, therefore, the drug is more likely to be absorbed. Report any adverse effects.
• Be sure to tell your doctor if you are pregnant. If large amounts of this drug are applied for prolonged periods, some of it will be absorbed and may cross the placenta. Although studies in humans have not been conducted, birth defects have been observed in the offspring of animals that were given large oral doses of this type of drug during pregnancy. Also, tell your doctor if you are breast-feeding an infant. If absorbed through the skin, small amounts of this type of drug pass into breast milk and may cause growth suppression or a decrease in natural adrenocorticosteroid production in the nursing infant.

Betapen-VK—see penicillin VK

Betatrex—see betamethasone valerate (topical)

Beta-Val—see betamethasone valerate (topical)

betaxolol (ophthalmic)

BRAND NAMES (Manufacturers)
Betoptic (Alcon)
Betoptic S (Alcon)
TYPE OF DRUG
Antiglaucoma ophthalmic solution
INGREDIENT
betaxolol

DOSAGE FORM
Ophthalmic drops (0.25% and 0.5% betaxolol)
STORAGE
Store at room temperature in a tightly closed container. Discard any outdated medication.

USES
Betaxolol is used to reduce pressure in the eye caused by glaucoma or other eye conditions. This medication belongs to a group of drugs known as beta blockers. When applied to the eye, betaxolol reduces pressure within the eye, perhaps by decreasing eye fluid (aqueous humor) production and by increasing the outflow of fluid from the eye.

TREATMENT
Wash your hands with soap and water before applying this drug. To avoid contamination of the drops, do not touch the tube portion of the dropper or let it touch your eye; do not wipe off or rinse the dropper after use.

To apply the drops, tilt your head back and pull down your lower eyelid with one hand to make a pouch below the eye. Drop the prescribed amount of medicine into this pouch and slowly close your eyes. Try not to blink. Keep your eyes closed, and place one finger at the corner of the eye next to your nose for a minute or two, applying slight pressure (this is done to prevent loss of medication into the nose and throat canal). Then wipe away any excess with a clean tissue. Since administering the drug is somewhat difficult, you may want to have someone else apply the drops for you.

If you miss a dose of this medication, apply the missed dose as soon as possible, then return to your regular dosing schedule. However, if it is almost time for the next dose, skip the dose you missed. Do not double the next dose.

SIDE EFFECTS
Minor. When you first apply this medication, it may sting or burn your eyes. This should stop in a few minutes. You may also notice sensitivity of your eyes to bright lights or sunlight. Wearing sunglasses and avoiding excessive exposure to sunlight may help relieve this sensitivity.
Major. Tell your doctor about any side effects that are persistent or particularly bothersome. IT IS ESPECIALLY IMPORTANT TO TELL YOUR DOCTOR about hives, irritation of the eye that lasts more than a few minutes after application, itching, or skin rash. Major side effects are rare when this product is used correctly. However, depression, fluid accumulation, insomnia, shortness of breath, or swelling of the feet may occur with this drug. If you have any of these symptoms, contact your doctor.

INTERACTIONS
Betaxolol may increase the side effects of reserpine and oral beta blockers. TELL YOUR DOCTOR about any medications you are currently taking.

WARNINGS
• Tell your doctor about unusual or allergic reactions you have had to any medications, especially to betax-

olol or to any other beta blocker (acebutolol, atenolol, carteolol, esmolol, labetalol, metoprolol, nadolol, penbutolol, pindolol, propranolol, and timolol).

• Be sure to tell your doctor if you now have or if you have ever had asthma, diabetes mellitus, heart failure, lung disease, slow or abnormal heartbeat, or thyroid disease.

• Before having surgery or any other medical or dental treatment, tell your doctor or dentist that you are taking this medication. Your doctor or dentist may want to gradually withdraw this medication prior to the procedure.

• Be sure to tell your doctor if you are pregnant. Although betaxolol appears to be safe in animals, studies in pregnant women have not been conducted. Also, tell your doctor if you are breast-feeding an infant. Small amounts of betaxolol will pass into breast milk.

betaxolol (systemic)

BRAND NAME (Manufacturer)
Kerlone (Searle)
TYPE OF DRUG
Beta-adrenergic blocking agent
INGREDIENT
betaxolol
DOSAGE FORM
Tablets (10 mg and 20 mg)
STORAGE
Betaxolol should be stored at room temperature in a tightly closed container.

USES
Betaxolol is prescribed for the treatment of high blood pressure. Betaxolol belongs to a group of medicines known as beta-adrenergic blocking agents or, more commonly, beta blockers. These drugs work by controlling impulses along certain nerve pathways. This results in a decreased workload for the heart.

TREATMENT
Betaxolol can be taken with a glass of water, with meals, immediately following meals, or on an empty stomach, depending on your doctor's instructions. It is important that you try to take the medication at the same time(s) each day.

Try not to miss any doses of this medication. If you do miss a dose of the medication, take the missed dose as soon as possible. However, if the next scheduled dose is within eight hours (if you are taking this medication only once a day) or within four hours (if you are taking this medication more than once a day), do not take the missed dose at all; just return to your regular dosing schedule. Do not double the next dose of the medication.

It is important to remember that betaxolol does not cure high blood pressure.

SIDE EFFECTS
Minor. Decreased sexual ability, diarrhea, fatigue, headache, indigestion, or nausea. These side effects should diminish as your body adjusts to the medication.

Major. Tell your doctor about any side effects that are persistent or particularly bothersome. IT IS ESPECIALLY IMPORTANT TO TELL YOUR DOCTOR about breathing difficulty or wheezing; cold hands or feet due to decreased blood circulation to the skin, fingers, and toes; confusion; dizziness; fever and sore throat; hair loss; hallucinations; light-headedness; mental depression; nightmares; reduced alertness; skin rash; swelling of the ankles, feet, or lower legs; or unusual bleeding or bruising.

INTERACTIONS
Betaxolol interacts with a number of other medications:
1. Indomethacin, other nonsteroidal anti-inflammatory agents, aspirin, or other salicylates may decrease the blood-pressure-lowering effects of beta blockers.
2. Calcium channel blockers (nifedipine, verapamil, and diltiazem) may be used with beta blockers such as betaxolol unless the patient has heart trouble. Very low blood pressure and heart failure have been observed in patients with impaired heart function who take beta blockers.
3. Side effects may also be increased if beta blockers are taken with epinephrine, phenylephrine, phenylpropanolamine, phenothiazine tranquilizers, reserpine, clonidine, prazosin, or monoamine oxidase (MAO) inhibitors. At least 14 days should separate the use of a beta blocker and the use of an MAO inhibitor.
4. Beta blockers may antagonize (work against) the effects of theophylline, aminophylline, albuterol, isoproterenol, metaproterenol, and terbutaline.
5. Beta blockers can also interact with insulin or oral antidiabetic agents—raising or lowering blood sugar levels or masking symptoms of low blood sugar.
6. The action of beta blockers may be increased if they are used with furosemide or hydralazine, which could have a negative effect.
7. Alcohol, barbiturates, and rifampin can decrease blood concentrations of this drug, which can result in a decrease in effectiveness.
8. If you are on both betaxolol and clonidine, and both of these medications are to be discontinued, it is recommended that the betaxolol be tapered off over several days before the gradual reduction of clonidine.
9. In patients who have congestive heart failure treated with digitalis glycosides (for example, digoxin or digitoxin), caution should be used as both betaxolol and digitalis products may slow heart conduction.

Before starting to take betaxolol, BE SURE TO TELL YOUR DOCTOR about any medications you are already taking, especially any of the medications listed above.

WARNINGS
• Tell your doctor about any unusual or allergic reactions you have had to any medications, especially to betaxolol or any other beta blocker (acebutolol, atenolol, carteolol, esmolol, labetolol, metoprolol, nadolol, penbutalol, pindolol, propranolol, and timolol).
• Tell your doctor if you now have or if you have ever had asthma, bronchitis, diabetes mellitus, heart block, heart failure, kidney disease, liver disease, peripheral vascular disease (poor circulation in the fingers or toes), severe bradycardia (slowed heart rate), or thyroid disease.

• Betaxolol therapy may increase the risk of cardiac failure in some patients. Report any abnormal heart function to your doctor.

• Patients with severe bronchospastic disease (such as asthma) should, in general, not receive beta blockers. Inform your physician if you experience breathing difficulties.

• In diabetics, betaxolol may block some of the warning signs of low blood sugar (hypoglycemia), such as rapid pulse rate, but not others, such as dizziness or sweating.

• You may want to check your pulse while taking this drug. If your pulse is much slower than your usual rate (or if it is less than 50 beats per minute), check with your doctor. A pulse that is too slow may cause circulation problems.

• This medication may affect your body's response to exercise. Ask your doctor what an appropriate amount of exercise would be for you.

• It is important that you do not stop taking this drug, without first checking with your doctor. Some conditions such as angina pectoris may become worse when the drug is stopped suddenly, and the danger of a heart attack is increased in some patients. Your doctor may want you to gradually reduce the amount of the drug you take before stopping completely. Make sure that you have enough medication on hand to last through vacations, and holidays.

• Tell your doctor or dentist that you are taking this drug before having surgery or any other medical or dental treatment. Often, this medication will be discontinued 48 hours prior to any major surgery.

• While taking this drug, do not use any over-the-counter (nonprescription) allergy, asthma, cough, cold, sinus, or diet preparations without first checking with your doctor or pharmacist. The combination of these medications with a beta blocker can result in high blood pressure.

• Betaxolol may reduce intraocular pressure and give a misleading negative glaucoma test.

• Be sure to tell your doctor if you are pregnant. Animal studies have shown that some beta blockers can cause problems in pregnancy when used at very high doses. Adequate studies have not been conducted in humans, but there has been some association between beta blockers used during pregnancy and low birth weight, breathing problems, and slow heart rate in the newborn. Also, tell your doctor if you are breast-feeding an infant. Although this medication has not been shown to cause problems in breast-fed infants, it may pass into breast milk, so caution is warranted.

• The safety of this medication has not been established in children.

bethanechol

BRAND NAMES (Manufacturers)
bethanechol chloride (various manufacturers)
Duvoid (Roberts)
Myotonachol (Glenwood)
Urabeth (Major)
Urecholine (Merck Sharp & Dohme)

TYPE OF DRUG
Cholinergic
INGREDIENT
bethanechol
DOSAGE FORM
Tablets (5 mg, 10 mg, 25 mg, and 50 mg)
STORAGE
Bethanechol should be stored at room temperature in a tightly closed container.

USES
Bethanechol is used to relieve retention of urine in the bladder. It acts on the nerves of the bladder to cause emptying.

TREATMENT
Bethanechol should be taken on an empty stomach one hour before or two hours after a meal. If it is taken soon after eating, nausea and vomiting may occur.

If you miss a dose and remember within an hour, take the missed dose immediately. If more than an hour has passed, do not take the missed dose at all; just return to your regular dosing schedule. Do not double the next dose.

SIDE EFFECTS
Minor. Abdominal cramps, belching, diarrhea, dizziness, excessive salivation, flushing of the skin, headache, nausea, sweating, or vomiting. These side effects should disappear as your body adjusts to the medication.

If you feel dizzy, sit or lie down for a while; get up slowly from a sitting or reclining position, and be careful on stairs.

Major. Tell your doctor about any side effects that are persistent or particularly bothersome. IT IS ESPECIALLY IMPORTANT TO TELL YOUR DOCTOR about chest pain, feeling faint, or shortness of breath.

INTERACTIONS
Bethanechol interacts with several other types of drugs:
1. Procainamide and quinidine can decrease the therapeutic effects of bethanechol.
2. Concurrent use of bethanechol and mecamylamine or trimethaphan can lead to a serious drop in blood pressure.

Before starting to take bethanechol, BE SURE TO TELL YOUR DOCTOR about any medications you are currently taking, especially any of those listed above.

WARNINGS
• Tell your doctor about unusual or allergic reactions you have had to any medications, especially to bethanechol.

• Before starting to take this medication, be sure to tell your doctor if you have ever had any of the following disorders: asthma, epilepsy, heart disease, high or low blood pressure, Parkinson's disease, stomach ulcers, thyroid disease, or an obstruction of the intestine or bladder.

• If this drug makes you dizzy, avoid taking part in any activity that requires alertness, such as driving a car or operating potentially dangerous equipment.

• Be sure to tell your doctor if you are pregnant. Although bethanechol appears to be safe during pregnancy, extensive studies in humans have not been conducted. Thus, bethanechol should only be administered during pregnancy if the benefits to the mother clearly outweigh potential risks to the fetus. Also, tell your doctor if you are breast-feeding. It is not known if small amounts of bethanechol pass into breast milk, so cautious use is warranted in nursing women.

bethanechol chloride—see bethanechol

Bethaprim DS—see sulfamethoxazole and trimethoprim combination

Betoptic—see betaxolol (ophthalmic)

Betoptic S—see betaxolol (ophthalmic)

Biaxin—see clarithromycin

Bleph-10—see sodium sulfacetamide (ophthalmic)

Blocadren—see timolol maleate (systemic)

Bonine—see meclizine

Brethaire—see terbutaline

Bontril PDM—see phendimetrazine

Bontril Slow-Release—see phendimetrazine

Brethine—see terbutaline

Brevicon—see oral contraceptives

Brexin L.A.—see pseudoephedrine and chlorpheniramine combination

Bricanyl—see terbutaline

---

bromocriptine

BRAND NAMES (Manufacturers)
Parlodel (Sandoz)
Parlodel SnapTabs (Sandoz)
TYPE OF DRUG
Dopamine agonist and antiparkinsonism agent
INGREDIENT
bromocriptine
DOSAGE FORMS
Tablets (2.5 mg)
Capsules (5 mg)
STORAGE
Bromocriptine should be stored at room temperature in a tightly closed, light-resistant container.

USES
This medication is used to treat the symptoms of Parkinson's disease and to decrease milk production in women who choose not to breast-feed their infants. Bromocriptine relieves the symptoms of Parkinson's disease by replacing a chemical (dopamine) that is diminished in the brains of these patients. Bromocriptine prevents milk production by blocking the action of the responsible hormone (prolactin).

TREATMENT
In order to avoid stomach irritation during therapy with bromocriptine, you can take the medication with food or with a full glass of water or milk.

If you miss a dose of this medication and remember within four hours, take the missed dose immediately. If more than four hours have passed, do not take the missed dose at all; just return to your regular dosing schedule. Do not double the next dose.

SIDE EFFECTS
Minor. Abdominal pain, constipation, diarrhea, dizziness, drowsiness, fatigue, headache, insomnia, light-headedness, loss of appetite, nasal congestion, nausea, or vomiting. These should disappear as your body adjusts to the drug.

Dizziness or fainting may occur, especially following the first dose. It is best, therefore, to take the first dose while lying down. If you feel dizzy or light-headed with later doses, sit or lie down; get up slowly; and be careful on stairs.

To relieve constipation, increase the amount of fiber in your diet (fresh fruits and vegetables, salads, bran, and whole-grain breads), exercise, and drink more water (unless your doctor directs you to do otherwise).
Major. Tell your doctor about any side effects that are persistent or particularly bothersome. IT IS ESPECIALLY IMPORTANT TO REPORT about abnormal, involuntary movements; anxiety; confusion; convulsions; depression; difficulty in swallowing; fainting; fluid retention; hallucinations; nervousness; nightmares; skin rash; shortness of breath; tingling in the hands or feet; or visual disturbances.

INTERACTIONS
Bromocriptine interacts with several other types of medications:
1. Phenothiazine tranquilizers, methyldopa, haloperidol, metoclopramide, reserpine, and monoamine oxidase (MAO) inhibitors decrease the beneficial effects of bromocriptine.
2. Dosages of antihypertensive medications may require adjustment when bromocriptine is started.

Before starting to take bromocriptine, BE SURE TO TELL YOUR DOCTOR about any medications you are currently taking, especially if you are taking any of those medications listed above.

WARNINGS
• Tell your doctor about unusual or allergic reactions you have had to any medications, especially to bromocriptine or ergotamine.
• Before starting treatment with this medication, be sure to tell your doctor if you now have or have ever had heart or blood vessel disease, kidney disease, liver disease, or mental disorders.

• If this drug makes you dizzy or drowsy, avoid tasks that require alertness, such as driving a car.

• Do not stop taking bromocriptine unless you first check with your doctor. Stopping the drug abruptly may lead to a worsening of your condition. Your doctor may want to reduce your dosage gradually to prevent this from occurring.

• Be sure to tell your doctor if you are pregnant. It is generally recommended that bromocriptine not be used during pregnancy because there have been reports of birth defects in both animals and humans whose mothers received the drug during pregnancy. Also, be sure to tell your doctor if you are breast-feeding an infant. Bromocriptine blocks milk production.

Bromophen T.D.—see phenylpropanolamine, phenylephrine, and brompheniramine combination

Bromphen—see brompheniramine

brompheniramine

BRAND NAMES (Manufacturers)
Bromphen (various manufacturers)
brompheniramine maleate (various manufacturers)
Diamine T.D. (Major)
Dimetane* (Robins)
Dimetane Extentabs* (Robins)
Veltane (Lannett)
*Available over-the-counter (without a prescription)

TYPE OF DRUG
Antihistamine

INGREDIENT
brompheniramine

DOSAGE FORMS
Tablets (4 mg and 8 mg)
Sustained-release tablets (8 mg and 12 mg)
Oral elixir (2 mg per 5-ml spoonful, with or without 3% alcohol)

STORAGE
Brompheniramine tablets and oral elixir should be stored at room temperature in tightly closed containers.

USES
This medication is an antihistamine (antihistamines block the action of histamine, a chemical released by the body during an allergic reaction). Brompheniramine is used to treat or prevent symptoms of allergy.

TREATMENT
To avoid stomach upset, take brompheniramine with food or with a full glass of milk or water (unless your doctor directs you to do otherwise).

The elixir form should be measured carefully with a specially designed 5-ml measuring spoon. An ordinary kitchen teaspoon is not accurate enough.

The sustained-release tablets should be swallowed whole. Breaking, chewing, or crushing them destroys their sustained-release activity and may increase side effects.

If you miss a dose, take the missed dose as soon as possible, unless it is almost time for your next dose. In that case, don't take the missed dose at all; just return to your regular dosing schedule. Do not double the next dose.

SIDE EFFECTS
Minor. Blurred vision; confusion; constipation; diarrhea; difficult or painful urination; dizziness; dry mouth, throat, or nose; headache; irritability; loss of appetite; nausea; restlessness; ringing or buzzing in the ears; stomach upset; or unusual increase in sweating. These side effects should disappear as your body adjusts to the medication.

This medication can cause increased sensitivity to sunlight. It is, therefore, important to avoid prolonged exposure to sunlight and sunlamps. Wear protective clothing, and use an effective sunscreen.

If you are constipated, increase the amount of fiber in your diet (fresh fruits and vegetables, salads, bran, and whole-grain breads), exercise, and drink more water (unless your doctor tells you not to do so.)

Chew sugarless gum, or suck on ice chips or a piece of hard candy to reduce mouth dryness.

If you feel dizzy or light-headed, sit or lie down for a while; get up slowly, and be careful on stairs.

Major. Tell your doctor about any side effects that are persistent or particularly bothersome. IT IS ESPECIALLY IMPORTANT TO TELL YOUR DOCTOR about a change in menstruation, clumsiness, feeling faint, flushing of the face, hallucinations, palpitations, rash, seizures, shortness of breath, sleeping disorders, sore throat or fever, tightness in the chest, unusual bleeding or bruising, or unusual tiredness or weakness.

INTERACTIONS
Brompheniramine interacts with several other drugs:
1. Concurrent use of it with central nervous system depressants (such as alcohol, barbiturates, benzodiazepine tranquilizers, muscle relaxants, narcotics, pain medications, and phenothiazine tranquilizers) or with tricyclic antidepressants can cause extreme drowsiness.
2. Monoamine oxidase (MAO) inhibitors (isocarboxazid, pargyline, phenelzine, and tranylcypromine) can increase the side effects of this medication. At least 14 days should separate the use of this drug and the use of an MAO inhibitor.
3. Brompheniramine can decrease the activity of oral anticoagulants (blood thinners, such as warfarin).

BE SURE TO TELL YOUR DOCTOR about any medications you are currently taking.

WARNINGS
• Tell your doctor about unusual or allergic reactions you have had to medications, especially to brompheniramine or to any other antihistamine (such as carbinoxamine, chlorpheniramine, clemastine, cyproheptadine, dexchlorpheniramine, dimenhydrinate, dimethindene, diphenhydramine, diphenylpyraline, doxylamine, hydroxyzine, promethazine, pyrilamine, terfenadine, trimeprazine, tripelennamine, and triprolidine).
• Tell your doctor if you now have or if you have ever had asthma, blood vessel disease, glaucoma, high blood

pressure, kidney disease, peptic ulcers, enlarged prostate gland, or thyroid disease.

• Brompheniramine can cause drowsiness or dizziness. Your ability to perform tasks that require alertness, such as driving a car or operating potentially dangerous machinery, may be decreased. Appropriate caution should be taken.

• Be sure to tell your doctor if you are pregnant. The effects of this medication during pregnancy have not been thoroughly studied in humans. Also, tell your doctor if you are breast-feeding an infant. Small amounts of brompheniramine pass into breast milk and may cause unusual excitement or irritability in nursing infants.

brompheniramine maleate—see brompheniramine

brompheniramine, phenylephrine, and phenylpropanolamine—see phenylpropanolamine, phenylephrine, and brompheniramine combination

Bromtapp Extended Tablets—see phenylpropanolamine, phenylephrine, and bromphiramine combination

Bronchial—see theophylline and guaifenesin combination

bronkodyl—see theophylline

bumetanide

BRAND NAME (Manufacturer)
Bumex (Roche)
TYPE OF DRUG
Diuretic and antihypertensive
INGREDIENT
bumetanide
DOSAGE FORM
Tablets (0.5 mg, 1 mg, and 2 mg)
STORAGE
Bumetanide should be stored at room temperature in a tightly closed, light-resistant container.

USES
Bumetanide is prescribed to treat high blood pressure. It is also used to reduce fluid accumulation in the body caused by conditions such as heart failure, cirrhosis of the liver, kidney disease, and the long-term use of some medications. This medication reduces fluid accumulation by increasing the elimination of salt and water through the kidneys.

TREATMENT
To decrease stomach irritation, you can take this medication with a glass of milk or with a meal (unless your doctor directs you to do otherwise). Try to take it at the same time every day. Avoid taking a dose after 6:00 P.M.; otherwise you may have to get up during the night to urinate.

If you miss a dose of this medication, take the missed dose as soon as possible, unless it is almost time for the

next one. In that case, do not take the missed dose at all; just wait until the next scheduled dose. Do not double the next dose.

This medication does not cure high blood pressure, but it will help to control the condition as long as you continue to take it.

SIDE EFFECTS
Minor. Blurred vision, constipation, cramps, diarrhea, dizziness, headache, loss of appetite, sore mouth, or stomach upset. As your body adjusts to the medication, these side effects should disappear.

This medication causes an increase in the amount of urine or frequency of urination when you first begin to take it. It may also cause you to have an unusual feeling of tiredness. These effects should lessen after several days.

This medication can cause increased sensitivity to sunlight. It is, therefore, important to avoid prolonged exposure to sunlight and sunlamps. Wear protective clothing, and use an effective sunscreen.

To relieve constipation, increase the amount of fiber in your diet (fresh fruits and vegetables, salads, bran, and whole-grain cereals and breads) and exercise (unless your doctor directs you to do otherwise).

To avoid dizziness or light-headedness when you stand, contract and relax the muscles of your legs for a few moments before rising. Do this by pushing one foot against the floor while raising the other foot slightly, alternating feet.
Major. Tell your doctor about any side effects that are persistent or particularly bothersome. IT IS ESPECIALLY IMPORTANT TO TELL YOUR DOCTOR about abdominal pain, confusion, difficulty in breathing, dry mouth, fainting, itching, joint pains, loss of appetite, mood changes, muscle pain and cramps, nausea, palpitations, rash, ringing in the ears, sore throat, thirst, tingling in the fingers and toes, unusual bleeding or bruising, vomiting, weakness, or yellowing of the eyes or skin.

INTERACTIONS
Bumetanide interacts with several other types of drugs:
1. It can increase the side effects of alcohol, barbiturates, narcotics, cephalosporin antibiotics, chloral hydrate, cortisone and cortisone-like steroids (such as dexamethasone, hydrocortisone, prednisone, and prednisolone), digoxin, digitalis, lithium, amphotericin B, cisplatin, mercaptopurine, and polymyxin B.
2. Probenecid and indomethacin may decrease the diuretic effectiveness of this medication.
Before taking bumetanide, BE SURE TO TELL YOUR DOCTOR about any medications you are currently taking, especially any of those listed above.

WARNINGS
•Tell your doctor about unusual or allergic reactions you have had to any medications, especially to bumetanide, other diuretics, or any other sulfa drugs, including oral antidiabetic medicines or sulfonamide antibiotics.
•Before you start taking this medication, tell your doctor if you now have or if you have ever had kidney disease or problems with urination, diabetes mellitus, gout, liver disease, or asthma.

•Bumetanide can cause potassium loss. Signs of potassium loss include dry mouth, thirst, weakness, muscle pain or cramps, nausea, and vomiting. If you experience any of these symptoms, call your doctor. Your doctor may want to have blood tests performed periodically in order to monitor your potassium levels. To help avoid potassium loss, take this medication with a glass of fresh or frozen orange or cranberry juice, or eat a banana every day. The use of a salt substitute also helps prevent potassium loss. Do not change your diet or use a salt substitute, however, before discussing it with your doctor. Too much potassium may also be dangerous.

•Before having surgery or any other medical or dental treatment, be sure to tell your doctor or dentist that you are taking bumetanide.

•In order to avoid dizziness or fainting while taking this medication, try not to stand for long periods of time; avoid drinking excessive amounts of alcohol; and avoid strenuous exercise in hot weather, as well as hot baths, showers, and saunas.

•If you have high blood pressure, do not take any over-the-counter (nonprescription) medication for weight control or for cough, cold, allergy, asthma, or sinus problems, unless you first check with your doctor.

•To prevent severe water loss (dehydration) while taking this medication, check with your doctor if you have any illness that causes severe or continuous nausea, vomiting, or diarrhea.

•This medication can raise blood sugar levels in diabetic patients. Therefore, blood sugar should be monitored carefully with blood or urine tests when this medication is being taken.

•Be sure to tell your doctor if you are pregnant. This drug crosses the placenta. Although studies in humans have not been conducted, adverse effects have been reported in the offspring of animals that were given large doses of this drug during pregnancy. Also, tell your doctor if you are breast-feeding an infant. Although problems in humans have not been reported, it is not known if bumetanide passes into breast milk.

Bumex—see bumetanide

---

bupropion

BRAND NAME (Manufacturer)
Wellbutrin (Burroughs Wellcome)
TYPE OF DRUG
Antidepressant
INGREDIENT
bupropion hydrochloride
DOSAGE FORM
Tablets (75 mg and 100 mg)
STORAGE
Store at room temperature in a tightly closed container.

USES
Bupropion is used to relieve the symptoms of mental depression in patients who cannot take other medications. The exact mechanism of action of bupropion is unknown, but it is thought to relieve depression by altering the concentration of certain chemicals that are necessary for nerve transmission in the brain.

TREATMENT
It is important to take your medication on a regular schedule as recommended by your physician. If you miss a dose and the next regular dose should be taken in less than six hours, skip the missed dose and take the next dose at the regularly scheduled time. Never double the dose.

The effects of this medication may not become apparent for several weeks.

SIDE EFFECTS
Minor. Constipation, decreased appetite, decreased sexual ability, diarrhea, dizziness, dry mouth, excessive sweating, fatigue, headache, irregular heartbeat, insomnia, nausea, sedation, or vomiting. These side effects should decrease or disappear as your body adjusts to the medication.

To relieve constipation, increase the amount of fiber in your diet (fresh fruits and vegetables, salads, bran, and whole-grain breads), exercise, and drink more water (unless your doctor directs you to do otherwise).

To decrease dry mouth, chew sugarless gum or suck on ice chips or hard candy.

To avoid dizziness or light-headedness when you stand, contract and relax the muscles in your legs for a few moments before rising from a sitting or reclining postion. Do this by pushing one foot against the floor while raising the other foot slightly, alternating feet so that you are "pumping" your legs in a pedaling motion.

Major. Tell your doctor about any side effects that are persistent or particularly bothersome. IT IS ESPECIALLY IMPORTANT TO TELL YOUR DOCTOR about agitation, blurred vision, movement disorders, rash, tremors, or seizures.

INTERACTIONS
1. Bupropion may decrease the effectiveness of carbamazepine, phenobarbital, or phenytoin, which may lead to increased seizures.

2. Bupropion can interact with monoamine oxidase (MAO) inhibitors. At least 14 days should separate the use of this drug and the use of an MAO inhibitor.

3. Bupropion may decrease the effectiveness of cimetidine.

4. Alcohol may increase the side effects of bupropion.

WARNINGS
• Tell your doctor about unusual or allergic reactions you have had to any medications, especially to bupropion.

• Tell your doctor if you now have or have ever had cataracts or vision problems, seizures or epilepsy, bulimia, anorexia nervosa, mania, liver or kidney disease, or respiratory disorders.

• This medication may make you tired or drowsy or affect your thinking ability. You should not operate potentially dangerous equipment or drive an automobile until you know how this drug affects you.

• Do not stop taking this medication abruptly or increase the dose unless directed by your physician. Stopping abruptly or increasing your dose in large amounts can lead to increased side effects.

• Do not take any over-the-counter (nonprescription) medication or new prescription drug without discussing it with your doctor or pharmacist. Many over-the-counter preparations and some prescription medications may interact with bupropion.

• Tell your doctor if you are pregnant. In high doses, bupropion has caused chromosomal changes in animals, but the effects in humans are unknown. Also, tell your doctor if you are breast-feeding an infant. This medication can pass into the breast milk and lead to adverse effects in the infant.

BuSpar—see buspirone

buspirone

BRAND NAME (Manufacturer)
BuSpar (Mead Johnson Pharm)
TYPE OF DRUG
Antianxiety agent
INGREDIENT
buspirone hydrochloride
DOSAGE FORM
Tablets (5 mg and 10 mg)
STORAGE
Buspirone should be stored at room temperature in a tightly closed container. Avoid exposure to high temperatures (greater than 86°F).

USES

Buspirone is prescribed as a treatment for the symptoms of anxiety. It is not yet understood exactly how this medication works. Buspirone has been shown to be effective in relieving symptoms of anxiety, but it is important that you try to identify and remove the cause of the anxiety as well.

TREATMENT

Buspirone should be taken exactly as directed by your doctor. It can be taken with food or a full glass of water if stomach upset occurs.

If you are taking this drug regularly and miss a dose, take the missed dose immediately if you remember within an hour. If more time has passed, however, skip the dose you missed and wait for the next scheduled dose. Do not double the dose.

SIDE EFFECTS

Minor. Diarrhea, dizziness, excitement, fatigue, headache, lightheadedness, nasal congestion, nausea, nervousness, sleeping problems, sweating, or weakness. These side effects should disappear as your body adjusts to this medication.

If you feel dizzy or light-headed, sit or lie down for a while; get up slowly from a sitting or reclining position, and be careful on stairs.

Major. Tell your doctor about any side effects that are persistent or particularly bothersome. IT IS ESPECIALLY IMPORTANT TO TELL YOUR DOCTOR about chest pain, confusion, feelings of anger, incoordination, muscle pain, numbness, rash, ringing in the ears, sore throat, tingling in your fingers or toes, or tremors.

INTERACTIONS

Although extensive studies have not yet been completed, buspirone may interact with several other medications.

To prevent oversedation, this drug should not be taken with alcohol or other central nervous system depressants (such as antihistamines, barbiturates, muscle relaxants, pain medicines, narcotics, medicines for seizures, phenothiazine tranquilizers, and antidepressants).

Before starting buspirone, BE SURE TO TELL YOUR DOCTOR about any medications you are currently taking, especially any of those listed above.

WARNINGS

• Before starting buspirone, be sure to tell your doctor about any unusual or allergic reactions you have had to any medications, especially to buspirone.

• Be sure to tell your doctor if you now have or if you have ever had kidney disease, liver disease, or any type of psychiatric disorder.

• Until you experience how this medication affects you, do not drive a car or operate potentially dangerous machinery.

• Be sure to tell your doctor if you are pregnant. Although buspirone does appear to be safe in animals, complete studies in pregnant women have not been conducted. Also, be sure to tell your doctor if you are breast-feeding an infant. Small amounts of buspirone have been shown to pass into the milk of animals.

busulfan

BRAND NAME (Manufacturer)
Myleran (Burroughs Wellcome)
TYPE OF DRUG
Antineoplastic (anticancer drug)
INGREDIENT
busulfan
DOSAGE FORM
Tablets (2 mg)
STORAGE
Busulfan should be stored at room temperature in a tightly closed container.

USES

Busulfan belongs to a group of drugs known as alkylating agents. It is used to treat leukemia. This medication works by binding to the rapidly growing cancer cells, preventing their multiplication and growth.

TREATMENT

Busulfan can be taken either on an empty stomach or with food or milk (as directed by your doctor).

The timing of the doses of this medication is important. Be sure you completely understand your doctor's instructions on how this medication should be taken.

If you miss a dose of this medication, do not take the missed dose at all; just return to your regular dosing schedule. Do not double the next dose.

SIDE EFFECTS

Minor. Diarrhea, dizziness, nausea, stomach upset, or vomiting. These side effects may disappear as your body adjusts to the medication. However, it is important to continue taking this medication despite any nausea or vomiting that may occur. Busulfan also causes hair loss, which is reversible when the medication is stopped.

If you feel dizzy, sit or lie down for a while; get up from a sitting or lying position slowly.

Major. Be sure to tell your doctor about any side effects that are persistent or particularly bothersome. IT IS ESPECIALLY IMPORTANT TO TELL YOUR DOCTOR about blurred vision, breast enlargement (in both sexes), chills, confusion, cough, darkening of the skin, difficulty in breathing, dry skin, fatigue, fever, itching, joint pain, loss of appetite, menstrual irregularities, mouth sores, muscle weakness, skin rash, sore throat, unusual bleeding or bruising, weight loss, or yellowing of the eyes or skin.

INTERACTIONS

Busulfan can increase the blood levels of uric acid, which can block the effectiveness of antigout medications (allopurinol, probenecid, sulfinpyrazone).

Before starting to take busulfan, BE SURE TO TELL YOUR DOCTOR about any medications you are currently taking, especially any antigout medication.

WARNINGS

• Tell your doctor about unusual or allergic reactions you have had to any medications, especially to busulfan.
• Before starting to take this medication, be sure to tell your doctor if you now have or if you have ever had blood disorders, chronic or recurrent infections, chicken pox or shingles, gout, or kidney stones.
• You should not receive any immunizations or vaccinations while taking this medication. Busulfan blocks the effectiveness of the vaccine and may result in infection.
• It is important to drink plenty of fluids (up to two or three quarts each day) while taking this medication, in order to prevent uric acid kidney stones from developing.
• Busulfan can lower your platelet count, thereby decreasing your body's ability to form blood clots. You should, therefore, be especially careful while brushing your teeth, flossing, or using toothpicks, razors, or fingernail scissors. Try to avoid falls and other injuries.
• Before having surgery or other medical or dental treatment, tell your doctor or dentist you are taking this drug.
• Busulfan can decrease fertility in both men and women.
• Be sure to tell your doctor if you are pregnant. Birth defects have been reported in both animals and humans whose mothers received busulfan during pregnancy. The risks should be discussed with your doctor. Also, tell your doctor if you are breast-feeding an infant. It is not known whether busulfan passes into breast milk.

butalbital with aspirin and caffeine—see aspirin, caffeine, and butalbital combination

Butazolidin—see phenylbutazone

Byclomine—see dicyclomine

Bydramine Cough Syrup—see diphenhydramine

Cafergot—see ergotamine and caffeine combination

Cafetrate—see ergotamine and caffeine combination

Calan—see verapamil

Calan SR—see verapamil

calcifediol

BRAND NAME (Manufacturer)
Calderol (Organon)
TYPE OF DRUG
Vitamin D analog
INGREDIENT
calcifediol (25-hydroxycholecalciferol)
DOSAGE FORM
Capsules (20 mcg and 50 mcg)
STORAGE
Calcifediol capsules should be stored at room temperature in a tightly closed, light-resistant container.

USES

Vitamin D is essential to many body systems, including bone structure, regulation of blood calcium levels, and heart and muscle contraction. Since vitamin D is activated in the kidneys, patients with chronic (long-term) kidney failure are unable to produce enough active vitamin D on their own. Calcifediol is one of the active forms of vitamin D. This medication is used to treat bone disease and hypocalcemia (low blood calcium levels) in patients on dialysis.

TREATMENT

Calcifediol can be taken either on an empty stomach or with food or milk (as directed by your doctor). The capsules should be swallowed whole; do not crush or chew them.

If you miss a dose of this drug, take the missed dose as soon as possible, unless it is almost time for the next dose. In that case, do not take the missed dose at all; return to your regular dosing schedule. Do not double the next dose.

SIDE EFFECTS

Minor. None, at the dosages normally prescribed.
Major. The side effects associated with calcifediol therapy are usually the result of too much medication (vitamin D toxicity). Tell your doctor about any side effects that are persistent or particularly bothersome. IT IS ESPECIALLY IMPORTANT TO TELL YOUR DOCTOR about

blurred vision, bone pain, constipation, dry mouth, headache, irritability, loss of appetite, mental disorders, metallic taste in the mouth, muscle pain, nausea, palpitations, runny nose, increased thirst, increased urination, vomiting, weakness, or weight loss.

INTERACTIONS

Calcifediol interacts with several types of medications:
1. The dosage of calcifediol may need to be altered if anticonvulsant medication (such as phenytoin, phenobarbital, and primidone) is started.
2. Cholestyramine, colestipol, and mineral oil can decrease the absorption of calcifediol from the gastrointestinal tract.
3. Use of magnesium-containing antacids along with calcifediol may cause high blood levels of magnesium.
4. Calcifediol may lower the effectiveness of verapamil.
　BE SURE TO TELL YOUR DOCTOR about any medications you are currently taking, especially any of those listed above.

WARNINGS

• Be sure to tell your doctor about unusual or allergic reactions you have had to any medications, especially to calcifediol, calcitriol, dihydrotachysterol, ergocalciferol, or vitamin D.
• Before starting to take this medication, be sure to tell your doctor if you now have or if you have ever had heart or blood vessel disease, hypercalcemia (high levels of calcium in the bloodstream), hyperphosphatemia (high levels of phosphate in the bloodstream), kidney disease, vitamin D intoxication, or sarcoidosis.
• Before taking over-the-counter (nonprescription) products that contain calcium, phosphates, magnesium, or vitamin D, consult your doctor. These ingredients can increase the side effects of calcifediol.
• Be sure to tell your doctor if you are pregnant. Although calcifediol (in normal doses) appears to be safe during pregnancy, extensive studies in humans have not been conducted. Birth defects have been reported in the offspring of animals that received large doses of this medication during pregnancy. Also, tell your doctor if you are breast-feeding an infant. Small amounts of calcifediol pass into breast milk.

Calciferol—see ergocalciferol (vitamin D)

calcitriol

BRAND NAME (Manufacturer)
Rocaltrol (Roche)
TYPE OF DRUG
Vitamin D analog
INGREDIENT
calcitriol (1.25-dihydroxycholecalciferol)
DOSAGE FORM
Capsules (0.25 mcg and 0.5 mcg)
STORAGE
Calcitriol should be stored at room temperature in a tightly closed, light-resistant container.

USES
Vitamin D is essential to bone structure, regulation of blood calcium levels, and heart and muscle contraction. Since vitamin D is activated in the kidneys, patients with chronic kidney failure are unable to produce enough active vitamin D on their own. Calcitriol is one of the active forms of vitamin D. This drug is used to treat bone disease and hypocalcemia (low blood calcium levels) in dialysis patients.

TREATMENT
Calcitriol can be taken either on an empty stomach or with food or milk (as directed by your doctor). The capsules should be swallowed whole; do not crush or chew them.
　If you miss a dose of this drug, take the missed dose as soon as possible, unless it is almost time for the next dose. In that case, do not take the missed dose at all; return to your regular dosing schedule. Do not double the next dose.

SIDE EFFECTS
Minor. None, at the dosages normally prescribed.
Major. Side effects result from too much medication (vitamin D toxicity). Tell your doctor about any side effects that are persistent or particularly bothersome. IT IS ESPECIALLY IMPORTANT TO TELL YOUR DOCTOR about appetite loss, blurred vision, bone pain, constipation, dry mouth, headache, irritability, mental disorders, metallic taste, muscle pain, nausea, palpitations, runny nose, increased thirst, increased urination, vomiting, weakness, or weight loss.

INTERACTIONS
Calcitriol interacts with several types of medications:
1. The dosage of calcitriol may need to be adjusted if anticonvulsant medication (phenytoin, phenobarbital, or primidone) is started.
2. Cholestyramine, colestipol, and mineral oil can decrease the absorption of calcitriol from the gastrointestinal tract.
3. Use of magnesium-containing antacids along with calcitriol may cause high blood levels of magnesium.
4. Calcitriol may lower the effectiveness of verapamil.
　BE SURE TO TELL YOUR DOCTOR about any medications you are currently taking, especially any of those listed above.

WARNINGS
• Be sure to tell your doctor about unusual or allergic reactions you have had to any medications, especially to calcitriol, calcifediol, dihydrotachysterol, ergocalciferol, or vitamin D.
• Before starting to take this drug, tell your doctor if you have ever had heart or blood vessel disease, hypercalcemia (high levels of blood calcium), hyperphosphatemia (high levels of blood phosphate), kidney disease, vitamin D intoxication, or sarcoidosis.
• Before taking any over-the-counter (nonprescription) products that contain calcium, phosphates, magnesium, or vitamin D, check with your doctor. These ingredients can increase the side effects of calcitriol.

• Be sure to tell your doctor if you are pregnant. Although calcitriol appears to be safe during pregnancy in humans, birth defects have been reported in the offspring of animals that received large doses during pregnancy. Also, tell your doctor if you are breast-feeding an infant. Studies have shown that small amounts of calcitriol may pass into breast milk.

CaldeCort Anti-Itch—see hydrocortisone (topical)

CaldeCort Light with Aloe—see hydrocortisone (topical)

Calderol—see calcifediol

Cam-ap-es—see hydralazine, hydrochlorothiazide, and reserpine combination

Capital with Codeine—see acetaminophen and codeine combination

Capoten—see captopril

Capozide—see captopril and hydrochlorothiazide

captopril

BRAND NAME (Manufacturer)
Capoten (Bristol-Meyers Squibb)
TYPE OF DRUG
Antihypertensive
INGREDIENT
captopril
DOSAGE FORM
Tablets (12.5 mg, 25 mg, 50 mg, and 100 mg)
STORAGE
Captopril should be stored at room temperature in a tightly closed container.

USES
Captopril is used to treat high blood pressure and congestive heart failure. It is a vasodilator (it dilates the blood vessels) that acts by blocking the production of chemicals that may be responsible for constricting or narrowing blood vessels.

TREATMENT
To obtain maximum benefit from captopril, you should take it on an empty stomach one hour before meals. In order to become accustomed to taking this medication, try to take it at the same time(s) every day.

It may be several weeks before you notice the full effects of this medication.

If you miss a dose of this medication, take the missed dose as soon as possible, unless it is almost time for the next dose. In that case, do not take the missed dose at all; just wait until the next scheduled dose. Do not double the dose.

Captopril does not cure high blood pressure, but it will help control the condition as long as you continue to take this drug.

SIDE EFFECTS
Minor. Abdominal pain, constipation, cough, diarrhea, dizziness, dry mouth, fatigue, flushing, headache, insomnia, loss of taste, loss of appetite, nausea, or vomiting. These side effects should disappear as your body adjusts to the medication.

This medication can increase your sensitivity to sunlight. It is, therefore, important to avoid prolonged exposure to sunlight and sunlamps. Wear protective clothing and sunglasses, and use an effective sunscreen.

To relieve constipation, increase the amount of fiber in your diet (fresh fruits and vegetables, salads, bran, and whole-grain breads), exercise, and drink more water (unless your doctor directs you to do otherwise).

To relieve mouth dryness, suck on ice chips or a piece of hard candy or chew sugarless gum.

To avoid dizziness or light-headedness when you stand, contract and relax the muscles of your legs for a few moments before rising. Do this by pushing one foot against the floor while raising the other foot slightly, alternating feet so that you are "pumping" your legs.
Major. Tell your doctor about any side effects that are persistent or particularly bothersome. IT IS ESPECIALLY IMPORTANT TO TELL YOUR DOCTOR about chest pain; chills; difficult or painful urination; fever; itching; mouth sores; palpitations; prolonged vomiting or diarrhea; rash; sore throat; swelling of the face, hands, or feet; tingling in the fingers or toes; unusual bleeding or bruising; or yellowing of the eyes or skin.

INTERACTIONS
Captopril interacts with several other types of medications:
1. Diuretics (water pills) and other antihypertensive medications can cause an excessive drop in blood pressure when combined with captopril (especially with the first dose).
2. The combination of captopril with spironolactone, triamterene, amiloride, potassium supplements, or salt substitutes can lead to hyperkalemia (dangerously high levels of potassium in the bloodstream).
3. Antineoplastic agents (anticancer drugs) or chloramphenicol can increase the bone marrow side effects of captopril.
4. Concurrent use of captopril and allopurinol can increase the risk of developing an allergic reaction.
5. Indomethacin can decrease the blood-pressure-lowering effects of captopril.
6. Captopril can delay the body's elimination of lithium. Concurrent use of captopril and lithium may cause lithium toxicity.

Before starting captopril, BE SURE TO TELL YOUR DOCTOR about any drugs you are taking, especially any of those listed above.

WARNINGS
• Tell your doctor about any reactions you have had to medications, especially to captopril or enalapril.
• Tell your doctor if you now have or if you have ever had aortic stenosis, blood disorders, kidney disease, kidney transplant, liver disease, systemic lupus erythematosus, or a heart attack or stroke.

• Be careful—excessive perspiration, dehydration, or prolonged vomiting or diarrhea can lead to an excessive drop in blood pressure while you are taking this medication. Contact your doctor if you have any of these symptoms.

• Before having surgery or other medical or dental treatment, tell your doctor you are taking this drug.

• The first few doses of this drug may cause dizziness. Try to avoid any sudden changes in posture.

• If you have high blood pressure, do not take any over-the-counter (nonprescription) medications for weight control, or for allergy, asthma, sinus, cough, or cold problems unless you first check with your doctor.

• Do not stop taking this medication unless you first consult your doctor. Stopping this drug abruptly may lead to a rise in blood pressure.

• Be sure to tell your doctor if you are pregnant. Captopril has been found to cause birth defects in the fetus if taken during the second or third trimester of pregnancy. Also tell your doctor if you are breast-feeding an infant. Captopril passes into breast milk. The effects of this drug on the infant have not been determined.

captopril and hydrochlorothiazide combination

BRAND NAME (Manufacturer)
Capozide (Squibb)
TYPE OF DRUG
Antihypertensive and diuretic
INGREDIENTS
captopril and hydrochlorothiazide
DOSAGE FORM
Tablets (25 mg captopril and 15 mg hydrochlorothiazide; 25 mg captopril and 25 mg hydrochlorothiazide; 50 mg captopril and 15 mg hydrochlorothiazide; 50 mg captopril and 25 mg hydrochlorothiazide)
STORAGE
Captopril and hydrochlorothiazide combination tablets should be stored at room temperature in a tightly closed container. This medication should be stored away from moisture and high heat (above 86°F).

USES
Captopril and hydrochlorothiazide combination is used to treat high blood pressure. Captopril is a vasodilator (it widens the blood vessels) that acts by blocking the production of chemicals that may be responsible for constricting blood vessels. Hydrochlorothiazide is a diuretic (water pill), which reduces body fluid accumulation by increasing the elimination of salt and water through the kidneys.

TREATMENT
To obtain the maximum benefit from this medication, take it on an empty stomach one hour before meals. In order to become accustomed to taking this medication, try to take it at the same time(s) every day.

Avoid taking a dose of this medication after 6:00 P.M.; otherwise, you may have to get up during the night to urinate.

It may be several weeks before you notice the full effects of this medication.

If you miss a dose of this medication, take the missed dose as soon as possible, unless it is almost time for the next dose. In that case, do not take the missed dose at all; just wait until the next scheduled dose. Do not double the dose.

Captopril and hydrochlorothiazide combination does not cure high blood pressure, but it will help to control the condition as long as you continue to take it.

SIDE EFFECTS
Minor. Abdominal pain, blurred vision, constipation, cough, cramping, diarrhea, dizziness, fatigue, flushing, headache, insomnia, loss of appetite, or loss of taste. These side effects should disappear as your body adjusts to this medication.

Hydrochlorothiazide can increase your sensitivity to sunlight. It is, therefore, important to avoid prolonged exposure to sunlight and sunlamps. Wear protective clothing and sunglasses, and use an effective sunscreen.

To relieve constipation, increase the amount of fiber in your diet (fresh fruits and vegetables, salads, bran, and whole-grain breads) and exercise (unless your doctor directs you to do otherwise).

To relieve mouth dryness, suck on ice chips or hard candy or chew sugarless gum.

To avoid dizziness or light-headedness when you stand, contract and relax the muscles of your legs for a few moments before rising. Do this by alternately pushing one foot against the floor while raising the other foot slightly, so that you are "pumping" your legs in a pedaling motion.

Major. Tell your doctor about any side effects that are persistent or particularly bothersome. IT IS ESPECIALLY IMPORTANT TO TELL YOUR DOCTOR about chest pain; chills; cough; difficult or painful urination; dry mouth; fever; hair loss; itching; mouth sores; muscle pain or cramps; nausea; palpitations; rash; shortness of breath; sore throat; swelling of the face, hands, or feet; thirst; tingling in the fingers or toes; unusual bleeding or bruising; vomiting; weakness; or yellowing of the eyes or skin.

INTERACTIONS
Captopril and hydrochlorothiazide combination can interact with several other types of medications:
1. The combination of captopril with spironolactone, triamterene, amiloride, potassium supplements, or salt substitutes can lead to hyperkalemia (dangerously high levels of potassium in the bloodstream).
2. Antineoplastic agents (anticancer drugs) and chloramphenicol can increase the bone marrow side effects of captopril.
3. Concurrent use of captopril and allopurinol can increase the risk of developing an allergic reaction.
4. Diuretics (water pills) and other antihypertensive medications can cause an excessive drop in blood pressure when combined with captopril (especially with the first dose).

5. Hydrochlorothiazide can decrease the effectiveness of oral anticoagulants, antigout medications, insulin, oral antidiabetic medicines, and methenamine.

6. Captopril can delay the body's elimination of lithium. Concurrent use of captopril and lithium may cause lithium toxicity.

7. Fenfluramine can increase the blood-pressure-lowering effects of hydrochlorothiazide (which can be dangerous).

8. Indomethacin can decrease the blood-pressure-lowering effects of captopril and hydrochlorothiazide, thereby counteracting the desired effects.

9. Cholestyramine and colestipol decrease the absorption of hydrochlorothiazide from the gastrointestinal tract. Hydrochlorothiazide should, therefore, be taken one hour before or four hours after a dose of cholestyramine or colestipol (if you have also been prescribed one of these drugs).

10. Hydrochlorothiazide may increase the side effects of amphotericin B, calcium supplements, cortisone and cortisone-like steroids (such as dexamethasone, hydrocortisone, prednisone, and prednisolone), digoxin, digitalis, lithium, quinidine, sulfonamide antibiotics, and vitamin D.

Before starting captopril and hydrochlorothiazide combination, BE SURE TO TELL YOUR DOCTOR about any medications you are currently taking.

WARNINGS

• Tell your doctor about unusual or allergic reactions you have had to any medications, especially to captopril or to hydrochlorothiazide or other diuretics (such as bendroflumethiazide, benzthiazide, chlorothiazide, chlorthalidone, cyclothiazide, hydroflumethiazide, methyclothiazide, metolozone, polythiazide, quinethazone, trichlormethiazide, and furosemide) or to sulfa medications (oral antidiabetic medications or sulfonamide antibiotics).

• Tell your doctor if you have ever had aortic stenosis, blood disorders, diabetes mellitus, gout, kidney disease or problems with urination, kidney transplant, liver disease, pancreatic disease, a heart attack, or systemic lupus erythematosus.

• Hydrochlorothiazide can cause potassium loss. Signs of potassium loss include dry mouth, thirst, weakness, muscle pain or cramps, nausea, and vomiting. If you experience any of these symptoms, call your doctor. To help prevent this problem, your doctor may have blood tests performed periodically to monitor your potassium levels. To help avoid potassium loss, take this medication with a glass of fresh or frozen orange juice or cranberry juice, or eat a banana every day. The use of a salt substitute also helps to prevent potassium loss. Do not change your diet or use a salt substitute, however, until you discuss it with your doctor. Too much potassium may also be dangerous.

• Limit your intake of alcoholic beverages while taking this medication, in order to prevent dizziness and light-headedness.

• If you have high blood pressure, do not take any over-the-counter (nonprescription) medications for weight control or for allergy, asthma, cough, cold, or sinus problems, unless your doctor directs you to do so.

• To prevent dehydration (severe water loss) while taking this medication, check with your doctor if you have any illness that causes severe or continuous diarrhea, nausea, or vomiting.

• This medication can raise blood sugar levels in diabetic patients. Therefore, sugar levels should be carefully monitored with blood or urine tests when this medication is started.

• Before having surgery or any other medical or dental treatment, be sure to tell your doctor or dentist that you are taking this medication.

• This drug may cause dizziness. Use caution while driving or operating potentially dangerous machinery.

•A "fixed-dose" drug like this is not generally the first choice in the treatment of high blood pressure. Usually, the patient first receives each ingredient singly. If there is an adequate response to the fixed dose contained in this product, it can then be substituted. The advantage of a combination product is increased convenience and (often) decreased cost.

• Do not stop taking this medication unless you first consult your doctor. Stopping this drug abruptly may lead to a rise in blood pressure.

• Be sure to tell your doctor if you are pregnant. Captopril has been found to cause birth defects in the fetus if taken during the second or third trimester of pregnancy. Hydrochlorothiazide can cause adverse effects in the newborn infant if it is given to the mother close to term. Also, tell your doctor if you are breast-feeding an infant. Although problems in humans have not been reported, small amounts of this drug can pass into breast milk, so caution is warranted.

Carafate—see sucralfate

---

carbamazepine

BRAND NAMES (Manufacturers)
carbamazepine (various manufacturers)
Epitol (Lemmon)
Tegretol (Geigy)
Tegretol Chewable (Geigy)
TYPE OF DRUG
Anticonvulsant
INGREDIENT
carbamazepine
DOSAGE FORMS
Tablets (200 mg)
Chewable tablets (100 mg)
Oral suspension (100 mg per 5-ml spoonful)
STORAGE
Carbamazepine tablets and oral suspension should be stored at room temperature in tightly closed containers.

USES

This medication is used for the treatment of seizure disorders and for relief of neuralgia (nerve pain). The mechanism of carbamazepine's antiseizure activity is unknown, but it is not related to other anticonvulsants.

Carbamazepine is not an ordinary pain reliever—it should not be used for minor aches or pains.

TREATMENT

Carbamazepine can be taken with food if stomach upset occurs, unless your doctor directs otherwise.

Carbamazepine works best when the level of medicine in your bloodstream is kept constant. It is best, therefore, to take it at evenly spaced intervals day and night. For example, if you are to take four doses a day, the doses should be spaced six hours apart.

Try not to miss any doses of this medication. If you do miss a dose, take the missed dose as soon as possible, unless it is almost time for the next dose. In that case, do not take the missed dose at all; just return to your regular dosing schedule. Do not double the next dose unless your doctor directs you to do so. If you are taking carbamazepine for a seizure disorder and you miss two or more doses, be sure to contact your doctor.

SIDE EFFECTS

Minor. Agitation; blurred vision; confusion; constipation; diarrhea; dizziness; drowsiness; dry mouth; headache; loss of appetite; muscle or joint pain; nausea; restlessness; sweating; vomiting; or weakness. These side effects should disappear over time and as your body adjusts to the medication.

This medication can increase your sensitivity to sunlight. It is, therefore, important to avoid prolonged exposure to sunlight and sunlamps. Wear protective clothing and sunglasses, and use an effective sunscreen.

To relieve constipation, increase the amount of fiber in your diet (fresh fruits and vegetables, salads, bran, and whole-grain breads), exercise, and drink more water (unless your doctor directs you to do otherwise).

To relieve mouth dryness, suck on ice chips or a piece of hard candy or chew sugarless gum.

If you feel dizzy or light-headed, sit or lie down for a while; get up slowly from a sitting or reclining position, and be careful on stairs.

Major. Be sure to tell your doctor about any side effects that are persistent or particularly bothersome. IT IS ESPECIALLY IMPORTANT FOR YOU TO TELL YOUR DOCTOR about abdominal pain, chills, depression, difficulty in breathing, difficulty in urinating, eye discomfort, fainting, fever, hair loss, hallucinations, impotence, loss of balance, mouth sores, nightmares, numbness or tingling sensations, palpitations, ringing in the ears, skin rash, sore throat, swelling of the hands and feet, twitching, unusual bleeding or bruising, or yellowing of the eyes or skin.

INTERACTIONS

Carbamazepine interacts with other types of medications:
1. Concurrent use of it with central nervous system depressants (such as alcohol, antihistamines, barbiturates, benzodiazepine tranquilizers, muscle relaxants, narcotics, pain medications, and phenothiazine tranquilizers) or with tricyclic antidepressants can cause extreme drowsiness.
2. Phenobarbital, phenytoin, and primidone can decrease blood levels and effectiveness of carbamazepine.

3. Isoniazid, propoxyphene, verapamil, cimetidine, troleandomycin, and erythromycin can increase the blood levels of carbamazepine, which can increase side effects.
4. The combination of lithium and carbamazepine can lead to central nervous system side effects.
5. Carbamazepine can decrease the effectiveness of phenytoin, oral anticoagulants (blood thinners, such as warfarin), doxycycline, oral contraceptives (birth control pills), ethosuximide, valproic acid, aminophylline, and theophylline.
6. The use of carbamazepine within 14 days of the use of a monoamine oxidase (MAO) inhibitor can lead to serious side effects.

Before you start to take carbamazepine, BE SURE TO TELL YOUR DOCTOR about any medications you are currently taking, especially any of those listed above.

WARNINGS

• Tell your doctor about unusual or allergic reactions you have had to any medications, especially to carbamazepine or to tricyclic antidepressants (such as amitriptyline, desipramine, doxepin, imipramine, protriptyline, or nortriptyline).
• Tell your doctor if you now have or if you have ever had bone marrow depression, blood disorders, difficulty urinating, glaucoma, heart or blood vessel disease, kidney disease, or liver disease.
• Before having surgery or any other medical or dental treatment, be sure to tell your doctor or dentist that you are taking this medication.
• If this medication makes you dizzy or drowsy, do not take part in any activity that requires alertness, such as driving a car or operating potentially dangerous equipment.
• If you are taking this medication to control a seizure disorder, do not stop taking it suddenly. If you stop abruptly, you may experience uncontrollable seizures.
• Be sure to tell your doctor if you are pregnant. Birth defects have been reported more often in infants whose mothers have seizure disorders. It is unclear if the increased risk of birth defects is associated with the disorder or with the anticonvulsant medications, such as carbamazepine, that are used to treat the condition. The risks and benefits of treatment should be discussed with your doctor. Also, tell your doctor if you are breast-feeding an infant. Small amounts of carbamazepine pass into breast milk.

carbenicillin

BRAND NAME (Manufacturer)
Geocillin (Roerig)
TYPE OF DRUG
Antibiotic
INGREDIENT
carbenicillin indanyl sodium
DOSAGE FORM
Tablets (382 mg)
STORAGE
Store at room temperature in a tightly closed container.

USES

Carbenicillin is used to treat infections of the urinary tract, respiratory tract, skin, abdomen, and the prostate gland. It acts by severely injuring the cell walls of the infecting bacteria, thereby preventing them from growing and multiplying. Carbenicillin kills susceptible bacteria but is not effective against viruses, parasites, or fungi.

TREATMENT

This drug should be taken on an empty stomach with a glass of water one hour before or two hours after a meal.

Carbenicillin works best when the level of medicine in your bloodstream is kept constant. It is best, therefore, to take the doses at evenly spaced intervals day and night. For example, if you are taking four doses a day, the doses should be spaced six hours apart.

If you miss a dose of this medication, take the missed dose immediately. However, if you do not remember to take the missed dose until it is almost time for your next dose, take it; space the following dose about halfway through the regular interval between doses; and then return to your regular schedule. Try not to skip any doses.

It is important to continue to take this medication for the entire time prescribed by your doctor (usually seven to 14 days), even if the symptoms of the infection disappear before the end of that period. If you stop taking the drug too soon, resistant bacteria are given the chance to continue growing, and the infection could recur.

SIDE EFFECTS

Minor. Diarrhea, heartburn, nausea, or vomiting. These side effects should disappear as your body adjusts to the medication.

Major. Tell your doctor about any side effects that are persistent or particularly bothersome. IT IS ESPECIALLY IMPORTANT TO TELL YOUR DOCTOR about bloating, chills, cough, darkened tongue, difficulty in breathing, fever, irritation of the mouth, muscle aches, rash, rectal or vaginal itching, severe diarrhea, or sore throat. Also, if your symptoms of infection seem to be getting worse rather than improving, you should contact your doctor.

INTERACTIONS

Carbenicillin interacts with other types of medications:
1. Probenecid can increase the blood concentrations and side effects of this medication.
2. Carbenicillin may decrease the effectiveness of oral contraceptives (birth control pills), and pregnancy could result. You should, therefore, use a different or additional form of birth control while taking this medication.

BE SURE TO TELL YOUR DOCTOR about any medications that you are currently taking, especially any of those listed above.

WARNINGS

• Tell your doctor about unusual or allergic reactions you have had to any drugs, especially to carbenicillin or penicillins or to cephalosporin antibiotics, penicillamine, or griseofulvin.
• Tell your doctor if you now have or if you have ever had allergies, asthma, bleeding problems, bowel disease, or kidney disease.

• This medication has been prescribed for your current infection only. Another infection later on, or one that someone else has, may require a different medicine. You should not give your medicine to other people, or use it for other infections, unless your doctor specifically directs you to do so.
• Diabetics taking carbenicillin should know that this drug can cause a false-positive sugar reaction with a Clinitest urine glucose test. To avoid this problem, while taking carbenicillin you should switch to Clinistix or Tes-Tape to test your urine for sugar.
• Be sure to tell your doctor if you are pregnant. Although carbenicillin appears to be safe during pregnancy, extensive studies in humans have not been conducted. Also, tell your doctor if you are breast-feeding an infant. Small amounts of this medication pass into breast milk and may temporarily alter the bacterial balance in the intestinal tract of the nursing infant, resulting in diarrhea.

Carbodec—see pseudoephedrine and carbinoxamine combination

Carbodec DM—see pseudoephedrine, carbinoxamine, and dextromethorphan combination

Cardec DM—see pseudoephedrine, carbinoxamine, and dextromethorphan combination

Cardec-S—see pseudoephedrine and carbinoxamine combination

Cardioquin—see quinidine

Cardizem—see diltiazem

Cardizem CD—see diltiazem

Cardizem SR—see diltiazem

---

carisoprodol

BRAND NAMES (Manufacturers)
carisoprodol (various manufacturers)
Rela (Schering)
Sodol (Major)
Soma (Wallace)
Soprodol (Schein)
TYPE OF DRUG
Muscle relaxant
INGREDIENT
carisoprodol
DOSAGE FORM
Tablets (350 mg)
STORAGE
Carisoprodol should be stored at room temperature in a tightly closed container.

USES

This medication is used to relieve painful muscle conditions. It should be used in conjunction with rest, physical therapy, and other measures to alleviate discomfort. It is not clear exactly how carisoprodol works, but it is thought to act as a central nervous system depressant. However, carisoprodol does not seem to act directly on the muscles of the body.

TREATMENT

In order to avoid stomach irritation, you can take carisoprodol with food or with a full glass of water or milk (unless your doctor directs you to do otherwise).

If you miss a dose of this medication and remember within an hour, take the missed dose immediately. If more than an hour has passed, do not take the missed dose at all; just return to your regular dosing schedule. Do not double the next dose of this drug.

SIDE EFFECTS

Minor. Dizziness, drowsiness, headache, hiccups, insomnia, nausea, stomach pain, or vomiting. These side effects should disappear as your body adjusts to the medication.

If you feel dizzy, sit or lie down for a while; get up slowly from a sitting or reclining position, and be careful on stairs.

Major. Tell your doctor about any side effects that are persistent or particularly bothersome. IT IS ESPECIALLY IMPORTANT TO TELL YOUR DOCTOR about agitation, depression, fainting, irritability, loss of coordination, palpitations, or tremors.

INTERACTIONS

Carisoprodol interacts with several other types of drugs: Concurrent use of it with other central nervous system depressants (such as alcohol, antihistamines, barbiturates, benzodiazepine tranquilizers, muscle relaxants, narcotics, pain medications, phenothiazine tranquilizers, and sleeping medications) or with tricyclic antidepressants can lead to extreme drowsiness.

BE SURE TO TELL YOUR DOCTOR about any medications you are currently taking, especially any listed above.

WARNINGS

• Tell your doctor about unusual or allergic reactions you have had to any medications, especially to carisoprodol, meprobamate, or tybamate.

• Before starting to take carisoprodol, tell your doctor if you now have or if you have ever had kidney disease, liver disease, or porphyria.

• If this drug makes you dizzy or drowsy, avoid taking part in any activity that requires alertness, such as driving a car or operating potentially dangerous equipment.

• Some of these products contain the color additive FD&C Yellow No. 5 (tartrazine), which can cause allergic-type reactions (rash, fainting, shortness of breath) in certain susceptible individuals.

• Carisoprodol has the potential for abuse and should be used with caution. Do not increase the dosage or stop taking the drug unless you first consult your doctor. If you have been taking carisoprodol for several months and you stop taking it abruptly, you could experience a withdrawal reaction. Your doctor may, therefore, want to decrease your dosage of the medication gradually.

• Be sure to tell your doctor if you are pregnant. Although carisoprodol appears to be safe during pregnancy, extensive studies have not been conducted in humans. Also, tell your doctor if you are breast-feeding an infant. This medication passes into breast milk and can cause excessive drowsiness and stomach upset in nursing infants.

Catapres—see clonidine

Catapres-TTS—see clonidine

Ceclor—see cefaclor

CeeNu—see lomustine

---

cefaclor

BRAND NAME (Manufacturer)
Ceclor (Lilly)
TYPE OF DRUG
Cephalosporin antibiotic
INGREDIENT
cefaclor
DOSAGE FORMS
Capsules (250 mg and 500 mg)
Oral suspension (125 mg, 187 mg, 250 mg, and 375 mg per 5-ml spoonful)
STORAGE
Cefaclor capsules should be stored at room temperature in a tightly closed container. The oral suspension form of this drug should be stored in the refrigerator in a tightly closed container. Any unused portion of the oral suspension should be discarded after 14 days because the drug loses its potency after that time. This medication should never be frozen.

USES

This medication is used to treat a wide variety of bacterial infections, including those of the middle ear, skin, upper and lower respiratory tract, and urinary tract. This drug acts by severely injuring the cell walls of the infecting bacteria, thereby preventing them from growing and multiplying. Cefaclor kills susceptible bacteria, but it is not effective against viruses, parasites, or fungi.

TREATMENT

Cefaclor can be taken either on an empty stomach or with food or milk (in order to avoid an upset stomach).

The contents of the suspension form of cefaclor tend to settle on the bottom of the bottle, so it is necessary to shake the container well to distribute the ingredients evenly and equalize the doses. Each dose should then be measured carefully with a specially designed 5-ml measuring spoon or with the dropper provided. An ordinary kitchen teaspoon is not accurate enough.

Cephalosporin antibiotics work best when the level of medicine in your bloodstream is kept constant. It is best, therefore, to take the doses at evenly spaced intervals day and night. For example, if you are to take three doses a day, the doses should be spaced eight hours apart.

If you miss a dose of this medication, take the missed dose immediately. If you do not remember to take the missed dose until it is almost time for your next dose, take it; space the following dose halfway through the regular interval between doses; then return to your regular dosing schedule. Try not to skip any doses.

It is important to continue to take this medication for the entire time prescribed by your doctor (usually seven to 14 days), even if the symptoms disappear before the end of that period. If you stop taking this drug too soon, resistant bacteria are given a chance to continue growing, and the infection could recur.

SIDE EFFECTS

Minor. Abdominal pain, diarrhea, dizziness, fatigue, headache, heartburn, loss of appetite, nausea, or vomiting. These side effects should disappear as your body adjusts to the medication.

If you feel dizzy, sit or lie down for a while; get up slowly from a sitting or reclining position, and be careful on stairs.

Major. Tell your doctor about any side effects that are persistent or particularly bothersome. IT IS ESPECIALLY IMPORTANT TO TELL YOUR DOCTOR about darkened tongue, difficulty in breathing, fever, itching, joint pain, rash, rectal or vaginal itching, severe diarrhea (which can be watery or can contain pus or blood), sore mouth, stomach cramps, tingling in the hands or feet, or unusual bleeding or bruising. Also, if symptoms of infection seem to be getting worse rather than improving, contact your doctor.

INTERACTIONS

Cefaclor interacts with several other types of medications:

1. Probenecid can increase the blood concentrations and side effects of this medication.

2. The side effects, especially effects on the kidneys, of furosemide, bumetanide, ethacrynic acid, colistin, vancomycin, polymyxin B, and aminoglycoside antibiotics can be increased by cefaclor.

BE SURE TO TELL YOUR DOCTOR about any medications you are currently taking, especially any listed above.

WARNINGS

• Tell your doctor about unusual or allergic reactions you have had to any medication, especially to cefaclor or other cephalosporin antibiotics (such as cefamandole, cephalexin, cephradine, cefadroxil, cefazolin, cefoperazone, cefotaxime, ceftizoxime, cephalothin, cephapirin, cefuroxime, and moxalactam) or to penicillin antibiotics.
• Tell your doctor if you now have or if you have ever had kidney disease.
• This medication has been prescribed for your current infection only. Another infection later on, or one that someone else has, may require a different medicine. You should not give your medication to other people or use it for other infections, unless your doctor specifically directs you to do so.
• Diabetics who are taking cefaclor should know that this medication can cause a false-positive sugar reaction with a Clinitest urine glucose test. To avoid this problem while taking cefaclor, you should switch to Clinistix or Tes-Tape to test your urine sugar content.
• Be sure to tell your doctor if you are pregnant. Although the cephalosporin antibiotics appear to be safe during pregnancy, extensive studies in humans have not been conducted. Also, tell your doctor if you are breast-feeding an infant. Small amounts of this medication pass into breast milk and may temporarily alter the bacterial balance in the intestinal tract of the nursing infant, resulting in diarrhea.

cefadroxil

BRAND NAMES (Manufacturers)
cefadroxil (various manufacturers)
Duricef (Mead Johnson)
Ultracef (Bristol)
TYPE OF DRUG
Cephalosporin antibiotic
INGREDIENT
cefadroxil
DOSAGE FORMS
Tablets (1 g)
Capsules (500 mg)
Oral suspension (125 mg, 250 mg, and 500 mg per each 5-ml spoonful)
STORAGE
Cefadroxil tablets and capsules should be stored at room temperature in tightly closed containers. The oral suspension form of this drug should be stored in the refrigerator in a tightly closed container. Any unused portion of the oral suspension should be discarded after 14 days because the drug loses its potency after that time. This medication should never be frozen.

USES

This medication is used to treat a wide variety of bacterial infections, including those of the middle ear, skin, upper and lower respiratory tract, and urinary tract. This drug acts by severely injuring the cell walls of the infecting bacteria, thereby preventing them from growing and multiplying. Cefadroxil kills susceptible bacteria, but it is not effective against viruses, parasites, or fungi.

TREATMENT

You can take cefadroxil either on an empty stomach or, to avoid stomach upset, with food or milk.

The contents of the suspension form of cefadroxil tend to settle on the bottom of the bottle, so it is necessary to shake the container well to distribute the ingredients evenly and equalize the doses. Each dose should then be measured carefully with a specially designed 5-ml measuring spoon or with the dropper provided. An ordinary kitchen teaspoon is not accurate enough.

Cephalosporin antibiotics work best when the level of medicine in your bloodstream is kept constant. It is best, therefore, to take the doses at evenly spaced intervals day and night. For example, if you are to take two doses a day, the doses should be spaced 12 hours apart.

If you miss a dose of this medication, take the missed dose immediately. However, if you do not remember to take the missed dose until it is almost time for your next dose, take it; space the following dose halfway through the regular interval between doses; then return to your regular schedule. Try not to skip any doses.

It is important to continue to take this medication for the entire time prescribed by your doctor (usually seven to 14 days), even if the symptoms disappear before the end of that period. If you stop taking this drug too soon, resistant bacteria could continue growing, and the infection could recur.

SIDE EFFECTS

Minor. Abdominal pain, diarrhea, dizziness, fatigue, headache, heartburn, loss of appetite, nausea, or vomiting. These side effects should disappear as you adjust to the drug.

If you feel dizzy, sit or lie down for a while; get up slowly from a sitting or reclining position, and be careful on stairs.

Major. Tell your doctor about any side effects that are persistent or particularly bothersome. IT IS ESPECIALLY IMPORTANT TO TELL YOUR DOCTOR about darkened tongue, difficulty in breathing, fever, itching, joint pain, rash, rectal or vaginal itching, severe diarrhea (which can be watery, or contain pus or blood), sore mouth, stomach cramps, tingling in the hands or feet, or unusual bleeding or bruising. Also, if your symptoms of infection seem to be getting worse rather than improving, contact your doctor.

INTERACTIONS

Cefadroxil interacts with several other types of medications:

1. Probenecid can increase the blood concentrations and side effects of this medication.

2. The side effects, especially effects on the kidneys, of furosemide, bumetanide, ethacrynic acid, colistin, vancomycin, polymyxin B, and aminoglycoside antibiotics can be increased by cefadroxil.

Before you start to take this medication, BE SURE TO TELL YOUR DOCTOR about any medications you are currently taking, especially any of those listed above.

WARNINGS

• Tell your doctor about unusual or allergic reactions you have had to any medication, especially to cefadroxil or other cephalosporin antibiotics (such as cefamandole, cephalexin, cefaclor, cephradine, cefazolin, cefoperazone, cefotaxime, ceftizoxime, cephalothin, cephapirin, cefoxitin, cefuroxime, and moxalactam) or to penicillin antibiotics.

• Tell your doctor if you have ever had kidney disease.

• This medication has been prescribed for your current infection only. Another infection later on, or one that someone else has, may require a different medicine. You should not give your medication to other people or use it for other infections, unless so directed by your doctor.

• Diabetics taking cefadroxil should know that this drug can cause a false-positive sugar reaction with a Clinitest urine glucose test. To avoid this problem, switch to Clinistix or Tes-Tape to test your urine for sugar.

• Be sure to tell your doctor if you are pregnant. Although the cephalosporin antibiotics appear to be safe during pregnancy, extensive studies in humans have not been conducted. Also, tell your doctor if you are breast-feeding an infant. Small amounts of this medication pass into breast milk and may temporarily alter the bacterial balance in the intestinal tract of the nursing infant, resulting in diarrhea.

Ceftin—see cefuroxime

cefuroxime

BRAND NAME (Manufacturer)
Ceftin (Allen & Hanburys)
TYPE OF DRUG
Cephalosporin antibiotic
INGREDIENT
cefuroxime axetil
DOSAGE FORM
Tablets (125 mg, 250 mg, and 500 mg)
STORAGE
Cefuroxime tablets should be stored at room temperature in a tightly closed container.

USES

This medication is used to treat a wide variety of bacterial infections, including those of the middle ear, upper and lower respiratory tract, skin, and urinary tract. This drug acts by severely injuring the cell walls of the infecting bacteria, thereby preventing them from growing and multiplying. Cefuroxime kills susceptible bacteria, but it is not effective against viruses, parasites, or fungi.

TREATMENT

Cefuroxime can be taken either on an empty stomach or with food or milk (in order to avoid an upset stomach). The tablets may be crushed and mixed with food (such as applesauce or ice cream); however, a strong, persistent, bitter taste may be noted.

Cephalosporin antibiotics work best when the level of medicine in your bloodstream is kept constant. It is best, therefore, to take the doses at evenly spaced intervals day and night. For example, if you are to take two doses a day, the doses should be spaced 12 hours apart.

If you miss a dose of this medication, take the missed dose immediately. If you do not remember to take the missed dose until it is almost time for your next dose, take it; space the following dose halfway through the regular interval between doses; then return to your regular dosing schedule. Try not to skip any doses.

It is important to continue to take this medication for the entire time prescribed by your doctor (usually seven to 14 days), even if the symptoms disappear before the end of that period. If you stop taking this drug too soon, resistant bacteria are given a chance to continue growing, and the infection could recur.

SIDE EFFECTS

Minor. Abdominal pain, diarrhea, dizziness, fatigue, headache, heartburn, loss of appetite, nausea, or vomiting. These side effects should disappear as your body adjusts to the medication.

If you feel dizzy, sit or lie down for a while; get up slowly from a sitting or reclining position, and be careful on stairs.

Major. Tell your doctor about any side effects that are persistent or particularly bothersome. IT IS ESPECIALLY IMPORTANT TO TELL YOUR DOCTOR about darkened tongue, difficulty in breathing, fever, itching, joint pain, rash, rectal or vaginal itching, severe diarrhea, sore mouth, stomach cramps, tingling in the hands or feet, or unusual bleeding or bruising. Also, if your symptoms of infection seem to be getting worse rather than improving, you should contact your doctor.

INTERACTIONS

Cefuroxime interacts with several other types of medications:

1. Probenecid can increase the blood concentrations and side effects of this medication.

2. The side effects, especially effects on the kidneys, of furosemide, bumetanide, ethacrynic acid, colistin, vancomycin, polymyxin B, and aminoglycoside antibiotics can be increased by cefuroxime.

BE SURE TO TELL YOUR DOCTOR about any medications you are currently taking, especially any listed above.

WARNINGS

• Tell your doctor about any unusual or allergic reactions you have had to any medication, especially to cefuroxime or other cephalosporin antibiotics (such as cefaclor, cefamandole, cephalexin, cephradine, cefadroxil, cefazolin, cefoperazone, cefotaxime, ceftizoxime, cephalothin, cephapirin, and moxalactam) or to penicillin antibiotics.

• Tell your doctor if you now have or if you have ever had kidney disease.

• This medication has been prescribed for your current infection only. Another infection later on, or one that someone else has, may require a different medicine. You should not give your medication to other people or use it for other infections, unless your doctor specifically directs you to do so.

• Diabetics taking cefuroxime should know that this drug can cause a false-positive sugar reaction with a Clinitest urine glucose test. To avoid this problem while taking cefuroxime, you should switch to Clinistix or Tes-Tape to test your urine sugar content.

• Be sure to tell your doctor if you are pregnant. Although the cephalosporin antibiotics appear to be safe during pregnancy, extensive studies in humans have not been conducted. Also, tell your doctor if you are breast-feeding an infant. Small amounts of this medication pass into breast milk and may temporarily alter the bacterial balance in the intestinal tract of the nursing infant, resulting in diarrhea.

Celestone—see betamethasone

Cena-K—see potassium chloride

Centrax—see prazepam

---

cephalexin

BRAND NAMES (Manufacturers)
cephalexin monohydrate (various manufacturers)
Keflet (Dista)
Keflex (Dista)
Keftab (Dista)
TYPE OF DRUG
Cephalosporin antibiotic
INGREDIENT
cephalexin
DOSAGE FORMS
Tablets (250 mg, 500 mg, and 1 g)
Capsules (250 mg and 500 mg)
Oral suspension (125 mg and 250 mg per 5-ml spoonful)
Pediatric oral suspension (100 mg per ml)
STORAGE
Cephalexin tablets and capsules should be stored at room temperature in tightly closed containers. The oral suspension forms of this drug should be stored in the refrigerator in tightly closed containers. Any unused portion of the oral suspension should be discarded after 14 days because the drug loses its potency after that time. This medication should never be frozen.

USES

This medication is used to treat a wide variety of bacterial infections, including those of the bones, middle ear, prostate, skin, upper and lower respiratory tract, and urinary tract. This drug acts by severely injuring the cell walls of the infecting bacteria, thereby preventing them from growing and multiplying. Cephalexin kills susceptible bacteria, but it is not effective against viruses, parasites, or fungi.

TREATMENT

You can take cephalexin either on an empty stomach or, to avoid stomach upset, with food or milk.

The contents of the suspension form of cephalexin tend to settle on the bottom of the bottle, so it is necessary to shake the container well to distribute the ingredients evenly and equalize the doses. Each dose should then be measured carefully with a specially designed 5-ml measuring spoon or with the dropper provided. An ordinary kitchen teaspoon is not accurate enough.

Cephalosporin antibiotics work best when the level of medicine in your bloodstream is kept constant. It is best, therefore, to take your doses of this medication at evenly spaced intervals throughout the day and night. For example, if you are to take four doses of the medication a day, the doses should be spaced six hours apart.

If you miss a dose, take the missed dose immediately. However, if you do not remember to take the missed dose until it is almost time for your next dose, take it;

space the following dose halfway through the regular interval between doses; then return to your regular schedule. Do not skip any doses.

It is important to continue to take this medication for the entire time prescribed by your doctor (usually seven to 14 days), even if the symptoms disappear before the end of that period. If you stop taking this drug too soon, resistant bacteria are given a chance to continue growing, and the infection could recur.

SIDE EFFECTS

Minor. Abdominal pain, diarrhea, dizziness, fatigue, headache, heartburn, loss of appetite, nausea, or vomiting. These side effects should disappear as your body adjusts to the medication.

If you feel dizzy, sit or lie down for a while; get up slowly from a sitting or reclining position, and be careful on stairs.

Major. Tell your doctor about any side effects that are persistent or particularly bothersome. IT IS ESPECIALLY IMPORTANT TO TELL YOUR DOCTOR about darkened tongue, difficulty in breathing, fever, itching, joint pain, rash, rectal or vaginal itching, severe diarrhea (which can be watery, or contain pus or blood), sore mouth, stomach cramps, tingling in the hands or feet, or unusual bleeding or bruising. Also, if your symptoms of infection seem to be getting worse rather than improving, you should contact your doctor.

INTERACTIONS

Cephalexin interacts with several other types of drugs:

1. Probenecid can increase the blood concentrations of this medication.

2. The side effects, especially effects on the kidneys, of furosemide, bumetanide, ethacrynic acid, colistin, vancomycin, polymyxin B, and aminoglycoside antibiotics can be increased by cephalexin.

BE SURE TO TELL YOUR DOCTOR about any medications you are currently taking, especially any of those listed above.

WARNINGS

• Tell your doctor about unusual or allergic reactions you have had to any medication, especially to cephalexin or other cephalosporin antibiotics (such as cefamandole, cephradine, cefaclor, cefadroxil, cefazolin, cefoperazone, cefotaxime, ceftizoxime, cephalothin, cephapirin, cefoxitin, cefuroxime, and moxalactam) or to penicillin antibiotics.

• Tell your doctor if you now have or if you have ever had kidney disease.

• This medication has been prescribed for your current infection only. Another infection later on, or one that someone else has, may require a different medicine. You should not give your medication to other people or use it for other infections, unless your doctor specifically directs you to do so.

• Diabetics taking cephalexin should know that this drug can cause a false-positive sugar reaction with a Clinitest urine glucose test. To avoid this problem while taking cephalexin, you should switch to Clinistix or Tes-Tape to test your urine for sugar.

• Be sure to tell your doctor if you are pregnant. Although the cephalosporin antibiotics appear to be safe during pregnancy, extensive studies in humans have not been conducted and cautious use is warranted. Also, tell your doctor if you are breast-feeding an infant. Small amounts of this medication pass into breast milk and may temporarily alter the bacterial balance in the intestinal tract of the nursing infant, resulting in diarrhea.

cephalexin monohydrate—see cephalexin

cephradine

BRAND NAMES (Manufacturers)
Anspor (Smith Kline & French)
cephradine (various manufacturers)
Velosef (Apothecon)
TYPE OF DRUG
Cephalosporin antibiotic
INGREDIENT
cephradine
DOSAGE FORMS
Capsules (250 mg and 500 mg)
Oral suspension (125 mg and 250 mg per 5-ml spoonful)
STORAGE
Cephradine capsules should be stored at room temperature in tightly closed containers. The oral suspension form of this drug should be stored in the refrigerator in a tightly closed container. Any unused portion of the oral suspension should be discarded after 14 days because the drug loses its potency after that time. This medication should never be frozen.

USES
This medication is used to treat a wide variety of bacterial infections, including those of the middle ear, prostate, skin, upper and lower respiratory tract, and urinary tract. This drug acts by severely injuring the cell walls of the infecting bacteria, thereby preventing them from growing and multiplying. Cephradine kills susceptible bacteria, but it is not effective against viruses, parasites, or fungi.

TREATMENT
You can take cephradine either on an empty stomach or, in order to avoid an upset stomach, with food or milk.

The contents of the suspension form of cephradine tend to settle on the bottom of the bottle; it is important to shake the container well to distribute the ingredients evenly and equalize the doses. Each dose should then be measured carefully with a specially designed 5-ml measuring spoon or with the dropper provided. An ordinary kitchen teaspoon is not accurate enough, and often kitchen teaspoons vary in size.

Cephalosporin antibiotics work best when the level of medicine in your bloodstream is kept constant. It is best, therefore, to take the doses at evenly spaced intervals day and night. For example, if you are to take four doses a day, the doses should be spaced six hours apart.

If you miss a dose of this medication, take the missed dose immediately. However, if you do not remember to take the missed dose until it is almost time for your next dose, take it and space the following dose halfway through the regular interval between doses; then return to your regular dosing schedule. It is important that you try not to skip any doses of this medication.

It is important to continue to take this medication for the entire time prescribed by your doctor (usually seven to 14 days), even if the symptoms disappear before the end of that period. If you stop taking this drug too soon, resistant bacteria are given a chance to continue growing, and the infection could recur.

SIDE EFFECTS

Minor. Abdominal pain, diarrhea, dizziness, fatigue, headache, heartburn, loss of appetite, nausea, or vomiting. These side effects should disappear as your body adjusts to the medication.

If you feel dizzy, sit or lie down for a while; get up slowly from a sitting or reclining position, and be careful on stairs.

Major. Tell your doctor about any side effects that are persistent or particularly bothersome. IT IS ESPECIALLY IMPORTANT TO TELL YOUR DOCTOR about darkened tongue, difficulty in breathing, fever, itching, joint pain, rash, rectal or vaginal itching, severe diarrhea (which can be watery, or contain pus or blood), sore mouth, stomach cramps, tingling in the hands or feet, or unusual bleeding or bruising. Also, if your symptoms of infection seem to be getting worse rather than improving, you should contact your doctor immediately.

INTERACTIONS

Cephradine interacts with several other types of medications:

1. Probenecid can increase the blood concentrations and side effects of this medication.

2. The side effects, especially effects on the kidneys, of furosemide, bumetanide, ethacrynic acid, colistin, vancomycin, polymyxin B, and aminoglycoside antibiotics can be increased by cephradine.

BE SURE TO TELL YOUR DOCTOR about any medications you are currently taking, especially any of the medications that are listed above.

WARNINGS

• Tell your doctor about unusual or allergic reactions you have had to any medication, especially to cephradine or other cephalosporin antibiotics (such as cefamandole, cephalexin, cefaclor, cefadroxil, cefazolin, cefoperazone, cefotaxime, ceftizoxime, cephalothin, cephapirin, cefoxitin, cefuroxime, and moxalactam) or to penicillin antibiotics.

• Tell your doctor if you now have or if you have ever had kidney disease.

• This medication has been prescribed for your current infection only. Another infection later on, or one that someone else has, may require a different medicine. You should not give your medication to other people or use it for other infections, unless your doctor specifically directs you to do so.

• Diabetics taking cephradine should know that this drug can cause a false-positive sugar reaction with a Clinitest urine glucose test. To avoid this problem while taking cephradine, you should switch to Clinistix or Tes-Tape.

• Be sure to tell your doctor if you are pregnant. Although the cephalosporin antibiotics appear to be safe during pregnancy, extensive studies in humans have not been conducted. Also, tell your doctor if you are breast-feeding. Small amounts of this medication pass into breast milk and may alter the bacterial balance in the intestinal tract of the nursing infant, resulting in diarrhea.

Cerespan—see papaverine

Cetacort—see hydrocortisone (topical)

Cetamide—see sodium sulfacetamide (ophthalmic)

Chemet—see succimer

Chenix—see chenodiol

chenodiol

BRAND NAME (Manufacturer)
Chenix (Reid-Rowell)
TYPE OF DRUG
Gallstone dissolver
INGREDIENT
chenodiol
DOSAGE FORM
Tablets (250 mg)
STORAGE
Chenodiol tablets should be stored at room temperature in a tightly closed container.

USES

This medication is used to dissolve gallstones in individuals who cannot tolerate surgery. Chenodiol is a naturally occurring bile acid that blocks the body's production of cholesterol. This action leads to gradual dissolution of cholesterol gallstones.

TREATMENT

In order to obtain the maximum benefit from this medication, you should take it with food or milk. It is important to continue taking this medication for the entire time prescribed by your doctor (usually six months to two years), even if your symptoms disappear. If you stop using this drug too soon, your symptoms could recur (the gallstones may not have completely dissolved).

If you miss a dose of this medication, take the missed dose as soon as possible, unless it is almost time for the next dose. In that case, do not take the missed dose at all; just return to your regular dosing schedule. Do not double the next dose.

SIDE EFFECTS

Minor. Constipation, diarrhea, gas, heartburn, loss of appetite, nausea, stomach cramps, or vomiting. These side effects should disappear as your body adjusts to the medication.

If diarrhea continues to be a problem, contact your doctor. Antidiarrheal medications may be effective for short periods, or your doctor may want to decrease your dose of chenodiol.

To relieve constipation, increase the amount of fiber in your diet (fresh fruits and vegetables, salads, bran, and whole-grain breads), exercise, and drink more water (unless your doctor directs you to do otherwise).

Major. Tell your doctor about any side effects that are persistent or particularly bothersome. IT IS ESPECIALLY IMPORTANT TO TELL YOUR DOCTOR about yellowing of the eyes or skin.

INTERACTIONS
Chenodiol may interact with several other types of medications:

1. Cholestyramine, colestipol, and aluminum-containing antacids can decrease the absorption of chenodiol from the gastrointestinal tract.

2. Estrogen-containing drugs, oral contraceptives (birth control pills), probucol, and clofibrate can counteract the effectiveness of chenodiol.

Before you start to take this medication, BE SURE TO TELL YOUR DOCTOR about any other medications you are currently taking, especially if you are taking any of those listed above.

WARNINGS
• Be sure to tell your doctor about any unusual or allergic reactions you have had to any medications, especially to chenodiol.
• Tell your doctor if you now have or if you have ever had biliary tract disease, blood vessel disease, colon cancer, inflammatory bowel disease, liver disease, or pancreatitis.
• Body weight and diet influence the formation and dissolution of gallstones. A high-fiber, low-fat diet and weight reduction are recommended to increase the effectiveness of chenodiol.
• Be sure to tell your doctor if you are pregnant. Although extensive studies in humans have not been conducted, this medication has caused birth defects in the offspring of animals that received large doses of it during pregnancy. Also, tell your doctor if you are breast-feeding. It is not known whether chenodiol passes into breast milk.

Cheracol—see codeine and guaifenesin combination

Cherapas—see hydralazine, hydrochlorothiazide, and reserpine combination

Children's Advil—see ibuprofen

Chlorafed (Half-Strength)—see pseudoephedrine and chlorpheniramine combination

Chlorafed HS Timecelles—see pseudoephedrine and chlorpheniramine combination

chloral hydrate

BRAND NAMES (Manufacturers)
Aquachloral Supprettes (Webcon)
chloral hydrate (various manufacturers)
Noctec (Squibb Mark)

TYPE OF DRUG
Sedative/hypnotic

INGREDIENT
chloral hydrate

DOSAGE FORMS
Capsules (250 mg and 500 mg)
Oral syrup (250 mg and 500 mg per 5-ml spoonful)
Suppositories (325 mg, 500 mg, and 650 mg)

STORAGE
Store at room temperature in a tightly closed, light-resistant container. This medication should never be frozen. The suppositories should be kept in the glass container in which they were dispensed.

USES
Chloral hydrate is used as a sleeping aid in the treatment of insomnia. It is also used as an anti-anxiety or pain medication before or after surgical procedures. Exactly how chloral hydrate works is not clearly understood, but it is known to be a central nervous system depressant.

TREATMENT
Chloral hydrate should be taken 15 to 30 minutes before bedtime.

In order to prevent stomach irritation, you should take chloral hydrate capsules with a full glass of water (unless your doctor directs you to do otherwise). The capsules should be swallowed whole to avoid their bad taste.

Each dose of the oral syrup should be measured carefully with a specially designed 5-ml measuring spoon. An ordinary kitchen teaspoon is not accurate enough. The syrup should then be mixed with at least one-half glass (four ounces) of a nonalcoholic beverage (to avoid stomach irritation and to mask the taste).

To insert the suppository form of this medication, first unwrap it and moisten it slightly with water (if the suppository is too soft, run cold water over it or refrigerate it for 30 minutes before you unwrap it). Lie down on your left side with your right knee bent. Push the suppository well into the rectum with your finger. Try to avoid having a bowel movement for at least an hour.

The use of this drug as a sleeping aid should be limited to two weeks. After that period, chloral hydrate loses its ability to induce and sustain sleep.

SIDE EFFECTS
Minor. Diarrhea, dizziness, drowsiness during the day, gas, headache, nausea, stomach irritation, unpleasant taste in the mouth, or vomiting. These side effects should disappear as your body adjusts to the medication.

If you feel dizzy or light-headed, sit or lie down for a while; get up slowly from a sitting or reclining position, and be careful on stairs.

Major. Tell your doctor about any side effects that are persistent or particularly bothersome. IT IS ESPECIALLY

IMPORTANT TO TELL YOUR DOCTOR about confusion, difficulty in breathing, disorientation, excitation, fatigue, feeling faint, hallucinations, hives or itching, loss of coordination, nightmares, skin rash, or yellowing of the eyes or skin.

INTERACTIONS

Chloral hydrate interacts with a number of other types of medications:

1. Concurrent use of chloral hydrate with other central nervous system depressants (such as alcohol, barbiturates, benzodiazepine tranquilizers, muscle relaxants, narcotics, pain medications, phenothiazine tranquilizers, and other sleeping medications) or with tricyclic antidepressants can lead to extreme drowsiness.

2. Chloral hydrate can increase the effects of oral anticoagulants (blood thinners, such as warfarin), which can lead to bleeding complications.

BE SURE TO TELL YOUR DOCTOR about any medications you are currently taking, especially any listed above.

WARNINGS

•Tell your doctor about unusual or allergic reactions you have had to any medications, especially to chloral hydrate or to triclofos.

•Before starting to take this medication, be sure to tell your doctor if you now have or if you have ever had gastritis, heart disease, inflammation of the esophagus, bowel, or rectum, kidney disease, liver disease, porphyria, or ulcers.

•If this drug makes you dizzy or drowsy, do not take part in any activity that requires alertness, such as driving an automobile or operating dangerous machinery or equipment.

•Some dosage forms of this drug contain the color additive FD&C Yellow No. 5 (tartrazine), which can cause allergic-type reactions (shortness of breath, fainting, rash) in susceptible individuals.

•This drug has the potential for abuse and must be used with caution. A tolerance to this medication develops quickly; do not increase the dosage or stop taking this drug unless you first consult your doctor. If you have been taking chloral hydrate for a long time or have been taking large doses, you may experience anxiety, muscle twitching, tremors, weakness, dizziness, nausea, vomiting, insomnia, or blurred vision when you stop taking it. Your doctor may, therefore, want to reduce your dosage of this medication gradually.

•Be sure to tell your doctor if you are pregnant. Although extensive studies in animals and humans have not been conducted, it is known that chloral hydrate crosses the placenta. Therefore, if it is used for prolonged periods during the last three months of pregnancy, there exists the possibility that the infant will be born with an addiction to the medication and will experience a withdrawal reaction (convulsions and irritability) at birth. Also, be sure to tell your doctor if you are currently breast-feeding an infant. Small amounts of chloral hydrate are known to pass into breast milk and may cause excessive drowsiness in the nursing infant.

chlorambucil

BRAND NAME (Manufacturer)
Leukeran (Burroughs Wellcome)
TYPE OF DRUG
Antineoplastic (anticancer drug)
INGREDIENT
chlorambucil
DOSAGE FORM
Tablets (2 mg)
STORAGE
Chlorambucil should be stored at room temperature in a tightly closed, light-resistant container.

USES

Chlorambucil belongs to a group of drugs known as alkylating agents. It is used to treat a variety of cancers. Chlorambucil works by binding to the rapidly growing cancer cells, preventing their multiplication and growth.

TREATMENT

Chlorambucil can be taken either on an empty stomach or with food or milk (as directed by your doctor).

The timing of the doses of this medication is important. Be sure you completely understand your doctor's instructions on how this medication should be taken.

If you miss a dose of this medication, take the missed dose as soon as possible, unless it is almost time for the next dose. In that case, do not take the missed dose at all; just return to your regular dosing schedule. Do not double the next dose.

SIDE EFFECTS

Minor. Nausea, stomach upset, or vomiting. These side effects may disappear as your body adjusts to this medication. It is important, however, to continue taking this medication despite any nausea and vomiting that may occur. Chlorambucil can also cause hair loss, which is reversible when the medication is stopped.

Major. Tell your doctor about any side effects that are persistent or particularly bothersome. IT IS ESPECIALLY IMPORTANT TO TELL YOUR DOCTOR about chills, convulsions, difficulty in breathing, fever, itching, joint pain, menstrual irregularities, mouth sores, skin rash, sore throat, unusual bleeding or bruising, or yellowing of the eyes or skin.

INTERACTIONS

Chlorambucil can increase the blood levels of uric acid, which can block the effectiveness of antigout medications (allopurinol, probenecid, sulfinpyrazone).

BE SURE TO TELL YOUR DOCTOR about any medications you are currently taking, especially any listed above.

WARNINGS

•Tell your doctor about unusual or allergic reactions you have had to any drugs, especially to chlorambucil or melphalan.

•Before starting to take this medication, be sure to tell your doctor if you now have or if you have ever had blood disorders, chronic or recurrent infections, gout, kidney stones, or seizures.

• You should not receive any immunizations or vaccinations while taking this medication. Chlorambucil blocks the effectiveness of the vaccine and may lead to overwhelming infection if a live-virus vaccine is administered.

• While you are taking this medication, it is important that you drink plenty of fluids to prevent the formation of uric acid kidney stones.

• Chlorambucil can lower your platelet count, which can decrease your body's ability to form blood clots. You should, therefore, be especially careful while brushing your teeth, flossing, or using toothpicks, razors, or fingernail scissors. Try to avoid falls and other injuries. Before having any surgery or other medical or dental treatment, be sure that your doctor or dentist knows that you are taking this medication.

• Chlorambucil can decrease fertility in both sexes.

• Be sure to tell your doctor if you are pregnant. Birth defects have been reported in both animals and humans whose mothers received chlorambucil during pregnancy. The risks should be discussed with your doctor. Also, tell your doctor if you are breast-feeding an infant. It is not known whether or not chlorambucil passes into breast milk.

chloramphenicol (systemic)

BRAND NAMES (Manufacturers)
chloramphenicol (various manufacturers)
Chloromycetin Kapseals (Parke-Davis)
TYPE OF DRUG
Antibiotic
INGREDIENT
chloramphenicol
DOSAGE FORMS
Capsules (250 mg)
Oral suspension (150 mg per 5-ml spoonful)
STORAGE
Chloramphenicol capsules and oral suspension should be stored at room temperature in tightly closed, light-resistant containers. This medication should never be frozen.

USES
This medication is an antibiotic that is used to treat a wide variety of bacterial infections. It attaches to the bacteria and blocks their production of protein, thereby preventing their growth and multiplication. Chloramphenicol kills susceptible bacteria, but it is not effective against viruses, parasites, or fungi.

TREATMENT
Chloramphenicol is most effective if it is taken on an empty stomach one hour before or two hours after a meal.

The suspension form of this medication should be shaken well just before measuring each dose. The contents tend to settle on the bottom of the bottle, so it is necessary to shake the container to distribute the ingredients evenly and equalize the doses. Each dose should then be measured carefully with a specially designed 5-ml measuring spoon. An ordinary kitchen teaspoon is not accurate enough.

Chloramphenicol works best when the level of medicine in your bloodstream is kept constant. It is best, therefore, to take the doses at evenly spaced intervals day and night. For example, if you are to take four doses a day, the doses should be spaced six hours apart.

Try not to miss any doses of this medication. If you do miss a dose, take it as soon as you remember. However, if you do not remember to take the missed dose until it is almost time for your next dose, take the missed dose immediately; space the following dose about halfway through the regular interval between doses; then continue with your regular dosing schedule.

It is important to continue to take this medication for the entire time prescribed by your doctor (usually seven to 14 days), even if the symptoms disappear before the end of that period. If you stop taking the drug too soon, resistant bacteria are given a chance to continue growing, and the infection could recur.

SIDE EFFECTS
Minor. Diarrhea, headache, nausea, or vomiting. These side effects should disappear as your body adjusts to the medication.

Major. Tell your doctor about any side effects that are persistent or particularly bothersome. IT IS ESPECIALLY IMPORTANT TO TELL YOUR DOCTOR about confusion, depression, fever, itching, mouth sores, skin rash, sore throat, sores on the tongue, tingling sensations, unusual bleeding or bruising, or unusual weakness. Also, if the symptoms of your infection seem to be getting worse rather than improving, you should contact your doctor.

INTERACTIONS
Chloramphenicol interacts with several other drugs:
1. It can increase the blood levels of dicumarol, phenytoin, phenobarbital, tolbutamide, and chlorpropamide, thereby leading to an increase in side effects.
2. Chloramphenicol can reduce the effectiveness of iron, vitamin B, and cyclophosphamide.
3. The blood levels and side effects of chloramphenicol may be increased by acetaminophen and penicillin.
4. Concurrent use of chloramphenicol and antineoplastic drugs (anticancer medicines), colchicine, gold, oxyphenbutazone, penicillamine, or phenylbutazone can lead to an increase in side effects, especially to the bone marrow.

BE SURE TO TELL YOUR DOCTOR about any medications you are currently taking, especially any of those listed above.

WARNINGS
• Tell your doctor about unusual or allergic reactions you have had to any drugs, especially to chloramphenicol.

• Before starting to take this medication, tell your doctor if you now have or if you have ever had anemia, bleeding disorders, kidney disease, liver disease, or porphyria.

• Diabetic patients should know that chloramphenicol can cause false-positive readings with the Clinitest urine glucose test. Switching to Clinistix or Tes-Tape to monitor urine glucose levels avoids this problem.

• Chloramphenicol has been prescribed for your current infection only. Another infection later on, or one that someone else has, may require a different medicine. You should not give your medication to other people or use it for other infections, unless your doctor specifically directs you to do so.

• Be sure to tell your doctor if you are pregnant. Chloramphenicol crosses the placenta. Although it appears to be safe during the early stages of pregnancy, chloramphenicol can cause serious side effects in a newborn infant if it is given to the mother late in pregnancy. Also, tell your doctor if you are breast-feeding an infant. Small amounts of chloramphenicol pass into breast milk and can cause serious side effects in nursing infants.

chlordiazepoxide

BRAND NAMES (Manufacturers)
chlordiazepoxide hydrochloride (various manufacturers)
Libritabs (Roche)
Librium (Roche)
Mitran (Hauck)
Reposans-10 (Wesley)
TYPE OF DRUG
Benzodiazepine sedative/hypnotic
INGREDIENT
chlordiazepoxide
DOSAGE FORMS
Capsules (5 mg, 10 mg, and 25 mg)
Tablets (5 mg, 10 mg, and 25 mg)
STORAGE
This medication should be stored at room temperature in tightly closed, light-resistant containers.

USES
Chlordiazepoxide is prescribed to treat the symptoms of anxiety and alcohol withdrawal. It is not clear exactly how this medicine works, but it may relieve anxiety by acting as a depressant of the central nervous system. This drug is used to relieve nervousness. It is effective for this purpose, but it is important to remove the cause of the anxiety as well.

TREATMENT
This medication should be taken exactly as directed by your doctor. It can be taken with food or a full glass of water if stomach upset occurs. Do not take this medication with a dose of antacids, since they may retard its absorption.

If you are taking this medication regularly and you miss a dose, take the missed dose immediately. If more than an hour has passed, however, skip the dose you missed and wait for the next scheduled dose. Do not double the dose.

SIDE EFFECTS
Minor. Bitter taste in the mouth, constipation, depression, diarrhea, dizziness, drowsiness (after a night's sleep),

dry mouth, excessive salivation, fatigue, flushing, headache, heartburn, loss of appetite, nausea, nervousness, sweating, or vomiting. As your body adjusts to the medicine, these side effects should disappear.

To relieve constipation, increase the fiber in your diet (fresh fruits and vegetables, salads, bran, and whole-grain breads), exercise, and drink more water (unless your doctor instructs you to do otherwise).

Dry mouth can be relieved by chewing sugarless gum or by sucking on ice chips.

If you feel dizzy, sit or lie down for a while; get up slowly from a sitting or reclining position, and be careful on stairs.

Major. Tell your doctor about any side effects that are persistent or particularly bothersome. IT IS ESPECIALLY IMPORTANT TO TELL YOUR DOCTOR about blurred or double vision, chest pain, difficulty in urinating, fainting, falling, fever, hallucinations, joint pain, mouth sores, nightmares, palpitations, rash, severe depression, shortness of breath, slurred speech, sore throat, uncoordinated movements, unusual excitement, unusual tiredness, or yellowing of the eyes or skin.

INTERACTIONS
Chlordiazepoxide interacts with several other drugs:
1. To prevent oversedation, this drug should not be taken with alcohol, other sedative drugs, central nervous system depressants (such as antihistamines, barbiturates, muscle relaxants, pain medicines, narcotics, medicines for seizures, and phenothiazine tranquilizers), or with antidepressants.
2. This medication may decrease the effectiveness of carbamazepine, levodopa, and oral anticoagulants (blood thinners) and may increase the effects of phenytoin.
3. Disulfiram, oral contraceptives (birth control pills), isoniazid, and cimetidine can increase the blood levels of chlordiazepoxide, which can lead to toxic effects.
4. Concurrent use of rifampin may decrease the effectiveness of chlordiazepoxide.

BE SURE TO TELL YOUR DOCTOR about any medications you are currently taking, especially any of the medications that are listed above.

WARNINGS
• Tell your doctor about unusual or allergic reactions you have had to any medications, especially to chlordiazepoxide or other benzodiazepine tranquilizers (such as alprazolam, clorazepate, diazepam, flurazepam, halazepam, lorazepam, oxazepam, prazepam, temazepam, and triazolam).
• Tell your doctor if you now have or if you have ever had liver disease, kidney disease, epilepsy, lung disease, myasthenia gravis, porphyria, sleep apnea, mental depression, or mental illness.
• This medicine can cause drowsiness. Avoid tasks that require alertness, such as driving a car or operating potentially dangerous machinery.
• Before having surgery or any other medical or dental treatment, tell your doctor or dentist that you are taking this drug.
• This medication has the potential for abuse and must be used with caution. Tolerance may develop quickly; do

not increase the dosage of the drug without first consulting your doctor. It is also important not to stop this drug suddenly if you have been taking it in large amounts or if you have used it for several weeks. Your doctor may want to reduce your dosage of this medication gradually.

• This is a safe drug when used properly. When it is combined with other sedative drugs or alcohol, however, serious side effects may develop.

• Be sure to tell your doctor if you are pregnant. This medicine may increase the chance of birth defects if it is taken during the first three months of pregnancy. In addition, too much use of this medicine during the last six months of pregnancy may lead to addiction of the fetus, resulting in withdrawal side effects in the newborn. Also, use of this medicine during the last weeks of pregnancy may cause excessive drowsiness, slowed heartbeat, and breathing difficulties in the infant. Tell your doctor if you are breast-feeding an infant. This medicine can pass into breast milk and cause excessive drowsiness, slowed heartbeat, and breathing difficulties in the nursing infant.

chlordiazepoxide and amitriptyline combination

BRAND NAMES (Manufacturers)
chlordiazepoxide and amitriptyline (various
 manufacturers)
Limbitrol DS (Roche)
TYPE OF DRUG
Benzodiazepine antianxiety and antidepressant
INGREDIENTS
chlordiazepoxide and amitriptyline
DOSAGE FORM
Tablets (5 mg chlordiazepoxide and 12.5 mg amitriptyline; 10 mg chlordiazepoxide and 25 mg amitriptyline)
STORAGE
Chlordiazepoxide and amitriptyline combination tablets should be stored at room temperature in a tightly closed, light-resistant container.

USES
Chlordiazepoxide and amitriptyline combination is used for the treatment of depression associated with anxiety. Amitriptyline belongs to a group of drugs referred to as tricyclic antidepressants. These medicines are thought to relieve depression by increasing the concentration of certain chemicals necessary for nerve transmission in the brain. It is not clear exactly how chlordiazepoxide works, but it may relieve anxiety by acting as a depressant of the central nervous system (brain and spinal cord).

TREATMENT
This medication combination should be taken exactly as your doctor prescribes. In order to avoid stomach upset, you can take this medication with food or with a full glass of milk or water (unless your doctor directs you to do otherwise). Do not take chlordiazepoxide and amitriptyline tablets with a dose of antacids—they retard absorption of this medication.

If you are taking this medication regularly and you miss a dose, take the missed dose as soon as possible, unless it is almost time for your next dose. In that case, do not take the missed dose at all; just return to your regular dosing schedule. Do not double the dose.

The benefits of therapy with this medication may not become apparent for two or three weeks.

SIDE EFFECTS
Minor. Agitation, anxiety, blurred vision, confusion, constipation, cramps, diarrhea, dizziness, drowsiness, dry mouth, fatigue, headache, heartburn, insomnia, loss of appetite, nausea, peculiar tastes in the mouth, restlessness, sweating, vomiting, weakness, or weight gain or loss. These side effects should disappear as your body adjusts to the medication.

This drug may cause increased sensitivity to sunlight, so avoid prolonged exposure to sunlight and sunlamps. Wear protective clothing and sunglasses, and use an effective sunscreen.

Amitriptyline may cause the urine to turn blue-green. This is a harmless effect.

Dry mouth can be relieved by chewing sugarless gum or you may choose to suck on ice chips or a piece of hard candy.

To relieve constipation, increase the amount of fiber in your diet (fresh fruits and vegetables, salads, bran, whole-grain breads), exercise, and drink more water (unless your doctor directs you to do otherwise).

To avoid dizziness or light-headedness when you stand, contract and relax the muscles of your legs for a few moments before rising. Do this by pushing one foot against the floor while raising the other foot slightly, alternating feet so that you are "pumping" your legs in a pedaling motion.

Major. Tell your doctor about any side effects that are persistent or particularly bothersome. IT IS ESPECIALLY IMPORTANT TO TELL YOUR DOCTOR about chest tightness, convulsions, difficult or painful urination, enlarged or painful breasts (in both sexes), fainting, fever, fluid retention, hair loss, hallucinations, impotence, mood changes, mouth sores, nervousness, nightmares, numbness in the fingers or toes, palpitations, ringing in the ears, skin rash, sore throat, tremors, uncoordinated movements or balance problems, unusual bleeding or bruising, or yellowing of the eyes or skin.

INTERACTIONS
Chlordiazepoxide and amitriptyline combination interacts with several other types of medications:
1. Extreme drowsiness can occur when this medicine is taken with central nervous system depressants (such as alcohol, antihistamines, barbiturates, other benzodiazepine tranquilizers, muscle relaxants, narcotics, pain medications, phenothiazine tranquilizers, and sleeping medications) or with other antidepressants.
2. Amitriptyline may decrease the effectiveness of antiseizure medications and may block the blood-pressure-lowering effects of clonidine and guanethidine.
3. Estrogen-containing drugs and oral contraceptives (birth control pills) can increase the side effects and reduce the effectiveness of amitriptyline.

4. Amitriptyline may increase the side effects of thyroid medication and over-the-counter (nonprescription) cough, cold, allergy, asthma, sinus, and diet medications.

5. The concurrent use of amitriptyline and monoamine oxidase (MAO) inhibitors should be avoided because the combination may result in fever, convulsions, or high blood pressure. At least 14 days should separate the use of this drug and the use of an MAO inhibitor.

6. Chlordiazepoxide may decrease the effectiveness of levodopa and oral anticoagulants (blood thinners) and may increase the effects of phenytoin.

7. Disulfiram, oral contraceptives (birth control pills), isoniazid, and cimetidine can increase the blood levels of chlordiazepoxide, which could possibly lead to toxic effects.

8. Concurrent use of rifampin may decrease the effectiveness of chlordiazepoxide and amitriptyline.

9. Cimetidine can decrease the elimination of amitriptyline from the body, which can increase the possibility of side effects.

BE SURE TO TELL YOUR DOCTOR about any medications you are currently taking, especially any of the medications that are listed above.

WARNINGS

• Tell your doctor about unusual or allergic reactions you have had to any medications, especially to chlordiazepoxide or other benzodiazepine tranquilizers (such as alprazolam, clorazepate, diazepam, flurazepam, halazepam, lorazepam, oxazepam, prazepam, temazepam, and triazolam), or to amitriptyline or other tricyclic antidepressants (such as desipramine, imipramine, nortriptyline, or doxepin).

• Tell your doctor if you have a history of alcoholism or if you have ever had asthma, high blood pressure, liver or kidney disease, lung disease, myasthenia gravis, heart disease, a heart attack, circulatory disease, stomach problems, intestinal problems, difficulty in urinating, enlarged prostate gland, epilepsy, glaucoma, thyroid disease, mental illness, or electroshock therapy.

• If this drug makes you dizzy or drowsy, do not take part in any activity that requires alertness, such as driving a car or operating potentially dangerous equipment.

• Before having surgery or any other medical or dental treatment, be sure to tell your doctor or dentist that you are taking this medication.

• The effects of this medication may last as long as seven days after you have stopped taking it. It is therefore important that you continue to observe all precautions during this period.

• This medication has the potential for abuse and must be used with caution. Tolerance develops quickly; do not increase the dosage of the drug unless you first consult your doctor. It is also important not to stop taking this drug suddenly, especially if it has been used in large amounts or has been used for longer than several weeks. Abruptly stopping this medication may cause nausea, headache, stomach upset, fatigue, or a worsening of your condition. Your doctor may want to reduce the dosage gradually.

• Be sure to tell your doctor if you are pregnant. Chlordiazepoxide may increase the chance of birth de-

fects if it is taken during the first three months of pregnancy. In addition, too much use of this medication during the last six months of pregnancy may lead to addiction of the fetus, resulting in withdrawal symptoms in the newborn. Use of this medication during the last weeks of pregnancy may cause excessive drowsiness, slowed heartbeat, and breathing difficulties in the newborn infant. Also, tell your doctor if you are breast-feeding an infant. This medicine may pass into breast milk and cause excessive drowsiness, slowed heartbeat, breathing difficulty, and irritability in the nursing infant.

chlordiazepoxide and clidinium combination

BRAND NAMES (Manufacturers)
chlordiazepoxide with clindinium bromide (various manufacturers)
Clindex (Rugby)
Clinoxide (Geneva Generics)
Clipoxide (Schein)
Librax (Roche)
Lidox (Major)
TYPE OF DRUG
Benzodiazepine antianxiety and anticholinergic
INGREDIENTS
Chlordiazepoxide and clidinium
DOSAGE FORM
Capsules (5 mg chlordiazepoxide and 2.5 mg clidinium)
STORAGE
Chlordiazepoxide and clidinium combination capsules should be stored at room temperature in a tightly closed, light-resistant container.

USES

Chlordiazepoxide and clidinium combination is used in conjunction with other drugs to treat peptic ulcer or irritable bowel syndrome. Clidinium is an anticholinergic agent that slows the activity of the gastrointestinal tract and reduces the production of stomach acid. Chlordiazepoxide belongs to a group of drugs known as benzodiazepine tranquilizers. It is not clear exactly how chlordiazepoxide works, but it may relieve anxiety by acting as a depressant of the central nervous system.

TREATMENT

You should take chlordiazepoxide and clidinium combination 30 to 60 minutes before meals. It can be taken with water or milk. Do not take it with antacids, since they may interfere with its absorption.

If you miss a dose of this medication, take the missed dose as soon as possible, unless it is almost time for you to take your next dose. In that case, do not take the missed dose at all; just return to your regular dosing schedule. Do not double the next dose.

SIDE EFFECTS

Minor. Blurred vision, change in your sense of taste, confusion, constipation, decreased sweating, depression, diarrhea, dizziness, drowsiness, dry mouth, fatigue, headache, insomnia, nausea, or vomiting. These side effects should disappear as your body adjusts to the medication.

This medication can cause increased sensitivity to sunlight. You should, therefore, avoid prolonged exposure to sunlight and sunlamps. Wear protective clothing and sunglasses, and use an effective sunscreen.

Dry mouth can be relieved by chewing sugarless gum or by sucking on ice chips or a piece of hard candy.

To relieve constipation, increase the amount of fiber in your diet (fresh fruits and vegetables, salads, bran, and whole-grain breads), exercise, and drink more water (unless your doctor directs you to do otherwise).

To avoid dizziness or light-headedness when you stand, contract and relax the muscles of your legs for a few minutes before rising. Do this by pushing one foot against the floor while raising the other foot slightly, alternating feet so that you are "pumping" your legs in a pedaling motion.

Major. Tell your doctor about any side effects that are persistent or particularly bothersome. IT IS ESPECIALLY IMPORTANT TO TELL YOUR DOCTOR about decreased sexual ability, difficulty in breathing, difficult or painful urination, excitation, fluid retention, hallucinations, palpitations, rash, sore throat, uncoordinated movements, or yellowing of the eyes or skin.

INTERACTIONS

This medication interacts with several other types of drugs:

1. Extreme drowsiness can occur when this medicine is taken with other central nervous system depressants (such as alcohol, antihistamines, barbiturates, muscle relaxants, narcotics, pain medications, phenothiazine tranquilizers, and sleeping medications) or with tricyclic antidepressants.

2. Chlordiazepoxide can decrease the effectiveness of carbamazepine, levodopa, and oral anticoagulants (blood thinners) and may increase the effects of phenytoin.

3. Disulfiram, oral contraceptives (birth control pills), isoniazid, and cimetidine can increase the blood levels of chlordiazepoxide, which could possibly lead to toxic effects.

4. Concurrent use of rifampin may decrease the effectiveness of chlordiazepoxide and clidinium.

5. Amantadine, haloperidol, phenothiazine tranquilizers, procainamide, quinidine, and tricyclic antidepressants may increase the side effects of clidinium.

Before starting to take this medication, BE SURE TO TELL YOUR DOCTOR about any medications you are currently taking, especially any of those listed above.

WARNINGS

• Tell your doctor if you have ever had unusual or allergic reactions to any medications, especially to chlordiazepoxide or other benzodiazepine tranquilizers (such as alprazolam, clorazepate, diazepam, flurazepam, halazepam, lorazepam, oxazepam, prazepam, temazepam, and triazolam) or to clidinium.

• Tell your doctor if you now have or if you have ever had glaucoma, obstructed bladder or intestine, enlarged prostate gland, heart disease, lung disease, liver disease,

kidney disease, ulcerative colitis, porphyria, high blood pressure, myasthenia gravis, epilepsy, thyroid disease, emotional instability, or hiatal hernia.

• This medication can decrease sweating and heat release from the body. You should, therefore, avoid becoming overheated by strenuous exercise in hot weather and should avoid taking hot baths, showers, and saunas.

• This medicine can cause drowsiness. Avoid tasks that require alertness, such as driving a car or operating potentially dangerous equipment.

• Before having surgery or any other medical or dental treatment, tell your doctor or dentist that you are taking this drug. This medication has the potential for abuse and must be used with caution. Tolerance develops quickly; do not increase the dosage unless you first consult your doctor. It is also important not to stop taking this drug suddenly if you have been using it in large amounts or for longer than several weeks. Your doctor may reduce the dosage gradually.

• This is a safe drug when used properly. When it is combined with other sedative drugs or alcohol, however, serious side effects may develop.

• Be sure to tell your doctor if you are pregnant. This medicine may increase the chance of birth defects if it is taken during the first three months of pregnancy. In addition, too much use of this medicine during the last six months of pregnancy may cause the baby to become dependent on it. This may result in withdrawal symptoms in the infant at birth. Use of this medicine during the last weeks of pregnancy may cause excessive drowsiness, slowed heartbeat, and breathing difficulties in the newborn infant. Also, tell your doctor if you are breast-feeding an infant. This medicine may pass into breast milk and cause excessive drowsiness, slowed heartbeat, and breathing difficulties in the nursing infant.

chlordiazepoxide hydrochloride—see chlordiazepoxide

chlordiazepoxide with clindinium bromide—see chlordiazepoxide and clindinium combination

---

chlorhexidine gluconate

BRAND NAME (Manufacturer)
Peridex (Procter & Gamble)
TYPE OF DRUG
Oral rinse
INGREDIENT
chlorhexidine as the gluconate salt
DOSAGE FORM
solution (0.12%)
STORAGE
This product should be stored at room temperature in a tightly closed, light-resistant container. Chlorhexidine gluconate solution should not be frozen.

USES

Chlorhexidine gluconate solution is prescribed by dentists for the treatment of gingivitis. Gingivitis is a medical term for inflammation of the gums characterized by redness, swelling, and bleeding upon probing. Although it is unknown exactly how the product works, it is believed to eliminate bacteria, which can cause dental plaque. Dental plaque is one of several causes of gingivitis.

TREATMENT
Treatment with chlorhexidine gluconate solution should begin following a thorough cleaning of your teeth by your dental practitioner.

Measure fluid ounce (as marked in the cap given with the product) of chlorhexidine gluconate solution, and swish in the mouth for at least 30 seconds. Do not dilute it in water or other liquids. It should be used full strength. Chlorhexidine gluconate solution should be used after brushing.

Do not swallow chlorhexidine gluconate solution following use. It should be expectorated (spit out) after rinsing the mouth.

SIDE EFFECTS
Minor. Irritation of the inside of the mouth can occur following use of this product. In addition, some patients may experience temporary taste disturbances. However, there have been no permanent taste disturbances reported with continued use of chlorhexidine.

Major. Be sure to tell your dentist about any side effects that are persistent or particularly bothersome. IT IS ESPECIALLY IMPORTANT TO TELL YOUR DENTIST about any inflammation and swelling of the parotid salivary gland.

Chlorhexidine may cause staining of the teeth and tongue. This staining will be more noticeable in patients who have a heavy accumulation of plaque. Usually, this staining is temporary and can be easily removed from most tooth surfaces with dental cleaning. Rarely, some persons, especially those with plaque, will have permanent stains.

INTERACTIONS
There do not appear to be any significant drug interactions with this medication. However, you should make sure your dentist knows about all the medications you are taking.

WARNINGS
• Tell your doctor about any reactions you have had to any drugs, especially to chlorhexidine gluconate solution.
• Chlorhexidine gluconate solution has not been fully evaluated in children under the age of 18. Therefore, the product should not be used by children in this age group.
• To determine the effectiveness of chlorhexidine use, it is advisable to have dental checkups at least every six months.
• Be sure to tell your dentist if you are pregnant or breast-feeding an infant. Scientific studies have not yet determined the effects of the administration of chlorhexidine to pregnant or nursing women or their babies. Therefore, use of this product during this time should be carefully considered.

Chloromycetin Kapseals—see chloramphenicol (systemic)

chlorothiazide

BRAND NAMES (Manufacturers)
chlorothiazide (various manufacturers)
Diachlor (Major)
Diurigen (Goldline)
Diuril (Merck Sharp & Dohme)
TYPE OF DRUG
Diuretic and antihypertensive
INGREDIENT
chlorothiazide
DOSAGE FORMS
Tablets (250 mg and 500 mg)
Oral suspension (250 mg per 5-ml spoonful; 0.5% alcohol)
STORAGE
Store at room temperature in a tightly closed container.

USES
Chlorothiazide is prescribed to treat high blood pressure. It is also used to reduce fluid accumulation in the body caused by conditions such as heart failure, cirrhosis of the liver, kidney disease, and the long-term use of some medications. It reduces fluid accumulation by increasing the elimination of salt and water through the kidneys.

TREATMENT
To decrease stomach irritation, you can take this medication with a glass of milk or with a meal (unless your doctor directs you to do otherwise). Try to take it at the same time every day. Avoid taking a dose after 6:00 P.M.; otherwise, you may have to get up during the night to urinate.

If you miss a dose of this medication, take the missed dose as soon as possible, unless it is almost time for the next dose. In that case, do not take the missed dose at all, just wait until the next scheduled dose. Do not double the dose.

This medication does not cure high blood pressure, but it will help to control the condition.

SIDE EFFECTS
Minor. Constipation, cramps, diarrhea, dizziness, drowsiness, headache, heartburn, loss of appetite, restlessness, or upset stomach. As your body adjusts to the medication, these side effects should disappear.

This medication can cause increased sensitivity to sunlight. Avoid prolonged exposure to sunlight or sunlamps. Wear protective clothing, and use effective sunscreen.

To relieve constipation, increase the amount of fiber in your diet (fresh fruits and vegetables, salads, bran, and whole-grain breads) and exercise (unless your doctor directs you to do otherwise).

To avoid dizziness or light-headedness when you stand, contract and relax the muscles of your legs for a few moments before rising. Do this by pushing one foot against the floor while raising the other foot slightly, alternating feet so that you are "pumping" your legs in a pedaling motion.

Major. Tell your doctor about any side effects that are persistent or particularly bothersome. IT IS ESPECIALLY-

IMPORTANT TO TELL YOUR DOCTOR about blurred vision, confusion, difficulty in breathing, dry mouth, excessive thirst, excessive weakness, fever, itching, joint pain, mood changes, muscle pains or spasms, nausea, palpitations, skin rash, sore throat, tingling in the fingers or toes, unusual bleeding or bruising, vomiting, or yellowing of the eyes or skin.

INTERACTIONS

Chlorothiazide diuretic and antihypertensive interacts with several other types of medications:

1. It may decrease the effectiveness of oral anticoagulants, antigout medications, insulin, oral antidiabetic medicines, and methenamine.

2. Fenfluramine can increase the blood-pressure-lowering effects of chlorothiazide, which can be dangerous.

3. Indomethacin can decrease the blood-pressure-lowering effects of chlorothiazide and counteract the desired effects.

4. Cholestyramine and colestipol decrease the absorption of this medication from the gastrointestinal tract. Chlorothiazide should, therefore, be taken one hour before or four hours after a dose of cholestyramine or colestipol (if you have also been prescribed one of these medications).

5. The side effects of amphotericin B, calcium, cortisone-like steroids (such as cortisone, dexamethasone, hydrocortisone, prednisone, and prednisolone), digoxin, digitalis, lithium, quinidine, sulfonamide antibiotics, and vitamin D may be increased by chlorothiazide.

BE SURE TO TELL YOUR DOCTOR about any medications you are currently taking.

WARNINGS

• Tell your doctor about unusual or allergic reactions you have had to any medications, especially to diuretics or any other sulfa drugs, including oral antidiabetic medications and sulfonamide antibiotics.

• Before you start taking chlorothiazide, tell your doctor if you now have or if you have ever had kidney disease or problems with urination, diabetes mellitus, gout, liver disease, asthma, pancreas disease, or systemic lupus erythematosus.

• Chlorothiazide can cause potassium loss. Signs of potassium loss include dry mouth, thirst, weakness, muscle pain or cramps, nausea, and vomiting. If you experience any of these symptoms, call your doctor. To help avoid potassium loss, take this drug with a glass of fresh or frozen orange or cranberry juice, or eat a banana every day. The use of a salt substitute also helps to prevent potassium loss. Do not change your diet or use a salt substitute, however, before discussing it with your doctor. Too much potassium can also be dangerous. Your doctor may want to have blood tests performed periodically to monitor your potassium levels.

• Limit your intake of alcoholic beverages while taking this medication, in order to prevent dizziness and light-headedness.

• If you have high blood pressure, do not take any over-the-counter (nonprescription) medications for weight control or for cough, cold, allergy, asthma, or sinus problems unless your doctor directs you to do so.

• To prevent dehydration (severe water loss) while taking this medication, check with your doctor if you have any illness that causes severe or continuous nausea, vomiting, or diarrhea.

• This medication can raise blood sugar levels in diabetic patients. Therefore, blood sugar should be carefully monitored by blood or urine tests when this medication is being taken.

• Be sure to tell your doctor if you are pregnant. Although studies in humans have not been conducted, chlorothiazide can cross the placenta and may cause adverse effects in the developing fetus. Also, tell your doctor if you are breastfeeding an infant. Although problems in humans have not been reported, small amounts of this drug can pass into breast milk, so caution is warranted.

chlorpromazine

BRAND NAMES (Manufacturers)

chlorpromazine hydrochloride (various manufacturers)
Ormazine (Hauck)
Sonazine (Cord)
Thorazine (Smith Kline & French)
Thorazine Spansules (Smith Kline & French)
Thor-Prom (Major)

TYPE OF DRUG

Phenothiazine tranquilizer

INGREDIENT

chlorpromazine hydrochloride

DOSAGE FORMS

Tablets (10 mg, 25 mg, 50 mg, 100 mg, and 200 mg)
Sustained-release capsules (30 mg, 75 mg, 150 mg, 200 mg, and 300 mg)
Oral concentrate (30 mg per ml and 100 mg per ml)
Oral syrup (10 mg per 5-ml spoonful)
Suppositories (25 mg and 100 mg)

STORAGE

The tablet and capsule forms of this drug should be stored at room temperature in tightly closed, light-resistant containers. The oral concentrate, oral syrup, and suppository forms of this drug should be stored in the refrigerator in tightly closed, light-resistant containers. If the oral concentrate or syrup turns to a slight yellow color, the medicine is still effective and can be used. However, if the oral concentrate or syrup changes color markedly or has particles floating in it, it should not be used; instead, it should be discarded down the sink. Chlorpromazine should never be frozen.

USES

Chlorpromazine is prescribed to treat the symptoms of certain types of mental illness, such as emotional symptoms of psychosis, the manic phase of manic-depressive illness, and severe behavioral problems in children. This medication is thought to relieve the symptoms of mental illness by blocking certain chemicals involved with nerve transmission in the brain.

Chlorpromazine may also be used to treat tetanus, porphyria, uncontrollable hiccups, anxiety before surgery, and nausea and vomiting (this medication works at the vomiting center in the brain to relieve nausea and vomiting).

TREATMENT
To avoid stomach irritation, take the tablet or capsule forms of this medication with a meal or with a glass of water or milk (unless your doctor directs you to do otherwise).

The sustained-release capsules should be taken whole; do not crush, break, or open them prior to swallowing. Breaking the capsule would release the medication all at once—defeating the purpose of the extended-release capsules.

Measure the oral syrup carefully with a specially designed 5-ml measuring spoon. An ordinary kitchen teaspoon is not accurate enough.

The oral concentrate form of this medication should be measured carefully with the dropper provided, then added to four ounces (one-half cup) or more of water, milk, or a carbonated beverage or to applesauce or pudding immediately prior to administration. Be careful that the serving size is not more than the patient is willing or able to drink or eat; otherwise, the full dose may not be consumed. To prevent possible loss of effectiveness, the medication should not be diluted in tea, coffee, or apple juice.

To use the suppository form of this medication, remove the foil wrapper and moisten the suppository with water (if the suppository is too soft to insert, refrigerate it for half an hour or run cold water over it before removing the wrapper). Lie on your left side with your right knee bent. Push the suppository into the rectum, pointed end first. Lie still for a few minutes. Try to avoid having a bowel movement for at least an hour.

If you miss a dose of this medication, take the missed dose as soon as possible, then return to your regular schedule. If it is almost time for the next dose, however, skip the one you missed and return to your regular schedule. Do not double the dose (unless your doctor directs you to do so).

Antacids and antidiarrheal medicines may decrease the absorption of this medication from the gastrointestinal tract. Therefore, at least one hour should separate doses of one of these medicines and chlorpromazine.

The full effects of this medication for the control of emotional or mental symptoms may not become apparent for two weeks after you start to take it.

SIDE EFFECTS
Minor. Blurred vision, constipation, decreased sweating, diarrhea, dizziness, drooling, drowsiness, dry mouth, fatigue, jitteriness, menstrual irregularities, nasal congestion, restlessness, tremors, vomiting, or weight gain. As your body adjusts to the medication, these side effects should disappear.

This medication can cause increased sensitivity to sunlight. It is, therefore, important to avoid prolonged exposure to sunlight or sunlamps. Wear protective clothing, and use an effective sunscreen.

Chlorpromazine can also cause discoloration of the urine to red, pink, or red-brown. This is a harmless effect.

If you are constipated, increase the amount of fiber in your diet (fresh fruits and vegetables, salads, bran, and whole-grain breads), exercise, and drink more water (unless your doctor directs you to do otherwise).

Chew sugarless gum or suck on ice chips or a piece of hard candy to reduce mouth dryness.

To avoid dizziness or light-headedness when you stand, contract and relax the muscles of your legs for a few moments before rising. Do this by pushing one foot against the floor while raising the other foot slightly, alternating feet so that you are "pumping" your legs in a pedaling motion.

Major. Tell your doctor about any side effects that are persistent or particularly bothersome. IT IS ESPECIALLY IMPORTANT TO TELL YOUR DOCTOR about breast enlargement (in both sexes); chest pain; convulsions; darkened skin; difficulty in swallowing or breathing; fainting; fever; impotence; involuntary movements of the face, mouth, jaw, or tongue; palpitations; rash; sleep disorders; sore throat; uncoordinated movements; unusual bleeding or bruising; visual disturbances; or yellowing of the eyes or skin.

INTERACTIONS
Chlorpromazine interacts with several types of drugs:
1. It can cause extreme drowsiness when combined with alcohol or other central nervous system depressants (such as barbiturates, benzodiazepine tranquilizers, muscle relaxants, narcotics, and pain medications) or with tricyclic antidepressants.
2. Chlorpromazine can decrease the effectiveness of amphetamines, guanethidine, anticonvulsants, and levodopa.
3. The side effects of cyclophosphamide, epinephrine, monoamine oxidase (MAO) inhibitors, phenytoin, and tricyclic antidepressants may be increased by this medication.
4. Chlorpromazine can increase the absorption of propranolol, which can increase the risks of side effects.
5. Lithium may increase the side effects and decrease the effectiveness of this medication.

Before starting to take chlorpromazine, BE SURE TO TELL YOUR DOCTOR about any medications you are currently taking, especially any of those listed above.

WARNINGS
• Tell your doctor about unusual or allergic reactions you have had to any medications, especially to chlorpromazine or any other phenothiazine tranquilizers (such as fluphenazine, mesoridazine, perphenazine, prochlorperazine, promazine, thioridazine, and trifluoperazine) or to loxapine.
• Tell your doctor if you have a history of alcoholism, or if you now have or ever had blood disease, bone marrow disease, brain disease, breast cancer, blockage in the urinary or digestive tract, drug-induced depression, epilepsy, high or low blood pressure, diabetes mellitus, glaucoma, heart or circulatory disease, liver disease, lung disease, Parkinson's disease, peptic ulcers, or an enlarged prostate gland.
• Tell your doctor about any recent exposure to a pesticide or an insecticide. Chlorpromazine may increase the side effects from the exposure.

• To prevent oversedation, avoid drinking alcoholic beverages while taking this medication.
• If this drug makes you dizzy or drowsy, avoid any activity that requires alertness. Be careful on stairs, and avoid getting up suddenly from a lying or sitting position.
• Before having surgery or any other medical or dental treatment, be sure to tell your doctor or dentist that you are taking this medication.
• Some of the side effects caused by this drug can be prevented by taking an antiparkinsonism drug. Discuss this with your doctor.
• This medication can decrease sweating and heat release from the body. You should, therefore, avoid becoming overheated by strenuous exercise in hot weather and should avoid taking hot baths, showers, and saunas.
• Do not stop taking this medication suddenly. If the drug is stopped abruptly, you may experience nausea, vomiting, stomach upset, headache, increased heart rate, insomnia, tremors, or a worsening of your condition. Your doctor may want to reduce the dosage gradually.
• If you are planning to have a myelogram or any other procedure in which dye will be injected into your spinal cord, tell your doctor that you are taking this medication.
• Avoid spilling the oral concentrate or oral syrup forms of this medication on your skin or clothing; it may cause redness and irritation of the skin.
• While you are being treated with this medication, do not take any over-the-counter (nonprescription) medications for weight control or for cough, cold, allergy, asthma, or sinus problems without first checking with your doctor. The combination of these medications with chlorpromazine may cause high blood pressure.
• Be sure to tell your doctor if you are pregnant. Small amounts of this medication cross the placenta. Although there are reports of safe use of this drug during pregnancy, there are also reports of liver disease and tremors in newborn infants whose mothers received this medication close to term. Also, tell your doctor if you are breast-feeding an infant. Small amounts of this medication pass into breast milk and may effect in the nursing infant.

chlorpromazine hydrochloride—see chlorpromazine

chlorpropamide

BRAND NAMES (Manufacturers)
chlorpropamide (various manufacturers)
Diabinese (Pfizer)
TYPE OF DRUG
Oral antidiabetic
INGREDIENT
chlorpropamide
DOSAGE FORM
Tablets (100 mg and 250 mg)
STORAGE
Store at room temperature in a tightly closed container.

USES
Chlorpropamide is used for the treatment of diabetes mellitus that appears in adulthood and cannot be managed by control of diet alone. This type of diabetes is known as non-insulin-dependent diabetes (sometimes called maturity-onset or Type II diabetes). Chlorpropamide lowers blood sugar by increasing the release of insulin from the pancreas.

TREATMENT
In order for this medication to work correctly, it must be taken as your doctor has directed. It is best to take this medicine at the same time each day in order to maintain a constant blood sugar level. It is important, therefore, to try not to miss any doses of this medication. If you do miss a dose, take it as soon as possible, unless it is almost time for the next dose. In that case, do not take the missed dose at all; just return to your regular dosing schedule. Do not double the next dose. Tell your doctor if you feel any side effects from missing a dose of this drug.

Diabetics who are taking oral antidiabetic medication may need to be switched to insulin if they develop diabetic coma, have a severe infection, are scheduled for major surgery, or become pregnant.

SIDE EFFECTS
Minor. Diarrhea, headache, heartburn, loss of appetite, nausea, stomach discomfort, stomach pain, or vomiting. These side effects usually disappear during treatment, as your body adjusts to the medication.

Chlorpropamide may increase your sensitivity to sunlight. Use caution during exposure to the sun. You may want to wear protective clothing and sunglasses. Use an effective sunscreen, and avoid exposure to sunlamps.
Major. If any side effects are persistent or particularly bothersome, it is important to notify your doctor. IT IS ESPECIALLY IMPORTANT TO TELL YOUR DOCTOR about dark urine, fatigue, itching of the skin, light-colored stools, sore throat and fever, unusual bleeding or bruising, or yellowing of the eyes or skin.

Chlorpropamide can also cause retention of body water, which in turn can lead to drowsiness; muscle cramps; seizures; swelling or puffiness of the face, hands, or ankles; and tiredness or weakness. IT IS IMPORTANT TO TELL YOUR DOCTOR if you notice any of these side effects.

INTERACTIONS
Chlorpropamide interacts with a number of medications:
1. Chloramphenicol, fenfluramine, guanethidine, insulin, miconazole, monoamine oxidase (MAO) inhibitors, oxyphenbutazone, oxytetracycline, phenylbutazone, probenecid, aspirin or other salicylates, sulfinpyrazone, or sulfonamide antibiotics, when combined with chlorpropamide, can lower blood sugar levels—sometimes to dangerously low levels.
2. Thyroid hormones, dextrothyroxine, epinephrine, phenytoin, thiazide diuretics (water pills), or cortisone-like medications (such as dexamethasone, hydrocortisone, and prednisone), when combined with chlorpropamide, can actually increase blood sugar levels.
3. Rifampin can decrease the blood levels of chlorpropamide, which can lead to a decrease in its effectiveness.

4. Antidiabetic medications can increase the effects of anticoagulants (blood thinners, such as warfarin), which can lead to bleeding complications.

5. Beta-blocking medications (acebutolol, atenolol, betaxolol, carteolol, esmolol, labetalol, metoprolol, nadolol, penbutolol, pindolol, propranolol, and timolol), combined with chlorpropamide, can result in either high or low blood sugar levels. Beta blockers can also mask the symptoms of low blood sugar, which can be dangerous.

6. Avoid drinking alcoholic beverages while taking this medication (unless otherwise directed by your doctor). Some patients who take this medicine suffer nausea, vomiting, dizziness, stomach pain, pounding headache, sweating, or redness of the face and skin when they drink alcohol. Also, large amounts of alcohol can lower blood sugar to dangerously low levels.

BE SURE TO TELL YOUR DOCTOR about any medications you are currently taking, especially any of those listed above.

WARNINGS

• It is important to tell your doctor if you have ever had unusual or allergic reactions to this medicine or to any sulfa medication (sulfonamide antibiotics, acetazolamide, diuretics {water pills}, or other oral antidiabetics).

• Tell your doctor if you now have or if you have ever had kidney disease, liver disease, severe infection, or thyroid disease.

• Follow the special diet that your doctor gave you. This is an essential part of controlling your blood sugar and is necessary in order for this medicine to work properly.

• Before having surgery or any other medical or dental treatment, be sure to tell your doctor or dentist that you are taking this medicine.

• Test for sugar in your urine as directed by your doctor. It is a convenient way to determine whether or not your diabetes is being controlled by this medicine.

• Eat or drink something containing sugar right away if you experience any symptoms of low blood sugar (such as anxiety, chills, cold sweats, cool or pale skin, drowsiness, excessive hunger, headache, nausea, nervousness, rapid heartbeat, shakiness, or unusual tiredness or weakness). It is important that your family and friends know the symptoms of low blood sugar and what to do if they observe any of these symptoms in you.

• Even if the symptoms of low blood sugar are corrected by eating or drinking sugar, it is important to contact your doctor as soon as possible after experiencing them. The blood-sugar-lowering effects of this medicine can last for hours, and the symptoms may return during this period. Good sources of sugar are orange juice, corn syrup, honey, sugar cubes, and table sugar. You are at greatest risk of developing low blood sugar if you skip or delay meals, exercise more than usual, cannot eat because of nausea or vomiting, or drink large amounts of alcohol.

• Be sure to tell your doctor if you are pregnant. Since extensive studies have not yet been conducted, it is not known whether this medication can cause problems when administered to a pregnant woman. Cautious use of this medication is thus warranted. It is also important to tell your doctor if you are currently breast-feeding an infant. It has been determined that this medicine passes into breast milk. For this reason this product is not recommended for use by a woman who is breast-feeding.

---

chlorprothixene

BRAND NAME (Manufacturer)
Taractan (Roche)
TYPE OF DRUG
Antipsychotic
INGREDIENT
chlorprothixene
DOSAGE FORMS
Tablets (10 mg, 25 mg, 50 mg, and 100 mg)
Oral suspension (100 mg as lactate and hydrochloride per 5-ml spoonful)
STORAGE
Store at room temperature in a tightly closed, light-resistant container. This medication should never be frozen.

USES
Chlorprothixene is prescribed to treat the symptoms of certain types of mental illness, such as emotional symptoms of psychosis. This medication is thought to relieve the symptoms of mental illness by blocking certain chemicals involved with nerve transmission in the brain.

TREATMENT
To avoid stomach irritation, you can take the tablet form of this medication with a meal or with a glass of water or milk (unless your doctor directs you to do otherwise).

Measure the oral suspension carefully with a specially designed 5-ml measuring spoon. An ordinary kitchen teaspoon is not accurate enough to ensure that you receive the proper dose of chlorprothixene.

Antacids and antidiarrheal medicines may decrease the absorption of this medication from the gastrointestinal tract. Therefore, it is very important to at least one hour should separate doses of chlorprothixene and one of these medicines.

If you miss a dose of this medication, take the missed dose as soon as possible and return to your regular schedule. If it is within two hours of your next dose, however, skip the dose you missed and return to your regular schedule. Do not double the dose (unless your doctor directs you to do so).

The full effects of this medication for the control of emotional or mental symptoms may not become apparent for two weeks after you start to take it.

SIDE EFFECTS
Minor. Blurred vision, constipation, decreased sweating, diarrhea, dizziness, drooling, drowsiness, dry mouth, fatigue, jitteriness, menstrual irregularities, nasal congestion, restlessness, tremors, vomiting, or weight gain. As your body adjusts to the medication, these side effects should disappear.

This medication can cause increased sensitivity to sunlight. It is, therefore, important to avoid prolonged exposure to sunlight and sunlamps. Wear protective clothing, and use an effective sunscreen.

Chlorprothixene can also cause discoloration of the urine to red, pink, or redbrown. This is a harmless effect.

If you are constipated, increase the amount of fiber in your diet (fresh fruits and vegetables, salads, bran, and whole-grain breads), exercise, and drink more water (unless your doctor directs you to do otherwise).

Chew sugarless gum or suck on ice chips or a piece of hard candy to reduce mouth dryness.

To avoid dizziness or light-headedness when you stand, contract and relax the muscles of your legs for a few moments before rising. Do this by pushing one foot against the floor while raising the other foot slightly, alternating feet so that you are "pumping" your legs.

Major. Tell your doctor about any side effects that are persistent or particularly bothersome. IT IS ESPECIALLY IMPORTANT TO TELL YOUR DOCTOR about breast enlargement (in both sexes); chest pain; convulsions; darkened skin; difficulty in swallowing or breathing; fainting; fever; impotence; involuntary movements of the face, mouth, jaw, or tongue; palpitations; rash; sleep disorders; sore throat; uncoordinated movements; unusual bleeding or bruising; visual disturbances; or yellowing of the eyes or skin.

INTERACTIONS

Chlorprothixene interacts with several other types of medications:

1. It can cause extreme drowsiness when combined with alcohol or other central nervous system depressants (such as barbiturates, benzodiazepine tranquilizers, muscle relaxants, narcotics, and pain medications) or with tricyclic antidepressants.

2. This medication can decrease the effectiveness of amphetamines, guanethidine, anticonvulsants, and levodopa.

3. The side effects of epinephrine, monoamine oxidase (MAO) inhibitors, and tricyclic antidepressants may be increased by this medication.

4. Lithium may increase the side effects and decrease the effectiveness of this medication.

Before starting to take chlorprothixene, BE SURE TO TELL YOUR DOCTOR about any medications you are currently taking, especially any of those listed above.

WARNINGS

• Tell your doctor about unusual or allergic reactions you have had to any medications, especially to chlorprothixene, thiothixene, or any phenothiazine tranquilizer.

• Tell your doctor if you have a history of alcoholism, or if you now have or have ever had blood disease, bone marrow disease, brain disease, breast cancer, blockage in the urinary or digestive tract, drug-induced depression, epilepsy, high or low blood pressure, glaucoma, heart or circulatory disease, liver disease, lung disease, Parkinson's disease, peptic ulcers, or an enlarged prostate gland.

• Avoid drinking alcoholic beverages while taking this medication, in order to prevent oversedation.

• If this medication makes you dizzy or drowsy, do not take part in any activity that requires alertness, such as driving a car or operating potentially dangerous equipment. Be careful on stairs, and avoid getting up suddenly from a lying or sitting position.

• Before having surgery or any other medical or dental treatment, be sure to tell your doctor or dentist that you are taking this medication.

• Some of the side effects caused by this drug can be prevented by taking an antiparkinsonism drug. Discuss this with your doctor.

• Chlorprothixene can decrease sweating and heat release from the body. You should, therefore, avoid becoming overheated by strenuous exercise in hot weather and avoid taking hot baths, showers, and saunas.

• Do not stop taking this medication suddenly. If the drug is stopped abruptly, you may experience nausea, vomiting, stomach upset, headache, increased heart rate, insomnia, tremulousness, or a worsening of your condition. Your doctor may want to reduce the dosage gradually.

• If you are planning to have a myelogram, or any other procedure in which dye will be injected into your spinal cord, tell your doctor that you are taking this medication.

• Avoid spilling the oral suspension form of this medication on your skin or clothing; it can cause redness and irritation of the skin.

• Chlorprothixene tablets contain the color additive FD&C Yellow No. 5 (tartrazine), which can cause allergic-type reactions (fainting, shortness of breath, or rash).

• While taking this medication, do not take any over-the-counter (nonprescription) drugs for weight control or for cough, cold, allergy, asthma, or sinus problems without checking with your doctor. The combination of these medications with chlorprothixene may cause high blood pressure.

• Be sure to tell your doctor if you are pregnant. Small amounts of this medication can cross the placenta. Although there are reports of safe use of this drug during pregnancy, there are also reports of liver disease and tremors in newborn infants whose mothers received this type of medication close to term. Also, tell your doctor if you are breast-feeding an infant. Small amounts of this medication pass into breast milk and may cause unwanted effects in the nursing infant.

chlorthalidone

BRAND NAMES (Manufacturers)
chlorthalidone (various manufacturers)
Hygroton (Rorer)
Hylidone (Major)
Thalitone (Boehringer Ingelheim)
TYPE OF DRUG
Diuretic and antihypertensive
INGREDIENT
chlorthalidone
DOSAGE FORM
Tablets (25 mg, 50 mg, and 100 mg)
STORAGE
Store at room temperature in a tightly closed container.

USES

Chlorthalidone is prescribed to treat high blood pressure. It is also used to reduce fluid accumulation in the body caused by conditions such as heart failure, cirrhosis of the liver, kidney disease, and the long-term use of some medications. This medication reduces fluid accumulation by increasing the elimination of salt and water through the kidneys.

TREATMENT

To decrease stomach irritation, you can take this medication with a glass of milk or with a meal (unless your doctor directs you to do otherwise). Try to take it at the same time every day. Avoid taking a dose after 6:00 P.M.; otherwise, you may have to get up during the night to urinate.

If you miss a dose of this medication, take the missed dose as soon as possible, unless it is almost time for the next dose. In that case, do not take the missed dose at all; just wait until the next scheduled dose. Do not double the dose.

This medication does not cure high blood pressure, but it will help to control the condition.

SIDE EFFECTS

Minor. Constipation, cramps, diarrhea, dizziness, drowsiness, headache, heartburn, loss of appetite, restlessness, or stomach upset. As your body adjusts to the medication, these side effects should disappear.

This medication can cause increased sensitivity to sunlight. Therefore, avoid prolonged exposure to sunlight and sunlamps. Wear protective clothing, and use an effective sunscreen.

To relieve constipation, increase the amount of fiber in your diet (fresh fruits and vegetables, salads, bran, and whole-grain breads) and exercise (unless your doctor directs you to do otherwise).

To avoid dizziness or light-headedness when you stand, contract and relax the muscles of your legs for a few moments before rising. Do this by pushing one foot against the floor while raising the other foot slightly, alternating feet so that you are "pumping" your legs in a pedaling motion.

Major. Tell your doctor about any side effects that are persistent or particularly bothersome. IT IS ESPECIALLY IMPORTANT TO TELL YOUR DOCTOR about any blurred vision, confusion, difficulty in breathing, dry mouth, excessive thirst, excessive weakness, fever, itching, joint pain, mood changes, muscle pains or spasms, nausea, palpitations, skin rash, sore throat, tingling in the fingers or toes, unusual bleeding or bruising, vomiting, or yellowing of the eyes or skin.

INTERACTIONS

Chlorthalidone interacts with several other types of drugs:
1. It may decrease the effectiveness of oral anticoagulants, antigout medications, insulin, oral antidiabetic medicines, and methenamine.
2. Fenfluramine can increase the blood-pressure-lowering effects of chlorthalidone, which can be dangerous.
3. Indomethacin can decrease the blood-pressure-lowering effects of chlorthalidone and counteract the desired effects.
4. Cholestyramine and colestipol decrease the absorption of this medication from the gastrointestinal tract.

Chlorthalidone should, therefore, be taken one hour before or four hours after a dose of cholestyramine or colestipol (if you have also been prescribed one of these medications).
5. The side effects of amphotericin B, calcium, cortisone-like steroids (such as cortisone, dexamethasone, hydrocortisone, prednisone and prednisolone), digoxin, digitalis, lithium, quinidine, sulfonamide antibiotics, and vitamin D may be increased by chlorthalidone.

BE SURE TO TELL YOUR DOCTOR about any medications you are currently taking, especially any of those listed above.

WARNINGS

• Tell your doctor about unusual or allergic reactions you have had to any drugs, especially to diuretics or any other sulfa drugs, including oral antidiabetics and sulfonamide antibiotics.
• Before you start taking chlorthalidone, tell your doctor if you now have or if you have ever had kidney disease or problems with urination, diabetes mellitus, gout, liver disease, asthma, pancreatic disease, or systemic lupus erythematosus.
• Chlorthalidone can cause potassium loss. Signs of potassium loss include dry mouth, thirst, weakness, muscle pain or cramps, nausea, and vomiting. If you experience any of these symptoms, call your doctor. To help avoid potassium loss, take this drug with a glass of fresh or frozen orange or cranberry juice, or eat a banana every day. The use of a salt substitute also helps to prevent potassium loss. Do not change your diet or use a salt substitute, however, before discussing it with your doctor. Too much potassium can also be dangerous. Your doctor may want to have blood tests performed periodically to monitor your potassium levels.
• Limit your intake of alcoholic beverages while taking this medication, to prevent dizziness and light-headedness.
• If you have high blood pressure, do not take any over-the-counter (nonprescription) medications for weight control or for cough, cold, allergy, asthma, or sinus problems unless your doctor directs you to do so.
• To prevent dehydration (severe water loss) while taking this medication, check with your doctor if you have any illness that causes severe or continuous nausea, vomiting, or diarrhea.
• This medication can raise blood sugar levels in diabetic patients. Therefore, blood sugar should be carefully monitored by blood or urine tests.
• Be sure to tell your doctor if you are pregnant. Although studies in humans have not been conducted, chlorthalidone can cross the placenta and may cause adverse effects in the developing fetus. Also, tell your doctor if you are breastfeeding an infant. Although problems in humans have not been reported, small amounts of this drug can pass into breast milk, so caution is warranted.

Chlor-Trimeton Decongestant—see pseudoephedrine and chlorpheniramine combination

Chlor-Trimeton Decongestant Repetabs—see pseudoephedrine and chlorpheniramine combination

Choledyl—see oxtriphylline

Choledyl SA—see oxtriphylline

cholestyramine

BRAND NAMES (Manufacturers)
Cholybar (Parke-Davis)
Questran (Bristol Labs)
Questran Light (Bristol Labs)
TYPE OF DRUG
Antihyperlipidemic (lipid-lowering drug)
INGREDIENT
cholestyramine
DOSAGE FORMS
Oral powder (4 gm of cholestyramine per 9 gm of powder or 4 gm of cholestyramine per 5 gm of powder)
Bar (4 gm of cholestyramine per bar)
STORAGE
Cholestyramine should be stored at room temperature in a tightly closed container.

USES
This medication is used to lower blood cholesterol and to treat itching associated with liver disease. Cholestyramine chemically binds to bile salts in the gastrointestinal tract and prevents the body from producing cholesterol.

TREATMENT
Cholestyramine is usually taken before meals. Each dose should be measured carefully, then placed on the surface of two to six ounces of a beverage (water, milk, fruit juice, or other noncarbonated beverage). The powder should be allowed to sit for one to two minutes without being stirred (to prevent lumpiness). The mixture should then be stirred and completely mixed (the powder does not completely dissolve). After the solution has been drunk, the glass should be refilled with the same beverage and this solution swallowed as well (this assures that the whole dose is taken). The powder can also be mixed with soup, applesauce, or crushed pineapple. You should never take cholestyramine dry; you might accidentally inhale the powder, which could irritate your throat and lungs. For the bar form of the drug, chew thoroughly. As with the powder, this should be followed with plenty of fluids.

If you miss a dose of this medication, take it as soon as possible, unless it is almost time for the next dose. In that case, do not take the missed dose at all; just return to your regular dosing schedule. Do not double the next dose.

Cholestyramine does not cure hypercholesterolemia (high blood cholesterol levels), but it will help to control the condition as long as you continue to take it.

SIDE EFFECTS
Minor. Anxiety, belching, constipation, diarrhea, dizziness, drowsiness, fatigue, gas, headache, hiccups, loss of appetite, nausea, stomach pain, vomiting, or weight loss or gain. These side effects should disappear as your body adjusts to the medication.

To relieve constipation, increase the amount of fiber in your diet (fresh fruits and vegetables, salads, bran, and whole-grain breads), exercise, and drink more water (unless your doctor directs you to do otherwise).

If you feel dizzy, sit or lie down for a while; get up slowly from a sitting or reclining position, and be careful on stairs.

Major. Tell your doctor about any side effects that are persistent or particularly bothersome. IT IS ESPECIALLY IMPORTANT TO TELL YOUR DOCTOR about backaches; bloody or black, tarry stools; difficult or painful urination; fluid retention; muscle or joint pains; rash or irritation of the skin, tongue, or rectal area; ringing in the ears; swollen glands; tingling sensations; unusual bleeding or bruising; or unusual weakness.

INTERACTIONS
Cholestyramine interferes with the absorption of a number of other drugs, including phenylbutazone, warfarin, thiazide diuretics (water pills), digoxin, penicillins, tetracycline, phenobarbital, folic acid, iron, thyroid hormones, cephalexin, clindamycin, trimethoprim, and fat-soluble vitamins (A, D, E, and K). The effectiveness of these medications will be decreased by cholestyramine. To avoid this interaction, take the other medications one hour before or four to six hours after a dose of cholestyramine.

BE SURE TO TELL YOUR DOCTOR about any medications you are currently taking, especially those listed above.

WARNINGS
• Tell your doctor about unusual or allergic reactions you have had to any medications, especially to cholestyramine.
• Tell your doctor if you now have or if you have ever had bleeding disorders, biliary obstruction, heart disease, hemorrhoids, gallstones or gallbladder disease, kidney disease, malabsorption, stomach ulcers, or an obstructed intestine.
• Cholestyramine should be used only in conjunction with diet, weight reduction, or correction of other conditions that could be causing high blood cholesterol levels.
• This product contains the color additive FD&C Yellow No. 5 (tartrazine), which can cause allergic-type reactions (fainting, rash, shortness of breath) in certain susceptible individuals.
• The color of cholestyramine powder may vary from batch to batch. This does not affect the effectiveness of the drug.
• Be sure to tell your doctor if you are pregnant. Although cholestyramine appears to be safe (because very little is absorbed into the bloodstream), extensive studies in humans during pregnancy have not been conducted. Also, tell your doctor if you are breast-feeding an infant. It is not known whether cholestyramine passes into breast milk. However, cholestyramine can decrease the absorption of some vitamins in the mother, which could result in decreased availability of the vitamins to the nursing infant.

Cholybar—see cholestyramine

Cibalith-S—see lithium

cimetidine

BRAND NAME (Manufacturer)
Tagamet (SK-Beecham)
TYPE OF DRUG
Gastric acid secretion inhibitor (decreases stomach acid)
INGREDIENT
cimetidine
DOSAGE FORMS
Tablets (200 mg, 300 mg, 400 mg, and 800 mg)
Oral liquid (300 mg per 5-ml spoonful, with 2. 8% alcohol)
STORAGE
Cimetidine tablets and oral liquid should be stored at room temperature in tightly closed, light-resistant containers. This medication should never be frozen. If cimetidine is not properly stored (especially if it is exposed to light or heat) it may develop a strong, unpleasant odor.

USES
Cimetidine is used to treat duodenal and gastric ulcers. It is also used in the long-term treatment of excessive stomach acid secretion and in the prevention of recurrent ulcers. It is also used to treat gastro-esophagal reflux (backflow of stomach contents into the esophagus), which can cause heartburn. Cimetidine works by blocking the effects of histamine in the stomach, which reduces stomach acid secretion.

TREATMENT
Take cimetidine with, or shortly after, meals and again at bedtime (unless your doctor directs otherwise).

The tablets should not be crushed or chewed, because cimetidine has a bitter taste and an unpleasant odor.

The oral liquid should be measured carefully with a specially designed 5-ml measuring spoon. An ordinary kitchen teaspoon is not accurate enough.

Antacids can block the absorption of cimetidine. If you are taking antacids as well as cimetidine, at least one hour should separate doses of the two medications.

If you miss a dose of cimetidine, take the missed dose as soon as possible, unless it is almost time for the next dose. In that case, do not take the missed dose at all; just return to your regular dosing schedule. Do not double the next dose.

SIDE EFFECTS
Minor. Diarrhea, dizziness, drowsiness, headache, or muscle pain. These side effects should disappear as your body adjusts to the medication.

If you feel dizzy, sit or lie down for a while; get up slowly from a sitting or reclining position, and be careful on stairs.

Major. Tell your doctor about any side effects that are persistent or particularly bothersome. IT IS ESPECIALLY IMPORTANT TO TELL YOUR DOCTOR about confu-
sion, fever, hair loss, enlarged or painful breasts (in both sexes), hallucinations, impotence, palpitations, rash, sore throat, unusual bleeding or bruising, weakness, or yellowing of the eyes or skin.

INTERACTIONS
Cimetidine interacts with other types of medications:
1. It can decrease the elimination, and thus increase the side effects, of theophylline, aminophylline, oxtriphylline, phenytoin, carbamazepine, beta blockers, benzodiazepine tranquilizers (such as clorazepate, chlordiazepoxide, diazepam, flurazepam, halazepam, and prazepam), tricyclic antidepressants, oral anticoagulants (blood thinners, such as warfarin), lidocaine, verapamil, quinidine, nifedipine, metronidazole, codeine, and morphine.
2. The combination of cimetidine and antineoplastic agents (anticancer drugs) may increase the risk of blood disorders.
3. The absorption of ketoconazole is decreased by cimetidine; at least two hours should separate doses of these two drugs.
4. Cimetidine may decrease the blood levels and effectiveness of digoxin.

BE SURE TO TELL YOUR DOCTOR about any medications you are currently taking, especially any of those listed above.

WARNINGS
• Tell your doctor about any unusual or allergic reactions you have had to medications, especially to cimetidine, famotidine, nizatidine, or ranitidine.
• Tell your doctor if you now have or if you have ever had arthritis, kidney disease, liver disease, or organic brain syndrome.
• Cimetidine can decrease the elimination of alcohol from the body, which can prolong its intoxicating effects.
• Cimetidine should be taken continuously for as long as your doctor prescribes. Stopping therapy early may be a cause of ineffective treatment.
• Cigarette smoking may block the beneficial effects of therapy with cimetidine.
• If this drug makes you dizzy or drowsy, do not take part in any activity that requires alertness, such as driving a car or operating potentially dangerous equipment.
• Be sure to tell your doctor if you are pregnant. Cimetidine appears to be safe during pregnancy; however, extensive testing has not been conducted. Also, tell your doctor if you are breast-feeding an infant. Small amounts of cimetidine pass into breast milk.

Cinobac—see cinoxacin

cinoxacin

BRAND NAME (Manufacturer)
Cinobac (Dista)
TYPE OF DRUG
Antibiotic
INGREDIENT
cinoxacin

DOSAGE FORM
Capsules (250 mg and 500 mg)
STORAGE
Cinoxacin capsules should be stored at room temperature in a tightly closed container.

USES

Cinoxacin is an antibiotic that is used to treat bacterial urinary tract infections. It chemically attaches to the bacteria, preventing their growth and multiplication. It kills susceptible bacteria, but it is not effective against viruses, parasites, or fungi.

TREATMENT

In order to prevent stomach irritation, you can take cinoxacin with food or with a full glass of water or milk (unless your doctor directs you to do otherwise).

Cinoxacin works best when the level of medicine in your urine is kept constant. It is best, therefore, to take the doses at evenly spaced intervals day and night. For example, if you are to take four doses a day, the doses should be spaced six hours apart.

Try not to miss any doses of this medication. If you do miss a dose, take it as soon as you remember. However, if you do not remember to take the missed dose until it is almost time for your next dose, take the missed dose immediately; space the following dose about halfway through the regular interval between doses; then continue with your regular dosing schedule.

It is important to continue to take this medication for the entire time prescribed by your doctor (usually seven to 14 days), even if the symptoms disappear before the end of that period. If you stop taking the drug too soon, resistant bacteria are given a chance to continue growing, and your infection could recur.

SIDE EFFECTS

Minor. Abdominal cramps, diarrhea, dizziness, headache, increased sensitivity of the eyes to light, insomnia, loss of appetite, nausea, nervousness, or rectal itching. These side effects should disappear as your body adjusts to the medication.

To relieve the increased sensitivity of your eyes to light, avoid prolonged exposure to sunlight and bright lights.
Major. Tell your doctor about any side effects that are persistent or particularly bothersome. IT IS ESPECIALLY IMPORTANT TO TELL YOUR DOCTOR about confusion, itching, rapid weight gain (three to five pounds within a week), ringing in the ears, skin rash, tingling sensations, visual disturbances, or yellowing of the eyes or skin. Also, if the symptoms of your infection do not improve within several days, contact your doctor.

INTERACTIONS

Probenecid blocks the excretion of cinoxacin into the urinary tract, decreasing its effectiveness.

BE SURE TO TELL YOUR DOCTOR about any medications you are currently taking, especially probenecid.

WARNINGS

Tell your doctor about unusual or allergic reactions you have had to any medications, especially to cinoxacin,

ciprofloxin, enoxacin, nalidixic acid, norfloxacin, or ofloxacin.

Tell your doctor if you now have or if you have ever had kidney disease or liver disease.

If this drug makes you dizzy, do not take part in any activity that requires alertness, such as driving a car or operating potentially dangerous equipment.

Cinoxacin has been prescribed for your current infection only. Another infection later on, or one that someone else has, may require a different medicine. Do not give your medicine to other people or use it for another infection unless your doctor specifically directs you to do so.

Be sure to tell your doctor if you are pregnant. Although cinoxacin use appears to be safe during pregnancy, extensive studies in humans have not been conducted. Also, tell your doctor if you are breast-feeding an infant. It is not known whether cinoxacin passes into breast milk.

Cin-Quin—see quinidine

Cipro—see ciprofloxacin

ciprofloxacin

BRAND NAME (Manufacturer)
Cipro (Miles)
TYPE OF DRUG
Antibiotic
INGREDIENT
ciprofloxacin
DOSAGE FORM
Tablets (250 mg, 500 mg, and 750 mg)
STORAGE
Ciprofloxacin tablets should be stored at room temperature in tightly closed containers away from direct light.

USES

Ciprofloxacin is an antibiotic that is used to treat a wide variety of bacterial infections. It chemically attaches to the bacteria and prevents their growth and multiplication. It is not effective against viruses, parasites, or fungi.

TREATMENT

Ciprofloxacin is best taken two hours after a meal with a full glass (8 ounces) of water. You should drink several additional glasses of water every day, unless your doctor directs you to do otherwise. Drinking extra water will help to prevent unwanted effects of ciprofloxacin.

Ciprofloxacin works best when the level of medicine in your bloodstream is kept constant. It is best, therefore, to take the doses at evenly spaced intervals day and night. For example, if you are to take two doses a day, the doses should be spaced 12 hours apart.

It is very important that you do not miss any doses of this medication. If you do miss a dose, take it as soon as you remember. However, if you do not remember to take the missed dose until it is almost time for your next dose, skip the missed dose and go back to your regular dosing schedule. Do not double the next dose.

Ciprofloxacin therapy may be required for four to six weeks or longer. It is important to continue to take this drug for the entire time prescribed, even if the symptoms of infection disappear before the end of that period. If you stop taking the drug too soon, resistant bacteria are given a chance to continue growing, and your infection could recur.

SIDE EFFECTS

Minor. Diarrhea, headache, light-headedness, nausea, stomach irritation, or vomiting. These side effects should disappear as your body adjusts to the medication.

Major. Tell your doctor about any side effects that are persistent or particularly bothersome. IT IS ESPECIALLY IMPORTANT TO TELL YOUR DOCTOR about blood in your urine, change in your vision, confusion, convulsions (seizures), agitation, dizziness, hallucinations, lower back pain, muscle or joint pain, pain or difficulty in urinating, restlessness, skin rash, tremor, unpleasant taste, unusual bleeding or bruising, or yellowing of the eyes or skin. Also, if the symptoms of your infection do not improve in several days, contact your doctor.

INTERACTIONS

Ciprofloxacin interacts with several other drugs:

1. Use of antacids with ciprofloxacin can decrease the absorption of this medicine. Do not take antacids within two hours of taking this medicine.

2. Use of sucralfate with ciprofloxacin can decrease the absorption of ciprofloxacin. Do not take a dose of sucralfate within two hours of a dose of ciprofloxacin unless directed to do so by your doctor.

3. Use of medicine containing theophylline along with ciprofloxacin can lead to increased bloodstream levels of theophylline and therefore to an increased chance of theophylline-related side effects.

4. Regular consumption of large quantities of caffeine-containing products (coffee, tea, or caffeine-containing soft drinks) with ciprofloxacin may lead to exaggerated or prolonged effects of caffeine. Your doctor may wish for you to restrict intake of caffeine during treatment.

5. Use of probenecid with ciprofloxacin can increase the bloodstream levels of ciprofloxacin and thus increase the risk of ciprofloxacin-related side effects.

Before starting to take ciprofloxacin, BE SURE TO TELL YOUR DOCTOR about any other medications you are currently taking, especially any of those listed above.

WARNINGS

• Tell your doctor about unusual or allergic reactions you have had to any medications, especially to ciprofloxacin, enoxacin, norfloxacin, cinoxacin, or nalidixic acid.

• Before starting to take this medication, be sure to tell your doctor if you now have or if you have ever had brain or spinal cord disease, epilepsy, kidney disease, or liver disease.

• To decrease the potential for harmful effects on your kidneys, you should increase your intake of fluids (non-alcoholic) unless your doctor directs you to do otherwise.

• Ciprofloxacin can cause dizziness or light-headedness, so patients taking this medicine should know how they react to this medicine before they operate an automobile or machinery, or engage in activities requiring alertness or coordination.

• This medicine can make your skin more sensitive to the sun. When you first begin taking this drug, avoid too much sun and do not use a sunlamp until you see how your skin responds to short periods of sun exposure. This is especially important if you tend to sunburn easily.

• Ciprofloxacin has been prescribed for your current infection only. Another infection later on, or one that someone else has, may require a different medicine. You should not give your medicine to other people or use it for other infections, unless your doctor specifically directs you to do so.

• Be sure to tell your doctor if you are pregnant. This drug is not recommended for use in pregnant women because it can result in serious adverse effects in the developing fetus. Also, tell your doctor if you are breast-feeding an infant. It is not known whether ciprofloxacin passes into breast milk.

---

clarithromycin

BRAND NAME (Manufacturer)
Biaxin (Abbott)
TYPE OF DRUG
Antibiotic
INGREDIENT
clarithromycin
DOSAGE FORM
Tablets (250 mg and 500 mg)
STORAGE
Clarithromycin tablets should be stored at room temperature in a tightly closed, light resistant container.

USES

Clarithromycin is used to treat a wide variety of bacterial infections including infections of the upper and lower respiratory tracts and skin. It acts by preventing the bacteria from manufacturing protein, which prevents their growth. Clarithromycin kills susceptible bacteria, but it is not effective against viruses, parasites, or fungi.

TREATMENT

Clarithromycin may be taken without regard to meals. If stomach upset should occur, clarithromycin may be taken with food or milk, unless your doctor tells you otherwise. The coated tablets should be swallowed whole; do not crush or chew these tablets.

Clarithromycin works best when the level of medicine in your bloodstream is kept constant. It is best, therefore, to take the doses at evenly spaced intervals, day and night. If you are to take two doses a day, the doses should be spaced 12 hours apart.

It is very important that you do not miss any doses of this medication. If you do miss a dose, take it as soon as you remember. However, if you do not remember to take the missed dose until it is almost time for your next dose, skip the missed dose and go back to you regular dosing schedule. Do not double the dose.

It is important to continue to take this medication for the entire time prescribed by your doctor (usually seven to 14 days), even if the symptoms disappear before the end of that period. If you stop taking the drug too soon, resistant bacteria are given a chance to continue growing and the infection could recur.

SIDE EFFECTS
Minor. Abdominal pain/discomfort, abnormal taste, diarrhea, dyspepsia, headache, nausea. These side effects should disappear as your body adjusts to the medication.
Major. Tell your doctor about any side effects that are persistent or particularly bothersome. IT IS ESPECIALLY IMPORTANT TO TELL YOUR DOCTOR about fever, hearing loss, rash, rectal or vaginal itching, or yellowing of the eyes or skin. Also, if your symptoms of infection seem to be getting worse rather than improving, you should contact your doctor.

INTERACTIONS
Clarithromycin can decrease the elimination of carbamazepine, aminophylline, theophylline, and oxtriphylline from the body, which can lead to serious side effects. Blood levels of digoxin and oral anticoagulants (blood thinners, such as warfarin) may also be increased by clarithromycin.

BE SURE TO TELL YOUR DOCTOR about any medications you are currently taking, especially any of those listed above.

WARNINGS
• Tell your doctor about any unusual or allergic reactions you have had to any medications, especially to clarithromycin, erythromycin, or azithromycin.
• Tell your doctor if you have now or have ever had kidney disease or liver disease.
• This medication has been prescribed for your current infection only. Another infection later on, or one that someone else has, may require a different medication. You should not give your medicine to other people or use it for another infection, unless your doctor specifically directs you to do so.
• Before having surgery or any other medical or dental treatment, be sure to tell your doctor or dentist that you are taking clarithromycin.
• Be sure to tell your doctor if you are pregnant. The effects of this medication during pregnancy have not been thoroughly studied in humans. Also, tell your doctor if you are breast-feeding an infant. It is not known whether clarithromycin passes into breast milk.

clemastine

BRAND NAMES (Manufacturers)
Tavist (Sandoz)
Tavist-1 (Sandoz)
TYPE OF DRUG
Antihistamine
INGREDIENT
clemastine fumarate

DOSAGE FORMS
Tablets (1.34 mg and 2.68 mg)
Oral syrup (0.67 mg per 5-ml spoonful, with 5. 5% alcohol)
STORAGE
Clemastine tablets and oral syrup should be stored at room temperature in tightly closed containers.

USES
This medication belongs to a group of drugs known as antihistamines (antihistamines block the action of histamine, a chemical that is released by the body during an allergic reaction). It is, therefore, used to treat or prevent symptoms of allergy.

TREATMENT
To avoid stomach upset, you can take clemastine with food or with a full glass of milk or water (unless your doctor directs you to do otherwise).

Each dose of the oral syrup should be measured carefully with a specially designed 5-ml measuring spoon. An ordinary kitchen teaspoon is not accurate enough.

If you miss a dose of this medication, take the missed dose as soon as possible, unless it is almost time for your next dose. In that case, do not take the missed dose at all; just return to your regular dosing schedule. Do not double the next dose.

SIDE EFFECTS
Minor. Blurred vision; confusion; constipation; diarrhea; difficult or painful urination; dizziness; drowsiness; dry mouth, throat, or nose; headache; irritability; loss of appetite; nausea; restlessness; ringing or buzzing in the ears; stomach upset; or unusual increase in sweating. These side effects should disappear as your body adjusts to the medication.

This medication can cause increased sensitivity to sunlight. It is, therefore, important to avoid prolonged exposure to sunlight and sunlamps. Wear protective clothing, and use an effective sunscreen.

If you are constipated, increase the amount of fiber in your diet (fresh fruits and vegetables, salads, bran, and whole-grain breads), exercise, and drink more water (unless your doctor tells you not to do so).

Chew sugarless gum or suck on ice chips or a piece of hard candy to reduce mouth dryness.

If you feel dizzy or light-headed, sit or lie down for a while; get up from a sitting or lying position slowly, and be careful on stairs.
Major. Tell your doctor about any side effects that are persistent or particularly bothersome. IT IS ESPECIALLY IMPORTANT TO TELL YOUR DOCTOR about change in menstruation, clumsiness, feeling faint, flushing of the face, hallucinations, palpitations, rash, seizures, shortness of breath, sleeping disorders, sore throat or fever, tightness in the chest, unusual bleeding or bruising, or unusual tiredness or weakness.

INTERACTIONS
Clemastine interacts with other types of medications:
1. Concurrent use of it with central nervous system depressants (such as alcohol, barbiturates, benzodiazepine

tranquilizers, muscle relaxants, narcotics, pain medications, and phenothiazine tranquilizers) or with tricyclic antidepressants can cause extreme drowsiness.

2. Monoamine oxidase (MAO) inhibitors (isocarboxazid, pargyline, phenelzine and tranylcypromine) can increase the side effects of this medication. At least 14 days should separate the use of this drug and the use of an MAO inhibitor.

3. Clemastine can also decrease the activity of oral anticoagulants (blood thinners, such as warfarin).

BE SURE TO TELL YOUR DOCTOR about any medications you are currently taking, especially any of the medications that are listed above.

WARNINGS

• Tell your doctor about unusual or allergic reactions you have had to any medications, especially to clemastine or to other antihistamines (such as astemizole, azatadine, brompheniramine, carbinoxamine, chlorpheniramine, cyproheptadine, dexchlorpheniramine, dimenhydrinate, dimethindene, diphenhydramine, diphenylpyraline, doxylamine, hydroxyzine, phenidamine, promethazine, pyrilamine, terfenadine, trimeprazine, tripelennamine, and triprolidine).

• Tell your doctor if you now have or if you have ever had asthma, blood vessel disease, glaucoma, high blood pressure, kidney disease, peptic ulcers, enlarged prostate gland, or thyroid disease.

• Clemastine can cause drowsiness or dizziness. Your ability to perform tasks that require alertness, such as driving a car or operating dangerous equipment, may be decreased. Appropriate caution should, be taken.

• Drinking alcoholic beverages can increase the sedative effects of clemastine.

• Be sure to tell your doctor if you are pregnant. The effects of this medication during pregnancy have not been thoroughly studied in humans. Also, tell your doctor if you are breast-feeding an infant. Small amounts of clemastine pass into breast milk and may cause unusual excitement or irritability in nursing infants.

Cleocin HCI—see clindamycin (systemic)

Cleocin Pediatric—see clindamycin (systemic)

Cleocin T—see clindamycin (topical)

clindamycin (systemic)

BRAND NAMES (Manufacturers)
Cleocin HCI (Upjohn)
Cleocin Pediatric (Upjohn)
clindamycin (various manufacturers)
TYPE OF DRUG
Antibiotic
INGREDIENT
clindamycin palmitate hydrochloride
DOSAGE FORMS
Capsules (75 mg, 150 mg, and 300 mg)
Oral suspension (75 mg per 5-ml spoonful)

STORAGE
Clindamycin capsules and oral suspension should be stored at room temperature in tightly closed containers. The oral suspension should not be refrigerated or frozen; when chilled, it thickens and becomes difficult to pour. The suspension form of this medication should be discarded after 14 days because it loses potency.

USES
Clindamycin is an antibiotic that is used to treat a wide variety of bacterial infections. It chemically attaches to the bacteria and prevents their growth and multiplication. Clindamycin kills susceptible bacteria, but it is not effective against viruses, parasites, or fungi.

TREATMENT
In order to prevent irritation to your esophagus (swallowing tube) or stomach, you should take clindamycin with food or a full glass of water or milk (unless your doctor directs you to do otherwise).

The suspension form of this medication should be shaken well just before measuring each dose. The contents tend to settle on the bottom of the bottle, so it is necessary to shake the container to distribute the ingredients evenly and equalize the doses. Each dose should then be measured carefully with a specially designed 5-ml measuring spoon. An ordinary kitchen teaspoon is not accurate enough.

Clindamycin works best when the level of medicine in your bloodstream is kept constant. It is best, therefore, to take the doses at evenly spaced intervals day and night. For example, if you are to take four doses a day, the doses should be spaced six hours apart.

Try not to miss any doses of this medication. If you do miss a dose, take it as soon as you remember. However, if you do not remember to take the missed dose until it is almost time for your next dose, take the missed dose immediately; space the following dose about halfway through the regular interval between doses; then continue with your regular dosing schedule.

It is important to continue to take this medication for the entire time prescribed by your doctor (usually seven to 14 days), even if your symptoms of infection disappear before the end of that period. If you stop taking the drug too soon, resistant bacteria are given a chance to continue growing, and your infection could recur.

SIDE EFFECTS
Minor. Diarrhea, loss of appetite, nausea, stomach or throat irritation, or vomiting. These side effects should disappear as your body adjusts to the medication. If the diarrhea becomes prolonged, CONTACT YOUR DOCTOR. Do not take antidiarrheal medicine.

Major. Tell your doctor about any side effects that are persistent or particularly bothersome. IT IS ESPECIALLY IMPORTANT TO TELL YOUR DOCTOR about bloody or pus-containing diarrhea, hives, itching, muscle or joint pain, skin rash, unusual bleeding or bruising, or yellowing of the eyes or skin. Also, if the symptoms of your infection do not improve in several days, contact your doctor. This medication may not be effective for your particular infection.

INTERACTIONS

Clindamycin should not interact with other medications if it is used according to directions.

WARNINGS

• Tell your doctor about unusual or allergic reactions you have had to any medications, especially to clindamycin or lincomycin.

• Before starting to take this medication, be sure to tell your doctor if you now have or if you have ever had colitis, kidney disease, or liver disease.

• Before having surgery or any other medical or dental treatment, be sure to tell your doctor or dentist that you are taking clindamycin.

• The capsule form of this medication contains the color additive FD&C Yellow No. 5 (tartrazine), which can cause allergic-type symptoms (fainting, shortness of breath, rash) in certain susceptible individuals.

• Clindamycin has been prescribed for your current infection only. Another infection later on, may require a different medicine. You should not give your medicine to other people or use it for other infections, unless your doctor specifically directs you to do so.

• Be sure to tell your doctor if you are pregnant. Although clindamycin appears to be safe during pregnancy, extensive studies in humans have not been conducted. Also, tell your doctor if you are breast-feeding an infant. Small amounts of clindamycin pass into breast milk.

clindamycin (topical)

BRAND NAME (Manufacturer)
Cleocin T (Upjohn)
TYPE OF DRUG
Antibiotic
INGREDIENT
clindamycin phosphate
DOSAGE FORMS
Topical solution (10 mg per ml)
Topical gel (1%)
Topical lotion (10 mg per ml)
STORAGE
Clindamycin topical solution, gel, or lotion should be stored at room temperature in a tightly closed container. It should be kept away from flames and heat because the solution is flammable (it contains alcohol).

USES

Clindamycin topical solution is used to treat acne vulgaris. It is an antibiotic that is thought to act by suppressing the growth of the bacteria *Propionibacterium acnes*. These bacteria are probably responsible for the formation of the acne sores.

TREATMENT

Before applying topical clindamycin, wash the affected area thoroughly with a mild soap and warm water. Then rinse well and pat dry. To avoid skin irritation from the alcohol, wait at least 30 minutes after washing or shaving before applying this medication.

The solution is packaged in a bottle with an applicator tip that can be used to apply the solution directly to the skin. Press the applicator tip firmly against your skin. The pressure applied determines the amount of medicine released. Use the applicator with a dabbing motion rather than a rolling motion. A thin film of medication should be applied to the entire area of skin affected by acne.

If you miss a dose of this medication, apply it as soon as possible, unless it is almost time for the next dose. In that case, do not apply the missed dose at all; just return to your regular dosing schedule.

Topical clindamycin does not cure acne, but it helps to control it as long as you continue to use the drug.

It is important to continue to apply this medication for the entire time prescribed by your doctor (which may be several months), even if your symptoms disappear in several days. If you stop applying the medication too soon, the bacteria are given a chance to continue growing, and your infection could recur.

If there is no improvement in your condition after six weeks of using this medication, check with your doctor. However, it may take up to 12 weeks before improvement in your acne is readily apparent.

SIDE EFFECTS

Minor. Diarrhea, dry skin, fatigue, headache, nausea, oily skin, or stomach irritation. These side effects should disappear as your body adjusts to the medication.

If diarrhea becomes severe or prolonged, CONTACT YOUR DOCTOR. Do not take any antidiarrheal medicine.

Major. Tell your doctor about any side effects that are persistent or particularly bothersome. IT IS ESPECIALLY IMPORTANT TO TELL YOUR DOCTOR about bloody or pus-containing diarrhea, increased urination, itching, sore throat, or swelling of the face.

INTERACTIONS

If you are using another topical medication as well as clindamycin, it is best to apply them at different times to increase effectiveness and reduce the chance of skin irritation.

Use of abrasive or medicated cleansers, medicated cosmetics, or any topical, alcohol-containing preparations (such as after-shave lotions or perfume) in conjunction with topical clindamycin can result in excessive skin dryness and irritation.

WARNINGS

• Tell your doctor about unusual or allergic reactions you have had to any drugs, especially to clindamycin or lincomycin.

• Tell your doctor if you have ever had colitis.

• Because this medication contains alcohol, it can cause skin irritation in sensitive areas. In addition, it has an unpleasant taste if it gets on the mouth or lips. You should avoid getting this medication in your eyes, nose, or mouth, or in the areas surrounding scratches or burns.

• You may continue to use cosmetics while applying this medication (unless otherwise directed by your doctor), but it is best to use only "water-based" cosmetics rather than ones with an oil base.

• Be sure to tell your doctor if you are pregnant. Although topical clindamycin appears to be safe during pregnancy, extensive studies in humans have not been conducted. Also, tell your doctor if you are breast-feeding an infant. It is not known whether topical clindamycin passes into breast milk.

Clindex—see chlordiazepoxide and clidinium combination

Clinoril—see sulindac

Clinoxide—see chlordiazepoxide and clidinium combination

Clipoxide—see chlordiazepoxide and clidinium combination

clofibrate

BRAND NAMES (Manufacturers)
Atromid-S (Ayerst)
clofibrate (various manufacturers)
TYPE OF DRUG
Antihyperlipidemic (lipid-lowering drug)
INGREDIENT
clofibrate
DOSAGE FORM
Capsules (500 mg)
STORAGE
Clofibrate should be stored at room temperature in a tightly closed, light-resistant container.

USES
Clofibrate is used to reduce fat (lipid) or cholesterol in the blood in patients with atherosclerosis (hardening of the arteries) and in patients having certain kinds of skin lesions caused by excessive fat levels in the blood. It is not clearly understood how clofibrate works, but it appears to decrease the body's production of cholesterol and fats.

Attempts are usually made to control serum fat levels with diet, exercise, weight loss, or control of diabetes before therapy with this drug is initiated.

TREATMENT
Clofibrate should be taken with food or immediately after a meal (unless your doctor directs you to do otherwise).

If you miss a dose of this medication, take the missed dose as soon as possible, unless it is almost time for the next dose. In that case, do not take the missed dose at all; just return to your regular dosing schedule. Do not double the next dose.

SIDE EFFECTS
Minor. Abdominal cramps, bloating, blurred vision, decreased sexual desire, diarrhea, dizziness, drowsiness, dry and brittle hair, dry skin, fatigue, gas, headache, increased sweating, itching, muscle cramps, nausea, sore mouth, vomiting, weakness, or weight gain. These side effects should disappear as your body adjusts to the medication.

If you feel dizzy, sit or lie down for a while; get up slowly from a sitting or reclining position, and be careful on stairs.

Major. Tell your doctor about any side effects that are persistent or particularly bothersome. IT IS ESPECIALLY IMPORTANT TO TELL YOUR DOCTOR about bloody or black, tarry stools; chest pain; difficult or painful urination; impotence; loss of hair; rash; palpitations; sore joints; tremors; or unusual bleeding or bruising.

INTERACTIONS
Clofibrate interacts with several other types of medications:
1. It can increase the side effects of oral anticoagulants (blood thinners, such as warfarin) and oral antidiabetic agents.
2. Rifampin can decrease the effectiveness of clofibrate.
3. Probenecid and furosemide can increase the side effects of clofibrate.

Before starting to take clofibrate, BE SURE TO TELL YOUR DOCTOR about any medications you are currently taking, especially any of those listed above.

WARNINGS
• Tell your doctor about unusual or allergic reactions you have had to any medications, especially to clofibrate.
• Before starting to take this medication, be sure to tell your doctor if you now have or if you have ever had diabetes mellitus, gallstones, heart disease, kidney disease, liver disease, stomach ulcers, or thyroid disease.
• Do not stop taking this medication without first checking with your doctor. Stopping this medication abruptly may lead to an increase in your blood fat levels. Your doctor may want you to follow a special diet to prevent this.
• Be sure to tell your doctor if you are pregnant. Clofibrate crosses the placenta and can build up in the body of the developing fetus. Because clofibrate has long-term effects on the body, you should not become pregnant for at least two months after you stop taking this drug. Also, tell your doctor if you are breast-feeding an infant. It is not known whether clofibrate passes into breast milk.

Clomid—see clomiphene

clomiphene

BRAND NAMES (Manufacturers)
Clomid (Merrell Dow)
Milophene (Milex)
Serophene (Serono)
TYPE OF DRUG
Fertility drug
INGREDIENT
clomiphene
DOSAGE FORM
Tablets (50 mg)
STORAGE
Clomiphene should be stored at room temperature in a tightly closed, light-resistant container.

USES

Clomiphene is used to treat infertility in women. This drug reverses some types of infertility in women by stimulating ovulation.

TREATMENT

Clomiphene can be taken either on an empty stomach or with food or milk, as directed by your doctor.

It is very important to follow your dosing schedule carefully. If you have any questions about how to take this medication, BE SURE TO CHECK WITH YOUR DOCTOR.

If you miss a dose of this medication, take the missed dose as soon as possible. If you do not remember until it is time for the next dose, double the dose, then return to your regular dosing schedule. If you miss more than one dose, CHECK WITH YOUR DOCTOR.

SIDE EFFECTS

Minor. Abdominal discomfort, bloating, dizziness, headache, insomnia, nausea, nervousness, or vomiting. These side effects should disappear as your body adjusts to the medication.

If you feel dizzy, sit or lie down for a while; get up slowly from a sitting or reclining position, and be careful on stairs.

Major. Tell your doctor about any side effects that are persistent or particularly bothersome. IT IS ESPECIALLY IMPORTANT TO TELL YOUR DOCTOR about breast tenderness, depression, fatigue, hair loss, hot flashes, pelvic pain, skin rash, or visual disturbances.

INTERACTIONS

Clomiphene should not interact with other medications if it is used according to directions.

WARNINGS

• Tell your doctor about unusual or allergic reactions you have had to any medications, especially to clomiphene.
• Before beginning to take clomiphene, tell your doctor if you now have or if you have ever had any of the following symptoms: abnormal vaginal bleeding, clotting problems, tumors or cysts of the uterus or ovaries, liver disease, or mental depression.
• If clomiphene makes you dizzy, do not take part in any activity that requires alertness, such as driving a car or operating potentially dangerous equipment, and take care going up and down stairs.
• While taking this medication, it is important to carefully follow your doctor's directions for recording your body temperature and for the timing of sexual intercourse.
• The risk of a multiple pregnancy is increased when clomiphene is used. This medication should not be taken if you are already pregnant. If you should become pregnant during treatment with clomiphene, tell your doctor immediately and, unless directed to do otherwise, discontinue the medication at once. It has been reported to cause birth defects in the offspring of animals that received large doses of clomiphene during pregnancy. Also, tell your doctor if you are breast-feeding an infant. It is not known whether clomiphene passes into breast milk.

clonazepam

BRAND NAME (Manufacturer)
Klonopin (Roche)
TYPE OF DRUG
Benzodiazepine anticonvulsant
INGREDIENT
clonazepam
DOSAGE FORM
Tablets (0.5 mg, 1 mg, and 2 mg)
STORAGE
Clonazepam should be stored at room temperature in a tightly closed, light-resistant container.

USES

This medication is used to treat certain seizure disorders. It is unclear exactly how clonazepam works to treat convulsions, but it appears to prevent the spread of seizures to all parts of the brain.

TREATMENT

This medication can be ingested either on an empty stomach or with food or milk. However, take it only as directed by your doctor.

Clonazepam works best when the level of medicine in your bloodstream is kept constant. It is best, therefore, to take the doses at evenly spaced intervals day and night. For example, if you are to take three doses a day, the doses should be spaced eight hours apart.

Try not to miss any doses of this medication. If you do miss a dose and remember within an hour, take the dose immediately. If more than an hour has passed, do not take the missed dose at all; just return to your regular dosing schedule. Do not double the next dose. If you miss two or more doses, CONTACT YOUR DOCTOR.

SIDE EFFECTS

Minor. Constipation, diarrhea, drowsiness, dry mouth, headache, increased appetite, insomnia, loss of appetite, nausea, runny nose, or weight loss or gain. These side effects should disappear as your body adjusts to the medication.

In order to relieve constipation, increase the amount of fiber in your diet (fresh fruits and vegetables, salads, bran, and whole-grain breads), exercise, and drink more water (unless your doctor directs you to do otherwise).

To relieve mouth dryness, chew sugarless gum or suck on ice chips or a piece of hard candy.

Major. Tell your doctor about any side effects that are persistent or particularly bothersome. IT IS ESPECIALLY IMPORTANT TO TELL YOUR DOCTOR about behavioral problems, confusion, depression, fever, fluid retention, hair loss, hallucinations, hysteria, increased or decreased urination, muscle weakness, palpitations, skin rash, slurred speech, sore gums, tremors, unusual bleeding or bruising, unusual body movements, or yellowing of the eyes or skin.

Clonazepam can also produce an increase in salivation, so it should be used cautiously by people who have swallowing difficulties. Contact your doctor if salivation becomes a problem.

INTERACTIONS

Clonazepam interacts with several other types of drugs:

1. Concurrent use of it with other central nervous system depressants (such as alcohol, antihistamines, barbiturates, benzodiazepine tranquilizers, muscle relaxants, narcotics, pain medications, phenothiazine tranquilizers, and sleeping medications) or with tricyclic antidepressants can cause extreme drowsiness.

2. Phenobarbital and phenytoin can decrease the blood levels and effectiveness of clonazepam.

3. Concurrent use of clonazepam and valproic acid can lead to increased seizure activity.

Before starting to take this medication, BE SURE TO TELL YOUR DOCTOR about any medications you are currently taking, especially any of those listed above.

WARNINGS

• Tell your doctor about unusual or allergic reactions you have had to any medications, especially to clonazepam or to other benzodiazepine tranquilizers (such as alprazolam, chlordiazepoxide, clorazepate, diazepam, flurazepam, halazepam, lorazepam, oxazepam, prazepam, temazepam, and triazolam).

• Tell your doctor if you now have or if you have ever had glaucoma, kidney disease, liver disease, or lung disease.

• If this drug makes you dizzy or drowsy, do not take part in any activity that requires alertness, such as driving a car or operating potentially dangerous equipment. Children should be careful while playing.

• Do not stop taking this medication unless you first check with your doctor. If you have been taking this medication for several months or longer, stopping the drug abruptly could lead to a withdrawal reaction and a worsening of your condition. Your doctor may, therefore, want to reduce your dosage of this medication gradually.

• Be sure to tell your doctor if you are pregnant. Although no harmful effects have been reported during pregnancy, extensive studies have not been conducted. The risks and benefits of clonazepam therapy during pregnancy should be discussed with your doctor. Also, tell your doctor if you are breast-feeding an infant. Small amounts of clonazepam pass into breast milk and may cause excessive drowsiness in nursing infants.

clonidine

BRAND NAMES (Manufacturers)
Catapres (Boehringer Ingelheim)
Catapres-TTS (Boehringer Ingelheim)
clonidine hydrochloride (various manufacturers)

TYPE OF DRUG
Antihypertensive

INGREDIENT
clonidine hydrochloride

DOSAGE FORMS
Tablets (0.1 mg, 0.2 mg, and 0.3 mg)
Transdermal patch (2. 5 mg, 5 mg, and 7. 5 mg per patch; release rate of clonidine is 0.1 mg, 0.2 mg, and 0.3 mg per 24 hours)

STORAGE
Clonidine tablets should be stored at room temperature in a tightly closed container. Do not remove a patch from its packaging until just before you apply it.

USES
This medication works on the central nervous system (brain and spinal cord) to prevent the release of chemicals responsible for maintaining high blood pressure.

TREATMENT
To avoid stomach irritation, you can take clonidine tablets with food or with a full glass of milk or water. In order to become accustomed to taking this medication, try to take it at the same time(s) every day.

Clonidine transdermal patches come with detailed patient instructions that should be carefully followed. Apply the patch to a hairless area of unbroken skin on the upper arm or chest. If the patch becomes loose before it is time to remove it (after seven days), apply adhesive tape over the patch to ensure good adhesion. To avoid skin irritation, apply each new patch to a different site.

If you miss a dose of clonidine tablets, take the missed dose as soon as possible, unless it is almost time for your next dose. In that case, do not take the missed dose at all; just return to your regular dosing schedule. Do not double the next dose. If you miss more than two doses of this medication, contact your doctor.

If you forget to remove the clonidine transdermal patch after seven days, remove the old patch as soon as you remember. Apply a new patch immediately to a different site.

Clonidine does not cure high blood pressure, but it will help control the condition as long as it is taken.

SIDE EFFECTS
Minor. Anxiety, constipation, decreased sexual desire, dizziness, drowsiness, dry eyes, dry mouth, fatigue, headache, insomnia, jaw pain, loss of appetite, nasal congestion, nausea, nervousness, or vomiting. These side effects should disappear as your body adjusts to the medication.

The patches can also cause burning, inflammation, itching, rash, or increased or decreased pigmentation of the skin at the site of application. TELL YOUR DOCTOR if the skin reactions persist or become bothersome.

To prevent constipation, increase the amount of fiber in your diet (fresh fruits and vegetables, salads, bran, and whole-grain breads), unless your doctor tells you not to.

To relieve mouth dryness, suck on ice chips or a piece of hard candy or chew sugarless gum.

"Artificial tears" eye drops may help relieve eye dryness.

To avoid dizziness or light-headedness when you stand, contract and relax the muscles of your legs for a few moments before rising. Do this by pushing one foot against the floor while raising the other foot slightly, alternating feet so that you are "pumping" your legs in a pedaling motion.

Major. Tell your doctor about any side effects that are persistent or particularly bothersome. IT IS ESPECIALLY

IMPORTANT TO TELL YOUR DOCTOR about chest pain; cold fingertips or toes; depression; difficulty in breathing; difficulty in urinating; enlarged, painful breasts (in both sexes); hair loss; hives; impotence; itching; nightmares; rash; swelling of the hands or feet; weight gain; or yellowing of the eyes or skin.

INTERACTIONS

Clonidine interacts with several other types of medications:

1. Concurrent use of clonidine with other central nervous system depressants (such as alcohol, antihistamines, barbiturates, benzodiazepine tranquilizers, muscle relaxants, narcotics, pain medications, phenothiazine tranquilizers, and sleeping medications) or with tricyclic antidepressants can cause extreme drowsiness.

2. Tricyclic antidepressants and anti-inflammatory agents (such as indomethacin) may block the blood-pressure-lowering effects of clonidine.

Before you start to take this medication, BE SURE TO TELL YOUR DOCTOR about any medications you are currently taking, especially any of those listed above.

WARNINGS

• Tell your doctor about any unusual or allergic reactions you have had to medications, especially to clonidine.

• Tell your doctor if you have ever had heart disease, kidney disease, depression, Raynaud's disease, or a heart attack or stroke.

• Before having surgery or any other medical or dental treatment, tell your doctor or dentist you are taking this drug.

• Do not take any over-the-counter (nonprescription) medications for weight control or for allergy, asthma, sinus, cough, or cold problems unless you first check with your doctor.

• If this drug makes you dizzy or drowsy, do not take part in any activity that requires alertness, such as driving a car or operating potentially dangerous equipment.

• Tolerance to this medication develops occasionally; consult your doctor if you feel that the drug is becoming less effective.

• Do not stop taking this medication without first consulting your doctor. If therapy with this drug is stopped abruptly, you may experience nervousness, agitation, headache, and a rise in blood pressure. Your doctor may, therefore, want to reduce your dosage of the drug gradually or start you on another medication.

• Make sure you have enough medication on hand to last through weekends, vacations, and holidays.

• Drinking alcoholic beverages, standing for prolonged periods, exercising, and hot weather can each increase the blood-pressure-lowering effects of clonidine and can cause fainting or dizziness.

• Be sure to tell your doctor if you are pregnant. Although clonidine appears to be safe in animals, extensive studies in humans during pregnancy have not been conducted. Also, tell your doctor if you are breast-feeding an infant. Small amounts of clonidine pass into breast milk.

clonidine hydrochloride—see clonidine

Clopra—see metoclopramide

clorazepate

BRAND NAMES (Manufacturers)
clorazepate (various manufacturers)
Tranxene-SD (Abbott)
Tranxene T-Tabs (Abbott)
TYPE OF DRUG
Benzodiazepine sedative/hypnotic
INGREDIENT
clorazepate
DOSAGE FORMS
Capsules (3.75 mg, 7.5 mg, and 15 mg)
Tablets (3.75 mg, 7.5 mg, 11.25 mg, 15 mg, and 22.5 mg)
STORAGE
This medication should be stored at room temperature in tightly closed, light-resistant containers.

USES
Clorazepate is prescribed to treat the symptoms of anxiety and sometimes to treat seizures and alcohol withdrawal symptoms. It is not clear exactly how this medicine works, but it may relieve anxiety by acting as a depressant of the central nervous system. Clorazepate is used to relieve nervousness. It is effective for this purpose, but it is important to remove the cause of the anxiety as well.

TREATMENT
This medication should be taken exactly as directed by your doctor. It can be taken with food or a full glass of water if stomach upset occurs. Do not take this medication with a dose of antacids, since they may retard its absorption.

If you are taking this medication regularly and you miss a dose, take the missed dose immediately if you remember within an hour. If more than an hour has passed, skip the dose you missed and wait for the next scheduled dose. Do not double the next dose.

SIDE EFFECTS
Minor. Bitter taste in the mouth, constipation, depression, diarrhea, dizziness, drowsiness (after a night's sleep), dry mouth, excessive salivation, fatigue, flushing, headache, heartburn, loss of appetite, nausea, nervousness, sweating, or vomiting. As your body adjusts to the medicine, these side effects should disappear.

To relieve constipation, increase the amount of fiber in your diet (fresh fruits and vegetables, salads, bran, and whole-grain breads), exercise, and drink more water (unless your doctor directs you to do otherwise).

Dry mouth can be relieved by chewing sugarless gum or by sucking on ice chips.

If you feel dizzy, sit or lie down for a while; get up slowly from a sitting or reclining position, and be careful on stairs.

Major. Tell your doctor about any side effects that are persistent or particularly bothersome. IT IS ESPECIALLY IMPORTANT TO TELL YOUR DOCTOR about blurred or double vision, chest pain, difficulty in urinating, fainting, falling, fever, joint pain, hallucinations, mouth sores, nightmares, palpitations, rash, severe depression, shortness of breath, slurred speech, sore throat, uncoordinated movements, unusual excitement, unusual tiredness, or yellowing of the eyes or skin.

INTERACTIONS
Clorazepate interacts with several other types of drugs:
1. To prevent oversedation, this drug should not be taken with alcohol or other sedative drugs, central nervous system depressants (such as antihistamines, barbiturates, muscle relaxants, pain medicines, narcotics, medicines for seizures, and phenothiazine tranquilizers), or with antidepressants.
2. This medication may decrease the effectiveness of carbamazepine, levodopa, and oral anticoagulants (blood thinners) and may increase the effects of phenytoin.
3. Disulfiram, oral contraceptives (birth control pills), isoniazid, and cimetidine can increase the blood levels of clorazepate, which can lead to increased sedation.
4. Concurrent use of rifampin may decrease the effectiveness of clorazepate.

BE SURE TO TELL YOUR DOCTOR about any medications you are currently taking, especially any of those listed above.

WARNINGS
• Tell your doctor about unusual or allergic reactions you have had to any medications, especially to clorazepate or other benzodiazepine tranquilizers (such as alprazolam, chlordiazepoxide, diazepam, flurazepam, halazepam, lorazepam, oxazepam, prazepam, temazepam, and triazolam).
• Tell your doctor if you now have or if you have ever had liver disease, kidney disease, epilepsy, lung disease, myasthenia gravis, porphyria, depression, or mental illness.
• This medicine can cause drowsiness. Avoid tasks that require alertness, such as driving a car or using potentially dangerous equipment. Also take care in going up and down stairs.
• This medication has the potential for abuse and must be used with caution. Tolerance may develop quickly; do not increase the dosage without first consulting your doctor. It is also important not to stop taking this drug suddenly if you have been taking it in large amounts or if you have used it for several weeks. Your doctor may want to reduce the dosage gradually.
• This is a safe drug when used properly. When it is combined with other sedative drugs or alcohol, however, serious side effects may develop.
• Be sure to tell your doctor if you are pregnant. This medicine may increase the chance of birth defects if it is taken during the first three months of pregnancy. In addition, too much use of this medicine during the last six months of pregnancy may cause the baby to become dependent on it. This may result in withdrawal symptoms in the newborn. Also, use of this medicine during the last weeks of pregnancy may cause excessive drowsiness, slowed heartbeat, and breathing difficulties in the newborn. Tell your doctor if you are breastfeeding an infant.

This medicine can pass into the breast milk and cause excessive drowsiness, slowed heartbeat, and breathing difficulties in the nursing infant.

clotrimazole (topical)

BRAND NAMES (Manufacturers)
Lotrimin (Schering)
Lotrimin AF* (Schering-Plough)
Mycelex (Miles)
Mycelex OTC* (Miles)
*Available without a prescription in 1% cream and 1% solution.
TYPE OF DRUG
Antifungal
INGREDIENT
clotrimazole
DOSAGE FORMS
Topical cream (1%)
Topical solution (1%)
Topical lotion (1%)
STORAGE
Store at room temperature in tightly closed containers. This medication should never be frozen.

USES
This medication is used to treat superficial fungal infections of the skin. Clotrimazole is an antifungal agent that is active against a broad range of fungi and yeasts. It acts by preventing the growth and multiplication of these organisms.

TREATMENT
Apply this medication in the morning and evening, unless your doctor directs you to do otherwise. Before applying clotrimazole, you should wash your hands. Then (unless otherwise directed) cleanse the affected area with soap and water. Pat the skin with a clean towel until it is almost dry. Gently massage a small amount of the cream, solution, or lotion over the entire area that is affected and the skin immediately surrounding this area. Do not bandage or cover the infection after applying the medication unless your doctor instructs you to do so. Wash your hands again after use.

Improvement in your condition may not become apparent for as much as a week after you begin treatment with this drug. However, you should be sure to complete the full course of therapy. If you stop using this drug too soon, resistant fungi are given a chance to continue growing, and the infection could recur. If your condition has not improved after four weeks of treatment with this medication, however, CONTACT YOUR DOCTOR. Clotrimazole may not be effective against the organism that is causing your infection.

If you miss a dose of this medication, apply the missed dose as soon as possible. If you do not remember until it is almost time for the next dose, however, do not apply the missed dose at all; just return to your regular dosing schedule. Do not use a double dose of the medication at the next application.

SIDE EFFECTS

Minor. You may experience some burning, itching, stinging, or redness when this drug is applied to the skin. These side effects should disappear as your body adjusts to the drug.

Major. Tell your doctor about any side effects that are persistent or particularly bothersome. IT IS ESPECIALLY IMPORTANT TO TELL YOUR DOCTOR about blistering, irritation, peeling of the skin, or swelling.

INTERACTIONS

Clotrimazole should not interact with other medications as long as it is used according to directions.

WARNINGS

• Tell your doctor about any unusual reactions you have had to medications, especially to clotrimazole.
• This medication has been prescribed for your current infection only. Another infection may require a different medication. Therefore, you should not give your medicine to other people or use it for other infections, unless your doctor specifically directs you to do so.
• Clotrimazole should not be used in or around the eyes.
• In order to avoid reinfection, keep the affected area clean and dry, wear freshly laundered clothing, and try to avoid wearing tight-fitting clothing.
• Be sure to tell your doctor if you are pregnant. Small amounts of clotrimazole may be absorbed through the skin. It should, therefore, be used cautiously, especially during the first three months of pregnancy. Also, tell your doctor if you are breast-feeding an infant. It is not known whether clotrimazole passes into breast milk.

clotrimazole (vaginal)

BRAND NAMES (Manufacturers)
Gyne-Lotrimin (Schering)*
Mycelex-G (Miles)
*Available without a prescription in 1% cream or 100 mg tablet.
TYPE OF DRUG
Antifungal
INGREDIENT
clotrimazole
DOSAGE FORMS
Vaginal cream (1%)
Vaginal tablets (100 mg and 500 mg)
STORAGE
Store at room temperature in a tightly closed container. This medication should never be frozen.

USES

This medication is used to treat fungal infections of the vagina. Clotrimazole is an antifungal agent that prevents the growth and multiplication of a wide range of fungi and yeast, including *Candida.*

TREATMENT

Clotrimazole vaginal cream and tablets are packaged with detailed directions for use. Follow these instructions carefully. An applicator will probably be provided for inserting the cream into the vagina. Use this medication at bedtime, unless otherwise directed by your doctor.

You should wash the area carefully prior to inserting the cream or tablet into the vagina.

If you begin to menstruate while being treated with clotrimazole, continue your regular dosing schedule.

If you miss a dose of this medication, insert the missed dose as soon as possible. However, if you do not remember until the following day, do not insert the missed dose at all; just return to your regular dosing schedule. Do not use a double dose of the medication at the next application.

It is important to continue to insert this medication for the entire time prescribed by your doctor—even if the symptoms disappear before the end of that period. If you stop using the drug too soon, resistant fungus could be given a chance to continue growing, and it is possible that your infection could recur.

SIDE EFFECTS

Minor. You may experience vaginal burning, itching, or irritation when this drug is inserted. This sensation should disappear as your body adjusts to the medication. Your sexual partner may also experience some burning or irritation.

Do not treat any side effects that occur in the area of the infection unless you first consult your doctor.

Major. Tell your doctor about any side effects that are persistent or particularly bothersome. IT IS ESPECIALLY IMPORTANT TO TELL YOUR DOCTOR about abdominal cramps, blistering, bloating, excessive irritation, painful urination, or peeling of the skin.

INTERACTIONS

Clotrimazole should not interact with other medications if it is used according to directions.

WARNINGS

• Tell your doctor about unusual or allergic reactions you have had to any medications, especially to clotrimazole.
• Tell your doctor if you have had other vaginal infections, especially if they have been resistant to treatment.
• To prevent reinfection, avoid sexual intercourse or ask your partner to use a condom until treatment is completed.
• There may be some vaginal drainage while using this medication; therefore, you may want to use a sanitary napkin or panty liner to prevent the staining of clothing. However, the use of tampons is not recommended since they may soak up too much of the medicine.
• Whenever possible, wear cotton panties rather than those made of nylon or other nonporous materials while being treated for a vaginal fungus infection. Also, in order to better prevent reinfection, always wear freshly laundered underclothes.
• If there is no improvement in your condition, or if irritation in the area continues after several days of treatment, CONTACT YOUR DOCTOR. This medication may be causing an allergic reaction, or it may not be effective against the organism causing your infection.

• This medication has been prescribed for your current infection only. Another infection that develops later on, or one that someone else has, may require a different medication. Therefore, you should not give your medication to other women or use it for other infections unless your doctor specifically directs you to do so.

• Tell your doctor if you are pregnant. Clotrimazole appears to be safe during pregnancy. However, extensive studies have not been conducted. In addition, your doctor may want to change the instructions on how you are to use this drug if you are pregnant. Also, tell your doctor if you are breast-feeding. It is not known whether this drug passes into breast milk.

cloxacillin

BRAND NAMES (Manufacturers)
cloxacillin sodium (various manufacturers)
Cloxapen (Beecham)
Tegopen (Bristol)
TYPE OF DRUG
Penicillin antibiotic
INGREDIENT
cloxacillin
DOSAGE FORMS
Capsules (250 mg and 500 mg)
Oral solution (125 mg per 5-ml spoonful)
STORAGE
Cloxacillin capsules should be stored at room temperature in a tightly closed container. The oral solution should be stored in the refrigerator in a tightly closed container. Any unused portion of the solution should be discarded after 14 days because the drug loses its potency after that time. This medication should never be frozen.

USES
Cloxacillin is used to treat a wide variety of bacterial infections, especially those caused by Staphylococcus bacteria. It acts by severely injuring the cell walls of the infecting bacteria, thereby preventing them from growing and multiplying. Cloxacillin kills susceptible bacteria, but it is not effective against viruses, parasites, or fungi.

TREATMENT
Cloxacillin should be taken on an empty stomach or with a glass of water one hour before or two hours after a meal. This medication should never be taken with fruit juices or carbonated beverages because the acidity of these drinks destroys the drug in the stomach.

The oral solution should be measured carefully with a specially designed 5-ml measuring spoon. An ordinary kitchen teaspoon is not accurate enough.

Cloxacillin works best when the level of medicine in your bloodstream is kept constant. Therefore, take the doses at evenly spaced intervals day and night. For example, if you are taking four doses a day, the doses should be spaced six hours apart.

If you miss a dose of this medication, take the missed dose immediately. However, if you do not remember to take the missed dose until it is almost time for your next dose, take it; space the following dose about halfway through the regular interval between doses; then return to your regular schedule. Try not to skip any doses.

It is important to continue to take this medication for the entire time prescribed by your doctor (usually seven to 14 days), even if the symptoms of the infection disappear before the end of that period. If you stop taking the drug too soon, resistant bacteria are given the chance to continue growing, and the infection could recur.

SIDE EFFECTS
Minor. Diarrhea, heartburn, nausea, or vomiting. These side effects should stop as your body adjusts to the drug.
Major. Tell your doctor about any side effects that are persistent or particularly bothersome. IT IS ESPECIALLY IMPORTANT TO TELL YOUR DOCTOR about bloating, chills, cough, darkened tongue, difficulty in breathing, fever, irritation of the mouth, muscle aches, rash, rectal or vaginal itching, severe diarrhea, or sore throat. Also, if your symptoms of infection seem to be getting worse rather than improving, you should contact your physician.

INTERACTIONS
Cloxacillin interacts with several other types of medications:
1. Probenecid can increase the blood concentrations and side effects of this medication.
2. Cloxacillin may decrease the effectiveness of birth control pills, and pregnancy could result. You should, therefore, use a different or additional form of birth control while taking this drug. Discuss this with your doctor.

BE SURE TO TELL YOUR DOCTOR about any medications you are currently taking, especially any listed above.

WARNINGS
• Tell your doctor about unusual or allergic reactions you have had to any medications, especially to cloxacillin or penicillins, cephalosporin antibiotics, penicillamine, or griseofulvin.
• Tell your doctor if you now have or if you have ever had kidney disease, asthma, or allergies.
• This medication has been prescribed for your current infection only. Another infection that develops later on, or one that someone else has, may require a different medicine. You should not give your medicine to other people to use or use your medication for other infections, unless your doctor specifically directs you to do so.
• Diabetics taking cloxacillin should know that this drug can cause a false-positive sugar reaction with a Clinitest urine glucose test. To avoid this problem, switch to Clinistix or Tes-Tape in order to test your urine for sugar.
• Be sure to tell your doctor if you are pregnant. Although cloxacillin appears to be safe during pregnancy, extensive studies in humans have not been conducted. Also, tell your doctor if you are breast-feeding an infant. Small amounts of this medication pass into breast milk and may temporarily alter the bacterial balance in the intestinal tract of the nursing infant, resulting in diarrhea.

cloxacillin sodium—see cloxacillin

Cloxapen—see cloxacillin

clozapine

BRAND NAME (Manufacturer)
Clozaril (Sandoz)
TYPE OF DRUG
Antipsychotic
INGREDIENT
clozapine
DOSAGE FORM
Tablets (25 mg and 100 mg)
STORAGE
Clozapine tablets should be stored at room temperature in the unit-dose packages provided by the manufacturer.

USES

Clozapine is prescribed for the treatment of schizophrenia in patients who have not been helped by or could not tolerate other medications. It is available only through pharmacies that agree to participate with your doctor in a program to monitor your blood. The program, which your doctor will arrange, provides a week's supply of the drug at the time that blood is drawn for testing.

TREATMENT

To avoid stomach irritation, you can take this medication with a meal or a glass of water or milk (unless your doctor directs you to do otherwise).

If you miss a dose of this medication, take the missed dose as soon as possible, then return to your regular dosing schedule. If it is almost time for the next dose, however, skip the one you missed and return to your regular schedule. Do not double the next dose (unless your doctor directs you to do otherwise).

The full effects of this medication for the control of emotional or mental symptoms may not become apparent for two weeks after you start to take it.

SIDE EFFECTS

Minor. Abdominal discomfort, constipation, dizziness, drowsiness, dry mouth, headache, heartburn, increased saliva production, light-headedness, nausea, vomiting, or weight gain. As your body adjusts to the medication, these side effects should disappear.

If you are constipated, increase the amount of fiber in your diet (fresh fruits and vegetables, salads, bran, and whole-grain breads), exercise, and drink more water (unless your doctor directs you to do otherwise).

Chew sugarless gum or suck on ice chips or a piece of hard candy to reduce mouth dryness.

To avoid dizziness or light-headedness when you stand, contract and relax the muscles of your legs for a few moments before rising. Do this by pushing one foot against the floor while raising the other foot slightly, alternating feet so that you are "pumping" your legs in a pedaling motion.

Major. Tell your doctor about any side effects that are persistent or particularly bothersome. IT IS ESPECIALLY IMPORTANT TO TELL YOUR DOCTOR about anxiety,

blurred vision, chest pain, chills, confusion, convulsions, difficulty in urinating, fainting, fever, increased sweating, loss of bladder control, mouth sores, muscle stiffness, nightmares, rapid heart rate, rash, restlessness, severe headache, sore throat, tremor, trouble sleeping, or unusual bleeding or bruising.

INTERACTIONS

Clozapine antipsychotic medication interacts with several other types of medications:

1. It can cause extreme drowsiness when combined with alcohol or other central nervous system (brain and spinal cord) depressants, such as barbiturates, benzodiazepine tranquilizers, muscle relaxants, phenothiazine tranquilizers, narcotics, and pain medications, or with tricyclic antidepressants.

2. Lithium may increase the side effects of this drug.

3. The effect of clozapine on blood cells may be increased by other drugs, such as antineoplastics (cancer medicine), antithyroid drugs, azathioprine, chloramphenicol, colchicine, flucytosine, interferon, and zidovudine.

4. The side effects of digoxin, phenytoin, and warfarin may be increased by this medication.

Before starting to take clozapine, BE SURE TO TELL YOUR DOCTOR about any other medications you are currently taking, especially if they are any of those listed above.

WARNINGS

• Be sure to tell your doctor about unusual or allergic reactions you have had to any medications, especially to clozapine.

• Tell your doctor if you have a history of alcoholism or if you now have or have ever had blood disease, depression, enlarged prostate, gastrointestinal problems, glaucoma, heart or circulatory disease, liver disease, or seizures.

• To avoid oversedation, avoid drinking alcoholic beverages while taking this medication.

• If this drug makes you dizzy or drowsy, do not take part in any activity that requires alertness, such as driving a car or operating potentially dangerous equipment. Be careful on stairs, and avoid getting up suddenly from a lying or sitting position.

• Do not stop taking this medication suddenly. Your doctor may want to gradually reduce the amount you are taking before stopping the drug. Be sure to consult your doctor before stopping this medication.

• It is very important that you have your blood tested weekly and that you have your doctor check your progress regularly. You can only receive the drug after your blood is drawn and a test is conducted. The results of your blood tests will assist your doctor in making safe dosage adjustments for you.

• Be sure to tell your doctor if you are pregnant. Although clozapine appears to be safe in animals, extensive studies in humans have not been conducted. Also, it is very important that you tell your doctor if you are breast-feeding an infant. Small amounts of this medication pass into breast milk.

Clozaril—see clozapine

codeine

BRAND NAMES (Manufacturers)
Codeine Phosphate (various manufacturers)
Codeine Sulfate (various manufacturers)
TYPE OF DRUG
Analgesic and cough suppressant
INGREDIENT
codeine
DOSAGE FORM
Tablets (15 mg, 30 mg, and 60 mg)
STORAGE
Codeine tablets should be stored at room temperature in a tightly closed, light-resistant container.

USES
Codeine is a narcotic analgesic that acts directly on the central nervous system (brain and spinal cord). It is used to relieve mild to moderate pain or to suppress coughing.

TREATMENT
In order to avoid stomach upset, you can take codeine with food or milk.

This drug works best if you take it at the onset of pain, rather than waiting until the pain becomes intense.

If you are taking this medication on a regular schedule and you miss a dose, take the missed dose as soon as possible, unless it is almost time for your next dose. In that case, do not take the missed dose at all; just return to your regular dosing schedule. Do not double the next dose.

SIDE EFFECTS
Minor. Constipation, dizziness, drowsiness, dry mouth, false sense of well-being, flushing, light-headedness, loss of appetite, nausea, painful or difficult urination, or sweating. These side effects should disappear as your body adjusts to the medication.

If you are constipated, increase the amount of fiber in your diet (fresh fruits and vegetables, salads, bran, and whole-grain breads), exercise, and drink more water (unless your doctor directs you to do otherwise).

Chew sugarless gum or suck on ice chips or a piece of hard candy to reduce mouth dryness.

If you feel dizzy, light-headed, or nauseated, sit or lie down for a while; get up from a sitting or lying position slowly, and be careful on stairs.
Major. Tell your doctor about any side effects that are persistent or particularly bothersome. IT IS ESPECIALLY IMPORTANT TO TELL YOUR DOCTOR about anxiety, breathing difficulties, excitation, fatigue, palpitations, rash, restlessness, sore throat and fever, tremors, or weakness.

INTERACTIONS
Codeine interacts with several other types of medications:

1. Concurrent use of this medication with other central nervous system depressants (such as alcohol, antihistamines, barbiturates, benzodiazepine tranquilizers, muscle relaxants, and phenothiazine tranquilizers) or with tricyclic antidepressants can cause extreme drowsiness.
2. A monoamine oxidase (MAO) inhibitor taken within 14 days of this medication can lead to unpredictable and severe side effects.
3. Cimetidine, combined with this medication, can cause confusion, disorientation, and shortness of breath.

BE SURE TO TELL YOUR DOCTOR about any medications you are currently taking.

WARNINGS
• Tell your doctor about unusual or allergic reactions you have had to medications, especially to codeine or to any other narcotic analgesics (such as hydrocodone, hydromorphone, meperidine, methadone, morphine, oxycodone, and propoxyphene).
• Tell your doctor if you now have or if you have ever had acute abdominal conditions, asthma, brain disease, colitis, epilepsy, gallstones or gallbladder disease, head injuries, heart disease, kidney disease, liver disease, lung disease, mental illness, emotional disorders, prostate disease, thyroid disease, or urethral stricture.
• If this drug makes you dizzy or drowsy, do not take part in any activity that requires alertness, such as driving a car or operating potentially dangerous equipment.
• Before having surgery or other medical or dental treatment, tell your doctor or dentist you are taking this drug.
• Because this product contains codeine, it has the potential for abuse and must be used with caution. Usually, it should not be taken on a regular schedule for longer than ten days (unless your doctor directs you to do so). Tolerance develops quickly; do not increase the dosage or stop taking the drug abruptly unless you first consult your doctor. If you have been taking large amounts of this medication for long periods, you may experience a withdrawal reaction (muscle aches, diarrhea, gooseflesh, runny nose, nausea, vomiting, shivering, trembling, stomach cramps, sleep disorders, irritability, weakness, excessive yawning, or sweating) when you stop taking it. Your doctor may, therefore, want to reduce the dosage gradually.
• Be sure to tell your doctor if you are pregnant. The effects of this medication during the early stages of pregnancy have not been thoroughly studied in humans. However, codeine, used regularly in large doses during the later stages of pregnancy, can result in addiction of the fetus, leading to withdrawal symptoms (irritability, excessive crying, tremors, fever, vomiting, diarrhea, sneezing, or excessive yawning) at birth. Also, tell your doctor if you are breast-feeding an infant. Small amounts of this medication may pass into breast milk and cause excessive drowsiness in the nursing infant.

codeine and guaifenesin combination

BRAND NAMES (Manufacturers)
Cheracol (Upjohn)
Guiatuss A.C. (various manufacturers)

Guiatussin with Codeine (Rugby)
Mytussin AC (PBI)
Nortussin with Codeine (Vortech)
Robitussin A-C (Robins)

TYPE OF DRUG
Cough suppressant and expectorant combination

INGREDIENT
codeine and guaifenesin

DOSAGE FORM
Oral syrup (10 mg codeine and 100 mg guaifenesin per 5-ml spoonful, with 3.5% or 4.75% alcohol)

STORAGE
Codeine and guaifenesin combination should be stored at room temperature in a tightly closed container.

USES

This medication is used to relieve coughs due to colds or infections or inflammation of the upper respiratory tract. Guaifenesin is an expectorant, which loosens bronchial secretions. Codeine is a narcotic cough suppressant, which acts on the cough center in the brain.

TREATMENT

You can take codeine and guaifenesin combination syrup either on an empty stomach or, to avoid stomach irritation, with food or milk (as directed by your doctor).

Each dose should be measured carefully with a specially designed 5-ml measuring spoon. An ordinary kitchen teaspoon is not accurate enough.

To help loosen the mucus in the bronchi, you should drink a glass of water after each dose.

If you miss a dose of this medication, take the missed one as soon as possible, unless it is almost time for the next dose. In that case, do not take the missed dose at all; just return to your regular dosing schedule. Do not double the next dose.

SIDE EFFECTS

Minor. Constipation, dizziness, drowsiness, nausea, restlessness, stomach upset, vomiting, or weakness. These side effects should disappear as your body adjusts to the medication.

If you feel dizzy, sit or lie down for a while; get up slowly from a sitting or reclining position, and be careful on stairs.

To relieve constipation, increase the amount of fiber in your diet (fresh fruits and vegetables, salads, bran, and whole-grain breads), exercise, and drink more water (unless your doctor directs you to do otherwise).
Major. Be sure to tell your doctor about any side effects that are persistent or particularly bothersome. IT IS ESPECIALLY IMPORTANT TO TELL YOUR DOCTOR about blurred vision; cold, clammy skin; confusion; difficulty in breathing; or fainting.

INTERACTIONS

Codeine and guaifenesin combination can interact with several other types of medications:
1. Concurrent use with other central nervous system depressants (such as alcohol, barbiturates, benzodiazepine tranquilizers, muscle relaxants, other narcotics, pain medications, phenothiazine tranquilizers, and sleeping medications) or with tricyclic antidepressants can lead to extreme drowsiness.
2. Use of a monoamine oxidase (MAO) inhibitor within 14 days of use of codeine and guaifenesin combination can lead to serious side effects.
3. Cimetidine combined with this medication can cause confusion, disorientation, and shortness of breath.

Before starting to take codeine and guaifenesin combination, BE SURE TO TELL YOUR DOCTOR about any medications you are currently taking.

WARNINGS

• Tell your doctor about unusual or allergic reactions you have had to any medications, especially to guaifenesin or codeine, or to other narcotics (such as hydrocodone, hydromorphone, meperidine, methadone, opium, oxycodone, propoxyphene, and pentazocine).
• Before starting to take this medication, be sure to tell your doctor if you now have or if you have ever had asthma, brain disease, enlarged prostate gland, gallstones or gallbladder disease, gastrointestinal diseases, heart disease, kidney disease, liver disease, lung disease, mental disorders, or thyroid disease.
• If this drug makes you dizzy or drowsy, do not take part in activities that require alertness, such as driving a car or operating potentially dangerous equipment. Be careful on stairs, and avoid getting up suddenly from a lying or sitting position.
• While you are taking this medication, drink several glasses of water a day to help loosen bronchial secretions, unless your doctor directs you to do otherwise.
• Because this product contains codeine, it has the potential for abuse and must be used with caution. Tolerance may develop quickly; you should not use it in higher doses or for longer periods than recommended by your doctor. If you have been taking it for longer than several weeks, do not stop taking it until you first check with your doctor. Stopping the drug abruptly can lead to a withdrawal reaction (body aches, diarrhea, gooseflesh, vomiting, restlessness, runny nose, sneezing, sweating, trembling, or excessive yawning). Your doctor may, therefore, want to reduce your dosage gradually.
• Be sure to tell your doctor if you are pregnant. Large amounts of codeine taken during pregnancy can lead to addiction in the developing fetus, resulting in withdrawal reactions in the newborn infant. Also, tell your doctor if you are breast-feeding an infant. Codeine may pass into breast milk and can cause extreme drowsiness in the nursing infant.

codeine and iodinated glycerol combination

BRAND NAMES (Manufacturers)
Iophen-C (various manufacturers)
Iotuss (Muro)
Par Glycerol C (Par)
Tussi-Organidin (Wallace)
Tussi-R-Gen (Goldline)

TYPE OF DRUG
Cough suppressant and expectorant combination
INGREDIENT
codeine and iodinated glycerol
DOSAGE FORM
Oral liquid (10 mg codeine and 30 mg iodinated glycerol per 5-ml spoonful)
STORAGE
Codeine and iodinated glycerol combination should be stored at room temperature in a tightly closed container. Avoid exposure of this medication to high temperatures.

USES
This drug is used to relieve coughs due to colds or infection or inflammation of the upper respiratory tract. Iodinated glycerol is an expectorant, which loosens bronchial secretions. Codeine is a narcotic cough suppressant, which acts on the cough center in the brain.

TREATMENT
You can take codeine and iodinated glycerol combination on an empty stomach or, to avoid stomach irritation, with food or milk (as directed by your doctor).

Each dose should be measured carefully with a specially designed 5-ml measuring spoon.

To help loosen the mucus in the bronchi, you should drink a glass of water after each dose.

If you miss a dose of this medication, take the missed one as soon as possible, unless it is almost time for the next dose. In that case, do not take the missed dose at all; just return to your regular dosing schedule. Do not double the next dose.

SIDE EFFECTS
Minor. Constipation, dizziness, drowsiness, nausea, restlessness, stomach upset, vomiting, or weakness. These side effects should disappear as your body adjusts to the medication.

If you feel dizzy, sit or lie down for a while; get up slowly from a sitting or reclining position, and be careful on stairs.

To relieve constipation, increase the amount of fiber in your diet (fresh fruits and vegetables, salads, bran, and whole-grain breads), exercise, and drink more water (unless your doctor directs you to do otherwise).
Major. Tell your doctor about any side effects that are persistent or particularly bothersome. IT IS ESPECIALLY IMPORTANT TO TELL YOUR DOCTOR about blurred vision; cold, clammy skin; confusion; difficulty in breathing; fainting; skin rash; or swollen lymph nodes.

INTERACTIONS
This drug can interact with other types of drugs:
1. Concurrent use with other central nervous system depressants (such as alcohol, barbiturates, benzodiazepine tranquilizers, muscle relaxants, other narcotics, pain medications, phenothiazine tranquilizers, and sleeping medications) or with tricyclic antidepressants can lead to extreme drowsiness.
2. Use of a monoamine oxidase (MAO) inhibitor within 14 days of use of codeine and iodinated glycerol combination can lead to serious side effects.

3. The iodine component of iodinated glycerol can increase the side effects of lithium on the thyroid gland. It can also increase the effects of antithyroid medications.
4. Cimetidine combined with this medication can cause confusion, disorientation, and shortness of breath.

BE SURE TO TELL YOUR DOCTOR about any medications you are currently taking.

WARNINGS
• Tell your doctor about unusual or allergic reactions you have had to any medications, especially to codeine, or to other narcotics (such as hydrocodone, hydromorphone, meperidine, methadone, opium, oxycodone, propoxyphene, and pentazocine), or to iodinated glycerol, iodine, or iodine-containing dyes.
• Before starting to take this medication, be sure to tell your doctor if you now have or if you have ever had acne, asthma, brain disease, cystic fibrosis, gallstones or gallbladder disease, gastrointestinal diseases, heart disease, kidney disease, liver disease, lung disease, mental disorders, enlarged prostate gland, or thyroid disease.
• If this drug makes you dizzy or drowsy, do not take part in activities that require alertness, such as driving a car or operating potentially dangerous equipment.
• While you are taking this medication, drink several glasses of water a day to help loosen bronchial secretions, unless your doctor directs you to do otherwise.
• Because this product contains codeine, it has the potential for abuse and must be used with caution. Tolerance may develop quickly; you should not use it in higher doses, or for longer periods, than recommended by your doctor. If you have been taking it for longer than several weeks, do not stop taking it until you first check with your doctor. Stopping the drug abruptly can lead to a withdrawal reaction (body aches, diarrhea, gooseflesh, vomiting, restlessness, runny nose, sneezing, sweating, trembling, or excessive yawning). Your doctor may, therefore, want to reduce your dosage gradually.
• Be sure to tell your doctor if you are pregnant. This medication should not be taken during pregnancy. Large amounts of codeine taken during pregnancy can lead to addiction in the developing fetus, resulting in withdrawal reactions in the newborn infant. Iodinated glycerol can cause goiter (an enlarged thyroid gland) in the developing fetus. Also, tell your doctor if you are breast-feeding an infant. Both codeine and iodinated glycerol can pass into the breast milk and cause side effects in the nursing infant.

Codeine Phosphate—see codeine

Codeine Sulfate—see codeine

Codimal-L.A.—see pseudoephedrine and chlorpheniramine combination

Codoxy—see aspirin and oxycodone combination

Cogentin—see benztropine

Co-Gesic—see acetaminophen and hydrocodone combination

colchicine

BRAND NAMES (Manufacturers)
colchicine (various manufacturers)
Colchicine (Abbott)
TYPE OF DRUG
Antigout
INGREDIENT
colchicine
DOSAGE FORM
Tablets (0.5 mg, 0.6 mg, and 0.65 mg)
STORAGE
Colchicine should be stored at room temperature in a tightly closed, light-resistant container.

USES

Colchicine is used to relieve the symptoms of a gout attack and to prevent further attacks. Colchicine prevents the movement of uric acid crystals, which are responsible for the pain in the joints that occurs during an attack of gout.

TREATMENT

Colchicine can be taken on an empty stomach or with food or a full glass of water or milk (as directed by your doctor).

If you are taking colchicine to control a gout attack, it is important that you understand how to take it and when it should be stopped. CHECK WITH YOUR DOCTOR.

If you miss a dose of this medication, take the missed dose as soon as possible, unless it is almost time for the next dose. In that case, do not take the missed dose at all; just return to your regular dosing schedule. Do not double the next dose.

SIDE EFFECTS

Minor. Abdominal pain, diarrhea, nausea, or vomiting. These side effects should disappear as your body adjusts to the medication.

Major. Tell your doctor about any side effects that are persistent or particularly bothersome. IT IS ESPECIALLY IMPORTANT TO TELL YOUR DOCTOR about difficult or painful urination, fever, loss of hair, muscle pain, persistent diarrhea, skin rash, sore throat, tingling in the hands or feet, or unusual bleeding or bruising.

INTERACTIONS

Colchicine interacts with several other types of medications:

1. It can decrease absorption of vitamin B.

2. The action of colchicine can be blocked by vitamin C and can be enhanced by sodium bicarbonate or ammonium chloride.

3. Colchicine can increase the drowsiness caused by central nervous system depressants.

BE SURE TO TELL YOUR DOCTOR about any medications you are currently taking.

WARNINGS

• Tell your doctor about unusual or allergic reactions you have had to any medications.

• Tell your doctor if you now have or if you have ever had blood disorders, gastrointestinal disorders, heart disease, kidney disease, or liver disease.

• Large amounts of alcohol can increase the blood levels of uric acid, which can decrease the effectiveness of colchicine. Alcohol ingestion should, therefore, be limited while you are taking this medication.

• Colchicine is not an analgesic (pain reliever) and does not relieve pain other than that of gout.

• Be sure to tell your doctor if you are pregnant. Colchicine is not recommended for use during pregnancy because it has been reported to cause birth defects in both animals and humans. Also, tell your doctor if you are breast-feeding an infant. It is not known whether colchicine passes into breast milk.

Colchicine—see colchicine

Colestid—see colestipol

colestipol

BRAND NAME (Manufacturer)
Colestid (Upjohn)
TYPE OF DRUG
Antihyperlipidemic (lipid-lowering drug)
INGREDIENT
colestipol
DOSAGE FORM
Oral granules (5 g per level 5-ml measuring spoon)
STORAGE
Colestipol should be stored at room temperature in a tightly closed container.

USES

This medication is used to lower cholesterol levels. It chemically binds to bile salts in the gastrointestinal tract and prevents the body from producing cholesterol.

TREATMENT

Colestipol is usually taken before meals. Each dose should be measured carefully with a specially designed 5-ml measuring spoon. An ordinary kitchen teaspoon is not accurate enough. The dose should then be added to at least three ounces of fluid (water, milk, fruit juice, or other carbonated or noncarbonated beverage). The mixture should be stirred and completely mixed (the granules do not completely dissolve). After the solution has been drunk, the glass should be refilled with the same beverage and this solution swallowed as well. This ensures that the whole dose is taken. The granules can also be mixed with soup, applesauce, or crushed pineapple. You should never take colestipol dry; you might accidentally inhale the granules, which could irritate your throat and lungs.

If you miss a dose of this drug, take the missed dose as soon as possible, unless it is almost time for the next dose. In that case, do not take the missed dose at all; just return to your regular dosing schedule. Do not double the next dose.

Colestipol does not cure hypercholesterolemia (high blood cholesterol levels), but it will help to control the condition as long as you continue to take it.

SIDE EFFECTS

Minor. Anxiety, belching, constipation, diarrhea, dizziness, drowsiness, fatigue, gas, headache, hiccups, loss of appetite, nausea, stomach pain, vomiting, or weight loss or gain. These side effects should disappear as your body adjusts to the medication.

To relieve constipation, increase the amount of fiber in your diet (fresh fruits and vegetables, salads, bran, and whole-grain breads), exercise, and drink more water (unless your doctor directs otherwise). A stool softener may also be helpful; ask your pharmacist to recommend one.

If you feel dizzy, sit or lie down for a while; get up slowly from a sitting or reclining position, and be careful on stairs.

Major. Tell your doctor about any side effects that are persistent or particularly bothersome. IT IS ESPECIALLY IMPORTANT TO TELL YOUR DOCTOR about backaches; bleeding gums; bloating; bloody or black, tarry stools; difficult or painful urination; muscle or joint pains; rash or irritation of the skin, tongue, or rectal area; ringing in the ears; swollen glands; tingling sensations; unusual bleeding or bruising; or unusual weakness.

INTERACTIONS

Colestipol interferes with the absorption of a number of other drugs, including phenylbutazone, warfarin, thiazide diuretics (water pills), digoxin, penicillins, tetracycline, phenobarbital, folic acid, iron, thyroid hormones, oral vancomycin, adrenocorticosteroids, and the fat-soluble vitamins (vitamins A, D, E, and K). The effectiveness of these medications will be decreased by colestipol. To avoid this interaction, take the other medications one hour before or four to six hours after a dose of colestipol.

BE SURE TO TELL YOUR DOCTOR about any medications you are currently taking, especially any of those listed above.

WARNINGS

• Tell your doctor if you have ever had unusual or allergic reactions to any type of drug, especially to colestipol.
• Before starting to take this drug, be sure to tell your doctor if you now have or if you have ever had bleeding disorders, biliary obstruction, heart disease, hemorrhoids, gallstones or gallbladder disease, kidney disease, malabsorptive disorders, stomach ulcers, or an obstructed intestine.
• Colestipol should be used only in conjunction with a carefully regulated diet, weight reduction, or correction of other conditions that could be causing high blood cholesterol levels.
• Be sure to tell your doctor if you are pregnant. Although colestipol appears to be safe (because none is absorbed into the bloodstream), extensive studies in humans during pregnancy have not been conducted. Also, be sure to tell your doctor if you are breast-feeding an infant. This medication can decrease absorption of some vitamins in the mother, which could result in decreased availability of the vitamins to the nursing infant.

Compazine—see prochlorperazine

Compazine Spansules—see prochlorperazine

Compoz—see diphenhydramine

Condrin-LA—see phenylpropanolamine and chlorpheniramine combination

Conex D.A.—see phenylpropanolamine and chlorpheniramine combination

conjugated estrogens—see estrogens, conjugated

Constant-T—see theophylline

Contac 12-Hour—see phenylpropanolamine and chlorpheniramine combination

Coracin—see hydrocortisone, polymyxin B, neomycin, and bacitracin combination (ophthalmic)

Cordran—see flurandrenolide (topical)

Cordran SP—see flurandrenolide (topical)

Corgard—see nadolol

Corque—see hydrocortisone and iodochlorhydroxyquin combination (topical)

Cortaid—see hydrocortisone (topical)

Cortatrigen Modified Ear Drops—see hydrocortisone, polymyxin B, and neomycin combination (otic)

Cort-Dome—see hydrocortisone (topical)

Cortef—see hydrocortisone (systemic)

Cortef Feminine Itch—see hydrocortisone (topical)

Cortin—see hydrocortisone and iodochlorhydroxyquin combination (topical)

Cortisporin Ophthalmic—see hydrocortisone, polymyxin B, neomycin, and bacitracin combination (ophthalmic)

Cortisporin Otic—see hydrocortisone, polymyxin B, and neomycin combination (otic)

cortisone acetate—see cortisone (topical)

cortisone (systemic)

BRAND NAMES (Manufacturers)
cortisone acetate (various manufacturers)
Cortone Acetate (Merck Sharp & Dohme)
TYPE OF DRUG
Adrenocorticosteroid hormone

INGREDIENT
cortisone
DOSAGE FORM
Tablets (5 mg, 10 mg, and 25 mg)
STORAGE
Cortisone tablets should be stored at room temperature in a tightly closed container.

USES
Your adrenal glands naturally produce certain cortisone-like chemicals. These chemicals are involved in various regulatory processes in the body (such as those involving fluid balance, temperature, and reaction to inflammation). Cortisone belongs to a group of drugs known as adrenocorticosteroids (or cortisone-like medications). It is used to treat a variety of disorders, including hormonal disorders; asthma; blood diseases; certain cancers; eye disorders; gastrointestinal disturbances, such as ulcerative colitis; respiratory diseases; and inflammations such as arthritis, dermatitis, and poison ivy. How this drug acts to relieve these disorders is not completely understood.

TREATMENT
In order to prevent stomach irritation, you can take cortisone with food or with milk.

If you are taking only one dose of this medication each day, try to take it before 9:00 A.M.

It is important to try not to miss any doses of cortisone. However, if you do miss a dose of this medication, follow these guidelines:

1. If you are taking it more than once a day, take the missed dose as soon as possible and return to your regular schedule. If it is already time for the next dose, double the dose.

2. If you are taking this medication once a day, take the dose you missed as soon as possible, unless you don't remember until the next day. In that case, do not take the missed dose at all; just follow your regular dosing schedule. Do not double the next dose.

3. If you are taking this drug every other day, take it as soon as you remember. If you missed the scheduled time by a whole day, take it when you remember, then skip a day before you take the next dose. Do not double the dose.

If you miss more than one dose of cortisone, CONTACT YOUR DOCTOR.

SIDE EFFECTS
Minor. Dizziness, false sense of well-being, fatigue, increased appetite, increased sweating, indigestion, menstrual irregularities, muscle weakness, nausea, reddening of the skin on the face, restlessness, sleep disorders, thinning of the skin, or weight gain. These side effects should disappear as your body adjusts to the medication.

To help avoid potassium loss while using this drug, you can take your dose with a glass of fresh or frozen orange juice, or eat a banana each day. The use of a salt substitute also helps to prevent potassium loss. Do not change your diet or take a salt substitute, however, before discussing it with your doctor.

Major. Tell your doctor about any side effects that are persistent or particularly bothersome. IT IS ESPECIALLY

IMPORTANT TO TELL YOUR DOCTOR about abdominal enlargement; acne or other skin problems; back or rib pain; bloody or black, tarry stools; blurred vision; convulsions; depression; eye pain; fever; glaucoma; growth impairment (in children); headaches; impaired healing of wounds; increased thirst and urination; mood changes; muscle wasting; nightmares; rapid weight gain (three to five pounds within a week); rash; severe abdominal pain; shortness of breath; sore throat; unusual bleeding or bruising; or unusual weakness.

INTERACTIONS
Cortisone interacts with several other types of medications:

1. Alcohol, aspirin, and anti-inflammatory medications (such as diflunisal, ibuprofen, indomethacin, ketoprofen, mefenamic acid, meclofenamate, naproxen, piroxicam, sulindac, and tolmetin) aggravate the stomach problems that may occur with use of this medication.

2. The dosage of oral anticoagulants (blood thinners, such as warfarin) and oral antidiabetic drugs or insulin may need to be altered when this medication is started or stopped.

3. The loss of potassium caused by cortisone can lead to serious side effects in individuals taking digoxin. Thiazide diuretics (water pills) and furosemide can increase the potassium loss caused by cortisone.

4. Phenobarbital, phenytoin, rifampin, and ephedrine can increase the elimination of cortisone from the body, thereby decreasing its effectiveness.

5. Oral contraceptives (birth control pills) and estrogen-containing drugs may decrease the elimination of this drug from the body, which can lead to an increase in side effects.

6. Cortisone can increase elimination of aspirin and isoniazid from the body, decreasing their effectiveness.

7. Cholestyramine and colestipol can chemically bind this medication in the stomach and gastrointestinal tract, preventing its absorption.

BE SURE TO TELL YOUR DOCTOR about any medications you are currently taking, especially any listed above.

WARNINGS
Tell your doctor about unusual or allergic reactions you have had to any medications, especially to cortisone or other adrenocorticosteroids (such as betamethasone, dexamethasone, hydrocortisone, methylprednisolone, paramethasone, prednisolone, prednisone, or triamcinolone).

Tell your doctor if you now have or if you have ever had bone disease, diabetes mellitus, emotional instability, glaucoma, fungal infections, heart disease, high blood pressure, high cholesterol levels, myasthenia gravis, peptic ulcers, osteoporosis, thyroid disease, tuberculosis, ulcerative colitis, kidney disease, or liver disease.

If you are using this medication for longer than a week, you may need to receive higher dosages if you are subjected to stress, such as serious infections, injury, or surgery. Discuss this with your doctor.

If you have been taking this drug for more than a week, do not stop taking it suddenly. If it is stopped suddenly, you may experience abdominal or back pain, dizziness,extreme weakness, fainting, fever, muscle or joint pain, nausea, vomiting, or shortness of breath. Your doctor may, therefore, want to reduce the dosage gradually. Never increase the dose or take the drug for longer than the prescribed time unless you first consult your doctor.

While you are taking this drug, you should not be vaccinated or immunized. This medication decreases the effectiveness of vaccines and can lead to infection if a live-virus vaccine is administered.

Before having surgery or any other medical or dental treatment, be sure to tell your doctor or dentist that you are taking this medication.

If you are taking this medication for prolonged periods of time, you should wear or carry an identification card or notice indicating that you are taking an adrenocorticosteroid drug.

Because this drug can cause glaucoma and cataracts with long-term use, your doctor may want you to have your eyes examined by an ophthalmologist periodically during treatment.

This medication can raise blood sugar levels in diabetic patients. Blood sugar should, therefore, be monitored carefully with blood or urine tests when this medication is being taken.

Be sure to tell your doctor if you are pregnant. This drug crosses the placenta. Although studies in humans have not been conducted, birth defects have been observed in the offspring of animals that were given large doses of this type of drug during pregnancy. Also, tell your doctor if you are breast-feeding an infant. Small amounts of this drug pass into breast milk and can cause growth suppression or a decrease in natural adrenocorticosteroid production in the nursing infant.

Cortizone-5—see hydrocortisone (topical)

Cortone Acetate—see cortisone (systemic)

Cortril—see hydrocortisone (topical)

Cotazym-S—see pancrelipase

Cotrim—see sulfamethoxazole and trimethoprim combination

Cotrim DS—see sulfamethoxazole and trimethoprim combination

Cotrim Pediatric—see sulfamethoxazole and trimethoprim combination

Coumadin—see warfarin

cromolyn sodium (inhalation)

BRAND NAME (Manufacturer)
Intal (Fisons)
TYPE OF DRUG
Antiallergic (antiasthmatic)
INGREDIENT
cromolyn

DOSAGE FORMS
Capsules (20 mg): for inhalation only
Solution (20 mg per 2-ml ampule): for inhalation only
Aerosol spray 8.1 g and 14. 2 g (800 mcg per spray): for inhalation only
STORAGE
Cromolyn sodium capsules and solution should be kept at room temperature in tightly closed, light-resistant storage containers. The container of the aerosol form is pressurized; it should, therefore, never be punctured or broken. It should also be stored away from heat and direct sunlight.

USES
This medication is used to prevent asthma attacks. It is not effective in relieving asthma symptoms once an attack has begun. It works by preventing release of the body chemicals that are thought to be responsible for the symptoms of asthma or allergy.

TREATMENT
Cromolyn sodium capsules are for inhalation only—they should NOT be swallowed. The medication is not effective if swallowed. This medication comes packaged with instructions for use of the capsules with the Spinhaler device. It is very important that you completely understand how to use this device. Consult your doctor or pharmacist if you have any questions about administering this medication.

The Spinhaler should be cleaned at least once a week. Take the Spinhaler apart and rinse it in clear, warm water. Do not use soap. Allow the inhaler to air-dry before you use it again. If properly cared for, the inhaler should last about six months.

The solution form of this medication should be used only with a power-operated nebulizer equipped with a face mask. The solution form should never be used with a hand-held nebulizer.

The aerosol form of this medication comes packaged with instructions for use. Read the instructions carefully; if you have any questions, check with your doctor or pharmacist. The aerosol can should be shaken well just before each dose is sprayed. The contents tend to settle on the bottom of the container, so it should be shaken to disperse the medication and equalize the doses. The 14.2 g container provides about 200 measured sprays, and the 8.1 g container provides about 112 measured sprays.

Cromolyn sodium is most effective when therapy is started before contact with allergens (the suspected offending agents causing your allergy), so if you expect to be exposed to something to which you know you are allergic, it is a good idea to start taking your medication first.

This medication will work most effectively when the level of medicine in your bloodstream is kept constant. It is best, therefore, that you try to take the doses at evenly spaced intervals throughout the day and night. For example, if you are to take four doses of this medication a day, the doses should be evenly spaced at six hour intervals.

If you are using another inhaler to open up the lungs (a bronchodilator), it should be used 20 to 30 minutes before using cromolyn sodium.

The full benefits of this medication may not become apparent for up to four weeks after you start to take it.

If you miss a dose of this medication and remember within an hour or so, take the missed dose immediately. If more than an hour has passed, however, do not take the missed dose at all; just return to your regular dosing schedule. Do not double the next dose of this medication.

SIDE EFFECTS

Minor. Cough, dizziness, drowsiness, headache, increased urination, nasal congestion, nasal itching, nausea, sneezing, stomach irritation, or tearing. These side effects should disappear as your body adjusts to the medication.

If you feel dizzy, sit or lie down for a while; get up slowly from a sitting or reclining position, and be careful on stairs.

This medication can cause mouth dryness, throat irritation, and hoarseness. Gargling and rinsing your mouth after each dose helps to prevent these effects.

Major. Tell your doctor about any side effects that are persistent or particularly bothersome. IT IS ESPECIALLY IMPORTANT TO TELL YOUR DOCTOR about itching, joint swelling or pain, nosebleeds, nose burning, painful or increased urination, rash, swelling of the face or eyes, swollen glands, or wheezing.

INTERACTIONS

Cromolyn sodium should not interact with other medications if it is used according to directions.

WARNINGS

• Tell your doctor about unusual or allergic reactions you have had to any drugs.
• Patients who are allergic to lactose, milk, or milk products may be allergic to the capsule form of this drug.
• Before starting to take this medication, tell your doctor if you now have or if you have ever had kidney or liver disease.
• Do not stop taking this medication unless you first check with your doctor. Stopping the drug abruptly may lead to a worsening of your condition.
• Be sure to tell your doctor if you are pregnant. Extensive safety studies in humans have not been conducted. Also, tell your doctor if you are breast-feeding an infant. It is not known whether this drug passes into breast milk.

cromolyn sodium (nasal)

BRAND NAME (Manufacturer)
Nasalcrom (Fisons)
TYPE OF DRUG
Antiallergic
INGREDIENT
cromolyn
DOSAGE FORM
Nasal solution (each spray delivers 5.2 mg)
STORAGE
Cromolyn sodium should be stored at room temperature in its original container.

USES

Cromolyn sodium nasal solution is used to prevent and treat allergic rhinitis (inflammation of the nasal passages resulting from allergies). Cromolyn sodium works by preventing the release of the body chemicals responsible for inflammation and swelling.

TREATMENT

This medication is for use within the nose only. The nasal passages should be cleared before administering the spray. You should inhale through the nose as you spray the solution. The container provides about 100 measured sprays.

This medication is most effective when therapy is started before contact with allergens (the suspected offending agents causing your allergy), so if you expect to be exposed to something to which you know you are allergic, it is a good idea to start taking your medication first.

This medication works best when the level of medicine in your bloodstream is kept constant. It is best, therefore, to take the doses at evenly spaced intervals day and night. For example, if you are to take four doses a day, the doses should be spaced six hours apart.

The maximum benefits of this medication may not become fully apparent for up to four weeks after you have started therapy.

If you miss a dose of this drug, take the missed dose as soon as possible, unless it is almost time for the next dose. In that case, do not take the missed dose at all; just return to your regular dosing schedule. Do not double the next dose.

SIDE EFFECTS

Minor. Bad taste in the mouth, headaches, irritation or stinging, nasal burning, postnasal drip, or sneezing. These side effects should stop as your body adjusts to the drug.
Major. Tell your doctor about any side effects that are persistent or particularly bothersome. IT IS ESPECIALLY IMPORTANT TO TELL YOUR DOCTOR about nosebleeds or skin rash.

INTERACTIONS

Cromolyn sodium should not interact with other medications if it is used according to directions.

WARNINGS

• Tell your doctor about unusual or allergic reactions you have had to any medication, especially to cromolyn sodium.
• Be sure to tell your doctor if you now have or if you have ever had kidney or liver disease.
• Do not stop taking this medication unless you first check with your doctor, even if the symptoms of your disorder disappear. Stopping the drug abruptly can lead to a worsening of your condition. Cromolyn sodium should be continued as long as you have contact with the substance causing your allergic symptoms.
• Be sure to tell your doctor if you are pregnant. Extensive safety studies in humans have not been conducted. Also, tell your doctor if you are breast-feeding an infant. It is not known whether cromolyn sodium passes into breast milk.

Cuprimine—see penicillamine

Curretab—see medroxyprogesterone

Cyclan—see cyclandelate

---

cyclandelate

BRAND NAMES (Manufacturers)
Cyclan (Major)
cyclandelate (various manufacturers)
Cyclospasmol (Wyeth)
TYPE OF DRUG
Vasodilator
INGREDIENT
cyclandelate
DOSAGE FORMS
Tablets (200 mg and 400 mg)
Capsules (200 mg and 400 mg)
STORAGE
Cyclandelate should be stored at room temperature in a tightly closed container.

USES

Cyclandelate is used to treat vascular (blood vessel) disease in the legs or brain. It acts directly on the muscle tissue of the blood vessels to increase the blood supply to various parts of the body.

TREATMENT

You can take cyclandelate on an empty stomach (unless your doctor gives you different instructions). However, if the drug causes stomach irritation, you may take it with food, milk, or antacids.

If you miss a dose of this medication, take the missed dose as soon as possible, unless it is almost time for the next dose. In that case, do not take the missed dose at all; just return to your regular dosing schedule. Do not double the next dose of this medication.

SIDE EFFECTS

Minor. Dizziness, drowsiness, flushing, headache, heartburn, stomach distress, or sweating. These side effects should disappear as your body adjusts to the medication.

If you feel dizzy, sit or lie down for a while; get up slowly from a sitting or reclining position, and be careful on stairs.
Major. Tell your doctor about any side effects that are persistent or particularly bothersome. IT IS ESPECIALLY IMPORTANT TO TELL YOUR DOCTOR about palpitations, skin rash, tingling in the hands or feet, or weakness.

INTERACTIONS

Cyclandelate does not interact with other medications if it is used according to directions.

WARNINGS

Tell your doctor about unusual or allergic reactions you have had to any medications, especially to cyclandelate.

Before starting to take this medication, tell your doctor if you have ever had angina, bleeding disorders, glaucoma, or a heart attack.

A government panel has recently reviewed the effectiveness of this medication in the treatment of leg cramps and hardening of the arteries and in the prevention of stroke. This drug may not be as effective as was once thought. Discuss this with your doctor.

Before taking any over-the-counter (nonprescription) cough, cold, allergy, asthma, sinus, or diet medication, check with your doctor or pharmacist. Some of these products can decrease the effectiveness of cyclandelate.

If this drug makes you dizzy or drowsy, do not take part in any activity that requires alertness, such as driving a car or operating potentially dangerous equipment.

The beneficial effects of this medication may be decreased by the nicotine in cigarettes. Try to stop smoking.

To prevent dizziness and fainting while taking this medication, avoid getting overheated by exercising strenuously in hot weather or by taking hot baths, showers, and saunas.

Be sure to tell your doctor if you are pregnant. Although cyclandelate appears to be safe during pregnancy, extensive studies in humans have not been conducted, and cautious use is warranted. Also, tell your doctor if you are breast-feeding an infant. It is not known whether cyclandelate passes into breast milk.

---

cyclobenzaprine

BRAND NAMES (Manufacturers)
cyclobenzaprine (various manufacturers)
Flexeril (Merck Sharp & Dohme)
TYPE OF DRUG
Muscle relaxant
INGREDIENT
cyclobenzaprine
DOSAGE FORM
Tablets (10 mg)
STORAGE
Cyclobenzaprine tablets should be stored at room temperature in a tightly closed container.

USES

Cyclobenzaprine is prescribed to relieve muscle pain and stiffness caused by injuries such as sprains or strains. It is not clear how this drug works, but it may block reflexes involved in producing and maintaining muscle spasms. It does not act directly on tense muscles.

TREATMENT

In order to avoid stomach irritation, you can take cyclobenzaprine with food or with a full glass of water or milk.

If you miss a dose of this medication and remember within an hour, take the missed dose; then return to your regular dosing schedule. If more than an hour has passed, do not take the missed dose at all; just return to your dosing schedule. Do not double the next dose.

SIDE EFFECTS
Minor. Abdominal pain, black tongue, blurred vision, constipation, diarrhea, dizziness, drowsiness, dry mouth, fatigue, indigestion, insomnia, loss of appetite, muscle pain, nausea, nervousness, sweating, unpleasant taste in the mouth, vomiting, or weakness. These side effects should disappear as your body adjusts to the medication.

If you are constipated, increase the amount of fiber in your diet (fresh fruits and vegetables, salads, bran, and whole-grain breads) and drink more water (unless your doctor directs you to do otherwise).

If you feel dizzy or light-headed, sit or lie down for a while; get up slowly from a sitting or reclining position, and be careful on stairs.

To relieve mouth dryness, chew sugarless gum, or suck on ice chips or hard candy.

Major. Tell your doctor about any side effects that are persistent or particularly bothersome. IT IS ESPECIALLY IMPORTANT TO TELL YOUR DOCTOR about confusion, depression, difficulty in urinating, disorientation, hallucinations, headache, itching, numbness in the fingers or toes, palpitations, rash, swelling of the face or tongue, tremors, or yellowing of your skin or eyes.

INTERACTIONS
Cyclobenzaprine interacts with several other types of drugs:

1. Concurrent use of cyclobenzaprine with other central nervous system depressants (such as alcohol, antihistamines, barbiturates, antianxiety medications, narcotics, pain medications, tranquilizers, and sleeping medications) or with tricyclic antidepressants can cause extreme drowsiness.

2. Cyclobenzaprine can block the blood-pressure-lowering effects of clonidine and guanethidine.

3. Use of this drug within 14 days of a monoamine oxidase (MAO) inhibitor (tranylcypromine, phenelzine, isocarboxazid, and pargyline) can lead to severe reactions and high blood pressure.

BE SURE TO TELL YOUR DOCTOR about any medications you are currently taking, especially those listed above.

WARNINGS
• Tell your doctor about unusual or allergic reactions you have had to medications, especially to cyclobenzaprine or to tricyclic antidepressants (such as amitriptyline, amoxapine, desipramine, doxepin, imipramine, nortriptyline, protriptyline, and trimipramine).

• Tell your doctor if you have ever had blood clots, epilepsy, heart disease, a heart attack, narrow-angle glaucoma, thyroid disease, or urinary retention.

• Use of cyclobenzaprine for periods longer than two to three weeks is not recommended because there is no evidence of benefit with prolonged use and because muscle spasm caused by sprain or strain is generally of short duration.

• This medication should not be taken as a substitute for rest, physical therapy, or other measures recommended by your doctor to treat your condition.

• If this medication makes you dizzy or drowsy or blurs your vision, do not take part in any activity that requires alertness, such as driving a car or operating potentially dangerous equipment.

• If you have been taking large doses of this medication for prolonged periods, you may experience nausea, headache, or fatigue when you stop taking it, until your body adjusts to the absence of the drug.

• Be sure to tell your doctor if you are pregnant. Although cyclobenzaprine appears to be safe during pregnancy, extensive studies in humans have not been conducted. Also, tell your doctor if you are breast-feeding an infant. It is not known whether cyclobenzaprine passes into breast milk.

cyclophosphamide

BRAND NAME (Manufacturer)
Cytoxan (Bristol Myers USP)
TYPE OF DRUG
Antineoplastic (anticancer drug)
INGREDIENT
cyclophosphamide
DOSAGE FORM
Tablets (25 mg and 50 mg)
STORAGE
Cyclophosphamide should be stored at room temperature in a tightly closed container.

USES
Cyclophosphamide belongs to a group of drugs known as alkylating agents or nitrogen mustards. It is used to treat a variety of cancers. Cyclophosphamide works by binding to the rapidly growing cancer cells, preventing their multiplication and growth. Cyclophosphamide has also been used as an immunosuppressant in order to treat severe rheumatoid arthritis.

TREATMENT
In order to obtain maximum benefit, you should take cyclophosphamide on an empty stomach. However, if stomach upset occurs, you can take it with food or milk (unless your doctor directs you to do otherwise).

The timing of the doses of this anticancer medication is important. Be sure you completely understand your doctor's instructions on how and when this medication should be taken. Try not to miss any doses.

If you miss a dose of this medication, do not take the missed dose at all; just return to your regular dosing schedule. Do not double the next dose.

SIDE EFFECTS
Minor. Diarrhea, loss of appetite, nausea, or vomiting. These side effects may disappear as your body adjusts to the medication. However, it is important to continue taking this medication despite the nausea and vomiting that may occur. Cyclophosphamide also causes hair loss, which is reversible when the medication is stopped.

Major. Tell your doctor about any side effects that are persistent or particularly bothersome. IT IS ESPECIALLY IMPORTANT TO TELL YOUR DOCTOR about blood in the urine, chills, cough, darkening of the skin or fingernails, difficult or painful urination, fever, menstrual irregularities, mouth sores, sore throat, unusual bleeding or bruising, or yellowing of the eyes or skin.

INTERACTIONS
This drug interacts with several other types of drugs:
1. It can decrease the absorption of digoxin from the gastrointestinal tract.
2. Phenobarbital can increase the side effects of cyclophosphamide.
3. Concurrent use of allopurinol, chloramphenicol, chlorpromazine, or thiazide diuretics (water pills) with cyclophosphamide can lead to bone marrow suppression.
4. It can increase the effect of warfarin (blood thinner).

Before starting to take this medication, BE SURE TO TELL YOUR DOCTOR about any medications you are currently taking, especially any of those listed above.

WARNINGS
• Tell your doctor about unusual or allergic reactions you have had to any medications, especially to cyclophosphamide.
• Before starting to take this medication, be sure to tell your doctor if you have ever had blood disorders, chronic or recurrent infections, gout, kidney disease, or liver disease.
• Before having surgery or any other medical or dental treatment, tell your doctor or dentist you are taking this drug.
• Cyclophosphamide tablets contain the color additive FD&C Yellow No. 5 (tartrazine), which can cause allergic-type reactions (fainting, shortness of breath, rash) in certain susceptible individuals.
• You should not receive any immunizations or vaccinations while taking this medication. Cyclophosphamide decreases the effectiveness of the vaccine and may result in an infection if a live-virus vaccine is administered.
• It is important to drink plenty of fluids (three quarts each day) while taking this medication. If the drug is allowed to concentrate in the bladder, it can cause bloody urine and can damage the kidneys or bladder.
• This medication can lower your platelet count, which can decrease your body's ability to form blood clots. You should, therefore, be especially careful while brushing your teeth, flossing, or using toothpicks, razors, or fingernail scissors. Try to avoid falls and other injuries.
• This drug can decrease fertility in both men and women.
• Be sure to tell your doctor if you are pregnant. Birth defects have been reported in both animals and humans whose mothers received cyclophosphamide during pregnancy. The risks should be discussed with your doctor. Also, tell your doctor if you are breast-feeding an infant. Since the drug passes into breast milk, a woman should stop breast-feeding before starting cyclophosphamide therapy.

Women of childbearing potential who are not already pregnant when treatment with cyclophosphamide is begun need to use some sort of birth control to prevent pregnancy from occurring. However, oral contraceptives (birth control pills) may not be recommended by your doctor since they may interfere with this medication. Consult with your physician about alternative methods of birth control.

Cyclospasmol—see cyclandetate

cyclosporine

BRAND NAME (Manufacturer)
Sandimmune (Sandoz)
TYPE OF DRUG
Immunosuppressant
INGREDIENT
cyclosporine
DOSAGE FORMS
Oral solution (100 mg per ml, with 12.5% alcohol)
Soft gelatin capsules (25 mg and 100 mg)
STORAGE
Cyclosporine oral solution and capsules should be stored in the original container at room temperature. This medication should never be refrigerated or frozen. Once the solution has been opened, it should be used within two months.

USES
Cyclosporine is used to prevent organ rejection after kidney, liver, and heart transplants. It is not clearly understood how cyclosporine works, but it appears to prevent the body's rejection of foreign tissue.

TREATMENT
To make it more palatable, the solution should be diluted with milk, chocolate milk, or orange juice (preferably at room temperature). The dose should be measured carefully with the dropper provided and placed in one of the fluids listed above. Use a glass container (cyclosporine chemically binds to wax-lined and plastic surfaces). Stir well and drink at once—do not allow the mixture to stand before drinking. Refill the glass with the same beverage and drink this solution to ensure that the whole dose is taken. The dropper should be wiped with a clean towel after use and stored in its container. If the dropper has been cleaned, make sure it is completely dry before using it again.

It is important not to miss any doses of this medication. If you do miss a dose, take the missed dose as soon as possible, unless it is almost time for the next dose. In that case, do not take the missed dose at all; just return to your regular dosing schedule. Do not double the next dose.

SIDE EFFECTS
Minor. Abdominal discomfort, diarrhea, flushing, headache, hiccups, leg cramps, loss of appetite, nausea, or vomiting. These side effects should disappear as your body adjusts to the medication.
Major. Tell your doctor about any side effects that are persistent or particularly bothersome. IT IS ESPECIALLY IMPORTANT TO TELL YOUR DOCTOR about acne; bleeding, tender, or enlarged gums; convulsions; difficult or painful urination; enlarged and painful breasts (in

both sexes); fever; hair growth; hearing loss; muscle pain; rapid weight gain (three to five pounds within a week); sore throat; tingling of the hands or feet; tremors; unusual bleeding or bruising; or yellowing of the eyes or skin.

INTERACTIONS
Cyclosporine interacts with several other types of drugs:
1. Carbamazepine, isoniazid, rifampin, phenytoin, phenobarbital, and trimethoprim/sulfamethoxazole can decrease the blood levels of cyclosporine, decreasing its effectiveness.
2. Cimetidine, diltiazem, erythromycin, ketoconazole, oral contraceptives, danazol, and amphotericin B can increase the blood levels of cyclosporine, which can lead to an increase in side effects.
3. Tell your doctor if you are currently taking corticosteroids, verapamil, or nonsteroidal anti-inflammatory drugs.

BE SURE TO TELL YOUR DOCTOR about any medications you are currently taking.

WARNINGS
• Tell your doctor about unusual or allergic reactions you have had to any medications, especially to cyclosporine or to polyoxyethylated castor oil.
• Before starting to take this medication, be sure to tell your doctor if you now have or if you have ever had hypertension (high blood pressure) or gastrointestinal disorders.
• Repeated laboratory tests are necessary while you are taking cyclosporine to ensure that you are receiving the correct dosage and to avoid liver and kidney damage.
• Certain cancers have occurred in patients receiving cyclosporine and other immunosuppressant drugs after transplantation. No causal effect has been established, however.
• Do not stop taking this medication without first consulting your doctor. If the drug is stopped abruptly, organ rejection may occur. Your doctor may, therefore, want to reduce your dosage gradually or start you on another drug if treatment with this drug is to be discontinued.
• Be sure to tell your doctor if you are pregnant. Although extensive studies in humans have not been conducted, cyclosporine has caused fetal damage when administered to animals. Also, tell your doctor if you are breast-feeding, because cyclosporine passes into breast milk.

Cycrin—see medroxyprogesterone

Cylert—see pemoline

cyproheptadine

BRAND NAMES (Manufacturers)
cyproheptadine hydrochloride (various manufacturers)
Periactin (Merck Sharp & Dohme)
TYPE OF DRUG
Antihistamine
INGREDIENT
cyproheptadine

DOSAGE FORMS
Tablets (4 mg)
Oral syrup (2 mg per 5-ml spoonful, with 5% alcohol)
STORAGE
Store at room temperature in a tightly closed container. Freezing of the oral syrup should be avoided.

USES
This medication belongs to a group of drugs known as antihistamines (antihistamines block the action of histamine, a chemical that is released by the body during an allergic reaction). It is used to treat or prevent symptoms of allergy.

TREATMENT
To avoid stomach upset, you can take cyproheptadine with food or with a full glass of milk or water (unless your doctor directs you to do otherwise).

The oral syrup should be measured carefully with a specially designed 5-ml measuring spoon. An ordinary kitchen teaspoon is not accurate enough.

If you miss a dose of this medication, take the missed dose as soon as possible, unless it is almost time for your next dose. If it is almost time for the next dose, do not take the missed dose at all; just return to your regular dosing schedule. Do not double the next dose.

SIDE EFFECTS
Minor. Blurred vision; confusion; constipation; diarrhea; difficult or painful urination; dizziness; dry mouth, throat, or nose; headache; increased or decreased appetite; irritability; nausea; restlessness; ringing or buzzing in the ears; stomach upset; or unusual increase in sweating. These side effects should disappear as your body adjusts to the medication.

This medication can cause increased sensitivity to sunlight. It is, therefore, important to avoid prolonged exposure to sunlight and sunlamps. Wear protective clothing and use an effective sunscreen.

If you are constipated, increase the amount of fiber in your diet (fresh fruits and vegetables, salads, bran, and whole-grain breads), exercise, and drink more water (unless your doctor directs you not to do so).

Chew sugarless gum or suck on ice chips or a piece of hard candy to reduce mouth dryness.

If you feel dizzy or light-headed, sit or lie down for a while; get up from a sitting or lying position slowly, and be careful on stairs.
Major. Tell your doctor about any side effects that are persistent or particularly bothersome. IT IS ESPECIALLY IMPORTANT TO TELL YOUR DOCTOR about change in menstruation, clumsiness, feeling faint, flushing of the face, hallucinations, palpitations, rash, seizures, shortness of breath, sleeping disorders, sore throat or fever, tightness in the chest, unusual bleeding or bruising, unusual tiredness or weakness, or yellowing of the eyes or skin.

INTERACTIONS
This drug interacts with several other types of drugs:
1. Concurrent use of this medication with other central nervous system depressants (such as alcohol, barbitu-

rates, benzodiazepine tranquilizers, muscle relaxants, narcotics, pain medications, and phenothiazine tranquilizers) or with tricyclic antidepressants can cause extreme drowsiness.

2. Monoamine oxidase (MAO) inhibitors (such as isocarboxazid, pargyline, phenelzine, and tranylcypromine) can increase the side effects of this medication.

BE SURE TO TELL YOUR DOCTOR about any medications you are currently taking.

WARNINGS

• Tell your doctor about unusual or allergic reactions you have had to any medications, especially to cyproheptadine or to other antihistamines (such as azatadine, astemizole, brompheniramine, carbinoxamine, chlorpheniramine, clemastine, cyproheptadine, dimenhydrinate, dimethindene, diphenhydramine, diphenylpyraline, doxylamine, hydroxyzine, phenidamine, promethazine, pyrilamine, terfenadine, trimeprazine, tripelennamine, and triprolidine).

• Tell your doctor if you now have or if you have ever had asthma, blood vessel disease, glaucoma, high blood pressure, kidney disease, peptic ulcers, enlarged prostate gland, or thyroid disease.

• Cyproheptadine can cause drowsiness or dizziness. Your ability to perform tasks that require alertness, such as driv-ing or operating potentially dangerous equipment, may be decreased.

• Be sure to tell your doctor if you are pregnant. The effects of this medication during pregnancy have not been thoroughly studied in humans. Also, tell your doctor if you are breast-feeding an infant. Small amounts of cyproheptadine pass into breast milk. The drug may also inhibit lactation.

cyproheptadine hydrochloride—see cyproheptadine

Cyronine—see liothyronine

Cytomel—see liothyronine

Cytotec—see misoprostal

Cytoxan—see cyclophosphamide

Dallergy-D—see pseudoephedrine and chlorpheniramine combination

Dalmane—see flurazepam

Damacet-P—see acetaminophen and hydrocodone combination

D-Amp—see ampicillin

Dantrium—see dantrolene

dantrolene

BRAND NAME (Manufacturer)
Dantrium (Norwich-Eaton)

TYPE OF DRUG
Muscle relaxant
INGREDIENT
dantrolene
DOSAGE FORM
Capsules (25 mg, 50 mg, and 100 mg)
STORAGE
Dantrolene should be stored at room temperature in a tightly closed container.

USES
This medication is used to relieve the spasticity caused by spinal cord injury, stroke, cerebral palsy, or multiple sclerosis. It works directly on muscles to prevent contraction. Dantrolene is also used prior to anesthesia to prevent malignant hyperthermia in patients known or suspected to be at risk for developing this complication.

TREATMENT
You can take dantrolene either on an empty stomach or with food or milk (as directed by your doctor). You can mix the contents of the capsule with fruit juice or another nonalcoholic beverage. Stir gently to mix the powder with the liquid and then take the dose immediately. Rinse the glass with a little more liquid and drink that as well.

If you miss a dose and remember within an hour, take the missed dose immediately. If more than an hour has passed, do not take the missed dose; just return to your regular dosing schedule. Do not double the next dose.

SIDE EFFECTS
Minor. Abnormal hair growth, alteration of taste, constipation, diarrhea, dizziness, drowsiness, excessive tearing, fatigue, headache, insomnia, loss of appetite, or stomach upset. These side effects should disappear as your body adjusts to the medication.

This medication can increase your sensitivity to sunlight. Avoid prolonged exposure to sunlight and sunlamps. Wear protective clothing and use an effective sunscreen.

To relieve constipation, increase the amount of fiber in your diet (fresh fruits and vegetables, salads, bran, and whole-grain breads), exercise, and drink more water (unless your doctor directs you to do otherwise).

If you feel dizzy, sit or lie down for a while; get up slowly from a sitting or reclining position, and be careful on stairs.

Major. Tell your doctor about any side effects that are persistent or particularly bothersome. IT IS ESPECIALLY IMPORTANT TO TELL YOUR DOCTOR about backaches; bloody or black, tarry stools; blurred vision; chills; confusion; convulsions; depression; difficult or painful urination; difficulty in breathing; difficulty in swallowing; feeling of suffocation; fever; increased urination; muscle pain; nervousness; palpitations; skin rash; speech disturbances; unusual weakness; or yellowing of the eyes or skin.

INTERACTIONS
Dantrolene interacts with several other types of drugs:
1. Concurrent use of dantrolene with central nervous system depressants (such as alcohol, antihistamines, barbi

turates, benzodiazepine tranquilizers, muscle relaxants, narcotics, pain medications, phenothiazine tranquilizers, and sleeping medications) or with tricyclic antidepressants can lead to extreme drowsiness.
2. Concurrent use of dantrolene and estrogen by women over 35 years of age can increase their risk of liver damage.

BE SURE TO TELL YOUR DOCTOR about any medications you are currently taking, especially any listed above.

WARNINGS
• Tell your doctor about unusual or allergic reactions you have had to any medications, especially to dantrolene.
• Before starting to take this medication, be sure to tell your doctor if you now have or if you have ever had heart disease, liver disease, or lung disease.
• Repeated laboratory tests are necessary while you are taking dantrolene to monitor changes that may indicate liver damage.
• If this drug makes you dizzy or drowsy or blurs your vision, do not take part in any activity that requires alertness, such as driving a car or operating potentially dangerous equipment.
• Be sure to tell your doctor if you are pregnant. Although extensive studies in humans have not been conducted, animal studies involving large doses of dantrolene have demonstrated adverse effects on the fetus. Also, tell your doctor if you are breast-feeding an infant. This drug is not recommended for nursing women.

Dapex—see phentermine

Darvocet-N 50—see acetaminophen and propoxyphene combination

Darvocet-N 100—see acetaminophen and propoxyphene combination

Darvon—see propoxyphene

Darvon Compound—see aspirin, caffeine, and propoxyphene combination

Darvon-N—see propoxyphene

Dazamide—see acetazolamide

Decadron—see dexamethasone (systemic)

Deconamine—see pseudoephedrine and chlorpheniramine combination

Deconamine SR—see pseudoephedrine and chlorpheniramine combination

Decongestabs—see phenylpropanolamine, phenylephrine, chlorpheniramine, and phenyltoloxamine combination

Dehist—see phenylpropanolamine and chlorpheniramine combination

Delacort—see hydrocortisone (topical)

Delta-Cortef—see prednisolone (systemic)

Deltasone—see prednisone (systemic)

Demazin—see phenylpropanolamine and chlorpheniramine combination

Demerol—see meperidine

Demulen—see oral contraceptives

Depakene—see valproic acid

Depakote—see valproic acid

Depen Titratable Tablets—see penicillamine

Deponit—see nitroglycerin (topical)

Dermacort—see hydrocortisone (topical)

DermiCort—see hydrocortisone (topical)

Dermolate Anti-Itch—see hydrocortisone (topical)

Dermolate Scalp-Itch—see hydrocortisone (topical)

Dermtex HC with aloe—see hydrocortisone (topical)

desipramine

BRAND NAMES (Manufacturers)
desipramine (various manufacturers)
Norpramin (Merrell Dow)
Pertofrane (Rorer)
TYPE OF DRUG
Tricyclic antidepressant
INGREDIENT
desipramine
DOSAGE FORMS
Capsules (25 mg and 50 mg)
Tablets (10 mg, 25 mg, 50 mg, 75 mg, 100 mg, and 150 mg)
STORAGE
Desipramine capsules and tablets should be stored at room temperature in tightly closed containers.

USES
Desipramine is used to relieve the symptoms of mental depression. This medication belongs to a group of drugs referred to as the tricyclic antidepressants. These medicines are thought to relieve depression by increasing the concentration of certain chemicals necessary for nerve transmission in the brain.

TREATMENT
This drug should be taken exactly as your doctor prescribes. You can take it with food to lessen stomach irritation, unless your doctor tells you otherwise.

If you miss a dose of this medication, take the missed dose as soon as possible, then return to your regular dosing schedule. If, however, the dose you missed was a once-a-day bedtime dose, do not take that dose in the morning; check with your doctor instead. If the dose is taken in the morning, it may cause some unwanted side effects. Never double the dose.

The effects of therapy with this medication may not become apparent for several weeks.

SIDE EFFECTS
Minor. Agitation, anxiety, blurred vision, confusion, constipation, cramps, diarrhea, dizziness, drowsiness, dry mouth, fatigue, heartburn, insomnia, loss of appetite, nausea, peculiar tastes in the mouth, restlessness, sweating, vomiting, weakness, or weight gain or loss. As your body adjusts to the medication, these side effects should disappear.

This medication may increase your sensitivity to sunlight. You should, therefore, avoid prolonged exposure to sunlight and sunlamps.

Dry mouth can be relieved by chewing sugarless gum or by sucking on ice chips or a piece of hard candy.

To relieve constipation, increase the amount of fiber in your diet (fresh fruits and vegetables, salads, bran, and whole-grain breads), exercise, and drink more water (unless your doctor directs you to do otherwise).

To avoid dizziness or light-headedness when you stand, contract and relax the muscles of your legs for a few moments before rising. Do this by pushing one foot against the floor while raising the other foot slightly, alternating feet so that you are "pumping" your legs.

Major. Tell your doctor about any side effects that are persistent or particularly bothersome. IT IS ESPECIALLY IMPORTANT TO TELL YOUR DOCTOR about chest pain, convulsions, difficulty in urinating, enlarged or painful breasts (in both sexes), fainting, fever, fluid retention, hair loss, hallucinations, headaches, impotence, mood changes, mouth sores, nervousness, nightmares, nosebleeds, numbness in the fingers or toes, palpitations, ringing in the ears, seizures, skin rash, sleep disorders, sore throat, tremors, uncoordinated movements or balance problems, unusual bleeding or bruising, or yellowing of the eyes or skin.

INTERACTIONS
Desipramine interacts with several other types of drugs:
1. Extreme drowsiness can occur when this medicine is taken with central nervous system depressants (such as alcohol, antihistamines, barbiturates, benzodiazepine tranquilizers, muscle relaxants, narcotics, pain medications, phenothiazine tranquilizers, and sleeping medications) or with other antidepressants.
2. Desipramine may decrease the effectiveness of anti-seizure medications.
3. It may block the blood-pressure-lowering effects of clonidine and guanethidine.
4. Cimetidine can decrease the elimination of desipramine from the body, increasing the possibility of side effects.
5. Birth control pills or estrogen-containing drugs can increase the side effects and reduce the effectiveness of the tricyclic antidepressants (including desipramine).

6. Tricyclic antidepressants may increase the side effects of thyroid medication and of over-the-counter (nonprescription) cough, cold, allergy, asthma, sinus, and diet drugs.
7. The concurrent use of tricyclic antidepressants and monoamine oxidase (MAO) inhibitors should be avoided, because the combination may result in fever, convulsions, or high blood pressure. At least 14 days should separate the use of this drug and the use of an MAO inhibitor.

BE SURE TO TELL YOUR DOCTOR about any medications you are currently.

WARNINGS
• Tell your doctor if you have had unusual or allergic reactions to medications, especially to desipramine or any of the other tricyclic antidepressants (such as amitriptyline, imipramine, doxepin, trimipramine, amoxapine, protriptyline, maprotiline, and nortriptyline).
• Tell your doctor if you have a history of alcoholism or if you have had asthma, high blood pressure, liver disease, kidney disease, heart disease, a heart attack, circulatory disease, stomach problems, intestinal problems, difficulty in urinating, enlarged prostate gland, epilepsy, seizures, glaucoma, thyroid disease, mental illness, or electroshock therapy.
• If this drug makes you dizzy or drowsy, do not take part in any activity that requires alertness, such as driving a car or operating potentially dangerous equipment.
• Before having surgery or other medical or dental treatment, tell your doctor or dentist about this drug.
• Do not stop taking this drug suddenly. Abruptly stopping it can cause nausea, headache, stomach upset, fatigue, or a worsening of your condition. Your doctor may want to reduce the dosage gradually.
• The effects of this medication may last as long as seven days after you have stopped taking it, so continue to observe all precautions during that period.
• The tablet form of this medication contains the color additive FD&C Yellow No. 5 (tartrazine), which can cause allergic-type symptoms (fainting, shortness of breath, rash) in certain susceptible individuals.
• Be sure to tell your doctor if you are pregnant. Problems in humans have not been reported; however, studies in animals have shown that this medication can cause side effects in the fetus when given to the mother in large doses during pregnancy. Also, tell your doctor if you are breast-feeding an infant. Small amounts of this drug can pass into breast milk, which may cause unwanted effects, such as irritability or sleeping problems, in the nursing infant.

Desoxyn—see methamphetamine

Desoxyn Gradumets—see methamphetamine

Desyrel—see trazodone

Desyrel Dividose—see trazodone

Dexacidin—see dexamethasone, neomycin, and polymixin B combination (ophthalmic)

Dexameth—see dexamethasone

dexamethasone (systemic)

BRAND NAMES (Manufacturers)
Decadron (Merck Sharp & Dohme)
Dexameth (Major)
dexamethasone (various manufacturers)
Dexone (Reid-Rowell)
Hexadrol (Organon)

TYPE OF DRUG
Adrenocorticosteroid hormone

INGREDIENT
dexamethasone

DOSAGE FORMS
Tablets (0.25 mg, 0.5 mg, 0.75 mg, 1 mg, 1.5 mg, 2 mg, 4 mg, and 6 mg)
Oral elixir (0.5 mg per 5-ml spoonful, with 5% alcohol)
Oral solution (0.5 mg per 5-ml spoonful)
Oral concentrate (0.5 mg per 0.5 ml, with 30% alcohol)

STORAGE
Dexamethasone should be stored at room temperature in a tightly closed container.

USES
Your adrenal glands naturally produce certain cortisone-like chemicals. These chemicals are involved in various regulatory processes in the body (such as those involving fluid balance, temperature, and reaction to inflammation). Dexamethasone belongs to a group of drugs known as adrenocorticosteroids (or cortisone-like medications). It is used to treat a variety of disorders, including endocrine and rheumatic disorders; asthma; blood diseases; certain cancers; eye disorders; gastrointestinal disturbances, such as ulcerative colitis; respiratory diseases; and inflammations such as arthritis, dermatitis, and poison ivy. How this drug acts to relieve these disorders is not completely understood.

TREATMENT
In order to prevent stomach irritation, you can take dexamethasone with food or milk.

If you are taking only one dose of this medication each day, try to take it before 9:00 A.M. This will mimic the body's normal production of this type of chemical.

The oral elixir and solution forms of this medication should be measured carefully with a specially designed 5-ml measuring spoon. An ordinary kitchen teaspoon is not accurate enough.

The oral concentrate may be diluted in juice, other liquids, or semi-solid foods like applesauce.

It is important to try not to miss any doses of dexamethasone. However, if you do miss a dose of this medication, follow these guidelines:
1. If you are taking this medication more than once a day, take the missed dose as soon as possible and return to your regular schedule. If it is already time for the next dose of medication, double the dose.
2. If you are taking this medication once a day, take the dose you missed as soon as possible, unless you don't

remember until the next day. In that case, do not take the missed dose at all, just follow your regular dosing schedule. Do not double the next dose.
3. If you are taking this drug every other day, take it as soon as you remember. If you missed the scheduled time by a whole day, take it when you remember, then skip a day before you take the next dose. Do not double the next dose.

If you miss more than one dose of dexamethasone, CONTACT YOUR DOCTOR.

SIDE EFFECTS
Minor. Dizziness, false sense of well-being, fatigue, increased appetite, increased sweating, indigestion, leg cramps, menstrual irregularities, muscle weakness, nausea, reddening of the skin on the face, restlessness, sleep disorders, thinning of the skin, or weight gain. These side effects should disappear as your body adjusts to the medication.

To help avoid potassium loss while using this drug, you can take your dose with a glass of fresh or frozen orange juice, or eat a banana each day. The use of a salt substitute also helps to prevent potassium loss. Check with your doctor before changing your diet or using a salt substitute.

Major. Tell your doctor about any side effects that are persistent or particularly bothersome. IT IS ESPECIALLY IMPORTANT TO TELL YOUR DOCTOR about abdominal enlargement or pain; acne or other skin problems; back or rib pain; bloody or black, tarry stools; blurred vision; convulsions; eye pain; fever and sore throat; growth impairment (in children); headaches; impaired healing of wounds; increased thirst and urination; mental depression; mood changes; muscle wasting; nightmares; peptic ulcers; rapid weight gain (three to five pounds within a week); rash; shortness of breath; unusual bleeding or bruising; or unusual weakness.

INTERACTIONS
This drug interacts with several other types of drugs:
1. Alcohol, aspirin, and anti-inflammatory medications (such as diclofenac, diflunisal, fenoprofen, flurbiprofen, ibuprofen, piroxicam, sulindac, and tolmetin) aggravate the stomach problems that may occur with use of this medication.
2. The dosage of oral anticoagulants (blood thinners, such as warfarin), oral antidiabetic drugs, or insulin may need to be altered when this medication is started or stopped.
3. The loss of potassium caused by this medication can lead to serious side effects in individuals taking digoxin.
4. Thiazide diuretics (water pills) can increase the potassium loss caused by dexamethasone.
5. Phenobarbital, phenytoin, rifampin, and ephedrine can increase the elimination of dexamethasone from the body, thereby decreasing its effectiveness.
6. Oral contraceptives (birth control pills) and estrogen-containing drugs may decrease the elimination of this drug from the body, which can lead to an increase in side effects.
7. Dexamethasone can increase the elimination of aspirin and isoniazid from the body, thereby decreasing the effectiveness of these two medications.

8. Cholestyramine and colestipol can chemically bind this medication in the stomach and gastrointestinal tract, preventing its absorption.

BE SURE TO TELL YOUR DOCTOR about any medications you are currently taking, especially any of those listed above.

WARNINGS

• Tell your doctor about unusual or allergic reactions you have had to any medications, especially to dexamethasone or other adrenocorticosteroids (such as alcometasone, amcinonide, betamethasone, clobetasol, clocortolone, cortisone, desonide, desoximetasone, diflorasone, flumethasone, fluocinolone, fluocinonide, fluorometholone, flurandrenolide, halcinonide, hydrocortisone, methylprednisolone, paramethasone, prednisolone, prednisone, and triamcinolone).

• Tell your doctor if you now have or if you have ever had bone disease, diabetes mellitus, emotional instability, glaucoma, fungal infections, heart disease, high blood pressure, high cholesterol levels, myasthenia gravis, peptic ulcers, osteoporosis, thyroid disease, tuberculosis, ulcerative colitis, kidney disease, or liver disease.

• If you are using this medication for longer than a week, you may need to receive higher doses if you are subjected to stress, such as serious infections, injury, or surgery. Discuss this with your doctor.

• If you have been taking this drug for more than one or two weeks, do not stop taking it suddenly. If it is stopped abruptly, you may experience abdominal or back pain, dizziness, extreme weakness, fainting, fever, muscle or joint pain, nausea, vomiting, or shortness of breath. Your doctor may, therefore, want to reduce the dosage gradually. Never increase the dosage or take the drug for longer than the prescribed time, unless you first consult your doctor.

• While you are taking this drug, you should not be vaccinated or immunized. This medication decreases the effectiveness of vaccines and can lead to infection if a live-virus vaccine is administered.

• Before having surgery or other medical or dental treatment, tell your doctor or dentist you are taking this drug.

• Because this drug can cause glaucoma and cataracts with long-term use, your doctor may want to have your eyes examined by an ophthalmologist periodically during treatment.

• If you are taking this medication for prolonged periods, you should wear or carry an identification card or notice stating that you are taking an adrenocorticosteroid.

• This drug can raise blood sugar levels in diabetic patients. Blood sugar should, therefore, be monitored carefully with blood or urine tests when this drug is being taken.

• Be sure to tell your doctor if you are pregnant. This drug crosses the placenta and may cause adverse effects in the fetus. Birth defects have been observed in the offspring of animals that were given large doses of this type of drug during pregnancy. Also, tell your doctor if you are breast-feeding an infant. Small amounts of this drug pass into breast milk and may cause growth suppression or a decrease in natural adrenocorticosteroid production in the nursing infant.

dexamethasone, neomycin, and polymyxin B combination (ophthalmic)

BRAND NAMES (Manufacturers)
AK-Trol (Akorn)
Dexacidin (Iolab Pharm)
Dexasporin (various manufacturers)
Infectrol (Bausch & Lomb)
Maxitrol (Alcon)
TYPE OF DRUG
Ophthalmic adrenocorticosteroid and antibiotic
INGREDIENTS
dexamethasone, neomycin, and polymyxin B
DOSAGE FORMS
Ophthalmic suspension (0.1% dexamethasone, 3.5 mg neomycin, and 10,000 units polymyxin B per ml)
Ophthalmic ointment (0.1% dexamethasone, 3.5 mg neomycin, and 10,000 units polymyxin B per gram)
STORAGE
The ophthalmic suspension and ointment should be stored at room temperature (never frozen) in tightly closed containers. If the suspension or ointment changes color, don't use the medication. A change in color indicates a loss of effectiveness.

USES
This medication is used for the short-term treatment of bacterial infections and inflammation of the eyes.

Your adrenal glands naturally produce certain cortisone-like chemicals. These chemicals are involved in various regulatory processes in the body (such as those involving fluid balance, temperature, and reaction to inflammation). Dexamethasone belongs to a group of drugs known as adrenocorticosteroids (or cortisone-like medications). It is used to relieve inflammation (redness, swelling, itching, and discomfort). How it does so is not completely understood.

Neomycin and polymyxin B are antibiotics, which act to prevent the growth and multiplication of infecting bacteria.

TREATMENT
Wash your hands with soap and water before using this medication. If you are using the suspension, shake the bottle well before measuring out the drops. The contents tend to settle on the bottom of the bottle, so it is necessary to shake the container to distribute the ingredients evenly and to equalize the doses.

In order to prevent contamination of the medicine, be careful not to touch the tube portion of the dropper, and do not let the dropper touch the eye.

Note that the bottle of the eye drops is not completely full. This is to allow control of the number of drops used.

To apply the drops, tilt your head back and pull down the lower eyelid with one hand to make a pouch below the eyeball. Drop the medicine into the pouch and slowly close your eyes. Do not blink. Place one finger at the corner of the eye next to your nose, applying slight pressure (this is done to prevent loss of medication through the duct that drains fluid from the surface of the eye into the nose and throat), and keep your eyes closed for a minute or two. If you think that the medicine did not get into your eye, repeat the process once. If you are using more than one type of eye drops, wait at least five minutes between doses of the two types drugs.

Follow the same general procedure for applying the ointment. Tilt your head back, pull down the lower eyelid, and squeeze the prescribed amount of ointment in a line along the pouch below the eyeball. Close your eyes, and place your finger at the corner of the eye near the nose for a minute or two. Do not rub your eyes. Wipe off excess ointment and the tip of the tube with clean tissues.

Since applying the medication is somewhat difficult to do, you may want someone else to apply it for you.

If you miss a dose of this drug, insert the drops or apply the ointment as soon as possible, unless it is almost time for the next application. In that case, do not use the missed dose at all; just return to your regular dosing schedule.

Your doctor may advise you to reduce the number of times you are applying this medication when the inflammation and infection begin to improve. Continue to take this medication for the entire time prescribed by your doctor, even if the symptoms of infection disappear then. If you stop applying the drug too soon, bacteria are given a chance to continue growing, and the infection could recur.

SIDE EFFECTS

Minor. Blurred vision, burning, or stinging. These side effects should disappear as your body adjusts to the drug.
Major. Tell your doctor about any side effects that are persistent or particularly bothersome. IT IS ESPECIALLY IMPORTANT TO TELL YOUR DOCTOR about disturbed or reduced vision; eye pain, itching, or swelling; headache; rash; or severe irritation.

INTERACTIONS

This medication should not interact with any other medications as long as it is used according to directions.

WARNINGS

• Tell your doctor about any reactions you have had to medications, especially to dexamethasone or other adrenocorticosteroids (such as alcometasone, amcinonide, betamethasone, clobetasol, clocortolone, cortisone, desonide, desoximetasone, diflorasone, flumethasone, fluocinolone, fluorometholone, flurandrenolide, halcinonide, hydrocortisone, methylprednisolone, prednisolone, prednisone, and triamcinolone), to polymyxin B, to neomycin, or to any related antibiotic (amikacin, gentamicin, kanamycin, netilmicin, paromomycin, streptomycin, and tobramycin).
• Tell your doctor if you have ever had fungal or viral infections of the eye, inner ear disease, kidney disease, or myasthenia gravis.
• If there is no change in your condition two or three days after starting to take this drug, contact your doctor. The drug may not be effective for your particular infection.

• Do not use this medication for longer than ten consecutive days unless your doctor directs you to do so. Prolonged use of this drug may result in glaucoma, secondary infection, cataracts, or eye damage. If you need to take this medication for several weeks, your doctor may want you to have an eye examination by an ophthalmologist.
• This medication has been prescribed for your current infection only. A subsequent infection may require a different medicine. Do not give this drug to other people or use it to treat other infections.
• Do not apply makeup to the affected eye.
• Be sure to tell your doctor if you are pregnant. When large amounts of dexamethasone are applied for prolonged periods, some of it is absorbed into the bloodstream. It may cross the placenta. Birth defects have been observed in the offspring of animals that were given large oral doses of this drug during pregnancy. Also, tell your doctor if you are breast-feeding an infant. If absorbed through the eye, small amounts of dexamethasone can pass into breast milk and may cause growth suppression or a decrease in natural adrenocorticosteroid production in the nursing infant.

Dexasporin—see dexamethasone, neomycin, and polymixin B combination (ophthalmic)

Dexchlor—see dexchlorpheniramine

dexchlorpheniramine

BRAND NAMES (Manufacturers)
Dexchlor (Henry Schein)
dexchlorpheniramine (various manufacturers)
Poladex (Major)
Polaramine (Schering)
Polaramine Repetabs (Schering)
TYPE OF DRUG
Antihistamine
INGREDIENT
dexchlorpheniramine
DOSAGE FORMS
Tablets (2 mg)
Repeat-action tablets (4 mg and 6 mg)
Oral syrup (2 mg per 5-ml spoonful, with 6% alcohol)
STORAGE
Dexchlorpheniramine tablets and oral syrup should be stored at room temperature in tightly closed containers.

USES

This medication belongs to a group of drugs known as antihistamines (antihistamines block the action of histamine, a chemical that is released by the body during an allergic reaction). It is used to treat or prevent symptoms of allergy.

TREATMENT

To avoid stomach upset, you can take dexchlorpheniramine with food or with a full glass of milk or water (unless your doctor directs you to do otherwise).

The syrup form of this medication should be measured carefully with a specially designed 5-ml measuring spoon. An ordinary kitchen teaspoon is not accurate enough for medical applications and does not ensure that you receive the proper dose.

The repeat-action tablet form of this medication should be swallowed whole. Breaking, chewing, or crushing these tablets destroys their sustained-release activity and may increase the side effects.

If you miss a dose of this medication, take the missed dose as soon as possible, unless it is almost time for your next dose. In that case, do not take the missed dose at all; just return to your regular dosing schedule. Do not double the next dose.

SIDE EFFECTS

Minor. Blurred vision; confusion; constipation; diarrhea; difficult or painful urination; dizziness; dry mouth, throat, or nose; headache; irritability; loss of appetite; nausea; rash; restlessness; ringing or buzzing in the ears; stomach upset; or unusual increase in sweating. These side effects should disappear as your body adjusts to the medication.

This medication can cause increased sensitivity to sunlight. It is, therefore, important to avoid prolonged exposure to sunlight and sunlamps. Wear protective clothing and use an effective sunscreen.

If you are constipated, increase the amount of fiber in your diet (fresh fruits and vegetables, salads, bran, and whole-grain breads), exercise, and drink more water (unless your doctor directs you to do otherwise).

If you experience mouth or throat dryness, you may wish to chew sugarless gum or suck on ice chips or a piece of hard candy to minimize these side effects.

If you feel dizzy or light-headed, sit or lie down for a while; get up from a sitting or lying position slowly, and be careful on stairs.

Major. Tell your doctor about any side effects that are persistent or particularly bothersome. IT IS ESPECIALLY IMPORTANT TO TELL YOUR DOCTOR about changes in menstruation, clumsiness, feeling faint, flushing of the face, hallucinations, seizures, shortness of breath, sleeping disorders, sore throat or fever, palpitations, tightness in the chest, unusual bleeding or bruising, or unusual tiredness or weakness.

INTERACTIONS

Dexchlorpheniramine interacts with several other types of medications:

1. Concurrent use of it with central nervous system depressants (such as alcohol, barbiturates, benzodiazepine tranquilizers, muscle relaxants, narcotics, pain medications, and phenothiazine tranquilizers) or with tricyclic antidepressants can cause extreme drowsiness.

2. Monoamine oxidase (MAO) inhibitors (such as isocarboxazid, pargyline, phenelzine, and tranylcypromine) can increase the side effects of this medication. At least 14 days should separate the use of this drug and the use of an MAO inhibitor.

BE SURE TO TELL YOUR DOCTOR about any medications you are currently taking, especially any of those listed above.

WARNINGS

• Tell your doctor about unusual or allergic reactions you have had to any medications, especially to dexchlorpheniramine or other antihistamines (such as astemizole, azatadine, brompheniramine, carbinoxamine, chlorpheniramine, clemastine, cyproheptadine, dimenhydrinate, dimethindene, diphenhydramine, diphenylpyraline, doxylamine, hydroxyzine, phenidamine, promethazine, pyrilamine, terfenadine, trimeprazine, tripelennamine, and triprolidine).

• Tell your doctor if you now have or if you have ever had asthma, blood vessel disease, glaucoma, high blood pressure, kidney disease, peptic ulcers, enlarged prostate gland, or thyroid disease.

• Dexchlorpheniramine can cause drowsiness or dizziness. Your ability to perform tasks that require alertness, such as driving a car or operating potentially dangerous equipment, may be decreased. Appropriate caution should, therefore, be taken.

• Be sure to tell your doctor if you are pregnant. The effects of this medication during pregnancy have not been thoroughly studied in humans. It is recommended that use of this drug be avoided during the last three months of pregnancy. Also, tell your doctor if you are breast-feeding an infant. Small amounts of dexchlorpheniramine pass into breast milk and may cause unusual excitement or irritability in nursing infants.

Dexedrine—see dextroamphetamine

Dexedrine Spansules—see dextroamphetamine

Dexone—see dexamethasone (systemic)

dextroamphetamine

BRAND NAMES (Manufacturers)
Dexedrine (Smith Kline & French)
Dexedrine Spansules (Smith Kline & French)
dextroamphetamine sulfate (various manufacturers)
Oxydess II (Vortech)
Spancap No. 1 (Vortech)

TYPE OF DRUG
Amphetamine

INGREDIENT
dextroamphetamine

DOSAGE FORMS
Tablets (5 mg and 10 mg)
Sustained-release capsules (5 mg, 10 mg, and 15 mg)

STORAGE
Dextroamphetamine tablets and capsules should be stored at room temperature in tightly closed containers.

USES
This medication is a central nervous system stimulant that increases mental alertness and decreases fatigue. It is used to treat narcolepsy (problems in staying awake) and abnormal behavioral syndrome in children (hyperkinetic syndrome or attention deficit disorder). The way this acts to control abnormal behavioral syndrome in children is not known.

Dextroamphetamine is also used as an appetite suppressant during the first few weeks of dieting (while you are trying to establish new eating habits). It is thought to relieve hunger by altering nerve impulses to the appetite control center in the brain. Its effectiveness as an appetite suppressant lasts only for short periods (three to 12 weeks), however.

TREATMENT

In order to avoid stomach upset, you can take dextroamphetamine with food or with a full glass of milk or water (unless your doctor directs you to do otherwise).

If this medication is being used to treat narcolepsy or abnormal behavioral syndrome in children, the first dose each day should be taken soon after awakening. Subsequent doses should be spaced at four- to six-hour intervals.

If this medication has been prescribed as a diet aid, it should be taken one hour before each meal.

The sustained-release form of this medication should be swallowed whole. Breaking, chewing, or crushing these capsules destroys their sustained-release activity and may increase the side effects.

In order to avoid difficulty in falling asleep, the last dose of this medication each day should be taken four to six hours before bedtime (tablets) or ten to 14 hours before bedtime (sustained-release capsules).

If you miss a dose of this medication, take the missed dose as soon as possible, unless it is almost time for your next dose. In that case, do not take the missed dose at all; just return to your regular dosing schedule. Do not double the next dose.

SIDE EFFECTS

Minor. Abdominal cramps, constipation, diarrhea, dizziness, dry mouth, false sense of well-being, insomnia, loss of appetite, irritability, nausea, overstimulation, restlessness, unpleasant taste in the mouth, or vomiting. These side effects should disappear as your body adjusts to the drug.

To prevent constipation, increase the amount of fiber in your diet (fresh fruits and vegetables, bran, salads, and whole-grain cereals and breads), exercise, and drink more water (unless your doctor directs you to do otherwise).

Dry mouth can be relieved by sucking on ice chips or a piece of hard candy or by chewing sugarless gum.

If you feel dizzy, sit or lie down for a while; get up from a sitting or lying position slowly.

Major. Tell your doctor about any side effects that are persistent or particularly bothersome. IT IS ESPECIALLY IMPORTANT TO TELL YOUR DOCTOR about blurred vision, confusion, fatigue, headaches, impotence, mental depression, nosebleeds, palpitations, rash, sweating, tightness in the chest, tremors, or uncoordinated movements.

INTERACTIONS

Dextroamphetamine interacts with several other types of medications:

1. Use of dextroamphetamine within 14 days of use of a monoamine oxidase (MAO) inhibitor (such as isocarboxazid, pargyline, phenelzine, and tranylcypromine) can result in high blood pressure and other side effects.

2. Barbiturate medications, certain tranquilizers (especially chlorpromazine), and tricyclic antidepressants can reverse the effect of this medication.

3. Amphetamines can decrease the blood-pressure-lowering effects of antihypertensive medications (especially guanethidine) and may alter dosage requirements for insulin and oral antidiabetic medication in diabetic patients.

4. The side effects of other central nervous system stimulants (such as caffeine, nonprescription appetite suppressants, and cough, sinus, allergy, asthma, or cold preparations) may be increased by dextroamphetamine.

5. Acetazolamide and sodium bicarbonate can decrease the elimination of the amphetamines from the body, thereby prolonging their duration of action.

BE SURE TO TELL YOUR DOCTOR about any medications you are currently taking, especially any listed above.

WARNINGS

• Tell your doctor about unusual or allergic reactions you have had to any medications, especially to dextroamphetamine or other central nervous system stimulants (such as albuterol, amphetamine, ephedrine, epinephrine, isoproterenol, metaproterenol, norepinephrine, phenylephrine, phenylpropanolamine, pseudoephedrine, and terbutaline).

• Tell your doctor if you have a history of drug abuse or if you have ever had problems with agitation, diabetes mellitus, glaucoma, heart or blood vessel disease, high blood pressure, or thyroid disease.

• Dextroamphetamine can mask the symptoms of extreme fatigue and can cause dizziness. Your ability to perform tasks that require alertness, such as driving a car or operating potentially dangerous equipment, may be decreased. Appropriate caution should, therefore, be taken.

• Before surgery or other medical or dental treatment, tell your doctor or dentist you are taking this drug.

• Dextroamphetamine is related to amphetamine and may be habit-forming when taken for long periods of time (both physical and psychological dependence can occur). Therefore, you should not increase the dosage of this medication or take it for longer than 12 weeks unless you first consult your doctor. It is also important that you not stop taking this medication abruptly; fatigue, sleep disorders, mental depression, nausea, vomiting, stomach cramps, or pain could occur. Your doctor may, therefore, want to decrease the dosage gradually in order to prevent these side effects.

• Some of these products contain the color additive FD&C Yellow No. 5 (tartrazine), which can cause allergic-type reactions (difficulty in breathing, fainting, rash, wheezing) in certain susceptible individuals.

• Be sure to tell your doctor if you are pregnant. Although side effects in humans have not been thoroughly studied, some of the amphetamines have caused heart, brain, and biliary tract abnormalities in the fetuses of animals that received large doses of these drugs during pregnancy. Also, tell your doctor if you are breast-feeding an infant. Small amounts of this drug pass into breast milk and can cause unwanted side effects in the nursing infant.

dextroamphetamine sulfate—see dextroamphetamine

dextromethorphan and iodinated glycerol combination

BRAND NAMES (Manufacturers)
Iophen DM (various manufacturers)
Torganic-DM (Major)
Tusside (Ortega)
Tussi-Organidin DM (Wallace)
Tussi-R-Gen DM (Goldline)

TYPE OF DRUG
Cough suppressant and expectorant combination

INGREDIENTS
dextromethorphan and iodinated glycerol

DOSAGE FORM
Oral liquid (10 mg dextromethorphan and 30 mg iodinated glycerol per 5-ml spoonful)

STORAGE
This medicine should be stored at room temperature in a tightly closed container. Avoid exposure of this medication to high temperatures during storage.

USES
Dextromethorphan and iodinated glycerol combination is used to relieve coughs due to colds or infections or inflammation of the upper respiratory tract. Iodinated glycerol is an expectorant, which loosens bronchial secretions. Dextromethorphan is a cough suppressant, which acts on the cough center in the brain.

TREATMENT
You can take dextromethorphan and iodinated glycerol combination either on an empty stomach or, to avoid stomach irritation, with food or milk (as directed by your doctor).

Each dose should be measured carefully with a specially designed 5-ml measuring spoon.

To help loosen the mucus in the bronchi, you should drink a glass of water after each dose.

If you miss a dose of this medication, take the missed dose as soon as possible, unless it is almost time for the next dose. In that case, do not take the missed dose at all; return to your regular dosing schedule. Do not double the dose.

SIDE EFFECTS
Minor. Drowsiness or stomach upset. These side effects should disappear as your body adjusts to this medication.

Major. Tell your doctor about any side effects that are persistent or particularly bothersome. IT IS ESPECIALLY IMPORTANT TO TELL YOUR DOCTOR about extreme weakness, skin rash, or swollen lymph nodes.

INTERACTIONS
This medicine can interact with other types of drugs:
1. Use with other central nervous system depressants (such as alcohol, barbiturates, benzodiazepine tranquil-izers, muscle relaxants, narcotics, pain medications, phenothiazine tranquilizers, and sleeping medications) or with tricyclic antidepressants can lead to drowsiness.
2. The iodine component of iodinated glycerol can increase the side effects of lithium on the thyroid gland. It can also increase the effects of antithyroid medications.
3. Use of dextromethorphan within 14 days of use of a monoamine oxidase inhibitor (such as isocarboxazid, pargyline, phenelzine, and tranylcypromine) can result in high blood pressure and other side effects.

Before starting this medication, BE SURE TO TELL YOUR DOCTOR about any medications you are currently taking, especially any of those listed above.

WARNINGS
• Tell your doctor about unusual or allergic reactions you have had to any medications, especially to dextromethorphan or to iodinated glycerol or iodine.
• Before starting to take this medication, be sure to tell your doctor if you now have or if you have ever had acne, cystic fibrosis, heart disease, or thyroid disease.
• If this drug makes you dizzy or drowsy, do not take part in activities that require alertness, such as driving a car or operating potentially dangerous equipment.
• While you are taking this medication, drink several glasses of water a day to help loosen bronchial secretions, unless your doctor directs you to do otherwise.
• Be sure to tell your doctor if you are pregnant. This medication should not be taken during pregnancy. Iodinated glycerol can cause goiter (an enlarged thyroid gland) in the developing fetus. Also, tell your doctor if you are breast-feeding an infant. Iodinated glycerol can pass into breast milk and cause side effects in the nursing infant.

DHT—see dihydrotachysterol

DiaBeta—see glyburide

Diabinese—see chlorpropamide

Diachlor—see chlorothiazide

Diamine T.D.—see brompheniramine

Diamox—see acetazolamide

Diamox Sequels—see acetazolamide

Diaqua—see hydrochlorothiazide

diazepam

BRAND NAMES (Manufacturers)
diazepam (various manufacturers)
Diazepam Intensol (Roxene)
Valium (Roche)
Valrelease (Roche)
Vazepam (Major)

TYPE OF DRUG
Sedative/hypnotic

INGREDIENT
diazepam
DOSAGE FORMS
Oral solution (5 mg per 5-ml spoonful)
Oral intensol solution (5 mg per ml)
Tablets (2 mg, 5 mg, and 10 mg)
Sustained-release capsules (15 mg)
STORAGE
This medication should be stored at room temperature in a tightly closed, light-resistant container.

USES
Diazepam is prescribed to treat symptoms of anxiety and sometimes to treat muscle spasms, convulsions, seizures, or alcohol withdrawal. It is not clear exactly how this medicine works, but it may relieve anxiety by acting as a depressant of the central nervous system (brain and spinal cord). Diazepam is currently used by many people to relieve nervousness. It is effective for this purpose for short periods, but it is important to try to remove the cause of the anxiety as well.

TREATMENT
The oral intensol solution should be mixed with a non-alcoholic liquid or semi-solid food such as water, juice, soda or soda-like beverages, applesauce, or pudding. Use only the calibrated dropper provided. Stir the liquid or food gently for a few seconds after adding the oral intensol solution. The entire amount of the mixture should be consumed immediately. Do not store prepared mixtures for future use. The tablet or capsule form of this medication should be taken exactly as directed by your doctor. It can be taken with food or a full glass of water if stomach upset occurs. Do not take this medication with a dose of antacids, since they may retard its absorption.

If you are taking this medication regularly and you miss a dose and remember within an hour, take the missed dose immediately. If more than an hour has passed, skip the dose you missed and wait for the next scheduled dose. Do not double the next dose.

SIDE EFFECTS
Minor. Bitter taste in the mouth, constipation, depression, diarrhea, dizziness, drowsiness (after a night's sleep), dry mouth, excessive salivation, fatigue, flushing, headache, heartburn, loss of appetite, nausea, nervousness, sweating, or vomiting. These side effects should disappear as your body adjusts to the medication.

To relieve constipation, increase the amount of fiber in your diet (fresh fruits and vegetables, salads, bran, and whole-grain breads), exercise, and drink more water (unless your doctor directs you to do otherwise).

Dry mouth can be relieved by chewing sugarless gum or by sucking on ice chips or hard candy.

If you feel dizzy, sit or lie down for a while; get up slowly from a sitting or reclining position, and be careful on stairs.

Major. Tell your doctor about any side effects that are persistent or particularly bothersome. IT IS ESPECIALLY IMPORTANT TO TELL YOUR DOCTOR about blurred or double vision, chest pain, difficulty in urinating, fainting, falling, fever, joint pain, hallucinations, mouth sores, nightmares, palpitations, rash, severe depression, shortness of breath, slurred speech, sore throat, uncoordinated movements, unusual excitement, unusual tiredness, or yellowing of the eyes or skin.

INTERACTIONS
This medication interacts with several other types of medications:

1. To prevent oversedation, this drug should not be taken with alcohol, other sedative drugs, or central nervous system depressants (such as antihistamines, barbiturates, muscle relaxants, pain medicines, narcotics, medicines for seizures, and tranquilizers), or with antidepressants.

2. This medication may decrease the effectiveness of carbamazepine, levodopa, and oral anticoagulants (blood thinners) and may increase the effects of phenytoin.

3. Disulfiram, oral contraceptives (birth control pills), isoniazid, fluoxetine, valproic acid, propranolol, metoprolol, and cimetidine can increase the blood levels of diazepam, which can lead to toxic effects.

4. Concurrent use of rifampin may decrease the effectiveness of diazepam.

BE SURE TO TELL YOUR DOCTOR about any medications you are currently taking, especially any of those listed above.

WARNINGS
• Tell your doctor about unusual or allergic reactions you have had to any medications, especially to diazepam or other benzodiazepine tranquilizers (such as alprazolam, flurazepam, halazepam, lorazepam, oxazepam, prazepam, temazepam, and triazolam).

• Tell your doctor if you now have or if you have ever had liver disease, kidney disease, epilepsy, lung disease, myasthenia gravis, porphyria, mental depression, or mental illness.

• This medicine can cause drowsiness. Avoid tasks that require alertness, such as driving a car or operating potentially dangerous machinery.

• This medication has the potential for abuse and must be used with caution. Tolerance may develop quickly; do not increase your dosage of the drug without first consulting your doctor. It is also important not to stop taking this drug suddenly if you have been taking it in large amounts or if you have used it for several weeks. Your doctor may want to reduce your dosage gradually.

• This is a safe drug when used properly. When it is combined with other sedative drugs or alcohol, however, serious side effects can develop.

• Be sure to tell your doctor if you are pregnant. This medicine may increase the chance of birth defects if it is taken during the first three months of pregnancy. In addition, too much use of this medicine during the last six months of pregnancy may cause the baby to become dependent on it, resulting in withdrawal side effects in the newborn. Also, use of this medicine during the last weeks of pregnancy may cause excessive drowsiness, slowed heartbeat, and breathing difficulties in the infant. Be sure to tell your doctor if you are breast-feeding an infant. This medication can pass into breast milk and cause excessive drowsiness, slowed heartbeat, and breathing difficulties in nursing infants.

Diazepam Intensol—see diazepam

diclofenac

BRAND NAME (Manufacturer)
Voltaren (Ciba-Geigy)
TYPE OF DRUG
Nonsteroidal anti-inflammatory analgesic
INGREDIENT
diclofenac
DOSAGE FORM
Enteric-coated tablets (25 mg, 50 mg, and 75 mg)
STORAGE
This medication should be stored in a tightly closed container at room temperature away from heat and direct sunlight.

USES
Diclofenac is used to treat the inflammation (pain, swelling, and stiffness) of arthritis and ankylosing spondylitis. Diclofenac has been shown to block the production of certain body chemicals, called prostaglandins, that may trigger pain. However, it is not yet fully understood how it works.

TREATMENT
You should take this medication on an empty stomach 30 to 60 minutes before meals or two hours after meals, so that it gets into your bloodstream quickly. To decrease stomach irritation, your doctor may want you to take this medication with food or antacids.

Do not break, crush, or chew the tablets before swallowing. They should be swallowed whole to lessen side effects.

It may take two weeks before you feel the full effects of this medication. Diclofenac does not cure arthritis or ankylosing spondylitis, but it will help to control the condition as long as you continue to take it.

It is important that you take diclofenac on schedule and do not miss any doses. If you do miss a dose, take it as soon as possible, unless it is almost time for your next dose. In that case, do not take the missed dose at all; just return to your regular dosing schedule. Do not double the next dose.

SIDE EFFECTS
Minor. Abdominal cramps, constipation, diarrhea, dizziness, headache, indigestion, or nausea. As your body adjusts to the drug, these side effects should disappear.

To relieve constipation, increase the amount of fiber in your diet (fresh fruits and vegetables, salads, bran, and whole-grain breads), exercise, and drink more water (unless your doctor directs you to do otherwise).

If you become dizzy, sit or lie down; get up slowly from a sitting or reclining position, and be careful on stairs.

Major. Tell your doctor about any side effects that are persistent or particularly bothersome. IT IS ESPECIALLY IMPORTANT TO TELL YOUR DOCTOR about bloody or black, tarry stools; blurred vision; confusion; difficult or painful urination; palpitations; a problem with hearing, or ringing or buzzing in your ears; skin rash, hives, or itching; stomach pain; swelling of the feet or hands; tightness in the chest; unexplained sore throat and fever; soreness of the tongue or mouth; unusual fatigue or weakness; unusual weight gain; wheezing or difficulty in breathing; or yellowing of the eyes or skin.

INTERACTIONS
Diclofenac interacts with several other types of medications:

1. Anticoagulants (blood thinners, such as warfarin) can lead to an increase in bleeding complications.
2. Aspirin, other salicylates, and other anti-inflammatory medications can increase stomach irritation. Aspirin may also decrease the effectiveness of diclofenac. Therefore, aspirin should not be used concurrently with diclofenac.
3. Diclofenac can decrease the elimination of digoxin, methotrexate, and lithium from the body, which can lead to serious side effects.
4. The activity of diuretics (water pills) and drugs to lower blood pressure (propranolol, metoprolol) may be inhibited by diclofenac.
5. Diclofenac may alter a diabetic patient's response to insulin, oral hypoglycemic agents, or antiseizure medication (phenytoin).

Before starting to take diclofenac, BE SURE TO TELL YOUR DOCTOR about any medications you are taking, especially any of those listed above.

WARNINGS
• Before you start to take this medication, it is important to tell your doctor if you have ever had unusual or allergic reactions to diclofenac or to any of the other chemically related drugs (aspirin, other salicylates, diflunisal, fenoprofen, flurbiprofen, indomethacin, ketoprofen, meclofenamate, mefenamic acid, naproxen, oxyphenbutazone, phenylbutazone, piroxicam, sulindac, or tolmetin).
• Tell your doctor if you now have or if you have ever had asthma, bleeding problems, colitis, stomach ulcers or other stomach problems, epilepsy, heart disease, high blood pressure, kidney disease, liver disease, mental illness, or Parkinson's disease.
• If diclofenac makes you dizzy or drowsy, do not take part in any activity that requires alertness, such as driving a car or operating potentially dangerous machinery.
• Because this drug can prolong your bleeding time, it is important to tell your doctor or dentist that you are taking this drug before having surgery or any other medical or dental treatment.
• Stomach problems are more likely to occur if you take aspirin regularly or drink alcohol while being treated with this medication. These should, therefore, be avoided (unless your doctor directs you to do otherwise).
• Be sure to tell your doctor if you are pregnant or planning to become pregnant. This medication can cause unwanted effects on the heart or blood flow of the fetus. Studies in animals have also shown that this medicine, if taken late in pregnancy, may increase the length of pregnancy, prolong labor, or cause other problems during delivery. Also tell your doctor if you are breast-feeding

an infant. Small amounts of diclofenac can pass into breast milk.

Dicloxacil—see dicloxacillin

dicloxacillin

BRAND NAMES (Manufacturers)
Dicloxacil (Goldline)
dicloxacillin sodium (various manufacturers)
Dycill (Beecham)
Dynapen (Bristol)
Pathocil (Wyeth)
TYPE OF DRUG
Penicillin antibiotic
INGREDIENT
dicloxacillin
DOSAGE FORMS
Capsules (125 mg, 250 mg, and 500 mg)
Oral suspension (62.5 mg per 5-ml spoonful)
STORAGE
Dicloxacillin capsules should be stored at room temperature in a tightly closed container. The oral suspension should be stored in the refrigerator in a tightly closed container. Any unused portion of the suspension should be discarded after 14 days because the drug loses its potency after that time. This medication should never be frozen.

USES
Dicloxacillin is used to treat a wide variety of bacterial infections, especially those caused by *Staphylococcus* bacteria. It acts by severely injuring the cell membranes of the infecting bacteria, thereby preventing them from growing and multiplying. Dicloxacillin kills susceptible bacteria, but it is not effective against viruses, parasites, or fungi.

TREATMENT
Dicloxacillin should be taken on an empty stomach or with a glass of water, one hour before or two hours after a meal. This medication should never be taken with fruit juices or carbonated beverages, because the acidity of these drinks destroys the drug in the stomach.

The suspension form of this medication should be shaken well just before measuring each dose. The contents tend to settle at the bottom of the bottle, so it is necessary to shake the container to distribute the ingredients evenly and equalize the doses. Each dose should then be measured carefully with a specially designed 5-ml measuring spoon. An ordinary kitchen teaspoon is not accurate enough.

Dicloxacillin works best when the level of medicine in your bloodstream is kept constant. It is best, therefore, to take the doses at evenly spaced intervals day and night. For example, if you are taking four doses a day, the doses should be spaced six hours apart.

If you miss a dose of this medication, take the missed dose immediately. However, if you do not remember to take the missed dose until it is almost time for your next dose, take it; space the following dose about halfway through the regular interval between doses; then return to your regular schedule. Try not to skip any doses.

It is important for you to continue to take this medication for the entire time prescribed by your doctor (usually seven to 14 days), even if the symptoms of your infection disappear before the end of that period. If you stop taking the drug too soon, bacteria are given a chance to continue growing, and the infection could recur.

SIDE EFFECTS
Minor. Diarrhea, heartburn, nausea, or vomiting. These side effects should disappear as your body adjusts to this particular drug.
Major. Tell your doctor about any side effects that are persistent or particularly bothersome. IT IS ESPECIALLY IMPORTANT TO TELL YOUR DOCTOR about bloating, chills, cough, darkened tongue, difficulty in breathing, fever, irritation of the mouth, muscle aches, rash, rectal or vaginal itching, severe diarrhea, or sore throat. In addition, if the symptoms of your infection seem to be getting worse rather than improving, you should contact your doctor.

INTERACTIONS
Dicloxacillin interacts with other types of medications:
1. Probenecid can increase the blood concentrations and side effects of this medication.
2. Dicloxacillin may decrease the effectiveness of oral contraceptives (birth control pills), and pregnancy could result. You should, therefore, use a different or additional form of birth control while taking this medication. Discuss this with your doctor.

BE SURE TO TELL YOUR DOCTOR about any medications you are currently taking, especially any of those listed above.

WARNINGS
• Tell your doctor about unusual or allergic reactions you have had to any medications, especially to dicloxacillin or penicillins, or to cephalosporin antibiotics, penicillamine, or griseofulvin.
• Tell your doctor if you now have or if you have ever had kidney disease, asthma, or allergies.
• This medication has been prescribed for your current infection only. Another infection later on, or one that someone else has, may require a different medicine. You should not give your medicine to other people or use it for other infections, unless your doctor specifically directs you to do so.
• Diabetics taking dicloxacillin should know that this drug can cause interference with a Clinitest urine glucose test. To avoid this problem while taking dicloxacillin, you should switch to Clinistix or Tes-Tape to test your urine for sugar.
• Be sure to tell your doctor if you are pregnant. Although dicloxacillin appears to be safe during pregnancy, extensive studies in humans have not been conducted. Also, tell your doctor if you are breast-feeding an infant. Small amounts of this medication pass into breast milk and may temporarily alter the bacterial balance in the intestinal tract of the nursing infant, resulting in diarrhea.

dicloxacillin sodium—see dicloxacillin

dicyclomine

BRAND NAMES (Manufacturers)
Bentyl (Lakeside Pharmaceutical)
Byclomine (Major)
dicyclomine hydrochloride (various manufacturers)
Di-Spaz (Vortech)
TYPE OF DRUG
Antispasmodic
INGREDIENT
dicyclomine
DOSAGE FORMS
Tablets (20 mg)
Capsules (10 mg and 20 mg)
Oral liquid (10 mg per 5-ml spoonful)
STORAGE
Dicyclomine tablets, capsules, and oral liquid should be stored at room temperature in tightly closed containers. This medication should never be frozen.

USES
Dicyclomine is used to treat gastrointestinal tract disorders and irritable bowel syndrome. Dicyclomine acts directly on the muscles of the gastrointestinal tract to decrease tone and slow their activity.

TREATMENT
Dicyclomine can be taken before or after meals. Consult your doctor for specific recommendations.

Antacids and antidiarrheal medicines may prevent absorption of this drug; therefore, at least one hour should separate doses of dicyclomine and one of these medications.

Measure the liquid form of dicyclomine carefully with a specially designed 5-ml measuring spoon. An ordinary kitchen teaspoon is not accurate enough. You can then dilute the oral liquid in other liquids to mask its taste.

If you miss a dose of this medication, do not take the missed dose at all; just return to your regular dosing schedule. Do not double the next dose.

SIDE EFFECTS
Minor. Bloating; blurred vision; confusion; constipation; dizziness; drowsiness; dry mouth, throat, and nose; headache; increased sensitivity to light; insomnia; loss of taste; nausea; nervousness; decreased sweating; vomiting; or weakness. These side effects should disappear as your body adjusts to the medication.

If you are constipated, increase the amount of fiber in your diet (fresh fruits and vegetables, salads, bran, and whole-grain breads), exercise, and drink more water (unless your doctor directs you to do otherwise).

Chew sugarless gum or suck on ice chips or a piece of hard candy to reduce mouth dryness.

Wear sunglasses if your eyes become sensitive to light.

To avoid dizziness or light-headedness when you stand, contract and relax the muscles of your legs for a few moments before rising. Do this by pushing one foot against the floor while raising the other foot slightly, alternating feet so that you are "pumping" your legs in a pedaling motion.

Major. Be sure to tell your doctor about any side effects that are persistent or particularly bothersome. IT IS ESPECIALLY IMPORTANT TO TELL YOUR DOCTOR about difficulty in urinating, fever, hallucinations, impotence, palpitations, rash, short-term memory loss, or sore throat.

INTERACTIONS
Dicyclomine does interact with several other types of medications:

1. It can cause extreme drowsiness when combined with central nervous system depressants (such as alcohol, antihistamines, barbiturates, benzodiazepine tranquilizers, muscle relaxants, narcotics, pain medications, and phenothiazine tranquilizers) or with tricyclic antidepressants.

2. Amantadine, antihistamines, haloperidol, monoamine oxidase (MAO) inhibitors, phenothiazine tranquilizers, procainamide, quinidine, and tricyclic antidepressants can increase the side effects of dicyclomine.

BE SURE TO TELL YOUR DOCTOR about any medications you are currently taking, especially those listed above.

WARNINGS
• Be sure to tell your doctor about unusual or allergic reactions you have had to any medications, especially to dicyclomine.

• Tell your doctor if you have ever had glaucoma; heart disease; hiatal hernia; high blood pressure; kidney, liver, or thyroid disease; myasthenia gravis; obstructed bladder; obstructed intestine; enlarged prostate gland; ulcerative colitis; or internal bleeding.

• If this medication makes you dizzy or drowsy or blurs your vision, do not take part in any activity that requires alertness, such as driving a car or operating potentially dangerous equipment. Be careful on stairs, and avoid getting up from a lying or sitting position suddenly.

• This drug can decrease sweating and heat release from the body. Avoid taking hot baths, showers, or saunas, and avoid getting overheated by exercising in hot weather.

• Before having surgery or other medical or dental treatment, tell your doctor or dentist you are taking this drug.

• Tell your doctor if you are pregnant. Although this drug appears to be safe during pregnancy, extensive studies in humans have not been conducted. Also, tell your doctor if you are breast-feeding an infant. Small amounts of dicyclomine pass into breast milk.

dicyclomine hydrochloride—see dicyclomine

diethylpropion

BRAND NAMES (Manufacturers)
diethylpropion hydrochloride (various manufacturers)
Tenuate (Lakeside Pharmaceutical)
Tenuate Dospan (Lakeside Pharmaceutical)
Tepanil (Riker)
Tepanil Ten-Tab (Riker)

TYPE OF DRUG
Anorectic
INGREDIENT
diethylpropion
DOSAGE FORMS
Tablets (25 mg)
Sustained-release tablets (75 mg)
STORAGE
Diethylpropion tablets should be stored at room temperature in tightly closed, light-resistant containers.

USES

Diethylpropion is used as an appetite suppressant during the first few weeks of dieting to help establish new eating habits. This medication is thought to relieve hunger by altering nerve impulses to the appetite control center in the brain. Its effectiveness lasts only for short periods (three to 12 weeks), however.

TREATMENT

You can take diethylpropion with a full glass of water one hour before meals (unless your doctor directs you to do otherwise).

In order to avoid difficulty in falling asleep, the last dose of this medication each day should be taken four to six hours before bedtime (regular tablets) or ten to 14 hours before bedtime (sustained-release tablets).

The sustained-release form of this medication should be swallowed whole. Breaking, chewing, or crushing these tablets destroys their sustained-release activity and may increase the side effects.

If you miss a dose, take the missed dose as soon as possible, unless it is almost time for your next dose. In that case, do not take the missed dose; just return to your regular dosing schedule. Do not double the next dose.

SIDE EFFECTS

Minor. Blurred vision, constipation, diarrhea, dizziness, dry mouth, euphoria, fatigue, insomnia, irritability, nausea, nervousness, restlessness, stomach pain, sweating, tremors, unpleasant taste in the mouth, or vomiting. These side effects should disappear as your body adjusts to the medication.

Dry mouth can be relieved by sucking on ice chips or a piece of hard candy or by chewing sugarless gum.

In order to prevent constipation, increase the amount of fiber in your diet (fresh fruits and vegetables, salads, bran, and whole-grain breads), exercise, and drink more water (unless your doctor directs you to do otherwise).
Major. Tell your doctor about any side effects that are persistent or particularly bothersome. IT IS ESPECIALLY IMPORTANT TO TELL YOUR DOCTOR about changes in sexual desire, chest pain, difficulty in urinating, enlarged breasts (in both sexes), fever, hair loss, headaches, impotence, menstrual irregularities, mental depression, mood changes, mouth sores, muscle pains, nosebleeds, palpitations, rash, or sore throat.

INTERACTIONS

Diethylpropion interacts with several other types of drugs:
1. Use of diethylpropion within 14 days of use of a monoamine oxidase (MAO) inhibitor (such as isocar-boxazid, pargyline, phenelzine, and tranylcypromine) can result in high blood pressure and other side effects.
2. Barbiturate medications and phenothiazine tranquilizers (especially chlorpromazine) can antagonize (act against) the appetite suppressant activity of this medication, decreasing its effectiveness.
3. Diethylpropion can decrease the blood-pressure-lowering effects of antihypertensive medications (especially guanethidine) and may alter some insulin and oral antidiabetic medication dosages requirement in some diabetic patients.
4. The side effects of other central nervous system stimulants (such as caffeine and nonprescription appetite suppressants and cough, allergy, asthma, sinus, and cold preparations) may be increased by this medication.

BE SURE TO TELL YOUR DOCTOR about any medications you are currently taking, especially any listed above.

WARNINGS

• Be sure to tell your doctor about unusual or allergic reactions you have had to any medications, especially to diethylpropion or other appetite suppressants (including benzphetamine, phendimetrazine, phenmetrazine, fenfluramine, mazindol, and phentermine), or to epinephrine, norepinephrine, ephedrine, amphetamine, dextroamphetamine, phenylephrine, phenylpropanolamine, pseudoephedrine, albuterol, metaproterenol, or terbutaline.
• Tell your doctor if you have a history of drug abuse, or if you have ever had angina, diabetes mellitus, emotional disturbances, glaucoma, heart or cardiovascular disease, high blood pressure, thyroid disease, or epilepsy.
• Diethylpropion can mask the symptoms of extreme fatigue and can cause dizziness or light-headedness. Your ability to perform tasks that require alertness, such as driving a car or operating potentially dangerous equipment, may be decreased. Appropriate caution should, therefore, be taken.
• Before surgery or other medical or dental treatment, tell your doctor or dentist you are taking diethylpropion.
• Diethylpropion is related to amphetamine and may be habit-forming when taken for long periods (both physical and psychological dependence can occur). Therefore, you should not increase the dosage of this drug or take it for longer than 12 weeks unless you first consult your doctor. It is also important that you not stop taking this drug abruptly if you have been taking large doses for a long time. Fatigue, sleep disorders, mental depression, nausea or vomiting, or stomach cramps or pain could occur. Your doctor may want to decrease your dosage gradually.
• Be sure to tell your doctor if you are pregnant. Although side effects in humans have not been thoroughly studied, some of the appetite suppressants such as, diethylpropion, have been shown to cause side effects in the fetuses of animals that received large doses during pregnancy. Also, tell your doctor if you are breast-feeding an infant. It is not known whether this medication passes into breast milk.

diethylpropion hydrochloride—see diethylpropion

diflunisal

BRAND NAME (Manufacturer)
Dolobid (Merck Sharp & Dohme)
TYPE OF DRUG
Nonsteroidal anti-inflammatory analgesic
INGREDIENT
diflunisal
DOSAGE FORM
Tablets (250 mg and 500 mg)
STORAGE
This medication should be stored in a closed container at room temperature, away from heat and direct sunlight.

USES

Diflunisal is used to treat the inflammation (pain, swelling, and stiffness) of osteoarthritis and muscle or skeletal injury. Diflunisal has been shown to block the production of certain body chemicals, called prostaglandins, that may trigger pain. However, it is not yet fully understood how diflunisal works.

TREATMENT

You should take this drug immediately after meals or with food in order to reduce stomach irritation. Do not break, crush, or chew the tablets before swallowing—they should be swallowed whole to lessen side effects and to maintain their benefits for a full 12 hours. Ask your doctor if you can take diflunisal with an antacid.

If you are taking diflunisal to relieve osteoarthritis, you must take it regularly, as directed by your doctor. It may take several days before you feel the full benefits of this medication. Diflunisal does not cure osteoarthritis, but it will help to control the condition as long as you continue to take the medication.

It is important to take diflunisal on schedule and not to miss any doses. If you do miss a dose of this medication, take the missed dose as soon as possible, unless more than six hours has passed. In that case, do not take the missed dose at all; just return to your regular dosing schedule. Do not double the next dose.

SIDE EFFECTS

Minor. Bloating, constipation, diarrhea, difficulty in sleeping, dizziness, drowsiness, headache, heartburn, indigestion, light-headedness, loss of appetite, nausea, nervousness, unusual sweating, or vomiting. As your body adjusts to the drug, these side effects should disappear.

To relieve constipation, increase the amount of fiber in your diet (fresh fruits and vegetables, salads, bran, and whole-grain breads), exercise, and drink more water (unless your doctor directs you to do otherwise).

If you become dizzy, sit or lie down for a while; get up slowly from a sitting or reclining position, and be careful on stairs.

Major. Tell your doctor about any side effects that are persistent or particularly bothersome. IT IS ESPECIALLY IMPORTANT TO TELL YOUR DOCTOR about bloody or black, tarry stools; blurred vision; confusion; depression; difficult or painful urination; difficulty in breathing; palpitations; ringing or buzzing in the ears or difficulty in hearing; skin rash, hives, or itching; stomach pain; swelling of the feet; tightness in the chest; unexplained sore throat and fever; unusual bleeding or bruising; unusual fatigue or weakness; unusual weight gain; wheezing; or yellowing of the eyes or skin.

INTERACTIONS

Diflunisal interacts with several other types of medications:

1. Anticoagulants (blood thinners, such as warfarin), in combination with diflunisal, can lead to an increase in bleeding complications.
2. Aspirin, salicylates, or other anti-inflammatory medications may cause increased stomach irritation.
3. Antacids can lower blood diflunisal concentrations, decreasing its effectiveness.
4. Diflunisal can increase the blood concentrations and side effects of acetaminophen.
5. Diflunisal can increase or decrease some effects of hydrochlorothiazide and furosemide.

BE SURE TO TELL YOUR DOCTOR about any medications you are currently taking, especially those listed above.

WARNINGS

• Before you take this medication, it is important to tell your doctor if you have ever had unusual or allergic reactions to diflunisal or any chemically related drug (including aspirin or other salicylates, diclofenac, fenoprofen, flurbiprofen, ibuprofen, indomethacin, ketoprofen, meclofenamate, mefenamic acid, naproxen, oxyphenbutazone, phenylbutazone, piroxicam, sulindac, or tolmetin).

• Before you take this medication, tell your doctor if you now have or if you have ever had bleeding problems, colitis, stomach ulcers or other stomach problems, epilepsy, heart disease, high blood pressure, asthma, kidney disease, liver disease, mental illness, or Parkinson's disease.

• Be sure to tell your doctor if this drug makes you dizzy or drowsy, do not take part in any activity that requires alertness, such as driving a car or operating potentially dangerous equipment.

• Because diflunisal can prolong your bleeding time, it is important to tell your doctor or dentist that you are taking this drug before having surgery or any other medical or dental treatment.

• Stomach problems are more likely to occur if you take aspirin regularly or drink alcohol while being treated with this medication. These should, therefore, be avoided (unless your doctor directs you to do otherwise).

• Be sure to tell your doctor if you are pregnant. Although studies in humans have not been conducted, unwanted side effects (defects in the spine and ribs) have been reported in the offspring of animals that received diflunisal during pregnancy. If taken during the last three months of pregnancy, this drug can cause heart problems in the fetus; it can also prolong labor. Also, tell your doctor if you are breast-feeding an infant. Because diflunisal can pass into breast milk, breast-feeding while taking this drug is not recommended.

digitoxin

BRAND NAME (Manufacturer)
digitoxin (various manufacturers)
TYPE OF DRUG
Cardiac glycoside
INGREDIENT
digitoxin
DOSAGE FORM
Tablets (0.1 mg and 0.2 mg)
STORAGE
Store at room temperature in a tightly closed container.

USES

Digitoxin belongs to a group of drugs known as digitalis glycosides. It is used to treat heart arrhythmias and congestive heart failure. Digitoxin improves the strength and efficiency of the heart and controls the heart rhythm.

TREATMENT

To avoid stomach irritation, take digitoxin with food, water, or milk (unless your doctor directs you to do otherwise).

In order to become accustomed to taking this medication, try to take it at the same time each day.

If you miss a dose of this medication, take the missed dose as soon as possible, unless it is almost time for the next dose. In that case, do not take the missed dose at all; just return to your regular dosing schedule. Do not double the next dose. If you miss two or more doses, check with your doctor.

Digitoxin does not cure heart failure, but it will help to control the condition as long as you continue to take it.

SIDE EFFECTS

Minor. Drowsiness, headache, loss of appetite, nausea, stomach upset, or vomiting. These side effects should disappear as your body adjusts to the medication.
Major. Tell your doctor about any side effects that are persistent or particularly bothersome. IT IS ESPECIALLY IMPORTANT TO TELL YOUR DOCTOR about bad dreams, blurred vision, breast enlargement (in both sexes), confusion, depression, disorientation, hallucinations, muscle weakness, palpitations, or tingling sensations.

INTERACTIONS

Digitoxin interacts with several other types of medications:
1. Barbiturates, phenytoin, aminoglutethimide, levodopa, penicillamine, phenylbutazone, and rifampin can decrease the blood levels and effectiveness of digitoxin.
2. The absorption of digitoxin from the gastrointestinal tract is reduced when it is taken with colestipol, cholestyramine, metoclopramide, antacids, neomycin, antineoplastic (anticancer) drugs, or sulfasalazine.
3. Tetracycline can increase the absorption of digitoxin from the gastrointestinal tract, which can increase the risk of side effects.
4. Spironolactone can unpredictably increase or decrease the side effects of digitoxin.
5. Concurrent use of quinidine, procainamide, hydrox-

ychloroquine, calcium, reserpine, ephedrine, or beta blockers (acebutolol, atenolol, betaxolol, carteolol, esmolol, labetalol, metoprolol, nadolol, penbutolol, pindolol, propranolol, and timolol) with digitoxin can lead to additive effects on the heart.
6. The dosage of digitoxin may require adjustment if therapy with thyroid hormones, methimazole, or propylthiouracil is started.
7. Concurrent use of digitoxin and quinidine, quinine, erythromycin, amiodarone, benzodiazepine tranquilizers, diltiazem, nifedipine, or verapamil can increase the blood levels and the side effects of digitoxin.

BE SURE TO TELL YOUR DOCTOR about any medications you are currently taking, especially those listed above.

WARNINGS

• Tell your doctor about unusual or allergic reactions you have had to medications, especially to digitoxin or any other digitalis glycoside.
• Before starting to take this medication, be sure to tell your doctor if you now have or if you have ever had blood electrolyte disorders (too much or too little calcium, magnesium, or potassium), heart disease, kidney disease, lung disease, liver disease, or thyroid disease.
• Before having surgery or any other medical or dental treatment, be sure to tell your doctor or dentist that you are taking this medication.
• Check with your doctor or pharmacist before taking any over-the-counter (nonprescription) allergy, asthma, cough, cold, diet, or sinus products. Some of these products can increase the side effects of digitoxin.
• Do not stop taking this medication unless you first check with your doctor. Stopping abruptly may lead to a worsening of your condition.
• While you are taking digitoxin, your doctor may want you to check your pulse every day. If your pulse is slower than your doctor has told you it should be or if the rhythm is irregular, CONTACT YOUR DOCTOR IMMEDIATELY.
• Be sure to tell your doctor if you are pregnant. Although digitoxin appears to be safe during pregnancy, extensive studies in humans have not been conducted. In addition, the dosage of digitoxin required to control your disorder may change during pregnancy. Also, tell your doctor if you are breast-feeding an infant. It is not known if digitoxin passes into breast milk.

digoxin

BRAND NAMES (Manufacturers)
digoxin (various manufacturers)
Lanoxicaps (Burroughs Wellcome)
Lanoxin (Burroughs Wellcome)
TYPE OF DRUG
Cardiac glycoside
INGREDIENT
digoxin
DOSAGE FORMS
Tablets (0.125 mg, 0.25 mg, and 0.5 mg)

Capsules (0.05 mg, 0.1 mg, and 0.2 mg)
Pediatric elixir (0.05 mg per ml, with 10% alcohol)

STORAGE

Digoxin tablets, capsules, and pediatric elixir should be stored at room temperature in tightly closed, light-resistant containers. This medication should never be frozen.

USES

Digoxin is used to treat heart arrhythmias and congestive heart failure. It works directly on the muscle of the heart to strengthen the heartbeat and improve heart rhythm and contraction.

TREATMENT

To avoid stomach irritation, take digoxin with water or with food. Try to take it at the same time every day.

Measure the dose of the pediatric elixir carefully with the dropper provided. An ordinary kitchen teaspoon is not accurate enough.

Antacids decrease the absorption of digoxin from the gastrointestinal tract. Therefore, if you are taking both digoxin and an antacid, the dose of digoxin should be taken one hour before or two hours after a dose of antacids.

Try not to miss any doses of this medication. If you do miss a dose, take the missed dose as soon as possible, unless it is almost time for the next dose. In that case, do not take the missed dose at all; just return to your regular dosing schedule. Do not double the next dose. If you miss more than two doses of digoxin, contact your doctor.

Digoxin does not cure congestive heart failure, but it will help to control the condition as long as you continue to take the medication.

SIDE EFFECTS

Minor. Apathy, diarrhea, drowsiness, headache, muscle weakness, or tiredness. These side effects should disappear as your body adjusts to the medication.

Major. Tell your doctor about any side effects that are persistent or particularly bothersome. IT IS ESPECIALLY IMPORTANT TO TELL YOUR DOCTOR about disorientation, enlarged and painful breasts (in both sexes), hallucinations, loss of appetite, mental depression, nausea, palpitations, severe abdominal pain, slowed heart rate, visual disturbances (such as blurred or yellow vision), or vomiting.

INTERACTIONS

Digoxin interacts with several other types of medications (interactions may vary depending upon the dosage form of digoxin being used):

1. Penicillamine, antiseizure medications, rifampin, amino-glutethimide, and levodopa can decrease the blood levels and, therefore, the effectiveness of digoxin.

2. Erythromycin, amiodarone, captopril, benzodiazepine tranquilizers, flecainide, tetracycline, hydroxychloroquine, ibuprofen, indomethacin, verapamil, nifedipine, diltiazem, quinidine, quinine, and spironolactone can increase the blood levels of digoxin, which can lead to an increase in side effects.

3. Thyroid hormone, propylthiouracil, and methimazole can change the dosage requirements of digoxin.

4. Antacids, kaolin-pectin, sulfasalazine, aminosalicylic acid, metoclopramide, antineoplastic agents (anticancer drugs), neomycin, colestipol, and cholestyramine can decrease the absorption of digoxin from the gastrointestinal tract, decreasing its effectiveness.

5. Calcium, tolbutamide, and reserpine can increase the side effects of digoxin.

6. Diuretics (water pills) and adrenocorticosteroids (cortisone-like medications) can cause hypokalemia (low potassium blood levels).

BE SURE TO TELL YOUR DOCTOR about any medications you are currently taking.

WARNINGS

• Tell your doctor about unusual or allergic reactions you have had to any medications, especially to digoxin, digitoxin, or any other digitalis glycoside.

• Tell your doctor if you now have or if you have ever had kidney disease, lung disease, thyroid disease, hypokalemia (low blood levels of potassium), or hypercalcemia (high blood levels of calcium).

• The pharmacologic activity of the different brands of this drug varies widely—the tablets dissolve in the stomach and bowel at different rates and to varying degrees. Because of this variability, it is important not to change brands of the drug without consulting your doctor.

• Meals high in bran fiber may reduce the absorption of digoxin from the gastrointestinal tract. Avoid these types of meals when taking your dose of medication.

• Your doctor may want you to take your pulse daily while you are using digoxin. Contact your doctor if your pulse becomes slower than what your doctor tells you is normal, or if it drops below 50 beats per minute.

• Before having surgery or any other medical or dental treatment, be sure to tell your doctor or dentist that you are taking this medication.

• Before taking any over-the-counter (nonprescription) asthma, allergy, cough, cold, sinus, or diet product, be sure to check with your doctor or pharmacist. Some of these drugs can increase the side effects of digoxin.

• Be sure to tell your doctor if you are pregnant. Although this drug appears to be safe during pregnancy, extensive studies in humans have not been conducted. In addition, the dosage of digoxin required to control your symptoms may change during pregnancy. Also, tell your doctor if you are breast-feeding an infant. Small amounts of digoxin pass into breast milk.

dihydrotachysterol

BRAND NAMES (Manufacturers)
dihydrotachysterol or DHT (Roxane)
Hytakerol (Winthrop)

TYPE OF DRUG
Vitamin D analog

INGREDIENT
dihydrotachysterol

DOSAGE FORMS
Tablets (0.125 mg, 0.2 mg, and 0.4 mg)
Capsules (0.125 mg)

Oral solution (0.25 mg per ml in oil)
Oral concentrate (0.2 mg per ml, with 20% alcohol)

STORAGE

Dihydrotachysterol tablets, capsules, oral solution, and oral concentrate should be stored at room temperature in tightly closed, light-resistant containers. This medication should never be frozen.

USES

Vitamin D is essential to many body systems (including muscle and heart function). Dihydrotachysterol is a vitamin D analog—it raises blood calcium levels. This medication is used to treat tetany and hypoparathyroidism, conditions characterized by low blood calcium levels.

TREATMENT

You can take dihydrotachysterol either on an empty stomach or with food or milk (as directed by your doctor).

Each dose of the oral solution form of this medication should be measured carefully with the dropper provided. The solution can then be swallowed directly or mixed with fruit juice, cereal, or other foods.

If you miss a dose of this medication, take the missed dose as soon as possible, unless it is almost time for the next dose. In that case, do not take the missed dose; just return to your regular dosing schedule. Do not double the dose.

SIDE EFFECTS

Minor. None, at the dosages normally prescribed.
Major. The side effects associated with dihydrotachysterol therapy are usually the result of too much medication (vitamin D intoxication). Tell your doctor about any side effects that are persistent or particularly bothersome. IT IS ESPECIALLY IMPORTANT TO TELL YOUR DOCTOR about blurred vision, bone pain, constipation, dry mouth, headache, increased thirst, increased urination, irritability, loss of appetite, mental disorders, metallic taste in the mouth, muscle pain, nausea, palpitations, runny nose, vomiting, weakness, or weight loss.

INTERACTIONS

This drug interacts with several other drugs.
1. If you are being treated for hypoparathyroidism, concurrent use of dihydrotachysterol and thiazide diuretics (water pills) can lead to hypercalcemia (high blood calcium levels).
2. The effects of this medication may be increased or decreased by digoxin, antacids, verapamil, or cholestyramine.

BE SURE TO TELL YOUR DOCTOR about any medications you are currently taking, especially any listed above.

WARNINGS

Tell your doctor about unusual or allergic reactions you have had to any medications, especially to dihydrotachysterol, calcitriol, calcifediol, ergocalciferol, or vitamin D.

Before starting to take this medication, it is very important that you tell your doctor if you now have or if you have ever had heart or blood vessel disease, hyper-calcemia, hyperphosphatemia, vitamin D intoxication, or sarcoidosis.

Before taking any over-the-counter (nonprescription) products that contain calcium, phosphates, magnesium, or vitamin D, check with your doctor. These ingredients can increase the side effects of dihydrotachysterol.

Dihydrotachysterol is more expensive than vitamin D products, but it is often prescribed instead of vitamin D because it is faster-acting and does not persist in the body once therapy is stopped.

Be sure to tell your doctor if you are pregnant. Although dihydrotachysterol has not been studied during pregnancy in humans, birth defects have been reported in the offspring of animals that received large doses of this medication during pregnancy. Also, tell your doctor if you are breast-feeding an infant. It is not known if this drug passes into breast milk.

Dilantin—see phenytoin

Dilantin Infatab—see phenytoin

Dilantin Kapseal—see phenytoin

Dilatrate-SR—see isosorbide dinitrate

Dilaudid—see hydromorphone

---

diltiazem

BRAND NAMES (Manufacturers)
Cardizem (Marion-Merrell Dow)
Cardizem CD (Marion-Merrell Dow)
Cardizem SR (Marion-Merrell Dow)

TYPE OF DRUG
Antianginal and antihypertensive

INGREDIENT
diltiazem

DOSAGE FORMS
Extended-release capsules (180 mg, 240 mg, and 300 mg)
Tablets (30 mg, 60 mg, 90 mg, and 120 mg)
Sustained-release capsules (60 mg, 90 mg, and 120 mg)

STORAGE
Diltiazem should be stored at room temperature in a tightly closed container.

USES

This medication is used to prevent the symptoms of angina (chest pain). It belongs to a group of drugs known as calcium channel blockers. It is unclear exactly how it does so, but diltiazem dilates the blood vessels of the heart and increases the amount of oxygen that reaches the heart muscle. This drug is also prescribed to lower blood pressure in patients with hypertension.

TREATMENT

If stomach irritation occurs, diltiazem can be taken either on an empty stomach or with meals, as directed by your doctor. The sustained-release capsules should be swallowed whole; chewing, crushing, or crumbling them destroys their controlled-release activity and possibly increases the side effects.

In order to become accustomed to taking this medication, try to take it at the same times each day.

However, Diltiazem does not relieve chest pain once the pain has begun; this medication should be used to prevent angina attacks.

If you miss a dose of this medication, take the missed dose as soon as possible, unless it is within four hours of the next scheduled dose. In that case, do not take the missed dose at all; just return to your regular dosing schedule. Do not double the next dose.

This medication does not cure angina, but it will help to control the condition as long as you continue to take it.

SIDE EFFECTS

Minor. Constipation, diarrhea, dizziness, drowsiness, headache, insomnia, light-headedness, nausea, nervousness, stomach upset, or vomiting. These side effects should disappear as your body adjusts to the medication.

This drug can increase your sensitivity to sunlight. Therefore, avoid prolonged exposure to sunlight and sunlamps. Wear protective clothing and sunglasses, and use an effective sunscreen.

If you feel dizzy or light-headed, sit or lie down for a while; get up slowly from a sitting or reclining position, and be careful on stairs. To avoid dizziness when you stand, relax and contract the muscles of your legs for a few moments before rising. Do this by pushing one foot against the floor while raising the other foot slightly, alternating feet so that you are "pumping" your legs in a pedaling motion.

To relieve constipation, increase the amount of fiber in your diet (fresh fruits and vegetables, salads, bran, and whole-grain breads), exercise, and drink more water (unless your doctor directs you to do otherwise).

Major. Tell your doctor about any side effects that are persistent or particularly bothersome. IT IS ESPECIALLY IMPORTANT TO TELL YOUR DOCTOR about confusion, depression, fainting, fatigue, flushing, fluid retention, hallucinations, palpitations, skin rash, tingling in the fingers or toes, unusual weakness, or yellowing of the eyes or skin.

INTERACTIONS

Diltiazem can interact with several other medications:
1. Diltiazem should be used cautiously with beta blockers (acebutolol, atenolol, betaxolol, carteolol, esmolol, labetalol, metoprolol, nadolol, penbutolol, propranolol, pindolol, and timolol), digitoxin, digoxin, or disopyramide. Side effects on the heart may be increased by the concurrent use of these medications.
2. Cimetidine can decrease the elimination of diltiazem from the body, which can increase the risk of side effects.
3. Diltiazem can increase the blood concentrations of carbamazepine and cyclosporine, which can increase the risk of side effects.

BE SURE TO TELL YOUR DOCTOR about any medications you are currently taking, especially any listed above.

WARNINGS

• Tell your doctor about unusual or allergic reactions you have had to any medications, especially to diltiazem.
• Be sure to tell your doctor if you now have or if you have ever had bradycardia (slow heartbeat), heart block, heart failure, kidney disease, liver disease, low blood pressure, or sick sinus syndrome.
• If this drug makes you dizzy or drowsy, avoid taking part in any activity that requires alertness, such as driving a car or operating potentially dangerous equipment.
• To prevent fainting while taking this drug, avoid drinking large amounts of alcohol. Also, avoid prolonged standing and strenuous exercise in hot weather.
• Be sure to tell your doctor if you are pregnant. Extensive studies in pregnant women have not been conducted, but birth defects have been reported in the offspring of animals that received large doses of diltiazem during pregnancy. It is also known that diltiazem passes into breast milk. If you are breast-feeding an infant while being treated with this medication, tell your doctor. Unless directed to do otherwise, breast-feeding is not recommended at this time.

Dimetane—see brompheniramine

Dimetane Extentabs—see brompheniramine

Dimetapp Extentabs—see phenylpropanolamine, phenylephrine, and brompheniramine combination

Diphenatol—see diphenoxylate and atropine combination

Diphen Cough Syrup—see diphenhydramine

diphenhydramine

BRAND NAMES (Manufacturers)
AllerMax (Pfeiffer)
Belix* (Halsey)
Benadryl* (Parke-Davis)
Benadryl Kapseals (Parke-Davis)
Benylin Cough Syrup* (Parke-Davis)
Bydramine Cough Syrup* (Major)
Compoz* (Jeffrey Martin)
Diphen Cough Syrup* (My-K Lab)
diphenhydramine hydrochloride (various manufacturers)
Dormarex 2* (Republic)
Hydramine* (Goldline)
Nervine Nighttime Sleep Aid* (Miles)
Nordryl (Vortech)
Nytol (Block)
Sleep-Eze 3* (Whitehall)
Sominex 2* (Beecham)
Tusstat (Century)
Twilite* (Pfeiffer)
Unisom Nighttime Sleep Aid (Leeming)
*Available over-the-counter (without a prescription)
TYPE OF DRUG
Antihistamine and sedative/hypnotic

INGREDIENT
diphenhydramine
DOSAGE FORMS
Tablets (50 mg)
Capsules (25 mg and 50 mg)
Elixir (12.5 mg per 5-ml spoonful, with 14% alcohol)
Oral syrup (12.5 mg per 5-ml spoonful, with 5% alcohol)
STORAGE
Store at room temperature in a tightly closed container.

USES
Diphenhydramine belongs to a group of drugs known as antihistamines (antihistamines block the action of histamine, a chemical that is released by the body during an allergic reaction). It is, therefore, used to treat or prevent symptoms of allergy. It is also used to treat motion sickness and Parkinson's disease, and it is used as a nighttime sleeping aid and nonnarcotic cough suppressant.

TREATMENT
To avoid stomach upset, take diphenhydramine with food, milk, or water (unless your doctor directs you otherwise).

The elixir and oral syrup forms of this medication should be measured carefully with a specially designed 5-ml measuring spoon. An ordinary teaspoon is not accurate enough.

If you miss a dose of this medication, take the missed dose as soon as possible, unless it is almost time for your next dose. In that case, do not take the missed dose at all; just return to your regular dosing schedule. Do not double the next dose.

SIDE EFFECTS
Minor. Blurred vision; confusion; constipation; diarrhea; dizziness; dry mouth, throat, or nose; headache; irritability; loss of appetite; nausea; restlessness; stomach upset; or unusual increase in sweating. These side effects should disappear as your body adjusts to the medication.

This medication can cause increased sensitivity to sunlight. It is, therefore, important to avoid prolonged exposure to sunlight and sunlamps. Wear protective clothing, and use an effective sunscreen.

If you are constipated, increase the amount of fiber in your diet (fresh fruits and vegetables, salads, bran, and whole-grain breads), exercise, and drink more water (unless your doctor tells you not to do so).

To reduce mouth dryness, chew sugarless gum or suck on ice chips or a piece of hard candy.

If you feel dizzy or light-headed, sit or lie down for a while; get up slowly from a sitting or reclining position, and be careful on stairs.

Major. Tell your doctor about any side effects that are persistent or particularly bothersome. IT IS ESPECIALLY IMPORTANT TO TELL YOUR DOCTOR about changes in menstruation, clumsiness, difficult or painful urination, feeling faint, flushing of the face, hallucinations, palpitations, ringing or buzzing in the ears, rash, seizures, shortness of breath, sleeping disorders, sore throat or fever, tightness in the chest, unusual bleeding or bruising, or unusual tiredness or weakness.

INTERACTIONS
Diphenhydramine interacts with several other types of medications:

1. Concurrent use of it with other central nervous system depressants (such as alcohol, barbiturates, benzodiazepine tranquilizers, muscle relaxants, narcotics, pain medications, and phenothiazine tranquilizers) or with tricyclic antidepressants can cause extreme drowsiness.

2. Monoamine oxidase (MAO) inhibitors (isocarboxazid, pargyline, phenelzine, and tranylcypromine) can increase the side effects of this medication. At least 14 days should separate the use of this drug and the use of an MAO inhibitor.

3. Diphenhydramine can also interfere with the activity of oral anticoagulants (blood thinners, such as warfarin) and decrease their effectiveness.

BE SURE TO TELL YOUR DOCTOR about any medications you are currently taking, especially any of those listed above.

WARNINGS
• Be sure to tell your doctor about unusual or allergic reactions you have had to any medications, especially to diphenhydramine or to any other antihistamine (such as astemizole, azatadine, brompheniramine, carbinoxamine, chlorpheniramine, clemastine, cyproheptadine, dexchlorpheniramine, dimenhydrinate, dimethindene, diphenylpyraline, doxylamine, hydroxyzine, phenindamine, promethazine, pyrilamine, terfenadine, trimeprazine, tripelennamine, and triprolidine).

• Tell your doctor if you now have or if you have ever had asthma, blood vessel disease, glaucoma, high blood pressure, kidney disease, peptic ulcers, enlarged prostate gland, or thyroid disease.

• Diphenhydramine can cause drowsiness or dizziness. Your ability to perform tasks that require alertness, such as driving a car or operating potentially dangerous equipment, may be decreased. Appropriate caution should, therefore, be taken.

• Be sure to tell your doctor if you are pregnant. The effects of this medication during pregnancy have not been thoroughly studied in humans. Also, tell your doctor if you are breast-feeding an infant. Small amounts of diphenhydramine pass into breast milk and may cause unusual excitement or irritability in nursing infants.

diphenhydramine hydrochloride—see diphenhydramine

---

diphenoxylate and atropine combination

BRAND NAMES (Manufacturers)
Diphenatol (Rugby)
diphenoxylate hydrochloride with atropine sulfate (various manufacturers)
Lofene (Lannett)
Logen (Goldline)
Lomanate (Barre)
Lomotil (Searle)

Lonox (Geneva Generics)
Low-Quel (Halsey)

TYPE OF DRUG

Antidiarrheal (antispasmodic and anticholinergic)

INGREDIENTS

diphenoxylate and atropine

DOSAGE FORMS

Tablets (2.5 mg diphenoxylate and 0.025 mg atropine)
Oral liquid (2.5 mg diphenoxylate and 0.025 mg atropine per 5-ml spoonful, with 15% alcohol)

STORAGE

Diphenoxylate and atropine combination tablets and oral liquid should be stored at room temperature in tightly closed, light-resistant containers. Neither form should be frozen.

USES

Diphenoxylate and atropine combination is used to treat severe diarrhea. Diphenoxylate is related to the narcotic analgesics and acts by slowing the movement of the gastrointestinal tract. Small amounts of atropine are added to this medication in order to prevent abuse of the narcotic diphenoxylate.

TREATMENT

In order to avoid stomach upset, you can take this medication with food or with a full glass of water or milk.

The oral liquid form of this medication should be measured carefully using a specially designed 5-ml measuring spoon. An ordinary kitchen teaspoon is not accurate enough.

If you miss a dose of this medication, do not take the missed dose at all; just return to your regular dosing schedule. Do not double the next dose.

SIDE EFFECTS

Minor. Blurred vision, constipation, dizziness, drowsiness, dry mouth, flushing, headache, loss of appetite, nervousness, sweating, or swollen gums. These side effects should disappear as your body adjusts to the medication.

To relieve mouth dryness, chew sugarless gum or suck on ice chips or a piece of hard candy.

If you feel dizzy or light-headed, sit or lie down for a while; get up slowly from a sitting or reclining position, and be careful on stairs.

Major. Tell your doctor about any side effects that are persistent or particularly bothersome. IT IS ESPECIALLY IMPORTANT TO TELL YOUR DOCTOR about abdominal pain, bloating, breathing difficulties, depression, difficult or painful urination, false sense of well-being, fever, hives, itching, numbness in the fingers or toes, palpitations, rash, severe nausea, vomiting, or weakness.

INTERACTIONS

This medication interacts with several other types of medications:

1. Concurrent use of this medication with central nervous system depressants (such as alcohol, antihistamines, barbiturates, benzodiazepine tranquilizers, muscle relaxants, narcotics, pain medications, and phenothiazine tranquilizers) or with tricyclic antidepressants can cause extreme drowsiness.

2. A monoamine oxidase (MAO) inhibitor (tranylcypromine, phenelzine, isocarboxazid, and pargyline) taken within 14 days of this medication can lead to unpredictable and severe side effects.

3. The side effects of the atropine component of this medication may be increased by amantadine, haloperidol, phenothiazine tranquilizers, procainamide, and quinidine.

BE SURE TO TELL YOUR DOCTOR about any medications you are currently taking, especially any of those listed above.

WARNINGS

• Tell your doctor about unusual or allergic reactions you have had to medications, especially to diphenoxylate or to atropine.

• Tell your doctor if you now have or if you have ever had drug-induced diarrhea, gallstones or gallbladder disease, glaucoma, heart disease, hiatal hernia, high blood pressure, kidney disease, liver disease, lung disease, myasthenia gravis, enlarged prostate gland, thyroid disease, or ulcerative colitis.

• If this medication makes you dizzy or drowsy, you should avoid taking part in any activity that requires alertness, such as driving a car or operating any potentially dangerous equipment.

• Before having surgery or any other medical or dental treatment, be sure to tell your doctor or dentist that you are taking this medication.

• Because this product contains diphenoxylate, it has the potential for abuse and must be used with caution. Tolerance develops quickly; do not increase the dosage or stop taking the drug unless you first consult your doctor. If you have been taking large amounts of this medication for long periods and then stop abruptly, you may experience a withdrawal reaction (muscle aches, diarrhea, gooseflesh, runny nose, nausea, vomiting, shivering, trembling, stomach cramps, sleep disorders, irritability, weakness, excessive yawning, or sweating). Your doctor may, therefore, want to reduce the dosage gradually.

• Check with your doctor if your diarrhea does not subside within two to three days. Unless your doctor specifically directs otherwise, you should not take this medication for more than five days.

• While taking this medication, drink lots of fluids to replace those lost with the diarrhea.

• Be sure to tell your doctor if you are pregnant. Although this medication has been shown to be safe in animals, its effects in humans during pregnancy have not been thoroughly studied. Also, tell your doctor if you are breastfeeding an infant. Small amounts of this medication may pass into breast milk and cause excessive drowsiness in nursing infants.

diphenoxylate hydrochloride with atropine sulfate—see diphenoxylate and atropine combination

Diphenylan—see phenytoin

Diprolene—see betamethasone dipropionate (topical)

Diprosone—see betamethasone dipropionate (topical)

dipyridamole

BRAND NAMES (Manufacturers)
dipyridamole (various manufacturers)
Persantine (Boehringer Ingelheim)
Pyridamole (Major)
TYPE OF DRUG
Antianginal
INGREDIENT
dipyridamole
DOSAGE FORM
Tablets (25 mg, 50 mg, and 75 mg)
STORAGE
Store at room temperature in a tightly closed container.

USES

Dipyridamole is used to prevent chronic chest pain (angina) due to heart disease. It relieves chest pain by dilating the blood vessels of the heart and providing more oxygen to the heart muscle. Dipyridamole is also used to prevent blood clot formation, especially in patients who have artificial heart valves.

TREATMENT

You should take this medication on an empty stomach with a full glass of water one hour before or two hours after a meal. If this drug upsets your stomach, check with your doctor to see if you can take it with food.

The full benefits of this medication may not become apparent for up to two to three months.

If you miss a dose of this medication, take the missed dose as soon as possible, unless it is within four hours of your next scheduled dose. In that case, do not take the missed dose at all; just return to your regular dosing schedule. Do not double the next dose.

SIDE EFFECTS

Minor. Dizziness, fatigue, flushing, headache, nausea, stomach cramps, or weakness. These side effects should disappear as your body adjusts to the medication.

To avoid dizziness or light-headedness when you stand, contract and relax the muscles of your legs for a few moments before rising. Do this by pushing one foot against the floor while raising the other foot slightly, alternating feet so that you are "pumping" your legs in a pedaling motion.
Major. Tell your doctor about any side effects that are persistent or particularly bothersome. IT IS ESPECIALLY IMPORTANT TO TELL YOUR DOCTOR about fainting, skin rash, or a worsening of your chest pain.

INTERACTIONS

Dipyridamole should not interact with other medications if it is used according to directions.

WARNINGS

• Tell your doctor about unusual or allergic reactions you have had to any medications, especially to dipyridamole.
• Tell your doctor if you have ever had low blood pressure.

• The effectiveness of dipyridamole in controlling chronic angina is controversial. This drug is more frequently prescribed to prevent blood clot formation, although use of dipyridamole for this purpose has not yet been approved by the Food and Drug Administration (FDA).
• This drug does not stop chest pain from angina that has already begun. It is used only to prevent such pain
• If this drug makes you dizzy, do not take part in any activity that requires alertness.
• Before having any surgery or other medical or dental treatment, be sure to tell your doctor or dentist that you are taking this medication.
• Be sure to tell your doctor if you are pregnant. Although this drug appears to be safe, extensive studies in humans during pregnancy have not been conducted. Also, tell your doctor if you are breast-feeding an infant. Small amounts of dipyridamole pass into breast milk.

disopyramide

BRAND NAMES (Manufacturers)
disopyramide (various manufacturers)
Napamide (Major)
Norpace (Searle)
Norpace CR (Searle)
TYPE OF DRUG
Antiarrhythmic
INGREDIENT
disopyramide
DOSAGE FORMS
Capsules (100 mg and 150 mg)
Sustained-release capsules (100 mg and 150 mg)
STORAGE
Disopyramide capsules should be stored at room temperature in tightly closed containers.

USES

Disopyramide is used for the treatment of heart arrhythmias. It corrects irregular heartbeats and helps to achieve a more normal rhythm.

TREATMENT

Disopyramide can be taken with or without food. Check with your doctor for a recommendation.

Try to take disopyramide at the same time(s) each day. This medication works best if the amount of the drug in your bloodstream is kept at a constant level. It is best, therefore, to take this medication at evenly spaced intervals day and night. For example, if you are to take it three times per day, the doses should be spaced eight hours apart.

Try not to miss any doses of this medication. If you do miss a dose and remember within two hours, take the missed dose as soon as possible. If more than two hours have passed, do not take the missed dose; just wait for your next scheduled dose. Do not double the next dose.

SIDE EFFECTS

Minor. Abdominal pain; aches and pain; blurred vision; constipation; decreased sweating; diarrhea; dizziness;

dry mouth, eyes, and throat; fatigue; gas; headache; impotence; loss of appetite; nausea; nervousness; or vomiting. These side effects should disappear as you adjust to the drug.

To relieve constipation, increase the amount of fiber in your diet (fresh fruits and vegetables, salads, bran, and whole-grain breads), exercise, and drink more water (unless your doctor directs you to do otherwise).

If you feel dizzy or light-headed, sit or lie down for a while; get up slowly from a sitting or reclining position.

To relieve mouth dryness, suck on ice chips or a piece of hard candy or chew sugarless gum.

"Artificial tears" eye drops may help to relieve eye dryness.

Major. Tell your doctor about any side effects that are persistent or particularly bothersome. IT IS ESPECIALLY IMPORTANT TO TELL YOUR DOCTOR about chest pain; depression; difficult or painful urination; enlarged, painful breasts (in both sexes); fainting; fever; muscle pain; muscle weakness; numbness or tingling sensations; palpitations; rash; shortness of breath; sore throat; swelling of the feet or ankles; weight gain; or yellowing of the eyes or skin.

INTERACTIONS
Disopyramide interacts with several other medications:
1. Phenytoin, rifampin, barbiturates, and glutethimide can decrease its effectiveness.
2. The combination of alcohol and disopyramide can lead to dizziness and hypoglycemia (low blood sugar levels). You should, therefore, avoid drinking alcoholic beverages while you are taking this medication.
3. The concurrent use of disopyramide and beta blockers (acebutolol, atenolol, betaxolol, carteolol, esmolol, labetalol, metoprolol, nadolol, penbutolol, pindolol, propranolol, and timolol) can have additive negative effects on the heart.
4. Disopyramide may interact with verapamil.

Before starting to take disopyramide, BE SURE TO TELL YOUR DOCTOR about any medications you are currently taking, especially any of those listed above.

WARNINGS
• Tell your doctor about unusual or allergic reactions you have had to any medications, especially to disopyramide.
• Tell your doctor if you now have or if you have ever had glaucoma, hypoglycemia (low blood sugar levels), hypokalemia (low blood potassium levels), kidney disease, liver disease, myasthenia gravis, urinary retention, or an enlarged prostate gland.
• If this drug makes you dizzy or drowsy or blurs your vision, do not take part in any activity that requires alertness, such as driving a car or operating potentially dangerous equipment.
• This medication can decrease sweating and heat release from the body. You should, therefore, avoid getting overheated by strenuous exercise in hot weather and should avoid taking hot baths, showers, and saunas.
• Before having surgery or any other medical or dental treatment, be sure to tell your doctor or dentist that you are taking this medication.

• Disopyramide can cause hypoglycemia. Signs of hypoglycemia include anxiety, chills, pale skin, headache, hunger, nausea, nervousness, shakiness, sweating, and weakness. If you experience this reaction, eat or drink something containing sugar, and CONTACT YOUR DOCTOR.
• Be sure to tell your doctor if you are pregnant. The effects of this medication during pregnancy have not been thoroughly studied in humans. It is known that disopyramide passes into breast milk. If you are breast-feeding an infant while being treated with this medication, tell your doctor. Unless directed to do otherwise, breast-feeding is not recommended during treatment with this medication.

Di-Spaz—see dicyclomine

disulfiram

BRAND NAMES (Manufacturers)
Antabuse (Wyeth-Ayerst)
disulfiram (various manufacturers)
TYPE OF DRUG
Antialcoholic
INGREDIENT
disulfiram
DOSAGE FORM
Tablets (250 mg and 500 mg)
STORAGE
Disulfiram should be stored at room temperature in a tightly closed, light-resistant container.

USES
Disulfiram is used as an aid to treat alcoholics who are strongly motivated to remain sober. Disulfiram blocks the breakdown of alcohol by the body, leading to an accumulation of the chemical acetaldehyde in the bloodstream. Buildup of acetaldehyde in the body can lead to a severe and very unpleasant reaction after alcohol consumption. Alcohol must, therefore, be avoided to prevent this reaction.

TREATMENT
Disulfiram can be taken either on an empty stomach or with food or milk (as directed by your doctor). The tablets can also be crushed and mixed with beverages (nonalcoholic).

If you miss a dose of this medication, take the missed dose as soon as possible, unless it is almost time for the next dose. In that case, do not take the missed dose at all; just return to your regular dosing schedule. Do not double the next dose.

SIDE EFFECTS
Minor. Drowsiness, fatigue, headache, metallic or garlic-like aftertaste, and restlessness. These side effects should disappear as your body adjusts to the medication.
Major. Tell your doctor about any side effects that are persistent or particularly bothersome. IT IS ESPECIALLY IMPORTANT TO TELL YOUR DOCTOR about blurred

vision, impotence, joint pain, mental disorders, skin rash, tingling sensations, or yellowing of the eyes or skin.

INTERACTIONS

Disulfiram interacts with several other types of medications:

1. It can increase the blood levels and side effects of diazepam, chlordiazepoxide, phenytoin, and oral anticoagulants (blood thinners, such as warfarin).

2. Concurrent use of disulfiram with isoniazid, antidepressants, metronidazole, or marijuana can lead to severe reactions.

BE SURE TO TELL YOUR DOCTOR about any medications you are currently taking, especially any of those listed above. Also, be sure to tell your doctor if you use marijuana.

WARNINGS

• Tell your doctor about unusual or allergic reactions you have had to any medications, especially to disulfiram, rubber, pesticides, or fungicides.

• Before starting to take this medication, be sure to tell your doctor if you have ever had brain damage, dermatitis, diabetes mellitus, epilepsy, heart disease, kidney disease, liver disease, mental disorders, or thyroid disease.

• It is important not to drink or to use any alcohol-containing preparations, medications, or foods (including beer, elixirs, tonics, wine, liquor, vinegar, sauces, aftershave lotions, liniments, or colognes) while taking this medication. Be sure to check the labels on any over-the-counter (nonprescription) products for their alcohol content, especially cough syrups, mouthwashes, and gargles.

• It is important that you understand the serious nature of the disulfiram-alcohol reaction. If you take disulfiram within 12 hours after ingesting alcohol or drink alcohol within two weeks after your last dose of disulfiram, you may experience blurred vision, chest pain, confusion, dizziness, fainting, flushing, headache, nausea, pounding heartbeat, sweating, vomiting, or weakness. The reaction usually occurs within five to ten minutes of drinking alcohol and can last from half an hour to two hours, depending on the dose of disulfiram and the quantity of alcohol ingested.

• If this drug makes you drowsy, do not take part in any activity that requires alertness, such as driving a car or operating potentially dangerous machinery. Also be careful when going up and down stairs.

• Be sure to tell your doctor if you are pregnant. Birth defects have been reported in both animals and humans whose mothers received disulfiram during pregnancy. It must also be kept in mind that alcohol, even in small amounts, can cause a variety of birth defects when ingested during pregnancy. Also, tell your doctor if you are breast-feeding an infant. It is not known if disulfiram passes into breast milk.

Ditropan—see oxybutynin

Diulo—see metolazone

Diurese—see trichlormethiazide

Diurigen—see chlorothiazide

Diuril—see chlorothiazide

Dizmiss—see meclizine

Dolacet—see acetaminophen and hydrocodone combination

Dolene—see propoxyphene

Dolene AP-65—see acetaminophen and propoxyphene combination

Dolene Compound-65—see aspirin, caffeine, and propoxyphene combination

Dolobid—see diflunisal

Dolophine—see methadone

Donnamor—see atropine, scopolamine, hyoscyamine, and phenobarbital combination

Donna-Sed—see atropine, scopolamine, hyoscyamine, and phenobarbital combination

Donnatal—see atropine, scopolamine, hyoscyamine, and phenobarbital combination

Dopar—see levodopa

Dorcol Children's Liquid Cold Formula—see pseudoephedrine and chlorpheniramine combination

Doriden—see glutethimide

Dormarex 2—see diphenhydramine

Doryx—see doxycycline

Doxaphene Compound—see aspirin, caffeine, and propoxyphene combination

doxepin

BRAND NAMES (Manufacturers)
Adapin (Pennwalt)
doxepin (various manufacturers)
Sinequan (Fisons)
TYPE OF DRUG
Tricyclic antidepressant
INGREDIENT
doxepin
DOSAGE FORMS
Capsules (10 mg, 25 mg, 50 mg, 75 mg, 100 mg, and 150 mg)
Oral concentrate (10 mg per ml)
STORAGE
Doxepin capsules and oral concentrate should be stored at room temperature in tightly closed containers. This medication should never be frozen.

USES

Doxepin is used to relieve the symptoms of mental depression. This medication belongs to a group of drugs referred to as the tricyclic antidepressants. These medicines are thought to relieve depression by increasing the concentration of certain chemicals necessary for nerve transmission in the brain.

TREATMENT

This medication should be taken exactly as your doctor prescribes. You can take it with food to lessen the chance of stomach irritation (unless your doctor tells you to do otherwise).

Each dose of the oral concentrate should be diluted in at least four ounces (half a glass) of water, milk, or fruit juice just prior to administration. Measure the correct amount carefully with the dropper provided. DO NOT mix the medication with grape juice or with carbonated beverages, since they may decrease the medicine's effectiveness.

If you miss a dose of this medication, take the missed dose as soon as possible, then return to your regular dosing schedule. If, however, the dose you missed was a once-a-day bedtime dose, do not take that dose in the morning; check with your doctor instead. If the dose is taken in the morning, it may cause some unwanted side effects. Never double the dose.

The antidepressant effects of therapy with this medication may not become apparent for two or three weeks.

SIDE EFFECTS

Minor. Blurred vision, constipation, cramps, diarrhea, dizziness, drowsiness, dry mouth, fatigue, indigestion, insomnia, loss of appetite, nausea, peculiar tastes in the mouth, restlessness, sweating, vomiting, weakness, or weight gain or loss. As your body adjusts to the medication, these side effects should disappear.

This drug may cause increased sensitivity to sunlight. Therefore, avoid prolonged exposure to sunlight and sunlamps. Wear protective clothing and use an effective sunscreen.

Dry mouth can be relieved by chewing sugarless gum or by sucking on ice chips or a piece of hard candy.

To relieve constipation, increase the amount of fiber in your diet (fresh fruits and vegetables, salads, bran, and whole-grain breads), exercise, and drink more water (unless your doctor directs you to do otherwise).

To avoid dizziness or light-headedness when you stand, contract and relax the muscles of your legs for a few moments before rising. Do this by pushing one foot against the floor while raising the other foot slightly, alternating feet so that you are "pumping" your legs in a pedaling motion.

Major. Tell your doctor about any side effects that are persistent or particularly bothersome. IT IS ESPECIALLY IMPORTANT TO TELL YOUR DOCTOR about agitation, anxiety, chest pain, confusion, convulsions, difficulty in urinating, enlarged or painful breasts (in both sexes), fainting, fever, fluid retention, hair loss, hallucinations, headaches, impotence, mood changes, mouth sores, nervousness, nightmares, numbness in the fingers or toes, palpitations, ringing in the ears, seizures, skin rash, sleep disorders, sore throat, a tendency to bleed or bruise, tremors, uncoordinated movements or balance problems, or yellowing of the eyes or skin.

INTERACTIONS

Doxepin interacts with a number of other types of medications:

1. Extreme drowsiness can occur when this medicine is taken with central nervous system depressants (such as alcohol, antihistamines, barbiturates, benzodiazepine tranquilizers, muscle relaxants, narcotics, pain medications, phenothiazine tranquilizers, and sleeping medications) or with other antidepressants.

2. Doxepin may decrease the effectiveness of antiseizure medications and may block the blood-pressure-lowering effects of clonidine and guanethidine.

3. Oral contraceptives (birth control pills) and estrogen-containing drugs can increase the side effects and reduce the effectiveness of the tricyclic antidepressants (including doxepin).

4. Cimetidine can decrease the elimination of doxepin from the body, which can increase the possibility that side effects will occur.

5. Tricyclic antidepressants may increase the side effects of thyroid medications and over-the-counter (nonprescription) cough, cold, allergy, asthma, sinus, and diet medications.

6. The concurrent use of this drug and monoamine oxidase (MAO) inhibitors should be avoided, because the combination may result in fever, convulsions, or high blood pressure. At least 14 days should separate the use of this drug and the use of an MAO inhibitor.

BE SURE TO TELL YOUR DOCTOR about any medications you are currently taking, especially any of those listed above.

WARNINGS

• Tell your doctor if you have had unusual or allergic reactions to any medications, especially to doxepin or any of the other tricyclic antidepressants (amitriptyline, imipramine, trimipramine, amoxapine, protriptyline, desipramine, maprotiline, and nortriptyline).

• Be sure to tell your doctor if you have a history of alcoholism or if you have ever had asthma, high blood pressure, liver or kidney disease, heart disease, a heart attack, circulatory disease, stomach problems, intestinal problems, difficulty in urinating, enlarged prostate gland, epilepsy, glaucoma, thyroid disease, mental illness, or electroshock therapy.

• If this drug makes you dizzy or drowsy, do not take part in any activity that requires alertness, such as driving a car or operating potentially dangerous equipment.

• Before having surgery or any other medical or dental treatment, be sure to tell your doctor or dentist that you are taking this medication.

• Do not stop taking this drug suddenly. Abruptly stopping it can cause nausea, headache, stomach upset, fatigue, or a worsening of your condition. Your doctor may want to reduce the dosage gradually.

• The effects of this medication may last as long as seven days after you have stopped taking it, so continue to observe all precautions during that period.

• Be sure to tell your doctor if you are pregnant. The effects of this drug during pregnancy have not been thoroughly studied in humans. Studies in animals have shown that this medication can cause side effects to the fetus if given to the mother in large doses during pregnancy. Also, tell your doctor if you are breast-feeding an infant. Small amounts of this drug can pass into breast milk and may cause unwanted effects in the nursing infant.

Doxy-Caps—see doxycycline

Doxychel Hyclate—see doxycycline

doxycycline

BRAND NAMES (Manufacturers)
AK-Ramycin (Akorn)
AK-Ratabs (Akorn)
Doryx (Parke-Davis)
Doxy-Caps (Edwards)
Doxychel Hyclate (Rachelle)
doxycycline (various manufacturers)
Doxy-Lemmon (Lemmon)
Vibramycin Hyclate (Pfizer)
Vibra Tabs (Pfizer)
TYPE OF DRUG
Tetracycline antibiotic
INGREDIENT
doxycycline
DOSAGE FORMS
Tablets (50 mg and 100 mg)
Capsules (50 mg and 100 mg)
Capsules, coated pellets (100 mg)
Oral suspension (25 mg per 5-ml spoonful)
Oral syrup (50 mg per 5-ml spoonful)
STORAGE
Doxycycline tablets, capsules, oral suspension, and oral syrup should be stored at room temperature in tightly closed, light-resistant containers. Any unused portion of the suspension should be discarded after 14 days because the drug loses its potency after that period. This medication should never be frozen.

USES
Doxycycline is used to treat a wide variety of bacterial infections and to prevent or treat traveler's diarrhea. It acts by inhibiting the growth of bacteria.

Doxycycline kills susceptible bacteria, but it is not effective against viruses or fungi.

TREATMENT
To avoid stomach upset, you can take this drug with food (unless your doctor directs you to do otherwise).

The suspension should be shaken well just before measuring each dose. The contents tend to settle on the bottom of the bottle, so it is necessary to shake the container to distribute the ingredients evenly and equalize the doses. Each dose of the oral suspension or oral syrup should be measured carefully with a specially designed 5-ml measuring spoon. An ordinary teaspoon is not accurate.

Do not mix the oral syrup form of this drug with other substances unless so directed by your doctor.

Doxycycline works best when the level of medicine in your bloodstream is kept constant. It is best, therefore, to take the doses at evenly spaced intervals day and night. For example, if you are to take two doses a day, the doses should be spaced 12 hours apart.

If you miss a dose of this medication, take the missed dose immediately. However, if you do not remember to take the missed dose until it is almost time for your next dose, take it; space the following dose about halfway through the regular interval between doses; then return to your regular dosing schedule. Try not to skip any doses.

It is very important that you take this drug for the entire time prescribed, even if the symptoms disappear before the end of that period. If you stop taking the drug too soon, resistant bacteria can continue to grow, and the infection could recur.

SIDE EFFECTS
Minor. Diarrhea, discoloration of the nails, dizziness, loss of appetite, nausea, stomach cramps and upset, or vomiting. These side effects should disappear as your body adjusts to the medication.

Doxycycline can increase your sensitivity to sunlight. You should, therefore, try to avoid prolonged exposure to sunlight and sunlamps. Wear protective clothing and sunglasses, and use an effective sunscreen.
Major. Tell your doctor about any side effects that are persistent or particularly bothersome. IT IS ESPECIALLY IMPORTANT TO TELL YOUR DOCTOR about darkened tongue, difficulty in breathing, joint pain, mouth irritation, rash, rectal or vaginal itching, sore throat and fever, unusual bleeding or bruising, or yellowing of the eyes or skin. Also, if your symptoms of infection seem to be getting worse rather than improving, you should contact your doctor.

INTERACTIONS
Doxycycline interacts with other types of medications:
1. It can increase the absorption of digoxin, which may lead to digoxin toxicity.
2. The gastrointestinal side effects (nausea, vomiting, stomach upset) of theophylline may be increased by doxycycline.
3. The dosage of oral anticoagulants (blood thinners, such as warfarin) may need to be adjusted when this medication is started.
4. Doxycycline may decrease the effectiveness of oral contraceptives (birth control pills), and pregnancy could result. You should, therefore, use a different or additional form of birth control while taking doxycycline. Discuss this with your doctor.
5. Barbiturates, carbamazepine, phenytoin, and antacids can lower the blood levels of doxycycline, decreasing its effectiveness.
6. Iron can bind to doxycycline in the gastrointestinal tract, which can decrease its absorption and, therefore, its effectiveness.

BE SURE TO TELL YOUR DOCTOR about any medications you are currently taking, especially any of those listed above.

WARNINGS

- Tell your doctor about unusual or allergic reactions you have had to any medications, especially to doxycycline, oxytetracycline, tetracycline, or minocycline.
- Tell your doctor if you now have or if you have ever had kidney or liver disease.
- Doxycycline can affect tests for syphilis; tell your doctor you are taking this medication if you are also being treated for this disease.
- Make sure that your prescription for this medication is marked with the drug's expiration date. The drug should be discarded after the expiration date. If doxycycline is used after it has expired, serious side effects (especially to the kidneys) could result.
- This medication has been prescribed for your current infection only. Another infection later on, or one that someone else has, may require a different medicine. You should not give your medicine to other people or use it for other infections, unless your doctor specifically directs you to do so.
- Be sure to tell your doctor if you are pregnant or if you are breast-feeding an infant. Doxycycline should not be used during pregnancy and breast-feeding. It crosses the placenta and passes into breast milk. This drug can cause permanent discoloration of the teeth and can inhibit tooth and bone growth if used during their development. Also, this drug should not be used by children less than eight years old.

Doxy-Lemmon—see doxycycline

Drisdol—see ergocalciferol (Vitamin D)

Drize—see phenylpropanolamine and chlorpheniramine combination

Drotic—see hydrocortisone, polymyxin B, and neomycin combination (otic)

Duotrate Plateau Caps—see pentaerythritol tetranitrate

Duradyne DHC—see acetaminophen and hydrocodone combination

Duralex—see pseudoephedrine and chlorpheniramine combination

Duraquin—see quinidine

Dura-Vent—see phenylpropanolamine and guaifenesin combination

Dura-Vent/A—see phenylpropanolamine and chlorpheniramine combination

Duricef—see cefadroxil

Duvoid—see bethanechol

Dyazide—see triamterene and hydrochlorothiazide combination

Dycill—see dicloxacillin

Dymelor—see acetohexamide

Dynacirc—see isradipine

Dynapen—see dicloxacillin

Dyrexan-OD—see phendimetrazine

Dyrenium—see triamterene

Earocol—see antipyrine, benzocaine, oxyquinoline, and glycerin combination

Easprin—see aspirin

Ecotrin—see aspirin

Edecrin—see ethacrynic acid

E.E.S. 200—see erythromycin

E.E.S. 400—see erythromycin

Elavil—see amitriptyline

Eldepryl—see selegiline

Elixomin—see theophylline

Elixophyllin—see theophylline

Empirin—see aspirin

Empirin with Codeine—see aspirin and codeine combination

E-Mycin—see erythromycin

---

enalapril

BRAND NAME (Manufacturer)
Vasotec (Merck Sharp & Dohme)
TYPE OF DRUG
Antihypertensive
INGREDIENT
enalapril
DOSAGE FORM
Tablets (2.5 mg, 5 mg, 10 mg, and 20 mg)
STORAGE
Store enalapril at room temperature in a tightly closed container.

USES

Enalapril is used to treat high blood pressure. It is a vasodilator (it widens the blood vessels) that acts by blocking the production of chemicals that may be responsible for constricting or narrowing the blood vessels.

TREATMENT

Enalapril can be taken either on an empty stomach or with food if it causes stomach irritation. To become accustomed to taking this medication, try to take it at the same time(s) every day.

It may be several weeks before you notice the full effects of this medication.

If you miss a dose of enalapril, take the missed dose as soon as possible, unless it is almost time for the next dose. In that case, do not take the missed dose at all; just wait until the next scheduled dose. Do not double the dose.

Enalapril does not cure high blood pressure, but it will help to control the condition as long as you continue to take the medication.

SIDE EFFECTS

Minor. Abdominal pain, cough, diarrhea, dizziness, drowsiness, fatigue, headache, heartburn, insomnia, nausea, nervousness, sweating, or vomiting. These side effects should disappear as your body adjusts to the medication.

To avoid dizziness when you stand, contract and relax the muscles of your legs for a few moments before rising. Do this by alternately pushing one foot against the floor while lifting the other foot slightly.

Major. Tell your doctor about any side effects that are persistent or particularly bothersome. IT IS ESPECIALLY IMPORTANT TO TELL YOUR DOCTOR about chest pain; difficulty in breathing; fainting; fever; itching; lightheadedness (especially during the first few days); muscle cramps; palpitations; rash; sore throat; swelling of the face, eyes, lips, or tongue; tingling in the fingers or toes; or yellowing of the eyes or skin.

INTERACTIONS

Enalapril interacts with several other types of medications:

1. Diuretics (water pills) and other antihypertensive medications can cause an excessive drop in blood pressure when they are combined with enalapril (especially with the first dose).

2. The combination of enalapril with spironolactone, triamterene, amiloride, potassium supplements, or salt substitutes can lead to hyperkalemia (dangerously high levels of potassium in the bloodstream).

Before starting to take enalapril, BE SURE TO TELL YOUR DOCTOR about any medications you are currently taking, especially any of those listed above.

WARNINGS

• Tell your doctor about unusual or allergic reactions you have had to any medications, especially to enalapril.

• Tell your doctor if you now have or if you have ever had blood disorders, heart failure, renal disease, or systemic lupus erythematosus.

• Excessive perspiration, dehydration, or prolonged vomiting or diarrhea can lead to an excessive drop in blood pressure while you are taking this medication. Contact your doctor if you have any of these symptoms.

• Before having surgery or other medical or dental treatment, tell your doctor or dentist you are taking this drug.

• If this drug makes you dizzy or drowsy, do not take part in any activity that requires alertness, such as driving a car or operating potentially dangerous equipment.

• If you have high blood pressure, do not take any over-the-counter (nonprescription) medications for weight control or for asthma, sinus, cough, cold, or allergy problems unless you first check with your doctor.

• Be sure to tell your doctor if you are pregnant. Drugs in the same class as enalapril have been shown to cause birth defects, including kidney damage, low blood pressure, improper skull development, and death, when taken in the second and third trimesters. Also, tell your doctor if you are breast-feeding an infant. It is not yet known if enalapril passes into human breast milk.

Endep—see amitriptyline

Enduron—see methyclothiazide

Enovil—see amitriptyline

Entex L.A.—see phenylpropanolamine and guaifenesin combination

Epifrin—see epinephrine (ophthalmic)

Epinal—see epinephrine (ophthalmic)

epinephrine (ophthalmic)

BRAND NAMES (Manufacturers)
Epifrin (Allergan)
Epinal (Alcon)
Eppy/N (Sola/Barnes-Hind)
Glaucon (Alcon)
TYPE OF DRUG
Antiglaucoma ophthalmic solution
INGREDIENT
epinephrine (adrenaline)
DOSAGE FORM
Ophthalmic solution (0.1%, 0.25%, 0.5%, 1%, and 2%)
STORAGE
Store at room temperature in a tightly closed, light-resistant container. This medication should never be frozen. The solution should be discarded if it turns brown or cloudy because this indicates deterioration and loss of potency.

USES

Epinephrine (ophthalmic) is used to treat glaucoma. It lowers the pressure in the eye by decreasing the production of aqueous humor (a particular fluid in the eye) and increasing its drainage.

TREATMENT

Wash your hands with soap and water before applying this medication. In order to avoid contamination of the eye drops, be careful not to touch the tube portion of the dropper or let it touch your eye; and DO NOT wipe off or rinse the dropper after each use.

To apply the eye drops, tilt your head back and pull down your lower eyelid with one hand to make a pouch below the eye. Drop the prescribed amount of medicine into this pouch and slowly close your eyes. Try not to blink. Keep your eyes closed, and place one finger at the corner of the eye next to your nose for a minute or two, applying slight pressure (this is done to prevent loss of the medication through the duct that drains fluid from the surface of the eye into the nose and throat). Then wipe away any excess with a clean tissue. Since the drops are somewhat difficult to apply, you may want to have someone else apply them for you.

If more than one type of eye drop has been prescribed for you, wait at least five minutes after applying epinephrine before using the other eye medication (to give the epinephrine time to work). However, if you are also using an eye drop that constricts your pupils, check with your doctor to see which drug should be applied first.

If you miss a dose of epinephrine, apply the missed dose as soon as possible, unless it is almost time for the next dose. In that case, do not apply the missed dose at all; just return to your regular dosing schedule. Do not double the next dose.

Epitol—see carbamazepine

E.P. Mycin—see oxytetracycline

Eppy/N—see epinephrine (ophthalmic)

Epromate—see meprobamate and aspirin combination

Equagesic—see meprobamate and aspirin combination

Equanil—see meprobamate

Equazine M—see meprobamate and aspirin combination

Eramycin—see erythromycin

ergocalciferol (vitamin D)

BRAND NAMES (Manufacturers)
Calciferol (Schwarz Pharma Kremers-Urban)
Drisdol (Winthrop)
vitamin D (various manufacturers)
TYPE OF DRUG
Vitamin
INGREDIENT
ergocalciferol
DOSAGE FORMS
Tablets (50,000 units)
Capsules (50,000 units)
Oral liquid (8,000 units per ml)*
*The oral liquid is available without a prescription.
STORAGE
Store at room temperature in a tightly closed, light-resistant container. This medication should never be frozen.

USES
Ergocalciferol is used to treat rickets, hypophosphatemia (low blood levels of phosphate), and hypoparathyroidism (underactive parathyroid gland). This medication is converted by the liver and kidney to the active form of vitamin D, a vitamin essential to many body systems (including bone and tooth structure, regulation of blood calcium levels, and heart and muscle contraction).

TREATMENT
Ergocalciferol can be taken either on an empty stomach or with food or milk (as directed by your doctor).

Each dose of the oral liquid form of this medication should be measured carefully with the dropper provided. The liquid can then be taken directly or mixed with fruit juice, cereal, or other foods.

If you miss a dose of this medication, take the missed dose as soon as possible, unless it is almost time for the next dose. In that case, do not take the missed dose at all; just return to your regular dosing schedule. Do not double the next dose.

SIDE EFFECTS
Minor. None, at the dosages normally prescribed.
Major. The side effects associated with ergocalciferol therapy are usually the result of too much medication (vitamin D intoxication). Tell your doctor about any side effects that are persistent or particularly bothersome. IT IS ESPECIALLY IMPORTANT TO TELL YOUR DOCTOR about blurred vision, bone pain, constipation, dry mouth, headache, increased thirst, increased urination, irritability, loss of appetite, metallic taste in the mouth, mental disorders, muscle pain, nausea, palpitations, runny nose, vomiting, weakness, or weight loss.

INTERACTIONS
Cholestyramine, colestipol, and mineral oil can decrease the absorption of ergocalciferol from the gastrointestinal tract, decreasing its effectiveness.

BE SURE TO TELL YOUR DOCTOR about any medications you are currently taking, especially any of those listed above.

WARNINGS
Tell your doctor about unusual or allergic reactions you have had to any medications, especially to ergocalciferol (vitamin D), calcitriol, calcifediol, or dihydrotachysterol.

Before starting to take this medication, be sure to tell your doctor if you now have or if you have ever had heart or blood vessel disease, hypercalcemia (high blood levels of calcium), hyperphosphatemia (high blood levels of phosphate), vitamin D intoxication, or sarcoidosis.

Before taking any over-the-counter (nonprescription) products that contain calcium, phosphates, magnesium, or vitamin D, check with your doctor. These ingredients can increase the side effects of ergocalciferol.

Some forms of this medication contain the color additive FD&C Yellow No. 5 (tartrazine), which can cause allergic-type symptoms (fainting, shortness of breath, rash) in certain susceptible individuals.

Be sure to tell your doctor if you are pregnant. Although the effects of this medication have not been thoroughly studied during human pregnancy, animal studies have shown that this medication can cause side effects to the fetus if given to the mother in large doses during pregnancy. Tell your doctor if you are breast-feeding an infant. It is not known if this drug passes into breast milk.

SIDE EFFECTS

Minor. Headache or transitory stinging on initial application. These side effects should disappear as your body adjusts to the medication.

Major. Tell your doctor about any side effects that are persistent or particularly bothersome. IT IS ESPECIALLY IMPORTANT TO TELL YOUR DOCTOR about blurred vision, eye pain, fainting, palpitations, sweating, or trembling.

INTERACTIONS

Epinephrine interacts with several other types of medications:

1. Concurrent use of epinephrine and monoamine oxidase (MAO) inhibitors or tricyclic antidepressants can lead to serious side effects. At least 21 days should, therefore, separate doses of epinephrine and either of these types of medications.

2. Digoxin can increase the side effects of epinephrine.

BE SURE TO TELL YOUR DOCTOR about any medications you are currently taking, especially any of those listed above.

WARNINGS

• Tell your doctor about unusual or allergic reactions you have had to any medications, especially to epinephrine.

• Tell your doctor if you are allergic to sulfites.

• Before starting to take this medication, be sure to tell your doctor if you now have or if you have ever had diabetes mellitus, heart or blood vessel disease, high blood pressure, a stroke, or thyroid disease.

• If this medication blurs your vision, try to avoid activities that require visual acuity, such as driving a car or operating potentially dangerous equipment.

• Epinephrine may occasionally cause discoloration of soft contact lenses. If you currently wear soft contact lenses, you should discuss with your doctor whether your medication or your contact lenses should be changed.

• Be sure to tell your doctor if you are pregnant. Although epinephrine (ophthalmic) appears to be safe during pregnancy, studies in humans have not been conducted. Also, tell your doctor if you are breast-feeding an infant. It is not known whether epinephrine passes into breast milk.

---

ergoloid mesylates

BRAND NAMES (Manufacturers)
ergoloid mesylates (various manufacturers)
Gerimal (Rugby)
Hydergine (Sandoz)
TYPE OF DRUG
Vasodilator
INGREDIENT
ergoloid mesylates
DOSAGE FORMS
Capsules, liquid (1 mg)
Oral tablets (0.5 mg and 1 mg)
Sublingual tablets (0.5 mg and 1 mg)
Oral liquid (1 mg per ml, with 30% alcohol)

STORAGE

Ergoloid mesylates capsules, tablets, and oral liquid should be stored at room temperature in tightly closed, light-resistant containers. Never freeze this medication.

USES

This medication is used to reduce the symptoms associated with senility. It is not clear how ergoloid mesylates work, but it is thought that they act by dilating (widening) the blood vessels, thus increasing blood flow to the brain.

TREATMENT

In order to avoid stomach irritation, you can take the capsules, tablets, or oral liquid with food or milk. Be sure to measure the dose of the liquid form of this medication carefully with the dropper provided.

The sublingual form of this medication must be placed under the tongue and allowed to dissolve completely. Try not to swallow for as long as possible, because the drug is more completely absorbed through the lining of the mouth than it is from the stomach. Do not drink any liquid, eat, or smoke for at least ten minutes after placing the tablet under the tongue.

If you miss a dose of this medication, take the missed dose as soon as possible, unless it is almost time for the next dose. In that case, do not take the missed dose at all; just return to your regular dosing schedule. Do not double the next dose.

It may take three or four weeks for the effects of this medication to become apparent.

SIDE EFFECTS

Minor. Blurred vision, dizziness, drowsiness, flushing, headache, irritation under the tongue (with the sublingual form only), light-headedness, loss of appetite, nasal congestion, nausea, stomach cramps, or vomiting. These side effects should disappear as your body adjusts to the medication.

If you feel dizzy or light-headed, sit or lie down for a while; get up slowly from a sitting or reclining position, and be careful on stairs.

Major. Tell your doctor about any side effects that are persistent or particularly bothersome. IT IS ESPECIALLY IMPORTANT TO TELL YOUR DOCTOR about a slowed heart rate.

INTERACTIONS

Ergoloid mesylates should not interact with other medications if they are used according to directions.

WARNINGS

• Tell your doctor about unusual or allergic reactions you have had to any medications, especially to ergoloid mesylates or ergot alkaloids (such as ergonovine, ergotamine, or bromocriptine).

• Before starting to take this medication, be sure to tell your doctor if you now have or if you have ever had liver disease, low blood pressure, porphyria, severe mental illness, or a slowed heart rate.

• Ergoloid mesylates may lessen your ability to adjust to the cold. Therefore, since you may experience increased sensitivity, do not expose your body to very cold temperatures for prolonged periods.

• Your doctor may want you to take your pulse daily while you are using this medication. Contact your doctor if your pulse becomes slower than normal or if it drops below 50 beats per minute.

• If this drug makes you dizzy or drowsy or blurs your vision, do not take part in any activity that requires alertness, such as driving a car or operating potentially dangerous equipment. Also, be carefull going up and down stairs.

• Some of these products contain the color additive FD&C Yellow No. 5 (tartrazine), which can cause allergic-type reactions (rash, shortness of breath, fainting) in certain susceptible individuals.

ergonovine

BRAND NAMES (Manufacturers)
ergonovine maleate (various manufacturers)
Ergotrate Maleate (Lilly)
TYPE OF DRUG
Uterine stimulant
INGREDIENT
ergonovine
DOSAGE FORM
Tablets (0.2 mg)
STORAGE
Ergonovine should be stored at room temperature in a tightly closed container.

USES
Ergonovine is used to prevent or treat postpartum (immediately after delivery) or postabortion uterine bleeding. This medication is usually administered for only a short period of time (usually 48 hours). It acts directly on the uterus to cause contractions and to constrict blood vessels.

TREATMENT
Ergonovine tablets can be taken either on an empty stomach or with food or milk (as directed by your doctor). For more rapid effect, the tablet can also be placed under the tongue to dissolve.

If you miss a dose of this medication, do not take the missed dose at all; just return to your regular dosing schedule. Do not double the next dose.

SIDE EFFECTS
Minor. Diarrhea, headache, nausea, or vomiting. These side effects should disappear as your body adjusts to the medication.

Major. Tell your doctor about any side effects that are persistent or particularly bothersome. IT IS ESPECIALLY IMPORTANT TO TELL YOUR DOCTOR about chest pain, confusion, convulsions, excitement, hallucinations, hives, itching, numbness or coldness of the fingers or toes, ringing in the ears, shortness of breath, skin rash, or tingling sensations—even if these side effects appear or continue after you stop taking ergonovine.

INTERACTIONS
Ergonovine should not interact with other medications if it is used according to directions.

WARNINGS
Tell your doctor about unusual or allergic reactions you have had to medications, especially to ergonovine or to any other ergot alkaloid (bromocriptine, ergotamine, ergoloid mesylates).

Before starting to take this medication, tell your doctor if you now have or if you have ever had hypocalcemia, heart disease, high blood pressure, kidney or liver disease, or peripheral vascular disease (poor circulation).

Be sure to tell your doctor if you are breast-feeding an infant. Ergonovine can pass into breast milk and may cause side effects in the nursing infant. It can also decrease milk production.

Ergonovine Maleate—see ergonvine

Ergostat—see ergotamine

Ergotrate Maleate—see ergovine

ergotamine

BRAND NAMES (Manufacturers)
Ergostat (Parke-Davis)
Medihaler Ergotamine (3M)
TYPE OF DRUG
Antimigraine (vasoconstrictor)
INGREDIENT
ergotamine
DOSAGE FORMS
Sublingual tablets (2 mg)
Aerosol (0.36 mg per spray)
STORAGE
This medication should be stored at room temperature in tightly closed, light-resistant containers.

The container of the aerosol is pressurized; it should, therefore, never be punctured or broken. It should also be stored away from heat and direct sunlight.

USES
This medication is used to treat migraine and cluster headaches. These headaches are thought to be caused by an increase in the diameter of the blood vessels in the head, which results in increased blood flow, increased pressure, and pain. Ergotamine is a vasoconstrictor; it acts by constricting (narrowing) the blood vessels.

TREATMENT
Take this medication as soon as you notice your migraine headache symptoms. If you wait until the headache is severe, the drug takes longer to work and may not be as effective.

After you take either of these forms of ergotamine, you should try to lie down in a quiet, dark room for at least two hours (in order to help the medication work). The drug usually takes effect in 30 to 60 minutes.

It is very important that you understand how often you can repeat a dose of this medication during an attack (usually every 30 to 60 minutes for the sublingual tablets, and every five minutes for the aerosol spray) and the maximum amount of medication you can take per day (usually three sublingual tablets or six inhalations). Five is generally the maximum number of sublingual tablets and 15 is about the maximum number of inhalations that can be taken in any one-week period. CHECK WITH YOUR DOCTOR if you have any questions.

The sublingual tablets should be placed under your tongue. DO NOT swallow these tablets—they are more efficiently absorbed through the lining of the mouth than from the gastrointestinal tract. Try not to eat, drink, chew, or smoke while the tablet is dissolving.

The aerosol form of this medication comes packaged with instructions for use. Read the directions carefully; if you have any questions, check with your doctor or pharmacist. The aerosol can should be shaken well just before each dose is sprayed. The contents tend to settle on the bottom of the container, so it should be shaken to disperse the medication and equalize the doses. The container provides about 60 measured sprays.

If you are on prolonged treatment with this drug and you miss a dose, take it as soon as you remember. Wait four hours to take the next dose. It is very important that you consult your doctor before you discontinue using this drug. Your doctor may want to reduce your dosage gradually.

SIDE EFFECTS
Minor. Diarrhea, dizziness, headache, nausea, vomiting, or sensation of cold hands and feet with MILD numbness or tingling. These side effects should disappear as your body adjusts to the medication.

The aerosol form of ergotamine can cause hoarseness or throat irritation. Gargling or rinsing your mouth out with water after taking the dose may help prevent this side effect.

Major. Tell your doctor about any side effects that are persistent or particularly bothersome. IT IS ESPECIALLY IMPORTANT TO TELL YOUR DOCTOR about chest pain; coldness, numbness, pain, tingling, or dark discoloration of the fingers or toes; confusion; fluid retention; itching; localized swelling; muscle pain; severe abdominal pain and swelling; or unusual weakness.

INTERACTIONS
Ergotamine interacts with several other types of medications:

1. Ergotamine interacts with amphetamines, ephedrine, epinephrine (adrenaline), pseudoephedrine, erythromycin, and troleandomycin. Such combinations can lead to increases in blood pressure or increased risk of adverse reaction to ergotamine.

2. Do not drink alcoholic beverages while you are taking this medication. Since alcohol dilates (widens) the blood vessels (which are already dilated during migraine headaches), drinking will only make your headache worse.

3. Nicotine and cocaine decrease the effectiveness of ergotamine and, therefore, make the headache worse.

4. The caffeine in tea, coffee, and cola drinks also interacts with this medication. It may actually help to relieve your headache.

BE SURE TO TELL YOUR DOCTOR about any medications or substances you are currently taking or using, especially any of those listed above.

WARNINGS
• Tell your doctor about unusual or allergic reactions you have had to any medications, especially to ergotamine or other ergot alkaloids (such as ergonovine or bromocriptine).

• Before starting to take this medication, be sure to tell your doctor if you now have or if you have ever had heart or blood vessel disease, high blood pressure, infections, kidney disease, liver disease, or thyroid disease.

• Avoid any foods to which you are allergic—they may make your headache worse.

• If this drug makes you dizzy or drowsy, do not take part in any activity that requires alertness, such as driving a car or operating potentially dangerous equipment.

• Try to avoid exposure to cold. Since this drug acts by constricting blood vessels throughout the body, your fingers and toes may become especially sensitive.

• Elderly patients are more sensitive to the effects of ergotamine. Consult your doctor if the side effects become bothersome.

• This medication should not be taken for longer periods or in higher doses than recommended by your doctor. Extended use of this drug can lead to serious side effects. In addition, tolerance can develop—higher doses would be required to obtain the same beneficial effects (at the same time increasing the risk of side effects).

• Be sure to tell your doctor if you are pregnant. Ergotamine can cause contractions of the uterus, which can harm the developing fetus. This drug should not be used during pregnancy. Also, tell your doctor if you are breast-feeding an infant. Ergotamine passes into breast milk and may cause vomiting, diarrhea, or convulsions in the nursing infant.

MONEY-SAVING TIP
Save the inhaler piece from the aerosol container. Refill units, which are less expensive, are available.

ergotamine and caffeine combination

BRAND NAMES (Manufacturers)
Cafergot (Sandoz)
Cafetrate (Schein)
Wigraine (Organon)
TYPE OF DRUG
Antimigraine (vasoconstrictor)
INGREDIENTS
ergotamine and caffeine
DOSAGE FORMS
Tablets (1 mg ergotamine, 100 mg caffeine)
Suppositories (2 mg ergotamine, 100 mg caffeine)

STORAGE

Ergotamine and caffeine combination tablets should be stored at room temperature in tightly closed, light-resistant containers. They should also be stored away from heat and direct sunlight.

The suppository form of this drug should be kept in the refrigerator (never frozen) in a closed container.

USES

This medication is used to treat migraine and cluster headaches. These headaches are thought to be caused by an increase in the diameter of the blood vessels in the head, which results in increased blood flow, increased pressure, and pain. Ergotamine is a vasoconstrictor: it acts by constricting (narrowing) the blood vessels. Caffeine helps in both the absorption of the drug from the gastrointestinal tract and in constricting blood vessels.

TREATMENT

It is best to take this medication as soon as you notice your migraine headache symptoms. If you wait until the headache becomes severe, the drug takes longer to work and may not be as effective.

After you take either of these forms of ergotamine and caffeine combination, you should try to lie down in a quiet, dark room for at least two hours (in order to help the medication work). The drug usually takes effect within 30 to 60 minutes.

It is very important that you understand how often you can repeat a dose of this medication during an attack (usually every 30 to 60 minutes) and the maximum number of tablets you can take per day (usually six tablets). Ten is generally the maximum number of tablets that can be taken in any one-week period. CHECK WITH YOUR DOCTOR if you have any questions.

The tablets should be swallowed with liquid. Take one tablet when you first notice your migraine headache symptoms. If necessary, take a second dose 30 to 60 minutes later to relieve your headache.

To use the suppository form of this medication, first unwrap it and moisten it slightly with water (if the suppository is too soft to insert, run cold water over it or refrigerate it for 30 minutes before you unwrap it). Lie down on your left side, with your right knee bent. Push the suppository well into the rectum with your finger. Try to avoid having a bowel movement for at least an hour to give the medication time to be absorbed. Insert one suppository when you first notice your migraine symptoms. If necessary, insert a second suppository one hour later for full relief of your migraine headache. Five is generally the maximum number of suppositories that can be taken in a one-week period.

If you are on prolonged treatment with this drug and you miss a dose, take it as soon as you remember. Wait four hours to take the next dose. It is very important that you consult your doctor before you discontinue using ergotamine and caffeine combination. Your doctor may want to reduce your dosage gradually.

SIDE EFFECTS

Minor. Diarrhea, dizziness, headache, nausea, nervousness or jitters, vomiting, or sensation of cold hands and feet with MILD numbness or tingling. These side effects should disappear as your body adjusts to the medication.
Major. Tell your doctor about any side effects that are persistent or particularly bothersome. IT IS ESPECIALLY IMPORTANT TO TELL YOUR DOCTOR about chest pain; coldness, numbness, pain, tingling, or dark discoloration of the fingers or toes; confusion; fluid retention; itching; localized swelling; muscle pain; severe abdominal pain and swelling; severe nausea or vomiting; or unusual weakness.

INTERACTIONS

Ergotamine and caffeine combination interacts with several other types of medications:
1. Ergotamine interacts with amphetamines, ephedrine, epinephrine (adrenaline), pseudoephedrine, erythromycin, and troleandomycin. Such combinations can lead to increases in blood pressure or increased risk of adverse reaction to ergotamine.
2. Do not drink alcoholic beverages while you are taking this medication. Since alcohol dilates (widens) the blood vessels, drinking will only make your headache worse.
3. Tobacco and cocaine decrease the effectiveness of ergotamine and can make the headache worse.
4. The caffeine in tea, coffee, and cola drinks also interacts with this medication.

BE SURE TO TELL YOUR DOCTOR about any medications or substances you are currently taking or using, especially any of those listed above.

WARNINGS

• Tell your doctor about unusual or allergic reactions you have had to medications, especially to ergotamine, caffeine, or any ergot alkaloid (ergonovine, ergoloid mesylates, and bromocriptine).
• Before starting to take ergotamine and caffeine combination, be sure to tell your doctor if you now have or if you have ever had heart or blood vessel disease, high blood pressure, infections, kidney disease, liver disease, or thyroid disease.
• Avoid any foods to which you are allergic—they may make your headache worse.
• If this drug makes you dizzy or drowsy, do not take part in any activity that requires alertness, such as driving a car or operating potentially dangerous equipment.
• Since this drug acts by constricting blood vessels throughout the body (not just in the head), your fingers and toes may become especially sensitive to the cold.
• Elderly patients are more sensitive to the effects of ergotamine.
• This medication should not be taken for longer periods or in higher doses than recommended by your doctor. Extended use of this drug can lead to serious side effects. In addition, your body can develop a tolerance to this medication—higher doses would be required to obtain the same beneficial effects and, at the same time, the risk of side effects would be increased.
• Be sure to tell your doctor if you are pregnant. This medication can cause contractions of the uterus, which can harm the developing fetus. This drug should not be used during pregnancy. Also, tell your doctor if you are

breast-feeding an infant. Ergotamine and caffeine combination passes into breast milk and may cause vomiting, diarrhea, irritability, or convulsions in the nursing infant.

Eridium—see phenazopyridine

Eryc—see erythromycin

EryPed—see erythromycin

Ery-Tab—see erythromycin

Erythrocin Stearate Filmtabs—see erythromycin

erythromycin

BRAND NAMES (Manufacturers)
E.E.S. 200 (Abbott)
E.E.S. 400 (Abbott)
E-Mycin (Boots)
Eramycin (Wesley)
Eryc (Parke-Davis)
EryPed (Abbott)
Ery-Tab (Abbott)
Erythrocin Stearate Filmtabs (Abbott)
Erythromycin Base (Abbott)
Ilosone (Dista)
Ilosone Pulvules (Dista)
PCE Dispertab (Abbott)
Robimycin (Robins)
Wyamycin S (Wyeth)
TYPE OF DRUG
Antibiotic
INGREDIENT
erythromycin
DOSAGE FORMS
Tablets (250 mg, 333 mg, and 500 mg)
Chewable tablets (200 mg)
Enteric-coated tablets (250 mg, 333 mg, and 500 mg)
Film-coated tablets (250 mg, 400 mg, and 500 mg)
Polymer-coated tablets (333 mg)
Capsules (250 mg)
Oral drops (100 mg per 2.5 ml)
Oral suspension (125 mg, 200 mg, 250 mg, and 400 mg per 5-ml spoonful)
STORAGE
Erythromycin tablets and capsules should be stored at room temperature in tightly closed, light-resistant containers. Erythromycin oral drops and oral suspension should be stored in the refrigerator in tightly closed, light-resistant containers. Any unused portion of the liquid forms should be discarded after 14 days. Erythromycin ethylsuccinate liquid does not need to be refrigerated; however, refrigeration helps to preserve the taste. This medication should never be frozen.

USES
Erythromycin is used to treat a wide variety of bacterial infections, including infections of the middle ear and the respiratory tract. It is also used to treat infections in persons who are allergic to penicillin. It acts by preventing the bacteria from manufacturing protein, which prevents their growth. It is not effective against viruses, parasites, or fungi.

TREATMENT
In order to prevent stomach upset, erythromycin coated tablets and erythromycin estolate or ethylsuccinate can be taken with food or milk. Other erythromycin products should be taken with a full glass of water, preferably on an empty stomach, one hour before or two hours after a meal.

The liquid forms should be taken undiluted.

Each dose of the oral drops should be measured carefully with the dropper provided.

The oral suspension form of this medication should be shaken well just before measuring each dose. The contents tend to settle on the bottom of the bottle, so it is necessary to shake the container to distribute the ingredients evenly and equalize the doses. Each dose should then be measured carefully with a specially designed 5-ml measuring spoon. An ordinary kitchen teaspoon is not accurate enough.

In order to prevent gastrointestinal side effects, the coated tablets and capsules should be swallowed whole; do not break, chew, or crush these products.

Erythromycin works best when the level of medicine in your bloodstream is kept constant. It is best, therefore, to take the doses at evenly spaced intervals day and night. For example, if you are to take four doses a day, the doses should be spaced six hours apart.

If you miss a dose of this medication, take the missed dose immediately. However, if you do not remember to take the missed dose until it is almost time for your next dose, take it; space the following dose about halfway through the regular interval between doses; then return to your regular schedule. Try not to skip any doses.

It is important to continue to take this medication for the entire time prescribed by your doctor (usually seven to 14 days), even if the symptoms disappear before the end of that period. If you stop taking this drug too soon, resistant bacteria continue growing, and the infection could recur.

SIDE EFFECTS
Minor. Abdominal cramps, diarrhea, fatigue, irritation of the mouth, loss of appetite, nausea, sore tongue, or vomiting. These side effects should disappear as your body adjusts to the medication.
Major. Tell your doctor about any side effects that are persistent or particularly bothersome. IT IS ESPECIALLY IMPORTANT TO TELL YOUR DOCTOR about fever, hearing loss, hives, rash, rectal or vaginal itching, or yellowing of the eyes or skin. Also, if your symptoms of infection seem to be getting worse rather than improving, you should contact your doctor.

INTERACTIONS
1. Erythromycin can decrease the elimination of aminophylline, oxtriphylline, theophylline, digoxin, oral anticoagulants (blood thinners, such as warfarin), and car-

bamazepine from the body, which can lead to serious side effects.

2. Therapy with erythromycin may increase the effects of methylprednisolone.

BE SURE TO TELL YOUR DOCTOR about any medications you are currently taking, especially any listed above.

WARNINGS

• Tell your doctor about unusual or allergic reactions you have had to any medications, especially to erythromycin.

• Be sure to tell your doctor if you have ever had liver disease.

• This drug has been prescribed for your current infection only. Another infection later on, or one that someone else has, may require a different drug. Do not give your medicine to other people or use it for other infections, unless your doctor specifically directs you to.

• Before having surgery or any other medical or dental treatment, be sure to tell your doctor or dentist that you are taking erythromycin.

• Not all erythromycin products are chemically equivalent. However, they all produce the same therapeutic effect. Discuss with your doctor or pharmacist which forms of erythromycin are appropriate for you, and then choose the least expensive product among those recommended.

• Some of these products contain the color additive FD&C Yellow No. 5 (tartrazine), which can cause allergic-type reactions (difficulty in breathing, rash, fainting) in certain susceptible individuals.

• Be sure to tell your doctor if you are pregnant. Although erythromycin appears to be safe during pregnancy, extensive studies in humans have not been conducted. Also, tell your doctor if you are breast-feeding an infant. Small amounts of this medication pass into breast milk and may temporarily alter the bacterial balance in the intestinal tract of the nursing infant, resulting in diarrhea.

erythromycin and sulfisoxazole combination

BRAND NAMES (Manufacturers)
Eryzole (Alra)
Pediazole (Ross)
TYPE OF DRUG
Antibiotic
INGREDIENTS
erythromycin and sulfisoxazole
DOSAGE FORM
Oral suspension (200 mg erythromycin and 600 mg sulfisoxazole per 5-ml spoonful)
STORAGE
Store in the refrigerator (never freeze) in a tightly closed container. Any unused portion of the erythromycin and sulfisoxazole combination should be discarded after the expiration date (usually after 14 days) because the drug loses its potency after that time.

USES

Erythromycin and sulfisoxazole combination is used to treat acute otitis media (middle ear infection) in children. Erythromycin acts by preventing the bacteria from manufacturing protein, thereby preventing their growth. Sulfisoxazole also acts by preventing production of nutrients that are required for growth of the infecting bacteria. Erythromycin and sulfisoxazole combination kills a wide range of susceptible bacteria, but it is not effective against viruses, parasites, or fungi.

TREATMENT

In order to avoid stomach upset, you can take this medication either with food or with a full glass of water or milk. You can also take it on an empty stomach.

The oral suspension should be shaken well just before measuring each dose. The contents tend to settle on the bottom of the bottle, so it is necessary to shake the container to distribute the ingredients evenly and equalize the doses. Each dose should then be measured carefully with a specially designed 5-ml measuring spoon. An ordinary kitchen teaspoon is not accurate enough.

This medication works best when the level of medicine in the bloodstream is kept constant. It is best, therefore, to take the doses at evenly spaced intervals day and night. For example, if you are to take four doses a day, the doses should be spaced six hours apart.

If you miss a dose of this medication, take the missed dose immediately. However, if you do not remember to take the missed dose until it is almost time for your next dose, take it; space the following dose about halfway through the regular interval between doses; then return to your regular schedule. Try not to skip any doses.

It is important to continue to take this medication for the entire time prescribed by your doctor (usually seven to 14 days), even if the symptoms disappear before the end of that period. If you stop taking the drug too soon, resistant bacteria are given a chance to continue growing, and the infection could recur.

SIDE EFFECTS

Minor. Diarrhea, dizziness, headache, loss of appetite, nausea, sleep disorders, sore mouth or tongue, or vomiting. These side effects should disappear as your body adjusts to the medication.

This medication can cause increased sensitivity to sunlight. It is, therefore, important to avoid prolonged exposure to sunlight and sunlamps. Wear protective clothing and sunglasses, and use an effective sunscreen. However, sunscreens containing para-aminobenzoic acid (PABA) interfere with the antibacterial activity of sulfisoxazole and should not be used.

If you feel dizzy, sit or lie down for a while; get up slowly from a sitting or reclining position, and be careful on stairs.

Major. Tell your doctor about any side effects that are persistent or particularly bothersome. IT IS ESPECIALLY IMPORTANT TO TELL YOUR DOCTOR about aching, or joint and muscle pain; convulsions; difficult or painful urination; difficulty in swallowing; hallucinations; mental depression; loss of hearing; redness, blistering, or peeling of the skin; itching; rash; sore throat and fever; uncoordinated movements; unusual bleeding or bruising; unusual tiredness; or yellowing of the eyes or skin. Also, if the symptoms of infection seem to be getting worse, contact your doctor.

INTERACTIONS
This medication interacts with several other types of drugs:

1. Erythromycin can decrease the elimination of aminophylline, oxtriphylline, theophylline, digoxin, oral anticoagulants (blood thinners, such as warfarin), and carbamazepine from the body, which can lead to serious side effects.

2. Sulfisoxazole can increase the active blood levels of oral anticoagulants (blood thinners, such as warfarin), oral antidiabetic agents, methotrexate, oxyphenbutazone, phenylbutazone, and phenytoin, which can lead to serious side effects.

3. Methenamine can increase the side effects to the kidneys caused by sulfisoxazole.

4. Probenecid and sulfinpyrazone can increase the blood levels of sulfisoxazole.

5. Erythromycin may increase the effects of methylprednisolone.

Before starting to take this medication, BE SURE TO TELL YOUR DOCTOR about any medications you are currently taking, especially any of those listed above.

WARNINGS
• Tell your doctor about unusual or allergic reactions you have had to any medications, especially to erythromycin, sulfisoxazole, any other sulfa medications (sulfonamide antibiotics, diuretics, dapsone, sulfoxone, oral antidiabetic medicines) or acetazolamide.

• Tell your doctor if you now have or if you have ever had glucose-6-phosphate dehydrogenase (G6PD) deficiency, kidney disease, liver disease, or porphyria.

• This medication has been prescribed for your current infection only. Another infection later on, or one that someone else has, may require a different medicine. You should not give your medicine to other people or use it for other infections, unless your doctor specifically directs you to do so.

• Be sure to tell your doctor if you are pregnant. Small amounts of erythromycin and sulfisoxazole cross the placenta. Although these antibiotics appear to be safe during pregnancy, extensive studies in humans have not been conducted. Also, tell your doctor if you are breast-feeding an infant. Small amounts of this medication pass into breast milk and may temporarily alter the bacterial balance in the intestinal tract of the infant, resulting in diarrhea. This medication should not be used in an infant less than two months of age in order to avoid side effects involving the liver.

Erythromycin Base—see erythromycin

Eryzole—see erythromycin and sulfisoxazole combination

Esidrix—see hydrochlorothiazide

Eskalith—see lithium

Eskalith CR—see lithium

Estinyl—see ethinyl estradiol

Estraderm—see estradiol (topical)

---

estradiol (topical)

BRAND NAME (Manufacturer)
Estraderm (Ciba)
TYPE OF DRUG
Estrogen
INGREDIENT
estradiol
DOSAGE FORM
Transdermal patch (delivers 0.05 mg or 0.1 mg per 24 hours)
STORAGE
Estradiol transdermal patches should be stored at room temperature in their original packages.

USES
Estradiol is a synthetic estrogen that is used to treat menopausal symptoms or other conditions associated with estrogen deficiency.

TREATMENT
Your prescription of estradiol will come with patient instructions. It is important that you follow the directions carefully.

Wash and dry your hands before and after applying the patch. Apply the patch to a clean, dry, hairless area of the skin on the trunk of the body or on the abdomen. Do not apply to the breasts. Avoid applying the patch over a cut or to any area of the body where tight clothes might rub against the patch and cause it to loosen. Apply the patch immediately after opening the packet and removing the protective liner. Press the patch firmly to the skin with the palm of your hand for about ten seconds. Make sure there is good contact of the patch to the skin, especially around the edges. Rotate the application sites on the skin, waiting at least one week before applying to the same site.

If the patch becomes loose or falls off, the same one can be reapplied. If necessary, however, a new patch can be applied. In either case, continue with your original treatment schedule.

If you miss an application of this medication, apply a new patch as soon as possible unless it is almost time for the next application. In that case, return to your regular schedule. Do not apply a double dose.

SIDE EFFECTS
Minor. Acne, abdominal cramping, abnormal vaginal bleeding, bloating, breast tenderness, change in sexual desire, darkening of the skin, diarrhea, dizziness, fluid retention, frequent or painful urination, hair loss, headache, nausea, nervousness, skin irritation at patch site, vomiting, or weight gain. These side effects should disappear as your body adjusts to the drug.

If you feel dizzy, sit or lie down for a while; get up slowly from a sitting or reclining position, and be careful on stairs.

Eating a full breakfast or having a midmorning snack may help to relieve the nausea and vomiting.

This medication can increase your sensitivity to sunlight. You should, therefore, try to avoid prolonged exposure to sunlight and sunlamps. Wear protective clothing and sunglasses, and use an effective sunscreen.

Major. Tell your doctor about any side effects that are persistent or particularly bothersome. IT IS ESPECIALLY IMPORTANT TO TELL YOUR DOCTOR about blurred vision, chest pain, convulsions, depression, itching, loss of coordination, pain or inflammation of the calves or thighs, shortness of breath, skin rash, slurred speech, or yellowing of the eyes or skin.

INTERACTIONS

Estradiol interacts with several other types of medications:

1. It can decrease the effectiveness of oral anticoagulants (blood thinners, such as warfarin).

2. Carbamazepine, phenobarbital, phenytoin, primidone, and rifampin can reduce the effectiveness of estradiol.

3. Estradiol can increase the side effects and decrease the effectiveness of tricyclic antidepressants.

BE SURE TO TELL YOUR DOCTOR about any medications you are currently taking.

WARNINGS

• Tell your doctor about unusual or allergic reactions you have had to any medications, especially to estradiol, other estrogens, or oral contraceptives.

• Tell your doctor if you now have or if you have ever had asthma, blood clot disorders, breast disease, depression, diabetes mellitus, epilepsy, endometriosis, gallstones or gallbladder disease, heart disease, high blood pressure, kidney disease, liver disease, migraine headaches, porphyria, or uterine tumors.

• Estrogens may cause a change in glucose tolerance in diabetic patients. Be sure to tell your doctor if you notice any abnormalities in your urine or blood glucose levels.

• Estrogens can change your blood's clotting ability, so be especially careful to avoid injuries.

• Although it is not known if estrogens can increase the risk of breast cancer, it is important that you examine your breasts regularly for lumps or discharge.

• If you notice tenderness, swelling, or bleeding of your gums, consult your doctor or dentist.

• Your doctor may schedule regular office visits to be sure your medication is working properly.

• Before having surgery or any other medical or dental treatment, be sure to tell your doctor or dentist that you are taking this medication.

• A package insert titled "Information for the Patient" should be dispensed with your prescription. It is important that you understand the possible risks and benefits of this medication. If you have any questions, check with your doctor or pharmacist.

• Cigarette smoking can greatly increase the risk of developing heart or blood vessel disorders while taking this medication. The risks increase with the amount of smoking and the age of the smoker.

• Be sure to tell your doctor if you are pregnant. If you suspect you are pregnant, discontinue use of the medication immediately. Estrogens have been shown to cause birth defects in the offspring of women who received these medications during pregnancy. Also, tell your doctor if you are breast-feeding an infant. Small amounts of estrogen pass into breast milk. Estradiol can also decrease milk production.

estrogens, conjugated

BRAND NAMES (Manufacturers)
conjugated estrogens (various manufacturers)
Premarin (Wyeth-Ayerst)
TYPE OF DRUG
Estrogen
INGREDIENTS
conjugated estrogens
DOSAGE FORM
Tablets (0.3 mg, 0.625 mg, 0.9 mg, 1.25 mg, and 2.5 mg)
STORAGE
These tablets should be stored at room temperature in a tightly closed container.

USES

Conjugated estrogens are a group of estrogen-like products obtained from natural sources (the urine of pregnant mares). They are used to treat menopausal symptoms, prostatic cancer, uterine bleeding, and some cases of breast cancer. They can also be used in replacement therapy for women who do not produce enough estrogen of their own.

TREATMENT

In order to avoid stomach irritation, you can take conjugated estrogens with food or immediately after a meal.

Follow your doctor's instructions carefully when you take this medication. Often, conjugated estrogens are prescribed to be taken for three-week periods, with one week off (in order to reduce potential side effects).

If you miss a scheduled dose of this medication, take the missed dose as soon as possible, unless it is almost time for the next dose. In that case, do not take the missed dose at all; just return to your regular dosing schedule. Do not double the next dose.

SIDE EFFECTS

Minor. Bloating, change in sexual desire, depression, diarrhea, dizziness, headache, loss of appetite, nausea, or vomiting. These side effects should disappear as your body adjusts to the medication.

This medication can increase your sensitivity to sunlight. You should, therefore, try to avoid prolonged exposure to sunlight and sunlamps. Wear protective clothing and sunglasses, and use an effective sunscreen.

If you feel dizzy or light-headed, sit or lie down for a while; get up slowly from a sitting or reclining position, and be careful on stairs.

Major. Tell your doctor about side effects that are persistent or particularly bothersome. IT IS ESPECIALLY IMPORTANT TO TELL YOUR DOCTOR about changes in menstrual patterns; chest pain; difficulty in breathing; eye pain; loss of coordination; lumps in the breast; painful urination; pain in the calves; skin color changes; slurred speech; sudden, severe headache; swelling of the feet or ankles; vision changes; weight gain or loss; or yellowing of eyes or skin.

INTERACTIONS
Conjugated estrogens interact with several other drugs:
1. Estrogens can decrease the effectiveness of oral anticoagulants (blood thinners, such as warfarin).
2. Carbamazepine, ampicillin, phenobarbital, phenytoin, primidone, and rifampin can increase the elimination of estrogen from the body, thus decreasing its effectiveness.
3. Estrogens can increase the side effects and decrease the effectiveness of the tricyclic antidepressants.

BE SURE TO TELL YOUR DOCTOR about any medications you are currently taking, especially those listed above.

WARNINGS
• Tell your doctor about unusual or allergic reactions you have had to any medications, especially to conjugated estrogens, to oral contraceptives (birth control pills), or to any other estrogen product.
• Before starting to take this drug, tell your doctor if you have ever had asthma, blood clot disorders, breast cancer, diabetes mellitus, endometriosis, epilepsy, gallbladder disease, heart disease, high blood pressure, hypercalcemia, kidney disease, liver disease, migraines, porphyria, uterine fibroid tumors, vaginal bleeding, or depression.
• Studies have shown that estrogens increase the risk of certain types of cancer. Ask your pharmacist for the brochure "Information for the Patient." It is important that you understand the possible risks and benefits of this medication. If you have any questions, check with your doctor or pharmacist.
• Although it is not known if estrogens can increase the risk of breast cancer, it is important that you examine your breasts regularly for lumps or discharge.
• If you notice tenderness, swelling, or bleeding of your gums, consult your doctor or dentist.
• Estrogens can cause a change in glucose tolerance in diabetic patients. If you are diabetic, be sure to tell your doctor if you notice any abnormalities in your urine or blood glucose levels.
• Do not change your brand of medication without the consent of your doctor. If your refill does not look the same, consult your doctor or pharmacist.
• Cigarette smoking increases the risk of serious side effects from estrogens. The risk increases with both age and the amount of smoking.
• If this medication makes you dizzy or light-headed, you should not take part in any activity that requires alertness, such as driving a car or operating potentially dangerous equipment.
• Estrogens can change your blood's clotting ability, so be especially careful to avoid injuries.
• Before having surgery or any other medical or dental treatment, be sure to tell your doctor or dentist that you are taking this medication.
• Be sure to tell your doctor if you are pregnant. If you suspect you are pregnant, discontinue use of this medication immediately. Several studies have shown that estrogens taken during pregnancy can cause birth defects. Also, tell your doctor if you are breast-feeding an infant. Estrogens pass into breast milk.

---

ethacrynic acid

BRAND NAME (Manufacturer)
Edecrin (Merck Sharp & Dohme)
TYPE OF DRUG
Diuretic and antihypertensive
INGREDIENT
ethacrynic acid
DOSAGE FORM
Tablets (25 mg and 50 mg)
STORAGE
Ethacrynic acid should be stored at room temperature in a tightly closed, light-resistant container.

USES
Ethacrynic acid is prescribed to treat high blood pressure. It is also used to reduce fluid accumulation in the body caused by conditions such as heart failure, cirrhosis of the liver, kidney disease, and the long-term use of some medications. This medication reduces fluid accumulation by increasing the elimination of salt and water through the kidneys.

TREATMENT
To decrease stomach irritation, you can take ethacrynic acid with a glass of milk or with a meal (unless your doctor directs you to do otherwise). Try to take it at the same time every day. Avoid taking a dose after 6:00 P.M.; otherwise, you may have to get up during the night to urinate.

If you miss a dose of this medication, take the missed dose as soon as possible, unless it is almost time for the next dose. In that case, do not take the missed dose at all; just return to your regular dosing schedule. Do not double the next dose.

This medication does not cure high blood pressure, but it will help to control the condition as long as you take it.

SIDE EFFECTS
Minor. Blurred vision, cramping, diarrhea, dizziness, headache, loss of appetite, sore mouth, or stomach upset. As your body adjusts to the medication, these side effects should disappear.

This medication will cause an increase in the amount of urine or in the frequency of urination when you first begin to take it. It may also cause you to have an unusual feeling of tiredness. These effects should lessen after several days.

To avoid dizziness or light-headedness when you stand, contract and relax the muscles of your legs for a few moments before rising. Do this by pushing one foot against the floor while raising the other foot slightly, alternating feet so that you are "pumping" your legs in a pedaling motion.

Major. Tell your doctor about any side effects that are persistent or particularly bothersome. IT IS ESPECIALLY IMPORTANT TO TELL YOUR DOCTOR about black, tarry stools; confusion; difficulty in breathing; dry mouth; fainting; increased thirst; itching; joint pains; loss of appetite; mood changes; muscle cramps; nausea; palpitations; rash; ringing in the ears; sore throat; severe abdominal pain; tingling in the fingers and toes; unusual bleeding or bruising; vomiting; watery diarrhea; weakness; or yellowing of the eyes or skin.

INTERACTIONS
Ethacrynic acid interacts with several other types of drugs:
1. It can increase the side effects of alcohol, barbiturates, narcotics, cephalosporin antibiotics, cortisone and cortisone-like steroids (such as dexamethasone, hydrocortisone, prednisone, and prednisolone), digoxin, digitalis, lithium, amphotericin B, heparin, and warfarin.
2. Probenecid and indomethacin may decrease the effectiveness of this medicine.
3. The effectiveness of antigout medications, insulin, and oral antidiabetic medications may be decreased by ethacrynic acid.

Before taking ethacrynic acid, BE SURE TO TELL YOUR DOCTOR about any medications you are currently taking, especially any of those listed above.

WARNINGS
Tell your doctor about unusual or allergic reactions you have had to any medications, especially to ethacrynic acid or other diuretics.

Before you start taking this medication, tell your doctor if you now have or if you have ever had kidney disease, problems with urination, systemic lupus erythematosis, or liver disease.

This drug can cause potassium loss. Signs of potassium loss include dry mouth, thirst, weakness, muscle pain or cramps, nausea, and vomiting. If you experience any of these symptoms, call your doctor. Your doctor may have blood tests performed periodically to monitor your potassium levels. To help avoid potassium loss, take this drug with a glass of fresh or frozen orange or cranberry juice, or eat a banana every day. The use of a salt substitute also helps to prevent potassium loss. Do not change your diet or use a salt substitute, however, before discussing it with your doctor. Too much potassium can also be dangerous.

To prevent severe water loss (dehydration) while taking this medication, check with your doctor if you have any illness that causes severe or continuous nausea, vomiting, or diarrhea.

Before having any kind of surgery or other medical or dental treatment, be sure to tell your doctor or dentist that you are taking ethacrynic acid.

To prevent dizziness, light-headedness, and fainting, get up from a sitting or lying position slowly, avoid standing for long periods of time, and avoid strenuous exercise and prolonged exposure to hot weather.

While taking this medication, limit your intake of alcoholic beverages in order to prevent dizziness or light-headedness.

If you have high blood pressure, do not take any over-the-counter (nonprescription) medication for weight control or for allergy, asthma, cough, cold, or sinus problems unless you first check with your doctor.

The elderly may be more sensitive to the medication.

Be sure to tell your doctor if you are pregnant. This drug crosses the placenta. Although studies in humans have not been conducted, adverse effects have been observed in the fetuses of animals that received large doses of this drug during pregnancy. Also, tell your doctor if you are breast-feeding an infant. Small amounts of this drug pass into breast milk.

ethinyl estradiol

BRAND NAMES (Manufacturers)
Estinyl (Schering)
Feminone (Upjohn)
TYPE OF DRUG
Estrogen
INGREDIENT
ethinyl estradiol
DOSAGE FORM
Tablets (0.02 mg, 0.05 mg, and 0.5 mg)
STORAGE
Ethinyl estradiol should be stored at room temperature in a tightly closed container.

USES
Ethinyl estradiol is a synthetic estrogen that is used to treat menopausal symptoms, certain types of breast cancer, and prostate cancer.

TREATMENT
To avoid stomach irritation, take ethinyl estradiol with food, milk, or water (unless your doctor directs otherwise).

If you miss a dose of this medication, take the missed dose as soon as possible, unless it is almost time for the next dose. In that case, do not take the missed dose at all; just return to your regular dosing schedule. Do not double the next dose.

SIDE EFFECTS
Minor. Abdominal cramping, abnormal vaginal bleeding, bloating, breast tenderness, darkening of the skin, diarrhea, dizziness, fluid retention, frequent or painful urination, headache, nausea, vomiting, or weight gain. These side effects should disappear as your body adjusts to the medication.

This medication can increase your sensitivity to sunlight. You should, therefore, try to avoid prolonged exposure to sunlight and sunlamps. Wear protective clothing and sunglasses, and use an effective sunscreen.

If you feel dizzy, sit or lie down for a while; get up slowly from a sitting or reclining position, and be careful on stairs.

Eating a full breakfast or having a midmorning snack may help to relieve the nausea and vomiting.

Major. Tell your doctor about any side effects that are persistent or particularly bothersome. IT IS ESPECIALLY IMPORTANT TO TELL YOUR DOCTOR about blurred vision, chest pain, convulsions, depression, hair loss, itching, pain or inflammation of the calves or thighs, shortness of breath, skin rash, or yellowing of the eyes or skin.

INTERACTIONS

Ethinyl estradiol interacts with other types of medications:

1. It can decrease the effectiveness of oral anticoagulants (blood thinners, such as warfarin).

2. Ampicillin, carbamazepine, phenobarbital, phenytoin, primidone, and rifampin can reduce the effectiveness of ethinyl estradiol.

3. Ethinyl estradiol can increase the side effects and decrease the effectiveness of tricyclic antidepressants.

BE SURE TO TELL YOUR DOCTOR about any medications you are currently taking, especially any listed above.

WARNINGS

• Tell your doctor about unusual or allergic reactions you have had to any medications, especially to ethinyl estradiol or other estrogens, or to oral contraceptives (birth control pills).

• Tell your doctor if you now have or if you have ever had asthma, blood clot disorders, breast disease, depression, diabetes mellitus, epilepsy, endometriosis, gallstones or gallbladder disease, heart disease, high blood pressure, kidney disease, liver disease, migraine headaches, porphyria, or uterine tumors.

• Some of these products contain the color additive FD&C Yellow No. 5 (tartrazine), which can cause allergic-type reactions (shortness of breath, fainting, rash) in certain susceptible individuals.

• Estrogens can change your blood's clotting ability, so be especially careful to avoid injuries.

• Estrogens can cause a change in glucose tolerance in diabetic patients. Be sure to tell your doctor if you notice any abnormalities in your urine or blood glucose levels.

• Before having surgery or any other medical or dental treatment, be sure to tell your doctor or dentist that you are taking this medication.

• A package insert titled "Information for the Patient" should be dispensed with your prescription. It is important that you understand the possible risks and benefits of this medication. If you have any questions, check with your doctor or pharmacist.

• Although it is not known if estrogens increase the risk of breast cancer, it is important that you examine your breasts regularly for lumps or discharge.

• Cigarette smoking can greatly increase the risk of developing heart or blood vessel disorders while taking this medication. The risks increase with the amount of smoking and the age of the smoker.

• Be sure to tell your doctor if you are pregnant. If you suspect you are pregnant, discontinue use of this medication immediately. Estrogens have caused birth defects in the offspring of women who received these medica-

tions during pregnancy. Also, tell your doctor if you are breast-feeding an infant. Small amounts of estrogen pass into breast milk. Ethinyl estradiol can also decrease milk production.

Ethon—see methyclothiazide

---

ethosuximide

BRAND NAME (Manufacturer)
Zarontin (Parke-Davis)
TYPE OF DRUG
Anticonvulsant
INGREDIENT
ethosuximide
DOSAGE FORMS
Capsules (250 mg)
Oral syrup (250 mg per 5-ml spoonful)
STORAGE
Ethosuximide capsules and oral syrup should be stored at room temperature in tightly closed, light-resistant containers. It should never be frozen. Discard any outdated medication.

USES

This medication is used to treat absence (petit mal) seizures. Although it is not exactly clear how it does so, ethosuximide seems to prevent seizure activity by decreasing the activity of certain chemicals (nerve transmitters) in the brain.

TREATMENT

To avoid stomach irritation, take ethosuximide with food, water, or milk (unless your doctor directs you otherwise).

Each dose of the oral syrup form of this medication should be measured carefully with a specially designed 5-ml measuring spoon. A kitchen teaspoon is not accurate enough.

Ethosuximide works best when the level of medicine in your bloodstream is kept constant. It is best, therefore, to take the doses at evenly spaced intervals day and night. For example, if you are to take three doses a day, the doses should be spaced eight hours apart.

It is important to try not to miss any doses of this medication. If you do miss a dose, and remember within four hours, take the missed dose immediately and then return to your normal schedule. If more than four hours have passed, do not take the missed dose at all; just return to your regular dosing schedule. Do not double the next dose.

SIDE EFFECTS

Minor. Constipation, diarrhea, dizziness, drowsiness, headache, hiccups, loss of appetite, nausea, stomach upset, or weight loss. These side effects should disappear as your body adjusts to the medication.

To relieve constipation, increase the amount of fiber in your diet (fresh fruits and vegetables, salads, bran, and whole-grain breads), exercise, and drink more water (unless your doctor directs you to do otherwise).

If you feel dizzy, sit or lie down for a while; get up slowly from a sitting or reclining position, and be careful on stairs.

Major. Tell your doctor about any side effects that are persistent or particularly bothersome. IT IS ESPECIALLY IMPORTANT TO TELL YOUR DOCTOR about blurred vision, confusion, depression, difficult or painful urination, false sense of well-being, fatigue, irritability, joint pains, loss of coordination, mental disorders, mood changes, nervousness, skin rash, swelling of the eyes or tongue, unusual bleeding or bruising, or vaginal bleeding.

INTERACTIONS

This drug can interact with several other types of drugs:

1. Tricyclic antidepressants, haloperidol, thiothixene, phenothiazine tranquilizers, and alcohol can increase the risk of seizures. Dosage adjustments of ethosuximide may be necessary when any of these medications are started.

2. Isoniazid can increase the side effects of ethosuximide.

 BE SURE TO TELL YOUR DOCTOR about any medications you are currently taking, especially any listed above.

WARNINGS

• Tell your doctor about unusual or allergic reactions you have had to any medications, especially to ethosuximide, methsuximide, or phensuximide.

• Tell your doctor if you now have or if you have ever had blood disorders, kidney disease, or liver disease.

• If this drug makes you dizzy or drowsy, do not take part in any activity that requires alertness, such as driving a car or operating potentially dangerous equipment. Children should be careful while playing.

• Before having surgery or any other medical or dental treatment, be sure to tell your doctor or dentist that you are taking ethosuximide.

• Do not stop taking this medication unless you first check with your doctor. Stopping the drug abruptly may lead to a worsening of your condition. Your doctor may want to reduce your dosage gradually or start you on another drug when treatment with ethosuximide is discontinued.

• Your doctor may schedule regular office visits, especially during the first few months of therapy, to be sure the drug is working properly.

• Be sure to tell your doctor if you are pregnant. Birth defects have been reported more often in infants whose mothers have seizure disorders. It is unclear if the increased risk of birth defects is associated with the disorder or with the anticonvulsant medications, such as ethosuximide, used to treat the condition. Also, tell your doctor if you are breast-feeding an infant. Ethosuximide passes into breast milk.

Etrafon—see perphenazine and amitriptyline combination

Exna—see benzthiazide

Glyceryl-T—see theophylline and guaifenesin combination

famotidine

BRAND NAME (Manufacturer)
Pepcid (Merck Sharp & Dohme)
TYPE OF DRUG
Gastric acid secretion inhibitor (decreases stomach acid)
INGREDIENT
famotidine
DOSAGE FORMS
Tablets (20 mg and 40 mg)
Oral suspension (40 mg per 5-ml spoonful)
STORAGE
Famotidine should be stored at room temperature (never frozen) in a tightly closed container. Avoid exposure of this medication to high temperatures during storage.

USES

Famotidine is used to treat active duodenal ulcers. It is also used in the long-term treatment of excessive stomach acid secretion (Zollinger-Ellison syndrome) and in the prevention of recurrent ulcers. Famotidine reduces stomach acid secretions by blocking the effects of histamine in the stomach.

TREATMENT

If you are taking a single daily dose of famotidine, it is best to take the dose at bedtime in order to obtain the maximum benefits from it. Antacids will not affect the activity of famotidine. Check with your doctor to see if you should be taking antacids as part of your ulcer treatment.

 The oral liquid should be measured carefully with a specially designed 5-ml measuring spoon. An ordinary kitchen teaspoon is not accurate enough to ensure that the proper dose will be taken.

 If you miss a dose of famotidine, take the missed dose as soon as possible, unless it is almost time for the next dose. In that case, do not take the missed dose at all; just return to your regular dosing schedule. Do not double the next dose.

SIDE EFFECTS

Minor. Abdominal pain, acne, change in taste, constipation, diarrhea, dizziness, dry mouth, dry skin, fatigue, flushing, headache, insomnia, loss of appetite, nausea, or vomiting. These side effects should disappear as your body adjusts to this drug.

 If you are constipated, exercise and drink more water (unless your doctor tells you not to do so).

 To reduce mouth dryness, chew sugarless gum or suck on ice chips or hard candy.

 If you feel dizzy or light-headed, sit or lie down for a while; get up slowly from a sitting or reclining position, and be careful on stairs.

Major. Tell your doctor about any side effects that are persistent or particularly bothersome. IT IS ESPECIALLY IMPORTANT TO TELL YOUR DOCTOR about anxiety, confusion, depression, fever, hair loss, hallucinations, itching, muscle or joint pain, palpitations, ringing in the ear, seizures, shortness of breath, tingling in the fingers or toes, or yellowing of the eyes or skin.

INTERACTIONS

No drug interactions with famotidine have yet been confirmed. It is still very important, however, to tell your doctor about all of the medications you are taking before starting famotidine.

WARNINGS

• Tell your doctor about any unusual or allergic reactions you have had to any medications, especially to famotidine or to the other gastric acid secretion inhibitors (cimetidine and ranitidine).

• Before starting famotidine, tell your doctor if you now have or if you have ever had kidney disease.

• Famotidine should be taken continuously for as long as your doctor prescribes. Stopping therapy early may be a cause of ineffective treatment.

• Cigarette smoking may interfere with the beneficial effects of famotidine.

• Aspirin, foods known to cause stomach upset, and certain drinks (such as those containing caffeine) may worsen your stomach irritation.

• If this drug makes you dizzy or drowsy, do not take part in any activity that requires alertness, such as driving a car or operating potentially dangerous equipment.

• Be sure to tell your doctor if you are pregnant. Studies in pregnant women have not been conducted. Also, tell your doctor if you are breast-feeding an infant. Small amounts of famotidine pass into animal milk.

Fastin—see phentermine

Fedahist—see pseudoephedrine and chlorpheniramine combination

Feldene—see piroxicam

Femazole—see metronidazole

Feminone—see ethinyl estradiol

fenfluramine

BRAND NAME (Manufacturer)
Pondimin (Robins)
TYPE OF DRUG
Anorectic
INGREDIENT
fenfluramine
DOSAGE FORM
Tablets (20 mg)
STORAGE
Fenfluramine should be stored at room temperature in a tightly closed, light-resistant container.

USES

Fenfluramine is used as an appetite suppressant during the first few weeks of dieting to help establish new eating habits. This medication is thought to relieve hunger by altering nerve impulses to the appetite control center in the brain. Its effectiveness lasts only for short periods (three to 12 weeks).

TREATMENT

You can take fenfluramine with a full glass of water, one hour before meals (unless your doctor directs you to do otherwise).

If you miss a dose of this medication, take the missed dose as soon as possible, unless it is almost time for your next dose. In that case, do not take the missed dose at all; just return to your regular dosing schedule. Do not double the next dose.

SIDE EFFECTS

Minor. Blurred vision, constipation, diarrhea, dizziness, dry mouth, euphoria, fatigue, frequent urination, headache, insomnia, irritability, nausea, nervousness, restlessness, stomach pain, sweating, unpleasant taste in the mouth, or vomiting. These side effects should disappear as your body adjusts to the medication.

Dry mouth can be relieved by sucking on ice chips or a piece of hard candy or by chewing sugarless gum.

In order to prevent constipation, increase the amount of fiber in your diet (fresh fruits and vegetables, salads, bran, and whole-grain breads), exercise, and drink more water (unless your doctor tells you not to do so).

Major. Tell your doctor about any side effects that are persistent or particularly bothersome. IT IS ESPECIALLY IMPORTANT TO TELL YOUR DOCTOR about changes in sexual desire, chest pain, difficulty in urinating, enlarged breasts (in both sexes), fever, hair loss, headaches, impotence, increased blood pressure, menstrual irregularities, mental depression, mood changes, mouth sores, muscle pains, nosebleeds, palpitations, rash, sore throat, or tremors.

INTERACTIONS

Fenfluramine anorectic medication interacts with several other types of medications:

1. Concurrent use of it with central nervous system depressants (such as alcohol, antihistamines, barbiturates, muscle relaxants, narcotics, pain medications, and phenothiazine tranquilizers) or with tricyclic antidepressants can cause extreme drowsiness.

2. Fenfluramine may alter insulin and oral antidiabetic medication dosage requirements in diabetic patients.

3. The blood-pressure-lowering effects of antihypertensive medications, especially guanethidine, reserpine, methyldopa, and diuretics (water pills), may be increased by this medication.

4. Use of fenfluramine within 14 days of a monoamine oxidase (MAO) inhibitor (isocarboxazid, pargyline, phenelzine, tranylcypromine) can result in high blood pressure and other side effects.

BE SURE TO TELL YOUR DOCTOR about any medications you are currently taking, especially those listed above.

WARNINGS

• Tell your doctor about unusual or allergic reactions you have had to any medications, especially to fenfluramine or other appetite suppressants (such as benzphetamine, phendimetrazine, diethylpropion, phenmetrazine, mazindol, and phentermine), or to epinephrine, norepinephrine, ephedrine, amphetamines,

dextroamphetamine, phenylephrine, phenylpropano-lamine, pseudoephedrine, albuterol, metaproterenol, or terbutaline.
• Tell your doctor if you have a history of drug abuse or alcoholism or if you have ever had angina, diabetes mellitus, emotional disturbances, glaucoma, heart or cardiovascular disease, high blood pressure, thyroid disease, epilepsy, or mental depression.
• Fenfluramine can mask the symptoms of extreme fatigue and can cause dizziness or light-headedness. Your ability to perform tasks that require alertness, such as driving a car or operating potentially dangerous equipment, may be decreased during therapy with this medication. Appropriate caution should also be taken when going up and down stairs.
• Before having surgery or any other medical or dental treatment, be sure to tell your doctor or dentist that you are taking this medication.
• Fenfluramine is related to amphetamine and may be habit-forming when taken for long periods of time (both physical and psychological dependence can occur). You should, therefore, not increase the dosage of this medication or take it for longer than 12 weeks, unless you first consult your doctor. It is also important that you not stop taking this medication abruptly. Fatigue, sleep disorders, mental depression, nausea, vomiting, stomach cramps, or pain could occur. Your doctor may want to decrease your dosage gradually in order to prevent these side effects.
• Fenfluramine can alter blood sugar levels in diabetic patients. Therefore, it is important to note that if you are diabetic and starting to take this medication, you should carefully monitor your blood or urine glucose levels for the first several days.
• Be sure to tell your doctor if you are pregnant. Although side effects in humans have not been studied, some of the appetite suppressants have been shown to cause side effects in the fetuses of animals that received large doses during pregnancy. Also, tell your doctor if you are breast-feeding an infant. It is not known whether this medication passes into breast milk.

fenoprofen

BRAND NAMES (Manufacturers)
fenoprofen (various manufacturers)
Nalfon (Dista)
Nalfon 200 (Dista)
TYPE OF DRUG
Nonsteroidal anti-inflammatory analgesic
INGREDIENT
fenoprofen
DOSAGE FORMS
Capsules (200 mg and 300 mg)
Tablets (600 mg)
STORAGE
This medication should be stored in tightly closed containers at room temperature away from heat and direct sunlight.

USES
Fenoprofen is used to treat the inflammation (pain, swelling, and stiffness) of certain types of arthritis, gout, bursitis, and tendinitis. Fenoprofen has been shown to block the production of certain body chemicals, called prostaglandins, that trigger pain. However, it is not yet fully understood how fenoprofen works.

TREATMENT
You should take this medication on an empty stomach 30 to 60 minutes before meals or two hours after meals, so that it gets into your bloodstream quickly. Since fenoprofen can cause stomach irritation, however, your doctor may want you to take this medicine with food or antacids.

If you are taking fenoprofen to relieve arthritis, you must take it regularly as directed by your doctor. It may take up to three weeks before you feel its full benefits. This medication does not cure arthritis, but it will help to control the condition as long as you continue to take it.

It is important to take fenoprofen on schedule and not to miss any doses. If you do miss a dose, take the missed dose as soon as possible, unless it is almost time for your next dose. In that case, do not take the missed dose at all; just return to your regular dosing schedule. Do not double the next dose.

SIDE EFFECTS
Minor. Bloating, constipation, diarrhea, difficulty in sleeping, dizziness, drowsiness, headache, heartburn, indigestion, light-headedness, loss of appetite, nausea, nervousness, soreness of the mouth, unusual sweating, or vomiting. As your body adjusts to the drug, these side effects should disappear.

To relieve constipation, increase the amount of fiber in your diet (fresh fruits and vegetables, salads, bran, and whole-grain breads), exercise, and drink more water (unless your doctor directs you to do otherwise).

If you become dizzy, sit or lie down for a while; get up slowly from a sitting or reclining position, and be careful on stairs.
Major. If any side effects are persistent or particularly bothersome, you should report them to your doctor. IT IS ESPECIALLY IMPORTANT TO TELL YOUR DOCTOR about bloody or black, tarry stools; blurred vision; confusion; depression; difficult or painful urination; difficulty in breathing; hearing difficulties; palpitations; ringing or buzzing in the ears; skin rash, hives, or itching; stomach pain; swelling of the feet; tightness in the chest; unexplained sore throat and fever; unusual bleeding or bruising; unusual fatigue or weakness; unusual weight gain; or yellowing of the eyes or skin.

INTERACTIONS
Fenoprofen interacts with several types of medications:
1. Anticoagulants (blood thinners, such as warfarin) can lead to an increase in bleeding complications.
2. Aspirin, salicylates, and other anti-inflammatory medications can lead to an increase in stomach irritation caused by fenoprofen.
3. Fenoprofen levels may be affected by concurrent use of phenobarbital.

4. Probenecid may increase blood levels of fenoprofen, which may increase the risk of side effects.

5. The action of beta blockers may be decreased by this drug.

BE SURE TO TELL YOUR DOCTOR about any medications you are currently taking, especially those listed above.

WARNINGS

• Tell your doctor if you have ever had unusual or allergic reactions to medications, especially to fenoprofen or any chemically related drug (such as aspirin or other salicylates, diclofenac, diflunisal, flurbiprofen, indomethacin, ibuprofen, oxyphenbutazone, piroxicam, sulindac, or tolmetin).

• Tell your doctor if you have ever had bleeding problems, colitis, ulcers or other stomach problems, epilepsy, heart disease, high blood pressure, asthma, kidney disease, liver disease, mental illness, or Parkinson's disease.

• If this drug makes you dizzy or drowsy, do not take part in any activity that requires alertness, such as driving a car or operating potentially dangerous equipment.

• Before having surgery or other medical or dental treatment, tell your doctor or dentist about this drug.

• Stomach problems are more likely to occur if you take aspirin regularly or drink alcohol while being treated with this medication. These should, therefore, be avoided (unless your doctor directs you to do otherwise).

• Be sure to tell your doctor if you are pregnant. Although studies in humans have not been conducted, unwanted heart side effects have been reported in the offspring of animals that received fenoprofen during pregnancy. Also, tell your doctor if you are breast-feeding an infant. Small amounts of this medication can pass into breast milk.

Festal II—see pancrelipase

Fiorgen PF—see aspirin, caffeine, and butalbital combination

Fiorinal—see aspirin, caffeine, and butalbital combination

Fiorinal with Codeine—see aspirin, caffeine, butalbital, and codeine combination

Flagyl—see metronidazole

Flexeril—see cyclobenzaprine

Florvite—see vitamins, multiple, with flouride

flunisolide (nasal)

BRAND NAME (Manufacturer)
Nasalide (Syntex)
TYPE OF DRUG
Nasal adrenocorticosteroid hormone
INGREDIENT
flunisolide

DOSAGE FORM
Nasal solution (25 mcg flunisolide per spray)
STORAGE
Flunisolide nasal solution should be stored at room temperature in a tightly closed container. Opened containers of this medication should be discarded after three months.

USES
Flunisolide nasal solution is used to relieve symptoms of rhinitis (inflammation of the nasal passages). How this drug acts to relieve these symptoms is not completely understood. Your adrenal glands naturally produce certain cortisone-like chemicals. These chemicals are involved in various regulatory processes in the body (such as those involving fluid balance, temperature, and reaction to inflammation). Flunisolide belongs to a group of drugs known as adrenocorticosteroids (or cortisone-like medications).

TREATMENT
Just before applying flunisolide nasal solution, clear your nasal passages of all secretions. Then carefully follow the patient instructions, which you should receive when your prescription is dispensed. The instructions will explain how to properly apply this medication. Do not increase the dose of flunisolide or increase the number of applications per day without first checking with your doctor.

If your doctor recommends that you use a nasal decongestant to clear your nasal passages, use the decongestant just before you apply flunisolide.

Relief from the symptoms of inflammation may not become apparent for up to three weeks after starting flunisolide. This drug does not cure the cause of inflammation, but it may help relieve the symptoms as long as you continue to use it. Therefore, its effectiveness depends on regular use while the condition is present. Your doctor may then recommend that you gradually decrease the number of daily doses as your condition improves.

If there is no improvement in your condition within three weeks after starting flunisolide, check with your doctor. He or she may want you to stop the medication. Try not to miss any doses of this medication.

If you do miss a dose, apply the dose as soon as possible, unless it is almost time for the next dose. In that case, do not apply the missed dose; just return to your regular dosing schedule. Do not double the next dose.

SIDE EFFECTS
Minor. Drying of nasal passages, headache, loss of smell or taste, nasal congestion, nasal irritation, nausea, nosebleeds, sneezing, sore throat, vomiting, or watery eyes. These side effects should disappear as your body adjusts to this medication. A mild, temporary burning or stinging sensation may occur after this medication is applied.
Major. Tell your doctor about any side effects that are persistent or particularly bothersome. IT IS ESPECIALLY IMPORTANT TO TELL YOUR DOCTOR about persistent burning or stinging after application.

INTERACTIONS
This medication should not interact with any other medications as long as it is used according to directions.

WARNINGS

• Tell your doctor about unusual or allergic reactions you have had to any medications, especially to flunisolide or other adrenocorticosteroids (such as amcinonide, beclomethasone, betamethasone, clocortolone, cortisone, desonide, desoximetasone, dexamethasone, diflorasone, flumethasone, fluocinolone, fluocinonide, fluorometholone, flurandrenolide, halcinonide, hydrocortisone, methylprednisolone, paramethasone, prednisolone, prednisone, and triamcinolone).
• Before starting flunisolide, tell your doctor if you now have or if you have ever had chicken pox, diabetes mellitus, or tuberculosis.
• Flunisolide can slow the healing of wounds. Therefore, tell your doctor about recent nasal surgery or injury, recurrent nosebleeds, or nasal ulcers.
• Tell your doctor if you are pregnant. Birth defects have been observed in the offspring of animals that were given large doses of this drug during pregnancy. Tell your doctor if you are breast-feeding . Small amounts of adrenocorticosteroids do pass into breast milk and may cause growth suppression or a decrease in natural adrenocorticosteroid production in the nursing infant.

fluocinolone (topical)

BRAND NAMES (Manufacturers)
fluocinolone acetonide (various manufacturers)
Fluonid (Herbert)
Flurosyn (Rugby)
Synalar (Syntex)
Synalar-HP (Syntex)
Synemol (Syntex)
TYPE OF DRUG
Adrenocorticosteroid hormone
INGREDIENT
fluocinolone
DOSAGE FORMS
Cream (0.01%, 0.025%, and 0.2%)
Ointment (0.025%)
Solution (0.01%)
STORAGE
Store at room temperature in a tightly closed container. This medication should never be frozen.

USES
Your adrenal glands naturally produce certain cortisone-like chemicals. These chemicals are involved in various regulatory processes in the body (such as those involving fluid balance, temperature, and reaction to inflammation). Fluocinolone belongs to a group of drugs known as adrenocorticosteroids (or cortisone-like medications). It is used to relieve the skin inflammation (redness, swelling, itching, and discomfort) associated with conditions such as dermatitis, eczema, and poison ivy. How this drug works is not completely understood.

TREATMENT
Before applying this medication, wash your hands. Then, unless your doctor gives you different instructions, gently wash the area of the skin where the medication is to be applied. With a clean towel, pat the area until it is almost dry; it should be slightly damp when you put the medicine on.

Apply a small amount of fluocinolone to the affected area in a thin layer. Do not bandage the area unless your doctor tells you to do so. If you are to apply an occlusive dressing (like kitchen plastic wrap), ask for instructions. Wash your hands again after application.

If you miss a dose of this medication, apply the missed dose as soon as possible, unless it is almost time for the next application. In that case, do not apply the missed dose at all; just return to your regular schedule. Do not put twice as much of the medication on your skin at the next application.

SIDE EFFECTS
Minor. Acne, burning, itching, rash, or skin dryness.

If the affected area is extremely dry or scaling, the skin may be moistened before applying the medication by soaking in water or by applying water with a clean cloth. The ointment form is probably better for dry skin.

A mild, temporary stinging sensation may occur after this medication is applied. If this persists, contact your doctor.

Major. Tell your doctor about any side effects that are persistent or particularly bothersome. IT IS ESPECIALLY IMPORTANT TO TELL YOUR DOCTOR about blistering, increased hair growth, irritation of the affected area, loss of skin color, secondary infection in the area being treated, or thinning of the skin with easy bruising.

INTERACTIONS
This medication should not interact with other medications as long as it is used according to directions.

WARNINGS
• Tell your doctor about unusual or allergic reactions you have had to any medications, especially to fluocinolone or any other adrenocorticosteroid (such as amcinonide, beclomethasone, betamethasone, clocortolone, cortisone, desonide, desoximetasone, dexamethasone, diflorasone, flumethasone, fluocinonide, fluorometholone, flurandrenolide, halcinonide, hydrocortisone, methylprednisolone, paramethasone, prednisolone, prednisone, and triamcinolone).
• Tell your doctor if you now have or if you have ever had blood vessel disease, chicken pox, diabetes mellitus, fungal infection, peptic ulcers, shingles, tuberculosis, tuberculosis of the skin, vaccinia, or any other type of infection, especially at the site currently being treated.
• If irritation develops while using this drug, immediately discontinue its use and notify your doctor.
• This product is not for use in the eyes, nose, or mouth; contact may result in side effects.
• Do not use this product with an occlusive wrap unless your doctor directs you to do so. Systemic absorption of this drug is increased if large areas of the body are treated, particularly if occlusive bandages are used. If it is necessary for you to use this drug under a wrap, follow your doctor's instructions exactly; do not leave the wrap in place longer than specified.

• If you are using fluocinolone on a child's diaper area, do not put tight-fitting diapers or plastic pants on the child. This could lead to increased systemic absorption of the drug and a possible increase in side effects.

• Be sure to tell your doctor if you are pregnant. If large amounts of this drug are applied for prolonged periods, some of it will be absorbed and may cross the placenta. Although studies in humans have not been conducted, birth defects have been observed in the offspring of animals that were given large oral doses of this type of drug during pregnancy. Also, tell your doctor if you are breast-feeding an infant. If absorbed through the skin, small amounts of this medication pass into breast milk and may cause growth suppression or a decrease in natural adrenocorticosteroid hormone production in the nursing infant.

fluocinolone acetonide—see fluocinolone (topical)

---

fluocinonide (topical)

BRAND NAMES (Manufacturers)
fluocinonide (various manufacturers)
Lidex (Syntex)
Lidex-E (Syntex)
Vasoderm (Taro)
Vasoderm E (Taro)
TYPE OF DRUG
Adrenocorticosteroid hormone
INGREDIENT
fluocinonide
DOSAGE FORMS
Ointment (0.05%)
Cream (0.05%)
Gel (0.05%)
Solution (0.05%, with 35% alcohol)
STORAGE
Fluocinonide ointment, cream, gel, and solution should be stored at room temperature in tightly closed containers. This medication should never be frozen.

USES
Your adrenal glands naturally produce certain cortisone-like chemicals. These chemicals are involved in various regulatory processes in the body (such as those involving fluid balance, temperature, and reaction to inflammation). Fluo-cinonide belongs to a group of drugs known as adrenocorticosteroids (or cortisone-like medications). It is used to relieve the skin inflammation (redness, swelling, itching, and discomfort) associated with conditions such as dermatitis, eczema, and poison ivy. How this drug works is not completely understood.

TREATMENT
Before applying this medication, wash your hands. Then, unless your doctor gives you different instructions, gently wash the area of the skin where the medication is to be applied. With a clean towel, pat the area almost dry; it should be slightly damp when you put the medicine on.

Apply a small amount of fluocinonide to the affected area in a thin layer. Do not bandage the area unless your doctor tells you to do so. If you are to apply an occlusive dressing (like kitchen plastic wrap), be sure you understand the instructions. Wash your hands again after application.

If you miss a dose of this medication, apply the missed dose as soon as possible, unless it is almost time for the next application. In that case, do not apply the missed dose at all; just return to your regular schedule. Do not double the next dose.

SIDE EFFECTS
Minor. Acne, burning sensation, itching, rash, or dry skin.

If the affected area is extremely dry or scaling, the skin may be moistened before applying the medication by soaking in water or by applying water with a clean cloth. The ointment form is probably better for dry skin.

A mild, temporary stinging sensation may occur after this medication is applied. If this persists, contact your doctor.

Major. Tell your doctor about any side effects that are persistent or particularly bothersome. IT IS ESPECIALLY IMPORTANT TO TELL YOUR DOCTOR about blistering, increased hair growth, irritation of the affected area, loss of skin color, secondary infection in the area being treated, or thinning of the skin with easy bruising.

INTERACTIONS
This medication should not interact with any other medications as long as it is used according to directions.

WARNINGS
• Tell your doctor about unusual or allergic reactions you have had to any medications, especially to fluocinonide or any other adrenocorticosteroid (such as amcinonide, betamethasone, clocortolone, cortisone, desonide, desoximetasone, dexamethasone, diflorasone, flumethasone, fluocinolone, fluorometholone, flurandrenolide, halcinonide, hydrocortisone, methylprednisolone, paramethasone, prednisolone, prednisone, and triamcinolone).

• Tell your doctor if you now have or if you have ever had blood vessel disease, chicken pox, diabetes mellitus, fungal infection, peptic ulcers, shingles, tuberculosis, tuberculosis of the skin, vaccinia, or any other type of infection, especially at the site currently being treated.

• If any type of irritation develops while using this drug, you should immediately discontinue use of the medication and notify your doctor.

• Fluocinonide is a topical medication. It is meant for use on the skin only. This product is not for use in the eyes, nose, or mouth; contact may result in side effects.

• Do not use this product with an occlusive wrap unless your doctor directs you to do so. Systemic absorption of this drug is increased if large areas of the body are treated, particularly if occlusive bandages are used. If it is necessary for you to use this drug under a wrap, follow your doctor's instructions exactly; do not leave the wrap in place longer than specified.

• If you are using fluocinonide on a child's diaper area, do not put tight-fitting diapers or plastic pants on the child. This may lead to increased systemic absorption of the drug and a possible increase in side effects.

• Be sure to tell your doctor if you are pregnant. If large amounts of this drug are applied for prolonged periods, some of it will be absorbed and may cross the placenta. Although studies in humans have not been conducted, birth defects have been observed in the offspring of animals that were given large oral doses of this type of drug during pregnancy. Also, tell your doctor if you are breast-feeding an infant. If absorbed through the skin, small amounts of fluocinonide pass into breast milk and may cause growth suppression or a decrease in natural adreno-corticosteroid hormone production in the nursing infant.

Fluonid—see fluocinolone (topical)

---

fluoxetine

BRAND NAME (Manufacturer)
Prozac (Dista)
TYPE OF DRUG
Cyclic antidepressant
INGREDIENT
fluoxetine
DOSAGE FORMS
Capsules (20 mg)
Liquid (20 mg per 5 ml spoonful)
STORAGE
Store at room temperature in a tightly closed container. Do not store in the bathroom. Heat or moisture can cause this medicine to break down.

USES
Fluoxetine is used to treat the symptoms of mental depression. It increases the concentration of certain chemicals necessary for nerve transmission in the brain.

TREATMENT
This medication should be taken exactly as prescribed by your doctor. In order to avoid stomach irritation, you can take fluoxetine with food or with a full glass of water (unless your doctor directs you to do otherwise).

The effects of therapy with this medication may not become apparent for one to three weeks.

If you miss a dose of this medicine, it is not necessary to make up the missed dose. Skip that dose and continue at the next scheduled time. You should never take a double dose to make up for one you missed.

SIDE EFFECTS
Minor. Agitation, change in vision, changes in taste, constipation, decreased appetite, decreased mental concentration, decreased sex drive, diarrhea, dizziness, drowsiness, dry mouth, fast heartbeat, flushing, frequent urination, headache, increased sweating, nausea, stomach cramps, stuffy nose, vomiting, or weight gain or loss.

Dry mouth can be relieved by chewing sugarless gum or sucking on hard candy.

To relieve constipation, increase the amount of fiber in your diet (fresh fruits and vegetables, salads, bran, and whole-grain breads), exercise, and drink more water (unless your doctor directs you to do otherwise).

To avoid dizziness when you stand, contract and relax the muscles of your legs for a few moments before rising.

Major. Tell your doctor about any side effects that are persistent or particularly bothersome. IT IS ESPECIALLY IMPORTANT TO TELL YOUR DOCTOR about anxiety, chills or fever, convulsions (seizures), enlarged lymph glands (swelling under jaw or in armpits or groin area), difficulty in breathing, joint or muscle pain, skin rash or hives, or swelling of the feet or lower legs.

INTERACTIONS
Fluoxetine interacts with a number of other types of drugs:
1. Extreme drowsiness can occur when this medicine is taken with central nervous system depressants (such as alcohol, antihistamines, barbiturates, benzodiazepine tranquilizers, muscle relaxants, narcotics, pain medications, phenothiazine tranquilizers, and sleeping medications) or with other antidepressants.
2. Fluoxetine may increase the effects of anticoagulants (blood thinners, such as warfarin) and certain heart medications (such as digitoxin).
3. Serious side effects may occur if a monoamine oxidase (MAO) inhibitor (such as furazolidone, isocarboxazid, pargyline, phenelzine, procarbazine, or tranylcypromine) is taken with fluoxetine. At least 14 days should separate the use of fluoxetine and the use of an MAO inhibitor.
4. Fluoxetine can increase agitation, restlessness, and stomach irritation when taken along with tryptophan.

Before starting to take fluoxetine, BE SURE TO TELL YOUR DOCTOR about any medications you are currently taking, especially any of those listed above.

WARNINGS
• Tell your doctor immediately if you develop a skin rash or hives while taking this medication, or if you have ever had an allergic reaction to fluoxetine.
• Tell your doctor if you have allergies to any substance, such as foods, sulfites or other preservatives, or dyes.
• Before starting to take this medication, be sure to tell your doctor if you have a history of alcoholism or if you have ever had a heart attack, asthma, circulatory disease, difficulty in urinating, electroshock therapy, enlarged prostate gland, epilepsy, glaucoma, high blood pressure, intestinal problems, liver or kidney disease, mental illness, stomach problems, or thyroid disease.
• If this drug makes you dizzy or drowsy, do not take part in any activity that requires alertness, such as driving a car or operating potentially dangerous equipment.
• Do not stop taking this drug suddenly. Abruptly stopping it can cause nausea, headache, stomach upset, or a worsening of your condition. Your doctor may want to reduce the dosage gradually.
• The elderly may be at increased risk for side effects. Use this drug cautiously, and report any mental status changes to your doctor immediately.
• The effects of this medication may persist for as long as five weeks after you stop taking it, so continue to observe all precautions during that period.
• Be sure to tell your doctor if you are pregnant. Although birth defects have not been documented in animal studies,

it is not known if fluoxetine is safe during human pregnancy. It is also not known if fluoxetine passes into breast milk, so be sure to tell your doctor if you are breast-feeding an infant.

fluphenazine

BRAND NAMES (Manufacturers)
Permitil (Schering)
Prolixin (Princeton)
TYPE OF DRUG
Phenothiazine tranquilizer
INGREDIENT
fluphenazine
DOSAGE FORMS
Tablets (1 mg, 2.5 mg, 5 mg, and 10 mg)
Oral concentrate (5 mg per ml, with 1% alcohol)
Oral elixir (2.5 mg per 5-ml spoonful, with 14% alcohol)
STORAGE
The tablet form should be stored at room temperature in a tightly closed, light-resistant container. The oral concentrate and the elixir forms should be stored in the refrigerator in tightly closed, light-resistant containers. If the concentrate or elixir turns slightly yellow, the medicine is still effective and can be used. However, if it changes color markedly or has particles floating in it, it should not be used; discard it down the sink. This drug should never be frozen.

USES
Fluphenazine is prescribed to treat the symptoms of certain types of mental illness, such as emotional symptoms of psychosis, the manic phase of manic-depressive illness, and severe behavioral problems in children and adults. This medication is thought to relieve the symptoms of mental illness by blocking certain chemicals involved with nerve transmission in the brain.

TREATMENT
To avoid stomach irritation, you can take the tablet or elixir form of this medication with a meal or with a glass of water or milk (unless your doctor directs you to do otherwise).

Measure the oral elixir carefully with a specially designed 5-ml measuring spoon. An ordinary kitchen teaspoon is not accurate enough.

The oral concentrate form of this medication should be measured carefully with the dropper provided, then added to four ounces (½ cup) or more of water, milk, or a cola-free, caffeine-free carbonated beverage or to applesauce or pudding immediately prior to administration. To prevent possible loss of effectiveness, the medication should not be diluted in tea, coffee, or apple juice.

Antacids and antidiarrheal medicines may decrease the absorption of this medication from the gastrointestinal tract. Therefore, at least one hour should separate doses of one of these medicines and fluphenazine.

The full effects of this medication for the control of emotional or mental symptoms may not become apparent until two weeks after you start to take it.

If you miss a dose of this medication, take the missed dose as soon as possible and return to your regular dosing schedule. If it is almost time for the next dose, however, skip the one you missed and return to your regular schedule. Do not double the dose (unless your doctor directs you to do so).

SIDE EFFECTS
Minor. Blurred vision, constipation, decreased sweating, diarrhea, dizziness, drooling, drowsiness, dry mouth, fatigue, jitteriness, menstrual irregularities, nasal congestion, restlessness, vomiting, or weight gain. As your body adjusts to the medication, these side effects should disappear.

Fluphenazine can also cause discoloration of the urine to red, pink, or red-brown. This is a harmless effect.

This drug can cause increased sensitivity to sunlight. Therefore, avoid prolonged exposure to sunlight and sunlamps. Wear protective clothing, and use an effective sunscreen.

If you are constipated, increase the amount of fiber in your diet (fresh fruits and vegetables, salads, bran, and whole-grain breads) and drink more water (unless your doctor directs you to do otherwise).

Chew sugarless gum or suck on ice chips or a piece of hard candy to reduce mouth dryness.

To avoid dizziness or light-headedness when you stand, contract and relax the muscles of your legs for a few moments before rising. Do this by pushing one foot against the floor while raising the other foot slightly, alternating feet so that you are "pumping" your legs in a pedaling motion.

Major. Tell your doctor about any side effects that are persistent or particularly bothersome. IT IS ESPECIALLY IMPORTANT TO TELL YOUR DOCTOR about breast enlargement (in both sexes); chest pain; convulsions; darkened skin; difficulty in swallowing or breathing; fainting; fever; impotence; involuntary movements of the face, mouth, jaw, tongue, or limbs; palpitations; rash; sleep disorders; sore throat; tremors; uncoordinated movements; unusual bleeding or bruising; visual disturbances; or yellowing of the eyes or skin. Also, tell your doctor if your original symptoms worsen or change after you begin taking fluphenazine.

INTERACTIONS
Fluphenazine interacts with several other types of medications:
1. It can cause extreme drowsiness when combined with alcohol or other central nervous system depressants (such as barbiturates, benzodiazepine tranquilizers, muscle relaxants, narcotics, and pain medications) or with tricyclic antidepressants.
2. Fluphenazine can decrease the effectiveness of amphetamines, guanethidine, anticonvulsants, and levodopa.
3. The side effects of epinephrine, monoamine oxidase (MAO) inhibitors, propranolol, phenytoin, and tricyclic antidepressants may be increased by this medication. At least 14 days should separate the use of this drug and the use of an MAO inhibitor.
4. Lithium may increase the side effects and decrease the effectiveness of this medication.

Before starting to take fluphenazine, BE SURE TO TELL YOUR DOCTOR about any medications you are currently taking, especially any of those listed above.

WARNINGS

• Tell your doctor about unusual or allergic reactions you have had to medications, especially to fluphenazine or any other phenothiazine tranquilizers (such as chlorpromazine, mesoridazine, perphenazine, prochlorperazine, promazine, thioridazine, and triflupromazine) or to loxapine.

• Tell your doctor if you have a history of alcoholism or if you now have or have ever had any blood disease, bone marrow disease, brain disease, breast cancer, blockage of the urinary or digestive tract, drug-induced depression, epilepsy, high or low blood pressure, diabetes mellitus, glaucoma, heart or circulatory disease, liver disease, lung disease, Parkinson's disease, peptic ulcers, or an enlarged prostate gland.

• Tell your doctor about any recent exposure to a pesticide or an insecticide. Fluphenazine may increase the side effects from the exposure.

• To prevent oversedation, avoid drinking alcoholic beverages while taking this medication.

• If this drug makes you dizzy or drowsy, do not take part in any activity that requires alertness, such as driving a car or operating potentially dangerous equipment. Be careful on stairs, and avoid getting up suddenly from a lying or sitting position.

• Prior to having surgery or any other medical or dental treatment, be sure to tell your doctor or dentist that you are taking this medication.

• Some of the side effects caused by this drug can be prevented by taking an antiparkinsonism drug. Discuss this with your doctor.

• This medication can decrease sweating and heat release from the body. You should, therefore, avoid getting overheated by strenuous exercise in hot weather and should avoid hot baths, showers, and saunas.

• Do not stop taking this medication suddenly. If the drug is stopped abruptly, you may experience nausea, vomiting, stomach upset, headache, increased heart rate, insomnia, tremors, or a worsening of your condition. Your doctor may want to reduce the dosage gradually.

• If you are planning to have a myelogram, or any other procedure in which dye will be injected into your spinal cord, tell your doctor that you are taking this medication.

• Avoid spilling the oral concentrate or elixir form of this medication on your skin or clothing; it may cause redness and irritation of the skin.

• While taking this medication, do not take any over-the-counter (nonprescription) medications for weight control or for cough, cold, allergy, asthma, or sinus problems without first checking with your doctor. The combination of these medications may cause high blood pressure.

• Some of these products contain the color additive FD&C Yellow No. 5 (tartrazine), which can cause allergic-type reactions (shortness of breath, rash, fainting) in certain susceptible individuals.

• A potentially permanent movement disorder called tardive dyskinesia may develop with the use of this medication. It is important to discuss this with your doctor and to report any unusual or uncontrolled movements.

• The elderly may be at greater risk for adverse effects when using this drug.

• Be sure to tell your doctor if you are pregnant. Small amounts of this medication cross the placenta. Although there are reports of safe use of this drug during pregnancy, there are also reports of liver disease and tremors in newborn infants whose mothers received this type of medication close to term. Also, tell your doctor if you are breast-feeding an infant. Small amounts of this medication pass into breast milk and may cause unwanted effects in the nursing infant.

flurandrenolide (topical)

BRAND NAMES (Manufacturers)
Cordran (Dista)
Cordran SP (Dista)
flurandrenolide (various manufacturers)
TYPE OF DRUG
Adrenocorticosteroid hormone
INGREDIENT
flurandrenolide
DOSAGE FORMS
Ointment (0.025% and 0.05%)
Cream (0.025% and 0.05%)
Lotion (0.05%)
Tape (4 mcg per square centimeter of tape)
STORAGE
Flurandrenolide ointment, cream, lotion, and tape should be stored at room temperature in tightly closed containers. This medication should never be frozen.

USES

Your adrenal glands naturally produce certain cortisone-like chemicals. These chemicals are involved in various regulatory processes in the body (such as those involving fluid balance, temperature, and reaction to inflammation). Flurandrenolide belongs to a group of drugs known as adrenocorticosteroids (or cortisone-like medications). It is used to relieve the skin inflammation (redness, swelling, itching, and discomfort) associated with conditions such as dermatitis, eczema, and poison ivy. How this drug acts to relieve these disorders is not completely understood.

TREATMENT

Before applying this medication, wash your hands. Then, unless your doctor gives you different instructions, gently wash the area of the skin where the medication is to be applied. With a clean towel, pat the area almost dry; it should be slightly damp when you put the medicine on.

If you are using the lotion form of this medication, shake the bottle well before pouring out the medicine. The contents tend to settle on the bottom of the bottle, so it is necessary to shake the container to distribute the ingredients evenly and equalize the doses. Apply a small amount of the medication to the affected area in a thin layer. Do not bandage the area unless your doctor tells you to do so. If you are to apply an occlusive dressing (like kitchen plastic wrap), be sure you understand the instructions.

When using the tape form of this medication, dry the skin thoroughly before applying the tape. Remove the tape from the package and cut a piece slightly larger than the area to be covered. Round off the corners. Pull the white paper from the transparent tape (be careful that the tape does not stick to itself). Press the tape into place, keeping the skin smooth. If ends of the tape loosen, they may be trimmed off and replaced with fresh tape. The tape should be cut, never torn.

If you miss a dose of this medication, apply the dose as soon as possible, unless it is almost time for the next application. In that case, do not apply the missed dose; just return to your regular schedule. Do not put twice as much of the medication on your skin at the next application.

SIDE EFFECTS
Minor. Acne, burning sensation, itching, rash, or skin dryness.

If the affected area is extremely dry or scaling, the skin may be moistened before applying the medication by soaking in water or by applying water with a clean cloth. The ointment form is probably better for dry skin.

A mild, temporary stinging sensation may occur after this medication is applied. If this persists, contact your doctor.

Major. Tell your doctor about any side effects that are persistent or particularly bothersome. IT IS ESPECIALLY IMPORTANT TO TELL YOUR DOCTOR about blistering, increased hair growth, irritation of the affected area, loss of skin color, secondary infection in the area being treated, or thinning of the skin with easy bruising.

INTERACTIONS
This medication does not interact with any other medications as long as it is used according to directions.

WARNINGS
Tell your doctor about unusual or allergic reactions you have had to medications, especially to flurandrenolide or any other adrenocorticosteroid (such as amcinonide, betamethasone, clocortolone, cortisone, desonide, desoximetasone, dexamethasone, diflorasone, flumethasone, fluocinolone, fluocinonide, fluorometholone, halcinonide, hydrocortisone, methylprednisolone, paramethasone, prednisolone, prednisone, and triamcinolone).

Tell your doctor if you now have or if you have ever had blood vessel disease, chicken pox, diabetes mellitus, fungal infection, peptic ulcers, shingles, tuberculosis, tuberculosis of the skin, vaccinia, or any other type of infection, especially at the site currently being treated.

If irritation develops while using this drug, immediately discontinue its use and notify your doctor.

This product is not for use in the eyes or mucous membranes; contact may result in side effects.

Do not use this product with an occlusive wrap unless your doctor directs you to do so. Systemic absorption of this drug is increased if extensive areas of the body are treated, particularly if occlusive bandages are used. If it is necessary for you to use this drug under a wrap, follow

your doctor's instructions exactly; do not leave the wrap in place longer than specified.

If you are using this medication on a child's diaper area, do not put tightfitting diapers or plastic pants on the child. This could lead to increased systemic absorption of the drug and a possible increase in side effects.

Be sure to tell your doctor if you are pregnant. If large amounts of this drug are applied for prolonged periods, some of it will be absorbed and may cross the placenta. Although studies in humans have not been conducted, birth defects have been observed in the offspring of animals that were given large oral doses of this type of drug during pregnancy. Also, tell your doctor if you are breast-feeding an infant. If absorbed through the skin, small amounts of flurandrenolide pass into breast milk and may cause decreased growth or a decrease in natural adrenocorticosteroid hormone production in the nursing infant.

flurazepam

BRAND NAMES (Manufacturers)
Dalmane (Roche)
flurazepam (various manufacturers)
TYPE OF DRUG
Benzodiazepine sedative/hypnotic
INGREDIENT
flurazepam
DOSAGE FORM
Capsules (15 mg and 30 mg)
STORAGE
This medication should be stored at room temperature in a tightly closed, light-resistant container.

USES
Flurazepam is prescribed to treat insomnia (including problems in falling asleep, waking during the night, and early morning wakefulness). It is not clear exactly how this medicine works, but it may relieve insomnia by acting as a depressant of the central nervous system (brain and spinal cord).

TREATMENT
Flurazepam should be taken ten to 15 minutes before bedtime. It can be taken with food or a full glass of water if stomach upset occurs. Do not take this medication with antacids, since they may slow its absorption from the gastrointestinal tract.

Your sleeping problem may improve the first night you take this medication, but it may take two or three nights before the effectiveness of flurazepam is noticed.

SIDE EFFECTS
Minor. Bitter taste in the mouth, constipation, depression, diarrhea, dizziness, daytime drowsiness, dry mouth, excessive salivation, fatigue, flushing, headache, heartburn, loss of appetite, nausea, nervousness, sweating, or vomiting. As your body adjusts to the medicine, these side effects should disappear.

To relieve constipation, increase the amount of fiber in your diet (fresh fruits and vegetables, salads, bran, and whole-grain breads), exercise more, and drink more water (unless your doctor directs you to do otherwise).

Dry mouth can be relieved by chewing sugarless gum or by sucking on ice chips.

If you feel dizzy while taking this medication, sit or lie down for a while; get up slowly from a sitting or reclining position, and be careful on stairs.

Major. Tell your doctor about any side effects that are persistent or particularly bothersome. IT IS ESPECIALLY IMPORTANT TO TELL YOUR DOCTOR about blurred or double vision, chest pain, fainting, falling, fever, hallucinations, joint pain, nightmares, palpitations, rash, severe depression, shortness of breath, slurred speech, sore throat, uncoordinated movements, unusual excitement, unusual tiredness, or yellowing of the eyes or skin.

INTERACTIONS
Flurazepam interacts with several other types of drugs:
1. To prevent oversedation, this drug should not be taken with alcohol, other sedative drugs, or central nervous system depressants (such as antihistamines, barbiturates, muscle relaxants, pain medicines, narcotics, drugs for seizures, phenothiazine tranquilizers) or with antidepressants.
2. This medication may decrease the effectiveness of levodopa and oral anticoagulants (blood thinners) and may increase the effects of phenytoin.
3. Disulfiram, oral contraceptives (birth control pills), isoniazid, and cimetidine can increase the blood levels of flurazepam, which can lead to increased side effects.
4. Concurrent use of rifampin or carbamazepine may decrease the effectiveness of flurazepam.

BE SURE TO TELL YOUR DOCTOR about any medications you are currently taking, especially any listed above.

WARNINGS
• Tell your doctor about any unusual or allergic reactions you have had to any medications, especially to flurazepam or other benzodiazepine tranquilizers (such as alprazolam, chlordiazepoxide, clorazepate, diazepam, halazepam, lorazepam, oxazepam, prazepam, temazepam, and triazolam).
• Tell your doctor if you now have or if you have ever had liver disease, kidney disease, epilepsy, lung disease, myasthenia gravis, porphyria, mental depression, or mental illness.
• Flurazepam can cause drowsiness. Avoid tasks that require alertness, such as driving a car or using potentially dangerous equipment.
• This medication has the potential for abuse and must be used with caution. Tolerance may develop quickly; do not increase the dosage of the drug without first consulting your doctor. It is also important not to stop taking this drug suddenly if you have been taking it in large amounts or if you have used it for several weeks. Your doctor may want to reduce the dosage gradually.
• This is a safe drug when used properly. When it is combined with other sedative drugs or with alcohol, however, serious side effects may develop.
• The elderly may be at increased risk for side effects, especially daytime drowsiness or confusion. Report any changes in mental status to your doctor immediately.

• Be sure to tell your doctor if you are pregnant. This type of medicine has been shown to increase the chance of birth defects if it is taken during the first three months of pregnancy. In addition, too much use of this medicine during the last six months of pregnancy may result in addiction of the fetus—leading to withdrawal side effects at birth. Also, use of this medicine during the last weeks of pregnancy may cause excessive drowsiness, slowed heartbeat, and breathing difficulties in the newborn. It is very important to tell your doctor if you are breast-feeding an infant. This medicine can pass into breast milk and cause excessive drowsiness, slowed heartbeat, and breathing difficulties in nursing infants.

flurbiprofen

BRAND NAME (Manufacturer)
Ansaid (Upjohn)
TYPE OF DRUG
Nonsteroidal anti-inflammatory analgesic
INGREDIENT
flurbiprofen
DOSAGE FORM
Tablets (50 mg and 100 mg)
STORAGE
This medication should be stored in a tightly closed container at room temperature away from heat and direct light.

USES
Flurbiprofen is used to treat the inflammation (pain, swelling, and stiffness) of arthritis and osteoarthritis. Flurbiprofen has been shown to block the production of certain body chemicals, called prostaglandins, that may trigger pain. However, it is not yet fully understood how flurbiprofen works.

TREATMENT
You should take this medication on an empty stomach 30 to 60 minutes before meals or two hours after meals, so that it gets into your bloodstream quickly. However, to decrease stomach irritation, your doctor may want you to take this medication with food or antacids. Always follow your doctor's directions.

It may take up to two weeks before you feel the full effects of this medication. Flurbiprofen does not cure arthritis or osteoarthritis, but it will help to control the condition as long as you continue to take it.

It is important to take flurbiprofen on schedule and not to miss any doses. If you do miss a dose, take it as soon as possible, unless it is almost time for your next dose. In that case, do not take the missed dose at all; just return to your regular dosing schedule. Do not double the next dose.

SIDE EFFECTS
Minor. Indigestion, diarrhea, abdominal pain, nausea, constipation, headache, or dizziness. As your body adjusts to the medication, these side effects should disappear.

To relieve constipation, increase the amount of fiber in your diet (fresh fruits and vegetables, salads, bran, and whole-grain breads), exercise, and drink more water (unless your doctor directs you to do otherwise).

If you become dizzy, sit or lie down for a while; get up slowly from a sitting or reclining position, and be careful on stairs.

Major. Tell your doctor about any side effects that are persistent or particularly bothersome. IT IS ESPECIALLY IMPORTANT TO TELL YOUR DOCTOR about bloody or black, tarry stools; blurred vision; confusion; difficult or painful urination; palpitations; a problem with hearing, or ringing or buzzing in your ears; skin rash, hives, or itching; stomach pain; swelling of the feet or hands; chest tightness; unexplained sore throat and fever; unusual bleeding or bruising; unusual weight gain; wheezing or difficulty in breathing; or yellowing of the eyes or skin.

INTERACTIONS

Flurbiprofen interacts with several other medications:
1. Anticoagulants (blood thinners, such as warfarin) can lead to an increase in bleeding complications.
2. Aspirin, other salicylates, and other anti-inflammatory medications can increase stomach irritation. Aspirin may also decrease the effectiveness of flurbiprofen; therefore, it should not be used concurrently with flurbiprofen.
3. Flurbiprofen may block the blood-pressure-lowering effects of beta-blocking drugs such as propranolol.
4. The activity of diuretics (water pills) may be inhibited by flurbiprofen.
5. Flurbiprofen may alter a diabetic patient's response to insulin or oral hypoglycemic agents.

Before starting to take flurbiprofen, BE SURE TO TELL YOUR DOCTOR about any medications you are currently taking, especially any of those listed above.

WARNINGS

• Before taking this medication, tell your doctor if you have ever had unusual or allergic reactions to flurbiprofen or to any of the other chemically related drugs (aspirin, other salicylates, diclofenac, diflunisal, fenoprofen, ibuprofen, indomethacin, ketoprofen, meclofenamate, mefenamic acid, naproxen, oxyphenbutazone, phenylbutazone, piroxicam, sulindac, or tolmetin).
• Tell your doctor if you now have or if you have ever had asthma, bleeding problems, epilepsy, heart disease, high blood pressure, kidney disease, liver disease, mental illness, or Parkinson's disease.
• If flurbiprofen makes you dizzy or drowsy, do not take part in any activity that requires alertness, such as driving a car or operating potentially dangerous machinery.
• Because this drug can prolong your bleeding time, it is important to tell your doctor or dentist that you are taking this drug before having surgery or any other medical or dental treatment.
• Stomach problems are more likely to occur if you take aspirin regularly or drink alcohol while being treated with this medication. These should, therefore, be avoided (unless your doctor directs you to do otherwise).
• The elderly may be at increased risk for side effects.
• Be sure to tell your doctor if you are pregnant or if you are planning to become pregnant. This medication can cause unwanted effects on the heart or blood flow of the fetus. Studies in animals have also shown that this medication, if taken late in pregnancy, may increase the length of pregnancy, prolong labor, or cause other problems during delivery. Also tell your doctor if you are breast-feeding an infant. Small amounts of flurbiprofen can pass into breast milk.

Flurosyn—see fluocinolone (topical)

Flutex—see triamcinolone (topical)

FoilleCort—see hydrocortisone (topical)

Fulvicin P/G—see griseofulvin

Fulvicin U/F—see griseofulvin

Fumide—see furosemide

Furadantin—see nitrofurantoin

Furalan—see nitrofurantoin

Furanite—see nitrofurantoin

furosemide

BRAND NAMES (Manufacturers)
Fumide (Everett)
furosemide (various manufacturers)
Lasix (Hoechst-Roussel)
TYPE OF DRUG
Diuretic (water pill) and antihypertensive
INGREDIENT
furosemide
DOSAGE FORMS
Tablets (20 mg, 40 mg, and 80 mg)
Oral solution (10 mg per ml, and 40 mg per 5 ml, with 0.02%, 0.2%, or 11.5% alcohol)
STORAGE
Furosemide tablets should be stored at room temperature in a tightly closed, light-resistant container. The oral solution should be stored in the refrigerator in a tightly closed, light-resistant container. This medication should never be frozen.

USES
Furosemide is prescribed to treat high blood pressure. It is also used to reduce fluid accumulation in the body caused by conditions such as heart failure, cirrhosis of the liver, kidney disease, and the long-term use of some medications. Furosemide reduces fluid accumulation by increasing the elimination of sodium and water through the kidneys.

TREATMENT
To decrease stomach irritation, you can take furosemide with a glass of milk or with a meal (unless your doctor directs you to do otherwise). Try to take it at the same time every day. Avoid taking a dose after 6:00 P.M.—this

will prevent you from having to get up during the night to urinate.

This medication does not cure high blood pressure, but it will help to control the condition, as long as you continue to take it.

If you miss a dose of this medication, take it as soon as possible, unless it is almost time for the next dose. In that case, do not take the missed dose at all; just wait until the next scheduled dose. Do not double the dose.

SIDE EFFECTS

Minor. Blurred vision, constipation, cramping, diarrhea, dizziness, headache, itching, loss of appetite, muscle spasms, nausea, sore mouth, stomach upset, vomiting, and weakness. As your body adjusts to the medication, these side effects should disappear.

This medication will cause an increase in the amount of urine or in your frequency of urination when you first begin to take it. It may also cause you to have an unusual feeling of tiredness. These effects should subside after several days.

Furosemide can cause increased sensitivity to sunlight. It is therefore important to avoid prolonged exposure to sunlight and sunlamps. Wear protective clothing, and use an effective sunscreen.

To avoid dizziness and light-headedness when you stand, contract and relax the muscles of your legs for a few moments before rising. Do this by pushing one foot against the floor while raising the other foot slightly, alternating feet so that you are "pumping" your legs in a pedaling motion.

Major. Tell your doctor about any side effects that are persistent or bothersome. IT IS ESPECIALLY IMPORTANT TO TELL YOUR DOCTOR about confusion, difficulty breathing, dry mouth, fainting, increased thirst, joint pains, loss of appetite, mood changes, muscle cramps, palpitations, rash, ringing in the ears, severe abdominal pain, sore throat, tingling in the fingers or toes, unusual bleeding or bruising, or yellowing of the eyes or skin.

INTERACTIONS

Furosemide interacts with several other drugs.

1. It can increase the side effects of alcohol, barbiturates, narcotics, cephalosporin antibiotics, chloral hydrate, cortisone-like steroids (such as cortisone, dexamethasone, hydrocortisone, prednisone, and prednisolone), digoxin, digitalis, lithium, amphotericin B, clofibrate, aspirin, and theophylline.

2. The effectiveness of antigout medications, insulin, and oral antidiabetic medications may be decreased by furosemide.

3. Phenytoin can decrease the absorption and effectiveness of furosemide.

4. Indomethacin can decrease the diuretic effects of furosemide.

Before taking furosemide, BE SURE TO TELL YOUR DOCTOR if you are taking any of the medicines listed above.

WARNINGS

• Tell your doctor about unusual or allergic reactions you have had to any medications, especially to diuret-ics, oral antidiabetic medicines, or sulfonamide antibiotics.

• Tell your doctor if you now have, or if you have ever had, kidney disease or problems with urination; diabetes mellitus; gout; liver disease; asthma; pancreas disease; or systemic lupus erythematosus (SLE).

• Furosemide can cause potassium loss. Signs of potassium loss include dry mouth, thirst, weakness, muscle pain or cramps, nausea, and vomiting. If you experience any of these symptoms, call your doctor. Your doctor may want to have blood tests performed periodically in order to monitor your blood potassium levels. To help avoid potassium loss, take this medication with a glass of fresh or frozen orange juice or cranberry juice, or eat a banana every day. The use of a salt substitute also helps to prevent potassium loss. Do not change your diet, however, before discussing it with your doctor. Too much potassium may also be dangerous.

• Before having any kind of surgery or other medical or dental treatment, be sure to tell your doctor or dentist that you are taking furosemide.

• To avoid dizziness, light-headedness, or fainting, get up from a sitting or lying position slowly; and avoid standing for long periods of time. You should also avoid strenuous exercise and prolonged exposure to hot weather.

• While taking this medication, limit your intake of alcoholic beverages, in order to prevent dizziness and light-headedness.

• If you have high blood pressure, do not take any over-the-counter (nonprescription) medications for weight control, or for cough, cold, asthma, allergy, or sinus problems, unless you first check with your doctor.

• To prevent severe water loss (dehydration) while taking this medication, check with your doctor if you have any illness that causes severe nausea, vomiting, or diarrhea.

• This medication can raise blood sugar levels in diabetic patients. Therefore, blood sugar should be monitored carefully with blood or urine tests when treatment with this medication is started.

• Be sure to tell your doctor if you are pregnant. This drug crosses the plaucenta. Although studies in humans have not been completed, adverse effects have been observed on the fetuses of animals who received large doses of this drug during pregnancy. Also, tell your doctor if you are breast-feeding an infant. Small amounts of furosemide pass into breast milk.

Gantanol—see sulfonamide antibiotics (oral)

Gantrisin—see sulfonamide antibiotics (oral)

---

gemfibrozil

BRAND NAME (Manufacturer)
Lopid (Parke-Davis)
TYPE OF DRUG
Antihyperlipidemic (lipid-lowering drug)
INGREDIENT
gemfibrozil

DOSAGE FORM
Tablets (600 mg)
STORAGE
Gemfibrozil capsules should be stored at room temperature in a tightly closed container.

USES
Gemfibrozil is used to treat hyperlipidemia (high blood fat levels) in patients who have not responded to diet, weight reduction, exercise, and control of blood sugar. It is not clear how gemfibrozil lowers blood lipid levels, but it is thought to decrease the body's production of certain fats.

TREATMENT
In order to maximize its effectiveness, gemfibrozil should be taken 30 minutes before meals.

If you miss a dose of this medication, take the missed dose as soon as possible, unless it is almost time for the next dose. In that case, do not take the missed dose; just return to your regular schedule. Do not double the dose.

SIDE EFFECTS
Minor. Constipation, diarrhea, dizziness, dry mouth, gas, headache, insomnia, loss of appetite, nausea, and stomach upset. These side effects should disappear in several days, as your body adjusts to the medication.

To relieve constipation, increase the amount of fiber in your diet (bran, salads, fresh fruits and vegetables, and whole-grain breads), exercise, and drink more water (unless your doctor directs you to do otherwise).

If you feel dizzy, sit or lie down awhile; get up slowly, and be careful on stairs.

To help relieve mouth dryness, chew sugarless gum or suck on ice chips.
Major. Tell your doctor about any side effects that are persistent or particularly bothersome. IT IS ESPECIALLY IMPORTANT TO TELL YOUR DOCTOR about back pain, blurred vision, fatigue, muscle cramps, rash, swollen or painful joints, tingling sensations, or yellowing of the eyes or skin.

INTERACTIONS
Gemfibrozil can increase the effects of oral anticoagulants (blood thinners, such as warfarin), which can lead to bleeding complications. BE SURE TO TELL YOUR DOCTOR if you are already taking a medication of this type.

WARNINGS
• Tell your doctor about unusual or allergic reactions you have had to any medications, especially to gemfibrozil.
• Before starting to take this medication, be sure to tell your doctor if you now have, or if you have ever had, biliary disorders; gallstones or gallbladder disease; kidney disease; or liver disease.
• If this drug makes you dizzy or blurs your vision, do not take part in activities that require alertness, such as driving a car or operating potentially dangerous equipment.
• Do not stop taking this medication unless you first check with your doctor. Stopping the drug abruptly may lead to a rapid increase in blood lipid (fats) and cholesterol levels.

Your doctor may therefore want to start you on a special diet or another medication when gemfibrozil is discontinued.
• Large doses of gemfibrozil administered to animals for prolonged periods of time have been associated with benign and malignant cancers. This association has not been observed in humans.
• Be sure to tell your doctor if you are pregnant. Although gemfibrozil appears to be safe during pregnancy, extensive studies in humans have not yet been completed. Also, tell your doctor if you are breast-feeding an infant. It is not known whether or not gemfibrozil passes into breast milk.

Genagesic—see acetaminophen and propoxyphene combination

Genamin—see phenylpropanolamine and chlorpheniramine combination

Gencold—see phenylpropanolamine and chlorpheniramine combination

Genpril—see ibuprofen

Geocillin—see carbenicillin

Geridium—see phenazopyridine

Gerimal—see ergoloid mesylates

Glaucon—see epinephrine (ophthalmic)

glipizide

BRAND NAME (Manufacturer)
Glucotrol (Roerig)
TYPE OF DRUG
Oral antidiabetic
INGREDIENT
glipizide
DOSAGE FORM
Tablets (5 mg and 10 mg)
STORAGE
This medication should be stored at room temperature in a tightly closed container.

USES
Glipizide is used for the treatment of diabetes mellitus (sugar diabetes), which appears in adulthood and cannot be managed by control of diet alone. This type of diabetes is known as non-insulin-dependent diabetes (sometimes called maturity-onset or Type II diabetes). Glipizide lowers blood sugar levels by increasing the release of insulin from the pancreas.

TREATMENT
This medication should be taken on an empty stomach 30 minutes before a meal (unless your doctor directs you to do otherwise).

It is important to try not to miss any doses of this medication. If you do miss a dose, take it as soon as possible, unless it is almost time for the next dose. In that case, do not take the missed dose at all; just return to your regular dosing schedule. Do not double the next dose. Tell your doctor if you feel any side effects from missing a dose of this drug.

Diabetics who are taking oral antidiabetic medication may need to be switched to insulin if they develop diabetic coma, have a severe infection, are scheduled for major surgery, or become pregnant.

SIDE EFFECTS

Minor. Diarrhea, headache, heartburn, loss of appetite, nausea, stomach pain, stomach discomfort, or vomiting. These side effects usually go away during treatment, as your body adjusts to the medicine.

Glipizide may increase your sensitivity to sunlight. It is therefore important to use caution during exposure to the sun. Use an effective sunscreen and avoid exposure to sunlamps.

Major. If any side effects are persistent or particularly bothersome, it is important to notify your doctor. IT IS ESPECIALLY IMPORTANT TO TELL YOUR DOCTOR about dark urine, fatigue, itching of the skin, light-colored stools, rash, sore throat and fever, unusual bleeding or bruising, or yellowing of the eyes or skin.

INTERACTIONS

Glipizide interacts with a number of other medications.
1. Chloramphenicol, guanethidine, insulin, monoamine oxidase (MAO) inhibitors, oxyphenbutazone, oxytetracycline, phenylbutazone, probenecid, aspirin or other salicylates, and sulfonamide antibiotics, when combined with glipizide, can lower blood sugar levels—sometimes to dangerously low levels.
2. Thyroid hormones; dextrothyroxine; epinephrine; phenytoin; thiazide diuretics (water pills); and cortisone-like medications (such as dexamethasone, hydrocortisone, prednisone), combined with glipizide, can actually increase blood sugar levels—just what you are trying to avoid.
3. Anti-diabetic medications can increase the effects of warfarin, which can lead to bleeding complications.
4. Beta-blocking medications (atenolol, metoprolol, nadolol, pindolol, propranolol, and timolol), combined with glipizide, can result in either high or low blood sugar levels. Beta-blockers can also mask the symptoms of low blood sugar, which can be dangerous.

BE SURE TO TELL YOUR DOCTOR if you are already taking any of the medications listed above.

WARNINGS

• It is important to tell your doctor if you have ever had any unusual or allergic reaction to this medicine or to any sulfa medication, including sulfonamide antibiotics, diuretics (water pills), or other oral antidiabetics.
• It is also important to tell your doctor if you now have, or if you have ever had, kidney disease, liver disease, severe infection, or thyroid disease.
• Avoid drinking alcoholic beverages while taking this medication (unless otherwise directed by your doctor).

Some patients who take this medicine suffer nausea, vomiting, dizziness, stomach pain, pounding headache, sweating, and redness of the face and skin when they drink alcohol. Also, large amounts of alcohol can lower blood sugar to dangerously low levels.
• Follow the special diet that your doctor gave you. This is an important part of controlling your blood sugar and is necessary in order for this medicine to work properly.
• Be sure to tell your doctor or dentist that you are taking this medicine before having any kind of surgery or other medical or dental treatment.
• Test for sugar in your urine as directed by your doctor. It is a convenient way to determine whether or not your diabetes is being controlled by this medicine.
• Eat or drink something containing sugar right away if you experience any symptoms of low blood sugar (such as anxiety, chills, cold sweats, cool or pale skin, drowsiness, excessive hunger, headache, nausea, nervousness, rapid heartbeat, shakiness, or unusual tiredness or weakness). It is also important that your family and friends know the symptoms of low blood sugar and what to do if they observe any of these symptoms in you.
• Check with your doctor as soon as possible—even if these symptoms are corrected by the sugar. The blood-sugar-lowering effects of this medicine can last for hours, and the symptoms may return during this period. Good sources of sugar are orange juice, corn syrup, honey, sugar cubes, and table sugar. You are at greatest risk of developing low blood sugar if you skip or delay meals, exercise more than usual, cannot eat because of nausea or vomiting, or drink large amounts of alcohol.
• Be sure to tell your doctor if you are pregnant. Studies have not yet been completed in humans, but studies in animals have shown that this medicine can cause birth defects. Also, tell your doctor if you are breast-feeding an infant. Small amounts of glipizide pass into breast milk.

Glucotrol—see glipizide

glutethimide

BRAND NAMES (Manufacturers)
Doriden (USV)
glutethimide (various manufacturers)
TYPE OF DRUG
Sedative/hypnotic (sleeping aid)
INGREDIENT
glutethimide
DOSAGE FORMS
Tablets (250 mg and 500 mg)
Capsules (500 mg)
STORAGE
Glutethimide tablets and capsules should be stored at room temperature in tightly closed containers.

USES

This medication is used for short-term treatment of insomnia. It is not clearly understood how glutethimide works to produce sleep, but it is a central nervous system depressant (a drug that slows the activity of the brain and spinal cord). This drug loses its effectiveness in producing and maintaining sleep after three to seven days of continuous treatment.

TREATMENT

You can take glutethimide tablets or capsules either on an empty stomach or, to avoid stomach irritation, with food or milk (unless your doctor directs you to do otherwise). The dose should be taken 15 to 30 minutes before bedtime.

SIDE EFFECTS

Minor. Drowsiness during the daytime; dizziness; a "hangover" feeling; headache; nausea; and vomiting. These side effects should disappear as your body adjusts to the medication.

If you feel dizzy, sit or lie down awhile; change positions slowly, and be careful on stairs.

Major. Tell your doctor about any side effects that are persistent or particularly bothersome. IT IS ESPECIALLY IMPORTANT TO TELL YOUR DOCTOR about blurred vision; clumsiness; confusion; convulsions; difficulty breathing; fever; hallucinations; muscle cramps; nightmares; skin rash; slurred speech; sore throat; trembling; unusual bleeding or bruising; or unusual weakness.

INTERACTIONS

Glutethimide interacts with a number of other medications.

1. Concurrent use of it with other central nervous system depressants (such as alcohol, antihistamines, barbiturates, benzodiazepine tranquilizers, muscle relaxants, narcotics, pain medications, phenothiazine tranquilizers, and other sleeping medications) or with tricyclic anti-depressants can lead to extreme drowsiness, and can be dangerous.

2. Glutethimide can decrease the blood levels and effectiveness of oral anti-coagulants (blood thinners, such as warfarin).

BE SURE TO TELL YOUR DOCTOR if you are already taking any of the medications listed above.

WARNINGS

Tell your doctor about unusual or allergic reactions you have had to any medications, especially to glutethimide.

Before starting to take this medication, be sure to tell your doctor if you now have, or if you have ever had, glaucoma; heart arrhythmias; kidney disease; severe pain; peptic ulcers; enlarged prostate gland; porphyria; or blockage of the intestines or urinary tract.

If this medication makes you drowsy or dizzy, or blurs your vision, do not take part in any activity that requires alertness, such as driving a car.

This medication has the potential for abuse. Therefore, it should not be used in higher doses or for longer periods than recommended by your doctor. If you have been taking glutethimide for longer than several weeks, check with your doctor before discontinuing it. Stopping abruptly can lead to a withdrawal reaction. Your doctor may want to reduce the dosage gradually to prevent this reaction.

Be sure to tell your doctor if you are pregnant. Extensive studies in pregnant women using glutethimide have not

yet been completed. However, it is known that large amounts of the drug taken during the last three months of pregnancy can cause the baby to become dependent on the medication, leading to withdrawal side effects at birth. Also, tell your doctor if you are breastfeeding an infant. Small amounts of glutethimide pass into breast milk and can cause extreme drowsiness in the nursing infant.

glyburide

BRAND NAMES (Manufacturers)
DiaBeta (Hoechst-Roussel)
Micronase (Upjohn)
TYPE OF DRUG
Oral antidiabetic
INGREDIENT
glyburide
DOSAGE FORM
Tablets (1.25 mg, 2.5 mg, and 5 mg)
STORAGE
This medication should be stored at room temperature in a tightly closed container.

USES

Glyburide is used for the treatment of diabetes mellitus (sugar diabetes) that appears in adulthood and cannot be managed by control of diet alone. This type of diabetes is known as non-insulin-dependent (sometimes called maturity-onset or Type II diabetes). Glyburide lowers blood sugar levels by increasing the release of insulin from the pancreas.

TREATMENT

In order for glyburide to work correctly, it must be taken as directed by your doctor. To maintain a constant blood sugar level, it is best to take this medication at the same time(s) each day. It is therefore important to try not to miss any doses of this medication. If you do miss a dose, take it as soon as possible, unless it is almost time for the next dose. In that case, do not take the missed dose at all; just return to your regular dosing schedule. Do not double the next dose. Tell your doctor if you feel any side effects from missing a dose of this drug.

It is important to note that diabetics who are taking oral antidiabetic medication may need to be switched to insulin if they develop diabetic coma, have a severe infection, are scheduled for major surgery, or become pregnant.

SIDE EFFECTS

Minor. Diarrhea, headache, heartburn, loss of appetite, nausea, vomiting, stomach pain, or stomach discomfort. The side effects from glyburide will most likely disappear during treatment, as your body adjusts to the medicine.

Glyburide may increase your sensitivity to sunlight. It is therefore important to use caution during exposure to the sun. You may want to wear protective clothing and sunglasses. Use an effective sunscreen and avoid exposure to sun lamps.

Major. If any side effects are persistent or particularly bothersome, it is important to notify your doctor. IT IS ESPECIALLY IMPORTANT TO TELL YOUR DOCTOR about dark urine, fatigue, itching of the skin, light-colored stools, rash, sore throat and fever, unusual bleeding or bruising, or yellowing of the eyes or skin.

INTERACTIONS
Glyburide interacts with a number of other medications.
1. Chloramphenicol, guanethidine, insulin, monoamine oxidase (MAO) inhibitors, oxyphenbutazone, oxytetracycline, phenylbutazone, probenecid, aspirin or other salicylates, and sulfonamide antibiotics, when combined with glyburide, can lower blood sugar levels—sometimes to dangerously low levels.
2. Thyroid hormones, dextrothyroxine, epinephrine, phenytoin, thiazide diuretics (water pills), and cortisone-like medications (such as dexamethasone, hydrocortisone, prednisone), combined with glyburide, can actually increase blood sugar levels.
3. Antidiabetic medications can increase the effects of warfarin, which can lead to bleeding complications.
4. Betablocking medications (atenolol, metoprolol, nadolol, pindolol, propranolol, and timolol), combined with glyburide, can result in either high or low blood sugar levels. Betablockers can also mask the symptoms of low blood sugar, which can be dangerous.

BE SURE TO TELL YOUR DOCTOR if you are already taking any of the medications listed above.

WARNINGS
• Tell your doctor if you have ever had unusual or allergic reactions to medications, especially to glyburide or to any sulfa medication, including sulfonamide antibiotics, diuretics (water pills), or other oral antidiabetics.
• Tell your doctor if you now have, or if you have ever had, kidney disease, liver disease, severe infection, or thyroid disease.
• Follow the special diet that your doctor gave you. This is an important part of controlling your blood sugar and is necessary in order for this medicine to work properly.
• Avoid drinking alcoholic beverages while taking this medication (unless otherwise directed by your doctor). Some patients who take this medicine suffer nausea, vomiting, dizziness, stomach pain, pounding headache, sweating, and redness of the face and skin when they drink alcohol. Also, large amounts of alcohol can lower blood sugar to dangerously low levels.
• Be sure to tell your doctor or dentist that you are taking this medication before having any kind of surgery or other medical or dental treatment.
• Test for sugar in your urine as directed by your doctor. It is a convenient way to determine whether or not your diabetes is being controlled by this medicine.
• Eat or drink something containing sugar right away if you experience any symptoms of low blood sugar (such as anxiety, chills, cold sweats, cool or pale skin, drowsiness, excessive hunger, headache, nausea, nervousness, rapid heartbeat, shakiness, or unusual tiredness or weakness). It is also important that your family and friends know the symptoms of low blood sugar and what to do if they observe any of these symptoms in you.

• Check with your doctor as soon as possible—even if these symptoms are corrected by the sugar. The blood-sugar-lowering effects of this medicine can last for hours, and the symptoms may return during this period. Good sources of sugar are orange juice, corn syrup, honey, sugar cubes, and table sugar. You are at greatest risk of developing low blood sugar if you skip or delay meals, exercise more than usual, cannot eat because of nausea or vomiting, or drink large amounts of alcohol.
• Be sure to tell your doctor if you are pregnant. Studies have not yet been completed in humans, but studies in animals have shown that this medication can cause birth defects.

Grifulvin V—see griseofulvin

Grisactin—see griseofulvin

Grisactin Ultra—see griseofulvin

griseofulvin

BRAND NAMES (Manufacturers)
Fulvicin P/G (Schering)
Fulvicin V/F (Schering)
Grifulvin V (Ortho Derm)
Grisactin (Wyeth-Ayerst)
Grisactin Ultra (Wyeth-Ayerst)
griseofulvin (various manufacturers)
Gris-PEG (Sandoz)
TYPE OF DRUG
Antifungal
INGREDIENT
griseofulvin
DOSAGE FORMS
Tablets (125 mg, 165 mg, 250 mg, 330 mg, and 500 mg)
Capsules (125 mg and 250 mg)
Oral suspension (125 mg per 5-ml teaspoonful)
STORAGE
Griseofulvin tablets, capsules, and oral suspension should be stored at room temperature in tightly closed containers. This medication should never be frozen.

USES
This medication is used to treat certain fungal infections of the skin and nails. Griseofulvin prevents the multiplication of susceptible fungi. It also enters the cells of skin, hair, and nails, and protects them from fungal invasion.

TREATMENT
In order to avoid stomach irritation, you can take griseofulvin with food or milk.

The oral suspension form of this medication should be shaken well, just before measuring each dose. The contents tend to settle on the bottom of the bottle, so it is necessary to shake the container to evenly distribute the ingredients and equalize the doses. Each dose should then be measured carefully with a specially designed, 5-ml measuring spoon. An ordinary kitchen teaspoon is not accurate enough.

If you miss a dose of this medication, take the missed dose as soon as possible, unless it is almost time for the next dose. In that case, do not take the missed dose at all; just return to your regular dosing schedule. Do not double the next dose.

It is important to continue to take this medication for the entire time prescribed by your doctor (perhaps six months or more), even if the symptoms disappear before the end of that period. If you stop taking this drug too soon, resistant fungi are given a chance to continue growing, and your infection could recur.

SIDE EFFECTS

Minor. Diarrhea, dizziness, fatigue, headache, insomnia, nausea, stomach upset, and vomiting. These side effects should disappear in several days, as your body adjusts to the medication.

If you feel dizzy, sit or lie down awhile; get up slowly.

This medication can increase your sensitivity to sunlight. You should therefore avoid prolonged exposure to sunlight and sunlamps. Wear protective clothing and sunglasses, and use an effective sunscreen.

Major. Tell your doctor about any side effects that are persistent or particularly bothersome. IT IS ESPECIALLY IMPORTANT TO TELL YOUR DOCTOR about confusion, itching, skin rash, sore throat, or a tingling of the hands or feet.

INTERACTIONS

Griseofulvin interacts with other types of medication.
1. It can increase the effects of alcohol, resulting in flushing and an increased heart rate.
2. Barbiturates can cause a decrease in the effectiveness of griseofulvin.
3. Griseofulvin can decrease the effectiveness of oral anticoagulants (blood thinners, such as warfarin).

Before starting to take griseofulvin, BE SURE TO TELL YOUR DOCTOR if you are already taking any of these other medications.

WARNINGS

• Tell your doctor about unusual or allergic reactions you have had to any medications, especially to griseofulvin, penicillins, cephalosporin antibiotics, or penicillamine.
• Before starting to take griseofulvin, be sure to tell your doctor if you now have, or if you have ever had, liver disease, porphyria, or systemic lupus erythematosus (SLE).
• If this drug makes you dizzy, do not take part in any activity that requires alertness, such as driving a car or operating potentially dangerous equipment.
• Observe good hygiene to control the source of infection and to prevent reinfection.
• Concurrent use of an appropriate topical antifungal medication may be necessary to help clear the infection.
• Be sure to tell your doctor if you are pregnant. Extensive studies in pregnant women have not yet been completed, but birth defects have been reported in animals whose mothers received large doses of griseofulvin during pregnancy. Also, tell your doctor if you are breast-feeding an infant. It is not known whether or not griseofulvin passes into breast milk.

Gris-PEG—see griseofulvin

Guaipax—see phenylpropanolamine and guaifenesin combination

---

guanadrel

BRAND NAME (Manufacturer)
Hylorel (Pennwalt)
TYPE OF DRUG
Anti-hypertensive
INGREDIENT
guanadrel as the sulfate salt
DOSAGE FORM
Tablets (10 mg and 25 mg)
STORAGE
Guanadrel tablets should be stored at room temperature, in a tightly closed container.

USES

Guanadrel is used to control high blood pressure. It works by blocking the action of the body chemicals responsible for increasing blood pressure.

TREATMENT

Guanadrel can be taken either on an empty stomach or, to avoid stomach irritation, with food or milk (as directed by your doctor). Try to take your doses at the same times each day, in order to become accustomed to taking this medication.

This medication does not cure high blood pressure, but it will help to control the condition.

If you miss a dose of this medication, take the missed dose as soon as possible, unless it is almost time for your next dose. In that case, do not take the missed dose at all; just return to your regular dosing schedule. Do not double the next dose.

SIDE EFFECTS

Minor. Constipation; diarrhea; dizziness; drowsiness; dry throat or mouth; fatigue; gas; headache; loss of appetite; nausea; sleep disorders; stomach upset; and weight gain or loss. These side effects should disappear in several weeks, as your body adjusts to the medication.

To relieve constipation, increase the amount of fiber in your diet (bran, salads, fresh fruits and vegetables, and whole-grain breads), and drink more water (unless your doctor directs you to do otherwise).

If you feel dizzy, sit or lie down awhile; change positions slowly, and be careful on stairs.

To help relieve mouth dryness, chew sugarless gum, or suck on ice chips or a piece of hard candy.

Major. Tell your doctor about any side effects that are persistent or particularly bothersome. IT IS ESPECIALLY IMPORTANT TO TELL YOUR DOCTOR about backache; blurred vision; chest pain; confusion; coughing; depression; fainting; impotence; increased urination; joint pain; leg cramps; mental disorders; mouth sores; palpitations; rapid weight gain (three to five pounds within a week); shortness of breath; or tingling sensations.

INTERACTIONS

Guanadrel interacts with several other types of drugs.

l. Concurrent use of guanadrel and alcohol can lead to fainting and extreme drowsiness.

2. Amphetamines, diet preparations, ephedrine, methylphenidate, phenothiazine tranquilizers, phenyl-propanolamine, and tricyclic anti-depressants can decrease the beneficial effects of guanadrel.

3. Concurrent use of guanadrel with monoamine oxidase (MAO) inhibitors can lead to serious side effects. At least one week should separate doses of these two types of medications.

TELL YOUR DOCTOR if you are already taking any of the medications listed above.

WARNINGS

Tell your doctor about unusual or allergic reactions you have had to any medications, especially to guanadrel.

Before starting to take this medication, be sure to tell your doctor if you now have, or if you have ever had, asthma, fevers, heart or blood vessel disease, peptic ulcers, pheochromocytoma, or a slowed heartbeat.

If this drug makes you dizzy or drowsy, or blurs your vision, avoid taking part in activities that require alertness.

Before having any surgery or other medical or dental treatment, be sure to tell your doctor or dentist that you are taking this medication.

Check with your doctor or pharmacist before taking any over-the-counter (non-prescription) asthma, allergy, cough, cold, diet, or sinus preparation. Some of these products can decrease the effectiveness of guanadrel.

To prevent feeling faint, you should avoid drinking alcoholic beverages. You should also avoid standing for prolonged periods, excessive exercising, and exposure to hot showers and saunas.

Be sure to tell your doctor if you are pregnant. Although guanadrel appears to be safe during pregnancy, extensive studies in humans have not yet been completed. Also, tell your doctor if you are breastfeeding an infant. It is not known whether or not guanadrel passes into breast milk.

guanabenz

BRAND NAME (Manufacturer)
Wytensin (Wyeth-Ayerst)
TYPE OF DRUG
Antihypertensive
INGREDIENT
guanabenz as the acetate salt
DOSAGE FORM
Tablets (4 mg and 8 mg)
STORAGE
Guanabenz should be stored at room temperature in a tightly closed, light-resistant container.

USES

This medication is used to control high blood pressure. It works by decreasing the release of chemicals in the brain that are responsible for increasing blood pressure.

TREATMENT

Guanabenz can be taken either on an empty stomach or, to avoid stomach irritation, with food or milk (as directed by your doctor).

Try to take the doses at the same times each day, so that you become accustomed to taking this medication. Your doctor may want you to take the last dose of the day at bedtime, in order to control blood pressure at night and to reduce daytime drowsiness.

Guanabenz does not cure high blood pressure, but it will help to control the condition as long as you continue to take it.

If you miss a dose of this medication, take the missed dose as soon as possible, unless it is almost time for your next dose. In that case, do not take the missed dose at all; just return to your regular dosing schedule. Do not double the next dose. If you miss more than two consecutive doses, contact your doctor as soon as possible.

SIDE EFFECTS

Minor. Constipation, diarrhea, dizziness, drowsiness, dry mouth, headache, nasal congestion, nausea, sleep disturbances, stomach upset, taste disorders, vomiting, and weakness. These side effects should disappear in several weeks, as your body adjusts to the medication.

To relieve constipation, increase the amount of fiber in your diet (bran, salads, fresh fruits and vegetables, and whole-grain breads), and drink more water (unless your doctor directs you to do otherwise).

If you feel dizzy or light-headed, sit or lie down awhile; get up from a sitting or lying position slowly, and be careful on stairs.

To help relieve mouth dryness, chew sugarless gum or suck on ice chips or a piece of hard candy.

Major. Tell your doctor about any side effects that are persistent or particularly bothersome. IT IS ESPECIALLY IMPORTANT TO TELL YOUR DOCTOR about anxiety, blurred vision, chest pain, depression, disturbances in sexual function, enlarged or painful breasts (in both sexes), increased urination, itching, loss of coordination, muscle aches, palpitations, rapid weight gain (three to five pounds within a week), shortness of breath, or skin rash.

INTERACTIONS

Concurrent use of guanabenz with central nervous system depressants (drugs that slow the activity of the brain and spinal cord), such as alcohol, antihistamines, barbiturates, benzodiazepine tranquilizers, muscle relaxants, narcotics, pain medications, phenothiazine tranquilizers, and sleeping medication, or with tricyclic antidepressants can lead to extreme drowsiness. BE SURE TO TELL YOUR DOCTOR if you are already taking any of these types of medication.

WARNINGS

• Tell your doctor about unusual or allergic reactions you have had to any medications, especially to guanabenz.

• Before starting to take this medication, be sure to tell your doctor if you now have, or if you have ever had, heart or blood vessel disease, kidney disease, or liver disease.

• If this medication makes you dizzy or drowsy, or blurs your vision, avoid taking part in activities that require alertness.

• Before having any surgery or other medical or dental treatment, be sure to tell your doctor or dentist that you are taking this medication.

• Do not stop taking guanabenz unless you first check with your doctor. If this drug is stopped abruptly, you may experience nervousness, agitation, headache, and a rise in blood pressure. Your doctor may therefore want to decrease your dosage.

• Check with your doctor or pharmacist before taking any over-the-counter (nonprescription) asthma, allergy, cough, cold, diet, or sinus preparations. Some of these products can reduce the effectiveness of guanabenz.

• Be sure to tell your doctor if you are pregnant. Although guanabenz appears to be safe during pregnancy, extensive studies in humans have not yet been completed. Studies on birth defects in animals have produced conflicting results. Also, tell your doctor if you are breast-feeding an infant. It is not known if guanabenz passes into breast milk.

guanethidine

BRAND NAME (Manufacturer)
Ismelin (Ciba)
TYPE OF DRUG
Anti-hypertensive
INGREDIENT
guanethidine as the sulfate salt
DOSAGE FORM
Tablets (10 mg and 25 mg)
STORAGE
Guanethidine should be stored at room temperature, in a tightly closed container.

USES

Guanethidine is used to control high blood pressure. It works by blocking the action of the chemicals responsible for increasing blood pressure.

TREATMENT

Guanethidine can be taken either on an empty stomach or, to avoid stomach irritation, with food or milk (as directed by your doctor). Try to take your doses at the same times each day, in order to become accustomed to taking this medication.

This medication does not cure high blood pressure, but it will help to control the condition, as long as you continue to take it.

If you miss a dose of this medication, take the missed dose as soon as possible, unless it is almost time for the next dose. In that case, do not take the missed dose at all; just return to your regular dosing schedule. Do not double the next dose.

SIDE EFFECTS

Minor. Diarrhea; dizziness; dry mouth; fatigue; nasal congestion; nausea; vomiting; weakness; and weight gain.

These side effects should disappear in several weeks, as your body adjusts to the medication.

If you feel dizzy, sit or lie down awhile; change positions slowly, and be careful on stairs.

To help relieve mouth dryness, chew sugarless gum, or suck on ice chips or a piece of hard candy.

Major. Tell your doctor about any side effects that are persistent or particularly bothersome. IT IS ESPECIALLY IMPORTANT TO TELL YOUR DOCTOR about blurred vision; chest pain; decreased sexual ability; depression; drooping eyelids; hair loss; increased urination; itching; muscle pain or tremors; rapid weight gain (three to five pounds within a week); skin rash; shortness of breath; or swollen or tender glands.

INTERACTIONS

Guanethidine interacts with several other types of drugs.
1. Concurrent use of guanethidine and alcohol can lead to fainting or extreme drowsiness.
2. Amphetamines, appetite suppressants, ephedrine, methylphenidate, phenothiazine tranquilizers, phenylpropanolamine, and tricyclic anti-depressants can decrease the beneficial effects of guanethidine.
3. Barbiturates, methotrimeprazine, narcotics, fenfluramine, and reserpine can increase the blood-pressure-lowering effects of guanethidine, which can be dangerous.
4. The dosage of oral anti-diabetic medications may need to be adjusted when guanethidine is started.
5. Concurrent use of guanethidine with monoamine oxidase (MAO) inhibitors can lead to serious side effects. At least one week should separate doses of these two types of medication.

BE SURE TO TELL YOUR DOCTOR if you are already taking any of the medications listed above in combination with guanethidine.

WARNINGS

Tell your doctor about unusual or allergic reactions you have had to any medications, especially to guanethidine.

Before starting to take this medication, be sure to tell your doctor if you now have, or if you have ever had, asthma; diabetes mellitus; fever; heart or blood vessel disease; kidney disease; liver disease; peptic ulcers,; pheochromocytoma; or a slowed heart rate.

If this medication makes you dizzy or drowsy, avoid taking part in activities that require alertness, such as driving a car or operating potentially dangerous equipment.

To prevent fainting while you are taking guanethidine, you should avoid drinking alcoholic beverages. You should also avoid standing for prolonged periods, excessive exercise, and exposure to hot showers and saunas.

Before having any surgery or other medical or dental treatment, be sure to tell your doctor or dentist that you are taking this medication.

Check with your doctor or pharmacist before taking any over-the-counter (non-prescription) asthma, allergy, cough, cold, diet, or sinus preparation. Some of these products can reduce the effectiveness of guanethidine.

Guanethidine 10 mg tablets contain F.D. & C. Yellow Dye No. 5 (tartrazine), which can cause allergic-type symptoms (fainting, shortness of breath, or rash) in certain susceptible individuals.

Be sure to tell your doctor if you are pregnant. Although guanethidine appears to be safe during pregnancy, extensive studies in humans have not yet been completed. Also, tell your doctor if you are breastfeeding an infant. It is not known whether or not guanethidine passes into breast milk.

Guiatuss A.C.—see codeine and guaifensin combination

Guiatussin with Codeine—see codeine and guaifensin combination

Gulfasin—see sulfonamide antibiotics (oral)

G-well—see lindane

Gynecort—see hydrocortisone (topical)

Gyne-Lotrimin—see clotrimazole (vaginal)

Habitrol—nicotine transdermal patch

halazepam

BRAND NAME (Manufacturer)
Paxipam (Schering)
TYPE OF DRUG
Sedative/hypnotic (anti-anxiety medication)
INGREDIENT
halazepam
DOSAGE FORM
Tablets (20 mg and 40 mg)
STORAGE
This medication should be stored at room temperature in a tightly closed, light-resistant container.

USES
Halazepam is prescribed to treat symptoms of anxiety. It is not clear exactly how this medicine works, but it may relieve anxiety by acting as a depressant of the central nervous system. Halazepam is currently used by many people to relieve nervousness. It is effective for this purpose for short periods, but it is important to try to remove the cause of the anxiety as well.

TREATMENT
This medication should be taken exactly as directed by your doctor. It can be taken with food or a full glass of water if stomach upset occurs. Do not take this medication with a dose of antacids, since they may retard its absorption from the gastrointestinal tract.

If you are taking this medication regularly and you miss a dose, take the missed dose immediately, if you remember within an hour. If more than an hour has passed, skip the dose you missed and wait for the next scheduled dose. Do not double the dose.

SIDE EFFECTS
Minor. Bitter taste in mouth; constipation; depression; diarrhea; dizziness; drowsiness (after a night's sleep); dry mouth; excess saliva; fatigue; flushing; headache; heart-

burn; loss of appetite; nausea; nervousness; sweating; and vomiting. As your body adjusts to the medicine, these effects should disappear.

Dry mouth can be relieved by chewing sugarless gum or by sucking on ice chips.

If you feel dizzy, sit or lie down awhile.

Major. Tell your doctor about any side effects that are persistent or particularly bothersome. IT IS ESPECIALLY IMPORTANT TO TELL YOUR DOCTOR about blurred or double vision; chest pain; severe depression; difficulty urinating; fainting; falling; fever; joint pain; hallucinations; mouth sores; nightmares; palpitations; rash; shortness of breath; slurred speech; sore throat; uncoordinated movements; unusual excitement; unusual tiredness; or yellowing of the eyes or skin.

INTERACTIONS
Halazepam interacts with several other medications.
1. To prevent over-sedation, it should not be taken with alcohol, other sedative drugs, central nervous system depressants (such as antihistamines, barbiturates, muscle relaxants, pain medicines, narcotics, medicines for seizures, phenothiazine tranquilizers), or with anti-depressants.
2. This medication may decrease the effectiveness of carbamazepine, levodopa, and oral anti-coagulants, and may increase the effects of phenytoin.
3. Disulfiram, isoniazid, and cimetidine can increase the blood levels of halazepam, which can lead to toxic effects.
4. Concurrent use of rifampin may decrease the effectiveness of halazepam.
If you are already taking any of the medications listed above, CONSULT YOUR DOCTOR about their use.

WARNINGS
Tell your doctor about unusual or allergic reactions you have had to medications, especially to halazepam or any other benzodiazepine tranquilizers (such as alprazolam, chlordiazepoxide, clorazepate, diazepam, flurazepam, lorazepam, oxazepam, prazepam, temazepam, or triazolam).

Tell your doctor if you now have, or if you have ever had, liver or kidney disease, epilepsy, lung disease, myasthenia gravis, porphyria, mental depression, or mental illness.

This medicine can cause drowsiness. You should therefore avoid tasks that require alertness, such as driving a car or using potentially dangerous machinery.

This medication has the potential for abuse and must be used with caution. Tolerance may develop quickly; do not increase the dosage without first consulting your doctor. It is also important not to stop taking this drug suddenly if you have been taking it in large amounts, or if you have used it for several weeks. Your doctor may want to reduce the dosage gradually.

This is a safe drug when used properly. When it is combined with other sedative drugs or alcohol, however, serious side effects can develop.

Be sure to tell your doctor if you are pregnant. This type of medicine may increase the chance of birth defects if it is taken during the first three months of pregnancy. In addition, too much use of this medicine during the last six months of pregnancy may result in addiction of the fetus, leading to withdrawal side effects in the newborn. Also, use of this medicine during the last weeks of pregnancy may cause excessive drowsiness, slowed heartbeat, and breathing difficulties in the infant. Tell your doctor if you are breastfeeding an infant. This medicine can pass into breast milk and cause excessive drowsiness, slowed heartbeat, and breathing difficulties in nursing infants.

---

halcinonide (topical)

BRAND NAMES (Manufacturers)
Halog (Westwood Squibb)
Halog-E (Westwood Squibb)
TYPE OF DRUG
Adrenocorticosteroid hormone
INGREDIENT
halcinonide
DOSAGE FORMS
Ointment (0.025% and 0.1%)
Cream (0.025% and 0.1%)
Solution (0.1%)
STORAGE
Halcinonide ointment, cream, and solution should be stored at room temperature in tightly closed containers. This medication should never be frozen.

USES
Your adrenal glands naturally produce certain cortisone-like chemicals. These chemicals are involved in various regulatory processes in the body (such as fluid balance, temperature, and reactions to inflammation). Halcinonide belongs to a group of drugs known as adrenocorticosteroids (or cortisone-like medications). It is used to relieve the skin inflammation (redness, swelling, itching, and discomfort) associated with conditions such as dermatitis, eczema, and poison ivy. How this drug acts to relieve these disorders is not completely understood.

TREATMENT
Before applying this medication, wash your hands. Then, unless your doctor gives you different instructions, gently wash the area of the skin where the medication is to be applied. With a clean towel, pat the area almost dry; it should be slightly damp when you put the medicine on.

Apply a small amount of the medication to the affected area in a thin layer. Do not bandage the area unless your doctor tells you to do so. If you are to apply an occlusive dressing (like kitchen plastic wrap), be sure you understand the instructions.

If you miss a dose of this drug, apply the dose as soon as possible, unless it is time for the next application. In that case, do not apply the missed dose, just return to your regular schedule. Do not double the dose.

SIDE EFFECTS
Minor. Acne, burning sensation, irritation of the affected area, itching, rash, and skin dryness.

If the affected area is extremely dry or scaling, the skin may be moistened before applying the medication by soaking in water or by applying water with a clean cloth. The ointment form is probably better for dry skin.

A mild, temporary stinging sensation may occur after this medication is applied. If this persists, contact your doctor.
Major. Tell your doctor about any side effects that are persistent or particularly bothersome. IT IS ESPECIALLY IMPORTANT TO TELL YOUR DOCTOR about blistering, increased hair growth, loss of skin color, secondary infection in the area being treated, or thinning of the skin with easy bruising.

INTERACTIONS
This medication does not interact with any other medications, as long as it is used according to directions.

WARNINGS
• Tell your doctor about unusual or allergic reactions you have had to medications, especially to halcinonide or any other adrenocorticosteroids (such as amcinonide, betamethasone, cortisone, desonide, desoximetasone, dexamethasone, flumethasone, fluocinolone, fluocinonide, fluorometholone, fluprednisolone, flurandrenolide, hydrocortisone, methylprednisolone, paramethasone, prednisolone, prednisone, or triamcinolone).
• Tell your doctor if you now have, or if you have ever had, blood vessel disease, chicken pox, diabetes mellitus, fungal infection, peptic ulcers, shingles, tuberculosis, tuberculosis of the skin, vaccinia, or any other type of infection, especially at the site currently being treated.
• If irritation develops while using this drug, immediately discontinue its use, and notify your doctor.
• This product is not for use in the eyes or mucous membranes. Exposure of this medication to the eye may result in ocular (to the eye) side effects.
• Do not use this product with an occlusive wrap unless your doctor directs you to do so. Systemic absorption of this drug is increased if occlusive bandages are used. If it is necessary for you to use this drug under a wrap, follow your doctors instructions exactly; do not leave the wrap in place longer than specified.
• If you are using this medication on a child's diaper area, do not put tight-fitting diapers or plastic pants on the child. This may lead to increased systemic absorption of the drug and a possible increase in side effects.
• Be sure to tell your doctor if you are pregnant. If large amounts of this drug are applied for prolonged periods, some of it will be absorbed and may cross the placenta. Although studies in humans have not yet been completed, birth defects have been observed in the offspring of animals who were given large oral doses of this type of drug during pregnancy. Also, tell your doctor if you are breastfeeding an infant. If absorbed through the skin, small amounts of halcinonide pass into breast milk and may cause growth suppression or a decrease in natural adrenocorticosteroid production in the nursing infant.

Halcion—see triazolam

Haldol—see haloperidol

Halog—see halcinonide (topical)

Halog-E—see halcinonide (topical)

haloperidol

BRAND NAMES (Manufacturers)
Haldol (McNeil CPC)
haloperidol (various manufacturers)
TYPE OF DRUG
Antipsychotic
INGREDIENT
haloperidol
DOSAGE FORMS
Tablets (0.5 mg, 1 mg, 2 mg, 5 mg, 10 mg, and 20 mg)
Oral concentrate (2 mg per ml)
STORAGE
Haloperidol tablets and oral concentrate should be stored at room temperature in a tightly closed, light-resistant container. This medication should never be frozen.

USES
Haloperidol is prescribed to treat the symptoms of certain types of mental illness, such as the emotional symptoms of psychosis, the manic phase of manic-depressive illness, Tourette's syndrome, and severe behavioral problems in children. This drug is thought to relieve symptoms of mental illness by blocking certain chemicals involved with nerve transmission in the brain.

TREATMENT
To avoid stomach irritation, you can take haloperidol tablets with a meal or with a glass of water or milk (unless your doctor directs you to do otherwise).

The oral form of this drug should be measured carefully with the dropper provided, then added to four ounces ($1/2$ cup) or more of water, milk, or a cola-free, caffeine-free carbonated beverage or to applesauce or pudding immediately prior to administration. To prevent possible loss of effectiveness, haloperidol should not be diluted with tea, coffee, caffeine-containing beverages, or apple juice.

If you miss a dose of this medication and remember within six hours, take the missed dose as soon as then return to your regular schedule. If more than six hours have passed, however, skip the missed dose and return to your regular dosing schedule. Do not double the next dose unless your doctor directs you to do so.

The full effects of haloperidol may not become apparent for two weeks after you start to take it.

SIDE EFFECTS
Minor. Blurred vision, constipation, decreased or increased sweating, diarrhea, dizziness, drooling, drowsiness, dry mouth, fatigue, headache, heartburn, jitteriness, loss of appetite, menstrual irregularities, nausea, restlessness, sleep disorders, vomiting, or weakness. As your body adjusts to the medication, these side effects should disappear.

This medication can cause increased sensitivity to sunlight. It is, therefore, important to avoid prolonged exposure to sunlight and sunlamps. Wear protective clothing and use an effective sunscreen.

If you are constipated, increase the amount of fiber in your diet (fresh fruits and vegetables, salads, bran, and whole-grain breads), exercise, and drink more water (unless your doctor directs you to do otherwise).

To reduce mouth dryness, chew sugarless gum or suck on ice chips or a piece of hard candy.

To avoid dizziness or light-headedness when you stand, contract and relax the muscles of your legs for a few moments before rising. Do this by pushing one foot against the floor while raising the other foot slightly, alternating feet so that you are "pumping" your legs in a pedaling motion.

Major. Tell your doctor about any side effects that are persistent or particularly bothersome. IT IS ESPECIALLY IMPORTANT TO TELL YOUR DOCTOR about aching joints and muscles; breast enlargement (in both sexes); chest pain; confusion; convulsions; difficulty in breathing or swallowing; difficulty in urinating; fainting; fever; fluid retention; hair loss; hallucinations; impotence; involuntary movements of the mouth, face, neck, tongue, or limbs; mouth sores; palpitations; skin darkening; skin rash; sore throat; tremors; unusual bleeding or bruising; visual disturbances; or yellowing of the eyes or skin.

INTERACTIONS
Haloperidol interacts with several other types of medications:

1. It can cause extreme drowsiness when combined with alcohol or other central nervous system depressants (such as antihistamines, barbiturates, benzodiazepine tranquilizers, muscle relaxants, narcotics, and pain medications) or with tricyclic antidepressants.

2. This drug can lessen the effectiveness of guanethidine and anticonvulsants (antiseizure medications).

3. Haloperidol may increase the side effects of epinephrine, lithium, and methyldopa.

Before starting to take haloperidol, BE SURE TO TELL YOUR DOCTOR about any medications you are currently taking, especially any of those listed above.

WARNINGS
• Tell your doctor about unusual or allergic reactions you have had to any medications, especially to haloperidol or to any other drugs used to treat mental illness.

• Tell your doctor if you now have or if you have ever had any blood disorders, blockage of the urinary tract, drug-induced depression, enlarged prostate gland, epilepsy, glaucoma, heart or circulatory disease, kidney disease, liver disease, lung disease, mental depression, Parkinson's disease, peptic ulcers, or thyroid disease.

• Avoid drinking alcoholic beverages while taking this medication in order to prevent oversedation.

•If this medication makes you dizzy or drowsy, do not take part in any activity that requires alertness, such as driving a car or operating potentially dangerous machinery. Be careful on stairs, and avoid getting up suddenly from a lying or sitting position.

• Prior to having surgery or any other medical or dental treatment, be sure to tell your doctor or dentist that you are taking this medication.

• Some of the side effects caused by this drug can be prevented by taking an antiparkinsonism drug. Discuss this with your doctor.

• This medication can decrease sweating and heat release from the body. You should, therefore, avoid getting overheated by strenuous exercise in hot weather and should avoid taking hot baths, showers, and saunas.

• Do not stop taking this medication suddenly. If the drug is stopped abruptly, you may experience nausea, vomiting, stomach upset, headache, increased heart rate, insomnia, tremors, or a worsening of your condition. Your doctor may want to reduce the dosage gradually.

• The elderly may be at increased risk for side effects. Watch closely for side effects or other changes, especially in mental status after taking haloperidol and report them to your doctor.

• If you are planning to have a myelogram or any other procedure in which dye is injected into the spinal cord, tell your doctor that you are taking this medication.

• Avoid spilling the oral concentrate form of this medication on your skin or clothing; it can cause redness and irritation of the skin.

• While taking haloperidol, do not take any over-the-counter (nonprescription) medications for weight control or for cough, cold, allergy, asthma, or sinus problems unless you first check with your doctor. The combination of these medications may cause high blood pressure.

• Haloperidol has the potential to cause a permanent movement disorder called tardive dyskinesia. It is important to discuss this with your doctor and to report any unusual or uncontrolled body movements.

• Some haloperidol formulations contain the color additive FD&C Yellow No. 5 (tartrazine), which can cause allergic-type reactions (rash, shortness of breath, fainting) in certain susceptible individuals.

• Be sure to tell your doctor if you are pregnant. A few cases of limb malformations have occurred in infants whose mothers had received haloperidol in combination with several other drugs during the first three months of pregnancy. Whether haloperidol was the cause is still not known. Also, tell your doctor if you are breast-feeding an infant. Small amounts of haloperidol pass into breast milk.

Haltran—see ibuprofen

Hemorrhoidal HC—see hydrocortisone, benzyl benzoate, bismuth resorcin compound, bismuth subgallate, zinc oxide, and Peruvian balsam combination (topical)

Hexadrol—see dexamethasone (systemic)

H-H-R—see hydralazine, hydrochlorothiazide, and reserpine combination

Hi-Cor—see hydrocortisone (topical)

Hiprex—see methenamine

Hismanal—see astemizole

Histalet—see pseudoephedrine and chlorpheniramine combination

Humulin L—see insulin

Humulin N—see insulin

Humulin R—see insulin

Hydergine—see ergoloid mesylates

---

hydralazine

BRAND NAMES (Manufacturers)
Alazine (Major)
Apresoline (Ciba)
hydralazine hydrochloride (various manufacturers)
TYPE OF DRUG
Antihypertensive
INGREDIENT
hydralazine
DOSAGE FORM
Tablets (10 mg, 25 mg, 50 mg, and 100 mg)
STORAGE
Hydralazine tablets should be stored at room temperature in a tightly closed, light-resistant container.

USES
This medication is used to treat high blood pressure or heart failure. Hydralazine is a vasodilator that directly relaxes the muscle of the blood vessels and allows the blood to flow at a lower force, which causes a lowering of blood pressure.

TREATMENT
In order to avoid stomach irritation while you are taking this medication, you can take your dose of hydralazine with food or with a glass of water or milk. To become accustomed to taking this medication, try to take it at the same time(s) each day. It may take up to two weeks before the full effects of this medication are observed.

Try not to miss any doses of this medication. If you do miss a dose, take the missed dose as soon as possible, unless it is almost time for the next dose. In that case, do not take the missed dose at all; just return to your regular dosing schedule. Do not double the next dose.

Hydralazine does not cure high blood pressure, but it will help to control the condition as long as you continue to take the medication.

SIDE EFFECTS
Minor. Constipation, diarrhea, dizziness, drowsiness, flushing, headache, light-headedness, loss of appetite, muscle cramps, nasal congestion, nausea, or vomiting. These minor side effects should disappear as your body adjusts to therapy with this medication.

To relieve constipation, increase the amount of fiber in your diet (fresh fruits and vegetables, salads, bran, and whole-grain breads), exercise, and drink more water (unless your doctor directs you to do otherwise).

If you feel dizzy or light-headed, sit or lie down for a while; get up slowly from a sitting or reclining position, and be careful on stairs. To avoid dizziness or light-headedness when you stand, contract and relax the muscles of your legs for a few moments before rising. Do this by pushing one foot against the floor while raising the other foot slightly, alternating feet so that you are "pumping" your legs in a pedaling motion.

Major. Tell your doctor about any side effects that are persistent or particularly bothersome. IT IS ESPECIALLY IMPORTANT TO TELL YOUR DOCTOR about anxiety, chest pain, confusion, cramping, depression, difficulty in urinating, fever, itching, numbness or tingling in the fingers or toes, palpitations, rapid weight gain (three to five pounds within a week), rash, shortness of breath, sore throat, tenderness in the joints and muscles, tiredness, unusual bleeding or bruising, or yellowing of the eyes or skin.

INTERACTIONS

Hydralazine interacts with several other types of drugs:

1. The combination of alcohol and hydralazine can lead to dizziness and fainting. You should, therefore, avoid drinking alcoholic beverages while taking this medication.

2. Used within 14 days of a monoamine oxidase (MAO) inhibitor, hydralazine can cause severe reactions.

Before you start to take hydralazine, BE SURE TO TELL YOUR DOCTOR about any medications you are currently taking, especially an MAO inhibitor.

WARNINGS

• Tell your doctor about any unusual or allergic reactions you have had to any medications, especially to hydralazine.

• Tell your doctor if you have ever had angina, heart disease, stroke, a heart attack, or kidney disease.

• To avoid dizziness or fainting, try not to stand for long periods of time, and avoid drinking alcohol. You should also try not to get overheated (avoid exercising strenuously in hot weather and avoid taking hot baths, showers, and saunas).

• If this drug makes you dizzy or drowsy, avoid taking part in any activities that require alertness, such as driving a car or operating potentially dangerous machinery.

• Before having surgery or any other medical or dental treatment, be sure to tell your doctor or dentist that you are taking this medication.

• Do not take any over-the-counter (nonprescription) allergy, asthma, sinus, cough, cold, or diet products unless you first consult your doctor or pharmacist. The combination of these medications with hydralazine may cause an increase in blood pressure.

• Some hydralazine formulations contain the color additive FD&C Yellow No. 5 (tartrazine), which can cause allergic-type reactions (rash, shortness of breath, fainting) in certain susceptible individuals.

• Do not stop taking this medication until you check with your doctor. If this drug is stopped abruptly, you could experience a sudden rise in blood pressure and other complications. Your doctor may, therefore, want to decrease your dosage gradually.

• Be sure to tell your doctor if you are pregnant. Although studies in humans have not been conducted, hydralazine crosses the placenta, and studies have shown that it causes birth defects in the offspring of animals that received large doses of it during pregnancy. Also, tell your doctor if you are breast-feeding an infant. It is not known whether hydralazine passes into breast milk.

hydralazine hydrochloride—see hydralazine

---

hydralazine, hydrochlorothiazide, and reserpine combination

BRAND NAMES (Manufacturers)
Cam-ap-es (Camall)
Cherapas (Kay)
H-H-R (Geneva Generics)
Ser-A-Gen (Goldline)
Seralazide (Lannett)
Ser-Ap-Es (Ciba)
Serpazide (Major)
Tri-Hydroserpine (Rugby)
Unipres (Solvay)

TYPE OF DRUG
Antihypertensive

INGREDIENTS
hydralazine, hydrochlorothiazide, and reserpine

DOSAGE FORM
Tablets (25 mg hydralazine, 15 mg hydrochlorothiazide, and 0.1 mg reserpine)

STORAGE
These tablets should be stored at room temperature in a tightly closed, light-resistant container.

USES

This drug is used to treat high blood pressure. Hydralazine is a vasodilator; it relaxes the muscles of the blood vessels, resulting in a lowering of blood pressure. Hydrochlorothiazide is a diuretic (water pill), which reduces body fluid accumulation by increasing the elimination of salt and water through the kidneys. Reserpine acts by depleting the body of certain chemicals that are responsible for maintaining high blood pressure.

TREATMENT

In order to avoid stomach irritation, you can take hydralazine, hydrochlorothiazide, and reserpine combination with food or with a full glass of water or milk. To become accustomed to taking this medication, try to take it at the same time(s) each day. Avoid taking a dose after 6:00 P.M.; otherwise, you may have to get up during the night to urinate.

If you miss a dose of this medication, take the missed dose as soon as possible, unless it is almost time for your next dose. In that case, do not take the missed dose at all; just return to your regular dosing schedule. Do not double the next dose.

Hydralazine, hydrochlorothiazide, and reserpine combination does not cure high blood pressure, but it will help to control the condition as long as you continue to take it.

The effects of this medication may not become apparent for up to two weeks after you start to take it.

SIDE EFFECTS

Minor. Abdominal pain, constipation, decrease in sexual desire, diarrhea, dizziness, flushing, loss of appetite, nasal congestion, or weight gain. These side effects should disappear as your body adjusts to the medication.

This medication can cause an increase in sensitivity to sunlight. It is, therefore, important to avoid prolonged exposure to sunlight and sunlamps. Wear protective clothing and sunglasses, and use an effective sunscreen.

To relieve constipation, increase the amount of fiber in your diet (fresh fruits and vegetables, salads, bran, and whole-grain breads) and exercise more (unless your doctor directs you to do otherwise).

To relieve mouth dryness, chew sugarless gum or suck on ice chips or a piece of hard candy.

If you feel dizzy or light-headed, sit or lie down for a while; get up slowly from a sitting or reclining position, and be careful on stairs. To avoid dizziness or light-headedness when you stand, contract and relax the muscles of your legs for a few moments before rising. Do this by pushing one foot against the floor while raising the other foot slightly, alternating feet so that you are "pumping" your legs in a pedaling motion.

Major. Tell your doctor about any side effects that are persistent or particularly bothersome. IT IS ESPECIALLY IMPORTANT TO TELL YOUR DOCTOR about anxiety; blurred vision; breast enlargement (in both sexes); chest pain; depression; difficulty in urinating; drowsiness; dry mouth; fainting; fatigue; fever; headaches; impotence; itching; joint pain; mood changes; muscle pain or spasms; nausea; nervousness; nightmares; palpitations; rapid weight gain (three to five pounds within a week); rash; shortness of breath; sore throat; swelling of the feet, ankles, or lower legs; thirst; tingling in the fingers or toes; tremors; unusual bleeding or bruising; vomiting; weakness; or yellowing of the eyes or skin.

INTERACTIONS

This medication interacts with several other types of drugs:

1. Concurrent use of it with central nervous system depressants (such as alcohol, antihistamines, barbiturates, benzodiazepine tranquilizers, muscle relaxants, narcotics, pain medications, phenothiazine tranquilizers, and sleeping medications) or with tricyclic antidepressants can cause extreme drowsiness.

2. The use of a monoamine oxidase (MAO) inhibitor within 14 days of this medication can lead to a severe reaction.

3. Tricyclic antidepressants can decrease the blood-pressure-lowering effects of reserpine. Reserpine can also decrease the effectiveness of levodopa and increase side effects (to the heart) of digoxin and quinidine.

4. Hydrochlorothiazide can decrease the effectiveness of warfarin, antigout medications, insulin, oral antidiabetic medicines, and methenamine.

5. Fenfluramine may increase the blood-pressure-lowering effects of hydrochlorothiazide (which can be dangerous).

6. Indomethacin may decrease the blood-pressure-lowering effects of hydrochlorothiazide, thereby counteracting the desired effects.

7. This medication should be taken one hour before or four hours after a dose of cholestyramine or colestipol (if you have also been prescribed one of these medications) because these medications can decrease the absorption of hydrochlorothiazide from the gastrointestinal tract.

8. Hydrochlorothiazide may increase the side effects of amphotericin B, calcium, adrenocorticosteroids (cortisone-like drugs), digitalis, digoxin, lithium, and vitamin D.

BE SURE TO TELL YOUR DOCTOR about any medications you are currently taking, especially any listed above.

WARNINGS

• Tell your doctor about unusual or allergic reactions you have had to any medications, especially to hydralazine, reserpine, or hydrochlorothiazide, or to any other sulfa drugs (other diuretics, oral antidiabetic medicines, or sulfonamide antibiotics).

• Before starting to take this medication, be sure to tell your doctor if you have ever had anuria (decreased urination), blood disorders, chest pain, diabetes mellitus, epilepsy, electroshock therapy, kidney disease, heart disease, liver disease, depression, gallstones or gallbladder disease, Parkinson's disease, peptic ulcers, stroke, systemic lupus erythematosus, or ulcerative colitis.

• Some of these products contain the color additive FD&C Yellow No. 5 (tartrazine), which can cause allergic-type reactions (rash, shortness of breath, fainting) in certain susceptible individuals.

• A doctor does not usually prescribe this drug or other "fixed-dose" products as the first choice in the treatment of high blood pressure. Generally, the patient first receives each ingredient singly. If the response is adequate to the fixed dose contained in this product, it can then be substituted. An advantage of a combination product is increased convenience.

• This drug can cause potassium loss. Signs of potassium loss include dry mouth, thirst, weakness, muscle pain or cramps, nausea, and vomiting. If you experience any of these symptoms, CONTACT YOUR DOCTOR. To help prevent this problem, your doctor may want to have blood tests performed to monitor your potassium levels. To avoid potassium loss, take this product with a glass of fresh or frozen orange or cranberry juice, or eat a banana every day. The use of a salt substitute also helps to prevent potassium loss. Do not change your diet or use a salt substitute, however, until you discuss it with your doctor. Too much potassium can also be dangerous.

• To prevent severe water loss (dehydration) while taking this medication, check with your doctor if you have any illness that causes severe or continuous nausea, vomiting, or diarrhea.

• Hydrochlorothiazide can raise blood sugar levels in diabetic patients. Blood sugar should, therefore, be monitored carefully (using blood or urine tests) when this medication is being taken.

• In order to prevent dizziness or fainting while taking this drug, try not to stand for long periods of time. You should also avoid drinking alcohol, and avoid becoming overheated by exercising strenuously in hot weather or by taking hot baths, showers, and saunas.

• If this drug makes you dizzy or drowsy, avoid taking part in any activity that requires alertness, such as driving a car or operating potentially dangerous machinery.

• Before having surgery or other medical or dental treatment, tell your doctor or dentist you are taking this drug.

• Before taking any over-the-counter (nonprescription) allergy, asthma, sinus, cough, cold, or diet products, check with your doctor or pharmacist. Some of these products can cause an increase in blood pressure.

• Do not stop taking this drug until you first check with your doctor. If this drug is stopped abruptly, you may experience a sudden rise in blood pressure. Your doctor may, therefore, want to decrease your dosage gradually.

• The elderly may be at increased risk for side effects, especially depression, confusion, or other mental changes. Report any such changes to your doctor.

•Tell your doctor if you are pregnant. Birth defects have been observed in the offspring of animals that received large doses of this drug during pregnancy. Also, tell your doctor if you are breast-feeding an infant. Small amounts of this drug pass into breast milk.

Hydramine—see diphenhydramine

Hydrex—see benzthiazide

Hydro-Chlor—see hydrochlorothiazide

hydrochlorothiazide

BRAND NAMES (Manufacturers)
Diaqua (Hauck)
Esidrix (Ciba)
hydrochlorothiazide (various manufacturers)
Hydro-Chlor (Vortech)
HydroDIURIL (Merck Sharp & Dohme)
Hydromal (Hauck)
Hydro-T (Major)
Hydro-Z 50 (Mayrand)
Hydrozide-50 (T.E. Williams)
Mictrin (EconoMed)
Oretic (Abbott)
Thiuretic (Warner-Chilcott)
TYPE OF DRUG
Diuretic and antihypertensive
INGREDIENT
hydrochlorothiazide
DOSAGE FORMS
Tablets (25 mg, 50 mg, and 100 mg)
Oral solution (50 mg per 5-ml spoonful)
Intensol oral solution (100 mg per ml)
STORAGE
This medication should be stored at room temperature in a tightly closed container.

USES
Hydrochlorothiazide is prescribed to treat high blood pressure (hypertension). It is also used to reduce fluid accumulation in the body caused by conditions such as heart failure, cirrhosis of the liver, kidney disease, and the long-term use of some medications. This medication reduces body fluid accumulation by increasing the elimination of salt and water through the kidneys.

TREATMENT
To decrease stomach irritation, you can take this medication with a glass of milk or with a meal (unless your doctor directs you to do otherwise). Each dose of the oral solution should be measured carefully with the dropper provided (Intensol solution) or a specially designed 5-ml measuring spoon. An ordinary kitchen teaspoon is not accurate enough. Try to take it at the same time every day. Avoid taking a dose after 6:00 P.M.; otherwise, you may have to get up during the night to urinate.

If you miss a dose of this medication, take the missed dose as soon as possible, unless it is almost time for the next dose. In that case, do not take the missed dose at all; just wait until the next scheduled dose. Do not double the dose.

This drug does not cure high blood pressure.

SIDE EFFECTS
Minor. Constipation, cramps, diarrhea, dizziness, drowsiness, headache, heartburn, loss of appetite, restlessness, or upset stomach. As your body adjusts to the medication, these side effects should disappear.

This drug can cause increased sensitivity to sunlight. Therefore, avoid prolonged exposure to sunlight and sunlamps. Wear protective clothing and use an effective sunscreen.

To relieve constipation, increase the amount of fiber in your diet (fresh fruits and vegetables, salads, bran, and whole-grain breads) and exercise more (unless your doctor directs you to do otherwise).

To avoid dizziness or light-headedness when you stand, contract and relax the muscles of your legs for a few moments before rising. Do this by pushing one foot against the floor while raising the other foot slightly, alternating feet so that you are "pumping" your legs in a pedaling motion.

Major. Tell your doctor about any side effects that are persistent or particularly bothersome. IT IS ESPECIALLY IMPORTANT TO TELL YOUR DOCTOR about blurred vision, confusion, difficulty in breathing, dry mouth, excessive thirst, excessive weakness, fever, itching, joint pain, mood changes, muscle pain or spasms, nausea, palpitations, skin rash, sore throat, tingling in the fingers or toes, vomiting, or yellowing of the eyes or skin.

INTERACTIONS
Hydrochlorothiazide interacts with several other types of medications:

1. It can decrease the effectiveness of oral anticoagulants, antigout medications, insulin, oral antidiabetic medicines, and methenamine.

2. Fenfluramine can increase the blood-pressure-lowering effects of hydrochlorothiazide (which can be dangerous).

3. Indomethacin can decrease the blood-pressure-lowering effects of hydrochlorothiazide, thereby counteracting the desired effects.

4. Cholestyramine and colestipol decrease the absorption of this medication from the gastrointestinal tract. Hydrochlorothiazide should, therefore, be taken one hour before or four hours after a dose of cholestyramine or colestipol (if you have also been prescribed one of these medications).

5. Hydrochlorothiazide may increase the side effects of amphotericin B, calcium, cortisone and cortisone-like steroids (such as dexamethasone, hydrocortisone, prednisone, or prednisolone), digoxin, digitalis, lithium, and vitamin D.

BE SURE TO TELL YOUR DOCTOR about any medications you are currently taking, especially any of those listed above.

WARNINGS

• Be sure to tell your doctor about unusual or allergic reactions you have had to any medications, especially to hydrochlorothiazide or other sulfa medications, including other diuretics, oral antidiabetic medications, and sulfonamide antibiotics.

• Be sure to tell your doctor if you now have or if you have ever had kidney disease or problems with urination, diabetes mellitus, gout, liver disease, asthma, pancreatic disease, or systemic lupus erythematosus.

• Hydrochlorothiazide can cause potassium loss. Signs of potassium loss include dry mouth, thirst, weakness, muscle pain or cramps, nausea, and vomiting. If you experience any of these symptoms, it is important that yiu call your doctor. To help avoid potassium loss, take this medication with a glass of fresh or frozen orange or cranberry juice, or eat a banana every day. The use of a salt substitute also helps to prevent potassium loss. Do not change your diet or use a salt substitute, however, before discussing it with your doctor. Too much potassium can also be dangerous. Your doctor may want you to have blood tests performed periodically in order to monitor your potassium levels while you are taking this drug.

• Limit your intake of alcoholic beverages while taking this medication to prevent dizziness and light-headedness.

• Becoming overheated can be hazardous while you are taking this medication. Avoid strenuous exercise in hot weather and do not take hot baths, showers, or saunas.

• If you have high blood pressure, do not take any over-the-counter (nonprescription) medications for weight control or for allergy, asthma, cough, cold, or sinus problems unless your doctor directs you to do so.

• To prevent dehydration (severe water loss) while taking this medication, check with your doctor if you have any illness that causes severe or continuous nausea, vomiting, or diarrhea.

• This medication can raise blood sugar levels in diabetic patients. Therefore, blood sugar should be carefully monitored by blood or urine tests when this medication is being taken.

• Before having surgery or any other medical or dental treatment, be sure to tell your doctor or dentist that you are taking this medication.

• Be sure to tell your doctor if you are pregnant. Hydrochlorothiazide can cross the placenta and may cause adverse effects on the developing fetus. Also, tell your doctor if you are breast-feeding an infant. Although problems in humans have not been reported, small amounts of this medication can pass into breast milk, so caution is warranted.

hydrocortisone (systemic)

BRAND NAMES (Manufacturers)
Cortef (Upjohn)
hydrocortisone (various manufacturers)
Hydrocortone (Merck Sharp & Dohme)
TYPE OF DRUG
Adrenocorticosteroid hormone
INGREDIENT
hydrocortisone (cortisol)
DOSAGE FORMS
Tablets (5 mg, 10 mg, and 20 mg)
Oral suspension (10 mg per 5-ml spoonful)
STORAGE
Store at room temperature in a tightly closed container. Never freeze this medication.

USES

Your adrenal glands naturally produce certain cortisone-like chemicals. These chemicals are involved in various regulatory processes in the body (such as those involving fluid balance, temperature, and reaction to inflammation). Hydrocortisone belongs to a group of drugs known as adrenocorticosteroids (or cortisone-like medications). It is used to treat a variety of disorders, including endocrine (hormonal) and rheumatic disorders; asthma; blood diseases; certain cancers; eye disorders; gastrointestinal disturbances, such as ulcerative colitis; respiratory diseases; and inflammations such as arthritis, dermatitis, poison ivy, and other allergic conditions. How this medication acts to relieve these disorders is not completely understood.

TREATMENT

In order to prevent stomach irritation, you can take hydrocortisone with food or milk.

If you are taking only one dose of this medication each day, try to take it before 9:00 A.M. This mimics the normal hormonal production in your body.

The oral suspension form of this medication should be shaken well just before measuring each dose. The contents tend to settle on the bottom of the bottle, so it is necessary to shake the container to distribute the ingredients evenly and equalize the doses. Each dose should then be measured carefully with a specially designed 5-ml measuring spoon. An ordinary kitchen teaspoon is not accurate enough.

It is important to try not to miss any doses of hydrocortisone. However, if you do miss a dose of this medication, follow these guidelines:

1. If you are taking ihydrocorizone more than once a day, take the missed dose as soon as possible, then return to your regular schedule. If it is already time for the next dose, double the dose.

2. If you are taking this medication once a day, take the dose you missed as soon as possible, unless you don't remember until the next day. In that case, do not take the missed dose at all; just follow your regular schedule. Do not double the next dose.

3. If you are taking this drug every other day, take the missed dose as soon as you remember. If you missed the scheduled dose by a whole day, take it when you remember and then skip a day before you take the next dose. Do not double the dose.

If you miss more than one dose of hydrocortisone, CONTACT YOUR DOCTOR.

SIDE EFFECTS

Minor. Dizziness, false sense of well-being, increased appetite, increased sweating, indigestion, menstrual irregularities, nausea, reddening and swelling of the skin on the face, restlessness, sleep disorders, or weight gain. These side effects should disappear as your body adjusts to the medication.

To help avoid potassium loss while using this drug, take your dose with a glass of fresh or frozen orange juice, or eat a banana each day. The use of a salt substitute also helps to prevent potassium loss. Check with your doctor before changing your diet or using a salt substitute.

Major. Tell your doctor about any side effects that are persistent or particularly bothersome. IT IS ESPECIALLY IMPORTANT TO TELL YOUR DOCTOR about abdominal (area around and above the waist) enlargement; acne or other skin problems; back or rib pain; bloody or black, tarry stools; blurred vision; convulsions; eye pain; fever and sore throat; growth impairment (in children); headaches; slow healing of wounds; increased thirst and urination; mental depression; mood changes; muscle wasting; muscle weakness; nightmares; rapid weight gain (three to five pounds within a week); rash; red lines across the abdomen; severe abdominal pain; shortness of breath; thinning of the skin; unusual bleeding or bruising; or unusual weakness.

INTERACTIONS

The systemic form of hydrocortisone adrenocorticosteroid hormone interacts with several other types of medications:

1. Alcohol, aspirin, and anti-inflammatory medications (such as diclofenac, diflunisal, flurbiprofen, ibuprofen, indomethacin, ketoprofen, mefenamic acid, meclofenamate, naproxen, piroxicam, sulindac, and tolmetin) aggravate the stomach problems that are common with use of this medication.

2. The dosage of oral anticoagulants (blood thinners, such as warfarin), oral antidiabetic drugs, or insulin may need to be adjusted when this medication is started or stopped.

3. The loss of potassium caused by hydrocortisone can lead to serious side effects in individuals taking digoxin. Also, thiazide diuretics (water pills) can increase the potassium loss caused by hydrocortisone.

4. Phenobarbital, phenytoin, rifampin, and ephedrine can increase the elimination of hydrocortisone from the body, thereby decreasing its effectiveness.

5. Oral contraceptives (birth control pills) and estrogen-containing drugs may decrease the elimination of this drug from the body, which can lead to an increase in side effects.

6. Hydrocortisone can increase the elimination of aspirin and isoniazid from the body, thereby decreasing the effectiveness of these two medications.

7. Cholestyramine and colestipol can chemically bind this medication in the stomach and gastrointestinal tract, preventing its absorption and decreasing its effectiveness.

BE SURE TO TELL YOUR DOCTOR about any medications you are currently taking, especially any of those listed above.

WARNINGS

• Tell your doctor about unusual or allergic reactions you have had to any medications, especially to hydrocortisone or other adrenocorticosteroids (such as betamethasone, cortisone, dexamethasone, fluocinolone, methylprednisolone, prednisolone, prednisone, and triamcinolone).

• Tell your doctor if you now have or if you have ever had bone disease, diabetes mellitus, emotional instability, glaucoma, fungal infections, heart disease, high blood pressure, high cholesterol levels, myasthenia gravis, peptic ulcers, osteoporosis, thyroid disease, tuberculosis, ulcerative colitis, kidney disease, or liver disease.

• If you are using this medication for longer than a week, you may need to receive higher dosages if you are subjected to stress, such as serious infections, injury, or surgery. Discuss this with your doctor.

• If you have been taking this drug for more than a week, do not stop taking it suddenly. If it is stopped suddenly, you may experience abdominal or back pain, dizziness, fainting, fever, muscle or joint pain, nausea, vomiting, shortness of breath, or extreme weakness. Your doctor may, therefore, want to reduce the dosage gradually. Never increase the dosage or take the drug for longer than the prescribed time, unless you first consult your doctor.

• While you are taking this drug, you should not be vaccinated or immunized. This medication decreases the effectiveness of vaccines and can lead to overwhelming infection if a live-virus vaccine is administered.

• Before having surgery or any other medical or dental treatment, be sure to tell your doctor or dentist that you are taking this medication.

• Because this drug can cause glaucoma and cataracts with long-term use, your doctor may want you to have your eyes examined by an ophthalmologist periodically during treatment.

• If you are taking this medication for prolonged periods, you should wear or carry an identification card or notice that clearly states that you are taking an adrenocorticosteroid medication.

• This medication can raise blood sugar levels in diabetic patients. Blood sugar levels should, therefore, be monitored carefully with blood or urine tests when this medication is being taken.

• Be sure to tell your doctor if you are pregnant. This drug crosses the placenta. Although studies in humans have not been conducted, birth defects have been observed in the offspring of animals that were given large doses of this drug during pregnancy. Also, tell your doctor if you are breast-feeding an infant. Small amounts of this drug pass into breast milk and may cause growth suppression or a decrease in natural adrenocorticosteroid hormone production in the nursing infant.

---

hydrocortisone (topical)

BRAND NAMES (Manufacturers)
Acticort 100 (Baker/Cummins)
Aeroseb-HC (Herbert)
Ala-Cort (Del-Ray)
Ala-Scalp (Del-Ray)
Bactine Hydrocortisone* (Miles)
CaldeCort Anti-Itch* (Fisons)
CaldeCort Light with Aloe* (Fisons)
Cetacort (Owen/Galderma)
Cortaid* (Upjohn)
Cort-Dome (Miles)
Cortef Feminine Itch* (Upjohn)
Cortizone-5* (Thompson)
Cortril (Pfizer)
Delacort* (Mericon)
Dermacort (Solvay)
DermiCort* (Republic Drug)
Dermolate Anti-Itch* (Schering)
Dermolate Scalp-Itch* (Schering)
Dermtex HC with aloe* (Pfeiffer)
FoilleCort* (Blistex)
Gynecort* (Combe)
Hi-Cor (C & M Pharmaceuticals)
hydrocortisone acetate (various manufacturers)
Hydro-Tex (Syosset)
Hydro-Tex* (Syosset)
Hytone (Dermik)
LactiCare-HC (Stiefel)
Lanacort* (Combe)
Locoid (Owen)
Nutracort (Owen)
Penecort (Herbert Labs)
Synacort (Syntex)
Texacort (GenDerm)
Westcort (Westwood)
*Available over-the-counter (without a prescription) in concentrations of 0.5% or less.

TYPE OF DRUG
Adrenocorticosteroid hormone

INGREDIENT
hydrocortisone

DOSAGE FORMS
Cream (0.1%, 0.2%, 0.25%, 0.5%, 1%, and 2.5%)
Ointment (0.1%, 0.2%, 0.5%, 1%, and 2.5%)
Lotion (0.25%, 0.5%, 1%, 2%, and 2.5%)
Gel (0.5%)
Pump spray (0.5%)
Aerosol (0.5%)

STORAGE
Hydrocortisone cream, ointment, lotion, gel, pump spray, and aerosol should be stored at room temperature in tightly closed containers. This medication should never be frozen.

The aerosol form of this medication is packaged under pressure. It should not be stored near heat or an open flame or in direct sunlight, and the container should never be punctured.

USES
Your adrenal glands naturally produce certain cortisone-like chemicals. These chemicals are involved in various regulatory processes in the body (such as those involving fluid balance, temperature, and reaction to inflammation). Hydrocortisone belongs to a group of drugs known as adrenocorticosteroids (or cortisone-like medications). It is used to relieve the skin inflammation (redness, swelling, itching, and discomfort) associated with conditions such as dermatitis, eczema, and poison ivy.

TREATMENT
Before applying this medication, wash your hands. Then, unless your doctor gives you different instructions, gently wash the area of the skin where the medication is to be applied. With a clean towel, pat the area almost dry; it should be slightly damp when you put the medicine on.

Apply a small amount of the medication to the affected area in a thin layer. Do not bandage the area unless your doctor tells you to do so. If you are to apply an occlusive dressing (like kitchen plastic wrap), be sure you understand the instructions. Wash your hands again after application.

If you are using the aerosol form, shake the can in order to disperse the medication evenly. Hold the can upright six to eight inches from the area to be sprayed, and spray the area for one to three seconds. DO NOT SMOKE while you are using the aerosol; the contents are under pressure and may explode when exposed to heat or flames.

If you miss a dose of this medication, apply the dose as soon as possible, unless it is almost time for the next application. In that case, do not apply the missed dose at all; just return to your regular dosing schedule. Do not double the next dose.

SIDE EFFECTS
Minor. Acne, burning sensation, itching, skin dryness, or rash.

If the affected area is extremely dry or scaling, the skin may be moistened before applying the medication by soaking in water or by applying water with a clean cloth. The ointment form is probably better for dry skin.

A mild stinging sensation may occur after this medication is applied. If this persists, contact your doctor.

Major. Tell your doctor about any side effects that are persistent or particularly bothersome. IT IS ESPECIALLY IMPORTANT TO TELL YOUR DOCTOR about blistering, increased hair growth, irritation of the affected area, loss of skin color, secondary infection in the area being treated, or thinning of the skin with easy bruising.

INTERACTIONS
This medication should not interact with other medications as long as it is used according to the directions given to you by your doctor or pharmacist.

WARNINGS

• Tell your doctor about unusual or allergic reactions you have had to any medications, especially to hydrocortisone or other adrenocorticosteroids (such as amcinonide, betamethasone, clocortolone, cortisone, desonide, desoximetasone, dexamethasone, diflorasone, flumethasone, fluocinolone, fluocinonide, flurandrenolide, halcinonide, methylprednisolone, paramethasone, prednisolone, prednisone, and triamcinolone).

• Tell your doctor if you now have or if you have ever had blood vessel disease, chicken pox, diabetes mellitus, fungal infections, peptic ulcers, shingles, tuberculosis, tuberculosis of the skin, vaccinia, or any other type of infection, especially at the site currently being treated.

• If any irritation develops while using hydrocortisone, immediately discontinue its use and notify your doctor.

• This product is not for use in the eyes, nose, or mouth; contact may result in side effects.

• Do not use this product with an occlusive wrap unless your doctor directs you to do so. Systemic absorption of hydrocortisone is increased if large areas of the body are treated, particularly if occlusive bandages are used. If it is necessary for you to use this drug under a wrap, follow your doctor's instructions exactly; do not leave the wrap in place longer than specified.

• If you are using this medication on a child's diaper area, do not put tight-fitting diapers or plastic pants on the child. This may lead to increased systemic absorption of the drug and a possible increase in side effects.

• In order to avoid freezing skin tissue when using the aerosol or pump spray form of hydrocortisone, make sure that you do not spray for more than three seconds; and hold the container at least six inches away from the skin.

• When using the aerosol or pump spray form of this medication on the face, cover your eyes, and do not inhale the spray (in order to avoid side effects).

• Be sure to tell your doctor if you are pregnant. If large amounts of this drug are applied for prolonged periods, some of it will be absorbed and may cross the placenta. Although studies in humans have not been conducted, birth defects have been observed in the offspring of animals that were given large oral doses of this drug during pregnancy. Also, tell your doctor if you are breast-feeding an infant. If absorbed through the skin, small amounts of hydrocortisone pass into breast milk and may cause growth suppression or a decrease in natural adrenocorticosteroid hormone production in the nursing infant.

hydrocortisone acetate—see hydrocortisone (topical)

hydrocortisone and iodochlorhydroxyquin combination (topical)

BRAND NAMES (Manufacturers)
Ala-Quin (Del-Ray)
Corque (Geneva Generics)
Cortin (C & M)

hydrocortisone with iodochlorhydroxyquin (various manufacturers)
Hysone (Hauck)
Lanvisone (Lannett)
Pedi-Cort V (Pedinol)
Pramosone (Ferndale)
Racet (Lemmon)
Vioform-Hydrocortisone (Ciba)
Vytone (Dermik)

TYPE OF DRUG
Adrenocorticosteroid hormone and anti-infective

INGREDIENTS
hydrocortisone and iodochlorydroxyquin

DOSAGE FORMS
Cream (0.5% hydrocortisone with1% or 3% iodochlorhydroxyquin; 1% hydrocortisone with 1% or 3% iodochlorhydroxyquin)
Ointment (1% hydrcortisone with 3% iodochlorhydroxyquin)

STORAGE
Hydrocortisone and iodochlorhydroxyquin combination cream and ointment shoukld be stored at room temperature in tightly closed, light-resistant containers. This medication should never be frozen.

USES
Your adrenal glands naturally produce certain cortisone-like chemicals. These chemicals are involved in various regulatory processes in the body (such as those involving fluid balance, temperature, and reactions to inflammation). Hydrocortisone belongs to a group of drugs known as adrenocorticosteroids (or cortisone-like medications). It is used to relieve the skin inflammation (redness, swelling, itching, and discomfort) associated with conditions such as dermatitis and eczema. How this drug acts to relieve inflammation is not completely understood. Iodochlorhydroxyquin is an antibiotic that acts to prevent the growth of the infecting bacteria or fungi.

TREATMENT
Before applying this medication, wash your hands. Then, unless your doctor gives you different instructions, gently wash the area of the skin where the drug is to be applied. With a clean towel, pat the area almost dry; it should be slightly damp when you put the drug on.

Apply a thin layer of the cream or ointment to the affected area. Do not bandage the area unless your doctor tells you to do so. If you are to apply an occlusive dressing (like kitchen plastic wrap), be sure you understand the instructions. Wash your hands again after application.

If you miss a dose of this drug, apply the dose as soon as possible, unless it is almost time for the next dose. In that case, do not apply the dose at all; just return to your schedule. Do not put twice as much of the medication on your skin at the next application.

It is important to continue to take the medication for the entire time prescribed by your doctor, even if the symptoms of infection disappear before the end of that period. If you stop applying the drug too soon, resistant bacteria are given a chance to continue growing, and the infection could recur.

SIDE EFFECTS

Minor. Acne, burning sensation, skin dryness, itching, or rash. These side effects should disappear as your body adjusts to the medication.

If the affected area is extremely dry or scaling, the skin may be moistened before applying the medication by soaking in water or by applying water with a clean cloth. The ointment form is probably better for dry skin.

A mild stinging sensation may occur after this medication is applied. If this persists, contact your doctor.

Major. Tell your doctor about any side effects that are persistent or particularly bothersome. IT IS ESPECIALLY IMPORTANT TO TELL YOUR DOCTOR about blistering, increased hair growth, irritation of the affected area, loss of skin color, secondary infection at the affected site, or thinning of the skin with easy bruising.

INTERACTIONS

This medication should not interact with other medications as long as it is used according to directions.

WARNINGS

• Tell your doctor about unusual or allergic reactions you have had to medications, especially to hydrocortisone or any other adrenocorticosteroid (such as amcinonide, betamethasone, clocortolone, cortisone, desonide, desoximetasone, dexamethasone, diflorasone, flumethasone, fluocinolone, fluocinonide, fluorometholone, flurandrenolide, methylprednisolone, prednisolone, prednisone, and triamcinolone), to iodochlorhydroxyquin, or to iodine.

• Tell your doctor if you now have or if you have ever had tuberculosis or viral or fungal infections of the skin.

• This product may affect the results of thyroid function tests. If you are scheduled to have such a test, be sure your doctor knows that you are using this medication.

• If additional irritation develops while using this drug, immediately discontinue its use and notify your doctor.

• This product is not for use in the eyes or mucous membranes; contact may result in side effects.

• Do not use this product with an occlusive wrap unless your doctor directs you to do so. Systemic absorption of this drug is increased if occlusive bandages are used. If it is necessary for you to use this drug under a wrap, follow your doctor's instructions exactly; do not leave the wrap in place longer than specified.

• If you are using this medication on a child's diaper area, do not put tight-fitting diapers or plastic pants on the child. This may lead to increased systemic absorption of the drug and a possible increase in side effects.

• This medication has been prescribed for your current infection only. Another infection later on, or one that someone else has, may require a different medicine. You should not give your medicine to other people or use it for other infections, unless your doctor specifically directs you to do so.

• Be sure to tell your doctor if you are pregnant. Birth defects have been observed in the offspring of animals that were given large oral doses of hydrocortisone during pregnancy. Also, tell your doctor if you are breastfeeding an infant. Small amounts of hydrocortisone pass into breast milk.

hydrocortisone, benzyl benzoate, bismuth resorcin compound, bismuth subgallate, zinc oxide, and Peruvian balsam combination (topical)

BRAND NAMES (Manufacturers)
Anumed HC (Major)
Anusol HC (Parke-Davis)
Hemorrhoidal HC (various manufacturers)
Rectacort (Century)

TYPE OF DRUG
Adrenocorticosteroid-containing hemorrhoidal and anorectal product

INGREDIENTS
hydrocortisone, benzyl benzoate, bismuth resorcin compound, bismuth subgallate, zinc oxide, and Peruvian balsam

DOSAGE FORMS
Rectal cream (0.5% hydrocortisone, 1.2% benzyl benzoate, 1.75% bismuth resorcin compound, 2.25% bismuth subgallate, 11% zinc oxide, and 1.8% Peruvian balsam)
Rectal suppositories (10 mg hydrocortisone, 1.2% benzyl benzoate, 1.75% bismuth resorcin compound, 2.25% bismuthsubgallate, 11% zinc oxide, and 1.8% Peruvian balsam per suppository)

STORAGE
The rectal cream should be stored at room temperature (never frozen) in a tightly closed container. The rectal suppositories should be stored in a cool, dry place or in the refrigerator.

USES
This combination medication is used to relieve the pain, itching, and discomfort arising from hemorrhoids and irritated anorectal tissues.

Your adrenal glands naturally produce certain cortisone-like chemicals. These chemicals are involved in various regulatory processes in the body (such as those involving fluid balance, temperature, and reaction to inflammation). Hydrocortisone belongs to a group of drugs known as adrenocorticosteroids (or cortisone-like drugs). Hydrocortisone is used to relieve inflammation (redness, swelling, itching, and discomfort). Zinc oxide is an astringent that causes shrinking and provides relief of irritation. The other ingredients provide a drying and softening effect.

TREATMENT
Wash your hands before applying this medication. To apply the rectal cream, first wash and dry the rectal area and then gently rub in a small amount of the cream. If you must insert the cream inside the rectum, attach the applicator tip to the opened tube. It may be helpful to

lubricate the applicator with a small amount of petroleum jelly to ease insertion. Insert the applicator tip into the rectum and squeeze the tube. Remove the applicator from the tube and wash it with hot water and soap; then thoroughly dry it before storing. Be sure to put the top back on the tube. Wash your hands again after application.

To insert the suppository, unwrap the suppository and moisten it slightly with water (if the suppository is too soft to insert, run cold water over it or refrigerate it for up to 30 minutes before you unwrap it). Lie down on your left side with your right knee bent. Push the suppository well into the rectum with your finger. Try not to have a bowel movement for at least an hour. Wash your hands again after application.

If you miss a dose of this medication, apply the cream or insert the suppository as soon as possible, unless it is almost time for the next application. In that case, do not use the missed dose at all; just wait until the next scheduled dose.

SIDE EFFECTS

Minor. Burning sensation upon application. The burning should disappear as your body adjusts to the medication.
Major. Tell your doctor about any side effects that are persistent or particularly bothersome. IT IS ESPECIALLY IMPORTANT TO TELL YOUR DOCTOR about any additional inflammation or infection at the site of application, as well as rectal pain, bleeding, leakage, itching, or blistering.

INTERACTIONS

This medication should not interact with any other medications as long as it is used according to the directions given to you by the doctor or pharmacist.

WARNINGS

• Tell your doctor about unusual or allergic reactions you have had to medications, especially to benzyl benzoate, bismuth resorcin compound, bismuth subgallate, Peruvian balsam, or to hydrocortisone or any other adrenocorticosteroid (such as amcinonide, betamethasone, clocortolone, cortisone, desonide, desoximetasone, dexamethasone, diflorasone, flumethasone, fluocinolone, fluocinonide, fluorometholone, flurandrenolide, halcinonide, methylprednisolone, paramethasone, prednisolone, prednisone, and triamcinolone).
• If additional irritation develops while using this drug, immediately discontinue its use and notify your doctor.
• You should not use this medication for more than seven consecutive days unless your doctor specifically directs you to do so.
• If this drug stains your clothing, the stain may be removed by washing with laundry detergent.
• Wearing a sanitary napkin may help to protect clothing and to keep the medication in the area.
• Be sure to tell your doctor if you are pregnant. If large amounts of hydrocortisone are applied for prolonged periods, some of it will be absorbed and may cross the placenta. Studies in humans have not been conducted, but birth defects have been observed in the offspring of animals that were given large oral doses of hydrocortisone

during pregnancy. Also, tell your doctor if you are breast-feeding an infant. If absorbed through the skin, small amounts of hydrocortisone pass into breast milk and may cause growth suppression or a decrease in natural adrenocorticosteroid hormone production in the nursing infant.

hydrocortisone, polymyxin B, and neomycin combination (otic)

BRAND NAMES (Manufacturers)
AK-Spore H.C. Otic (Akorn)
Cortatrigen Modified Ear Drops (Goldline)
Cortisporin Otic (Burroughs Wellcome)
Drotic (Ascher)
Ortega-Otic M (Ortega)
Otocort (Lemmon)
Otomycin-Hpn Otic (Misemer)
TYPE OF DRUG
Otic adrenocorticosteroid and antibiotic
INGREDIENTS
hydrocortisone, polymyxin B, and neomycin
DOSAGE FORMS
Otic solution (1% hydrocortisone, 10,000 units polymyxin B, and 5 mg neomycin per ml)
Otic suspension (1% hydrocortisone, 10,000 units polymyxin B, and 5 mg neomycin per ml)
STORAGE
The medication should be stored at room temperature (never frozen) in tightly closed, light-resistant containers.

USES

This medication is used to treat superficial bacterial infections of the outer ear. Your adrenal glands naturally produce certain cortisone-like chemicals. These chemicals are involved in various regulatory processes in the body (such as those involving fluid balance, temperature, and reaction to inflammation). Hydrocortisone belongs to a group of drugs known as adrenocorticosteroids (or cortisone-like medications). It is used to relieve inflammation (redness, swelling, itching, pain). Polymyxin B and neomycin are antibiotics, which act to prevent the growth and multiplication of the infecting bacteria.

TREATMENT

For accuracy, and in order to avoid contamination, another person should insert the ear drops if possible.

To warm the drops before administration, roll the bottle back and forth between your hands. DO NOT place the bottle in boiling water; high temperatures destroy the medication.

Before administration, the suspension form of this medication should be shaken well. The contents tend to settle on the bottom of the bottle, so it is necessary to shake the container to distribute the ingredients evenly and equalize the doses.

To administer the ear drops, tilt the head to one side with the affected ear turned upward. Grasp the earlobe and gently pull it upward and back to straighten the ear canal. (If administering ear drops to a child, gently pull the earlobe downward and back.) Fill the dropper and place the prescribed number of drops into the ear. Be careful not to touch the dropper to the ear canal, since the dropper can easily become contaminated. Keep the ear tilted upward for about five minutes. Your doctor may want you to put a piece of cotton soaked with the medication into your ear to keep the medicine from leaking out. To avoid contamination, DO NOT wash or wipe the dropper after you use it.

If you miss a dose, administer as soon as possible, unless it is almost time for the next dose. In that case, don't use the missed dose at all; return to your regular dosing schedule.

It is important to continue to take this medication for the entire time prescribed by your doctor, even if the symptoms of infection disappear before the end of that period. If you stop using the drug too soon, resistant bacteria are given a chance to continue growing, and the infection could recur.

SIDE EFFECTS
Minor. Burning sensation upon application. The burning should disappear as your body adjusts to the medication.
Major. Tell your doctor about any side effects that are persistent or particularly bothersome. IT IS ESPECIALLY IMPORTANT TO TELL YOUR DOCTOR about itching, rash, redness, or swelling at the site of application.

INTERACTIONS
This medication should not interact with any other medications as long as it is used according to directions.

WARNINGS
• Tell your doctor about unusual or allergic reactions you have had to medications, especially to hydrocortisone or any other adrenocorticosteroids (such as amcinonide, betamethasone, clocortolone, cortisone, desonide, desoximetasone, dexamethasone, diflorasone, flumethasone, fluocinolone, fluocinonide, fluorometholone, flurandrenolide, halcinonide, methylprednisolone, prednisolone, prednisone, and triamcinolone), to polymyxin B, or to neomycin or any related antibiotic (such as amikacin, colistimethate, colistin, gentamicin, kanamycin, netilmicin, paromycin, streptomycin, tobramycin, or viomycin).
• Tell your doctor if you now have or if you have ever had viral or fungal infections of the ear, a punctured eardrum, myasthenia gravis, or kidney disease.
• Do not use this medication for longer than ten consecutive days, unless your doctor directs you to do so. If there is no change in your condition within two or three days after starting to take this medication, contact your doctor. The medication may not be effective for the type of infection you have.
• This medication has been prescribed for your current infection only. Another infection later on, or one that someone else has, may require a different medicine. You should not give your medicine to other people or use it for other infections, unless your doctor specifically directs you to do so.

• Be sure to tell your doctor if you are pregnant. If large amounts of hydrocortisone are applied for prolonged periods, some of it will be absorbed and may cross the placenta. Studies in humans have not been conducted, but birth defects have been observed in the offspring of animals that were given large oral doses of hydrocortisone during pregnancy. Also, tell your doctor if you are breast-feeding an infant. If absorbed through the skin, small amounts of the drug pass into breast milk and may cause growth suppression or a decrease in natural adrenocorticosteroid hormone production in the infant.

hydrocortisone, polymyxin B, neomycin, and bacitracin combination (ophthalmic)

BRAND NAMES (Manufacturers)
Coracin (Hauck)
Cortisporin Ophthalmic (Burroughs Wellcome)
Triple Antibiotic with HC (various manufacturers)
Triple-Gen (Goldline)
TYPE OF DRUG
Ophthalmic adrenocorticosteroid and antibiotic
INGREDIENTS
hydrocortisone, polymyxin B, neomycin, and bacitracin (ointment only)
DOSAGE FORMS
Ophthalmic drops (1% hydrocortisone; 10,000 units polymyxin B; 0.5% neomycin; and 0.001% thimerosal per ml)
Ophthalmic ointment (1% hydrocortisone; 10,000 units polymyxin B; 0.5% neomycin; 400 units bacitracin)
STORAGE
This medication should be stored at room temperature (never frozen) in tightly closed containers. If the drops or ointment change color, do not use the medication. A change in color signifies a loss of effectiveness.

USES
This medication is used for the short-term treatment of bacterial infections of the eyes.

Your adrenal glands naturally produce certain cortisone-like chemicals. These chemicals are involved in various regulatory processes in the body (such as those involving fluid balance, temperature, and reaction to inflammation). Hydrocortisone belongs to a group of drugs known as adrenocorticosteroids (or cortisone-like medications). It is used to relieve inflammation (redness, swelling, itching, and discomfort). How it does so is not completely understood.

Polymyxin B, neomycin, and bacitracin are antibiotics, which act to prevent the growth and multiplication of infecting bacteria. Thimerosal is a preservative.

TREATMENT
Wash your hands with soap and water before using this medication. If you are using the drops, shake the bottle well before measuring out the drops. The contents tend to

settle on the bottom of the bottle, so it is necessary to shake the container to distribute the ingredients evenly and equalize the doses.

To prevent contamination of the medicine, do not touch the tube portion of the dropper or let it touch the eye.

Note that the bottle of the eye drops is not completely full. This is to allow control of the number of drops used.

To apply the drops, tilt your head back and pull down the lower eyelid with one hand to make a pouch below the eye. Drop the prescribed amount of medicine into the pouch and slowly close your eyes. Try not to blink. Keep your eyes closed, and place one finger at the corner of the eye next to your nose for a minute or two, applying a slight pressure (this is done to prevent loss of medication through the duct that drains fluid from the surface of the eye into the nose and throat). Then wipe away any excess with a clean tissue. If you don't think the medicine got into your eye, repeat the process once. If you are using more than one type of eye drop, wait at least five minutes between doses of the two types of medication.

Follow the same general procedure for applying the ointment. Tilt your head back, pull down the lower eyelid, and squeeze the ointment in a line along the pouch below the eye. Close your eyes, and place your finger at the corner of the eye near the nose for a minute or two. Do not rub your eyes. Wipe off excess ointment and the tip of the tube with clean tissues.

Since applying the medication is somewhat difficult to do, you may want someone else to apply it for you.

If you miss a dose of this medication, insert the drops or apply the ointment as soon as possible, unless it is almost time for the next application. In that case, do not use the missed dose at all; just wait until the next scheduled dose.

It is important to continue to take this medication for the entire time prescribed by your doctor, even if the symptoms of infection disappear before the end of that period. If you stop applying the drug too soon, resistant bacteria are given a chance to continue growing, and the infection could recur.

SIDE EFFECTS

Minor. Blurred vision, burning, or stinging. These side effects should disappear as your body adjusts to the medication.

Major. Tell your doctor about any side effects that are persistent or particularly bothersome. IT IS ESPECIALLY IMPORTANT TO TELL YOUR DOCTOR about disturbed or reduced vision; eye pain, itching, or swelling; headache; rash; continued burning; or severe irritation.

INTERACTIONS

This medication should not interact with other medications as long as it is used according to the directions given to you by your doctor or pharmacist.

WARNINGS

• Tell your doctor about unusual or allergic reactions you have had to any medications, especially to hydrocortisone or other adrenocorticosteroids (such as amcinonide, betamethasone, clocortolone, cortisone, desonide, desoximetasone, dexamethasone, diflorasone,

flumethasone, fluocinolone, fluorometholone, flurandrenolide, halcinonide, methylprednisolone, prednisolone, prednisone, and triamcinolone) or to polymyxin B, neomycin, bacitracin, or any related antibiotic (amikacin, colistimethate, colistin, gentamicin, kanamycin, neomycin, netilmicin, paromycin, streptomycin, tobramycin, or viomycin), or to thimerosal or other mercury compounds.

• Tell your doctor if you now have or if you have ever had fungal or viral infections of the eye, cataracts, glaucoma, inner ear disease, kidney disease, or myasthenia gravis.

• Tell your doctor if you wear contact lenses. Your doctor may suggest that you wear eyeglasses until the infection is gone.

• If there is no change in your condition two or three days after starting to take this medication, contact your doctor. The medication may not be effective for your particular infection.

• Do not use this drug for longer than ten consecutive days, unless your doctor directs you to. Prolonged use of this drug may result in glaucoma, secondary infection, cataracts, or eye damage. If you need to take this drug for as long as six weeks, your doctor may want you to have an eye examination by an ophthalmologist.

• This medication has been prescribed for your current infection only. Another infection later on, or one that a family member or friend has, may require a different medicine. You should not give your medicine to other people or use it for other infections, unless your doctor specifically directs you to do so.

• In order to allow your eye infection to clear, you should not apply makeup to the affected eye during treatment with this medication.

• Be sure to tell your doctor if you are pregnant. When large amounts of hydrocortisone are applied for prolonged periods, some of it is absorbed into the bloodstream. It may cross the placenta. Studies in humans have not been conducted, but birth defects have been observed in the offspring of animals that were given large oral doses of hydrocortisone during pregnancy. Also, tell your doctor if you are breast-feeding. If absorbed through the skin, small amounts of hydrocortisone pass into breast milk and may cause growth suppression or a decrease in natural adrenocorticosteroid hormone production in the nursing infant.

Hydrocortone—see hydrocortisone (systemic)

HydroDIURIL—see hydrochlorothiazide

Hydrogesic—see acetaminophen and hydrocodone combination

Hydromal—see hydrochlorothiazide

hydromorphone

BRAND NAMES (Manufacturers)
Dilaudid (Knoll)
hydromorphone hydrochloride (various manufacturers)

TYPE OF DRUG
Analgesic
INGREDIENT
hydromorphone
DOSAGE FORMS
Tablets (1 mg, 2 mg, 3 mg, and 4 mg)
Suppositories (3 mg)
STORAGE
Hydromorphone tablets should be stored at room temperature in a tightly closed, light-resistant container. The suppositories should be stored in the refrigerator.

USES
Hydromorphone is a narcotic analgesic that acts directly on the central nervous system (brain and spinal cord). It is used to relieve moderate to severe pain.

TREATMENT
In order to avoid stomach upset, you can take hydromorphone tablets with food or milk.

To use the suppository, remove the foil wrapper and moisten the suppository with water (if the suppository is too soft to insert, refrigerate it for half an hour or run cold water over it before removing the wrapper). Lie on your left side with your right knee bent. Push the suppository into the rectum, pointed end first. Lie still for a few minutes. Try to avoid having a bowel movement for at least an hour.

Hydromorphone works best if you take it at the onset of pain, rather than when the pain becomes intense.

If you are taking this medication on a regular schedule and you miss a dose, take the missed dose as soon as possible, unless it is almost time for your next dose. In that case, do not take the missed dose at all; just return to your regular dosing schedule. Do not double the next dose.

SIDE EFFECTS
Minor. Constipation, dizziness, drowsiness, dry mouth, false sense of well-being, flushing, light-headedness, loss of appetite, nausea, or sweating. These side effects should disappear as your body adjusts to the medication.

If you are constipated, increase the amount of fiber in your diet (fresh fruits and vegetables, salads, bran, and whole-grain breads), exercise, and drink more water (unless your doctor directs you to do otherwise).

Chew sugarless gum or suck on ice chips or a piece of hard candy to reduce mouth dryness.

If you feel dizzy or light-headed, sit or lie down for a while; get up from a sitting or lying position slowly, and be careful on stairs.

Major. Tell your doctor about any side effects that are persistent or particularly bothersome. IT IS ESPECIALLY IMPORTANT TO TELL YOUR DOCTOR about anxiety, confusion, continued constipation, difficult or painful urination, difficulty in breathing, excitability, fatigue, rash, restlessness, sore throat and fever, tremors, or weakness.

INTERACTIONS
Hydromorphone interacts with several other types of drugs:

1. Concurrent use of it with other central nervous system depressants (such as alcohol, antihistamines, barbiturates, benzodiazepine tranquilizers, muscle relaxants, and phenothiazine tranquilizers) or with tricyclic antidepressants can cause extreme drowsiness.

2. A monoamine oxidase (MAO) inhibitor taken within 14 days of this medication can lead to unpredictable and severe side effects.

BE SURE TO TELL YOUR DOCTOR about any medications you are currently taking, especially those listed above.

WARNINGS
• Tell your doctor about unusual or allergic reactions you have had to any medications, especially to hydromorphone or to any other narcotic analgesics (such as codeine, hydrocodone, meperidine, methadone, morphine, oxycodone, and propoxyphene).

• Tell your doctor if you now have or if you have ever had acute abdominal conditions, asthma, brain disease, colitis, epilepsy, gallstones or gallbladder disease, head injuries, heart disease, kidney disease, liver disease, lung disease, mental illness, emotional disorders, prostate disease, thyroid disease, or urethral stricture.

• If this drug makes you dizzy or drowsy, do not take part in any activity that requires alertness, such as driving a car or operating potentially dangerous machinery.

• Before having surgery or any other medical or dental treatment, be sure to tell your doctor or dentist that you are taking this medication.

• Hydromorphone has the potential for abuse and must be used with caution. Usually, you should not take it on a regular schedule for longer than ten days (unless your doctor directs you to do so). Tolerance develops quickly; do not increase the dosage or stop taking the drug abruptly, unless you first consult your doctor. If you have been taking large amounts of this medication for long periods, you may experience a withdrawal reaction (muscle aches, diarrhea, gooseflesh, runny nose, nausea, vomiting, shivering, trembling, stomach cramps, sleep disorders, irritability, weakness, excessive yawning, or sweating). Your doctor may, therefore, want to reduce the dosage gradually.

• The elderly may be more sensitive to side effects, especially constipation, mental effects, or breathing problems. Report any such effects to your doctor.

• Be sure to tell your doctor if you are pregnant. The effects of this medication during the early stages of pregnancy have not been thoroughly studied in humans. However, hydromorphone used regularly in large doses during the later stages of pregnancy can result in addiction of the fetus, leading to withdrawal symptoms (irritability, excessive crying, tremors, fever, vomiting, diarrhea, sneezing, or excessive yawning) at birth. Also, be sure to tell your doctor if you are breast-feeding an infant. Small amounts of this medication may pass into breast milk and cause excessive drowsiness in the nursing infant.

hydromorphone hydrochloride—see hydromorphone

Hydro-T—see hydrochlorothiazide

Hydro-Tex—see hydrocortisone (topical)

hydroxyzine

BRAND NAMES (Manufacturers)
Anxanil (EconoMed)
Atarax (Roerig)
hydroxyzine hydrochloride (various manufacturers)
hydroxyzine pamoate (various manufacturers)
Vistaril (Pfizer)
TYPE OF DRUG
Antihistamine and sedative/hypnotic
INGREDIENT
hydroxyzine
DOSAGE FORMS
Tablets (10 mg, 25 mg, 50 mg, and 100 mg)
Capsules (25 mg, 50 mg, and 100 mg)
Oral syrup (10 mg per 5-ml spoonful, with 0.5% alcohol)
Oral suspension (25 mg per 5-ml spoonful)
STORAGE
Hydroxyzine tablets, capsules, oral syrup, and oral suspension should be stored at room temperature in tightly closed, light-resistant containers. This medication should never be frozen.

USES
Hydroxyzine belongs to a group of drugs known as antihistamines (antihistamines block the action of histamine, which is a chemical that is released by the body during an allergic reaction). This medication is used to treat or prevent symptoms of allergy. It is also used as a sleeping aid and to relieve the symptoms of anxiety and tension.

TREATMENT
To avoid stomach upset, you can take hydroxyzine with food or with a full glass of milk or water (unless your doctor directs you to do otherwise).

The oral suspension form of this medication should be shaken well just before measuring each dose. The contents tend to settle on the bottom of the bottle, so it is necessary to shake the container to distribute the ingredients evenly and equalize the doses. Each dose of the oral syrup or oral suspension should be measured carefully with a specially designed 5-ml measuring spoon. An ordinary kitchen teaspoon is not accurate enough for medical purposes.

If you miss a dose of this medication, take the missed dose as soon as possible, unless it is almost time for your next dose. In that case, don't take the missed dose at all; just return to your regular dosing schedule. Do not double the next dose.

SIDE EFFECTS
Minor. Drowsiness or dry mouth. These side effects should disappear as your body adjusts to the medication.

Dry mouth can be relieved by chewing sugarless gum or by sucking on ice chips or a piece of hard candy.
Major. Tell your doctor about any side effects that are persistent or particularly bothersome. IT IS ESPECIALLY IMPORTANT TO TELL YOUR DOCTOR about convulsions, feeling faint, irritability, mental confusion, rash, or trembling or shakiness.

INTERACTIONS
Hydroxyzine can interact with other types of drugs:
Concurrent use of it with other central nervous system depressants (such as alcohol, barbiturates, benzodiazepine tranquilizers, muscle relaxants, narcotics, pain medications, and phenothiazine tranquilizers) or with tricyclic antidepressants can cause extreme drowsiness.

BE SURE TO TELL YOUR DOCTOR about any medications you are currently taking, especially any listed above.

WARNINGS
• Tell your doctor about allergic or unusual reactions you have had to medications, especially to hydroxyzine or to any other antihistamines (such as azatadine, brompheniramine, carbinoxamine, chlorpheniramine, clemastine, cyproheptadine, dexchlorpheniramine, dimenhydrinate, dimethindene, diphenhydramine, diphenylpyraline, doxylamine, promethazine, pyrilamine, trimeprazine, tripelennamine, and triprolidine).
• Hydroxyzine can cause drowsiness or dizziness. Your ability to perform tasks that require alertness, such as driving a car or operating potentially dangerous machinery, may be decreased. Appropriate caution should, therefore, be taken.
• Elderly patients may be more sensitive to side effects, especially drowsiness, confusion, and irritability. Report any such effects to your doctor.
• Be sure to tell your doctor if you are pregnant. The effects of this medication during pregnancy have not been thoroughly studied in humans. Also, tell your doctor if you are breast-feeding an infant. Small amounts of hydroxyzine pass into breast milk.

hydroxyzine hydrochloride—see hydroxyzine

hydroxyzine pamoate—see hydroxyzine

Hydro-Z 50—see hydrochlorothiazide

Hydrozide-50—see hydrochlorothiazide

Hygroton—see chlorthalidone

Hylidone—see chlorthalidone

Hylorel—see guanadrel

Hyosophen—see atropine, scopolamine, hyoscyamine, and phenobarbital combination

Hy-Phen—see acetaminophen and hydrocodone combination

Hysone—see hydrocortisone and iodochlorhydroxyquin combination (topical)

Hytakerol—see dihydrotachysterol

Hytone—see hydrocortisone (topical)

Ibuprin—see ibuprofen

ibuprofen

BRAND NAMES (Manufacturers)
Aches-N-Pain* (Lederle)
Advil* (Whitehall)
Children's Advil (Whitehall)
Genpril* (Goldline)
Haltran* (Roberts)
Ibuprin* (Thompson Medical)
ibuprofen (various manufacturers)
Medipren* (McNeil CPC)
Midol 200* (Glenbrook)
Motrin (Upjohn)
Motrin IB* (Upjohn)
Nuprin* (Bristol-Myers)
Pamprin-IB* (Chattem)
PediaProfen (McNeil CPC)
Rufen (Boots)
Trendar* (Whitehall)
*Available over-the-counter (without a prescription) as 200-mg tablets.

TYPE OF DRUG
Nonsteroidal anti-inflammatory analgesic

INGREDIENT
ibuprofen

DOSAGE FORMS
Tablets (200 mg, 300 mg, 400 mg, 600 mg, and 800 mg)
Oral suspension (100 mg per 5-ml spoonful)

STORAGE
Store in a tightly closed, light-resistent container at room temperature. This medication should never be frozen.

USES
Ibuprofen is used to treat the inflammation (pain, swelling, stiffness) of certain types of arthritis, gout, bursitis, and tendinitis. It is also used to treat painful menstruation. Ibuprofen has been shown to block production of certain body chemicals, called prostaglandins, that may trigger pain.

TREATMENT
You should take this medication on an empty stomach 30 to 60 minutes before meals or two hours after meals, so that it gets into your bloodstream quickly. However, to decrease stomach irritation, your doctor may want you to take the medication with food or antacids.

The oral suspension form of this medication should be shaken well just before measuring each dose. The contents tend to settle on the bottom of the bottle, so it is necessary to shake the container to distribute the ingredients evenly and equalize the doses. Each dose of the oral syrup or oral suspension should be measured carefully with a specially designed 5-ml measuring spoon. An ordinary kitchen teaspoon is not accurate enough.

If you are taking ibuprofen to relieve arthritis, you must take it regularly as directed by your doctor. It may take up to two weeks before you feel the full effects of this medication. Ibuprofen does not cure arthritis, but it will help to control the condition as long as you continue to take it.

It is important to take ibuprofen on schedule and not to miss any doses. If you do miss a dose, take it as soon as possible, unless it is almost time for your next dose. In that case, don't take the missed dose at all; just return to your regular dosing schedule. Do not double the next dose.

SIDE EFFECTS
Minor. Bloating, constipation, diarrhea, difficulty in sleeping, dizziness, drowsiness, headache, heartburn, indigestion, light-headedness, loss of appetite, nausea, nervousness, soreness of the mouth, unusual sweating, or vomiting. As your body adjusts to the drug, these side effects should disappear.

To relieve constipation, increase the amount of fiber in your diet (fresh fruits and vegetables, salads, bran, and whole-grain breads), exercise, and drink more water (unless your doctor directs you to do otherwise).

If you become dizzy or light-headed, sit or lie down for a while; get up slowly from a sitting or reclining position, and be careful on stairs.

Major. If any side effects are persistent or particularly bothersome, you should report them to your doctor. IT IS ESPECIALLY IMPORTANT TO TELL YOUR DOCTOR about bloody or black, tarry stools; blurred vision; confusion; depression; difficult or painful urination; palpitations; a problem with hearing; ringing or buzzing in your ears; skin rash, hives, or itching; stomach pain; swelling of the feet; tightness in the chest; unexplained sore throat and fever; unusual bleeding or bruising; unusual fatigue or weakness; unusual weight gain; wheezing or difficulty in breathing; or yellowing of the eyes or skin.

INTERACTIONS
Ibuprofen interacts with several other types of medications:
1. Anticoagulants (blood thinners, such as warfarin) can lead to an increase in bleeding complications.
2. Aspirin, other salicylates, and other anti-inflammatory medications can increase stomach irritation. Aspirin may also decrease the effectiveness of ibuprofen.
3. Ibuprofen can interact with diuretics (water pills).
4. Probenecid may increase blood levels of ibuprofen, which may increase the risk of side effects.
5. The action of beta blockers may be decreased by this drug.

BE SURE TO TELL YOUR DOCTOR about any medications you are currently taking, especially any listed above.

WARNINGS
• Before you start to take this medication, it is important to tell your doctor if you have ever had unusual or allergic reactions to ibuprofen, or to any of the other chemically related drugs (aspirin, other salicylates, diclofenac, diflunisal, fenoprofen, flurbiprofen, indomethacin, ketoprofen, meclofenamate, mefenamic acid, naproxen, oxyphenbutazone, phenylbutazone, piroxicam, sulindac, or tolmetin).
• Tell your doctor if you now have or if you have ever had bleeding problems, colitis, stomach ulcers or other stomach problems, epilepsy, heart disease, high blood pressure, asthma, kidney disease, liver disease, mental illness, or Parkinson's disease.

• If ibuprofen makes you dizzy or drowsy, do not take part in any activity that requires alertness.

• Because this drug can prolong bleeding time, tell your doctor or dentist you are taking this drug before having surgery or other medical or dental treatment.

• Stomach problems are more likely to occur if you take aspirin regularly or drink alcohol while being treated with this medication. These should, therefore, be avoided (unless your doctor directs you to do otherwise).

• The elderly may be at increased risk for experiencing side effects of this drug.

• Be sure to tell your doctor if you are pregnant. This type of medication can cause unwanted effects to the heart or blood flow of the fetus. Studies in animals have also shown that this type of medicine, if taken late in pregnancy, may increase the length of pregnancy, prolong labor, or cause other problems during delivery. Also, tell your doctor if you are breast-feeding an infant. Small amounts of ibuprofen can pass into breast milk.

Iletin I—see insulin

Iletin II—see insulin

Ilosone—see erythromycin

Ilosone Pulvules—see erythromycin

Ilozyme—see pancrelipase

imipramine

BRAND NAMES (Manufacturers)
imipramine hydrochloride (various manufacturers)
Janimine (Abbott)
Tipramine (Major)
Tofranil (Geigy)
Tofranil-PM (Geigy)
TYPE OF DRUG
Tricyclic antidepressant
INGREDIENT
imipramine
DOSAGE FORMS
Tablets (10 mg, 25 mg, and 50 mg)
Capsules (75 mg, 100 mg, 125 mg, and 150 mg)
STORAGE
Store at room temperature in a tightly closed container.

USES
Imipramine is used to relieve the symptoms of mental depression. This medication belongs to a group of drugs referred to as tricyclic antidepressants. These medicines are thought to relieve depression by increasing the concentration of certain chemicals necessary for nerve transmission in the brain. This medication is also used to treat enuresis (bed-wetting) in children six to 12 years of age.

TREATMENT
Imipramine should be taken exactly as your doctor prescribes. It can be taken with water or with food to lessen the chance of stomach irritation, unless your doctor tells you to do otherwise.

If you miss a dose of this medication, take the missed dose as soon as possible, then return to your regular dosing schedule. If, however, the dose you missed was a once-a-day bedtime dose, do not take that dose in the morning; check with your doctor instead. If the dose is taken in the morning, it may cause unwanted side effects. Never double the dose.

The effects of therapy with this medication may not become apparent for two or three weeks.

SIDE EFFECTS
Minor. Agitation, anxiety, blurred vision, confusion, constipation, cramps, diarrhea, dizziness, drowsiness, dry mouth, fatigue, heartburn, insomnia, loss of appetite, nausea, peculiar tastes in the mouth, restlessness, sweating, vomiting, weakness, or weight gain or loss. As your body adjusts to the medication, these side effects should disappear.

This drug may cause increased sensitivity to sunlight. Therefore, avoid prolonged exposure to sunlight and sunlamps. Wear protective clothing, and use an effective sunscreen.

Dry mouth caused by therapy with this medication can be relieved by chewing sugarless gum or by sucking on ice chips or a piece of hard candy.

To relieve constipation, increase the amount of fiber in your diet (fresh fruits and vegetables, salads, bran, and whole-grain breads), exercise, and drink more water (unless your doctor directs you to do otherwise).

To avoid dizziness or light-headedness when you stand, contract and relax the muscles of your legs for a few moments before rising. Do this by pushing one foot against the floor while raising the other foot slightly, alternating feet so that you are "pumping" your legs in a pedaling motion.

Major. Tell your doctor about any side effects that are persistent or particularly bothersome. IT IS ESPECIALLY IMPORTANT TO TELL YOUR DOCTOR about chest pains, convulsions, difficulty in urinating, enlarged or painful breasts (in both sexes), fainting, fever, fluid retention, hair loss, hallucinations, headaches, impotence, mood changes, mouth sores, nervousness, nightmares, numbness in the fingers or toes, palpitations, ringing in the ears, seizures, skin rash, sleep disorders, sore throat, tremors, uncoordinated movements or balance problems, unusual bleeding or bruising, or yellowing of the eyes or skin.

INTERACTIONS
Imipramine interacts with a number of other types of medications:
1. Extreme drowsiness can occur when this medicine is taken with central nervous system depressants (such as alcohol, antihistamines, barbiturates, benzodiazepine tranquilizers, muscle relaxants, narcotics, pain medications, phenothiazine tranquilizers, and sleeping medications) or with other tricyclic antidepressants.
2. Imipramine may decrease the effectiveness of antiseizure medications and may block the blood-pressure-lowering effects of clonidine and guanethidine.

3. Oral contraceptives (birth control pills) and estrogen-containing drugs can increase the side effects and reduce the effectiveness of the tricyclic antidepressants (including imipramine).

4. Cimetidine can decrease the breakdown of imipramine in the body, thus increasing the possibility of side effects.

5. Tricyclic antidepressants may increase the side effects of thyroid medication and of over-the-counter (nonprescription) cough, cold, allergy, asthma, sinus, and diet medications.

6. The concurrent use of tricyclic antidepressants and monoamine oxidase (MAO) inhibitors should be avoided, because the combination may result in fever, convulsions, or high blood pressure. At least 14 days should separate the use of this drug and the use of an MAO inhibitor.

BE SURE TO TELL YOUR DOCTOR about any medications you are currently taking, especially those listed above.

WARNINGS

• Tell your doctor if you have had unusual or allergic reactions to any medications, especially to imipramine or any of the other tricyclic antidepressants (such as amitriptyline, doxepin, trimipramine, amoxapine, protriptyline, desipramine, maprotiline, and nortriptyline).

• Tell your doctor if you have a history of alcoholism or if you have ever had asthma, high blood pressure, liver or kidney disease, heart disease, a heart attack, circulatory disease, stomach problems, intestinal problems, difficulty in urinating, enlarged prostate gland, epilepsy, glaucoma, thyroid disease, mental illness, or electroshock therapy.

• If the use of imipramine makes you dizzy or drowsy, do not take part in any activity that requires alertness, such as driving a car or operating potentially dangerous machinery.

• Before having surgery or any other medical or dental treatment, tell your doctor or dentist you are taking this drug.

• Do not stop taking this drug suddenly. Stopping it abruptly can cause nausea, headache, stomach upset, fatigue, or a worsening of your condition. Your doctor may want to reduce the dosage gradually.

• The effects of this medication may last as long as seven days after you stop taking it, so continue to observe all precautions during that period.

• Some of these products contain the color additive FD&C Yellow No. 5 (tartrazine), which can cause allergic-type reactions (skin rash, fainting, difficulty in breathing) in certain susceptible individuals.

• The elderly may be at increased risk for experiencing side effects. Report any such effects, especially dizziness, drowsiness, dry mouth, difficulty urinating, or mental confusion to your doctor.

• Be sure to tell your doctor if you are pregnant. Adverse effects have been observed in the fetuses of animals that were given large doses of this drug during pregnancy. Also, tell your doctor if you are breast-feeding an infant. Small amounts of this drug can pass into breast milk and may cause unwanted effects in nursing infants.

imipramine hydrochloride—see imipramine

Imodium—see loperamide

Imuran—see azathioprine

indapamide

BRAND NAME (Manufacturer)
Lozol (Rorer)
TYPE OF DRUG
Diuretic and antihypertensive
INGREDIENT
indapamide
DOSAGE FORM
Tablets (2.5 mg)
STORAGE
Store at room temperature in a tightly closed container.

USES
Indapamide is prescribed to treat high blood pressure. It is also used to reduce fluid accumulation in the body caused by conditions such as heart failure, cirrhosis of the liver, kidney disease, and the long-term use of some drugs. This drug reduces fluid accumulation by increasing the elimination of salt and water through the kidneys.

TREATMENT
To decrease stomach irritation, you can take indapamide with a glass of milk or with a meal (unless your doctor directs you to do otherwise). Try to take it at the same time every day. Avoid taking a dose after 6:00 P.M.; otherwise, you may have to get up during the night to urinate.

If you miss a dose of this medication, take the missed dose as soon as possible, unless it is almost time for the next dose. In that case, do not take the missed dose at all; just wait until the next scheduled dose. Do not double the dose.

This medication does not cure high blood pressure, but it will help to control the condition as long as you continue to take it.

SIDE EFFECTS
Minor. Constipation, cramps, diarrhea, dizziness, drowsiness, headache, heartburn, loss of appetite, restlessness, or upset stomach. As your body adjusts to the medication, these side effects should disappear.

This drug can cause increased sensitivity to sunlight. Therefore, avoid prolonged exposure to sunlight and sunlamps. Wear protective clothing, and use an effective sunscreen.

To relieve constipation, increase the amount of fiber in your diet (fresh fruits and vegetables, salads, bran, and whole-grain breads) and exercise more (unless your doctor directs you to do otherwise).

To avoid dizziness or light-headedness when you stand, contract and relax the muscles of your legs for a few moments before rising. Do this by pushing one foot against the floor while raising the other foot slightly, alternating feet so that you are "pumping" your legs in a pedaling motion.

Major. Tell your doctor about any side effects that are persistent or particularly bothersome. IT IS ESPECIALLY IMPORTANT TO TELL YOUR DOCTOR about blurred vision, confusion, difficulty in breathing, dry mouth, excessive thirst, excessive weakness, fever, itching, joint pain, mood changes, muscle pain or spasms, nausea, palpitations, skin rash, sore throat, tingling in the fingers or toes, unusual bleeding or bruising, vomiting, or yellowing of the eyes or skin.

INTERACTIONS
Indapamide interacts with several other types of medications:

1. It may decrease the effectiveness of oral anticoagulants, antigout medications, insulin, oral antidiabetic medicines, and methenamine.

2. Fenfluramine can increase the blood-pressure-lowering effects of indapamide (which can be dangerous).

3. Indomethacin can decrease the blood-pressure-lowering effects of indapamide, thereby counteracting the desired effects.

4. Cholestyramine and colestipol can decrease the absorption of this medication from the gastrointestinal tract. Indapamide should, therefore, be taken one hour before or four hours after a dose of cholestyramine or colestipol (if you have also been prescribed one of these drugs).

5. Indapamide may increase the side effects of amphotericin B, calcium, cortisone and cortisone-like steroids (such as dexamethasone, hydrocortisone, prednisone, and prednisolone), digoxin, digitalis, lithium, and vitamin D.

BE SURE TO TELL YOUR DOCTOR about any medications you are currently taking, especially any of those listed above.

WARNINGS
• Tell your doctor about unusual or allergic reactions you have had to any medications, especially to indapamide or any other sulfa drugs, including other diuretics, oral antidiabetic medications, and sulfonamide antibiotics.

• Tell your doctor if you now have or if you have ever had kidney disease or problems with urination, diabetes mellitus, gout, liver disease, asthma, pancreatic disease, or systemic lupus erythematosus.

• Indapamide can cause potassium loss. Signs of potassium loss include dry mouth, thirst, weakness, muscle pain or cramps, nausea, and vomiting. If you experience any of these symptoms, call your doctor. To help avoid potassium loss, take this drug with a glass of fresh or frozen orange juice or cranberry juice, or eat a banana every day. The use of a salt substitute also helps to prevent potassium loss. Do not change your diet or use a salt substitute, however, before discussing it with your doctor. Too much potassium can also be dangerous. Your doctor may want to have blood tests performed periodically to monitor your potassium levels.

• In order to avoid dizziness or fainting while taking this medication, try not to stand for long periods of time; avoid drinking excessive amounts of alcohol; and avoid getting overheated (do not perform strenuous exercise in hot weather or take hot baths, showers, or saunas).

• If you have high blood pressure, do not take any over-the-counter (nonprescription) medications for weight control or for allergy, asthma, cough, cold, or sinus problems unless your doctor directs you to do so.

• To prevent dehydration (severe water loss) while taking this medication, check with your doctor if you have any illness that causes severe or continuous nausea, vomiting, or diarrhea.

• This medication can raise blood sugar levels in diabetic patients. Therefore, blood sugar levels should be carefully monitored by blood or urine tests when this medication is being taken.

• Be sure to tell your doctor if you are pregnant. Studies in humans have not been conducted, but adverse effects have been observed in the fetuses of animals that received large doses of this drug during pregnancy. Also, tell your doctor if you are breast-feeding an infant. Although problems in humans have not been reported, small amounts of this medication can pass into breast milk, so caution is warranted.

Inderal—see propranolol

Inderal LA—see propranolol

Inderide—see propranolol and hydrochlorothiazide combination

Inderide LA—see propranolol and hydrochlorothiazide combination

Indocin—see indomethacin

Indocin SR—see indomethacin

indomethacin

BRAND NAMES (Manufacturers)
Indocin (Merck Sharp & Dohme)
Indocin SR (Merck Sharp & Dohme)
indomethacin (various manufacturers)
TYPE OF DRUG
Nonsteroidal anti-inflammatory analgesic
INGREDIENT
indomethacin
DOSAGE FORMS
Capsules (25 mg and 50 mg)
Extended-release capsules (75 mg)
Oral suspension (25 mg per 5-ml spoonful, with 1% alcohol)
Rectal suppositories (50 mg)
STORAGE
Indomethacin capsules, oral suspension, and rectal suppositories should be stored in closed containers at room temperature away from heat and direct sunlight. The rectal suppositories can also be stored in the refrigerator.

USES
Indomethacin is used to treat the inflammation (pain, swelling, and stiffness) of certain types of arthritis, gout,

bursitis, and tendinitis. Indomethacin has been shown to block the production of certain body chemicals, called prostaglandins, that may trigger pain. However, it is not yet fully understood how indomethacin works.

TREATMENT

You should take this drug immediately after meals or with food, in order to reduce stomach irritation. Ask your doctor if you can take indomethacin with an antacid.

Do not chew or crush the extended—release capsules; they should be swallowed whole. Breaking the capsule would release the medication all at once—defeating the purpose of the extended-release dosage form.

The suspension form of this medication should be shaken well just before measuring each dose. The contents tend to settle on the bottom of the bottle, so it is necessary to shake the container to distribute the ingredients evenly and equalize the doses. Each dose should be measured carefully with a specially designed 5-ml measuring spoon. An ordinary kitchen teaspoon is not accurate enough.

To use the rectal suppository form of this medication, remove the foil wrapper, and moisten the suppository with water. If the suppository is too soft to insert, refrigerate it for 30 minutes or run cold water over it before removing the foil wrapper. Lie on your left side with your right knee bent. Push the suppository into the rectum, pointed end first. Lie still for a few minutes. Try to avoid having a bowel movement for at least one hour.

It is important to take indomethacin on schedule and not to miss any doses. If you do miss a dose, take the missed dose as soon as possible, unless more than an hour has passed. In that case, do not take the missed dose at all; just return to your regular dosing schedule. Do not double the next dose.

This drug does not cure arthritis, but will help to control the condition as long as you continue to take it. It may take up to four weeks before you feel the full benefits of this medication.

SIDE EFFECTS

Minor. Bloating, constipation, diarrhea, difficulty in sleeping, dizziness, drowsiness, headache, heartburn, indigestion, light-headedness, loss of appetite, nausea, nervousness, soreness of the mouth, unusual sweating, or vomiting. As you adjust to the drug, the side effects should disappear.

To relieve constipation, increase the amount of fiber in your diet (fresh fruits and vegetables, salads, bran, and whole-grain breads), exercise, and drink more water (unless your doctor directs you to do otherwise).

If you become dizzy, sit or lie down for a while; get up slowly from a sitting or reclining position, and be careful on stairs.

Major. Tell your doctor about any side effects that are persistent or particularly bothersome. IT IS ESPECIALLY IMPORTANT TO TELL YOUR DOCTOR about bloody or black, tarry stools; blurred vision; confusion; depression; difficult or painful urination; palpitations; a problem with hearing; ringing or buzzing in the ears; skin rash, hives, or itching; stomach pain; swelling of the feet; rectal irritation; tightness in the chest; unexplained sore

throat and fever; unusual bleeding or bruising; unusual fatigue or weakness; unusual weight gain; wheezing or difficulty in breathing; or yellowing of the eyes or skin.

INTERACTIONS

Indomethacin interacts with several other types of drugs:
1. Use of anticoagulants (blood thinners, such as warfarin) can lead to an increase in bleeding complications.
2. Anti-inflammatory medications such as aspirin, salicylates, and diflunisal can cause increased stomach irritation when used while taking this drug.
3. Indomethacin can decrease the elimination of lithium from the body, possibly resulting in lithium toxicity.
4. Indomethacin may interfere with the blood-pressure-lowering effects of captopril, enalapril, or beta-blocking medications (acebutolol, atenolol, betaxolol, carteolol, esmolol, labetalol, metoprolol, nadolol, penbutolol, pindolol, propranolol, timolol).
5. Indomethacin can interfere with the diuretic effects of furosemide and thiazide-type diuretics (water pills).
6. Indomethacin can alter the effects of the potassium-sparing diuretics (such as amiloride, spironolactone, or triamterene).
7. The concurrent use of triamterene and indomethacin can result in kidney problems.
8. Probenecid can increase the amount of indomethacin in the bloodstream when both drugs are being taken.

BE SURE TO TELL YOUR DOCTOR about any medications you are currently taking, especially those listed above.

WARNINGS

• Tell your doctor if you have ever had unusual or allergic reactions to any medications, especially to indomethacin or any chemically related drugs.
• Before taking indomethacin, tell your doctor if you now have or if you have ever had bleeding problems, colitis, stomach ulcers or other stomach problems, epilepsy, heart disease, high blood pressure, asthma, kidney disease, liver disease, mental illness, or Parkinson's disease.
• If indomethacin makes you dizzy or drowsy, do not take part in any activity that requires alertness, such as driving a car or operating potentially dangerous machinery.
• If you will be taking this medication for a long period of time, your doctor may want to have your eyes examined periodically by an ophthalmologist. Some visual problems have been known to occur with long-term indomethacin use. Your doctor might want to keep a careful watch for these.
• Stomach problems are more likely to occur if you take aspirin regularly or drink alcohol while being treated with this medication. These should therefore be avoided (unless your doctor directs you to do otherwise).
• The elderly may be at increased risk for experiencing side effects of this drug.
• Be sure to tell your doctor if you are pregnant. Studies in animals have shown that indomethacin can cause unwanted effects in offspring, including lower birth weights, slower development of bones, nerve damage, and heart damage. If taken late in pregnancy, the drug can also prolong labor. Studies in humans have not been conducted.

Also, tell your doctor if you are breast-feeding. Small amounts of indomethacin can pass into breast milk, so caution is warranted.

Infectrol—see dexamethasone, neomycin, and polymyxin B combination (opthalmic)

Insulatard NPH—see insulin

insulin

BRAND NAMES (Manufacturers)
Humulin L (Lilly)
Humulin N (Lilly)
Humulin R (Lilly)
Iletin I (Lilly)
Iletin II (Lilly)
Insulatard NPH (Novo Nordisk)
Mixtard (Novo Nordisk)
Novolin (Novo Nordisk)
Velosulin (Novo Nordisk)

TYPE OF DRUG
Antidiabetic

INGREDIENT
insulin

DOSAGE FORM
Injectable (all types) (100 units/ml)
Injectable (regular) (100 units/ml, 500 units/ml)
This drug is available only as an injectable (if swallowed, it is destroyed by stomach acid). Various types of insulin provide different times of onset and durations of action (see below).

Insulin type	Onset of action (in hours)	Duration of action (in hours)
Regular insulin	½	6
Insulin zinc suspension, prompt (Semilente)	1½	14
Isophane insulin (NPH)	1	24
Insulin zinc suspension (Lente)	1	24
Protamine zinc insulin (PZI)	6	36
Insulin zinc suspension, extended (Ultralente)	6	36

STORAGE
After opening, keep most forms (except 500 units/ml strength) at room temperature if used in six months. Refrigerate unopened vials. Never freeze insulin.

USES
Insulin is a hormone that is normally produced by the pancreas; it functions in the regulation of blood sugar levels. This medication is used to treat diabetes mellitus (sugar diabetes) a disorder that results from an inability of the pancreas to produce enough insulin. Injectable insulin is used only to treat those patients whose blood sugar levels cannot be controlled by diet or by oral antidiabetic medications.

TREATMENT
Your doctor, nurse, dietitian, or pharmacist will show you how to inject insulin, using a specially marked hypodermic syringe. This medication is packaged with printed instructions that should be carefully followed.

You may prefer to use presterilized disposable needles and syringes, which are used once and then discarded. If you use a glass syringe and metal needle, you must sterilize them before reuse.

Make sure that the insulin you are using is exactly the kind your doctor ordered and that its expiration date has not passed.

Do not shake the bottle; tip it gently, end to end, to mix. ALWAYS CHECK THE DOSE in the syringe at least twice before injecting it.

Clean the site of the injection thoroughly with an antiseptic, such as rubbing alcohol.

Change the site of the injection daily, and avoid injecting cold insulin.

NEVER use a vial of insulin if there are lumps in it. Make your insulin injection a regular part of your schedule, so that you do not miss any doses. Ask your doctor what to do if you have to take a dose later than the scheduled time.

SIDE EFFECTS
Minor. Insulin can cause redness and rash at the site of injection. Try to rotate injection sites in order to avoid this reaction.
Major. Be sure to tell your doctor about any side effects that are persistent or particularly bothersome. IT IS ESPECIALLY IMPORTANT TO TELL YOUR DOCTOR about palpitations, fainting, shortness of breath, skin rash, or sweating.

Too much insulin can cause hypoglycemia (low blood sugar), which can lead to anxiety, chills, cold sweats, drowsiness, fast heart rate, headache, loss of consciousness, nausea, nervousness, tremors, unusual hunger, or unusual weakness. If you experience these symptoms, eat a quick source of sugar (such as table sugar, orange juice, honey, or a nondiet cola). You should also tell your doctor that you have had this reaction.

Too little insulin can cause symptoms of hyperglycemia (high blood sugar), such as confusion, drowsiness, dry skin, fatigue, flushing, frequent urination, fruit-like breath odor, loss of appetite, or rapid breathing. If you experience any of these symptoms, contact your doctor; he or she may want to modify your dosing schedule or change your insulin dosage.

INTERACTIONS
Insulin interacts with several other types of medications:
1. Insulin can increase digoxin's side effects to the heart.
2. Oral contraceptives (birth control pills), adrenocorticosteroids (cortisone-like medicines), danazol, dextrothyroxine, furosemide, ethacrynic acid, thyroid hor-

mone, thiazide diuretics (water pills), phenytoin, or nicotine (from smoking) can increase insulin requirements.

3. Monoamine oxidase (MAO) inhibitors, phenylbutazone, fenfluramine, guanethidine, disopyramide, sulfinpyrazone, tetracycline, alcohol, anabolic steroids, or large doses of aspirin can increase the effects of insulin, leading to hypoglycemia.

4. Beta blockers (acebutolol, atenolol, betaxolol, carteolol, esmolol, labetalol, metoprolol, nadolol, penbutolol, pindolol, propranolol, timolol) may prolong the effects of insulin and mask the signs of hypoglycemia.

BE SURE TO TELL YOUR DOCTOR about any medications you are currently taking, especially any of those listed above.

WARNINGS

• Tell your doctor about unusual or allergic reactions you have had to any medications, especially to insulin.

• Before starting to take this medication, be sure to tell your doctor if you now have or if you have ever had high fevers, infections, kidney disease, liver disease, thyroid disease, or severe nausea and vomiting.

• If your doctor prescribes two types of insulin to achieve better glucose control and recommends mixing the insulin into one syringe, always draw the regular insulin (clear) into the syringe first.

• Some insulin mixtures won't interact with each other for some time. Others react quickly and require immediate injection. Consult your doctor or pharmacist about this.

• Make sure that your friends and family are aware of the symptoms of an insulin reaction and know what to do should they observe any of the symptoms in you.

• Carry a card or wear a bracelet that identifies you as a diabetic.

• Always have insulin and syringes available.

• When traveling, always carry an ample supply of your diabetic needs and, if possible, a prescription for insulin and syringes. Carry insulin and syringes on your person; baggage can be lost, delayed, or stolen.

• Do not store insulin in your car's glove compartment.

• To avoid the possibility of hypoglycemia (low blood sugar levels), you should eat on a regular schedule and should avoid skipping meals.

• Before having surgery or other medical or dental treatment, tell your doctor or dentist you are taking insulin.

• Check with your doctor or pharmacist before taking any over-the-counter (nonprescription) cough, cold, diet, allergy, asthma, or sinus medications. Some of these products affect blood sugar levels.

• If you become ill—if you catch a cold or the flu or become nauseated—your insulin requirements may change. Consult your doctor.

• Be sure to tell your doctor if you are pregnant. Insulin dosing requirements often change during pregnancy.

Intal—see cromolyn sodium (inhalation)

Ionamin—see phentermine

Iophen-C—see codeine and iodinated glycerol combination

Iophen DM—see dextromethorphan and iodinated glycerol combination

Iotuss—see codeine and iodinated glycerol combination

ipecac

BRAND NAME (Manufacturer)
Ipecac (various manufacturers)
Note: This product is available without a prescription.
TYPE OF DRUG
Emetic
INGREDIENT
ipecac
DOSAGE FORM
Oral syrup (with 1.5% or 2% alcohol)
STORAGE
Store at room temperature in a tightly closed container.

USES
Ipecac is for emergency use to treat drug overdose or poisoning. Ipecac works on the stomach and on the vomiting center in the brain to produce vomiting.

TREATMENT
Before administering ipecac, call a poison control center, emergency room, or physician for advice. You must administer ipecac with adequate amounts of water ($1/2$ glass for infants less than 1 year old; 1 to 2 glasses for children and adults) for adequate fluid in the stomach. If vomiting does not occur within 20 minutes after a second dose has been given, call again IMMEDIATELY for instructions.

SIDE EFFECTS
Minor. Ipecac can cause diarrhea, drowsiness, nausea, or vomiting that continues for more than 30 minutes. These side effects should disappear within several hours.
Major. Be sure to tell your doctor about any side effects that are persistent or particularly bothersome. IT IS ESPECIALLY IMPORTANT TO TELL YOUR DOCTOR about aching or stiffness of the muscles, difficulty in breathing, palpitations, stomach cramps or pain, or weakness as soon as possible.

INTERACTIONS
Ipecac oral syrup should not be administered with milk or with carbonated beverages; these fluids may affect how quickly ipecac works. Activated charcoal absorbs ipecac. If both activated charcoal and ipecac oral syrup are to be used, give the activated charcoal only after successful vomiting has been produced by the ipecac.

WARNINGS
• Vomiting is not the proper treatment in all cases of possible poisoning; ipecac should NOT be used if gasoline, oils, kerosene, acids, alkalies (lye), corrosives, or strychnine has been swallowed, since vomiting of these substances may cause seizures, additional throat burns, or pneumonia.

• Ipecac should probably not be used if the poisoned patient is losing consciousness, has no gag reflex, is in shock, is having seizures, or has heart disease unless directed by a health professional.

• Muscle and heart disorders and at least one death have been reported as a result of the chronic use of ipecac by young women who were using it to induce vomiting.

• Ipecac is available over-the-counter (nonprescription) and can be purchased from most pharmacies. Mothers should have a one-ounce bottle of ipecac for each child in the house. Always call a poison control center, emergency room, or physician for instructions BEFORE administering ipecac.

• Be sure to tell your doctor if the overdose or poisoning victim is pregnant. Although ipecac appears to be safe, studies in pregnant women have not been done.

Iso-Bid—see isosorbide dinitrate

Isoclor—see pseudoephedrine and chlorpheniramine combination

Isoclor Timesules—see pseudoephedrine and chlorpheniramine combination

Isollyl Improved—see aspirin, caffeine, and butalbital combination

Ismelin—see guanethidine

isoniazid

BRAND NAMES (Manufacturers)
isoniazid (various manufacturers)
Laniazid (Lannett)
Nydrazid (Apothecon)
TYPE OF DRUG
Antitubercular
INGREDIENT
isoniazid
DOSAGE FORMS
Tablets (50 mg, 100 mg, and 300 mg)
Oral syrup (50 mg per 5-ml spoonful)
STORAGE
Store at room temperature in a tightly closed, light-resistant container. This medication should never be frozen.

USES
Isoniazid is used to prevent and treat tuberculosis. It acts by severely injuring the cell structure of tuberculosis bacteria, thereby preventing them from growing and multiplying.

TREATMENT
In order to avoid stomach irritation, you can take isoniazid with food or a full glass of water or milk (unless your doctor directs you to do otherwise).

Antacids prevent the absorption of isoniazid from the gastrointestinal tract, so they should not be taken within an hour of a dose of isoniazid.

Each dose of the oral syrup should be measured carefully with a specially designed 5-ml measuring spoon. An ordinary kitchen teaspoon is not accurate enough for medical purposes.

It is important to continue to take this medication for the entire time prescribed by your doctor, even if your symptoms disappear before the end of that period. If you stop taking the drug too soon, your infection could recur.

It is common for therapy to last for at least six months and, at times, for as long as two years.

Try not to miss any doses of this medication. If you do miss a dose, take the missed dose as soon as possible, unless it is almost time for the next dose. In that case, do not take the missed dose at all; just return to your regular dosing schedule. Do not double the next dose.

SIDE EFFECTS
Minor. Abdominal pain, dizziness, heartburn, nausea, or vomiting. These side effects should disappear as your body adjusts to the medication.

If you feel dizzy, sit or lie down for a while; get up slowly from a sitting or reclining position, and be careful on stairs.

Major. Tell your doctor about any side effects that are persistent or particularly bothersome. IT IS ESPECIALLY IMPORTANT TO TELL YOUR DOCTOR about blurred vision, breast enlargement (in both sexes), chills, darkening of the urine, eye pain, fever, malaise, memory impairment, numbness or tingling in the fingers or toes, rash, unusual bleeding or bruising, vision changes, weakness, or yellowing of the eyes or skin.

Your doctor may want to prescribe vitamin B_6 (pyridoxine) to prevent the numbness and tingling. However, do not take vitamin B_6 without consulting your doctor.

INTERACTIONS
Isoniazid interacts with several other types of medications:

1. Concurrent use of isoniazid and alcohol can lead to decreased effectiveness of isoniazid and increased side effects on the liver.

2. The combination of isoniazid and cycloserine can result in dizziness or drowsiness.

3. The combination of isoniazid and disulfiram can lead to dizziness, loss of coordination, irritability, and insomnia.

4. Isoniazid can decrease the breakdown of phenytoin and carbamazepine in the body, which can lead to an increase in side effects from phenytoin and carbamazepine.

5. Isoniazid can decrease the effectiveness of ketoconazole.

6. In combination, rifampin and isoniazid can increase the risk of liver damage. However, this is a commonly prescribed combination.

7. The effectiveness of isoniazid may be decreased by adrenocorticosteroids (cortisone-like medicines).

8. The side effects of benzodiazepine tranquilizers or meperidine may be increased by isoniazid.

BE SURE TO TELL YOUR DOCTOR about any medications you are currently taking, especially those listed above.

WARNINGS
• Tell your doctor about unusual or allergic reactions you have had to any medications, especially to isoniazid, ethionamide, pyrazinamide, or niacin (vitamin B_3).

• Before starting to take this medication, be sure to tell your doctor if you have a history of alcoholism, or if you now have or ever had kidney disease, liver disease, or seizures.

• If this drug makes you dizzy, avoid tasks that require alertness, such as driving a car.

• Your doctor may want you to have periodic eye examinations while taking this medication, especially if you begin to have vison side effects.

• Isoniazid can interact with several foods (skipjack fish, tuna, yeast extracts, sauerkraut juice, sausages, and certain cheeses), leading to severe reactions. You should, therefore, avoid eating these foods while being treated with isoniazid.

• Diabetics using Clinitest urine glucose tests may get erroneously high sugar readings while they are taking isoniazid. Temporarily changing to Clinistix or Tes-Tape urine tests avoids this problem.

• Be sure to tell your doctor if you are pregnant. Although isoniazid appears to be safe during pregnancy, it does cross the placenta. Extensive studies in pregnant women have not been conducted. Also, tell your doctor if you are breastfeeding an infant. Small amounts of isoniazid pass into breast milk.

Isoptin—see verapamil

Isoptin SR—see verapamil

Isopto Carpine—see pilocarpine (ophthalmic)

Isopto Cetamide—see sodium sulfacetamide (ophthalmic)

Isordil Tembids—see isosorbide dinitrate

Isordil Titradose—see isosorbide dinitrate

---

isosorbide dinitrate

BRAND NAMES (Manufacturers)
Dilatrate-SR (Reed & Carnrick)
Iso-Bid (Geriatric)
Isordil Tembids (Wyeth-Ayerst)
Isordil Titradose (Wyeth-Ayerst)
isosorbide dinitrate (various manufacturers)
Isotrate Timecelles (Hauck)
Sorbitrate (ICI Pharma)
Sorbitrate SA (ICI Pharma)
TYPE OF DRUG
Antianginal
INGREDIENT
isosorbide dinitrate
DOSAGE FORMS
Tablets (5 mg, 10 mg, 20 mg, 30 mg, and 40 mg)
Chewable tablets (5 mg and 10 mg)
Sublingual tablets (2.5 mg, 5 mg, and 10 mg)
Sustained-release tablets (40 mg)
Sustained-release capsules (40 mg)
STORAGE
Isosorbide dinitrate tablets and capsules should be stored in a cool, dry place. This medication loses potency when exposed to heat or moisture.

USES
Isosorbide dinitrate is a vasodilator that relaxes the muscle of the blood vessels, leading to an increase in the oxygen supply to the heart. It is used to relieve (chewable and sublingual tablets) or to prevent (oral tablets and capsules) angina (chest pain). The chewable and sublingual tablets act quickly; they can be used to relieve chest pain after it has begun. The oral tablets and capsules do not act quickly; they are used only to prevent angina attacks.

TREATMENT
Take the chewable or sublingual forms of this medication at the first sign of an angina attack. DO NOT WAIT for the attack to become severe. Then sit down. These tablets are absorbed more completely through the lining of the mouth than from the stomach. Your mouth should be empty when you take these tablets. Do not eat, drink, or smoke with a tablet in your mouth. If the pain of an attack continues, you can take another tablet after five minutes, and a third tablet after another five minutes. If three tablets provide no relief within 15 minutes, CONTACT YOUR DOCTOR IMMEDIATELY or go to the nearest hospital.

The chewable tablet should be chewed for at least two minutes before swallowing.

Place the sublingual tablet under the tongue or against the cheek and allow it to dissolve—DO NOT CHEW OR SWALLOW IT. Do not swallow until the drug is dissolved, and do not rinse your mouth for several minutes (this gives a greater opportunity for the drug to be absorbed through the lining of the mouth).

The regular tablets and the sustained-release forms of this medication should be taken with a full glass of water on an empty stomach. The sustained-release forms should be swallowed whole. Breaking, crushing, or chewing these tablets or capsules destroys their sustained-release activity and possibly increases the side effects.

If you are taking this medication on a regular schedule, try not to miss any doses. If you do miss a dose, take the missed dose as soon as possible, unless it is within two hours of the next dose (or six hours for the sustained-release forms). In that case, do not take the missed dose at all; return to your regular dosing schedule. Do not double the next dose.

Some doctors may recommend using this medication to prevent an anginal attack before expected physical or emotional stress. Discuss this with your doctor.

SIDE EFFECTS
Minor. Dizziness, flushing, headache, light-headedness, nausea, or vomiting. These side effects should disappear as your body adjusts to the medication.

If you feel dizzy or light-headed, sit or lie down for a while; get up slowly from a sitting or reclining position, and be careful on stairs. To avoid dizziness or light-headedness when you stand, contract and relax the muscles of your legs for a few moments before rising. Do this by pushing one foot against the floor while raising the other foot slightly, alternating feet so that you are "pumping" your legs in a pedaling motion.

Acetaminophen may help relieve headaches caused by this medication.

Major. Tell your doctor about any side effects that are persistent or particularly bothersome. IT IS ESPECIALLY IMPORTANT TO TELL YOUR DOCTOR about fainting spells, palpitations, rash, restlessness, sweating, or unusual weakness.

INTERACTIONS

Isosorbide dinitrate can interact with other types of drugs:

1. Isosorbide dinitrate, in combination with alcohol, can lead to dizziness and fainting.

2. Over-the-counter (nonprescription) sinus, allergy, cough, cold, asthma, and diet products can block the antiangina effects of isosorbide dinitrate.

BE SURE TO TELL YOUR DOCTOR about any medications you are currently taking, especially any of those listed above.

WARNINGS

• Tell your doctor about unusual or allergic reactions you have had to any medications, especially to isosorbide dinitrate or to any other nitrate-containing drugs (such as nitroglycerin).

• Before starting to take this medication, tell your doctor if you have ever had severe anemia, glaucoma, a heart attack, or thyroid disease.

• Before using this medication to relieve chest pain, be certain that the pain arises from the heart and is not due to a muscle spasm or to indigestion. If your chest pain is not relieved by use of this drug, or if pain arises from a different location or differs in severity, CONSULT YOUR DOCTOR IMMEDIATELY.

• If this drug makes you dizzy or light-headed, do not take part in any activity that requires alertness, such as driving a car or operating potentially dangerous machinery.

• Before having surgery or any other medical or dental treatment, be sure to tell your doctor or dentist that you are taking this medication.

• Tolerance to this medication may develop. If the drug begins to lose its effectiveness, contact your doctor.

• Isosorbide dinitrate should not be discontinued unless you first consult your doctor. Stopping the drug abruptly may lead to further chest pain. Your doctor may, therefore, want to decrease your dosage gradually.

• If you have frequent diarrhea, you may not be absorbing the sustained-release form of this medication. Discuss this with your doctor.

• Be sure to tell your doctor if you are pregnant. Although this drug appears to be safe, extensive studies in pregnant women have not been conducted. Also, tell your doctor if you are breast-feeding an infant. It is not known whether isosorbide dinitrate passes into breast milk.

Isotrate Timecelles—see isosorbide dinitrate

isotretinoin

BRAND NAME (Manufacturer)
Accutane (Roche)
TYPE OF DRUG
Acne preparation
INGREDIENT
isotretinoin
DOSAGE FORM
Capsules (10 mg, 20 mg, and 40 mg)
STORAGE
Isotretinoin should be stored at room temperature in a tightly closed, light-resistant container.

USES

This medication is used to treat severe cystic acne. It is not clearly understood how isotretinoin works, but it decreases the production of sebum (a skin oil) and dries up the acne lesions.

TREATMENT

An information leaflet is packaged with this product. Be sure to read it carefully.

Isotretinoin should be taken with meals to obtain maximum benefit.

It may take one to two months before the maximum effects of this medication are observed.

If you miss a dose of this medication, take the missed dose as soon as possible, and then return to your regular dosing schedule. However, if you do not remember until it is time for your next dose, double the next dose, and then return to your regular dosing schedule.

SIDE EFFECTS

Minor. Changes in skin color, drowsiness, dry lips or mouth, fatigue, fluid retention, headache, indigestion, inflammation of the eyelids, inflammation of the lips, irritation of the eyes, or thinning of the hair. These side effects may disappear as your body adjusts to the medication.

You may notice a worsening of your acne for the first few days of treatment.

This medication can cause increased sensitivity to sunlight. Therefore, avoid prolonged exposure to sunlight and sunlamps. You should wear protective clothing and sunglasses, and also use an effective sunscreen.

To relieve mouth dryness, chew sugarless gum or suck on ice chips or a piece of hard candy. If there is no relief within two weeks, consult your doctor.

Major. Tell your doctor about any side effects that are persistent or particularly bothersome. IT IS ESPECIALLY IMPORTANT TO TELL YOUR DOCTOR about black, tarry stools; bruising; burning or tingling sensation of the skin; changes in the menstrual cycle; depression; dizziness; hives; muscle pain; peeling of the palms and soles; rash; visual disturbances; or weight loss.

INTERACTIONS

This medication interacts with the following substances:

1. The concurrent use of alcohol and isotretinoin can lead to an increase in blood lipid (fat) levels, which can be dangerous.

2. Vitamin A and isotretinoin together can result in additive toxic effects.

BE SURE TO TELL YOUR DOCTOR about any medications you are currently taking, especially vitamin A.

WARNINGS
• Tell your doctor about unusual or allergic reactions you have had to any medications, especially to isotretinoin, vitamin A, or the preservative parabens.
• Before starting to take this medication, tell your doctor if you now have or if you have ever had diabetes mellitus (sugar diabetes) or hyperlipidemia (high blood lipid levels).
• If this drug makes you drowsy, do not take part in any activity that requires alertness, such as driving a car or operating potentially dangerous machinery.
• Be sure to tell your doctor if you are pregnant. Isotretinoin has been shown to cause birth defects in humans. An effective form of birth control should be used by women of child-bearing age while they are taking this drug and for at least one month before and after they stop taking it. Within two weeks of starting this drug, women should have a blood pregnancy test. If the test is negative, the drug will be started on the second or third day of the next normal menstrual period. Women should have a pregnancy test each month while they take this medication. All women must also sign an informed-consent sheet. Also, tell your doctor if you are breast-feeding an infant. It is not known whether this drug passes into breast milk.

isradipine

BRAND NAME (Manufacturer)
Dynacirc (Sandoz)
TYPE OF DRUG
Antianginal (calcium channel blocker) and antihypertensive
INGREDIENT
isradipine
DOSAGE FORM
Capsules (2.5 mg and 5 mg)
STORAGE
Isradipine should be stored at room temperature in a tightly closed container, out of the reach of children and away from moisture and direct light.

USES
Isradipine is used to treat high blood pressure. It belongs to a group of drugs known as calcium channel blockers, which are useful for several cardiovascular conditions. Calcium channel blockers are less likely than beta-blockers or thiazide diuretics to have adverse effects on plasma lipids or blood glucose control in hypertensive patients with diabetes, asthma, or hardening of the arteries. It is not fully understood how isradipine works, but by blocking calcium, it relaxes and prevents spasms of the blood vessels of the heart and reduces the oxygen needs of the heart muscle. Isradipine is also a potent vasodilator that relaxes the muscle tissue of the blood vessels, thereby lowering blood pressure.

TREATMENT
If you miss a dose of this medication, take the missed dose as soon as possible, unless it is almost time for the next dose. In that case, do not take the missed dose at all; just return to your regular dosing schedule. Do not double the next dose. If you have a heart condition and have been taking isradipine regularly, isradipine should not should be stopped suddenly as this may worsen your symptoms of heart disease.

This medication does not cure high blood pressure, but it will help to control the condition as long as you continue to take it. It may take several weeks to develop its full effect.

SIDE EFFECTS
Minor. Constipation, dizziness, flushing of the face, headaches, increased heart rate, nervousness, painful extremeties, rash, stomach upset, and swollen ankles.

To relieve constipation, increase the amount of fiber in your diet (fresh fruits and vegetables, salads, bran, and whole-grain breads), exercise, and drink more water (unless your doctor directs you to do otherwise).
Major. Tell your doctor about any side effects that are persistent or particularly bothersome. IT IS ESPECIALLY IMPORTANT TO TELL YOUR DOCTOR about changes in menstruation, confusion, depression, fainting, fatigue, hair loss, itching, loss of balance, palpitations, rapid weight gain (three to five pounds within a week), recurrent infections, shortness of breath, swelling of the hands or feet, tremors, or unusual weakness.

INTERACTIONS
Isradipine may increase the blood pressure lowering effect of beta blockers, especially if there is a pre-existing heart condition. Isradipine may also increase the blood levels of the beta blocker, propranolol.

Other drugs that may interact with isradipine are adenosine, calcium supplements, chlorpromazine, cimetidine, digoxin, fentanyl used in conjunction with anesthesia, phenylbutazone, prazosin, and tolbutamide.

WARNINGS
• Tell your doctor about unusual or allergic reactions you have had to any medications, especially to isradipine.
• Before starting to take this medication, be sure to tell your doctor if you now have or if you have ever had any type of heart disease, kidney disease, liver disease, low blood pressure, or a slowed heartbeat.
• Your doctor may want you to check your pulse regularly while you are taking this medication. If your heart rate drops below 50 beats per minute, contact your doctor.
• If you experience angina symptoms, stopping this medication abruptly may lead to a worsening of your chest pain. Your doctor may, therefore, want to reduce your dosage gradually or have you switch to another medication when isradipine is discontinued.
• In order to prevent dizziness or light-headedness while taking this medication, try not to stand for long periods of time, avoid drinking alcoholic beverages, and try not to become overheated. Avoid exercising strenuously in hot weather, and do not take hot baths, showers, and saunas.

• Be sure to tell your doctor if you are pregnant. There are some indications that israpidine may cause birth defects in animals, but conclusive studies in humans have not been conducted. Also tell your doctor if you are breast-feeding an infant. It is not known whether isradipine passes into breast milk.

Janimine—see imipramine

Kaochlor—see potassium chloride

Kaon—see potassium chloride

Kato—see potassium chloride

Kay Ciel—see potassium chloride

K-Dur—see potassium chloride

Keflet—see cephalexin

Keflex—see cephalexin

Keftab—see cephalexin

Kenacort—see triamcinolone (systemic)

Kenalog—see triamcinolone (topical)

Kenalog-H—see triamcinolone (topical)

Kerlone—see betaxolol (systemic)

ketoprofen

BRAND NAME (Manufacturer)
Orudis (Wyeth-Ayerst)
TYPE OF DRUG
Nonsteroidal anti-inflammatory analgesic
INGREDIENT
ketoprofen
DOSAGE FORM
Capsules (25 mg, 50 mg, and 75 mg)
STORAGE
Store at room temperature in a tightly closed container.

USES

Ketoprofen is used to treat rheumatoid arthritis and osteoarthritis. Ketoprofen has been shown to block the production of certain body chemicals, called prostaglandins, that trigger pain and inflammation. However, it is not yet fully understood how ketoprofen works.

TREATMENT

Ketoprofen should be taken immediately after meals or with food in order to reduce stomach irritation. Check with your doctor about taking ketoprofen with an antacid.

Take ketoprofen on schedule and try not to miss any doses. If you do miss a dose, take the missed dose as soon as possible, unless it is almost time for the next dose. In that case, do not take the missed dose at all; just re-turn to your regular dosing schedule. Do not double the next dose.

Ketoprofen does not cure arthritis, but it will help to control symptoms as long as you take the drug.

SIDE EFFECTS

Minor. Abdominal pain, changes in taste, constipation, decreased or increased appetite, diarrhea, dizziness, drowsiness, dry mouth, excessive salivation, fatigue, flushing, gas, headache, heartburn, increased heart rate, increased thirst, nausea, nosebleeds, sweating, vomiting, or weight change. These side effects should disappear as your body adjusts to this medication.

Ketoprofen may cause increased sensitivity to sunlight. It is, therefore, important to avoid prolonged exposure to sunlight and sunlamps. Wear protective clothing and sunglasses, and use an effective sunscreen.

To relieve constipation, increase the amount of fiber in your diet (fresh fruits and vegetables, salads, bran, and whole-grain breads), exercise, and drink more water (unless your doctor directs you to do otherwise).

If you become dizzy, sit or lie down; get up slowly from a sitting or reclining position, and be careful on stairs.

Major. Tell your doctor about any side effects that are persistent or particularly bothersome. IT IS ESPECIALLY IMPORTANT TO TELL YOUR DOCTOR about black or tarry stools, chills, confusion, decreased or painful urination, hair loss, itching, memory loss, mouth sores, muscle pains, palpitations, rash, shortness of breath, swelling of the feet, tingling in the fingers or toes, unusual bleeding or bruising, unusual weight gain, visual disturbances, or yellowing of the eyes or skin.

INTERACTIONS

Ketoprofen interacts with several other types of medications:
1. Ketoprofen can increase the risk of bleeding complications with anticoagulants (blood thinners, such as warfarin).
2. Ketoprofen can interfere with the diuretic effects of furosemide and thiazidetype diuretics (water pills).
3. Aspirin can alter the blood levels and elimination of ketoprofen from the body.
4. Probenecid can increase the blood levels of ketoprofen, which can lead to an increased chance of side effects.
5. The action of beta blockers may be affected by this drug.

BE SURE TO TELL YOUR DOCTOR about any medications you are currently taking, especially those listed above.

WARNINGS

• Tell your doctor about any unusual or allergic reactions you have had to any medications, especially to ketoprofen or to any other chemically related drugs, including aspirin, other salicylates, diclofenac, diflunisal, fenoprofen, flurbiprofen, ibuprofen, indomethacin, meclofenamate, mefenamic acid, naproxen, oxyphenbutazone, phenylbutazone, piroxicam, sulindac, or tolmetin.
• Before taking ketoprofen, tell your doctor if you now have or if you have ever had anemia, bleeding problems,

gastrointestinal diseases, heart failure, hypertension, kidney disease, liver disease, or ulcers.
• If ketoprofen makes you dizzy or drowsy, do not take part in any activity that requires alertness, such as driving a car or operating potentially dangerous machinery.
• If vision problems develop while taking this medication, your doctor may refer you to an ophthalmologist.
• Stomach problems are more likely to occur if you take aspirin regularly or drink alcohol while being treated with this medication.
• Before having surgery or any other medical or dental treatment, be sure to tell your doctor or dentist that you are taking this medication. Your doctor or dentist may recommend stopping ketoprofen for several days prior to surgery, to decrease the risk of bleeding complications.
• The elderly may be at increased risk of experiencing some of the side effects of this medication.
• Be sure to tell your doctor if you are pregnant. Although ketoprofen appears to be safe in animals, studies in pregnant women have not been conducted. Ketoprofen should be avoided late in pregnancy because it can alter fetal heart circulation. Also tell your doctor if you are breast-feeding an infant. It is not yet known whether ketoprofen passes into human breast milk.

Kinesed—see atropine, scopolamine, hyoscyamine, and phenobarbital combination

Klonopin—see clonazepam

K-Lor—see potassium chloride

Klorvess—see potassium chloride

Klotrix—see potassium chloride

K-Lyte/Cl—see potassium chloride

Kolyum—see potassium chloride

Kronofed-A Jr.—see pseudoephedrine and chlorpheniramine combination

Kronofed-A Kronocaps—see pseudoephedrine and chlorpheniramine combination

K-Tab—see potassium chloride

Ku-Zyme—see pancrelipase

Kwell—see lindane

labetalol

BRAND NAMES (Manufacturers)
Normodyne (Schering)
Trandate (Allen & Hanburys)
TYPE OF DRUG
Alpha/beta-adrenergic blocking agent
INGREDIENT
labetalol

DOSAGE FORM
Tablets (100 mg, 200 mg, and 300 mg)
STORAGE
Labetalol should be stored at room temperature in a tightly closed container.

USES
Labetalol is used to treat high blood pressure. Labetalol belongs to a group of medicines known as beta-adrenergic blocking agents or, more commonly, beta blockers. These drugs work by controlling impulses along certain nerve pathways.

TREATMENT
Labetalol can be taken either on an empty stomach or with food or milk (as directed by your doctor). In order to become accustomed to taking this medication, try to take it at the same time(s) each day.

If you miss a dose of this medication, take the missed dose as soon as possible, unless it is almost time for your next dose. In that case, do not take the missed dose at all; just wait until the next scheduled dose. Do not double the dose.

Labetalol does not cure high blood pressure, but it will help control the condition.

SIDE EFFECTS
Minor. Abdominal pain; change in taste; diarrhea; dizziness; drowsiness; dryness of the eyes, mouth, and skin; fainting; fatigue; headache; heartburn; light-headedness; nasal congestion; nausea; numbness or tingling of the fingers or toes; scalp tingling; or vomiting. These side effects should disappear as your body adjusts to this medication.

If you are extra-sensitive to the cold, be sure to dress warmly during cold weather.

Plain, nonmedicated eye drops (artificial tears) may help to relieve eye dryness.

Sucking on ice chips or chewing sugarless gum helps to relieve mouth and throat dryness.

To avoid dizziness or light-headedness when you stand, contract and relax the muscles of your legs for a few moments before rising. Do this by alternately pushing one foot against the floor while raising the other foot slightly, so that you are "pumping" your legs in a pedaling motion.
Major. Tell your doctor about any side effects that are persistent or particularly bothersome. IT IS ESPECIALLY IMPORTANT TO TELL YOUR DOCTOR about cold hands or feet (due to decreased blood circulation to skin, fingers, and toes), confusion, depression, difficult or painful urination, impotence, itching, muscle cramps, rapid weight gain (three to five pounds within a week), rash, sore throat and fever, unusual bleeding or bruising, vision disturbances, wheezing or difficulty in breathing, or yellowing of the eyes or skin.

INTERACTIONS
This medication interacts with several other types of drugs:
1. Indomethacin, aspirin, and other salicylates may decrease the blood-pressure-lowering effects of beta blockers.

2. Concurrent use of beta blockers and calcium channel blockers (diltiazem, nifedipine, verapamil) or disopyramide can lead to heart failure or very low blood pressure. However, there may be times when your doctor may decide that multiple medications are necessary.

3. Cimetidine can increase the blood concentrations of labetalol, which can result in greater side effects.

4. Side effects may also be increased when beta blockers are taken with clonidine, digoxin, epinephrine, chlorpromazine, furosemide, hydralazine, phenylephrine, phenylpropanolamine, phenothiazine tranquilizers, prazosin, reserpine, or monoamine oxidase (MAO) inhibitors. At least 14 days should separate the use of a beta blocker and an MAO inhibitor.

5. Beta blockers may antagonize (work against) the effects of theophylline, aminophylline, albuterol, isoproterenol, metaproterenol, and terbutaline.

6. Beta blockers can also interact with insulin or oral antidiabetic agents, raising or lowering blood sugar levels or masking the symptoms of low blood sugar.

7. Concurrent use of tricyclic antidepressants and labetalol can increase the risk of tremors.

8. Halothane anesthesia and nitroglycerin can increase the blood-pressurelowering effects of labetalol.

TELL YOUR DOCTOR about any drugs you are currently taking, especially those listed above.

WARNINGS

• Before you start taking this medication, it is important for you to tell your doctor about any unusual or allergic reaction you have had to any medications, especially to labetalol or to any other beta blocker (acebutolol, atenolol, betaxolol, carteolol, esmolol, metoprolol, nadolol, penbutolol, pindolol, propranolol, timolol).

• Tell your doctor if you now have or if you have ever had asthma, bronchitis, diabetes mellitus, heart block, heart failure, liver disease, pheochromocytoma, poor circulation in fingers and toes, or a slow heartbeat.

• You may want to check your pulse while taking this medication. If your pulse is much slower than your usual rate (or if it is less than 50 beats per minute), check with your doctor. A pulse rate that is too slow may cause circulation problems.

• This drug may affect your body's response to exercise. Ask your doctor how much exercise is appropriate given your state of health.

• Do not stop taking this medicine without first checking with your doctor. Some conditions may become worse when the medicine is stopped suddenly, and the danger of a heart attack is increased in some patients. Your doctor may want you to gradually reduce the amount of medicine you take before stopping completely. Have enough medicine on hand to last through vacations, holidays, and weekends.

• Before undergoing surgery or any other medical or dental treatment, tell your physician or dentist that you are taking this medicine. Often, this medication will be discontinued 48 hours prior to any major surgery.

• Labetalol can cause decreased alertness, dizziness, drowsiness, and light-headedness. Exercise caution while driving a car or using any potentially dangerous machinery.

• While taking this medicine, do not use any over-the-counter allergy, asthma, cough, cold, sinus, or diet preparation without first checking with your pharmacist or doctor. The combination of these medicines with a beta blocker can result in high blood pressure.

• Be sure to tell your doctor if you are pregnant. Although labetalol appears to be safe in animals, studies in pregnant women have not been conducted. Also, tell your doctor if you are breast-feeding an infant. Small amounts of labetalol may pass into breast milk.

LactiCare-HC—see hydrocortisone (topical)

Lanacort—see hydrocortisone (topical)

Laniazid—see isoniazid

Lanophyllin—see theophylline

Lanophyllin GG—see theophylline and guaiferesin combination

Lanorinal—see aspirin, caffeine, and butalbital combination

Lanoxicaps—see digoxin

Lanoxin—see digoxin

Lanvisone—see hydrocortisone and iodochlorhydroxyquin combination (topical)

Larodopa—see levodopa

Lasix—see furosemide

Ledercillin VK—see penicillin VK

Leukeran—see chlorambucil

levodopa

BRAND NAMES (Manufacturers)
Dopar (Norwich Eaton)
Larodopa (Roche)
TYPE OF DRUG
Antiparkinsonism agent
INGREDIENT
levodopa
DOSAGE FORMS
Tablets (100 mg, 250 mg, and 500 mg)
Capsules (100 mg, 250 mg, and 500 mg)
STORAGE
Levodopa tablets and capsules should be stored at room temperature in tightly closed, light-resistant containers.

USES

Levodopa is used to treat the symptoms of Parkinson's disease. It is converted in the body to dopamine, a chemical in the brain that is diminished in patients with Parkinson's disease.

TREATMENT

In order to avoid stomach irritation, you can take levodopa with food or with a full glass of milk or water (unless your doctor directs you to do otherwise).

You may not observe significant benefit from this drug for two to three weeks after starting to take it.

If you miss a dose, take the missed dose as soon as possible, unless it is within two hours of the next scheduled dose. In that case, do not take the missed dose at all; just return to your regular dosing schedule. Do not double the next dose.

SIDE EFFECTS

Minor. Abdominal pain, anxiety, bitter taste in the mouth, constipation, diarrhea, dizziness, dry mouth, fatigue, flushing, gas, headache, hiccups, hoarseness, increased hand tremors, increased sexual interest, increased sweating, insomnia, loss of appetite, nausea, offensive body odor, salivation, vision changes, vomiting, weakness, or weight gain. These side effects may disappear as your body adjusts to the medication.

Levodopa can cause a darkening of your urine or sweat. This is a harmless effect.

To relieve constipation, increase the amount of fiber in your diet (fresh fruits and vegetables, salads, bran, and whole-grain breads), drink more water, and exercise (unless your doctor directs you to do otherwise).

If you feel dizzy, sit or lie down for a while; get up slowly from a sitting or reclining position, and be careful on stairs.

To relieve mouth dryness, chew sugarless gum or suck on ice chips or a piece of hard candy.

Major. Tell your doctor about any side effects that are persistent or particularly bothersome. IT IS ESPECIALLY IMPORTANT TO TELL YOUR DOCTOR about bloody or black, tarry stools; confusion; convulsions; depression; fainting; false sense of well-being; loss of coordination; loss of hair; nightmares; painful erection; palpitations; rapid weight gain (three to five pounds within a week); skin rash; visual disturbances; uncontrolled movements; or unusual weakness.

INTERACTIONS

Levodopa interacts with several other types of medications:

1. The dosage of antihypertensive drugs may require adjustment when levodopa is started.

2. The effectiveness of levodopa may be decreased by benzodiazepine tranquilizers, phenothiazine tranquilizers, haloperidol, thiothixene, phenytoin, papaverine, and reserpine.

3. Methyldopa can increase or decrease the side effects of therapy with levodopa.

4. Use of levodopa and a monoamine oxidase (MAO) inhibitor within 14 days of each other can lead to severe side effects.

5. Levodopa can increase the side effects of tricyclic antidepressants, ephedrine, and amphetamines.

6. Antacids may alter the absorption of levodopa from the gastrointestinal tract.

7. Pyridoxine (vitamin B) can decrease the effectiveness of levodopa.

BE SURE TO TELL YOUR DOCTOR about any medications you are currently taking, especially those listed above.

WARNINGS

• Tell your doctor about unusual or allergic reactions you have had to any medications, especially to levodopa.

• Before starting to take this medication, be sure to tell your doctor if you now have or if you have ever had asthma, diabetes mellitus, difficulty in urinating, epilepsy, glaucoma, heart disease, hormone disorders, kidney disease, liver disease, lung disease, melanoma (a type of skin cancer), mental disorders, or peptic ulcers.

• Some of these products contain the color additive FD&C Yellow No. 5 (tartrazine), which can cause allergic-type symptoms (difficulty in breathing, faintness, or rash) in certain susceptible individuals.

• If levodopa makes you dizzy or blurs your vision, avoid activities that require alertness, such as driving a car or operating potentially dangerous machinery.

• Notify your doctor if you start to experience any uncontrolled movements of the limbs or face while taking this medication.

• Before having surgery or any other medical or dental treatment, be sure to tell your doctor or dentist that you are taking this medication.

• Levodopa can cause erroneous readings of urine glucose and ketone tests. Diabetic patients should not change their medication dosage unless they first check with their doctor.

• Pyridoxine (vitamin B) can decrease the effectiveness of levodopa. Persons taking levodopa should avoid taking this vitamin and should avoid foods rich in pyridoxine (including beans, bacon, avocados, liver, dry skim milk, oatmeal, sweet potatoes, peas, and tuna).

• Be sure to tell your doctor if you are pregnant. Although levodopa appears to be safe in humans, birth defects have been reported in the offspring of animals that were administered large doses during pregnancy. Also, tell your doctor if you are breast-feeding an infant. Levodopa passes into breast milk and can cause side effects in nursing infants.

Levothroid—see levothyroxine

---

levothyroxine

BRAND NAMES (Manufacturers)
Levothroid (R-P Roerer)
levothyroxine sodium (various manufacturers)
Levoxine (Daniels)
Synthroid (Boots)
TYPE OF DRUG
Thyroid hormone
INGREDIENT
levothyroxine
DOSAGE FORM
Tablets (0.025 mg, 0.05 mg, 0.075 mg, 0.088 mg, 0.1 mg, 0.112 mg, 0.125 mg, 0.15 mg, 0.175 mg, 0.2 mg, and 0.3 mg)

STORAGE
Levothyroxine tablets should be stored at room temperature in a tightly closed, light-resistant container.

USES
Levothyroxine is prescribed to replace natural thyroid hormones that are absent because of a disorder of the thyroid gland. It is also used to help decrease the size of enlarged thyroid glands and to treat thyroid cancer. This product is prepared synthetically (artificially) but is exactly like the natural thyroid hormone that is produced by the human body.

TREATMENT
Levothyroxine tablets should be taken on an empty stomach with a full glass of water. If the drug upsets your stomach, ask your doctor if you can take it with food or milk.

In order to get used to taking this drug, try to take it at the same time each day. Try not to miss any doses. If you do miss a dose of this drug, take it as soon as possible, unless it is almost time for the next dose. In that case, do not take the missed dose at all; just return to your regular dosing schedule. Do not double the next dose. If you miss more than one or two doses, contact your doctor.

SIDE EFFECTS
Minor. Constipation; dry, puffy skin; fatigue; headache; listlessness; or weight gain. These effects are symptoms of an underactive thyroid. They should disappear after your body adjusts to the medication. It could take several weeks for the medication to take effect. Consult your doctor if these symptoms persist.

Major. Tell your doctor about any side effects that are persistent or particularly bothersome. Most of the major side effects associated with this drug are the result of too large a dose. The dosage of this medication may need to be adjusted if you experience any of the following side effects: chest pain, diarrhea, fever, heat intolerance, insomnia, irritability, leg cramps, menstrual irregularities, muscle aches, nervousness, palpitations, shortness of breath, sweating, trembling, or weight loss. CHECK WITH YOUR DOCTOR.

INTERACTIONS
Levothyroxine interacts with several other types of drugs:
1. Dosing requirements for digoxin, insulin, or oral antidiabetic agents may change when levothyroxine is used.
2. The effects of oral anticoagulants (blood thinners, such as warfarin) may be increased by levothyroxine, which could lead to bleeding complications.
3. Cholestyramine and colestipol prevent the body's absorbtion of levothyroxine. At least four hours should separate doses of levothyroxine and one of these drugs.
4. Oral contraceptives (birth control pills) and estrogen-containing drugs may change dosage requirements.
5. Phenobarbital may decrease the effects of levothyroxine; but tricyclic antidepressants and over-the-counter (nonprescription) allergy, asthma, cough, cold, sinus, and diet medications may increase its side effects.

BE SURE TO TELL YOUR DOCTOR about any medications you are currently taking, especially any listed above.

WARNINGS
• Tell your doctor about unusual or allergic reactions you have had to any medications, especially to thyroid hormone, levothyroxine, or liothyronine or to any other substances such as foods, preservatives, or dyes.
• Tell your doctor if you now have or if you have ever had angina pectoris, diabetes mellitus, heart disease, high blood pressure, kidney disease, or an underactive adrenal or pituitary gland.
• If you have an underactive thyroid gland, you may need to take this medication for life. You should not stop taking it unless you first check with your doctor.
• Before having surgery or any other medical or dental treatment, be sure to tell your doctor or dentist that you are taking levothyroxine.
• Over-the-counter allergy, asthma, cough, cold, sinus, and diet medications can increase the side effects of levothyroxine. Therefore, check with your doctor or pharmacist before taking ANY of these products.
• Although many thyroid products are on the market, they are not all bioequivalent; that is, they may not all be absorbed into the bloodstream at the same rate or have the same overall activity. DON'T CHANGE BRANDS of this drug without first consulting your doctor or pharmacist to make sure you are receiving an equivalent product.
• Some of these products contain the color additive FD&C Yellow No. 5 (tartrazine), which can cause allergic-type reactions (fainting, rash, difficulty in breathing) in certain susceptible individuals.
• Tell your doctor if you are pregnant. Levothyroxine does not readily cross the placenta, and the drug appears to be safe during pregnancy. However, your dosing of levothyroxine may change during pregnancy. Also, tell your doctor if you are breast-feeding an infant.

levothyroxine sodium—see levothyroxine

Levoxine—see levothyroxine

Librax—see chlordiazepoxide and clidinium combination

Libritabs—see chlordiazepoxide

Librium—see chlordiazepoxide

Lidex—see fluocinonide (topical)

Lidex-E—see fluocinonide (topical)

Lidox—see chlordiazepoxide and clidinium combination

Limbitrol DS—see chlordiazepoxide and amitriptyline combination

lindane

BRAND NAMES (Manufacturers)
G-well (Goldline)
Kwell (Reed & Carnrick)

lindane (various manufacturers)
Scabene (Stiefel)
TYPE OF DRUG
Pediculicide and scabicide
INGREDIENT
lindane (formerly known as gamma benzene hexachloride)
DOSAGE FORMS
Cream (1%)
Lotion (1%)
Shampoo (1%)
STORAGE
Lindane should be stored at room temperature in tightly closed containers. This medication should never be frozen.

USES
This medication is used to eliminate crab lice, head lice, and scabies. Lindane is a central nervous system (brain and spinal cord) stimulant, which causes convulsions and death of the parasites (at the dosage generally used, it is not harmful to humans). Lindane cream and lotion are used to treat only scabies infestations. Lindane shampoo is used to treat only lice infestations.

TREATMENT
Complete directions for the use of these products are supplied by the manufacturers. Be sure to ask your doctor or pharmacist for these directions, and follow the instructions carefully.

If you are applying this medication to another person, you should wear plastic or rubber gloves on your hands in order to avoid absorption of this drug through the skin.

The lotion form of this medication should be shaken well before each dose is measured. The contents of the lotion tend to settle on the bottom of the bottle, so the bottle must be shaken in order to distribute the medication evenly and equalize the doses.

Be sure to rinse off this product according to the directions. If it is not rinsed off COMPLETELY, too much of the medication will be absorbed.

SIDE EFFECTS
Minor. Rash or skin irritation upon application.
Major. Tell your doctor about any side effects that are persistent or particularly bothersome. The serious side effects associated with this medication (clumsiness, convulsions, irritability, muscle cramps, palpitations, restlessness, unsteadiness, unusual nervousness, or vomiting) are due to absorption of this drug through the skin. This should not happen if the product is used according to directions. CONTACT YOUR DOCTOR if you experience any of these symptoms.

INTERACTIONS
Do not use other skin preparations (lotions, ointments, or oils). They increase the absorption of this product through the skin, which can lead to serious side effects.

WARNINGS
• Tell your doctor about unusual or allergic reactions you have had to any medications, especially to lindane.

• This product should NOT be used on the face. If you do get lindane in your eyes, it should be flushed out immediately. In order to decrease the amount of drug absorbed through the skin, avoid using this product on any open wounds, cuts, or sores.
• Lice are easily transmitted from one person to another. All family members (and sexual partners) should be carefully examined. Personal items (clothing, towels) should be machine-washed using the "hot" temperature cycle and then dried. No unusual cleaning measures are required. Combs, brushes, and other washable items may be soaked in boiling water for one hour.
• After using the shampoo for head lice, you must remove the dead nits (eggs). Use a fine-tooth comb to remove them from your hair, or mix a solution of equal parts of water and vinegar and apply it to the affected area. Rub the solution in well. After several minutes, shampoo with your regular shampoo and then brush your hair. This process should remove all nits.
• Be sure to tell your doctor if you are pregnant. Lindane is absorbed through the skin and may cause central nervous system side effects in the mother and in the developing fetus. Also, tell your doctor if you are breast-feeding an infant. Lindane probably passes into breast milk and may cause central nervous system side effects in nursing infants.

Lioresal—see baclofen

liothyronine

BRAND NAMES (Manufacturers)
Cyronine (Major)
Cytomel (Smith Kline & French)
liothyronine (various manufacturers)
TYPE OF DRUG
Thyroid hormone
INGREDIENT
liothyronine
DOSAGE FORM
Tablets (5 mcg, 25 mcg, and 50 mcg)
STORAGE
Liothyronine should be stored at room temperature in a tightly closed container.

USES
Liothyronine is a synthetic form of natural thyroid hormone. It has all of the pharmacologic activities of the natural substance. This medication is used to replace thyroid hormone in patients who cannot produce enough of their own.

TREATMENT
Liothyronine can be taken either on an empty stomach or with food or a full glass of water or milk, as directed by your doctor.

In order for you to become accustomed to taking this medication, try to take it at the same time each day.

If you miss a dose of this medication, take the missed dose as soon as possible, unless it is almost time for the next dose. In that case, do not take the missed dose at all; just return to your regular dosing schedule. Do not double the next dose.

SIDE EFFECTS

Minor. Abdominal cramps, diarrhea, headache, insomnia, or nausea. These side effects may disappear as your body adjusts to the medication.

Major. Tell your doctor about any side effects that are persistent or particularly bothersome. Most of the serious side effects of this medication are the result of too high a dose. These include chest pain, fever, intolerance to heat, menstrual irregularities, nervousness, palpitations, skin rash, sweating, tremors, and weight loss. CONTACT YOUR DOCTOR if you experience any of these symptoms.

INTERACTIONS

Liothyronine interacts with several other types of medications:

1. It can increase the effects of oral anticoagulants (blood thinners, such as warfarin), which can lead to bleeding complications.

2. The dosage of digoxin, insulin, or oral antidiabetic medicines may require adjustment when liothyronine is started.

3. Cholestyramine decreases the absorption of liothyronine from the gastrointestinal tract. Therefore, at least four to five hours should separate doses of these medications.

4. Liothyronine may increase the side effects of tricyclic antidepressants.

Before starting to take this medication, BE SURE TO TELL YOUR DOCTOR about any medications you are currently taking, especially any of those listed above.

WARNINGS

Tell your doctor about unusual or allergic reactions you have had to any medications, especially to liothyronine, thyroid hormone, or levothyroxine.

Before starting to take this medication, be sure to tell your doctor if you now have or if you have ever had an underactive adrenal gland, diabetes mellitus, heart or blood vessel disease, or an underactive pituitary gland.

Before having surgery or any other medical or dental treatment, be sure to tell your doctor or dentist that you are taking this medication.

Because liothyronine is replacing natural thyroid hormone, you may need to take this medication for the rest of your life.

Do not stop taking this medication unless you first check with your doctor. Stopping this medication may result in worsening of your condition.

Do not take any over-the-counter (nonprescription) cough, cold, allergy, asthma, sinus, or diet medications without first checking with your doctor or pharmacist. Some of these products can increase the side effects of liothyronine.

The elderly may be at increased risk of experiencing side effects of this medication.

Be sure to tell your doctor if you are pregnant. Your dosage of liothyronine may need to be adjusted during pregnancy. Also, tell your doctor if you are breastfeeding an infant. Small amounts of liothyronine pass into breast milk.

Liquid Pred—see prednisone (systemic)

---

lisinopril

BRAND NAMES (Manufacturers)
Prinivil (Merck Sharp & Dohme)
Zestril (Stuart)
TYPE OF DRUG
Antihypertensive
INGREDIENT
lisinopril
DOSAGE FORM
Tablets (5 mg, 10 mg, 20 mg, and 40 mg)
STORAGE
Store this medication away from heat, direct light, or moisture.

USES

Lisinopril is currently approved for the treatment of hypertension (high blood pressure). It is also being investigated for the treatment of heart failure. Lisinopril is a vasodilator (it widens the blood vessels) that acts by blocking the production of chemicals that may be responsible for constricting blood vessels.

TREATMENT

The duration of action of lisinopril permits once-a-day dosing. Lisinopril can be taken either on an empty stomach or with food if it causes stomach irritation.

If you miss a dose of this medication, take the missed dose as soon as possible, unless it is almost time for the next dose. In that case, do not take the missed dose at all; just wait until the next scheduled dose. Do not double the dose.

In some patients it may require two to four weeks of therapy to achieve maximum therapeutic benefit.

Lisinopril does not cure high blood pressure, but it will help to control the condition as long as you take it.

SIDE EFFECTS

Minor. Dizziness; headache; fatigue; diarrhea; nasal congestion; or dry, hacking cough.

To avoid dizziness or light-headedness when you stand, contract and relax the muscles of your legs for a few moments before rising. Do this by pushing one foot against the floor while raising the other foot slightly, alternating feet so that you are "pumping" your legs in a pedaling motion.

Major. Tell your physician about any effects that are persistent or bothersome. IT IS ESPECIALLY IMPORTANT TO TELL YOUR DOCTOR about chest pain; chills; difficult or painful urination; fever; itching; mouth sores; palpitations; prolonged vomiting or diarrhea; rash; shortness of breath; sore throat; swelling of the face, hands, or feet; tingling in the fingers or toes; unusual bleeding or bruising; or yellowing of the eyes or skin.

INTERACTIONS

1. Lisinopril tends to cause retention of potassium in the body. Many salt substitutes contain potassium chloride and should only be used with the advice of your physician. Caution should also be observed with low-salt foods, some of which may contain significant amounts of potassium. Other medications such as the diuretics (water pills), triamterene, spironolactone, or amiloride may cause potassium retention. Use of these medications together with lisinopril may lead to excessive levels of potassium in the blood.

2. The anti-inflammatory drug indomethacin may reduce the effectiveness of lisinopril.

3. Excessive hypotension (low blood pressure) may occur when starting lisinopril in patients on diuretics.

BE SURE TO TELL YOUR DOCTOR about any medications you are currently taking, especially those listed above.

WARNINGS

• Tell your doctor about unusual or allergic reactions you have had to any medications, especially to lisinopril, captopril, or enalapril.

• Tell your doctor if you have any other medical problems, such as diabetes, heart disease, kidney disease, liver disease, or systemic lupus erythematosus.

• Tell your doctor if you experience light-headedness, which may be a symptom of excessive hypotension (low blood pressure). This is especially likely to occur during the first few days of therapy. If fainting occurs, stop the drug and consult with your physician.

• Excessive perspiration or dehydration may cause an excessive fall in blood pressure.

• Report any evidence of infections (such as sore throat or fever) to your physician.

• If you have high blood pressure, do not take any over-the-counter (nonprescription) medication for weight control, or for allergy, asthma, sinus, cough, or cold problems unless you first check with your doctor.

• Because lisinopril is eliminated from the body through the kidneys, be sure to report to your physician any symptoms of kidney disease, such as difficulty in urinating.

• Before having surgery or any other medical or dental treatment, be sure to tell your doctor or dentist that you are taking this medication.

• Be sure to tell your doctor if you are pregnant or plan to become pregnant. Studies in animals, in which administered doses far exceeded those used in humans, have shown a decrease in the number of successful pregnancies. Also tell your doctor if you are breast-feeding an infant. It is not known whether lisinopril passes into breast milk.

Lithane—see lithium

lithium

BRAND NAMES (Manufacturers)
Cibalith-S (Ciba)
Eskalith (Smith Kline & French)
Eskalith CR (Smith Kline & French)
Lithane (Miles Pharmaceutical)
lithium carbonate (various manufacturers)
lithium citrate (various manufacturers)
Lithobid (Ciba)
Lithonate (Reid-Rowell)
Lithotabs (Reid-Rowell)

TYPE OF DRUG
Antimanic (mood stabilizer)

INGREDIENT
lithium

DOSAGE FORMS
Tablets (300 mg)
Extended-release tablets (300 mg and 450 mg)
Capsules (150 mg, 300 mg, and 600 mg)
Syrup (300 mg per 5-ml spoonful, with 0.3% alcohol)

STORAGE
Lithium tablets, capsules, and syrup should be stored at room temperature away from heat and direct sunlight. The syrup should not be frozen. Do not store the medication in the bathroom cabinet, because moisture may cause the breakdown of lithium. Do not keep these medications beyond the expiration date.

USES
Lithium is a medication used to treat manic-depressive illness by controlling the manic (excited) phase of the illness and by reducing the frequency and severity of depression. Manic-depressive patients often experience unstable emotions ranging from excitement to hostility to depression. The mechanism of the mood-stabilizing effect of lithium is unknown, but it appears to work on the central nervous system to control emotions.

TREATMENT
Lithium should be taken exactly as directed by your doctor. The effectiveness of this medication depends upon the amount of lithium in your bloodstream. Therefore, the medication should be taken every day at regularly spaced intervals in order to keep a constant amount of lithium in your bloodstream.

The syrup form must be measured carefully with a specially designed 5-ml measuring spoon. An ordinary kitchen teaspoon is not accurate enough.

If you miss a dose of this medication, take it as soon as possible. However, if it is within two hours (six hours for extended-release tablets) of your next scheduled dose, skip the missed dose and return to your regular schedule. Do not take more than one dose at a time.

If you are taking the long-acting or slow-release form of lithium, swallow the tablet or capsule whole. Do not break, crush, or chew before swallowing.

An improvement in your condition may not be observed for up to several weeks after you start to take this drug.

SIDE EFFECTS
Minor. Acne, bloating, diarrhea, drowsiness, increased frequency of urination, increased thirst, nausea, trembling of the hands, weight gain, or weakness or tiredness. These side effects should disappear as your body adjusts to this medication.

Major. Blurred vision, clumsiness, confusion, convulsions, difficulty in breathing, dizziness, fainting, palpitations, severe trembling, and slurred speech are possible effects of too much drug in the bloodstream. Dry, rough skin; hair loss; hoarseness; swelling of the feet or lower legs; swelling of the neck; unusual sensitivity to the cold; unusual tiredness; or unusual weight gain may be the result of low thyroid function caused by the medication. CHECK WITH YOUR DOCTOR IMMEDIATELY if any of these side effects appear.

INTERACTIONS
Lithium interacts with a number of other types of medications:

1. Aminophylline, caffeine, verapamil, acetazolamide, sodium bicarbonate, dyphylline, oxtriphylline, and theophylline can increase the elimination of lithium from the body, thus decreasing its effectiveness.

2. Diuretics (water pills), especially hydrochlorothiazide, chlorothiazide, chlorthalidone, triamterene and hydrochlorothiazide combination, and furosemide may cause lithium toxicity by delaying the body's lithium elimination.

3. Captopril, chlorpromazine and other phenothiazine tranquilizers, ibuprofen, indomethacin, naproxen, and piroxicam can also slow lithium elimination.

4. Lithium can increase the side effects of haloperidol and other medications for mental illness.

5. Phenytoin, methyldopa, carbamazepine, and tetracycline can increase the side effects of lithium.

6. Drinking large amounts of caffeine-containing coffees, teas, or colas may reduce the effectiveness of lithium by increasing its elimination from the body through the urine.

BE SURE TO TELL YOUR DOCTOR about any medications you are currently taking, especially any of those listed above.

WARNINGS
• Tell your doctor about unusual or allergic reactions you have had to any medications, especially to lithium.
• Tell your doctor if you now have or if you have ever had diabetes mellitus, epilepsy, heart disease, kidney disease, Parkinson's disease, or thyroid disease.
• Elderly patients may be more sensitive to lithium's side effects.
• In order to maintain a constant level of lithium in your bloodstream, it is important to drink two to three quarts of water or other fluids each day and not to change the amount of salt in your diet, unless your doctor specifically directs you to do so.
• The loss of large amounts of body fluid (from prolonged vomiting or diarrhea or from heavy sweating due to hot weather, fever, exercise, saunas, or hot baths) can result in increased lithium levels in the blood, which can lead to an increase in side effects.
• The toxic dose of lithium is very close to the therapeutic dose, so it is extremely important to follow your correct dosing schedule. Diarrhea, drowsiness, lack of coordination, muscular weakness, and vomiting may be signs of toxicity. If these symptoms occur for any length of time or begin shortly after taking a dose, inform your doctor.

• Lithium is not recommended for use during pregnancy, especially during the first three months, because of possible effects on the thyroid and heart of the developing fetus. Also, tell your doctor if you are breast-feeding. Lithium also passes into breast milk and may cause side effects in the nursing infant.
• If this drug makes you drowsy or dizzy, do not take part in any activities that require alertness, such as driving a car or operating potentially dangerous machinery.

lithium carbonate—see lithium

lithium citrate—see lithium

Lithobid—see lithium

Lithonate—see lithium

Lithotabs—see lithium

Locoid—see hydrocortisone (topical)

Loestrin—see oral contraceptives

Lofene—see diphenoxylate and atropine combination

Logen—see diphenoxylate and atropine combination

Lomanate—see diphenoxylate and atropine combination

Lomotil—see diphenoxylate and atropine combination

---

lomustine

BRAND NAME (Manufacturer)
CeeNU (Bristol)
TYPE OF DRUG
Antineoplastic (anticancer drug)
INGREDIENT
lomustine
DOSAGE FORM
Capsules (10 mg, 40 mg, and 100 mg)
STORAGE
Lomustine should be stored at room temperature in a tightly closed container.

USES
This medication belongs to a group of drugs known as nitrosourea alkylating agents. It is used to treat a variety of cancers. Lomustine is thought to work by binding to the rapidly growing cancer cells, preventing their multiplication and growth.

TREATMENT
To help prevent nausea, you should take lomustine on an empty stomach (unless your doctor directs otherwise).

The patient is usually required to take this medication as a single dose once a week. The total weekly dose consists of a number of capsules of different strengths and colors, which are all taken at the same time. The timing of each weekly dose is very important; be sure you completely understand your doctor's instructions on how and when this medication should be taken.

SIDE EFFECTS

Minor. Nausea and vomiting may occur three to six hours after taking a dose of lomustine; these symptoms usually last less than 24 hours. The use of lomustine may also cause hair loss, which is reversible when the medication is stopped.

Major. Tell your doctor about any side effects that are persistent or particularly bothersome. IT IS ESPECIALLY IMPORTANT TO TELL YOUR DOCTOR about chills, confusion, decreased coordination, difficult or painful urination, disorientation, fever, itching, loss of appetite, lethargy, mouth sores, sore throat, unusual bleeding or bruising, weakness, or yellowing of the eyes or skin. These side effects may even appear several weeks after the last dose is taken.

INTERACTIONS

Lomustine should not interact with other medications if it is used according to directions.

WARNINGS

Tell your doctor about unusual or allergic reactions you have had to any medications, especially to lomustine, carmustine, or streptozocin.

Before starting to take this medication, be sure to tell your doctor if you now have or if you have ever had blood disorders, chronic or recurrent infections, or kidney disease.

Before having surgery or any other medical or dental treatment, be sure to tell your doctor or dentist that you are taking this medication.

You should not receive any immunizations or vaccinations while taking this medication. Lomustine blocks the effectiveness of vaccines, which could result in an overwhelming infection if a live-virus vaccine is administered. Be sure to tell your doctor you are taking lomustine before you are given any immunizations or vaccinations.

Lomustine can lower your platelet count, which can decrease your body's ability to form blood clots. You should, therefore, be especially careful while brushing your teeth, flossing, or using toothpicks, razors, or fingernail scissors. Try to avoid falls and other injuries. Your doctor may also order periodic laboratory tests to monitor your blood.

Lomustine can decrease fertility in both men and women.

Tell your doctor if you are pregnant. Lomustine has been reported to cause birth defects in both animals and humans whose mothers received the drug during pregnancy. The risks should be discussed with your doctor. Also, tell your doctor if you are breast-feeding an infant. Small amounts of lomustine pass into breast milk.

Loniten—see minoxidil (systemic)

Lonox—see diphenoxylate and atropine combination

Lo/Ovral—see oral contraceptives

loperamide

BRAND NAME (Manufacturer)
Imodium (Janssen)
TYPE OF DRUG
Antidiarrheal
INGREDIENT
loperamide
DOSAGE FORMS
Capsules (2 mg)
Oral liquid (1 mg per 5-ml spoonful)*
*Available over-the-counter (without a prescription)
STORAGE
Loperamide capsules and liquid should be stored at room temperature in tightly closed containers. This medication should never be frozen.

USES

Loperamide is used to treat acute and chronic diarrhea and to reduce the volume of discharge in patients who have ileostomies. It acts by slowing the movement of the gastrointestinal tract and decreasing the passage of water and other substances into the bowel.

TREATMENT

In order to avoid stomach upset, you can take loperamide with food or with a full glass of water or milk.

If you miss a dose of this medication, do not take the missed dose at all; just return to your regular dosing schedule. Do not double the next dose.

SIDE EFFECTS

Minor. Constipation, dizziness, drowsiness, dry mouth, fatigue, loss of appetite, nausea, or vomiting. These effects should disappear as your body adjusts to the drug.

To relieve constipation, exercise and drink more water (unless your doctor directs you to do otherwise).

To reduce mouth dryness, chew sugarless gum or suck on ice chips or a piece of hard candy.

If you feel dizzy or light-headed, sit or lie down for a while; get up from a sitting or lying position slowly, and be careful on stairs.

Major. Tell your doctor about any side effects that are persistent or particularly bothersome. IT IS ESPECIALLY IMPORTANT TO TELL YOUR DOCTOR about abdominal bloating or pain, fever, rash, or sore throat.

INTERACTIONS

Loperamide should not interact with any other drugs.

WARNINGS

• Tell your doctor about unusual or allergic reactions you have had to any medications.
• Tell your doctor if you now have or if you have ever had colitis, diarrhea caused by infectious organisms, drug-induced diarrhea, liver disease, dehydration, or conditions in which constipation must be avoided (such as hemorrhoids, diverticulitis, heart or blood vessel disorders, or blood clotting disorders).
• If this drug makes you dizzy or drowsy, do not take part in any activity that requires alertness.

• Before having surgery or any other medical or dental treatment, be sure to tell your doctor or dentist that you are taking this medication.

• Check with your doctor if your diarrhea does not subside within three days. Unless your doctor prescribes otherwise, do not take this drug for more than ten days at a time.

• While taking this medication, drink lots of fluids to replace those lost because of diarrhea.

• Be sure to tell your doctor if you are pregnant. The effects of this medication during pregnancy have not been thoroughly studied in humans. Also, tell your doctor if you are breast-feeding an infant. It is not known whether loperamide passes into breast milk.

Lopid—see gemfibrozil

Lopressor—see metoprolol

Lopurin—see allopurinol

lorazepam

BRAND NAMES (Manufacturers)
Ativan (Wyeth)
lorazepam (various manufacturers)
TYPE OF DRUG
Benzodiazepine sedative/hypnotic
INGREDIENT
lorazepam
DOSAGE FORM
Tablets (0.5 mg, 1 mg, and 2 mg)
STORAGE
This medication should be stored at room temperature in a tightly closed, light-resistant container.

USES

Lorazepam is prescribed to treat symptoms of anxiety and anxiety associated with depression. It is not clear exactly how this medicine works, but it may relieve anxiety by acting as a depressant of the central nervous system (brain and spinal cord). This medication is currently used by many people to relieve nervousness. It is effective for this purpose for short periods, but it is important to try to remove the cause of the anxiety as well.

TREATMENT

Lorazepam should be taken exactly as your doctor directs. It can be taken with food or a full glass of water if stomach upset occurs. Do not take this medication with a dose of antacids, since they may slow its absorption from the gastrointestinal tract.

If you are taking this medication regularly and you miss a dose, take the missed dose immediately if you remember within an hour. If more than an hour has passed, skip the dose you missed and wait for the next scheduled dose. Do not double the dose.

SIDE EFFECTS

Minor. Bitter taste in the mouth, constipation, diarrhea, dizziness, drowsiness (after a night's sleep), dry mouth, fatigue, flushing, headache, heartburn, excessive salivation, loss of appetite, nausea, nervousness, sweating, or vomiting. As your body adjusts to the medication, these side effects should disappear.

To relieve constipation, increase the amount of fiber in your diet (fresh fruits and vegetables, salads, bran, and whole-grain breads), exercise, and drink more water (unless your doctor directs you to do otherwise).

Dry mouth can be relieved by chewing sugarless gum or by sucking on ice chips.

If you feel dizzy, sit or lie down for a while; get up slowly from a sitting or reclining position, and be careful on stairs.

Major. Tell your doctor about any side effects that are persistent or particularly bothersome. IT IS ESPECIALLY IMPORTANT TO TELL YOUR DOCTOR about blurred or double vision, chest pain, depression, difficulty in urinating, fainting, falling, fever, joint pain, hallucinations, memory problems, mouth sores, nightmares, palpitations, rash, shortness of breath, slurred speech, sore throat, uncoordinated movements, unusual excitement, unusual tiredness, or yellowing of the eyes or skin.

INTERACTIONS

Lorazepam interacts with several other types of medications:

1. To prevent oversedation, this drug should not be taken with alcohol, other sedative drugs, or central nervous system depressants (such as antihistamines, barbiturates, muscle relaxants, pain medicines, narcotics, medicines for seizures, and phenothiazine tranquilizers) or with antidepressants.

2. This medication may decrease the effectiveness of carbamazepine, levodopa, and oral anticoagulants (blood thinners) and may increase the effects of phenytoin.

3. Disulfiram, cimetidine, and isoniazid can increase the blood levels of lorazepam, which can lead to toxic effects.

4. Concurrent use of rifampin may decrease the effectiveness of lorazepam.

BE SURE TO TELL YOUR DOCTOR about any medications you are currently taking, especially any listed above.

WARNINGS

• Tell your doctor about unusual or allergic reactions you have had to any medications, especially to lorazepam or other benzodiazepine tranquilizers (such as alprazolam, chlordiazepoxide, clorazepate, diazepam, flurazepam, halazepam, midazolam, oxazepam, prazepam, temazepam, and triazolam).

• Tell your doctor if you now have or if you have ever had liver disease, kidney disease, epilepsy, lung disease, myasthenia gravis, porphyria, mental depression, or mental illness.

• This medicine can cause drowsiness. Avoid tasks that require alertness, such as driving a car or using potentially dangerous machinery.

• This medication has the potential for abuse and must be used with caution. Tolerance may develop quickly; do not increase the dosage without first consulting your doctor. It is also important not to stop this drug suddenly if you have been taking it in large amounts or if you have used it for several weeks. Your doctor may want to reduce the dosage gradually.

• This is a safe drug when used properly. When it is combined with other sedative drugs or alcohol, however, serious side effects can develop.

• Be sure to tell your doctor if you are pregnant. This medicine may increase the chance of birth defects if it is taken during the first three months of pregnancy. In addition, too much use of this medicine during the last six months of pregnancy may cause the fetus to become dependent on it, resulting in withdrawal side effects in the newborn. Also, use of this drug during the last weeks of pregnancy may cause drowsiness, slowed heartbeat, and breathing difficulties in the newborn. Tell your doctor if you are breast-feeding. This drug can pass into the breast milk and cause drowsiness, slowed heartbeat, and breathing difficulties in the nursing infant.

Lorelco—see probucol

Lortab 5—see acetaminophen and hydrocodone combination

Lotrimin—see clotrimazole (topical)

Lotrimin AF—see clotrimazole (topical)

Lotrisone—see betamethasone dipropionate and clotrimazole combination (topical)

---

lovastatin

BRAND NAME (Manufacturer)
Mevacor (Merck Sharp & Dohme)
TYPE OF DRUG
Antihyperlipidemic (lipid-lowering drug)
INGREDIENT
lovastatin
DOSAGE FORM
Tablets (20 mg)
STORAGE
This medication should be stored at room temperature in a tightly closed, light-resistant container. Exposure to heat or moisture may cause this drug to break down.

USES
Lovastatin is used to treat hyperlipidemia (high blood fat levels). It is prescribed in conjunction with nondrug therapies, such as diet modification and regular exercise, in an attempt to regulate lipid and cholesterol levels. Lovastatin chemically interferes with an enzyme in the body that is responsible for synthesizing cholesterol. This decreases the LDL (low-density lipoprotein) type of cholesterol, which has been associated with coronary heart disease and atherosclerosis.

TREATMENT
This medication should be taken exactly as prescribed by your doctor. If you are to take the drug once a day, it is best to take the drug in the evening. Lovastatin can be

taken with meals or a full glass of water if stomach upset occurs.

While using this medication, try to develop a set schedule for taking it. If you miss a dose and remember within a few hours, take the missed dose and resume your regular schedule. If many hours have passed, skip the dose you missed and then take your next dose as scheduled. Do not double the dose.

SIDE EFFECTS
Minor. Abdominal pain or cramps, constipation, diarrhea, gas, nausea, or stomach pain. These effects may be relieved by taking lovastatin with a meal, adding fiber to your diet, or using mild stool softeners.

Major. Tell your doctor about any side effects that are persistent or particularly bothersome. IT IS ESPECIALLY IMPORTANT TO TELL YOUR DOCTOR about blurred vision (or any other visual changes or difficulties) or muscle pain or tenderness, especially with malaise or fever.

INTERACTIONS
There do not appear to be any significant drug interactions with this medication. However, you should make sure your doctor knows all the medications you are taking.

WARNINGS
• Tell your doctor about unusual or allergic reactions you have had to any medications.

• Tell your doctor if you have ever had liver disease, heart disease, stroke, or disorders of the digestive tract.

• In preliminary studies with lovastatin, some patients were found to develop eye-related problems during treatment. Although these findings are inconclusive, and it has not yet been determined whether lovastatin is involved in such occurrences, it is advisable to have regular checkups with your ophthalmologist and inform him/her of your use of this drug.

• This drug should not be taken if you are pregnant or breast-feeding an infant.

Low-Quel—see diphenoxylate and atropine combination

---

loxapine

BRAND NAMES (Manufacturers)
Loxitane (Lederle)
Loxitane C (Lederle)
TYPE OF DRUG
Antipsychotic
INGREDIENT
loxapine
DOSAGE FORMS
Capsules (5 mg, 10 mg, 25 mg, and 50 mg)
Oral concentrate (25 mg per ml)

STORAGE
Loxapine capsules and oral concentrate should be stored at room temperature (never frozen) in tightly closed containers. If the oral concentrate turns slightly yellowish,

the drug is still effective and can be used. However, if the oral concentrate changes color markedly or has particles floating in it, it shouldn't be used; rather, it should instead be discarded down the sink.

USES
Loxapine is prescribed to treat the symptoms of mental illness, such as the emotional symptoms of psychosis. This medication is thought to relieve the symptoms of mental illness by blocking certain chemicals involved with nerve transmission in the brain.

TREATMENT
To avoid stomach irritation, you can take the tablet form of loxapine with a meal or with a glass of water or milk (unless your doctor directs you to do otherwise.)

The oral concentrate form of this medication should be measured carefully with the dropper provided and diluted in eight ounces (a full cup) or more of orange or grapefruit juice immediately prior to administration.

If you miss a dose of this medication, take the missed dose as soon as possible and return to your regular dosing schedule. If it is almost time for the next dose, however, skip the one you missed and then return to your regular schedule. Do not double the dose unless you are directed to do so by your doctor.

Antacids and antidiarrheal medicines can decrease the absorption of this medication from the gastrointestinal tract. Therefore, at least one hour should separate doses of one of these medicines and loxapine.

The full effects of this medication for the control of emotional or mental symptoms may not become apparent for two weeks after you start to take it.

SIDE EFFECTS
Minor. Blurred vision, constipation, decreased sweating, diarrhea, dizziness, drooling, drowsiness, dry mouth, fatigue, jitteriness, menstrual irregularities, nasal congestion, restlessness, vomiting, or weight gain. As your body adjusts to the medication, these side effects should disappear.

This medication can cause increased sensitivity to sunlight. It is, therefore, important to avoid prolonged exposure to sunlight and sunlamps. Wear protective clothing, and use an effective sunscreen.

If you are constipated, increase the amount of fiber in your diet (fresh fruits and vegetables, salads, bran, and whole-grain breads), exercise, and drink more water (unless your doctor directs you to do otherwise).

To reduce mouth dryness, chew sugarless gum or suck on ice chips or a piece of hard candy.

To avoid dizziness or light-headedness when you stand, contract and relax the muscles of your legs for a few moments before rising. Do this by pushing one foot against the floor while raising the other foot slightly, alternating feet so that you are "pumping" your legs in a pedaling motion.

Major. Tell your doctor about any side effects that are persistent or particularly bothersome. IT IS ESPECIALLY IMPORTANT TO TELL YOUR DOCTOR about breast enlargement (in both sexes); chest pain; convulsions; darkened skin; difficulty in swallowing or breathing; fainting;

fever; impotence; involuntary movements of the face, mouth, jaw, or tongue; palpitations; rash; sleep disorders; sore throat; tremors; uncoordinated movements; unusual bleeding or bruising; visual disturbances; or yellowing of the eyes or skin.

INTERACTIONS
Loxapine can interact with a number of other types of medications:

1. It can cause extreme drowsiness when combined with alcohol or other central nervous system depressants (such as barbiturates, benzodiazepine tranquilizers, muscle relaxants, narcotics, and pain medications) or with tricyclic antidepressants.

2. This medication can cause a decrease in the effectiveness of amphetamines, guanethidine, anticonvulsants, and levodopa.

3. The side effects of epinephrine, monoamine oxidase (MAO) inhibitors, and tricyclic antidepressants may be increased when combined with this medication. At least 14 days should separate the use of this drug and the use of an MAO inhibitor.

BE SURE TO TELL YOUR DOCTOR about any medications you are currently taking, especially any of those listed above.

WARNINGS
• Tell your doctor about unusual or allergic reactions you have had to any medications, especially to loxapine or to any phenothiazine tranquilizer.

• Tell your doctor if you have a history of alcoholism or if you now have or ever had heart or circulatory disease, epilepsy, glaucoma, liver disease, Parkinson's disease, enlarged prostate gland, or blockage of the urinary tract.

• Avoid drinking alcoholic beverages while taking this medication, in order to prevent oversedation.

• If this medication makes you dizzy or drowsy, do not take part in any activity that requires alertness, such as driving a car or operating potentially dangerous machinery. Be careful on stairs, and avoid getting up suddenly from a lying or sitting position.

• Prior to having surgery or any other medical or dental treatment, be sure to tell your doctor or dentist that you are taking loxapine.

• Some of the side effects caused by this drug can be prevented by taking an antiparkinsonism drug. Discuss this with your doctor.

• This medication can decrease sweating and heat release from the body. Therefore, avoid getting overheated by strenuous exercise in hot weather, and avoid taking hot baths, showers, and saunas.

• This medication has the potential to cause a permanent movement disorder called tardive dyskinesia. Therefore, be sure to report any uncontrolled movements of the body to your doctor.

• Do not stop taking this medication suddenly. If the drug is stopped abruptly, you may experience nausea, vomiting, stomach upset, headache, increased heart rate, insomnia, tremors, or worsening of your condition. Your doctor may want to reduce the dosage gradually.

• If you are planning to have a myelogram, or any other procedure in which dye is injected into the area surrounding the spinal cord, tell your doctor that you are taking this medication.

• Avoid spilling the oral concentrate form of this medication on your skin or clothing; it can cause redness and irritation of the skin.

• While you are taking this prescription medication, do not take any over-thecounter (nonprescription) medication or preparation for weight control or for cough, cold, asthma, allergy, or sinus problems unless you first check with your doctor. The combination of these two types of medications can cause high blood pressure.

• Elderly patients may be at increased risk of experiencing side effects of this medication.

• Be sure to tell your doctor if you are pregnant. Small amounts of this medication will cross the placenta. Although there are reports of safe use of this type of drug during pregnancy, there are also reports of liver disease and tremors in newborn infants whose mothers received this type of medication close to term. Also, tell your doctor if you are breast-feeding an infant. Small amounts of this medication pass into breast milk and may cause unwanted effects in the nursing infant.

Loxitane—see loxapine

Loxitane C—see loxapine

Lozol—see indapamide

Ludiomil—see maprotiline

Lysodren—see mitotane

Macrodantin—see nitrofurantoin

Malatal—see atropine, scopolamine, hyoscyamine, and phenobarbital combination

Mandameth—see methenamine

Mandelamine—see methenamine

maprotiline

BRAND NAME (Manufacturer)
Ludiomil (Ciba)
TYPE OF DRUG
Tetracyclic antidepressant
INGREDIENT
maprotiline
DOSAGE FORM
Tablets (25 mg, 50 mg, and 75 mg)
STORAGE
Maprotiline tablets should be stored at room temperature in a tightly closed container.

USES

Maprotiline is used to relieve the symptoms of mental depression. This medication is a tetracyclic antidepressant. It is related to a group of drugs referred to as the tricyclic antidepressants. These medicines are thought to relieve depression by increasing the concentration of certain chemicals necessary for nerve transmission in the brain.

TREATMENT

This medication should be taken exactly as your doctor prescribes. It can be taken with water or food to lessen the chance of stomach irritation, unless your doctor tells you to do otherwise.

If you miss a dose of this medication, take the missed dose as soon as possible, then return to your regular dosing schedule. However, if the dose you missed was a once-a-day bedtime dose, do not take that dose in the morning; check with your doctor instead. If the dose is taken in the morning, it may cause some unwanted side effects. Never double the dose.

The effects of therapy with this medication may not become apparent for two or three weeks.

SIDE EFFECTS

Minor. Anxiety, blurred vision, confusion, constipation, diarrhea, dizziness, drowsiness, dry mouth, fatigue, heartburn, insomnia, loss of appetite, nausea, peculiar tastes in the mouth, restlessness, sweating, vomiting, weakness, or weight gain or loss. As your body adjusts to the medication, these side effects should disappear.

This medication can cause increased sensitivity to sunlight. Avoid prolonged exposure to sunlight and sunlamps. Wear protective clothing, and use an effective sunscreen.

Mouth dryness can be relieved by chewing sugarless gum or by sucking on ice chips or a piece of hard candy.

To relieve constipation, increase the amount of fiber in your diet (fresh fruits and vegetables, salads, bran, and whole-grain breads), exercise, and drink more water (unless your doctor directs you to do otherwise).

To avoid dizziness or light-headedness when you stand, contract and relax the muscles of your legs for a few moments before rising. Do this by pushing one foot against the floor while raising the other foot slightly, alternating feet so that you are "pumping" your legs.

Major. Tell your doctor about any side effects that are persistent or particularly bothersome. IT IS ESPECIALLY IMPORTANT TO TELL YOUR DOCTOR about agitation, chest pain, convulsions, cramps, difficulty in urinating, enlarged or painful breasts (in both sexes), fainting, fever, fluid retention, hair loss, hallucinations, headaches, impotence, mood changes, mouth sores, nervousness, nightmares, numbness in the fingers or toes, palpitations, ringing in the ears, seizures, skin rash, sleep disorders, sore throat, tremors, uncoordinated movements or balance problems, unusual bleeding or bruising, or yellowing of the eyes or skin.

INTERACTIONS

Maprotiline interacts with other types of medications:
1. Extreme drowsiness can occur when this medicine is taken with central nervous system depressants (such as alcohol, antihistamines, barbiturates, benzodiazepine tranquilizers, muscle relaxants, narcotics, pain medications, phenothiazine tranquilizers, and sleeping medications) or with other antidepressants.

2. Maprotiline may decrease the effectiveness of anti-seizure medications and may block the blood-pressure-lowering effects of clonidine and guanethidine.

3. Oral contraceptives (birth control pills) and estrogen-containing drugs can increase the side effects and reduce the effectiveness of tricyclic antidepressants and maprotiline.

4. Tetracyclic antidepressants may increase the side effects of thyroid medication and over-the-counter (nonprescription) allergy, cough, cold, asthma, sinus, and diet medications.

5. The concurrent use of tetracyclic antidepressants and monoamine oxidase (MAO) inhibitors should be avoided, because the combination may result in fever, convulsions, or high blood pressure. At least 14 days should separate the use of this drug and the use of an MAO inhibitor.

Before starting to take maprotiline, BE SURE TO TELL YOUR DOCTOR about any medications you are currently taking, especially any of those listed above.

WARNINGS

• Tell your doctor if you have had unusual or allergic reactions to any medications, especially to maprotiline or any of the tricyclic antidepressants (such as amitriptyline, imipramine, doxepin, trimipramine, amoxapine, protriptyline, desipramine, and nortriptyline).

• Tell your doctor if you have a history of alcoholism or if you have ever had asthma, high blood pressure, liver or kidney disease, heart disease, a heart attack, circulatory disease, stomach problems, intestinal problems, difficulty in urinating, enlarged prostate gland, epilepsy, glaucoma, thyroid disease, mental illness, or electroshock therapy.

• If this drug makes you dizzy or drowsy, do not take part in any activity that requires alertness, such as driving a car or operating potentially dangerous machinery.

• Before having surgery or other medical or dental treatment, tell your doctor or dentist about this drug.

• Do not stop taking this drug suddenly. Abruptly stopping it can cause nausea, headache, stomach upset, fatigue, or a worsening of your condition. Your doctor may want to reduce the dosage gradually.

• The effects of this medication may last as long as seven days after you have stopped taking it, so continue to observe all precautions during that period. Be sure to tell your doctor if the effects continue past that time.

• Elderly patients may be at increased risk of experiencing side effects of this medication.

• Be sure to tell your doctor if you are pregnant. Problems in humans have not been reported; however, studies in animals have shown that this type of medication can cause side effects in the fetus if given to the mother in large doses during pregnancy. Also, be sure to tell your doctor if you are breast-feeding an infant. It is possible small amounts of this drug will pass into breast milk and cause unwanted side effects, such as irritability or sleeping problems, in the nursing infant.

Marbaxin—see methocarbamol

Marnal—see aspirin, caffeine, and butalbital combination

Matulane—see procarbazine

Maxitrol—see dexamethasone, neomycin, and polymyxin B combination (ophthalmic)

Maxivate—see betamethasone dipropionate

Maxolon—see metoclopramide

Maxzide—see triamterene and hydrochlorothiazide combination

---

mazindol

BRAND NAMES (Manufacturers)
Mazanor (Wyeth)
Sanorex (Sandoz)
TYPE OF DRUG
Anorectic (appetite suppressant)
INGREDIENT
mazindol
DOSAGE FORM
Tablets (1 mg and 2 mg)
STORAGE
Mazindol should be stored at room temperature in a tightly closed container.

USES

Mazindol is used as an appetite suppressant during the first few weeks of dieting, to help establish new eating habits. This medication is thought to relieve hunger by altering nerve impulses to the appetite control center in the brain. Its effectiveness lasts only for short periods (three to 12 weeks), however.

TREATMENT

Mazindol can be taken with a full glass of water one hour before meals (unless your doctor directs you to do otherwise).

If you miss a dose of this medication, take the missed dose as soon as possible, unless it is almost time for your next dose. In that case, do not take the missed dose at all; just return to your regular dosing schedule. Do not double the next dose.

In order to avoid difficulty in falling asleep, the last dose of this medication each day should be taken four to six hours before bedtime (for the 1mg tablet) or ten to 14 hours before bedtime (for the 2-mg tablet).

SIDE EFFECTS

Minor. Constipation, diarrhea, dizziness, dry mouth, false sense of well-being, fatigue, insomnia, irritability, nausea, nervousness, restlessness, stomach pain, sweating, tremors, unpleasant taste in the mouth, or vomiting. These side effects should disappear as your body adjusts to the drug.

Dry mouth can be relieved by sucking on ice chips or a piece of hard candy or by chewing sugarless gum.

In order to prevent constipation, increase the amount of fiber in your diet (fresh fruits and vegetables, salads, bran, and whole-grain breads), exercise, and drink more water (unless your doctor directs you to do otherwise).

Major. Tell your doctor about any side effects that are persistent or particularly bothersome. IT IS ESPECIALLY IMPORTANT TO TELL YOUR DOCTOR about blurred vision, changes in sexual desire, chest pain, difficulty in urinating, enlarged breasts (in both sexes), fever, hair loss, headaches, impotence, increased blood pressure, menstrual irregularities, mental depression, mood changes, mouth sores, muscle pains, palpitations, rash, sore throat, or unusual bleeding or bruising.

INTERACTIONS

Mazindol interacts with several other types of medications:

1. Use of this medication within 14 days of a monoamine oxidase (MAO) inhibitor (such as isocarboxazid, pargyline, phenelzine, and tranylcypromine) can result in high blood pressure and other side effects.

2. Barbiturate medications and phenothiazine tranquilizers (especially chlorpromazine) can antagonize (act against) the appetite-suppressant activity of this medication.

3. Mazindol can decrease the blood-pressure-lowering effects of antihypertensive medications (especially guanethidine) and may alter insulin and oral antidiabetic medication dosage requirements in diabetic patients.

4. The side effects of other central nervous system stimulants, such as caffeine, over-the-counter (nonprescription) appetite suppressants or sinus, cough, cold, asthma, and allergy preparations, may be increased by the concurrent use of this medication.

Before starting to take mazindol, BE SURE TO TELL YOUR DOCTOR about any medications you are currently taking, especially any of those listed above.

WARNINGS

Tell your doctor about unusual or allergic reactions you have had to any medications, especially to mazindol or other appetite suppressants (such as benzphetamine, phendimetrazine, diethylpropion, fenfluramine, phenmetrazine, and phentermine) or to epinephrine, norepinephrine, ephedrine, amphetamines, dextroamphetamine, phenylephrine, phenylpropanolamine, pseudoephedrine, albuterol, metaproterenol, or terbutaline.

Tell your doctor if you have a history of drug abuse or if you have ever had angina, diabetes mellitus, emotional disturbances, glaucoma, heart or cardiovascular disease, high blood pressure, or thyroid disease.

Mazindol can mask the symptoms of extreme fatigue and can cause dizziness or light-headedness. Your ability to perform tasks that require alertness, such as driving a car or operating potentially dangerous machinery, may be decreased. Appropriate caution should, therefore, be taken.

Before having surgery or any other medical or dental treatment, be sure to tell your doctor or dentist that you are taking this medication.

Mazindol is related to amphetamine and may be habit-forming when taken for long periods of time (both physical and psychological dependence can occur). Therefore,

you should not increase the dosage of this medication or take it for longer than 12 weeks unless you first consult your doctor. It is also important that you not stop taking this medication abruptly. Fatigue, sleep disorders, mental depression, nausea or vomiting, or stomach cramps or pain can occur while your body adjusts to discontinuation of this medication. Your doctor may want to decrease the dosage gradually in order to prevent these side effects.

Mazindol should not be used in children less than 12 years of age.

There is no specific information about the use of appetite suppressants such as this medication in the elderly.

Be sure to tell your doctor if you are pregnant. Although studies in humans have not been conducted, it is known that some of the appetite suppressants cause side effects in the offspring of animals that receive large doses of these drugs during pregnancy. Also, tell your doctor if you are breast-feeding an infant. It is not known whether this medication passes into breast milk.

Mazanor—see Mazindol

Measurin—see aspirin

meclizine

BRAND NAMES (Manufacturers)
Antivert (Roerig)
Antivert/25 (Roerig)
Antivert/50 (Roerig)
Antrizine (Major)
Bonine* (Pfipharmecs)
Dizmiss* (Bowman)
meclizine hydrochloride (various manufacturers)
Ru-Vert-M (Reid-Provident)
Wehvert* (Hauck)
*Available over-the-counter (without a prescription)
TYPE OF DRUG
Antiemetic
INGREDIENT
meclizine
DOSAGE FORMS
Tablets (12. 5 mg, 25 mg, and 50 mg)
Chewable tablets (25 mg)
STORAGE
Store at room temperature in a tightly closed container.

USES
Meclizine is used to provide symptomatic relief of dizziness and to prevent or relieve dizziness, nausea, and vomiting due to motion sickness. It is thought to relieve dizziness and vomiting by altering nerve transmission in the balance and vomiting centers in the brain.

TREATMENT
To avoid stomach upset, take meclizine with food, milk, or water (unless your doctor directs you to do otherwise).

The chewable tablets should be chewed for at least two minutes in order to obtain the full benefit of this drug.

If you are taking meclizine to prevent motion sickness, you should take it one hour before traveling.

If you miss a dose of this medication, take the missed dose as soon as possible, unless it is almost time for your next dose. In that case, do not take the missed dose at all; just return to your regular dosing schedule. Do not double the next dose.

SIDE EFFECTS
Minor. Confusion; constipation; diarrhea; dizziness; dry mouth, throat, or nose; headache; irritability; loss of appetite; nausea; restlessness; or stomach upset. These side effects should disappear as your body adjusts to the medication.

If you are constipated, increase the amount of fiber in your diet (fresh fruits and vegetables, salads, bran, and whole-grain breads), exercise, and drink more water (unless your doctor tells you not to do so).

Chew sugarless gum or suck on ice chips or a piece of hard candy to reduce mouth dryness.

Major. Tell your doctor about any side effects that are persistent or particularly bothersome. IT IS ESPECIALLY IMPORTANT TO TELL YOUR DOCTOR about blurred vision, change in menstruation, clumsiness, decreased blood pressure, difficult or painful urination, feeling faint, flushing of the face, hallucinations, palpitations, ringing or buzzing in the ears, rash, seizures, shortness of breath, sleeping disorders, sore throat or fever, tightness in the chest, unusual bleeding or bruising, unusual increase in sweating, or unusual tiredness or weakness.

INTERACTIONS
1. Meclizine interacts with several other types of medications: Concurrent use of it with other central nervous system depressants (such as alcohol, barbiturates, benzodiazepine tranquilizers, muscle relaxants, narcotics, pain medications, and phenothiazine tranquilizers) or with tricyclic antidepressants can cause extreme drowsiness.

2. If you take meclizine on a regular basis and also take large amounts of aspirin (for example, for arthritis pain relief), tell your doctor. The effects of too much aspirin (ringing in the ears) may be masked by meclizine.

BE SURE TO TELL YOUR DOCTOR about any medications you are currently taking, especially those listed above.

WARNINGS
• Tell your doctor about allergic or unusual reactions you have had to any medications, especially to meclizine, cyclizine, or buclizine.

• Tell your doctor if you now have or if you have ever had asthma, blood vessel disease, glaucoma, high blood pressure, kidney disease, peptic ulcers, enlarged prostate gland, or thyroid disease.

• Meclizine can cause drowsiness or dizziness. Your ability to perform tasks that require alertness, such as driving a car or operating potentially dangerous machinery, may be decreased. Appropriate caution should, therefore, be taken.

• Meclizine should be given to children under age 12 years only under the supervision of a doctor.

• The elderly may be especially sensitive to side effects such as dry mouth.

• Be sure to tell your doctor if you are pregnant. The effects of this medication during pregnancy have not been thoroughly studied in humans. Also, tell your doctor if you are breast-feeding an infant. Small amounts of meclizine pass into breast milk and may cause unusual excitement or irritability in nursing infants.

meclizine hydrochloride—see meclizine

meclofenamate

BRAND NAMES (Manufacturers)
meclofenamate sodium (various manufacturers)
Meclomen (Parke-Davis)
TYPE OF DRUG
Nonsteroidal anti-inflammatory analgesic
INGREDIENT
meclofenamate
DOSAGE FORMS
Tablets (50 mg and 100 mg)
Capsules (50 mg and 100 mg)
STORAGE
This medication should be stored in a tightly closed container at room temperature, away from heat and direct sunlight.

USES
Meclofenamate is used as a short-term treatment for the pain and inflammation (pain, swelling, stiffness) of certain types of arthritis, gout, bursitis, and tendinitis. Meclofenamate has been shown to block the production of certain body chemicals, called prostaglandins, that may trigger pain. However, it is not yet fully understood how meclofenamate works.

TREATMENT
If this medication upsets your stomach, you can take it with food, milk, or antacids (unless your doctor recommends otherwise). If stomach irritation continues, check with your doctor.

It is important to take meclofenamate on schedule and not to miss any doses. If you do miss a dose, take it as soon as possible, unless it is almost time for your next dose. In that case, do not take the missed dose at all; just return to your regular dosing schedule. Do not double the next dose.

If you are taking meclofenamate to relieve arthritis, you must take it regularly, as directed by your doctor. It may take up to three weeks before you feel the full benefits of this medication.

This medication does not cure arthritis, but it will help to control the condition as long as you continue to take it.

SIDE EFFECTS
Minor. Bloating, constipation, diarrhea, difficulty in sleeping, dizziness, drowsiness, headache, heartburn, indigestion, light-headedness, loss of appetite, nausea, nervousness, soreness of the mouth, unusual sweating, or

vomiting. As your body adjusts to the drug, these side effects should disappear.

To relieve constipation, increase the amount of fiber in your diet (fresh fruits and vegetables, salads, bran, and whole-grain breads), exercise, and drink more water (unless your doctor directs you to do otherwise).

If you become dizzy, sit or lie down for a while; get up slowly from a sitting or reclining position, and be careful on stairs.

Major. If any side effects are persistent or particularly bothersome, you should report them to your doctor. IT IS ESPECIALLY IMPORTANT TO TELL YOUR DOCTOR about bloody or black, tarry stools; blurred vision; confusion; depression; difficult or painful urination; palpitations; a problem with hearing; ringing or buzzing in the ears; severe diarrhea; severe sunburn; shortness of breath; skin rash, hives, or itching; stomach pain; swelling of the feet; tightness in the chest; wheezing or difficulty in breathing; unexplained sore throat and fever; unusual bleeding or bruising; unusual fatigue or weakness; unusual weight gain; or yellowing of the eyes or skin.

INTERACTIONS

Meclofenamate interacts with several other types of medications:

1. Anticoagulants (blood thinners), such as warfarin, taken at the same time as meclofenamate can lead to an increase in bleeding complications.

2. Concurrent use of aspirin, salicylates, or other anti-inflammatory medications can increase stomach irritation.

3. Probenecid may increase blood levels of meclofenamate, which may increase the risk of side effects.

4. The action of beta blockers may be decreased by this drug.

5. This drug can interact with diuretics (water pills).

BE SURE TO TELL YOUR DOCTOR about any medications you are currently taking, especially any of those listed above.

WARNINGS

Tell your doctor if you have ever had unusual or allergic reactions to meclofenamate or any of the other chemically related drugs (aspirin, other salicylates, diclofenac, diflunisal, fenoprofen, flurbiprofen, ibuprofen, indomethacin, ketoprofen, mefenamic acid, naproxen, oxyphenbutazone, phenylbutazone, piroxicam, sulindac, or tolmetin).

Before taking meclofenamate, it is important to tell your doctor if you now have or if you have ever had bleeding problems, colitis, stomach ulcers or other stomach problems, epilepsy, heart disease, high blood pressure, asthma, kidney disease, liver disease, mental illness, or Parkinson's disease.

If this drug makes you dizzy or drowsy, do not take part in any activity that requires alertness, such as driving a car or operating potentially dangerous machinery.

Because this drug can prolong your bleeding time, it is important to tell your doctor or dentist that you are taking this drug before having surgery or any other medical or dental treatment.

Stomach problems are more likely to occur if you take aspirin regularly or drink alcohol while being treated with this medication. These should, therefore, be avoided (unless your doctor directs you to do otherwise).

The elderly may be at increased risk of experiencing side effects from this drug.

The safety and effectiveness of this drug in children below the age of 14 has not been established.

Be sure to tell your doctor if you are pregnant. Studies have shown that meclofenamate can cause unwanted effects (including slower development of bones and heart damage) in the offspring of animals that received this drug during pregnancy. If taken late in pregnancy, meclofenamate can also prolong labor. Also, tell your doctor if you are breast-feeding an infant. Small amounts of meclofenamate pass into breast milk.

Meclofenamate sodium—see meclofenamate

Meclomen—see meclofenamate

Medihaler Ergotamine—see ergotamine

Medipren—see ibuprofen

Medrol—see methylprednisolone (systemic)

---

medroxyprogesterone

BRAND NAMES (Manufacturers)
Amen (Carnrick)
Curretab (Reid-Provident)
Cycrin (Ayerst)
medroxyprogesterone acetate (various manufacturers)
Provera (Upjohn)
TYPE OF DRUG
Progesterone
INGREDIENT
medroxyprogesterone
DOSAGE FORM
Tablets (2.5 mg, 5 mg, and 10 mg)
STORAGE
These tablets should be stored at room temperature in a tightly closed container.

USES

Medroxyprogesterone is a synthetic progesterone (progesterone is a female hormone that is naturally produced by the body) that is used to treat abnormal menstrual bleeding, difficult menstruation, or lack of menstruation. It can be used for other conditions as determined by your doctor.

TREATMENT

This medication may cause stomach irritation. To avoid or minimize this side effect, you can take medroxyprogesterone with food or immediately after a meal.

If you miss a dose of this medication, take the missed dose as soon as possible, unless it is almost time for the next dose. In that case, do not take the missed dose at all; just return to your regular dosing schedule. Do not double the next dose of the medication.

SIDE EFFECTS

Minor. Acne, dizziness, hair growth, headache, nausea, or vomiting. These side effects should disappear as your body adjusts to the medication.

This medication can increase your sensitivity to sunlight. Avoid prolonged exposure to sunlight and sunlamps. Wear protective clothing and use an effective sunscreen.

This medication may cause tenderness, swelling, or bleeding of the gums. Brushing and flossing your teeth regularly may prevent this. Also, you should see your dentist regularly while you are taking this medicine.

If you feel dizzy or light-headed, sit or lie down for a while; get up slowly from a sitting or reclining position, and be careful on stairs.

Major. Tell your doctor about any side effects that are persistent or particularly bothersome. IT IS ESPECIALLY IMPORTANT TO TELL YOUR DOCTOR about breast tenderness; change in menstrual patterns; chest pain; depression; fainting; hair loss; itching; pain in the calves; rapid weight gain (three to five pounds within a week); rash; slurred speech; sudden, severe headache; swelling of the feet or ankles; unusual vaginal bleeding; or yellowing of the eyes or skin.

INTERACTIONS

Medroxyprogesterone should not interact with other medications if it is used according to directions.

WARNINGS

• Tell your doctor about unusual or allergic reactions you have had to any medications, especially to medroxyprogesterone, progestin, or progesterone.
• Before starting this drug, tell your doctor if you have ever had cancer of the breast or genitals, clotting disorders, diabetes mellitus, depression, epilepsy, gallbladder disease, asthma, heart disease, kidney disease, liver disease, migraines, porphyria, stroke, or vaginal bleeding.
• A package insert should come with this drug. Read it carefully, and ask your doctor if you have any questions.
• If this drug makes you dizzy or drowsy, do not take part in any activities that require alertness, such as driving a car or operating potentially dangerous machinery.
• Be sure to tell your doctor if you are pregnant. Medroxyprogesterone should not be used during the first four months of pregnancy because it has been shown to cause birth defects. Since hormones have long-term effects on the body, medroxyprogesterone should be stopped at least three months before you attempt to become pregnant. Also, tell your doctor if you are breast-feeding an infant. Small amounts of medroxyprogesterone pass into breast milk.

medroxyprogesterone acetate—see
    medroxyprogesterone

mefenamic acid

BRAND NAME (Manufacturer)
Ponstel (Parke-Davis)

TYPE OF DRUG
Nonsteroidal anti-inflammatory analgesic
INGREDIENT
mefenamic acid
DOSAGE FORM
Capsules (250 mg)
STORAGE
This medication should be stored in a tightly closed container at room temperature away from heat and direct sunlight.

USES

Mefenamic acid is used to treat painful menstruation. Mefenamic acid has been shown to block the production of certain body chemicals, called prostaglandins, that may trigger pain. However, it is not yet fully understood how it works.

TREATMENT

Mefenamic acid should be taken with food or antacids to lessen stomach irritation (unless your doctor recommends otherwise). Take this medication only as directed by your doctor. Do not take more of it or take it more often; and do not take it for longer than seven days at a time, unless your doctor tells you to do so. Taking too much of this medicine or using it for long periods of time may increase your chances of experiencing serious side effects.

It is important to take mefenamic acid on schedule and not to miss any doses. If you do miss a dose, take it as soon as possible, unless it is almost time for your next dose. In that case, do not take the missed dose at all; just return to your regular dosing schedule. Do not double the next dose.

SIDE EFFECTS

Minor. Bloating, constipation, diarrhea, difficulty in sleeping, dizziness, drowsiness, headache, heartburn, indigestion, light-headedness, loss of appetite, nausea, nervousness, soreness of the mouth, unusual sweating, or vomiting. As your body adjusts to the drug, these side effects should disappear.

To relieve constipation, increase the amount of fiber in your diet (fresh fruits and vegetables, salads, bran, and whole-grain breads), exercise, and drink more water (unless your doctor directs you to do otherwise).

If you become dizzy, sit or lie down for a while; get up slowly from a sitting or reclining position, and be careful on stairs. Avoid operating a car or potentially dangerous equipment.

Major. If any side effects are persistent or particularly bothersome, you should report them to your doctor. IT IS ESPECIALLY IMPORTANT TO TELL YOUR DOCTOR about bloody or black, tarry stools; blurred vision; confusion; depression; difficult or painful urination; palpitations; a problem with hearing; ringing or buzzing in the ears; severe diarrhea; skin rash, hives, or itching; stomach pain; swelling of the feet; tightness in the chest, shortness of breath, or wheezing; unexplained sore throat and fever; unusual bleeding or bruising; unusual fatigue or weakness; unusual weight gain; or yellowing of the eyes or skin.

INTERACTIONS

Mefenamic acid interacts with several other medications:

1. Anticoagulants (blood thinners) such as warfarin can lead to an increase in bleeding complications if taken at the same time as mefenamic acid.

2. Concurrent use with aspirin, salicylates, or other anti-inflammatory medications can increase stomach irritation. Aspirin may also decrease the effectiveness of mefenamic acid.

3. Probenecid may increase blood levels of mefenamic acid, which may increase the risk of side effects.

4. The action of beta blockers may be decreased by this medication.

5. The drug can interact with diuretics (water pills).

BE SURE TO TELL YOUR DOCTOR about any medications you are currently taking, especially any listed above.

WARNINGS

• Tell your doctor if you have ever had unusual or allergic reactions to any medications, especially to mefenamic acid or to any of the other chemically related drugs (aspirin, other salicylates, diclofenac, diflunisal, fenoprofen, flurbiprofen, ibuprofen, meclofenamate, indomethacin, ketoprofen, naproxen, oxyphenbutazone, phenylbutazone, piroxicam, sulindac, or tolmetin).

• Before taking mefenamic acid, it is important to tell your doctor if you now have or if you have ever had asthma, bleeding problems, colitis, stomach ulcers or other stomach problems, epilepsy, heart disease, high blood pressure, kidney disease, liver disease, mental illness, or Parkinson's disease.

• If this drug makes you dizzy or drowsy, do not take part in any activity that requires alertness, such as driving a car or operating potentially dangerous machinery.

• Because mefenamic acid can prolong your bleeding time, it is important to tell your doctor or dentist that you are taking this drug before having surgery or any other medical or dental treatment.

• If you experience severe diarrhea while taking this medication, check with your doctor immediately. Do not take this medication again unless you first check with your doctor, because severe diarrhea can occur each time you take it.

• Stomach problems are more likely to occur if you take aspirin regularly or drink alcohol while being treated with this medication. These should, therefore, be avoided (unless your doctor directs you to do otherwise).

• If this drug is to be given to a child under 12 years of age, discuss the risks as well as the benefits with your doctor.

• Be sure to tell your doctor if you are pregnant. This type of medication may cause unwanted effects on the heart or blood flow in the fetus. Also, studies in animals have shown that this type of medicine, if taken late in pregnancy, can increase the length of pregnancy, prolong labor, and cause other problems during delivery. Mefenamic acid has not been shown to cause birth defects in animals; however, studies in humans have not been conducted. Also, tell your doctor if you are breastfeeding. Small amounts of mefenamic acid pass into breast milk.

Mellaril—see thioridazine

meperidine

BRAND NAMES (Manufacturers)
Demerol (Winthrop-Breon)
meperidine hydrochloride (various manufacturers)
TYPE OF DRUG
Analgesic
INGREDIENT
meperidine
DOSAGE FORMS
Tablets (50 mg and 100 mg)
Syrup (50 mg per 5-ml spoonful)
STORAGE
Store at room temperature in a tightly closed, light-resistant container. This medication should never be frozen.

USES

Meperidine is a narcotic analgesic (pain reliever) that acts directly on the central nervous system (brain and spinal cord). It is used to relieve moderate to severe pain.

TREATMENT

In order to avoid stomach upset, you can take meperidine with food or milk. It works most effectively if you take it at the onset of pain, rather than waiting until the pain becomes intense.

Measure the syrup form of this medication carefully with a specially designed 5ml measuring spoon. An ordinary kitchen teaspoon is not accurate enough. Each dose of the syrup should be diluted in four ounces (half a glass) of water in order to avoid the numbness of the mouth and throat that this medication can cause.

If you are taking this medication on a regular schedule and you miss a dose, take the missed dose as soon as possible, unless it is almost time for your next dose. In that case, do not take the missed dose at all; just return to your regular dosing schedule. Do not double the next dose.

SIDE EFFECTS

Minor. Constipation, dizziness, drowsiness, dry mouth, false sense of well-being, flushing, light-headedness, loss of appetite, nausea, rash, or sweating. These side effects should disappear as your body adjusts to the medication.

If you are constipated, increase the amount of fiber in your diet (fresh fruits and vegetables, salads, bran, and whole-grain breads), exercise, and drink more water (unless your doctor directs you to do otherwise).

Chew sugarless gum or suck on ice chips or a piece of hard candy to reduce mouth dryness associated with the use of this medication.

If you feel dizzy or light-headed, sit or lie down for a while; get up from a sitting or lying position slowly, and be careful on stairs.

Major. Tell your doctor about any side effects that are persistent or particularly bothersome. IT IS ESPECIALLY IMPORTANT TO TELL YOUR DOCTOR about anxiety, breathing difficulties, excitability, fatigue, painful or difficult urination, restlessness, sore throat and fever, tremors, or weakness.

INTERACTIONS
Meperidine interacts with several other types of medications:

1. Concurrent use of this medication with other central nervous system depressants (such as alcohol, antihistamines, barbiturates, benzodiazepine tranquilizers, muscle relaxants, and phenothiazine tranquilizers) or with tricyclic antidepressants can cause extreme drowsiness.

2. A monoamine oxidase (MAO) inhibitor taken within 14 days of this medication can lead to unpredictable and severe side effects.

3. The combination of cimetidine and meperidine can cause confusion, disorientation, and shortness of breath.

BE SURE TO TELL YOUR DOCTOR about any medications you are currently taking, especially any listed above.

WARNINGS
• Tell your doctor about unusual or allergic reactions you have had to any drugs, especially to meperidine or to any other narcotic analgesic (such as codeine, hydrocodone, hydromorphone, methadone, morphine, oxycodone, and propoxyphene).

• Tell your doctor if you now have or if you have ever had acute abdominal conditions, asthma, brain disease, colitis, epilepsy, gallstones or gallbladder disease, head injuries, heart disease, kidney disease, liver disease, lung disease, mental illness, emotional disorders, enlarged prostate gland, thyroid disease, or urethral stricture.

• If this drug makes you dizzy or drowsy, do not take part in any activity that requires alertness, such as driving a car or operating potentially dangerous machinery. Take special care going up and down stairs.

• Before having surgery or any other medical or dental treatment, tell your doctor or dentist about this drug.

• Meperidine has the potential for abuse and must be used with caution. Usually, it should not be taken on a regular schedule for longer than ten days (unless your doctor directs you to do so). Tolerance develops quickly; do not increase the dosage or stop taking the drug abruptly unless you first consult your doctor. If you have been taking large amounts of this medication or have been taking it for a long period of time, you may experience withdrawal symptoms (muscle aches, diarrhea, gooseflesh, runny nose, nausea, vomiting, shivering, trembling, stomach cramps, sleep disorders, irritability, weakness, excessive yawning, or sweating) when you stop taking it. Your doctor may, therefore, want to reduce your dosage gradually.

• Tell your doctor if you are pregnant. The effects of this drug during the early stages of pregnancy have not been thoroughly studied in humans. However, the use of meperidine regularly in large doses during the later stages of pregnancy can result in addiction of the fetus. Also, tell your doctor if you are breast-feeding. Small amounts of this drug may pass into breast milk and cause excessive drowsiness in the nursing infant.

meperidine hydrochloride—see meperidine

Mephyton—see vitamin K

Mepro-analgesic—see meprobamate and aspirin combination

---

meprobamate

BRAND NAMES (Manufacturers)
Equanil (Wyeth)
meprobamate (various manufacturers)
Meprospan (Wallace)
Miltown (Wallace)
TYPE OF DRUG
Sedative/hypnotic
INGREDIENT
meprobamate
DOSAGE FORMS
Tablets (200 mg, 400 mg, and 600 mg)
Capsules (400 mg)
Sustained-release capsules (200 mg and 400 mg)
STORAGE
Meprobamate tablets and capsules should be stored at room temperature in tightly closed containers.

USES
Meprobamate is used to relieve anxiety or tension and is also prescribed as a sleeping aid. It is not exactly clear how meprobamate works, but it is thought to act as a central nervous system (brain and spinal cord) depressant.

TREATMENT
In order to avoid stomach irritation, you can take meprobamate with food or with a full glass of water or milk.

The sustained-release capsules should be swallowed whole. Breaking, chewing, or crushing these capsules destroys their sustained-release activity.

If you are taking this medication on a regular schedule and you miss a dose, take the missed dose immediately if you remember within an hour. If more than an hour has passed, skip the dose you missed and wait for the next scheduled dose. Do not double the dose.

SIDE EFFECTS
Minor. Diarrhea, dizziness, drowsiness, dry mouth, headache, nausea, vomiting, or weakness. These side effects should disappear as your body adjusts to the medication.

If you feel dizzy while taking this medication, sit or lie down for a while; get up slowly from a sitting or reclining position, and be careful on stairs.

To relieve mouth dryness, chew sugarless gum or suck on ice chips or a piece of hard candy.

Major. Tell your doctor about any side effects that are persistent or particularly bothersome. IT IS ESPECIALLY IMPORTANT TO TELL YOUR DOCTOR about blurred vision, clumsiness, confusion, convulsions, difficulty in breathing, difficult or painful urination, fainting, false sense of well-being, fever, nightmares, numbness or tingling, palpitations, rapid weight gain (three to five pounds within a week), rash, slurred speech, sore throat, unusual bleeding or bruising, or unusual weakness.

INTERACTIONS

Concurrent use of meprobamate with other central nervous system depressants (such as alcohol, antihistamines, barbiturates, benzodiazepine tranquilizers, muscle relaxants, narcotics, pain medications, phenothiazine tranquilizers, and sleeping medications) or with tricyclic antidepressants can cause extreme drowsiness.

BE SURE TO TELL YOUR DOCTOR about any medications you are currently taking, especially any listed above.

WARNINGS

Tell your doctor about any unusual or allergic reactions you have had to medications, especially to meprobamate, carbromal, carisoprodol, mebutamate, or tybamate.

Before starting to take this medication, be sure to tell your doctor if you have a history of drug abuse or if you now have or have ever had epilepsy, kidney disease, liver disease, or porphyria.

If this drug causes dizziness or drowsiness, avoid tasks that require alertness, such as driving a car or operating potentially dangerous machinery.

This drug has the potential for abuse and must be used with caution. Tolerance develops quickly; do not increase the dosage unless you first consult your doctor.

Do not stop taking this drug abruptly if you have been taking it for two or three months. Stopping abruptly can lead to a withdrawal reaction. Your doctor may, therefore, want to reduce your dosage gradually.

Some of these products contain the color additive FD&C Yellow No. 5 (tartrazine), which can cause allergic-type reactions (rash, fainting, shortness of breath) in certain susceptible individuals.

Be sure to tell your doctor if you are pregnant. Meprobamate has been reported to cause birth defects when taken during the first three months of pregnancy. Also, tell your doctor if you are breast-feeding an infant. Meprobamate passes into breast milk and can cause excessive drowsiness in the nursing infant.

meprobamate and aspirin combination

BRAND NAMES (Manufacturers)

aspirin and meprobamate combination (various manufacturers)
Epromate (Major)
Equagesic (Wyeth)
Equazine M (Rugby)
Mepro-analgesic (United Research)
Meprobamate Compound (Interstate)
Mepro Compound (Schein)
Meprogese (Geneva Generics)
Meprogesic Q (various manufacturers)
Micrainin (Wallace)

TYPE OF DRUG

Sedative and analgesic

INGREDIENTS

meprobamate and aspirin

DOSAGE FORM

Tablets (200 mg meprobamate and 325 mg aspirin)

STORAGE

Meprobamate and aspirin combination tablets should be stored at room temperature in a tightly closed, light-resistant container. Moisture can cause aspirin to decompose.

USES

Meprobamate and aspirin combination is used to relieve tension headaches and pain in muscles or joints associated with tension or anxiety. It is unclear exactly how meprobamate works to relieve anxiety and tension, but it appears to be a central nervous system (brain and spinal cord) depressant.

TREATMENT

In order to avoid stomach irritation, you can take meprobamate and aspirin combination with food or with a full glass of water or milk (unless your doctor directs otherwise).

If you are taking this medication on a regular schedule and you miss a dose, take the missed dose as soon as possible, unless it is almost time for the next dose. In that case, do not take the missed dose at all; just return to your regular dosing schedule. Do not double the next dose.

SIDE EFFECTS

Minor. Abdominal pain, diarrhea, dizziness, drowsiness, dry mouth, fatigue, headache, light-headedness, nausea, vomiting, or weakness. These side effects should disappear as your body adjusts to the medication.

If you feel dizzy or light-headed, sit or lie down for a while; get up slowly from a sitting or reclining position, and be careful on stairs.

Major. Tell your doctor about any side effects that are persistent or particularly bothersome. IT IS ESPECIALLY IMPORTANT TO TELL YOUR DOCTOR about blurred vision, buzzing in the ears, chest tightness, clumsiness, confusion, convulsions, difficult or painful urination, fainting, false sense of well-being, fever, headache, loss of coordination, mental depression, nightmares, numbness or tingling, palpitations, rapid weight gain, shortness of breath, skin rash, slurred speech, sore throat, unusual bleeding or bruising, or unusual weakness.

INTERACTIONS

This medicine interacts with other types of drugs:
1. Concurrent use of meprobamate with other central nervous system depressants (such as alcohol, antihistamines, barbiturates, benzodiazepine tranquilizers, muscle relaxants, narcotics, pain medications, phenothiazine tranquilizers, and sleeping medications) or with tricyclic antidepressants may cause extreme drowsiness.
2. Aspirin can increase the effects of blood thinners, such as warfarin, thereby leading to a possible increase in bleeding complications.

3. The antigout effects of probenecid and sulfinpyrazone may be blocked by aspirin.

4. Aspirin can increase the gastrointestinal side effects of anti-inflammatory medications, including nonsteroidal anti-inflammatory drugs, alcohol, phenylbutazone, and adrenocorticosteroids (cortisone-like medicines).

5. Ammonium chloride, methionine, and furosemide can increase the side effects of aspirin; and acetazolamide, methazolamide, antacids, and phenobarbital can decrease the effectiveness of aspirin.

6. Aspirin can increase the side effects of methotrexate, penicillin, thyroid hormone, phenytoin, sulfinpyrazone, naproxen, valproic acid, insulin, and oral antidiabetic medicines.

7. It can decrease the effects of spironolactone.

BE SURE TO TELL YOUR DOCTOR about any medications you are currently taking, especially those listed above.

WARNINGS

• Tell your doctor about unusual or allergic reactions you have had to any medications, especially to meprobamate, carbromal, carisoprodol, mebutamate, tybamate, aspirin, methyl salicylate (oil of wintergreen), diclofenac, diflunisal, fenoprofen, flurbiprofen, ibuprofen, indomethacin, ketoprofen, meclofenamate, mefenamic acid, naproxen, piroxicam, sulindac, or tolmetin.

• Before starting to take meprobamate and aspirin combination, be sure to tell your doctor if you have a history of drug abuse or if you now have or have ever had asthma, bleeding disorders, congestive heart failure, diabetes, epilepsy, glucose-6-phosphate dehydrogenase (G6PD) deficiency, gout, hemophilia, high blood pressure, kidney disease, liver disease, nasal polyps, peptic ulcers, porphyria, or thyroid disease.

• Before having surgery or any other medical or dental treatment, be sure to tell your doctor or dentist that you are taking aspirin. Treatment with aspirin is usually discontinued five to seven days before surgery, to prevent bleeding complications.

• If this drug makes you dizzy or drowsy, avoid taking part in any activity that requires alertness, such as driving a car or operating potentially dangerous machinery.

• The use of aspirin in children (about 16 years of age or less) with the flu or chicken pox has been associated with a rare, life-threatening condition called Reye's syndrome. Aspirin-containing products should, therefore, not be given to children with signs of infection.

• Diabetic patients should know that large doses of aspirin (greater than eight 325-mg tablets per day) can cause erroneous readings on urine glucose tests. Diabetics should, therefore, check with their doctor before changing their insulin dosage while they are taking this medication.

• Meprobamate is a potentially habit-forming medication. It should, therefore, be used with caution. If this drug is being used for several months, tolerance to it may develop. Do not stop taking the drug unless you first consult your doctor. A withdrawal reaction could result from stopping this medication abruptly. Your doctor may, therefore, want to reduce your dosage of the medication gradually.

• Because meprobamate and aspirin combination contains aspirin, additional medications that contain aspirin should not be administered without your doctor's approval. Check the labels on any over-the-counter (non-prescription) pain, sinus, allergy, asthma, cough, and cold products you might be taking to see if they contain aspirin.

• Be sure to tell your doctor if you are pregnant. Meprobamate can cause birth defects if taken during the first three months of pregnancy. In addition, large doses of aspirin taken close to term may prolong labor and may cause bleeding complications in the mother and heart problems in the infant. Also, tell your doctor if you are breast-feeding an infant. Both meprobamate and aspirin pass into breast milk.

Meprobamate Compound—see meprobamate and aspirin combination

Mepro Compound—see meprobamate and aspirin combination

Meprogese—see meprobamate and aspirin combination

Meprogesic Q—see meprobamate and aspirin combination

Meprospan—see meprobamate

---

mesoridazine

BRAND NAME (Manufacturer)
Serentil (Boehringer Ingelheim)
TYPE OF DRUG
Phenothiazine tranquilizer
INGREDIENT
mesoridazine
DOSAGE FORMS
Tablets (10 mg, 25 mg, 50 mg, and 100 mg)
Oral concentrate (25 mg per ml, with 0.61% alcohol)
STORAGE
The tablet form of this medicine should be stored at room temperature in a tightly closed, light-resistant container. The oral concentrate form of this medication should be stored in the refrigerator in a tightly closed, lightresistant container. If the oral concentrate turns slightly yellow, the medicine is still effective and can be used. However, if the oral concentrate changes color markedly or has particles floating in it, it should not be used; rather, it should be discarded down the sink. This medication should never be frozen.

USES

Mesoridazine is prescribed to treat certain types of mental illness, such as psychosis, the manic phase of manic-depressive illness, and severe behavioral problems in children. This medication is thought to relieve the symptoms of mental illness by blocking certain chemicals involved in nerve transmission in the brain. Mesoridazine may also be used to treat anxiety.

TREATMENT

To avoid stomach irritation during treatment with mesoridazine, you can take the tablet form of this medication with a meal or with a glass of water or milk (unless your doctor directs you to do otherwise).

The oral concentrate form of this medication should be measured carefully with the dropper provided and then added to four ounces (cup) or more of water, milk, or a carbonated beverage or to applesauce or pudding immediately prior to administration. To prevent possible loss of effectiveness, the medication should not be diluted in tea, coffee, or apple juice.

If you miss a dose of this medication, take the missed dose as soon as possible, unless it is almost time for the next dose. In that case, do not take the missed dose at all; just return to your regular dosing schedule. Do not double the next dose (unless your doctor directs you to do so).

The full effects of this medication for the control of emotional or mental symptoms may not become apparent for two weeks after you start to take it.

SIDE EFFECTS

Minor. Constipation; decreased sweating; diarrhea; discoloration of the urine to red, pink, or red-brown; dizziness; drooling; drowsiness; dry mouth; fatigue; jitteriness; menstrual irregularities; nasal congestion; restlessness; vomiting; or weight gain. As your body adjusts to the medication, these side effects should disappear.

This medication can cause increased sensitivity to sunlight. It is, therefore, important to avoid prolonged exposure to sunlight and sunlamps. Wear protective clothing, and use an effective sunscreen.

If you are constipated, increase the amount of fiber in your diet (fresh fruits and vegetables, salads, bran, and whole-grain breads), exercise, and drink more water (unless your doctor directs you to do otherwise).

Chew sugarless gum or suck on ice chips or a piece of hard candy to reduce mouth dryness.

To avoid dizziness or light-headedness when you stand, contract and relax the muscles of your legs for a few moments before rising. Do this by pushing one foot against the floor while raising the other foot slightly, alternating feet so that you are "pumping" your legs in a pedaling motion.

Major. Tell your doctor about any side effects that are persistent or particularly bothersome. IT IS ESPECIALLY IMPORTANT TO TELL YOUR DOCTOR about blurred vision; breast enlargement (in both sexes); chest pain; convulsions; darkened skin; difficulty in swallowing or breathing; fainting; fever; impotence; involuntary movements of the face, mouth, jaw, or tongue; palpitations; rash; sleep disorders; sore throat; tremors; uncoordinated movements; unusual bleeding or bruising; visual disturbances; or yellowing of the eyes or skin.

INTERACTIONS

Mesoridazine interacts with several other types of medications:

1. It can cause extreme drowsiness when combined with alcohol, other central nervous system depressants (such as barbiturates, benzodiazepine tranquilizers, muscle relaxants, narcotics, and pain medications), or tricyclic antidepressants.

2. Mesoridazine can decrease the effectiveness of amphetamines, guanethidine, and levodopa.

3. The combination of mesoridazine with antiarrhythmic agents such as quinidine may result in impaired heart function.

4. The effects of epinephrine, monoamine oxidase (MAO) inhibitors, propranolol, phenytoin, and tricyclic antidepressants may be increased when combined with this medication.

5. Lithium may increase the side effects and decrease the effectiveness of this medication.

6. Antacids and antidiarrheal medicines may decrease the absorption of mesoridazine from the gastrointestinal tract. Therefore, at least one hour should separate doses of one of these medicines and mesoridazine.

Before starting this drug, BE SURE TO TELL YOUR DOCTOR about any drugs you are currently taking.

WARNINGS

Tell your doctor about unusual or allergic reactions you have had to any medications, especially to mesoridazine or any other phenothiazine tranquilizers (such as chlorpromazine, fluphenazine, perphenazine, prochlorperazine, promazine, thioridazine, trifluoperazine, and triflupromazine) or to loxapine.

Tell your doctor if you have a history of alcoholism or if you now have or have ever had any blood disease, bone marrow disease, brain disease, breast cancer, blockage in the urinary or digestive tract, drug-induced depression, epilepsy, high or low blood pressure, diabetes mellitus, glaucoma, heart or circulatory disease, liver disease, lung disease, Parkinson's disease, peptic ulcers, or an enlarged prostate gland.

Tell your doctor about any recent exposure to a pesticide or an insecticide. Mesoridazine may increase the side effects from the exposure.

To prevent oversedation, avoid drinking alcoholic beverages while taking this medication.

If this medication makes you dizzy or drowsy, do not take part in any activity that requires alertness, such as driving a car or operating potentially dangerous machinery. Be careful on stairs.

Prior to having surgery or any other medical or dental treatment, be sure to tell your doctor or dentist that you are taking this medication.

Mesoridazine can decrease sweating and heat release from the body. You should, therefore, avoid becoming overheated by strenuous exercise in hot weather and avoid taking hot baths, showers, and saunas.

Do not stop taking this medication suddenly. If the drug is stopped abruptly, you may experience nausea, vomiting, stomach upset, headache, increased heart rate, insomnia, tremors, or worsening of your condition. Your doctor may want to reduce the dosage gradually.

If you are planning to have a myelogram, or any other procedure in which dye is injected into your spinal cord, tell your doctor that you are taking this medication.

Avoid spilling the oral concentrate form of this medication on your skin or clothing; it may cause redness and irritation of the skin.

While taking this medication, do not take any over-the-counter (nonprescription) medication for weight control or for cough, cold, allergy, asthma, or sinus problems without first checking with your doctor. The combination of these drugs with mesoridazine may cause high blood pressure.

Be sure to tell your doctor if you are pregnant. Small amounts of this medication cross the placenta. Although there are reports of safe use of this drug during pregnancy, there are also reports of liver disease and tremors in newborn infants whose mothers received this type of medication close to term. Also, tell your doctor if you are breast-feeding an infant. Small amounts of this medication pass into breast milk and may cause unwanted effects in the nursing infant.

Metahydrin—see trichlormethiazide

Metandren—see methyltestosterone

Metaprel—see metaproternol

metaproterenol

BRAND NAMES (Manufacturers)
Alupent (Boehringer Ingelheim)
Metaprel (Dorsey)
TYPE OF DRUG
Bronchodilator
INGREDIENT
metaproterenol
DOSAGE FORMS
Tablets (10 mg and 20 mg)
Oral syrup (10 mg per 5-ml spoonful)
Inhalation aerosol (each spray delivers 0.65 mg)
Solution for nebulization (0.6% and 5%)
STORAGE
Metaproterenol tablets and oral syrup should be stored at room temperature in tightly closed, light-resistant containers. The solution for nebulization should be stored in the refrigerator. The inhalation aerosol should be stored at room temperature away from excessive heat—the contents are pressurized, and the container can explode if heated. Metaproterenol syrup and solution should not be used if they turn brown or contain particles.

USES
Metaproterenol is used to relieve wheezing and shortness of breath caused by lung diseases such as asthma, bronchitis, and emphysema. This drug acts directly on the muscles of the bronchi (breathing tubes) to relieve bronchospasm (muscle contractions of the bronchi), thereby allowing air to move to and from the lungs.

TREATMENT
In order to lessen stomach upset, you can take metaproterenol tablets or oral syrup with food (unless your doctor directs you to do otherwise).

The oral syrup form of this medication should be measured carefully with a specially designed 5-ml measuring spoon. An ordinary kitchen teaspoon is not accurate enough.

The inhalation aerosol form of this medication is usually packaged with an instruction sheet. Read the directions carefully before using this medication. The container should be shaken well just before each use. The contents tend to settle on the bottom, so it is necessary to shake the container to distribute the ingredients evenly and equalize the doses. If more than one inhalation is necessary, wait at least one full minute between doses, so that you receive the full benefit of the first dose.

If you miss a dose of this medication and remember within an hour, take it; then follow your regular schedule for the next dose. If you miss the dose by more than an hour or so, just wait until the next scheduled dose. Do not double the dose.

If you are also using an aerosol corticosteroid (such as beclomethasone, dexamethasone, or triamcinolone), use the metaproterenol inhalation first and wait about five minutes before using the corticosteroid inhalation, unless otherwise directed by your doctor. This will allow the corticosteroid inhalation to better reach your lungs.

SIDE EFFECTS
Minor. Anxiety, dizziness, headache, flushing, irritability, insomnia, loss of appetite, muscle cramps, nausea, nervousness, restlessness, sweating, vomiting, weakness, or dryness or irritation of the mouth or throat (from the inhalation aerosol). These side effects should disappear as your body adjusts to the medication.

To help prevent dryness and irritation of the mouth or throat, rinse your mouth with water after each dose of the inhalation aerosol.

In order to avoid difficulty in falling asleep, check with your doctor to see if you can take the last dose of this medication several hours before bedtime each day.

If you feel dizzy, sit or lie down for a while; get up from a sitting or lying position slowly.
Major. Tell your doctor about any side effects that are persistent or particularly bothersome. IT IS ESPECIALLY IMPORTANT TO TELL YOUR DOCTOR about chest pain, difficult breathing, difficult or painful urination, palpitations, rash, or tremors.

INTERACTIONS
Metaproterenol interacts with several other types of medications:
1. Beta blockers (acebutolol, atenolol, betaxolol, carteolol, esmolol, labetalol, metoprolol, nadolol, penbutolol, pindolol, propranolol, timolol) antagonize (act against) this medication, decreasing its effectiveness.
2. Monoamine oxidase (MAO) inhibitors, tricyclic antidepressants, antihistamines, levothyroxine, and over-the-counter (nonprescription) cough, cold, allergy, asthma, diet, and sinus medications may increase the side effects of metaproterenol. At least 14 days should separate the use of this drug and the use of an MAO inhibitor.
3. There may be a change in the dosage requirements of insulin or oral antidiabetic medications when metaproterenol is started.
4. The blood-pressure-lowering effects of guanethidine may be decreased by this medication.

5. The use of metaproterenol with other bronchodilator drugs (either oral or inhaled) can have additive side effects. Discuss this with your doctor.

BE SURE TO TELL YOUR DOCTOR about any medications you are currently taking, especially any of the medications that are listed above.

WARNINGS

• Tell your doctor about unusual or allergic reactions you have had, especially to metaproterenol or any related drug (such as albuterol, amphetamines, ephedrine, epinephrine, isoproterenol, norepinephrine, phenylephrine, phenylpropanolamine, pseudoephedrine, and terbutaline).

• Tell your doctor if you now have or if you have ever had diabetes, glaucoma, high blood pressure, epilepsy, heart disease, enlarged prostate gland, or thyroid disease.

• This medication can cause dizziness. Your ability to perform tasks that require alertness, such as driving a car or operating potentially dangerous machinery, may be decreased. Appropriate caution should, therefore, be taken.

• Before having surgery or any other medical or dental treatment, be sure to tell your doctor or dentist that you are taking this medication.

• Do not exceed the recommended dosage of this medication. Excessive use may lead to an increase in side effects or a loss of effectiveness.

• Try to avoid contact of the aerosol with your eyes.

• Do not puncture, break, or burn the aerosol container. The contents are under pressure and may explode.

• Contact your doctor if you do not respond to the usual dose of this medication. It may be a sign of worsening asthma, which may require additional therapy.

• Be sure to tell your doctor if you are pregnant. The effects of this medication during pregnancy have not been thoroughly studied in humans. Also, tell your doctor if you are breast-feeding an infant. It is not known whether this drug passes into breast milk.

Metezole—see metronidazole

---

methadone

BRAND NAMES (Manufacturers)
Dolophine (Lilly)
methadone hydrochloride (various manufacturers)
TYPE OF DRUG
Analgesic
INGREDIENT
methadone
DOSAGE FORMS
Tablets (5 mg, 10 mg, and 40 mg)
Oral solution (5 mg and 10 mg per 5-ml spoonful, with 8% alcohol, 10 mg per 10-ml spoonful, and 10 mg per 1-ml spoonful)
STORAGE
Methadone analgesic tablets and oral solution should be stored at room temperature in tightly closed, light-resistant containers.

USES
Methadone is a narcotic analgesic (pain reliever) that acts directly on the central nervous system (brain and spinal cord). It is used to relieve moderate to severe pain. It is also used to detoxify narcotic addicts and to provide temporary maintenance treatment for them.

TREATMENT
To avoid stomach upset, take methadone with food or milk. This medication is most effective if you take it at the onset of pain, rather than when the pain becomes intense.

Measure the dose of the solution form of this medication carefully with a specially designed 5-ml measuring spoon. An ordinary kitchen teaspoon is not accurate enough.

If you are taking this medication on a regular schedule and you miss a dose, take the missed dose as soon as possible, unless it is almost time for your next dose. In that case, do not take the missed dose at all; just return to your regular dosing schedule. Do not double the next dose.

SIDE EFFECTS
Minor. Constipation, dizziness, drowsiness, dry mouth, false sense of well-being, light-headedness, loss of appetite, nausea, or sweating. These side effects should disappear as your body adjusts to the medication.

If you are constipated, increase the amount of fiber in your diet (fresh fruits and vegetables, salads, bran, and whole-grain breads), exercise, and drink more water (unless your doctor directs you to do otherwise).

Chew sugarless gum or suck on ice chips or a piece of hard candy to reduce mouth dryness.

If you feel dizzy or light-headed, sit or lie down for a while; get up from a sitting or lying position slowly, and be careful on stairs. Take special care when operating potentially dangerous equipment.

Major. Tell your doctor about any side effects that are persistent or particularly bothersome. IT IS ESPECIALLY IMPORTANT TO TELL YOUR DOCTOR about anxiety, breathing difficulties, excitability, fainting, fatigue, flushing, painful or difficult urination, palpitations, pinpoint pupils of eyes, rash, restlessness, sore throat and fever, tremors, or weakness.

INTERACTIONS
Methadone interacts with several other types of medications:

1. Concurrent use of it with other central nervous system depressants (such as alcohol, antihistamines, barbiturates, benzodiazepine tranquilizers, muscle relaxants, and phenothiazine tranquilizers) or with tricyclic antidepressants can cause extreme drowsiness.

2. A monoamine oxidase (MAO) inhibitor taken within 14 days of this medication can lead to unpredictable and severe side effects.

3. Rifampin and phenytoin can decrease the blood levels and effectiveness of methadone.

4. The combination of cimetidine and this medication can cause confusion, disorientation, and shortness of breath.

BE SURE TO TELL YOUR DOCTOR about any medications you are currently taking, especially any listed above.

WARNINGS

• Tell your doctor about unusual or allergic reactions you have had to any medications, especially to methadone or to any other narcotic analgesic.

• Tell your doctor if you now have or if you have ever had acute abdominal conditions, asthma, brain disease, colitis, epilepsy, gallstones or gallbladder disease, head injuries, heart disease, kidney disease, liver disease, lung disease, mental illness, emotional disorders, enlarged prostate gland, thyroid disease, or urethral stricture.

• If this drug makes you dizzy or drowsy, do not take part in any activity that requires alertness, such as driving a car or operating potentially dangerous machinery.

• Before having surgery or any other medical or dental treatment, be sure to tell your doctor or dentist that you are taking this medication.

• Methadone has the potential for abuse and must be used with caution. Usually, it should not be taken on a regular schedule for longer than ten days (unless your doctor directs you to do so). Tolerance develops quickly; do not increase the dosage or stop taking the drug abruptly unless you first consult your doctor. If you have been taking large amounts of this medication or if you have been taking it for long periods of time, you may experience withdrawal symptoms (muscle aches, diarrhea, gooseflesh, runny nose, nausea, vomiting, shivering, trembling, stomach cramps, sleep disorders, irritability, weakness, excessive yawning, or sweating) when you stop taking it. Your doctor may, therefore, want to reduce the dosage gradually.

• Be sure to tell your doctor if you are pregnant. The effects of this medication during the early stages of pregnancy have not been thoroughly studied in humans. However, regular use of methadone in large doses during the later stages of pregnancy can result in addiction of the fetus, leading to withdrawal symptoms (irritability, excessive crying, tremors, fever, vomiting, diarrhea, sneezing, or excessive yawning) at birth. Also, tell your doctor if you are breast-feeding an infant. Small amounts of this medication may pass into breast milk and cause excessive drowsiness in the nursing infant.

methadone hydrochloride—see methadone

methamphetamine

BRAND NAMES (Manufacturers)
Desoxyn (Abbott)
Desoxyn Gradumets (Abbott)
TYPE OF DRUG
Amphetamine
INGREDIENT
methamphetamine
DOSAGE FORMS
Tablets (5 mg)
Sustained-release tablets (5 mg, 10 mg, and 15 mg)

STORAGE
Methamphetamine should be stored at room temperature in a tightly closed container.

USES
This medication is a central nervous system stimulant that increases mental alertness and decreases fatigue. It is used to treat narcolepsy (a disorder involving uncontrollable desires to sleep or actual sleep attacks that occur in a rapid and unpredictable manner) and abnormal behavioral syndrome in children (hyperkinetic syndrome or attention deficit disorder). The way this medication acts to control abnormal behavioral syndrome in children is not clearly understood.

Methamphetamine is also used as an appetite suppressant during the first few weeks of dieting (while you are trying to establish new eating habits). It is thought to relieve hunger by altering nerve impulses to the appetite control center in the brain. Its effectiveness as an appetite suppressant lasts for only short periods (three to 12 weeks), however.

TREATMENT
In order to avoid stomach upset, you can take methamphetamine with food or with a full glass of milk or water (unless your doctor directs you to do otherwise).

If this medication is being used to treat narcolepsy or abnormal behavioral syndrome in children, the first dose each day should be taken soon after awakening. Subsequent doses should be spaced at four- to six-hour intervals.

If this medication has been prescribed as a diet aid, it should be taken one hour before each meal.

The sustained-release form of this medication should be swallowed whole. Breaking, chewing, or crushing these tablets destroys their sustained-release activity and may increase the side effects.

In order to avoid difficulty in falling asleep, the last dose of this medication each day should be taken four to six hours before bedtime (tablets) or ten to 14 hours before bedtime (sustained-release tablets).

If you miss a dose of this drug, take the missed dose as soon as possible, unless it is time for your next dose. In that case, do not take the missed dose at all; just return to your regular dosing schedule. Do not double the next dose.

SIDE EFFECTS
Minor. Abdominal cramps, constipation, diarrhea, dizziness, dry mouth, false sense of well-being, insomnia, irritability, loss of appetite, nausea, restlessness, unpleasant taste in the mouth, or vomiting. These side effects should disappear as your body adjusts to the medication.

In order to prevent constipation, increase the amount of fiber in your diet (fresh fruits and vegetables, salads, bran, and whole-grain breads), exercise, and drink more water (unless your doctor directs you to do otherwise).

Dry mouth can be relieved by sucking on ice chips or a piece of hard candy or by chewing sugarless gum.

If you feel dizzy, sit or lie down for a while; get up from a sitting or lying position slowly, and be careful on stairs.

Major. Tell your doctor about any side effects that are persistent or particularly bothersome. IT IS ESPECIALLY IMPORTANT TO TELL YOUR DOCTOR about blurred vision, confusion, fatigue, headaches, impotence, mental depression, palpitations, rash, sweating, tightness in the chest, tremors, or uncoordinated movements.

INTERACTIONS
Methamphetamine interacts with several other types of medications:

1. Use of it within 14 days of a monoamine oxidase (MAO) inhibitor (isocarboxazid, pargyline, phenelzine, tranylcypromine) can result in high blood pressure and other side effects.

2. Barbiturate medications, phenothiazine tranquilizers (especially chlorpromazine), and tricyclic antidepressants can antagonize (act against) this medication.

3. Amphetamines (such as methamphetamine) can decrease the blood-pressure-lowering effects of antihypertensive medication (especially guanethidine) and may alter insulin and oral antidiabetic medication dosage requirements in diabetic patients.

4. The side effects of other central nervous system stimulants, such as caffeine, over-the-counter (nonprescription) appetite suppressants, and asthma, allergy, cough, sinus, or cold preparations may be increased by methamphetamine.

5. Acetazolamide and sodium bicarbonate can decrease the elimination of methamphetamine from the body, thereby prolonging its action and increasing the risk of side effects.

BE SURE TO TELL YOUR DOCTOR about any medications you are currently taking, especially any of those listed above.

WARNINGS
Tell your doctor about unusual or allergic reactions you have had to any medications, especially to methamphetamine or other central nervous system stimulants (such as albuterol, amphetamine, dextroamphetamine, ephedrine, isoproterenol, metaproterenol, norepinephrine, phenylephrine, phenylpropanolamine, pseudoephedrine, and terbutaline).

Tell your doctor if you have a history of drug abuse or if you have ever had problems with agitation, diabetes mellitus, glaucoma, heart or blood vessel disease, high blood pressure, or thyroid disease.

Methamphetamine can mask the symptoms of extreme fatigue and can cause dizziness. Your ability to perform tasks that require alertness, such as driving a car or operating potentially dangerous machinery, may be decreased. Appropriate caution should, therefore, be taken.

Before having surgery or any other medical or dental treatment, be sure to tell your doctor or dentist that you are taking this medication.

Methamphetamine is related to amphetamine and may be habit-forming when taken for long periods of time (both physical and psychological dependence can occur). Therefore, you should not increase the dosage of this medication or take it for longer than 12 weeks, unless you first consult your doctor. It is also important that you not stop taking this medication abruptly; fatigue, sleep

disorders, mental depression, nausea, vomiting, stomach cramps, or pain could occur. Your doctor may, therefore, want to reduce your dosage gradually.

Some of these products contain the color additive FD&C Yellow No. 5 (tartrazine), which can cause allergic-type reactions (rash, fainting, difficulty in breathing) in certain susceptible individuals.

Long-term methamphetamine use in children may cause unwanted effects on growth. The benefits and risks of the drug should be thoroughly discussed before treatment begins.

Be sure to tell your doctor if you are pregnant. Although side effects in humans have not been studied, some of the amphetamines can cause heart, brain, and biliary tract abnormalities in the fetuses of animals that receive large doses of these drugs during pregnancy. Also, tell your doctor if you are breastfeeding an infant. Small amounts of this type of drug pass into breast milk and can cause excessive stimulation in nursing infants.

methenamine

BRAND NAMES (Manufacturers)
Hiprex (Merrell Dow)
Mandameth (Major)
Mandelamine (Parke-Davis)
methenamine hippurate (various manufacturers)
methenamine mandelate (various manufacturers)
Urex (Riker)

TYPE OF DRUG
Antibiotic

INGREDIENT
methenamine

DOSAGE FORMS
Tablets (500 mg and 1 g)
Enteric-coated tablets (500 mg and 1 g).
Oral suspension (250 mg and 500 mg per 5-ml spoonful)
Oral granules (1 g packets)

STORAGE
Methenamine tablets, oral suspension, and granules should be stored at room temperature in tightly closed containers. This medication should never be frozen.

USES
Methenamine is used to prevent and treat bacterial infections of the urinary tract.

TREATMENT
In order to avoid stomach irritation, you should take methenamine with food or with a full glass of water or milk (unless your doctor directs you to do otherwise).

The oral suspension form of this medication should be shaken well just before measuring each dose. The contents tend to settle on the bottom of the bottle, so it is necessary to shake the container to distribute the ingredients evenly and equalize the doses. Each dose should then be measured carefully with a specially designed 5-ml measuring spoon. An ordinary kitchen teaspoon is not accurate enough.

The enteric-coated tablets should be swallowed whole. Breaking, crushing, or chewing these tablets increases their gastrointestinal side effects.

If you are taking the oral granules, the contents of the packet should be dissolved in two to four ounces of water just before you take the dose.

Try not to miss any doses of this medication. If you do miss a dose, take it immediately. However, if you do not remember to take the missed dose until it is almost time for your next dose, take the missed dose immediately; space the following dose about halfway through the regular interval between doses; and then continue with your regular dosing schedule.

It is important to continue to take this medication for the entire time prescribed by your doctor (usually seven to 14 days), even if the symptoms disappear before the end of that period. If you stop taking the drug too soon, resistant bacteria are given a chance to continue growing, and the infection could recur.

This medication works best when your urine is acidic (ph 5.5 or below). You may want to talk to your doctor about testing the acidity of your urine before you begin treatment with methenamine.

SIDE EFFECTS

Minor. Abdominal cramps, diarrhea, headache, loss of appetite, nausea, or vomiting. These side effects should disappear as your body adjusts to the medication.

Major. Tell your doctor about any side effects that are persistent or particularly bothersome. IT IS ESPECIALLY IMPORTANT TO TELL YOUR DOCTOR about difficulty in breathing, difficult or painful urination, itching, mouth sores, rapid weight gain (three to five pounds within a week), shortness of breath, or skin rash.

INTERACTIONS

Methenamine interacts with several other types of medications:

1. Sodium bicarbonate, antacids, acetazolamide, and diuretics (water pills) can decrease the effectiveness of methenamine by preventing its conversion to formaldehyde.

2. Methenamine can increase the side effects (to the kidneys) of sulfonamide antibiotics.

Before starting to take methenamine, BE SURE TO TELL YOUR DOCTOR about any medications you are currently taking, especially any of those listed above.

WARNINGS

• Tell your doctor about unusual or allergic reactions you have had to any medications, especially to methenamine.

• Before starting to take methenamine, be sure to tell your doctor if you now have or if you have ever had dehydration, kidney disease, or liver disease.

• Some of these products contain the color additive FD&C Yellow No. 5 (tartrazine), which can cause allergic-type reactions (fainting, rash, shortness of breath) in certain susceptible individuals.

• This medication has been prescribed for your current infection only. Another infection later on, or one that someone else has, may require a different medicine. You should not give your medicine to other people or use it for other infections, unless your doctor specifically directs you to do so.

• If the symptoms of your infection do not improve in several days, CONTACT YOUR DOCTOR.

• In order for this medication to work properly, it is necessary that your urine remain acidic. You should, therefore, avoid foods that cause the urine to become alkaline such as milk products. Your doctor may also want you to take vitamin C to help keep the urine acidic.

• Be sure to tell your doctor if you are pregnant. Although methenamine appears to be safe during pregnancy, it does cross the placenta, and extensive studies have not been conducted. Also, tell your doctor if you are breastfeeding an infant. Small amounts of methenamine pass into breast milk.

methenamine hippurate—see methenamine

methenamine mandelate—see methenamine

methocarbamol

BRAND NAMES (Manufacturers)
Marbaxin (Vortech)
methocarbamol (various manufacturers)
Robaxin (Robins)
TYPE OF DRUG
Muscle relaxant
INGREDIENT
methocarbamol
DOSAGE FORM
Tablets (500 mg and 750 mg)
STORAGE
Methocarbamol should be stored at room temperature in a tightly closed container.

USES

This medication is used to relieve the discomfort of painful muscle aches and spasms. It should be used in conjunction with rest, physical therapy, and other measures that your doctor may prescribe. It is not clear exactly how methocarbamol works, but it is thought to relieve muscle spasms by acting as a central nervous system (brain and spinal cord) depressant.

TREATMENT

Methocarbamol can be taken either on an empty stomach or with food or a full glass of water or milk (as directed by your doctor). These tablets can be crushed and mixed with food or liquid if you have trouble swallowing them.

If you miss a dose of this medication and remember within an hour, take the missed dose immediately. If more than an hour has passed, do not take the missed dose; just return to your regular dosing schedule. Do not double the next dose.

SIDE EFFECTS

Minor. Dizziness, drowsiness, headache, light-headedness, metallic taste in the mouth, nausea, or stomach upset. These side effects should disappear as your body adjusts to the medication.

This medication can cause the urine to darken to brown, black, or green. This is a harmless effect.

If you feel dizzy or light-headed, sit or lie down for a while; get up slowly from a sitting or reclining position, and be careful on stairs. Be especially careful when driving an automobile or operating potentially dangerous equipment.

Major. Tell your doctor about any side effects that are persistent or particularly bothersome. IT IS ESPECIALLY IMPORTANT TO TELL YOUR DOCTOR about fainting, fatigue, fever, flushing, nasal congestion, skin rash, uncoordinated movements, or visual disturbances.

INTERACTIONS
Methocarbamol interacts with several other types of medications:

1. Concurrent use of methocarbamol with other central nervous system depressants (such as alcohol, antihistamines, barbiturates, benzodiazepine tranquilizers, muscle relaxants, narcotics, pain medications, phenothiazine tranquilizers, and sleeping medications) or with tricyclic antidepressants can cause extreme drowsiness.

2. Methocarbamol can decrease the effectiveness of pyridostigmine.

Before starting to take methocarbamol, BE SURE TO TELL YOUR DOCTOR about any medications you are currently taking, especially any of those listed above.

WARNINGS
• Tell your doctor about unusual or allergic reactions you have had to any medications, especially to methocarbamol.

• Before starting to take this medication, be sure to tell your doctor if you now have or if you have ever had brain disease.

• If this drug makes you dizzy or drowsy, avoid taking part in any activity that requires mental alertness, such as driving a car or operating potentially dangerous machinery.

• Be sure to tell your doctor if you are pregnant. Although methocarbamol appears to be safe, extensive studies in humans have not been conducted. Also, tell your doctor if you are breast-feeding an infant. Small amounts of methocarbamol pass into breast milk.

methotrexate

BRAND NAME (Manufacturer)
Methotrexate (Lederle)
TYPE OF DRUG
Antineoplastic (anticancer drug), antipsoriatic
INGREDIENT
methotrexate
DOSAGE FORM
Tablets (2.5 mg)
STORAGE
Methotrexate should be stored at room temperature in a tightly closed container.

USES
Methotrexate is used to treat certain types of cancer and severe psoriasis. It works by slowing the growth rate of rapidly proliferating cells.

TREATMENT
In order to avoid stomach irritation, you can take methotrexate with food or with a full glass of water or milk (unless your doctor directs you to do otherwise).

Try not to miss any doses of this medication. If you do miss a dose, take the missed dose as soon as possible, unless it is almost time for the next dose. In that case, do not take the missed dose at all; just return to your regular dosing schedule. Do not double the next dose. If you miss more than two doses in a row, CONTACT YOUR DOCTOR.

SIDE EFFECTS
Minor. Abdominal distress, fatigue, loss of appetite, nasal congestion, nausea, or vomiting. These side effects should disappear as your body adjusts to the medication. Methotrexate also causes hair loss, which is reversible when the medication is stopped.

This medication can increase your sensitivity to sunlight. You should, therefore, try to avoid prolonged exposure to sunlight and sunlamps. Wear protective clothing and sunglasses, and use an effective sunscreen.

Major. Tell your doctor about any side effects that are persistent or particularly bothersome. IT IS ESPECIALLY IMPORTANT TO TELL YOUR DOCTOR about back pain, blurred vision, convulsions, diarrhea, difficult or painful urination, drowsiness, fever, headache, itching, menstrual changes, mouth sores, rash, severe abdominal pain, skin color changes, unusual bleeding or bruising, or yellowing of the eyes or skin.

INTERACTIONS
Methotrexate interacts with several other types of medications:

1. Concurrent use of alcohol and methotrexate can lead to an increased risk of liver damage.

2. Methotrexate can block the effectiveness of antigout medications.

3. Phenylbutazone, probenecid, phenytoin, tetracycline, aspirin, chloramphenicol, salicylates, naproxen, ketoprofen, and sulfonamide antibiotics can increase the blood levels of methotrexate, which can lead to an increase in serious side effects.

4. Methotrexate can increase the effects of the blood thinner warfarin, which can lead to bleeding complications.

5. Folic acid vitamins may decrease the effect of this medication.

Before starting to take methotrexate, BE SURE TO TELL YOUR DOCTOR about any medications you are currently taking, especially any of those listed above.

WARNINGS
• Tell your doctor about unusual or allergic reactions you have had to any medications, especially to methotrexate.

• Before starting to take this medication, be sure to tell your doctor if you now have or if you have ever had

blood disorders, gout, infection, kidney disease, liver disease, or inflammation of the gastrointestinal tract.
• If this drug makes you dizzy or drowsy, be careful going up and down stairs, and do not take part in any activity that requires alertness, such as driving a car or operating potentially dangerous machinery.
• While you are taking methotrexate, you should drink plenty of fluids so that you urinate often (unless your doctor directs you to do otherwise). This helps prevent kidney and bladder problems during therapy.
• You should not be immunized or vaccinated while taking methotrexate. The vaccination or immunization will not be effective and may lead to an infection if a live-virus vaccine is used.
• Methotrexate is a potent medication that can cause serious side effects. Your doctor will, therefore, want to monitor your therapy carefully with blood tests.
• Be sure to tell your doctor if you are pregnant. Methotrexate has been shown to cause birth defects or death of the fetus. Effective contraception should be used during treatment and for at least eight weeks after treatment is stopped. Also, tell your doctor if you are breastfeeding an infant. Methotrexate passes into breast milk and can cause side effects in nursing infants.

methyclothiazide

BRAND NAMES (Manufacturers)
Aquatensen (Wallace)
Enduron (Abbott)
Ethon (Major)
methyclothiazide (various manufacturers)
TYPE OF DRUG
Diuretic and antihypertensive
INGREDIENT
methyclothiazide
DOSAGE FORM
Tablets (**2.** 5 mg and 5 mg)
STORAGE
This medication should be stored at room temperature in a tightly closed container.

USES
Methyclothiazide is prescribed to treat high blood pressure. It is also used to reduce fluid accumulation in the body caused by certain conditions, such as heart failure, cirrhosis of the liver, and kidney disease, and by the long-term use of some medications. This medication reduces fluid accumulation by increasing the elimination of salt and water through the kidneys.

TREATMENT
This medication can be taken with a glass of milk or with a meal to decrease stomach irritation (unless your doctor directs you to do otherwise). Try to take it at the same time every day. Avoid taking a dose after 6:00 P.M.; otherwise, you may have to get up during the night to urinate.
If you miss a dose of this medication, take the missed dose as soon as possible, unless it is almost time for the next dose. In that case, do not take the missed dose at all; just wait until the next scheduled dose. Do not double the dose.
This medication does not cure high blood pressure, but it will help to control the condition as long as you continue to take it.

SIDE EFFECTS
Minor. Constipation, cramps, diarrhea, dizziness, drowsiness, headache, heartburn, loss of appetite, restlessness, or upset stomach. As your body adjusts to the medication, these side effects should disappear.
This medication can cause increased sensitivity to sunlight. It is, therefore, important to avoid prolonged exposure to sunlight and sunlamps. Wear protective clothing, and use an effective sunscreen.
To relieve constipation, increase the amount of fiber in your diet (fresh fruits and vegetables, salads, bran, and whole-grain breads) and exercise more (unless your doctor directs you to do otherwise).
To avoid dizziness or light-headedness when you stand, contract and relax the muscles of your legs for a few moments before rising. Do this by pushing one foot against the floor while raising the other foot slightly, alternating feet so that you are "pumping" your legs in a pedaling motion.
Major. Tell your doctor about any side effects that are persistent or particularly bothersome. IT IS ESPECIALLY IMPORTANT TO TELL YOUR DOCTOR about blurred vision, confusion, difficulty in breathing, dry mouth, excessive thirst, excessive weakness, fainting, fever, itching, joint pain, mood changes, muscle pain or spasms, nausea, palpitations, skin rash, sore throat, tingling in the fingers or toes, unusual bleeding or bruising, vomiting, or yellowing of the eyes or skin.

INTERACTIONS
Methyclothiazide interacts with several other types of medications:
1. It may decrease the effectiveness of oral anticoagulants, antigout medications, insulin, oral antidiabetic medicines, and methenamine.
2. Fenfluramine can increase the blood-pressure-lowering effects of methyclothiazide (which can be dangerous to your health).
3. Indomethacin can decrease the blood-pressure-lowering effects of methyclothiazide, thereby counteracting the desired effects.
4. Cholestyramine and colestipol decrease the absorption of this medication from the gastrointestinal tract. Methyclothiazide should, therefore, be taken one hour before or four hours after a dose of cholestyramine or colestipol (if one of those medications has also been prescribed).
5. The side effects of amphotericin B, calcium, cortisone and cortisone-like steroids (such as dexamethasone, hydrocortisone, prednisone, and prednisolone), digitalis, digoxin, lithium, quinidine, sulfonamide antibiotics, and vitamin D may be increased by methyclothiazide.
BE SURE TO TELL YOUR DOCTOR about any medications you are currently taking, especially any listed above.

WARNINGS

Tell your doctor about unusual or allergic reactions you have had to any medications, especially to methyclothiazide or any other sulfa drug, including other diuretics, oral antidiabetic medications, or sulfonamide antibiotics.

Before you start taking methyclothiazide, tell your doctor if you now have or if you have ever had kidney disease or problems with urination, diabetes mellitus, gout, liver disease, asthma, pancreatic disease, or systemic lupus erythematosus.

Methyclothiazide can cause potassium loss. Signs of potassium loss include dry mouth, thirst, weakness, muscle pain or cramps, nausea, and vomiting. If you experience any of these symptoms, call your doctor. To help avoid potassium loss, take this drug with a glass of fresh or frozen orange juice or cranberry juice or eat a banana every day. The use of a salt substitute also helps to prevent potassium loss. Do not change your diet or use a salt substitute, however, before discussing it with your doctor. Too much potassium can also be dangerous. Your doctor may want to have blood tests performed periodically in order to monitor your potassium levels.

In order to avoid dizziness or fainting while taking this medication, try not to stand for long periods of time; avoid drinking excessive amounts of alcohol; and try not to get overheated (avoid strenuous exercise in hot weather and do not take hot baths, showers, and saunas).

Do not take any over-the-counter (nonprescription) medications for weight control or for cough, cold, allergy, asthma, or sinus problems, unless your doctor directs you to do so. Some of these products can cause an increase in blood pressure.

To prevent dehydration (severe water loss) while taking this medication, check with your doctor if you have any illness that causes severe or continuous nausea, vomiting, or diarrhea.

This medication can raise the blood sugar level in diabetic patients. Therefore, blood sugar levels should be carefully monitored by blood or urine tests when this medication is being taken.

Be sure to tell your doctor if you are pregnant. Methyclothiazide can cross the placenta and may cause adverse effects in the developing fetus. Also, tell your doctor if you are breast-feeding an infant. Although problems in humans have not been reported, small amounts of this drug can pass into breast milk, so caution is warranted.

---

methyldopa

BRAND NAMES (Manufacturers)
Aldomet (Merck Sharp & Dohme)
Amodopa (Major)
methyldopa (various manufacturers)
TYPE OF DRUG
Antihypertensive
INGREDIENT
methyldopa
DOSAGE FORMS
Tablets (125 mg, 250 mg, and 500 mg)

Oral suspension (250 mg per 5-ml spoonful, with 1% alcohol)
STORAGE
Store at room temperature in a tightly closed, light-resistant container. This drug should never be frozen.

USES

Methyldopa is used to treat high blood pressure. It is not clear exactly how methyldopa works, but it is thought to act on the central nervous system (brain and spinal cord) to prevent the release of chemicals responsible for maintaining high blood pressure.

TREATMENT

In order to prevent stomach irritation, you can take methyldopa with food or a full glass of water or milk. Try to take it at the same time(s) each day (unless your doctor directs you to do otherwise).

The oral suspension should be shaken well before each dose is measured. The contents tend to settle to the bottom of the bottle, so the bottle should be shaken to distribute the medication evenly and equalize the doses. Each dose should then be measured carefully with a specially designed 5-ml measuring spoon. An ordinary kitchen teaspoon is not accurate enough.

Methyldopa does not cure high blood pressure, but it will help to control the condition as long as you take it.

If you miss a dose of this medication, take the missed dose as soon as possible, unless it is almost time for the next dose. In that case, do not take the missed dose at all; just return to your regular dosing schedule. Do not double the next dose.

SIDE EFFECTS

Minor. Bloating, constipation, diarrhea, dizziness, drowsiness, dry mouth, gas, headache, light-headedness, loss of appetite, nasal congestion, nausea, vomiting, or weakness. These side effects should disappear as your body adjusts to the medication.

To relieve constipation, increase the amount of fiber in your diet (fresh fruits and vegetables, salads, bran, and whole-grain breads), exercise, and drink more water (unless your doctor directs you to do otherwise).

If you feel dizzy or light-headed, sit or lie down for a while; get up slowly from a sitting or reclining position, and be careful on stairs. To avoid dizziness or light-headedness when you stand, contract and relax the muscles of your legs for a few moments before rising. Do this by pushing one foot against the floor while raising the other foot slightly, alternating feet so that you are "pumping" your legs in a pedaling motion.

Major. Tell your doctor about any effects that are persistent or bothersome. IT IS ESPECIALLY IMPORTANT TO TELL YOUR DOCTOR about abdominal distention, blurred vision, breast enlargement (in both sexes), chest pain, confusion, decreased sexual ability, depression, difficulty in breathing, fainting, fatigue, fever, inflamed salivary glands, insomnia, nightmares, numbness or tingling, rapid weight gain (three to five pounds within a week), severe stomach cramps, sore joints, sore or "black" tongue, tremors, unusual bleeding or bruising, unusual body movements, or yellowing of the eyes or skin.

INTERACTIONS

Methyldopa interacts with several other types of drugs:

1. It can increase or decrease the antiparkinsonism effects of levodopa.

2. The use of a monoamine oxidase (MAO) inhibitor within 14 days of methyldopa can cause headaches, severe hypertension, and hallucinations.

3. The combination of methyldopa and methotrimeprazine can cause a severe drop in blood pressure; methyldopa and haloperidol can cause irritability; methyldopa and phenoxybenzamine can cause urinary retention; and methyldopa and alcohol can cause dizziness and fainting.

4. The effects of methyldopa may be increased by verapamil and fenfluramine.

5. Methyldopa can also increase the side effects of tolbutamide and lithium.

6. Methyldopa may increase the effects of norepinephrine and phenylpropanolamine, which may increase blood pressure.

Before starting to take methyldopa, BE SURE TO TELL YOUR DOCTOR about any medications you are currently taking, especially any of those listed above.

WARNINGS

• Tell your doctor about unusual or allergic reactions you have had to any medications, especially to methyldopa.

• Before starting to take this medication, be sure to tell your doctor if you now have or if you have ever had anemia, angina, kidney disease, liver disease, mental depression, Parkinson's disease, or stroke.

• In order to avoid dizziness or fainting while you are taking this medication, try not to stand for long periods of time; avoid drinking excessive amounts of alcohol; and try not to get overheated (avoid strenuous exercise in hot weather and do not take hot baths, showers, and saunas).

• If this drug makes you dizzy or drowsy, avoid taking part in any activity that requires alertness, such as driving a car or operating potentially dangerous machinery.

• Before surgery or other medical or dental treatment, be sure that you tell your doctor or dentist you are taking this medication.

• Before taking any over-the-counter (nonprescription) allergy, asthma, sinus, cough, cold, or diet product, check with your doctor or pharmacist. Some of these products can cause an increase in blood pressure.

• Do not stop taking this medication unless you first check with your doctor. If this drug is stopped abruptly, you could experience a sudden rise in blood pressure. Your doctor may, therefore, want to decrease your dosage gradually.

• If you have an unexplained fever, especially during the first two or three weeks after starting to take this medication, CONTACT YOUR DOCTOR. Fever can be a sign of a serious reaction to methyldopa.

• Occasionally, during the second or third month of therapy, drug tolerance may develop. If you notice a decrease in effectiveness of methyldopa, contact your doctor.

• Before donating blood or receiving a blood transfusion, be sure that the doctor knows you are taking this medication. It can cause changes in your blood cells.

• Aldomet suspension contains sodium bisulfite, which may cause allergic-type reactions (hives, itching, wheezing) in certain susceptible persons.

• Be sure to tell your doctor if you are pregnant. Although this drug appears to be safe, extensive studies in women during pregnancy have not been conducted. Also, tell your doctor if you are breast-feeding an infant. Small amounts of methyldopa pass into breast milk.

methyldopa and hydrochlorothiazide combination

BRAND NAMES (Manufacturers)
Aldoril (Merck Sharp & Dohme)
methyldopa and hydrochlorothiazide combination (various manufacturers)

TYPE OF DRUG
Antihypertensive and diuretic

INGREDIENTS
methyldopa and hydrochlorothiazide

DOSAGE FORM
Tablets (250 mg methyldopa and 15 mg hydrochlorothiazide; 250 mg methyldopa and 25 mg hydrochlorothiazide; 500 mg methyldopa and 30 mg hydrochlorothiazide; 500 mg bmethyldopa and 50 mg hydrochlorothiazide)

STORAGE
These tablets should be stored at room temperature in a tightly closed container.

USES
Methyldopa and hydrochlorothiazide combination is used to treat high blood pressure. It is not exactly clear how methyldopa works, but it is thought to act on the central nervous system (brain and spinal cord) to prevent the release of chemicals responsible for maintaining high blood pressure. Hydrochlorothiazide is a diuretic (water pill), which reduces fluid accumulation by increasing the elimination of salt and water through the kidneys.

TREATMENT
To avoid stomach irritation, you can take methyldopa and hydrochlorothiazide combination with food or with a full glass of water or milk (unless your doctor directs you to do otherwise). In order to become accustomed to taking this medication, try to take it at the same time(s) each day. Avoid taking a dose after 6:00 P.M.; otherwise, you may have to get up during the night to urinate.

Methyldopa and hydrochlorothiazide combination does not cure high blood pressure, but it will help to control the condition as long as you continue to take it.

If you miss a dose of this medication, take the missed dose as soon as possible, unless it is almost time for the next dose. In that case, do not take the missed dose at all; return to your regular dosing schedule. Do not double the dose.

SIDE EFFECTS

Minor. Bloating, constipation, diarrhea, dizziness, drowsiness, gas, headache, light-headedness, loss of appetite, nasal congestion, or increased urination. These effects should disappear as your body adjusts to the drug.

This medication can increase your sensitivity to sunlight. You should, therefore, avoid prolonged exposure to sunlight and sunlamps. Wear protective clothing and sunglasses, and use an effective sunscreen.

To relieve constipation, increase the amount of fiber in your diet (fresh fruits and vegetables, salads, bran, and whole-grain breads) and exercise (unless your doctor directs you to do otherwise).

If you feel dizzy or light-headed, sit or lie down for a while; get up slowly from a sitting or reclining position, and be careful on stairs. To avoid dizziness or light-headedness when you stand, contract and relax the muscles of your legs for a few moments before rising. Do this by pushing one foot against the floor while raising the other foot slightly, alternating feet.

Major. Tell your doctor about any side effects that are persistent or particularly bothersome. IT IS ESPECIALLY IMPORTANT TO TELL YOUR DOCTOR about abdominal distention, blurred vision, breast enlargement (in both sexes), chest pain, confusion, decreased sexual ability, depression, difficulty in breathing, dry mouth, fainting, fatigue, fever, inflamed salivary glands, insomnia, joint pains, muscle pains or spasms, nausea, nightmares, numbness or tingling, rapid weight gain (three to five pounds within a week), severe stomach cramps, sore or "black" tongue, swelling of the feet or ankles, thirst, tremors, unusual bleeding or bruising, unusual body movements, vomiting, weakness, or yellowing of the eyes or skin.

INTERACTIONS

This medicine interacts with other types of drugs:

1. Methyldopa can either increase or decrease the antiparkinsonism effects of levodopa.

2. The use of a monamine oxidase (MAO) inhibitor within 14 days of methyldopa can cause headaches, severe hypertension, and hallucinations.

3. The combination of methyldopa and methotrimeprazine can cause a severe drop in blood pressure; methyldopa and haloperidol can cause irritability; methyldopa and phenoxybenzamine can cause urinary retention; and methyldopa and alcohol can cause dizziness and fainting.

4. The effects of methyldopa may be increased by verapamil and fenfluramine, which may have a negative effect.

5. Methyldopa can increase the side effects of tolbutamide and lithium.

6. Methyldopa may increase the effects of norepinephrine and phenylpropanolamine, which may increase blood pressure.

7. Hydrochlorothiazide can decrease the effectiveness of oral anticoagulants (blood thinners, such as warfarin), antigout medications, insulin, oral antidiabetic medications, and methenamine.

8. Fenfluramine may increase the blood-pressure-lowering effects of hydrochlorothiazide, and indomethacin may decrease its blood-pressure-lowering effects.

9. Cholestyramine and colestipol can decrease the absorption of hydrochlorothiazide from the gastrointestinal tract. Therefore, this medication should be taken one hour before or four hours after a dose of either of these other drugs.

10. The side effects of amphotericin B, calcium, adrenocorticosteroids (cortisone-like medicines), digitalis, digoxin, lithium, quinidine, sulfonamide antibiotics, and vitamin D may be increased by hydrochlorothiazide.

BE SURE TO TELL YOUR DOCTOR about any medications you are currently taking.

WARNINGS

• Tell your doctor about unusual or allergic reactions you have had to medications, especially to methyldopa or hydrochlorothiazide or to any other sulfa medication (diuretics, oral antidiabetic medicines, sulfonamide antibiotics, dapsone, or sulfone).

• Before starting to take this medication, be sure to tell your doctor if you have ever had anemia, angina, diabetes mellitus, gout, kidney disease, liver disease, mental depression, Parkinson's disease, pancreatitis, or stroke.

• A doctor generally does not prescribe this drug or other "fixed-dose" products as the first choice in the treatment of high blood pressure. The patient should initially receive each ingredient singly. If the response is adequate to the dose contained in this product, it can then be substituted. The advantage of a combination product is its increased convenience.

• This medication can cause potassium loss. Signs of potassium loss include dry mouth, thirst, weakness, muscle pain or cramps, nausea, and vomiting. If you experience any of these symptoms, CONTACT YOUR DOCTOR. To help prevent this problem, your doctor may want to have blood tests performed periodically to monitor your potassium levels. To help avoid potassium loss, take this medication with a glass of fresh or frozen orange juice or cranberry juice or eat a banana every day. The use of a salt substitute also helps to prevent potassium loss. Do not change your diet or use a salt substitute, however, until you discuss it with your doctor. Too much potassium can also be dangerous.

• To prevent severe water loss (dehydration) while taking hydrochlorothiazide, check with your doctor if you have any illness that causes severe or continuous nausea, vomiting, or diarrhea.

• Hydrochlorothiazide can raise blood sugar levels in diabetic patients. Blood sugar should, therefore, be monitored carefully when this medication is being taken.

• In order to avoid dizziness or fainting while taking this medication, try not to stand for long periods of time; avoid drinking excessive amounts of alcohol; and try not to get overheated (avoid strenuous exercise in hot weather and do not take hot baths, showers, and saunas).

• If this drug makes you dizzy or drowsy, avoid taking part in any activity that requires alertness.

• Before having surgery or any other medical or dental treatment, be sure to tell your doctor or dentist that you are taking this medication.

• Before taking any over-the-counter (nonprescription) allergy, asthma, sinus, cough, cold, or diet product, check with your doctor or pharmacist.

• Do not stop taking this medication unless you first check with your doctor. If this drug is stopped abruptly, you could experience a sudden rise in blood pressure. Your doctor may, therefore, want to decrease your dosage gradually.

• If you have an unexplained fever, especially during the first two to three weeks after starting to take this medication, CONTACT YOUR DOCTOR. Fever can be a sign of a serious reaction to methyldopa.

•Tolerance to this drug can develop, usually during the second or third month of therapy. If you notice a decrease in effectiveness of this drug, contact your doctor.

• Before donating blood or receiving a blood transfusion, be sure you let the doctor know that you are taking this medication. Methyldopa can cause a change in the blood cells.

• Be sure to tell your doctor if you are pregnant. Methyldopa and hydrochlorothiazide cross the placenta and may cause adverse effects in the developing fetus. Also, tell your doctor if you are breast-feeding an infant. Small amounts of both of these drugs pass into breast milk.

methylphenidate

BRAND NAMES (Manufacturers)
methylphenidate hydrochloride (various manufacturers)
Ritalin (Ciba)
Ritalin-SR (Ciba)
TYPE OF DRUG
Adrenergic
INGREDIENT
methylphenidate
DOSAGE FORMS
Tablets (5 mg, 10 mg, and 20 mg)
Sustained-release tablets (20 mg)
STORAGE
Methylphenidate should be stored at room temperature in tightly closed, light-resistant containers.

USES
Methylphenidate is a central nervous system (brain and spinal cord) stimulant that increases mental alertness and decreases fatigue. It is used in the treatment of narcolepsy (a disorder involving uncontrollable desires to sleep or actual sleep attacks that occur in a rapid and unpredictable manner), mild depression, and abnormal behavioral syndrome in children (hyperkinetic syndrome or attention deficit disorder). The way this medication works in abnormal behavioral syndrome in children is not clearly understood.

TREATMENT
In order to avoid stomach upset, you can take methylphenidate with food or with a full glass of water or milk (unless your doctor directs you to do otherwise).

If methylphenidate is being used to treat narcolepsy or abnormal behavioral syndrome in children, the first dose should be taken soon after awakening.

In order to avoid difficulty in falling asleep, the last dose of the regular tablets should be taken four to six hours before bedtime each day (the sustained-release tablets should be taken at least eight hours before bedtime).

The sustained-release tablets should be swallowed whole. Chewing, crushing, or breaking these tablets destroys their sustained-release activity and may increase the side effects.

If you miss a dose, take the missed dose as soon as possible, unless it is almost time for your next dose. In that case, do not take the missed dose; just return to your regular dosing schedule. Do not double the next dose.

SIDE EFFECTS
Minor. Abdominal pain, dizziness, drowsiness, dry mouth, headache, insomnia, loss of appetite, nausea, nervousness, vomiting, or weakness. These side effects should disappear as your body adjusts to the medication.

Dry mouth can be relieved by sucking on ice chips or a piece of hard candy or by chewing sugarless gum.

If you feel dizzy, sit or lie down for a while; get up from a sitting or lying position slowly, and be careful on stairs.

Major. Tell your doctor about any side effects that are persistent or particularly bothersome. IT IS ESPECIALLY IMPORTANT TO TELL YOUR DOCTOR about chest pain, fever, hair loss, hallucinations, hives, joint pain, mood changes, palpitations, rash, seizures, sore throat, uncoordinated movements, or bleeding or bruising.

INTERACTIONS
Methylphenidate interacts with several other types of medications:
1. Use of it within 14 days of a monoamine oxidase (MAO) inhibitor (such as isocarboxazid, pargyline, phenelzine, tranylcypromine) can result in severe high blood pressure.
2. Methylphenidate can decrease the blood-pressure-lowering effects of antihypertensive medications (especially guanethidine).
3. Acetazolamide and sodium bicarbonate can decrease the elimination of methylphenidate from the body, thereby prolonging its action and increasing the risk of side effects.
4. Methylphenidate can decrease the elimination and increase the side effects of oral anticoagulants (blood thinners, such as warfarin), tricyclic antidepressants (such as amitriptyline, desipramine, imipramine, and nortriptyline), anticonvulsants (such as phenytoin, phenobarbital, and primidone), and phenylbutazone.

Before starting to take this medication, BE SURE TO TELL YOUR DOCTOR about any medications you are currently taking, especially any of those listed above.

WARNINGS
• Tell your doctor about unusual or allergic reactions you have had to any medications, especially to methylphenidate.
• Tell your doctor if you have ever had epilepsy, glaucoma, high blood pressure, motor tics, Tourette's syndrome, anxiety, agitation, depression, or tension.

• Methylphenidate can mask the symptoms of extreme fatigue and can cause dizziness. Your ability to perform tasks that require alertness, such as driving a car or operating potentially dangerous machinery, may be decreased. Appropriate caution should, therefore, be taken. A child taking methylphenidate should be careful while engaging in physical activity.

• Before having surgery or any other medical or dental treatment, be sure to tell your doctor that you are taking this medication.

• Methylphenidate is related to amphetamine and may be habit-forming when taken for long periods of time (both physical and psychological dependence can occur). You should not increase the dosage of this medication or take it for longer than the prescribed time unless you first consult your doctor. It is also important that you not stop taking this medication abruptly; fatigue, sleep disorders, mental depression, nausea, vomiting, or stomach cramps or pain could occur. Your doctor may want to decrease the dosage gradually in order to prevent these side effects.

• Methylphenidate can slow growth in children. Therefore, if this medication is being taken by a child, your doctor may recommend drug-free periods during school holidays and summer vacations. Growth spurts often occur during these drug-free periods.

• Children may be more sensitive to certain side effects such as loss of appetite, stomach pain, trouble sleeping, and weight loss.

• If cocaine is being used now or was used in the past, taking methylphenidate may cause severe nervousness, irritability, trouble sleeping, or possibly irregular heartbeat or seizures.

• Be sure to tell your doctor if you are pregnant. Effects of this drug during pregnancy have not been thoroughly studied in either humans or animals. Also, tell your doctor if you are breast-feeding an infant. Small amounts of methylphenidate may pass into breast milk.

methylphenidate hydrochloride—see methylphenidate

---

methylprednisolone (systemic)

BRAND NAMES (Manufacturers)
Medrol (Upjohn)
methylprednisolone (various manufacturers)
TYPE OF DRUG
Adrenocorticosteroid hormone
INGREDIENT
methylprednisolone
DOSAGE FORM
Tablets (2 mg, 4 mg, 8 mg, 16 mg, 24 mg, and 32 mg)
STORAGE
Store at room temperature in a tightly closed container.

USES

Your adrenal glands naturally produce certain cortisone-like chemicals. These chemicals are involved in various regulatory processes in the body (such as those involving fluid balance, temperature, and reactions to inflam-

mation). Methylprednisolone belongs to a group of drugs known as adrenocorticosteroids (or cortisone-like medications). It is used to treat a variety of disorders, including endocrine and rheumatic disorders; asthma; blood diseases; certain cancers; eye disorders; gastrointestinal disturbances, such as ulcerative colitis; respiratory diseases; and inflammations, such as arthritis, dermatitis, and poison ivy. How this drug acts to relieve these disorders is not completely understood.

TREATMENT

In order to prevent stomach irritation, you can take methylprednisolone with food or milk.

If you are taking only one dose of this medication each day, try to take it before 9:00 A.M. This will mimic the body's normal production of this type of chemical.

It is important to try not to miss any doses of methylprednisolone. However, if you do miss a dose of this medication, follow these guidelines:

1. If you are taking this medication more than once a day, take the missed dose as soon as possible and return to your regular schedule. If it is already time for the next dose, double the dose.

2. If you are taking this medication once a day, take the dose you missed as soon as possible, unless you don't remember until the next day. In that case, do not take the missed dose at all; just follow your regular schedule. Do not double the next dose.

3. If you are taking this drug every other day, take it as soon as you remember. If you missed the scheduled time by a whole day, take it when you remember, and then skip a day before you take the next dose. Do not double the dose.

If you miss more than one dose, CONTACT YOUR DOCTOR IMMEDIATELY.

SIDE EFFECTS

Minor. Dizziness, false sense of well-being, increased appetite, increased susceptibility to infections, increased sweating, indigestion, menstrual irregularities, nausea, reddening of the skin on the face, restlessness, sleep disorders, or weight gain. These side effects should disappear as your body adjusts to the medication.

Major. Tell your doctor about any side effects that are persistent or particularly bothersome. IT IS ESPECIALLY IMPORTANT TO TELL YOUR DOCTOR about abdominal enlargement; abdominal pain; acne or other skin problems; back or rib pain; bloody or black, tarry stools; blurred vision; convulsions; eye pain; fever and sore throat; growth impairment (in children); headaches; impaired healing of wounds; increased thirst and urination; mental depression; mood changes; muscle wasting; muscle weakness; nightmares; rapid weight gain (three to five pounds within a week); rash; shortness of breath; thinning of the skin; unusual bleeding or bruising; and unusual weakness.

INTERACTIONS

Methylprednisolone interacts with several other types of medications:

1. Alcohol, aspirin, and anti-inflammatory medications (diclofenac, diflunisal, fenoprofen, flurbiprofen, ibuprofen, indomethacin, ketoprofen, mefenamic acid, meclofenamate, naproxen, piroxicam, sulindac, or tolmetin) aggravate the stomach problems that are common with use of this medication.

2. The dosage of oral anticoagulants (blood thinners, such as warfarin), oral antidiabetic medications, or insulin may need to be altered when this therapy with systemic methylprednisolone is started or stopped.

3. The loss of potassium caused by methylprednisolone can lead to serious side effects in individuals taking digoxin. Thiazide diuretics (water pills) can increase the potassium loss caused by methylprednisolone.

4. Phenobarbital, phenytoin, rifampin, and ephedrine can increase the elimination of methylprednisolone from the body, thereby decreasing its effectiveness.

5. Oral contraceptives (birth control pills) and estrogen-containing drugs may decrease the elimination of this medication from the body, which can lead to an increase in side effects.

6. Methylprednisolone can increase the elimination of aspirin and isoniazid, thereby decreasing the effectiveness of these two medications.

7. Cholestyramine and colestipol can chemically bind this medication in the stomach and gastrointestinal tract and prevent its absorption.

BE SURE TO TELL YOUR DOCTOR about any medications you are currently taking, especially any of those listed above.

WARNINGS

• Tell your doctor about unusual or allergic reactions you have had to any medications, especially to methylprednisolone or other adrenocorticosteroids (such as betamethasone, cortisone, dexamethasone, hydrocortisone, paramethasone, prednisolone, prednisone, and triamcinolone).

• Tell your doctor if you now have or if you have ever had bone disease, diabetes mellitus, emotional instability, glaucoma, fungal infections, heart disease, high blood pressure, high cholesterol levels, myasthenia gravis, peptic ulcers, osteoporosis, thyroid disease, tuberculosis, ulcerative colitis, kidney disease, or liver disease.

• To help avoid potassium loss while using this drug, take your dose with a glass of fresh or frozen orange juice or eat a banana each day. The use of a salt substitute also helps to prevent potassium loss. Check with your doctor before using a salt substitute.

• If you are using this medication for longer than a week, you may need to have your dosage adjusted if you are subjected to stress, such as serious infections, injury, or surgery. Discuss this with your doctor.

• If you have been taking this drug for more than a week, do not stop taking it suddenly. If it is stopped suddenly, you may experience abdominal or back pain, dizziness, fainting, fever, muscle or joint pain, nausea, vomiting, shortness of breath, or extreme weakness. Your doctor may, therefore, want to reduce the dosage gradually. Never increase the dosage or take the drug for longer than the prescribed time, unless you first consult your doctor.

• While you are taking methylprednisolone, you should not be vaccinated or immunized. This medication decreases the effectiveness of vaccines and can lead to overwhelming infection if a live-virus vaccine is administered.

• Before having surgery or medical or dental treatment, be sure to tell your doctor or dentist about this drug.

• Because this drug can cause glaucoma and cataracts with long-term use, your doctor may want you to have your eyes examined by an ophthalmologist periodically during treatment.

• If you are taking this medication for prolonged periods, you should wear or carry a notice or identification card stating that you are taking an adrenocorticosteroid.

• This medication can raise blood sugar levels in diabetic patients. Blood sugar levels should, therefore, be monitored carefully with blood or urine tests when this medication is being taken.

• Some of these products contain the color additive FD&C Yellow No. 5 (tartrazine), which can cause allergic-type reactions in certain susceptible individuals.

• Be sure to tell your doctor if you are pregnant. This drug crosses the placenta. Although studies in humans have not been conducted, birth defects have been observed in the fetuses of animals that were given large doses of this type of drug during pregnancy. Also, tell your doctor if you are breast-feeding an infant. Small amounts of methylprednisolone pass into breast milk and may cause growth suppression or a decrease in natural adrenocorticosteroid production in the nursing infant.

methyltestosterone

BRAND NAMES (Manufacturers)
Android (Brown)
Metandren (Ciba)
methyltestosterone (various manufacturers)
Oreton Methyl (Schering)
Testred (ICN)
Virilon (Star)

TYPE OF DRUG
Androgen

INGREDIENT
methyltestosterone

DOSAGE FORMS
Oral tablets (10 mg and 25 mg)
Buccal tablets (5 mg and 10 mg)
Capsules (10 mg)

STORAGE
Methyltestosterone should be stored at room temperature in a tightly closed container.

USES

This medication is a synthetic androgen (male hormone) that is used to treat conditions such as delayed puberty, eunuchism, or impotence in males whose bodies cannot produce enough testosterone on their own. The medication may be used to treat breast cancer in women whose breast tumor responds to hormone treatment.

TREATMENT

In order to avoid stomach irritation, you can take methyltestosterone oral tablets or capsules with food or with a full glass of water or milk (unless your doctor directs you to do otherwise).

The buccal tablet form of methyltestosterone is meant to be absorbed through the lining of the mouth, rather than swallowed. The tablet should be placed between your gum and cheek and allowed to dissolve slowly. Do not eat, drink, chew, or smoke while the tablet is dissolving.

If you miss a dose of this medication, take the missed dose as soon as possible, unless it is almost time for the next dose. In that case, do not take the missed dose at all; just return to your regular dosing schedule. Do not double the next dose of the medication.

SIDE EFFECTS
Minor. Decrease or increase in sexual desire, diarrhea, headache, loss of appetite, nausea, stomach irritation, sleeping difficulties, or vomiting. These side effects should disappear as your body adjusts to the medication.
Major. Tell your doctor about any side effects that are persistent or particularly bothersome. IT IS ESPECIALLY IMPORTANT TO TELL YOUR DOCTOR about acne; black, bloody, or tarry stools; breast enlargement or tenderness; flushing; frequent or continuous erection; hair loss or growth; hoarseness or deepening of the voice; increased urination; shortness of breath; skin rash; swelling of the hands or feet; sore throat; tiredness; unusual bleeding or bruising; or yellowing of the eyes or skin.

INTERACTIONS
Methyltestosterone interacts with several other types of medications:
1. It can increase the effects of oral anticoagulants (blood thinners, such as warfarin), which can lead to bleeding complications.
2. Diabetic patients should know that methyltestosterone can lower blood sugar levels. The dosage of oral antidiabetic medication or insulin may, therefore, require adjustment when this medication is being taken.
3. Concurrent use of methyltestosterone and adrenocorticosteroids (cortisone-like medications) can lead to fluid retention.

Before starting to take methyltestosterone, BE SURE TO TELL YOUR DOCTOR about any medications you are currently taking, especially any of those listed above.

WARNINGS
Tell your doctor about unusual or allergic reactions you have had to any medications, especially to methyltestosterone or to any other androgen (such as fluoxymesterone or testosterone).

Before starting to take this medication, be sure to tell your doctor if you now have or if you have ever had breast cancer, fluid retention, heart disease, hypercalcemia (high blood calcium levels), kidney disease, liver disease, or prostate disorders.

Although androgens have been used by athletes to increase muscle strength, there is no conclusive evidence that these drugs increase athletic performance. There is also some question as to their safety.

High-dose methyltestosterone therapy may cause infertility in males.

Some of these products contain the color additive FD&C Yellow No. 5 (tartrazine), which can cause allergic-type reactions (fainting, rash, shortness of breath) in certain susceptible individuals.

Be sure to tell your doctor if you are pregnant. If methyltestosterone is taken by a pregnant woman, it can cause masculine characteristics in the developing fetus, such as increased body hair. (Note: This does NOT affect the sex of the fetus, which is determined at conception.) Also, tell your doctor if you are breast-feeding an infant. Methyltestosterone passes into breast milk and can cause masculinization of the nursing infant.

Meticorten—see prednisone (systemic)

metoclopramide

BRAND NAMES (Manufacturers)
Clopra (Quantum)
Maxolon (Beecham)
metoclopramide (various manufacturers)
Reglan (Robins)
TYPE OF DRUG
Dopamine antagonist and antiemetic
INGREDIENT
metoclopramide
DOSAGE FORMS
Tablets (5 mg and 10 mg)
Oral syrup (5 mg per 5-ml spoonful)
STORAGE
Metoclopramide tablets and oral syrup should be stored at room temperature in tightly closed containers. Do not freeze the syrup form of this medication.

USES
This medication is used to relieve the symptoms associated with diabetic gastric stasis or gastric reflux and to prevent nausea and vomiting. Metoclopramide acts directly on the vomiting center in the brain to prevent nausea and vomiting. It also increases the movement of the stomach and intestines.

TREATMENT
To obtain the best results from treatment, you should take metoclopramide tablets or syrup 30 minutes before a meal and at bedtime.

Each dose of the syrup should be measured carefully with a specially designed 5-ml measuring spoon. An ordinary kitchen teaspoon is not accurate enough.

If you miss a dose of this medication, take the missed dose as soon as possible, unless it is almost time for the next dose. In that case, do not take the missed dose at all; just return to your regular dosing schedule. Do not double the next dose.

SIDE EFFECTS
Minor. Diarrhea, dizziness, drowsiness, dry mouth, fatigue, headache, insomnia, nausea, restlessness, or weakness. These side effects should disappear as your body adjusts to the medication.

If you feel dizzy or light-headed, sit or lie down for a while; get up slowly from a sitting or reclining position, and be careful on stairs.

To relieve mouth dryness, chew sugarless gum or suck on ice chips or a piece of hard candy.

Major. Tell your doctor about any side effects that are persistent or particularly bothersome. IT IS ESPECIALLY IMPORTANT TO TELL YOUR DOCTOR about anxiety; confusion; depression; disorientation; involuntary movements of the eyes, face, or limbs; muscle spasms; rash; or trembling of the hands.

INTERACTIONS

Metoclopramide interacts with several types of drugs:

1. Concurrent use of metoclopramide with other central nervous system depressants (such as alcohol, antihistamines, barbiturates, muscle relaxants, narcotics, pain medications, phenothiazine tranquilizers, benzodiazepine tranquilizers, and sleeping medications) or with tricyclic antidepressants can cause extreme drowsiness.

2. Narcotic analgesics may block the effectiveness of metoclopramide.

3. Metoclopramide can block the effectiveness of bromocriptine. It can also decrease the absorption of cimetidine and digoxin from the gastrointestinal tract, decreasing their effectiveness.

4. Metoclopramide can increase the absorption of acetaminophen, tetracycline, levodopa, and alcohol.

5. Diabetic patients should know that dosage requirements of insulin may change when metoclopramide is being taken.

Before starting to take metoclopramide, BE SURE TO TELL YOUR DOCTOR about any medications you are currently taking, especially any of those listed above.

WARNINGS

• Tell your doctor about unusual or allergic reactions you have had to any medications, especially to metoclopramide, procaine, or procainamide.

• Before starting to take metoclopramide, be sure to tell your doctor if you now have or if you have ever had epilepsy, kidney disease, liver disease, intestinal bleeding or blockage, Parkinson's disease, or pheochromocytoma.

• If this drug makes you dizzy or drowsy, do not take part in any activities that require alertness, such as driving a car or operating potentially dangerous machinery.

• Be sure to tell your doctor if you are pregnant. Extensive studies in women during pregnancy have not been conducted. Also, tell your doctor if you are breast-feeding an infant. Metoclopramide passes into breast milk.

metolazone

BRAND NAMES (Manufacturers)
Diulo (Searle)
Microx (Pennwalt)
Zaroxolyn (Pennwalt)
TYPE OF DRUG
Diuretic and antihypertensive

INGREDIENT
metolazone
DOSAGE FORM
Tablets (2.5 mg, 5 mg, and 10 mg)
STORAGE
This medication should be stored at room temperature in a tightly closed container.

USES

Metolazone is prescribed to treat high blood pressure. It is also used to reduce fluid accumulation in the body caused by conditions such as heart failure, cirrhosis of the liver, kidney disease, and the long-term use of some medications. Metolazone reduces fluid accumulation by increasing the elimination of salt and water through the kidneys.

TREATMENT

To decrease stomach irritation, you can take this medication with a glass of milk or with a meal (unless your doctor directs you to do otherwise). Try to take it at the same time every day. Avoid taking a dose after 6:00 P.M.; otherwise, you may have to get up during the night to urinate.

If you miss a dose of this medication, take the missed dose as soon as possible, unless it is almost time for the next dose. In that case, do not take the missed dose at all; just wait until the next scheduled dose. Do not double the dose.

This medication does not cure high blood pressure, but it will help to control the condition as long as you take it.

SIDE EFFECTS

Minor. Constipation, cramps, diarrhea, dizziness, drowsiness, headache, heartburn, loss of appetite, restlessness, or upset stomach. As your body adjusts to the medication, these side effects should disappear.

This medication can cause increased sensitivity to sunlight. It is, therefore, important to avoid prolonged exposure to sunlight and sunlamps. Wear protective clothing, and use an effective sunscreen.

To relieve constipation, increase the amount of fiber in your diet (fresh fruits and vegetables, salads, bran, and whole-grain breads) and exercise more (unless your doctor directs you to do otherwise).

To avoid dizziness or light-headedness when you stand, contract and relax the muscles of your legs for a few moments before rising. Do this by pushing one foot against the floor while raising the other foot slightly, alternating feet so that you are "pumping" your legs in a pedaling motion. Also, be very careful going up and down the stairs.

Major. Tell your doctor about any side effects that are persistent or particularly bothersome. IT IS ESPECIALLY IMPORTANT TO TELL YOUR DOCTOR about blurred vision, confusion, difficulty in breathing, dry mouth, excessive thirst, excessive weakness, fever, itching, joint pain, mood changes, muscle spasms, nausea, palpitations, skin rash, sore throat, tingling in the fingers or toes, unusual bleeding or bruising, vomiting, or yellowing of the eyes or skin.

INTERACTIONS

Metolazone interacts with several other types of drugs:

1. It may decrease the effectiveness of oral anticoagulants, antigout medications, insulin, oral antidiabetic medicines, and methenamine.

2. Fenfluramine can increase the blood-pressure-lowering effects of metolazone (which can be dangerous).

3. Indomethacin can decrease the blood-pressure-lowering effects of metolazone, and counteract the desired effects.

4. Cholestyramine and colestipol decrease the absorption of this medication from the gastrointestinal tract. Metolazone should, therefore, be taken one hour before or four hours after a dose of cholestyramine or colestipol (if you have also been prescribed one of these medications).

5. The side effects of amphotericin B, calcium, cortisone and cortisone-like steroids (such as dexamethasone, hydrocortisone, prednisone, and prednisolone), digitalis, digoxin, lithium, quinidine, sulfonamide antibiotics, and vitamin D may be increased when these drugs are taken concurrently with metolazone.

Before starting to take metolazone, BE SURE TO TELL YOUR DOCTOR about any medications you are currently taking, especially any of those listed above.

WARNINGS

• Tell your doctor about unusual or allergic reactions you have had to any medications, especially to metolazone or to any other sulfa drugs, including other diuretics, oral antidiabetic medications, or sulfonamide antibiotics.

• Tell your doctor if you now have or if you have ever had kidney disease or problems with urination, diabetes mellitus, gout, liver disease, asthma, pancreatic disease, or systemic lupus erythematosus.

• Metolazone can cause potassium loss. Signs of potassium loss include dry mouth, thirst, weakness, muscle pain or cramps, nausea, and vomiting. If you experience any of these symptoms, call your doctor. To help avoid potassium loss, take this drug with a glass of fresh or frozen orange juice or cranberry juice, or eat a banana every day. The use of a salt substitute also helps to prevent potassium loss. Do not change your diet or use a salt substitute, however, before discussing it with your doctor. Too much potassium can also be dangerous. Your doctor may want to have blood tests performed periodically to monitor your potassium levels.

• Limit your intake of alcoholic beverages while taking this medication, in order to prevent dizziness.

• Do not take any over-the-counter (nonprescription) medications for weight control or for cough, cold, allergy, asthma, or sinus problems unless your doctor directs you to do so. Some of these products can increase blood pressure.

• To prevent dehydration (severe water loss) while taking this medication, check with your doctor if you have any illness that causes severe or continuous nausea, vomiting, or diarrhea.

• This medication can raise blood sugar levels in diabetic patients. Therefore, blood sugar levels should be carefully monitored by blood or urine tests when this medication is being taken.

• Be sure to tell your doctor if you are pregnant. Metolazone can cross the placenta and may cause adverse effects in the fetus. Also, tell your doctor if you are breast-feeding an infant. Although problems in humans have not been reported, small amounts of this drug can pass into breast milk, so caution is warranted.

---

metoprolol

BRAND NAME (Manufacturer)
Lopressor (Geigy)
TYPE OF DRUG
Beta-adrenergic blocking agent
INGREDIENT
metoprolol
DOSAGE FORM
Tablets (50 mg and 100 mg)
STORAGE
Metoprolol should be stored at room temperature in a tightly closed, light-resistant container.

USES

Metoprolol is used to treat high blood pressure and angina (chest pain) and to prevent additional heart attacks in heart attack patients. Metoprolol belongs to a group of medicines known as beta-adrenergic blocking agents or, more commonly, beta blockers. These drugs work by controlling nerve impulses along certain nerve pathways.

TREATMENT

Metoprolol can be taken with a glass of water, with meals, immediately following meals, or on an empty stomach, depending on your doctor's instructions. Try to take the medication at the same time(s) each day.

Try not to miss any doses of this medicine. If you do miss a dose of the medication, take the missed dose as soon as possible. However, if the next scheduled dose is within eight hours (if you are taking this medicine only once a day) or within four hours (if you are taking this medicine more than once a day), do not take the missed dose of the medication at all; just return to your regular dosing schedule. Do not double the next dose of the medication.

It is important to remember that metoprolol does not cure high blood pressure, but it will help to control the condition as long as you continue to take it.

SIDE EFFECTS

Minor. Anxiety; cold hands or feet (due to decreased blood circulation to the skin, fingers, and toes); constipation; decreased sexual ability; diarrhea; difficulty in sleeping; drowsiness; dryness of the eyes, mouth, and skin; headache; nausea; nervousness; stomach discomfort; tiredness; or weakness. These side effects should disappear during treatment, as your body adjusts to the medicine.

If you are extra-sensitive to the cold, be sure to dress warmly during cold weather.

To relieve constipation, increase the amount of fiber in your diet (fresh fruits and vegetables, salads, bran, and whole-grain breads) and exercise more (unless your doctor directs you to do otherwise).

Plain, nonmedicated eye drops (artificial tears) may help to relieve eye dryness.

Chew sugarless gum or suck on ice chips or a piece of hard candy to relieve mouth or throat dryness.

Major. Tell your doctor about any side effects that are persistent or particularly bothersome. IT IS ESPECIALLY IMPORTANT TO TELL YOUR DOCTOR about breathing difficulty or wheezing, confusion, dizziness, fever and sore throat, hair loss, hallucinations, light-headedness, mental depression, nightmares, numbness or tingling of the fingers or toes, rapid weight gain (three to five pounds within a week), reduced alertness, skin rash, swelling, or unusual bleeding or bruising.

INTERACTIONS

Metoprolol interacts with several other types of medications:

1. Indomethacin, aspirin, or other salicylates may decrease the blood-pressure-lowering effects of beta blockers.

2. Concurrent use of beta blockers and calcium channel blockers or disopyramide can lead to heart failure or very low blood pressure.

3. Cimetidine and oral contraceptives (birth control pills) can increase the blood concentrations of metoprolol, which can result in greater side effects.

4. Alcohol, barbiturates, and rifampin can decrease the effectiveness of metoprolol.

5. Side effects may be increased if beta blockers are taken with clonidine, digoxin, epinephrine, phenylephrine, phenylpropanolamine, phenothiazine tranquilizers, prazosin, or monoamine oxidase (MAO) inhibitors. At least 14 days should separate the use of a beta blocker and the use of an MAO inhibitor.

6. Beta blockers may antagonize (work against) the effects of theophylline, aminophylline, albuterol, isoproterenol, metaproterenol, and terbutaline.

7. Beta blockers can also interact with insulin or oral antidiabetic agents, raising or lowering blood sugar levels and masking the symptoms of low blood sugar.

8. The action of beta blockers may be increased if they are used with chlorpromazine, furosemide, or hydralazine, which may have a negative effect.

BE SURE TO TELL YOUR DOCTOR about any medications you are currently taking, especially any listed above.

WARNINGS

• Tell your doctor if you have ever had unusual or allergic reactions to any drugs, especially to metoprolol or any other beta blocker (acebutolol, atenolol, carteolol, esmolol, labetalol, nadolol, penbutolol, pindolol, propranolol, or timolol).

• Tell your doctor if you now have or have ever had allergies, asthma, hay fever, eczema, slow heartbeat, bronchitis, diabetes mellitus, emphysema, heart or blood vessel disease, kidney disease, liver disease, thyroid disease, or poor circulation in the fingers or toes.

• You may want to check your pulse while taking this medication. If your pulse is much slower than your usual rate (or if it is less than 50 beats per minute), check with your doctor. A pulse rate that is too slow may cause circulation problems.

• This medicine may affect your body's response to exercise. Make sure you discuss with your doctor a safe amount of exercise for your medical condition.

• It is important that you do not stop taking this medicine without first checking with your doctor. Some conditions may become worse when the medicine is stopped suddenly, and the danger of a heart attack is increased in some patients. Your doctor may want you to reduce gradually the amount of medicine you take before stopping completely to minimize the potential risks. Make sure that you have enough medicine on hand to last through vacations, holidays, and weekends.

• Before having surgery or any other medical or dental treatment, tell your doctor or dentist that you are taking metoprolol. Often, this medication will be discontinued 48 hours prior to any major surgery.

• Metoprolol can cause dizziness, drowsiness, light-headedness, or decreased alertness. Exercise caution while driving a car or using any potentially dangerous machinery.

• While taking this medicine, do not use any over-the-counter (nonprescription) allergy, asthma, cough, cold, sinus, or diet preparation without first checking with your pharmacist or doctor. Some of these medicines can result in high blood pressure when taken at the same time as a beta blocker.

• Be sure to tell your doctor if you are pregnant. Animal studies have shown that some beta blockers, when used in very high doses, can cause problems in pregnancy. Adequate studies have not been conducted in humans, but there has been some association between beta blockers used during pregnancy and low birth weight, as well as breathing problems and slow heart rate in newborn infants. However, other reports have shown no effects on newborn infants. Also, tell your doctor if you are breast-feeding an infant. Although this medicine has not been shown to cause problems in breast-fed infants, some of the medicine may pass into breast milk, so caution is warranted.

Metra—see phendimetrazine

MetroGel—see metronidazole

metronidazole

BRAND NAMES (Manufacturers)
Femazole (Major)
Flagyl (Searle)
Metezole (Glenwood)
MetroGel (Curatab)
metronidazole (various manufacturers)
Metryl (Lemmon)
Protostat (Ortho)
Satric (Savage)
TYPE OF DRUG
Antibiotic and antiparasitic

INGREDIENT
metronidazole
DOSAGE FORMS
Tablets (250 mg and 500 mg)
Topical gel (0.75%)
STORAGE
Metronidazole should be stored at room temperature in a tightly closed, light-resistant container. The topical gel form of this medication should never be frozen.

USES
Metronidazole is used to treat a wide variety of infections, including infections of the vagina, urinary tract, lower respiratory tract, bones, joints, intestinal tract, and skin. It is also used topically to treat acne rosacea. It acts by killing bacteria or parasites.

TREATMENT
In order to avoid stomach irritation, you should take metronidazole with food or with a full glass of water or milk (unless your doctor directs you to do otherwise).

Metronidazole works best when the level of medicine in your bloodstream is kept constant. It is best, therefore, to take the doses at evenly spaced intervals day and night. For example, if you are to take three doses a day, the doses should be spaced eight hours apart.

Try not to miss any doses of this medication. If you do miss a dose, take the missed dose as soon as possible, unless it is almost time for the next dose. In that case, do not take the missed dose at all; just return to your regular dosing schedule. Do not double the next dose.

It is important to continue to take this medication for the entire time prescribed by your doctor (usually seven to 14 days), even if the symptoms disappear before the end of that period. If you stop taking the drug too soon, resistant bacteria and parasites are given a chance to continue growing, and the infection could recur.

SIDE EFFECTS
Minor. Abdominal cramps, constipation, decreased sexual interest, diarrhea, dizziness, dry mouth, headache, insomnia, irritability, joint pain, loss of appetite, metallic taste in the mouth, nasal congestion, nausea, restlessness, or vomiting. These side effects should disappear as your body adjusts to the medication.

To relieve constipation, increase the amount of fiber in your diet (fresh fruits and vegetables, salads, bran, and whole-grain breads), exercise, and drink more water (unless your doctor directs you to do otherwise).

If you feel dizzy, sit or lie down for a while.

To relieve mouth dryness, chew sugarless gum or suck on ice chips or a piece of hard candy.

Major. Tell your doctor about any side effects that are persistent or particularly bothersome. IT IS ESPECIALLY IMPORTANT TO TELL YOUR DOCTOR about confusion, convulsions, flushing, hives, itching, joint pain, loss of bladder control, mouth sores, numbness or tingling in the fingers or toes, rash, sense of pressure inside your abdomen, unexplained sore throat and fever, or unusual weakness. Also, if your symptoms of infection seem to be getting worse rather than improving, you should contact your doctor.

INTERACTIONS
Metronidazole interacts with several other types of medications:

1. Concurrent use of alcohol and metronidazole can lead to a severe reaction (abdominal cramps, nausea, vomiting, headache, and flushing), the severity of which is dependent upon the amount of alcohol ingested.

2. Concurrent use of disulfiram and metronidazole can lead to confusion.

3. The effects of oral anticoagulants (blood thinners, such as warfarin) may be increased by metronidazole, which can lead to bleeding complications.

4. Barbiturates can increase the breakdown of metronidazole, which can decrease its effectiveness.

5. Cimetidine can decrease the breakdown of metronidazole, which can increase the chance of side effects.

BE SURE TO TELL YOUR DOCTOR about any medications you are currently taking, especially any of those listed above.

WARNINGS
• Tell your doctor about unusual or allergic reactions you have had to any medications.

• Before starting to take this medication, be sure to tell your doctor if you now have or if you have ever had blood disorders, a central nervous system (brain or spinal cord) disease, or liver disease.

• When metronidazole is used to treat a vaginal infection, sexual partners should receive concurrent therapy in order to prevent reinfection. In addition, sexual intercourse should be avoided or condoms should be used until treatment is completed.

• This medication has been prescribed for your current infection only. Another infection later on, or one that someone else has, may require different drug therapy. Therefore, you should not give your medicine to other people or use it for other infections, unless your doctor specifically directs you to do so.

• If this drug makes you dizzy, avoid tasks that require alertness, such as driving a car or operating potentially dangerous machinery.

• Before having surgery or any other medical or dental treatment, be sure to tell your doctor or dentist that you are taking this medication.

• Be sure to tell your doctor if you are pregnant. Although metronidazole appears to be safe, it does cross the placenta, and extensive studies in pregnant women have not been conducted. Also, tell your doctor if you are breast-feeding an infant. Metronidazole passes into breast milk.

Metryl—see metronidazole

Mevacor—see lovastatin

mexiletine

BRAND NAME (Manufacturer)
Mexitil (Boehringer Ingelheim)
TYPE OF DRUG
Antiarrhythmic

INGREDIENT
mexiletine
DOSAGE FORM
Capsules (150 mg, 200 mg, and 250 mg)
STORAGE
Mexiletine should be stored at room temperature in a tightly closed container. It should not be exposed to high temperatures.

USES

Mexiletine is used to treat arrhythmias (irregular heart rhythms). This medication works through the suppression of irregular heartbeats and the establishment of a more normal rhythm.

TREATMENT

Mexiletine can be taken with meals or an antacid to decrease stomach irritation.

Try to take mexiletine at the same times each day. This medication is most effective when the amount of the drug in your bloodstream is kept at a constant level. Mexiletine should, therefore, be taken at evenly spaced intervals day and night. For example, if you are supposed to take mexiletine three times per day, the doses should be spaced eight hours apart. Your doctor can determine the best dose of mexiletine for you by measuring the amount in your blood. You may need periodic blood tests for this reason.

If you miss a dose of this medication and remember within four hours (if you are taking it three times per day) or within six hours (if you are taking it two times per day), take the missed dose and then return to your regular dosing schedule. If more than that time has passed, do not take the missed dose; just return to your regular dosing schedule. Do not double the next dose.

SIDE EFFECTS

Minor. Abdominal pain, altered taste, changes in appetite, constipation, diarrhea, dizziness, dry skin, fatigue, fluid accumulation, headaches, heartburn, hiccups, hot flashes, light-headedness, nausea, nervousness, sleeping problems, slowed heart rate, sweating, vomiting, or weakness. These side effects should disappear as your body adjusts to the medication.

You may experience constipation when taking this drug. To relieve constipation, increase the amount of fiber in your diet (fresh fruits and vegetables, salads, bran, and whole-grain breads), exercise, and drink more water (unless your doctor directs you to do otherwise).

If you become dizzy, sit or lie down for a while; get up slowly from a sitting or reclining position, and be careful on stairs.

Major. Tell your doctor about any side effects that are persistent or particularly bothersome. IT IS ESPECIALLY IMPORTANT TO TELL YOUR DOCTOR about black or tarry stools, chest pain, confusion, coordination difficulties, depression, difficult or painful urination, fainting, fever, hair loss, impotence, palpitations, psychological changes, rash, ringing in the ears, seizures, shortness of breath, speech difficulties, tingling or numbness in the hands or feet, trembling of the hands, or visual disturbances.

INTERACTIONS

Mexiletine interacts with several other types of medications:

1. Acetazolamide, sodium bicarbonate, or high doses of antacids can decrease the elimination of mexiletine from the body, which can increase the risks of side effects.
2. Cimetidine can increase the blood levels of mexiletine, which can increase the risks of side effects.
3. Phenytoin, rifampin, and phenobarbital can decrease the blood levels of mexiletine, which can decrease its effectiveness.

Before starting mexiletine, BE SURE TO TELL YOUR DOCTOR about any medications you are currently taking, especially any of those listed above.

WARNINGS

• Tell your doctor about any unusual or allergic reactions you have had to any medications, especially to mexiletine.
• Before taking mexiletine, tell your doctor if you now have or if you have ever had heart block, heart failure, liver disease, low blood pressure, or seizures.
• If this drug makes you dizzy or light-headed, do not take part in any activity that requires alertness, such as driving a car.
• Before having surgery or any other medical or dental treatment, be sure to tell your doctor or dentist that you are taking mexiletine.
• Do not take any over-the-counter (nonprescription) asthma, allergy, sinus, cough, cold, or diet preparation without first checking with your pharmacist or doctor.
• Do not stop taking this drug without first consulting your doctor. Stopping antiarrhythmics abruptly may cause a serious change in the activity of your heart. Your doctor may, therefore, want to reduce your dosage gradually.
• Be sure to tell your doctor if you are pregnant. Although mexiletine appears to be safe in animals, studies in pregnant women have not been conducted. Also, tell your doctor if you are breast-feeding an infant. Small amounts of mexiletine pass into human breast milk.

Mexitil—see mexiletine

---

miconazole (vaginal)

BRAND NAMES (Manufacturers)
Monistat 3 (Ortho)*
Monistat 7 (Ortho)*
Monistat Dual-Pak (Ortho)*
*Available without a prescription.
TYPE OF DRUG
Vaginal antifungal agent
INGREDIENT
miconazole
DOSAGE FORMS
Vaginal cream (2%)
Lotion (2%)
Vaginal suppositories (100 mg and 200 mg)
STORAGE
Store at room temperature in a tightly closed container.

USES

Miconazole is used to treat fungal infections of the vagina. This medication is an antifungal agent that prevents the growth and multiplication of the yeast-like fungus *Candida.*

TREATMENT

Miconazole vaginal cream and suppositories are packaged with detailed directions for use. Follow these instructions carefully. An applicator will probably be provided.

You should wash the vaginal area carefully prior to inserting the cream or suppository.

If you begin to menstruate while being treated with miconazole, continue with your regular dosing schedule.

If you miss a dose, insert the missed dose as soon as possible. However, if you do not remember until the following day, do not insert the missed dose at all; just return to your regular dosing schedule. Do not double the dose.

It is important to continue to insert this medication for the entire time prescribed by your doctor, even if the symptoms disappear before the end of that time. If you stop using the drug too soon, your infection could recur.

Usually, one three-day or one seven-day course of miconazole is sufficient. However, it may be repeated if your doctor determines that *Candida* is still causing your infection.

SIDE EFFECTS

Minor. You may experience vaginal burning, itching, or irritation when this drug is inserted. This sensation should disappear as your body adjusts to the medication.

Do not treat any side effects that occur in the area of the infection unless you first consult your doctor.

Major. Tell your doctor about any side effects that are persistent or particularly bothersome. IT IS ESPECIALLY IMPORTANT TO TELL YOUR DOCTOR about headache, hives, pelvic cramps, or skin rash.

INTERACTIONS

Miconazole (vaginal) does not interact with other medications if it is used according to directions.

WARNINGS

• Tell your doctor about unusual or allergic reactions you have had to any medications, especially to miconazole.

• Tell your doctor if you have had other vaginal infections, especially if they have been resistant to treatment.

• To prevent reinfection, avoid sexual intercourse or ask your partner to use a condom until treatment is complete.

• There may be some vaginal drainage while you are using this medication; therefore, you may want to use a sanitary napkin or panty liner to prevent the staining of clothing.

• Wear cotton panties rather than those made of nylon or other nonporous materials while being treated for a fungal infection of the vagina. Also, in order to prevent reinfection, always wear freshly laundered underclothes.

• If there is no improvement in your condition, or if irritation in the area continues after several days of treatment, CONTACT YOUR DOCTOR. This medication may be causing an allergic reaction, or it may not be effective against the organism causing your infection.

• Miconazole has been prescribed for your current infection only. Another infection later on, or one that someone else has, may require a different medication. You should not give your medication to other women or use it for other infections you might have, unless your doctor specifically directs you to do so.

• Be sure to tell your doctor if you are pregnant. Small amounts of miconazole have been shown to be absorbed from the vagina, so caution should be used when using this medication. In addition, your doctor may want to change the instructions on how you are to insert this medication if you are pregnant. Also, tell your doctor if you are breast-feeding an infant. It is not known whether miconazole passes into breast milk.

Micrainin—see meprobamate and aspirin combination

Micro-K—see potassium chloride

Micro-K Extencaps—see potassium chloride

Micronase—see glyburide

Microsulfon—see sulfonamide antibiotics (oral)

Microx—see metolazone

Mictrin—see hydrochlorothiazide

Midamor—see amiloride

Midol 200—see ibuprofen

Millazine—see thioridazine

Milophene—see clomiphene

Miltown—see meprobamate

Minipress—see prazosin

Minocin—see minocycline

minocycline

BRAND NAME (Manufacturer)
Minocin (Lederle)
TYPE OF DRUG
Antibiotic
INGREDIENT
minocycline
DOSAGE FORMS
Capsules (50 mg and 100 mg)
Tablets (50 mg and 100 mg)
Oral suspension (50 mg per 5-ml spoonful, with 5% alcohol)
STORAGE
Minocycline should be stored at room temperature in tightly closed, light-resistant containers.

USES

Minocycline is used to treat a wide range of bacterial infections and to prevent meningococcal meningitis. It acts by preventing the growth of bacteria. This drug kills susceptible bacteria, but it is not effective against viruses or fungi.

TREATMENT

To avoid stomach upset, you can take this medication with food (unless your doctor directs you to do otherwise).

The suspension form of this medication should be shaken well just before measuring each dose. The contents tend to settle on the bottom of the bottle, so it is necessary to shake the container to distribute the ingredients evenly and equalize the doses. Each dose should be measured carefully with a specially designed 5-ml measuring spoon. An ordinary kitchen teaspoon is not accurate enough.

Minocycline works best when the level of medicine in your bloodstream is kept constant. It is best, therefore, to take the doses at evenly spaced intervals day and night. For example, if you are to take two doses a day, the doses should be spaced 12 hours apart.

If you miss a dose of this medication, take the missed dose immediately. However, if you do not remember to take the missed dose until it is almost time for your next dose, take it; space the following dose about halfway through the regular interval between doses; then return to your regular dosing schedule. Try not to skip any doses.

It is important to continue to take this medication for the entire time prescribed by your doctor, even if the symptoms disappear before the end of that period. If you stop taking the drug too soon, resistant bacteria are given a chance to continue growing, and the infection could recur.

SIDE EFFECTS

Minor. Diarrhea, dizziness, headache, light-headedness, loss of appetite, nausea, stomach cramps and upset, vomiting, or discoloration of the nails. These side effects should disappear as your body adjusts to the medication.

Minocycline can increase your sensitivity to sunlight. You should, therefore, try to avoid prolonged exposure to sunlight and sunlamps. Wear protective clothing and sunglasses, and use an effective sunscreen.

If you feel dizzy or light-headed, sit or lie down for a while; get up from a sitting or lying position slowly, and be careful on stairs.

Major. Tell your doctor about any side effects that are persistent or particularly bothersome. IT IS ESPECIALLY IMPORTANT TO TELL YOUR DOCTOR about darkened tongue, difficulty in breathing, joint pain, mouth irritation, rash, rectal or vaginal itching, sore throat and fever, unusual bleeding or bruising, or yellowing of the eyes or skin. Also, if your symptoms of infection seem to be getting worse rather than improving, you should contact your doctor.

INTERACTIONS

Minocycline interacts with several other types of medications:

1. It can increase the absorption of digoxin, which may lead to digoxin toxicity.

2. The gastrointestinal side effects (nausea, vomiting, and stomach upset) of theophylline may be increased by minocycline.

3. The dosage of oral anticoagulants (blood thinners, such as warfarin) may need to be adjusted when this medication is started.

4. Minocycline may decrease the effectiveness of oral contraceptives (birth control pills), and pregnancy could result. You should, therefore, use a different or additional form of birth control while taking minocycline. Discuss this with your doctor.

5. Antacids, calcium channel blockers, and iron may decrease the effects of this drug if they are taken at the same time. Two to three hours should separate doses of these medications and minocycline.

BE SURE TO TELL YOUR DOCTOR about any medications you are currently taking.

WARNINGS

• Tell your doctor about unusual or allergic reactions you have had to any medications, especially to minocycline or to oxytetracycline, doxycycline, or tetracycline.

• Tell your doctor if you now have or if you have ever had kidney or liver disease.

• Minocycline can cause dizziness or light-headedness. Your ability to perform tasks that require alertness, such as driving a car or operating potentially dangerous machinery, may be decreased. Appropriate caution should, therefore, be taken.

• Minocycline can affect tests for syphilis; tell your doctor you are taking this medication if you are also being treated for this disease.

• Make sure that your prescription for this medication is marked with the expiration date. The drug should be discarded after the expiration date. If the drug is used after this date, serious side effects (especially to the kidneys) could result.

• This medication has been prescribed for your current infection only. Another infection later on, or one that someone else has, may require a different medicine. You should not give your medicine to other people or use it for other infections, unless your doctor specifically directs you to do so.

• Be sure to tell your doctor if you are pregnant or if you are breast-feeding an infant. Minocycline crosses the placenta and passes into breast milk. In addition, it should not be used for infants or for children less than eight years of age. This drug can cause permanent discoloration of the teeth and can inhibit tooth and bone growth if used during their development.

Minodyl—see minoxidil (systemic)

minoxidil (systemic)

BRAND NAMES (Manufacturers)
Loniten (Upjohn)
Minodyl (Quantum)

TYPE OF DRUG
Antihypertensive
INGREDIENT
minoxidil
DOSAGE FORM
Tablets (2.5 mg and 10 mg)
STORAGE
Minoxidil should be stored at room temperature in a tightly closed container.

USES
In its oral tablet form, minoxidil is prescribed by doctors to treat high blood pressure. This medication lowers blood pressure by dilating (widening) the blood vessels in the body.

TREATMENT
Minoxidil can be taken either on an empty stomach or with food or a full glass of water or milk (as directed by your doctor or pharmacist).

In order to become accustomed to taking this medication, try to take it at the same time(s) each day.

Minoxidil does not cure high blood pressure, but it will help to control the condition as long as you continue to take the medication.

If you miss a dose of this medication, take the missed dose as soon as possible, unless it is almost time for your next dose. In that case, do not take the missed dose at all; just return to your regular dosing schedule. Do not double the next dose.

SIDE EFFECTS
Minor. Fatigue, flushing, headache, nausea, or vomiting. These side effects should disappear as your body adjusts to the medication.
Major. Tell your doctor about any side effects that are persistent or particularly bothersome. IT IS ESPECIALLY IMPORTANT TO TELL YOUR DOCTOR about abnormal hair growth, breast tenderness (in both sexes), chest pain, difficult or painful urination, darkening of the skin, palpitations, rapid weight gain (three to five pounds within a week), skin rash, or unusual bleeding or bruising.

INTERACTIONS
Concurrent use of minoxidil and guanethidine can cause a severe drop in blood pressure.

BE SURE TO TELL YOUR DOCTOR about any medications you are currently taking, especially if you are taking guanethidine.

WARNINGS
• Tell your doctor about unusual or allergic reactions you have had to any medications, especially to minoxidil.
• Before starting to take this medication, be sure to tell your doctor if you have ever had angina, heart failure, a heart attack, kidney disease, pericardial effusions, pheochromocytoma, or a stroke.
• Do not take any over-the-counter (nonprescription) cough, cold, allergy, asthma, sinus, or diet medications unless you first check with your doctor or pharmacist. Some of these products can increase your blood pressure.

• Do not stop taking minoxidil unless you first check with your doctor. Stopping the drug abruptly may lead to a worsening of your high blood pressure. Your doctor may, therefore, want to reduce your dosage gradually or start you on another medication when you stop taking minoxidil in order to prevent this from occurring.
• Be sure to tell your doctor if you are pregnant. Birth defects have been reported in the offspring of animals that received large doses of minoxidil during pregnancy. Also, tell your doctor if you are breast-feeding an infant. Minoxidil passes into breast milk, and it is recommended that a woman taking this medication should not breast-feed.

minoxidil (topical)

BRAND NAME (Manufacturer)
Rogaine (Upjohn)
TYPE OF DRUG
Hair growth stimulant
INGREDIENT
minoxidil
DOSAGE FORM
2% solution (20 mg per ml); 60 ml bottle
STORAGE
Minoxidil topical solution should be stored at room temperature in a tightly closed container. It should be kept away from heat or flames because the solution is flammable (it contains alcohol).

USES
Minoxidil topical solution is used to stimulate hair growth in men who are balding. The drug seems to exert its maximum effect at the crown of the head. The exact way that it works is not known, but it may stimulate hair growth by improving the blood supply to the hair follicles.

TREATMENT
Before applying topical minoxidil, the hair and scalp should be dry. To avoid skin irritation from the alcohol contained in this product, wait at least 30 minutes after washing or shaving before applying this medication to the scalp. The evening dose of medication should be applied at least 30 minutes before bedtime for more complete absorption of the medication into the scalp. This will prevent the medication from rubbing onto the pillowcase.

Complete directions for the use of this product are supplied with the medication. Be sure to ask your doctor or pharmacist for these directions, and follow the instructions carefully. The solution is packaged with three applicators that can be used to apply the solution directly to the scalp. Apply 1 ml to the balding areas of the scalp twice daily (in the morning and evening), unless directed to do otherwise by your doctor. Six sprays with either of the spray applicators deliver a 1-ml dose. The rub-on applicator delivers a 1-ml dose when the bottle is squeezed to fill the top chamber to the black line. The full amount in the chamber should then be applied to the scalp. The total daily dosage should not exceed 2 ml. If finger tips are used to apply the solution, wash hands afterwards to avoid spreading the medication to the eyes or other parts of the body.

Two daily applications for up to 4 months may be required before evidence of hair regrowth is observed. The onset and degree of hair regrowth may be variable among different patients treated with this medicine. If hair regrowth occurs, two daily applications are necessary for additional and continued hair growth (unless your doctor directs otherwise).

First hair growth may be soft, downy, colorless hair that is barely visible. After further treatment, the new hair should be the same color and thickness as the other hair on the scalp.

If one or two applications are missed, restart twice daily applications and return to the usual schedule. Do not attempt to make up for missed doses.

It is important to continue to use this medication for the entire time prescribed by your doctor, even if hair growth does not appear within several months.

If there is no hair growth after at least four months or more, consult with your doctor, as this medication may not be effective for you.

SIDE EFFECTS

Minor. Diarrhea, dry skin/scalp, flaking, itching, local redness, nausea, or vomiting. These side effects should disappear as your body adjusts to the medication.
Major. Tell your doctor about any side effects that are persistent or particularly bothersome. IT IS ESPECIALLY IMPORTANT TO TELL YOUR DOCTOR about back pain, chest pain, cough, cold, dizziness, faintness, light-headedness, rapid heart beat, fluid retention, headache, weight gain, or worsening of hair loss.

INTERACTIONS

Use of abrasive or medicated cleansers, medicated cleaners, medicated cosmetics, or any topical, alcohol-containing preparations (such as after-shave lotions or cologne) along with topical minoxidil solution can result in excessive skin dryness and irritation.

WARNINGS

• Tell your doctor about unusual or allergic reactions you have had to any medications, especially to minoxidil.
• Before starting to use this medication, be sure to tell your doctor if you now have or if you have ever had heart disease, high blood pressure, or skin problems, such as dermatitis or local abrasions.
• Because this medication contains alcohol, it can cause skin irritation to sensitive areas. You should, therefore, avoid getting this medication in your eyes, nose, or mouth, or in areas surrounding scratches or burns.
• Do not apply minoxidil to other areas of the body because absorption of the drug may be increased and the risk of side effects may become greater; do not use along with other topical medication on your scalp, unless directed to do so by your doctor.
• Avoid inhaling the spray mist.
• If treatment is stopped, new hair growth will probably be shed within a few months.
• More frequent applications or use of larger doses (more

than 1 ml twice daily) will not speed up the process of hair growth and may increase the possibility of side effects.

misoprostol

BRAND NAME (Manufacturer)
Cytotec (Searle)
TYPE OF DRUG
Prostaglandin E1 analog (gastrointestinal protective agent)
INGREDIENT
misoprostol
DOSAGE FORM
Tablets (200 mcg)
STORAGE
Store at room temperature in a tightly closed container.

USES

Misoprostol is used to prevent stomach ulcers in people who are taking nonsteroidal anti-inflammatory drugs (NSAIDs). NSAIDs (such as aspirin, carprofen, diclofenac, diflunisal, fenoprofen, flurbiprofen, ibuprofen, indomethacin, ketoprofen, meclofenamate, mefenamic acid, naproxen, phenylbutazone, piroxicam, salsalate, sulindac, or tolmetin) are frequently prescribed to treat pain or arthritis. NSAIDs have been shown to cause ulcers in some patients. Misoprostol belongs to a group of chemicals called prostaglandins, which protect the stomach by decreasing the secretion of acid and increasing the secretion of mucus.

TREATMENT

This medication should be taken with meals and at bedtime, unless otherwise directed by your doctor.

If you miss a dose, take the missed dose as soon as possible, unless it is almost time for your next dose. If that is the case, do not take the missed dose at all; just return to your regular dosing schedule. Never take a double dose.

Misoprostol treatment should continue for as long as you take a NSAID. This medication should be taken exactly as prescribed by your doctor.

SIDE EFFECTS

Minor. Abdominal pain, change in appetite, constipation, diarrhea, flatulence, gas and bloating, heartburn, menstrual cramps and abnormal bleeding, nausea, or vomiting.
Major. Tell your doctor about any side effects that are persistent or particularly bothersome. IT IS ESPECIALLY IMPORTANT TO TELL YOUR DOCTOR ABOUT chest pain, difficulty in breathing, postmenopausal vaginal bleeding, or rash.

INTERACTIONS

Antacids decrease the absorption of misoprostol into the bloodstream. However, antacids do not appear to decrease the beneficial effects of misoprostol in preventing ulcers. Consult your doctor before using antacids with this product.

Before starting to take misoprostol, BE SURE TO TELL YOUR DOCTOR about any other medications you are currently taking.

WARNINGS

• Misoprostol should not be taken by anyone with a history of allergy to prostaglandins.

• Tell your doctor immediately if you develop a rash while taking this medication.

• Women should notify their doctors immediately if they experience any abnormal vaginal bleeding while taking this medication.

• Women of child-bearing age must use extreme caution not to become pregnant while taking misoprostol. This medication may cause miscarriage. Miscarriages caused by misoprostol may be incomplete, which could lead to potentially dangerous bleeding. ANY WOMAN WHO IS PREGNANT OR PLANS TO BECOME PREGNANT SHOULD NOT TAKE MISOPROSTOL. If you are taking misoprostol and discover that you are pregnant, stop taking the drug immediately and call your doctor.

• Nursing mothers should not take misoprostol. The body converts it to misoprostol acid, which can pass into breast milk and cause diarrhea in the nursing infant.

mitotane

BRAND NAME (Manufacturer)
Lysodren (Bristol)
TYPE OF DRUG
Antineoplastic (anticancer drug)
INGREDIENT
mitotane
DOSAGE FORM
Tablets (500 mg)
STORAGE
Mitotane should be stored at room temperature in a tightly closed, lightresistant container.

USES

This medication is used to treat cancer of the adrenal gland and Cushing's syndrome (overactive adrenal gland) in patients on whom surgery cannot be performed. Mitotane directly suppresses the activity of the adrenal gland.

TREATMENT

Initial therapy with mitotane often occurs in the hospital until the dosage is stabilized. Mitotane is potent medication. The dosage is usually adjusted to an individual's needs and tolerance. Be sure you understand your doctor's instructions on how this medication should be taken.

Mitotane tablets can be taken either on an empty stomach or, to reduce stomach irritation, with food or milk (unless your doctor directs you to do otherwise).

Try not to miss any doses of this medication. If you do miss a dose, take the missed dose as soon as possible, unless it is almost time for the next dose. In that case, do not take the missed dose at all; just return to your regular dosing schedule. Do not double the next dose.

SIDE EFFECTS

Minor. Diarrhea, dizziness, drowsiness, loss of appetite, nausea, or vomiting. These side effects should disappear as your body adjusts to the medication. However, it is important to continue taking this medication despite the nausea and vomiting that may occur.

Mitotane can also cause hair loss (which is reversible when the medication is discontinued).

If you feel dizzy, sit or lie down for a while; get up slowly from a sitting or reclining position, and be careful on stairs.

Major. Tell your doctor about any side effects that are persistent or particularly bothersome. IT IS ESPECIALLY IMPORTANT TO TELL YOUR DOCTOR about blurred vision, depression, difficult or painful urination, fainting, flushing, lethargy, muscle aches, or skin rash.

INTERACTIONS

Mitotane interacts with several other types of medications:

1. Concurrent use of it with central nervous system depressants (such as alcohol, antihistamines, barbiturates, benzodiazepine tranquilizers, muscle relaxants, narcotics, pain medications, phenothiazine tranquilizers, and sleeping medications) or with tricyclic antidepressants can cause extreme drowsiness.

2. Mitotane can decrease the effectiveness of adrenocorticosteroids (cortisonelike medications).

BE SURE TO TELL YOUR DOCTOR about any medications you are currently taking, especially any of those listed above.

WARNINGS

Tell your doctor about unusual or allergic reactions you have had to any medications, especially to mitotane.

Before starting to take this medication, be sure to tell your doctor if you now have or if you have ever had chronic infections or liver disease.

If this medication makes you dizzy, drowsy, or tired or blurs your vision, avoid any activity that requires alertness, such as driving a car or operating potentially dangerous machinery.

Do not stop taking this medication unless you first check with your doctor. The effects of mitotane on the adrenal glands last several weeks after the drug is stopped.

Mitotane can impair your body's response to injury, stress, illness, and infection. If you experience injury, stress, illness, or infection while taking this medication, or shortly after you stop taking it (within several weeks), check with your doctor. You may need to take supplemental adrenal hormone during this period.

Before having surgery or any other medical or dental treatment, be sure to tell your doctor or dentist that you are taking this medication.

Be sure to tell your doctor if you are pregnant. Extensive studies of mitotane in pregnant women have not been conducted. The risks should be discussed with your doctor. Also, tell your doctor if you are breast-feeding an infant. It is not known whether mitotane passes into breast milk.

Mitran—see chlordiazepoxide

Mixtard—see insulin

Modicon—see oral contraceptives

Moduretic—see amiloride and hydrochlorothiazide combination

Monistat 3—see miconazole (vaginal)

Monistat 7—see miconazole (vaginal)

Monistat Dual-Pak—see miconazole (vaginal)

morphine

BRAND NAMES (Manufacturers)
morphine sulfate (various manufacturers)
MS Contin (Purdue-Frederick)
MSIR (Purdue-Frederick)
RMS (Upsher-Smith)
Roxanol (Roxane)
Roxanol SR (Roxane)
TYPE OF DRUG
Analgesic
INGREDIENT
morphine
DOSAGE FORMS
Tablets (15 mg and 30 mg)
Sustained-release tablets (30 mg and 60 mg)
Oral solution (10 mg and 20 mg per 5-ml spoonful, with 10% alcohol; 20 mg per ml)
Rectal suppositories (5 mg, 10 mg, and 20 mg)
STORAGE
Morphine tablets and oral solution should be stored at room temperature in tightly closed, light-resistant containers. The rectal suppositories should be stored in the refrigerator.

USES
Morphine is a narcotic analgesic that acts directly on the central nervous system (brain and spinal cord). It is used to relieve moderate to severe pain.

TREATMENT
In order to avoid stomach upset, you can take morphine with food or milk. This medication works most effectively if you take it at the onset of pain, rather than waiting until the pain becomes intense.

The solution form of this medication can be mixed with fruit juices to improve the taste. Measure each dose carefully with a specially designed 5-ml measuring spoon or with the dropper provided. An ordinary kitchen teaspoon is not accurate enough.

The sustained-release tablets should be swallowed whole. Chewing, crushing, or crumbling the tablets destroys their sustained-release activity and possibly increases the side effects.

To use the suppository form of this medication, remove the foil wrapper and moisten the suppository with water (if the suppository is too soft to insert, refrigerate it for half an hour or run cold water over it before removing the wrapper). Lie on your left side with your right knee bent. Push the suppository into the rectum, pointed end first. Lie still for a few minutes. Try to avoid having a bowel movement for at least an hour (to give the medication time to be absorbed).

If you are taking this drug on a regular schedule and you miss a dose, take the missed dose as soon as possible, unless it is almost time for your next dose. In that case, do not take the missed dose at all; just return to your regular dosing schedule. Do not double the next dose.

SIDE EFFECTS
Minor. Constipation, dizziness, drowsiness, dry mouth, false sense of well-being, flushing, light-headedness, loss of appetite, nausea, rash, or sweating. These side effects should disappear as your body adjusts to the medication.

If you are constipated, increase the amount of fiber in your diet (fresh fruits and vegetables, salads, bran, and whole-grain breads), exercise, and drink more water (unless your doctor directs you to do otherwise).

Chew sugarless gum or suck on ice chips to reduce mouth dryness.

If you feel dizzy or light-headed, sit or lie down for a while; get up from a sitting or lying position slowly.
Major. Tell your doctor about any side effects that are persistent or particularly bothersome. IT IS ESPECIALLY IMPORTANT TO TELL YOUR DOCTOR about anxiety, difficulty in breathing, excitation, fainting, fatigue, painful or difficult urination, palpitations, restlessness, sore throat and fever, tremors, or weakness.

INTERACTIONS
Morphine interacts with several other types of drugs:
1. Concurrent use of it with other central nervous system depressants (such as alcohol, antihistamines, barbiturates, benzodiazepine tranquilizers, muscle relaxants, and phenothiazine tranquilizers) or with tricyclic antidepressants can cause extreme drowsiness.
2. A monoamine oxidase (MAO) inhibitor taken within 14 days of this medication can lead to unpredictable and severe side effects.
3. The depressant effects of morphine can be dangerously increased by chloral hydrate, glutethimide, beta blockers, and furazolidone.
4. The combination of cimetidine and morphine can cause confusion, disorientation, and shortness of breath.

BE SURE TO TELL YOUR DOCTOR about any medications you are currently taking, especially any of those listed above.

WARNINGS
• Tell your doctor about unusual or allergic reactions you have had to any medications, especially to morphine or to other narcotic analgesics (such as codeine, hydrocodone, hydromorphone, meperidine, methadone, oxycodone, and propoxyphene).
• Tell your doctor if you now have or if you have ever had acute abdominal conditions, asthma, brain disease, colitis, epilepsy, gallstones or gallbladder disease, head injuries, heart disease, kidney disease, liver disease, lung disease, mental illness, emotional disorders, enlarged prostate gland, thyroid disease, or urethral stricture.

• If this drug makes you dizzy or drowsy, do not take part in any activity that requires alertness, such as driving a car or operating potentially dangerous machinery.

• Before having surgery or any other medical or dental treatment, be sure to tell your doctor or dentist that you are taking this medication.

• Morphine has the potential for abuse and must be used with caution. Usually, it should not be taken for longer than ten days (unless your doctor directs you to do so). Tolerance develops quickly; do not increase the dosage or stop taking the drug abruptly, unless you first consult your doctor. If you have been taking large amounts of this drug, or if you have been taking it for long periods of time, you may experience a withdrawal reaction (muscle aches, diarrhea, gooseflesh, runny nose, nausea, vomiting, shivering, trembling, stomach cramps, sleep disorders, irritability, weakness, excessive yawning, or sweating) when you stop taking it. Your doctor may, therefore, want to reduce the dosage gradually.

• Be sure to tell your doctor if you are pregnant. The effects of this medication during the early stages of pregnancy have not been thoroughly studied in humans. However, regular use of morphine in large doses during the later stages of pregnancy can result in addiction of the fetus, leading to withdrawal symptoms (irritability, excessive crying, tremors, fever, vomiting, diarrhea, sneezing, or excessive yawning) at birth. Also, tell your doctor if you are breast-feeding an infant. Small amounts of this medication may pass into breast milk and cause excessive drowsiness in the nursing infant.

morphine sulfate—see morphine

Motrin—see ibuprofen

Motrin IB—see ibuprofen

MS Contin—see morphine

MSIR—see morphine

multiple sulfonamides—see sulfonamide antibiotics (oral)

Multi-Vita Drops with Fluoride—see vitamins, multiple, with fluoride

Mycadec DM—see pseudoephedrine, carbinoxamine, and dextromethorphan combination

Mycelex—see clotrimazole (topical)

Mycelex OTC—see clotrimazole (topical)

Mycelex-G—see clotrimazole (vaginal)

Mycitracin ophthalmic—see neomycin, polymyxin B, and bacitracin or gramicidin combination (ophthalmic)

Mycostatin—see nystatin

Myco Triacet—see triamcinolone, neomycin, nystatin, and gramicidin combination (topical)

Myfedrine Plus—see pseudoephedrine and chlorpheniramine combination

Myidone—see primidone

Myleran—see busulfan

Myminic—see phenylpropanolamine and chlorpheniramine combination

Myotonachol—see bethanechol

Myproic acid—see valproic acid

Mysoline—see primidone

Mytussin AC—see codeine and guaifenesin combination

nadolol

BRAND NAME (Manufacturer)
Corgard (Princeton Pharm.)
TYPE OF DRUG
Beta-adrenergic blocking agent
INGREDIENT
nadolol
DOSAGE FORM
Tablets (20 mg, 40 mg, 80 mg, 120 mg, and 160 mg)
STORAGE
Nadolol should be stored at room temperature in a tightly closed, light-resistant container.

USES
Used to treat high blood pressure and angina pectoris (chest pain). It belongs to a group of medicines known as beta-adrenergic blocking agents or, more commonly, beta blockers. These drugs work by controlling nerve impulses along certain nerve pathways.

TREATMENT
Nadolol can be taken with a glass of water, with meals, immediately following meals, or on an empty stomach, depending on your doctor's instructions. Try to take the medication at the same time(s) each day.

Try not to miss any doses of this medicine. If you do miss a dose, take the missed dose as soon as possible. However, if the next scheduled dose is within eight hours (if you are taking this medicine only once a day) or within four hours (if you are taking this medicine more than once a day), do not take the missed dose at all; just return to your regular dosing schedule. Do not double the next dose.

Nadolol does not cure high blood pressure, but it will help control your condition as long as you take it.

SIDE EFFECTS
Minor. Anxiety; cold hands or feet (due to decreased blood circulation to the skin, fingers, and toes); constipation; decreased sexual ability; diarrhea; difficulty in sleeping; drowsiness; dryness of the eyes, mouth, and skin; headache; nausea; nervousness; stomach discom-

fort; tiredness; or weakness. These side effects should disappear during treatment, as your body adjusts to the medication.

If you are extra-sensitive to the cold, be sure to dress warmly during cold weather.

To relieve constipation, increase the amount of fiber in your diet (fresh fruits and vegetables, salads, bran, and whole-grain breads), exercise, and drink more water (unless your doctor directs you to do otherwise).

Plain, nonmedicated eye drops (artificial tears) may help to relieve eye dryness.

Sucking on ice chips or chewing sugarless gum helps to relieve mouth or throat dryness.

Major. Tell your doctor about any side effects that are persistent or particularly bothersome. IT IS ESPECIALLY IMPORTANT TO TELL YOUR DOCTOR about breathing difficulty or wheezing, confusion, dizziness, fever and sore throat, hair loss, hallucinations, light-headedness, mental depression, nightmares, numbness or tingling of the fingers or toes, rapid weight gain (three to five pounds within a week), reduced alertness, swelling, skin rash, or unusual bleeding or bruising.

INTERACTIONS

Nadolol interacts with several other types of medications:

1. Indomethacin, aspirin, or other salicylates may decrease the blood-pressure-lowering effects of beta blockers.

2. Concurrent use of beta blockers and calcium channel blockers (diltiazem, nifedipine, verapamil) or disopyramide can potentially lead to heart failure or very low blood pressure.

3. Side effects may be increased when nadolol is taken with cimetidine, clonidine, digoxin, epinephrine, phenylephrine, phenylpropanolamine, phenothiazine tranquilizers, prazosin, or monoamine oxidase (MAO) inhibitors. At least 14 days should separate the use of a beta blocker and an MAO inhibitor.

4. Alcohol, barbiturates, and rifampin may decrease the blood concentrations of beta blockers, which can result in a decrease in effectiveness.

5. Beta blockers may antagonize (work against) the effects of theophylline, aminophylline, albuterol, isoproterenol, metaproterenol, and terbutaline.

6. Beta blockers can also interact with insulin or oral antidiabetic agents, raising or lowering blood sugar levels or masking the symptoms of low blood sugar.

7. The concurrent use of nadolol and reserpine can have additive blood-pressure-lowering effects and can slow the heartbeat.

8. The action of beta blockers may be increased if they are used with chlorpromazine, furosemide, hydralazine, or oral contraceptives (birth control pills), which may have a negative effect.

BE SURE TO TELL YOUR DOCTOR about any medications you are currently taking, especially any of those listed above.

WARNINGS

• Tell your doctor if you have ever had unusual or allergic reactions to any medications, especially to nadolol or any other beta blocker (acebutolol, atenolol, carteolol, esmolol, labetalol, metoprolol, penbutolol, pindolol, propranolol, or timolol).

• Tell your doctor if you now have or if you have ever had allergies, asthma, hay fever, eczema, slow heartbeat, bronchitis, diabetes mellitus, emphysema, heart or blood vessel disease, kidney disease, liver disease, thyroid disease, or poor circulation in the fingers or toes.

• You may want to check your pulse regularly while you are taking this medication. If your pulse is much slower than your usual rate (or if it is less than 50 beats per minute), check with your doctor. A pulse rate that is too slow may cause circulation problems.

• This medicine may affect your body's response to exercise. Make sure you discuss with your doctor a safe amount of exercise for your medical condition.

• It is important that you do not stop taking this medicine without first checking with your doctor. Some conditions may become worse when the medicine is stopped suddenly, and the danger of a heart attack is increased in some patients. Your doctor may want you to gradually reduce the amount of medicine you take before stopping completely. Make sure that you have enough medicine on hand to last through vacations, holidays, and weekends.

• Before having surgery or any other medical or dental treatment, be sure to tell your physician or dentist that you are taking nadolol. Often, this medication will be discontinued 48 hours prior to any major surgery.

• Nadolol can cause dizziness, drowsiness, light-headedness, or decreased alertness. You should, therefore, use caution while driving a car or operating any potentially dangerous machinery.

• While taking this medicine, do not use any over-the-counter (nonprescription) allergy, asthma, cough, cold, sinus, or diet preparations unless you first check with your pharmacist or doctor. Some of these medicines can result in high blood pressure when combined with a beta blocker.

• Be sure to tell your doctor if you are pregnant. Animal studies have shown that some beta blockers can cause problems in pregnancy when used at very high doses. Adequate studies have not been conducted in humans, but there has been some association between beta blockers used during pregnancy and low birth weight, as well as breathing problems and slow heart rate in newborn infants. However, other reports have shown no effects on newborn infants. Also, tell your doctor if you are breast-feeding an infant. Although this medicine has not been shown to cause problems in breast-fed infants, some of the medicine may pass into breast milk, so caution is warranted.

nafcillin

BRAND NAME (Manufacturer)
Unipen (Wyeth)
TYPE OF DRUG
Penicillin antibiotic
INGREDIENT
nafcillin

DOSAGE FORMS
Tablets (500 mg)
Capsules (250 mg)
Oral solution (250 mg per 5-ml spoonful)

STORAGE
Nafcillin tablets and capsules should be stored at room temperature in tightly closed containers. The oral solution should be stored in the refrigerator in a tightly closed container. Any unused portion of the solution should be discarded after 14 days because the drug loses its potency after that time. This medication should never be frozen.

USES
Nafcillin is used to treat a wide variety of bacterial infections, especially those caused by Staphylococcus bacteria. It acts by severely injuring the cell membranes of the infecting bacteria, thereby preventing them from growing and multiplying. Nafcillin kills susceptible bacteria, but it is not effective against viruses, parasites, or fungi.

TREATMENT
Nafcillin should be taken on an empty stomach or with a glass of water one hour before or two hours after a meal. This medication should never be taken with fruit juices or carbonated beverages because the acidity of these drinks destroys the drug in the stomach.

The oral solution should be measured carefully with a specially designed 5-ml measuring spoon. An ordinary kitchen teaspoon is not accurate enough.

Nafcillin works best when the level of medicine in your bloodstream is kept constant. It is best, therefore, to take the doses at evenly spaced intervals day and night. For example, if you are taking four doses a day, the doses should be spaced six hours apart.

If you miss a dose of this medication, take the missed dose immediately. However, if you do not remember to take the missed dose until it is almost time for your next dose, take it; space the following dose about halfway through the regular interval between doses; and then return to your regular dosing schedule. Try not to skip any doses.

Take this drug for the entire time prescribed by your doctor (usually seven to 14 days), even if your symptoms disappear before the end of that period. If you stop taking the drug too soon, resistant bacteria are given a chance to continue growing, and the infection could recur.

SIDE EFFECTS
Minor. Diarrhea, heartburn, nausea, or vomiting. These side effects should disappear as your body adjusts to the medication.

Major. Tell your doctor about any side effects that are persistent or particularly bothersome. IT IS ESPECIALLY IMPORTANT TO TELL YOUR DOCTOR about bloating, chills, cough, darkened tongue, difficult or painful urination, difficulty in breathing, fever, irritation of the mouth, muscle aches, rash, rectal or vaginal itching, severe diarrhea, sore throat, or yellowing of the skin or eyes. Also, if your symptoms of infection seem to be getting worse rather than improving, you should contact your doctor.

INTERACTIONS
Nafcillin interacts with several other types of medications:

1. Probenecid can increase the blood concentrations of this medication.

2. Nafcillin may decrease the effectiveness of oral contraceptives (birth control pills), and pregnancy could result. You should, therefore, use another form of birth control while taking this medication. Discuss this with your doctor.

BE SURE TO TELL YOUR DOCTOR about any medications you are currently taking, especially those listed above.

WARNINGS
Tell your doctor about unusual or allergic reactions you have had to any medications, especially to nafcillin, penicillins, cephalosporin antibiotics, penicillamine, or griseofulvin.

Tell your doctor if you now have or if you have ever had kidney disease, asthma, or allergies.

This medication has been prescribed for your current infection only. Another infection later on, or one that someone else has, may require a different medicine. You should not give your medicine to other people or use it for other infections, unless your doctor specifically directs you to do so.

Diabetics taking nafcillin should know that this drug can cause a false-positive sugar reaction with a Clinitest urine glucose test. To avoid this problem while taking nafcillin, you should switch to Clinistix or Tes-Tape to test your urine for sugar.

Be sure to tell your doctor if you are pregnant. Although nafcillin appears to be safe during pregnancy, extensive studies in humans have not been conducted. Also, tell your doctor if you are breast-feeding an infant. Small amounts of this medication pass into breast milk and may temporarily alter the bacterial balance in the intestinal tract of the nursing infant, resulting in diarrhea.

Naldecon—see phenylpropanolamine, phenylephrine, chlorpheniramine, and phenyltoloxamine combination

Naldelate—see phenylpropanolamine, phenylephrine, chlorpheniramine, and phenyltoloxamine combination

Nalfon—see fenoprofen

Nalfon 200—see fenoprofen

Nalgest—see phenylpropanolamine, phenylephrine, chlorpheniramine, and phenyltoloxamine combination

nalidixic acid

BRAND NAME (Manufacturer)
NegGram (Winthrop)

TYPE OF DRUG
Antibiotic

INGREDIENT
nalidixic acid

DOSAGE FORMS
Tablets (250 mg, 500 mg, and 1,000 mg)
Oral suspension (250 mg per 5-ml spoonful)
STORAGE
Nalidixic acid tablets and suspension should be stored at room temperature in tightly closed containers. This medication should never be frozen.

USES
Nalidixic acid is an antibiotic that is used to treat bacterial urinary tract infections. It works by preventing the growth and multiplication of susceptible bacteria. This medication is not effective against viruses, parasites, or fungi.

TREATMENT
In order to avoid stomach irritation, you can take nalidixic acid with food or with a full glass of water or milk (unless your doctor directs you to do otherwise).

The suspension form of this medication should be shaken well just before measuring each dose. The contents tend to settle on the bottom of the bottle, so it is necessary to shake the container to distribute the ingredients evenly and equalize the doses. Each dose should then be measured carefully with a specially designed 5-ml measuring spoon. An ordinary kitchen teaspoon is not accurate enough to ensure that you receive the proper dose.

Nalidixic acid works best when the level of medicine in your bloodstream and urine is kept constant. It is best, therefore, to take the doses at evenly spaced intervals day and night. For example, if you are to take four doses a day, the doses should be spaced six hours apart.

Try not to miss any doses of this medication. If you do miss a dose, take it as soon as you remember. However, if it is almost time for your next dose, take the missed dose immediately; space the following dose about halfway through the regular dosing interval; and then continue with your regular dosing schedule.

It is important to continue to take this medication for the entire time prescribed by your doctor (usually seven to 14 days), even if the symptoms disappear before the end of that period. If you stop taking the drug too soon, resistant bacteria are given a chance to continue growing, and your infection could recur.

SIDE EFFECTS
Minor. Abdominal pain, diarrhea, dizziness, drowsiness, headache, nausea, vomiting, or weakness. These side effects should disappear as your body adjusts to the medication.

This medication can increase your sensitivity to sunlight. You should, therefore, avoid prolonged exposure to sunlight and sunlamps. Wear protective clothing and sunglasses, and use an effective sunscreen.

If you feel dizzy, sit or lie down for a while; get up slowly from a sitting or reclining position, and be careful on stairs.
Major. Tell your doctor about any side effects that are persistent or particularly bothersome. IT IS ESPECIALLY IMPORTANT TO TELL YOUR DOCTOR about convulsions, itching, joint pain, skin rash, tingling sensations, unusual bleeding or bruising, visual disturbances, or yellowing of the eyes or skin.

INTERACTIONS
This drug can interact with several other types of drugs:
1. Nalidixic acid can increase the effects of oral anticoagulants, which can lead to bleeding complications.
2. Nitrofurantoin can reduce the effectiveness of this drug.

BE SURE TO TELL YOUR DOCTOR about any medications you are currently taking, especially any listed above.

WARNINGS
• Tell your doctor about unusual or allergic reactions you have had to any medications, especially to nalidixic acid or to cinoxacin or norfloxacin.
• Before starting to take this medication, be sure to tell your doctor if you now have or if you have ever had brain disorders, epilepsy, kidney disease, or liver disease.
• If this drug makes you dizzy or drowsy, do not take part in any activity that requires alertness, such as driving a car or operating potentially dangerous machinery.
• This drug has been prescribed for your current infection only. Another infection later on, or one that someone else has, may require a different medicine. You should not give your medication to other people or use it for other infections, unless your doctor specifically directs you to do so.
• Diabetic patients should know that nalidixic acid can cause false-positive readings of Clinitest urine glucose tests. Temporarily changing to Clinistix or Tes-Tape urine glucose tests avoids this problem. CHECK WITH YOUR DOCTOR before adjusting the dosage of your antidiabetic medication.
• If the symptoms of your infection do not improve within several days after starting this medication, CHECK WITH YOUR DOCTOR. Nalidixic acid may not be effective against the organism causing your infection.
• Be sure to tell your doctor if you are pregnant. Although nalidixic acid may cross the placenta, it appears to be safe during pregnancy. However, extensive studies in humans have not been conducted. Also, tell your doctor if you are breast-feeding an infant. Small amounts of nalidixic acid pass into breast milk.

Napamide—see disopyramide

Napril—see pseudoephedrine and chlorpheniramine combination

Naprosyn—see naproxen

---

naproxen

BRAND NAMES (Manufacturers)
Anaprox (Syntex)
Anaprox DS (Syntex)
Naprosyn (Syntex)
TYPE OF DRUG
Nonsteroidal anti-inflammatory analgesic

INGREDIENT
naproxen (Naprosyn)
naproxen as the sodium salt (Anaprox)
DOSAGE FORMS
Tablets (250 mg, 375 mg, and 500 mg {Naprosyn};
  275 mg and 550 mg {Anaprox})
Oral suspension (125 mg per 5-ml spoonful {Naprosyn})
STORAGE
This medication should be stored in a tightly closed container at room temperature, away from heat and direct sunlight.

USES
Naproxen is used to treat the inflammation (pain, swelling, and stiffness) of certain types of arthritis, gout, bursitis, and tendinitis. Naproxen is also used to treat painful menstruation. Naproxen has been shown to block the production of certain body chemicals, called prostaglandins, that may trigger pain. However, it is not yet fully understood how naproxen works.

TREATMENT
You should take this medication on an empty stomach 30 to 60 minutes before meals or two hours after meals, so that it gets into your bloodstream quickly. However, to decrease stomach irritation, your doctor may want you to take the medicine with food or antacids.

It is important to take naproxen on schedule and not to miss any doses. If you do miss a dose, take it as soon as possible, unless it is almost time for your next dose. In that case, do not take the missed dose at all; just return to your regular dosing schedule. Do not double the next dose.

If you are taking naproxen to relieve arthritis, you must take it regularly, as directed by your doctor. It may take up to four weeks before you feel the full benefits of this medication. This medication does not cure arthritis, but it will help to relieve the condition as long as you continue to take it.

SIDE EFFECTS
Minor. Bloating, constipation, diarrhea, difficulty in sleeping, dizziness, drowsiness, headache, heartburn, indigestion, light-headedness, loss of appetite, nausea, nervousness, soreness of the mouth, unusual sweating, and vomiting. As your body adjusts to the medication, these side effects should disappear.

To relieve constipation, increase the amount of fiber in your diet (fresh fruits and vegetables, salads, bran, and whole-grain breads), exercise, and drink more water (unless your doctor directs you to do otherwise).

If you become dizzy, sit or lie down for a while; get up slowly from a sitting or reclining position, and be careful on stairs.

Major. Tell your doctor about any side effects that are persistent or particularly bothersome. IT IS ESPECIALLY IMPORTANT TO TELL YOUR DOCTOR about bloody or black, tarry stools; blurred vision; confusion; depression; palpitations; ringing or buzzing in the ears or a problem with hearing; shortness of breath or wheezing; skin rash, hives, or itching; stomach pain; sudden decrease in amount of urine; swelling of the feet; tightness in the chest; unexplained sore throat and fever; unusual bleeding or bruising; unusual fatigue or weakness; unusual weight gain; or yellowing of the eyes or skin.

INTERACTIONS
Naproxen interacts with several other types of medications:

1. Concurrent use of anticoagulants (blood thinners, such as warfarin) can lead to an increase in bleeding complications.

2. Aspirin, salicylates, or other anti-inflammatory medications can cause increased stomach irritation when used concurrently with naproxen.

3. Naproxen can decrease the elimination of lithium and methotrexate from the body, resulting in possible toxicity from these medications.

4. Naproxen may interfere with the blood-pressure-lowering effects of beta-blocking medications (such as acebutolol, atenolol, betaxolol, carteolol, esmolol, labetalol, metoprolol, nadolol, penbutolol, pindolol, propranolol, and timolol).

5. This medication can also interfere with the diuretic effects of furosemide and thiazide-type diuretics.

6. Probenecid can increase the amount of naproxen in the bloodstream when both drugs are being taken.

Before starting to take this medication, BE SURE TO TELL YOUR DOCTOR about any medications you are currently taking, especially any of those listed above.

WARNINGS
• Before you take this medication, it is important to tell your doctor if you have ever had unusual or allergic reactions to any medications, especially to naproxen or any of the other chemically related drugs (including aspirin, other salicylates, carprofen, diclofenac, diflunisal, fenoprofen, flurbiprofen, indomethacin, ketoprofen, meclofenamate, mefenamic acid, oxyphenbutazone, phenylbutazone, piroxicam, sulindac, or tolmetin).

• Before taking this medication, it is important to tell your doctor if you now have or if you have ever had bleeding problems, colitis, stomach ulcers or other stomach problems, asthma, epilepsy, heart disease, high blood pressure, kidney disease, liver disease, mental illness, or Parkinson's disease.

• If naproxen makes you dizzy or drowsy, do not take part in any activity that requires alertness, such as driving a car or operating potentially dangerous machinery.

• Because this drug can prolong your bleeding time, it is important to tell your doctor or dentist that you are taking this drug before having surgery or any other medical or dental treatment.

• Stomach problems are more likely to occur if you take aspirin regularly or drink alcohol while being treated with this medication. You should avoid taking frequent doses of aspirin or drinking alcohol while undergoing treatment with this medication (unless your doctor tells you otherwise).

• Be sure to tell your doctor if you are pregnant. Naproxen analgesic may cause unwanted effects on the heart or blood flow of the fetus. Studies in animals have shown that taking naproxen late in pregnancy may increase the length of pregnancy, prolong labor, or cause other problems during delivery. Also, be sure to tell your doctor if you are currently breast-feeding an infant. Small amounts of this medication have been shown to pass into breast milk.

Naptrate—see pentaerythritol tetranitrate

Naqua—see trichlormethiazide

Nardil—see phenelzine

Nasalcrom—see cromolyn sodium (nasal)

Nasalide—see flunisolide (nasal)

Naturetin—see bendroflumethiazide

Navane—see thiothixene

ND Clear T.D.—see pseudoephedrine and chlorpheniramine combination

NegGram—see nalidixic acid

Nembutal—see pentobarbital

---

neomycin, polymyxin B, and bacitracin or gramicidin combination (ophthalmic)

BRAND NAMES (Manufacturers)
AK-Spore (Akorn)
Mycitracin ophthalmic (Upjohn)
neomycin, polymyxin B, and bacitracin or gramicidin combination (various manufacturers)
Neomycin, Polymyxin B, and Gramicidin (Rugby)
Neosporin (Burroughs Wellcome)
TYPE OF DRUG
Ophthalmic antibiotic
INGREDIENTS
neomycin, polymyxin B, and bacitracin (ointment only) or gramicidin (drops only)
DOSAGE FORMS
Ophthalmic drops (1.75 mg neomycin, 10,000 units polymyxin B, and 0.025 mg gramicidin per ml)
Ophthalmic ointment (3.5 mg neomycin, 10,000 units polymyxin B, and 400 units or 500 units bacitracin per gm)
STORAGE
The ophthalmic drops and ointment should be stored at room temperature in tightly closed containers. This medication should never be frozen.

USES
This medication combination is used to treat bacterial infections of the eye. It is an antibiotic combination that is effective against a wide range of bacteria. The medication combination acts by preventing the production of nutrients that are required for growth of the infecting bacteria. This medication is not effective against infections caused by viruses or fungi.

TREATMENT
Wash your hands with soap and water before using this medication. In order to prevent contamination of the medication, be careful not to touch the tube portion of the dropper, and do not let the dropper touch your eye.

Note that the bottle of eye drops is not completely full. This is to allow control of the number of drops dispensed. To apply the eye drops, tilt your head back and pull down the lower eyelid with one hand to make a pouch below the eye. Drop the prescribed amount of medicine into this pouch and slowly close your eyes. Try not to blink. Keep your eyes closed, and place one finger at the corner of the eye next to your nose for a minute or two, applying slight pressure (this is done to prevent loss of medication through the duct that drains fluid from the surface of the eye into the nose and throat). Then wipe away any excess with a clean tissue. If you don't think the medicine got into the eye, repeat the process once. If you are using more than one kind of eye drop, wait at least five minutes before applying the other medication(s).

Follow the same general procedure for the ointment. Tilt your head back, pull down your lower eyelid, and squeeze the ointment in a line along the pouch below the eye. Close the eye and place your finger at the corner of the eye near the nose for a minute or two. Do not rub your eyes. Wipe off excess ointment and the tip of the tube with clean tissues.

Since this medication is somewhat difficult to apply, you may prefer to have someone else apply it for you.

If you miss a dose of this medication, insert the drops or apply the ointment as soon as possible, unless it is almost time for the next application. In that case, do not use the missed dose; just return to your regular dosing schedule.

Continue using this medicine for the entire time prescribed by your doctor, even if the symptoms disappear. If you stop too soon, the infection could recur.

SIDE EFFECTS
Minor. Blurred vision, burning, or stinging. These side effects should disappear as your body adjusts to the drug.
Major. Tell your doctor about any side effects that are persistent or particularly bothersome. IT IS ESPECIALLY IMPORTANT TO TELL YOUR DOCTOR about disturbed or reduced vision and about itching, rash, redness, or swelling in or around your eyes (other than the original symptoms of your infection). Also, if the infection seems to be getting worse rather than improving, contact your doctor.

INTERACTIONS
This medication should not interact with other medications as long as it is used according to directions.

WARNINGS
• Tell your doctor about unusual or allergic reactions you have had to any medications, especially to neomycin, bacitracin, polymyxin B, gramicidin, or any related antibiotics (such as amikacin, colistimethate, colistin, gen-

tamicin, kanamycin, netilmicin, paromomycin, streptomycin, tobramycin, and viomycin).

• Tell your doctor if you now have or if you have ever had kidney disease, an injured cornea, inner ear disease, or myasthenia gravis.

• Do not use this medication for longer than ten consecutive days unless your doctor directs you to do so. Prolonged use of this drug may result in eye damage. If you need to use this medication for six weeks or longer, your doctor may want you to have an eye examination.

• This medication has been prescribed for your current infection only. Another infection later on may require a different medicine. You should not give your medicine to other people or use it for other infections, unless your doctor specifically directs you to do so.

• In order to allow your eye infection to clear, do not apply makeup to the affected eye.

• Tell your doctor if you are pregnant. The effects of this drug during pregnancy have not been studied.

Neomycin, Polymyxin B, and Gramicidin—see neomycin, polymyxin B, and bacitracin or gramicidin combination (ophthalmic)

Neosporin—see neomycin, polymyxin B, and bacitracin or gramicidin combination (ophthalmic)

Neotrizine—see sulfonamide antibiotics (oral)

Nervine Nighttime Sleep Aid—see diphenhydramine

New-Decongest—see phenylpropanolamine, phenylephrine, chlorpheniramine, and phenyltoloxamine combination

Niazide—see trichlormethiazide

Nicoderm—nicotine transdermal patch

Nicorette—see nicotine gum

nicotine gum

BRAND NAME (Manufacturer)
Nicorette (Merrell Dow)
TYPE OF DRUG
A "stop smoking" aid
INGREDIENT
nicotine
DOSAGE FORM
Chewing gum (2 mg)
STORAGE
This medication should be kept in its original, child-resistant packaging until it is ready to be chewed.

USES

Nicotine gum is used as a temporary aid for smoking cessation programs. It helps control the symptoms of nicotine withdrawal (irritability, headache, fatigue, insomnia) and thus helps you to concentrate on overcoming the psychological and social aspects of your smoking habit.

TREATMENT

Use nicotine gum when you feel the urge to smoke. Keep the gum with you at all times. Place it where you usually keep your cigarettes. Whenever you feel that you want to smoke, put one piece of gum into your mouth. Chew the gum very slowly, until you taste it or feel a slight tingling in your mouth. As soon as you get the taste of the gum, stop chewing. After the taste or tingling is almost gone (after about one minute), chew slowly again until you taste the gum. Then stop chewing again. The gum should be chewed slowly for 30 minutes to release most of the nicotine. You should not expect the gum to give you the same quick satisfaction that smoking does. Do not drink caffeine-containing beverages while chewing a piece of nicotine gum.

Most people find that ten to 12 pieces of gum per day are enough to control their urge to smoke. Depending on your needs, you can adjust the rate of chewing and the time between pieces. Do not chew more than 30 pieces per day (unless your doctor directs you to do so).

The risk of smoking again is highest in the first few months, so it is important that you follow your smoking cessation program and use nicotine gum as directed during this period.

SIDE EFFECTS

Minor. Because of its nicotine content, the gum does not taste like ordinary chewing gum. It has a peppery taste. During the first several days of chewing the nicotine gum, you may experience mouth sores, jaw muscle aches, headaches, and increased salivation. These side effects should disappear as you continue to use the gum.

If you chew the gum too fast, you may feel effects similar to those experienced when people inhale a cigarette for the first time or when they smoke too fast. These effects include constipation, coughing, dizziness, dry mouth, gas pains, hiccups, hoarseness, insomnia, light-headedness, nausea, redness of the face, sneezing, stomach pain, stomach upset, throat and mouth irritation, and vomiting. Most of these side effects can be controlled by chewing the gum more slowly.

Major. If any of the side effects are persistent or particularly bothersome, report them to your doctor. IT IS ESPECIALLY IMPORTANT TO TELL YOUR DOCTOR about signs of too much nicotine (cold sweats, confusion, difficulty in breathing, disturbed hearing or vision, faintness, marked weakness, palpitations, or seizures).

If you accidently swallow a piece of gum, you should not experience adverse effects. The nicotine is released by chewing and is absorbed primarily in the mouth.

INTERACTIONS

Smoking cessation, with or without nicotine gum, may affect blood levels of certain medications (including aminophylline, caffeine, glutethimide, imipramine, pentazocine, phenacetin, propoxyphene, and theophylline).

Nicotine can reduce the diuretic effects of furosemide and lessen the blood-pressure-lowering effects of beta blockers.

BE SURE TO TELL YOUR DOCTOR about any medications you are currently taking, especially any listed above.

WARNINGS

• Tell your doctor if you have recently had a heart attack or if you have ever had heart palpitations or arrhythmias, angina, active temporomandibular (jaw) joint disease, cardiovascular disease, endocrine (hormone) disease, thyroid problems, pheochromocytoma, diabetes mellitus, high blood pressure, peptic ulcers, mouth or throat inflammation, or dental problems.

• Be sure to tell your doctor if you are pregnant. Nicotine (from the gum or from cigarette smoke) can cause fetal harm. Also, tell your doctor if you are breast-feeding an infant. Small amounts of nicotine can pass into breast milk.

nicotine transdermal patch

BRAND NAMES (Manufacturers)
Habitrol (Basel)
Nicoderm (Marion Merrell Dow)
Nicotrol (Warner-Lambert)
ProStep (Lederle)

TYPE OF DRUG
A "stop smoking" aid

INGREDIENT
nicotine

DOSAGE FORM
Transdermal patches (5 mg, 7 mg, 10 mg, 11 mg, 14 mg, 15 mg, 21 mg, 22 mg)

STORAGE
This medication should be kept in its original, child-resistant packaging until ready to be applied to the skin. After use, the patch should be disposed of carefully, as the nicotine patches contain a large quantity of residual nicotine that may be harmful to children or pets.

USES
Nicotine patches are used as a temporary aid to smoking cessation programs. They help to control the symptoms of nicotine withdrawal (irritability, headache, fatigue, insomnia) and thus help you to concentrate on overcoming the psychological and social aspects of your smoking habit. Over time the dose of nicotine delivered from the patch is lowered until you are gradually weaned off nicotine.

TREATMENT
It is important to STOP SMOKING when therapy with nicotine patches is started. If you continue to smoke and use the nicotine patches, you are increasing the amount of nicotine in your blood and may be more likely to experience side effects. The nicotine patch should be applied daily to a non-hairy, clean, dry skin site on the upper trunk (chest, back, stomach) or upper outer arm. After 24 hours, the used patch should be removed and a new patch applied to a different site on your body. Try to change the patch at the same time every day, as this may prevent you from forgetting to apply a new patch. Depending on the type of nicotine patch your doctor prescribes and the severity of your withdrawal symptoms, you may be using the patches daily for six weeks to 12 weeks in order to help you stop smoking.

The risk of smoking again is highest in the first few months after using nicotine patches. Follow your smoking cessation program to prevent smoking "relapse."

SIDE EFFECTS
Minor. Abnormal dreams, diarrhea, difficulty sleeping, dry mouth, mood changes, skin rash, swelling, hives, burning or itching at the patch site, and sweating. These side effects should disappear as your body adjusts to the medication.

Major. If any of the side effects are persistent or particularly bothersome, report them to your doctor or pharmacist. IT IS ESPECIALLY IMPORTANT TO TELL YOUR DOCTOR about signs of too much nicotine (cold sweats, confusion, diarrhea, difficulty in breathing, disturbed hearing or vision, nervousness, nightmares, marked weakness, muscle palpitations, severe itching, or rash and seizures).

INTERACTIONS
Smoking cessation, with or without nicotine patches, may affect blood levels of certain medications (including aminophylline, caffeine, furosemide, imipramine, insulin, labetalol, pentazocine, prazosin, propoxyphene, and theophylline. Nicotine can also lessen the blood-pressure-lowering effects of beta blockers, such as propranolol. BE SURE TO TELL YOUR DOCTOR about any medications you are currently taking, especially those listed above.

WARNINGS
• Tell your doctor if you have recently had a heart attack. It is also important to tell your doctor if you now have or if you have ever had heart palpitations or irregular heartbeat, angina, heart disease, hormone imbalances, kidney problems, thyroid problems, pheochromocytoma, diabetes mellitus, high blood pressure, or stomach ulcers.

• Be sure to tell your doctor if you are pregnant. Nicotine (from the patches or from cigarette smoke) can cause fetal harm. Also, tell your doctor if you are breast-feeding an infant. Small amounts of nicotine can pass into breast milk.

Nicotrol—see nicotine transdermal patch

nifedipine

BRAND NAMES (Manufacturers)
Adalat (Miles)
Procardia (Pfizer)
Procardia XL (Pfizer)

TYPE OF DRUG
Antianginal

INGREDIENT
nifedipine

DOSAGE FORM
Capsules (10 mg, 20 mg, 30 mg, 60 mg, and 90 mg)

STORAGE
Nifedipine capsules should be stored at room temperature in a tightly closed, light-resistant container.

USES

This medication is used to treat various types of angina (chest pain). Nifedipine belongs to a group of drugs known as calcium channel blockers. By blocking calcium, nifedipine relaxes and prevents spasms of the blood vessels of the heart and reduces the oxygen needs of the heart muscle.

TREATMENT

Nifedipine should be taken on an empty stomach with a full glass of water one hour before or two hours after a meal (unless your doctor directs you to do otherwise). These capsules should be swallowed whole to obtain maximum benefit.

If you miss a dose of this medication, take the missed dose as soon as possible, unless it is within two hours of your next scheduled dose. In that case, do not take the missed dose at all; just return to your regular dosing schedule. Do not double the next dose.

SIDE EFFECTS

Minor. Bloating, cough, dizziness, flushing, gas, giddiness, headache, heartburn, heat sensation, nasal congestion, nausea, nervousness, sleep disturbances, sweating, or weakness. These side effects should disappear as your body adjusts to the medication.

If you feel dizzy or light-headed, sit or lie down for a while; get up slowly from a sitting or reclining position, and be careful on stairs. To avoid dizziness or light-headedness when you stand, contract and relax the muscles of your legs for a few moments before rising. Do this by pushing one foot against the floor while raising the other foot slightly, alternating feet so that you are "pumping" your legs in a pedaling motion.

Major. Tell your doctor about any side effects that are persistent or particularly bothersome. IT IS ESPECIALLY IMPORTANT TO TELL YOUR DOCTOR about blurred vision, chills, confusion, difficulty in breathing, fainting, fever, fluid retention, impotence, mood changes, muscle cramps, palpitations, rash, sore throat, or tremors.

INTERACTIONS

Nifedipine interacts with several other types of medications:

1. Nifedipine can increase the active blood levels of digoxin, warfarin, phenytoin, and quinine, which can lead to an increase in side effects.

2. The combination of nifedipine and beta blockers (acebutolol, atenolol, betaxolol, carteolol, esmolol, labetalol, metoprolol, nadolol, penbutolol, pindolol, propranolol, or timolol) can lead to a severe drop in blood pressure.

3. Nifedipine can lower quinidine blood levels, which can decrease its effectiveness.

4. Cimetidine can decrease the breakdown of nifedipine in the body, which can increase the risk of side effects.

Before starting to take nifedipine, BE SURE TO TELL YOUR DOCTOR about any medications you are currently taking, especially any of those listed above.

WARNINGS

• Tell your doctor about unusual or allergic reactions you have had to any medications, especially to nifedipine.

• Tell your doctor if you have ever had heart disease, kidney disease, low blood pressure, or liver disease.

• If this drug makes you dizzy or drowsy, do not take part in any activity that requires alertness, such as driving a car or operating potentially dangerous machinery.

• Before having surgery or any other medical or dental treatment, tell your doctor or dentist you are taking this drug.

• Do not stop taking this medication unless you first consult your doctor. Stopping this medication abruptly may lead to severe chest pain. Your doctor may, therefore, want to decrease your dosage gradually.

• Be sure to tell your doctor if you are pregnant. Nifedipine has been shown to cause birth defects in the offspring of animals that received large doses of it during pregnancy. This medication has not been studied in pregnant women. Also, tell your doctor if you are breast-feeding an infant. It is not known whether nifedipine passes into breast milk.

Nilstat—see nystatin

Nitro-Bid—see nitroglycerin (topical)

Nitro-Bid Plateau Caps—see nitroglycerin (systemic)

Nitrocine Timecaps—see nitroglycerin (systemic)

Nitrodisc—see nitroglycerin (topical)

Nitro-Dur—see nitroglycerin (topical)

Nitrofan—see nitrofurantoin

nitrofurantoin

BRAND NAMES (Manufacturers)
Furadantin (Norwich-Eaton)
Furalan (Lannett)
Furanite (Major)
Macrodantin (Norwich-Eaton)
Nitrofan (Major)
nitrofurantoin (various manufacturers)

TYPE OF DRUG
Antibiotic

INGREDIENT
nitrofurantoin

DOSAGE FORMS
Tablets (50 mg and 100 mg)
Capsules (25 mg, 50 mg, and 100 mg)
Oral suspension (25 mg per 5-ml spoonful)

STORAGE
Nitrofurantoin tablets, capsules, and oral suspension should be stored at room temperature in tightly closed, light-resistant containers. Never freeze this medication.

USES

Nitrofurantoin is used to treat bacterial infections of the urinary tract (bladder and kidneys). It kills susceptible bacteria by breaking down their cell membranes and interfering with their production of vital nutrients.

TREATMENT

In order to avoid stomach irritation and to increase the effectiveness of this drug, you can take it with a meal or with a glass of water or milk.

The tablets and capsules should be swallowed whole to obtain maximum benefit.

The oral suspension form of this medication should be shaken well just before measuring each dose. The contents tend to settle on the bottom of the bottle, so it is necessary to shake the container in order to distribute the ingredients evenly and equalize the doses. Each dose of the medication should then be measured carefully with a specially designed 5-ml measuring spoon. An ordinary kitchen teaspoon is not accurate enough to measure your dose of the medication. You can then dilute the dose with water, milk, fruit juice, or infant's formula to mask the unpleasant taste.

Nitrofurantoin works best when the level of medicine in your urine is kept constant. It is best, therefore, to take the doses at evenly spaced invervals day and night. For example, if you are to take three doses a day, the doses should be spaced eight hours apart.

If you miss a dose of this medication, take the missed dose immediately. However, if you do not remember to take the missed dose until it is almost time for your next dose, take it; space the following dose about halfway through the regular interval between doses; then return to your regular dosing schedule. Try not to skip any doses.

It is important to continue to take this medication for the entire time prescribed by your doctor (usually seven to 14 days), even if the symptoms disappear before the end of that period. If you stop taking the drug too soon, resistant bacteria are given a chance to continue growing, and the infection could recur.

SIDE EFFECTS

Minor. Abdominal cramps, diarrhea, dizziness, drowsiness, loss of appetite, nausea, or vomiting. These side effects should disappear as your body adjusts to the medication.

Nitrofurantoin can cause your urine to change color (to rust-yellow or brown). This is a harmless effect, but it may stain your underclothing. The color change will disappear after you stop taking the drug.

If this drug makes you dizzy, sit or lie down; get up slowly, and be careful on stairs.

Major. Tell your doctor about any side effects that are persistent or particularly bothersome. IT IS ESPECIALLY IMPORTANT TO TELL YOUR DOCTOR about chest pain, chills, cough, difficulty in breathing, fainting, fever, hair loss, irritation of the mouth, muscle aches, numbness or tingling, rash, rectal or vaginal itching, unusual bleeding or bruising, weakness, or yellowing of the eyes or skin. Also, if your symptoms or infection seem to be getting worse rather than improving, you should contact your doctor.

INTERACTIONS

Nitrofurantoin interacts with other types of medications:
1. Probenecid and sulfinpyrazone can decrease the effectiveness and increase the side effects of nitrofurantoin.
2. Certain antacids (magnesium trisilicate) can decrease the absorption of nitrofurantoin from the gastrointestinal tract.

Before starting to take nitrofurantoin, BE SURE TO TELL YOUR DOCTOR about any medications you are currently taking, especially any of those listed above.

WARNINGS

• Tell your doctor about unusual or allergic reactions you have had to any medications, especially to nitrofurantoin, nitrofurazone, or furazolidone.
• Be sure to tell your doctor if you now have or if you have ever had anemia, diabetes mellitus, electrolyte abnormalities, glucose-6-phosphate dehydrogenase (G6PD) deficiency, kidney disease, lung disease, nerve damage, or vitamin B deficiencies.
• If this drug makes you dizzy or drowsy, do not take part in any activity that requires alertness, such as driving a car.
• Before surgery or other medical or dental treatment, tell your doctor or dentist you are taking this drug.
• Diabetics should know that nitrofurantoin can cause false-positive results with some urine sugar tests (for example, Clinitest). Be sure to check with your doctor before adjusting your insulin dose.
• This medication has been prescribed for your current infection only. Another infection later on, or one that someone else has, may require a different medicine. You should not give your medicine to other people or use it for other infections, unless your doctor specifically directs you to do so.
• Be sure to tell your doctor if you are pregnant. Nitrofurantoin should not be used close to term. It may cause anemia in the newborn infant. Nitrofurantoin should not be used in an infant less than one month of age. Also, tell your doctor if you are breast-feeding an infant. Nitrofurantoin passes into the breast milk.

Nitrogard—see nitroglycerin (systemic)

Nitroglycerin—see nitroglycerin (systemic)

---

nitroglycerin (systemic)

BRAND NAMES (Manufacturers)
Nitro-Bid Plateau Caps (Marion)
Nitrocine Timecaps (Schwarz Pharma)
Nitrogard (Parke-Davis)
Nitroglycerin (Lilly)
Nitroglyn (Key)
Nitrolingual (Rorer)
Nitrong (Wharton)
Nitrostat (Parke-Davis)
TYPE OF DRUG
Antianginal
INGREDIENT
nitroglycerin
DOSAGE FORMS
Sustained-release tablets (2.6 mg, 6.5 mg, and 9 mg)
Sustained-release capsules (2.5 mg, 6.5 mg, and 9 mg)
Sublingual tablets (0.15 mg, 0.3 mg, 0.4 mg, and 0.6 mg)

Buccal tablets, controlled release (1 mg, 2 mg, and 3 mg)
Oral spray (6.4 mg per dose)
STORAGE
Nitroglycerin tablets, capsules, and oral spray should be stored in a tightly capped bottle in a cool, dry place.

The sublingual tablets should be kept in their original glass container. A small, temporary supply of tablets can also be stored in a stainless-steel container that is now available. The pendant-type container, which can be worn around your neck, is a convenient storage place for an emergency supply. NEVER store them in the refrigerator or the bathroom medicine cabinet, because the drug may lose its potency.

USES
This medication is used to treat angina (chest pain). Nitroglycerin is a vasodilator, which relaxes the muscles of the blood vessels, causing an increase in the oxygen supply to the heart.

The oral tablets and capsules do not act quickly; they are used to prevent chest pain. The sublingual tablets and oral spray act quickly and can be used to relieve chest pain after it has started.

TREATMENT
You should take the sustained-release tablets or capsules with a full glass of water on an empty stomach one hour before or two hours after a meal. The tablets and capsules should be swallowed whole. Chewing, crushing, or breaking them destroys their sustained-release activity and possibly increases the side effects.

NEVER chew or swallow the sublingual or buccal tablets. The sublingual tablet and oral spray forms of the drug are absorbed directly through the lining of the mouth. The sublingual tablet should be allowed to dissolve under the tongue or against the cheek.

To use the spray, remove the plastic cover on the container. Then, without shaking the container, spray the medication onto or under the tongue. Try not to inhale the spray. Close your mouth after each spray, and try to avoid swallowing right away. Nitroglycerin spray loses its effectiveness if it is swallowed.

Take one tablet or one or two spray doses at the first sign of chest pain. Sit down while you are waiting for the medicine to take effect. Do not eat, drink, or smoke while nitroglycerin is in your mouth. Try not to swallow while nitroglycerin is dissolving, and do not rinse your mouth afterward. Sublingual nitroglycerin or nitroglycerin spray should start working in one to three minutes. If there is no relief, take another tablet in five minutes. IF YOU TAKE THREE TABLETS OR THREE SPRAY DOSES WITHOUT ANY SIGN OF IMPROVEMENT, CALL A DOCTOR IMMEDIATELY OR GO TO A HOSPITAL EMERGENCY ROOM. As a preventive measure, take a nitroglycerin sublingual tablet or a spray dose five or ten minutes before heavy exercise, exposure to high altitudes or extreme cold, or any other potentially stressful situation. Be sure to carry some nitroglycerin sublingual tablets or oral spray with you at ALL times.

The buccal tablet should be placed between the upper lip and the gum on either side of the front teeth or between the cheek and the gum. The tablet is held in place by a sticky gel seal that develops once the tablet is in contact with saliva. If you wear dentures, the tablet can be placed anywhere between the cheek and the gum. Avoid drinking hot liquids or touching the tablet with your tongue. This can cause the tablet to dissolve faster and could increase the risk of side effects. If the tablet is swallowed by mistake, replace it with another tablet. Nitroglycerin buccal tablets lose their effectiveness when swallowed. Try not to take the buccal tablet at bedtime in order to avoid inadvertently swallowing and choking on the tablet while you are sleeping.

If you miss a dose of the sustained-release tablets or capsules, take the missed dose as soon as possible, unless it is more than halfway through the interval between doses. In that case, do not take the missed dose at all; just return to your regular dosing schedule. Do not double the next dose.

SIDE EFFECTS
Minor. Dizziness, flushing of the face, headache, lightheadedness, nausea, vomiting, or weakness. These side effects should disappear as your body adjusts to the medication.

If you feel dizzy or light-headed, sit or lie down for a while; get up slowly from a sitting or reclining position, and be careful on stairs. To avoid dizziness or light-headedness when you stand, contract and relax the muscles of your legs for a few moments before rising. Do this by pushing one foot against the floor while raising the other foot slightly, alternating feet so that you are "pumping" your legs in a pedaling motion.

Acetaminophen may help to relieve headaches.
Major. Tell your doctor about any side effects that are persistent or particularly bothersome. IT IS ESPECIALLY IMPORTANT TO TELL YOUR DOCTOR about diarrhea, fainting, palpitations, rash, or sweating.

INTERACTIONS
Nitroglycerin can interact with other types of medications:
1. The combination of alcohol and nitroglycerin can lead to dizziness and fainting.
2. Nitroglycerin can increase the side effects of the tricyclic antidepressants.

Before starting to take nitroglycerin, BE SURE TO TELL YOUR DOCTOR about any medications you are currently taking, especially tricyclic antidepressants.

WARNINGS
• Tell your doctor about unusual or allergic reactions you have had to any medications, especially to nitroglycerin or isosorbide dinitrate.
• Before starting to take this medication, be sure to tell your doctor if you now have or if you have ever had anemia, glaucoma, a head injury, low blood pressure, or thyroid disease or if you have recently had a heart attack.
• If this drug makes you dizzy or light-headed, do not take part in any activity that requires alertness, such as driving a car or operating potentially dangerous machinery.
• Before surgery or other medical or dental treatment, tell your doctor or dentist you are taking this drug.

• Tolerance may develop to this medication within one to three months. If it seems to lose its effectiveness, contact your doctor.

• You should not discontinue use of nitroglycerin (if you have been taking it on a regular basis) unless you first consult your doctor. Stopping the drug abruptly may lead to further chest pain. Your doctor may, therefore, want to decrease your dosage gradually.

• If you have frequent diarrhea, you may not be absorbing the sustained-release form of this medication. Discuss this with your doctor.

• While taking this medication, do not take any over-the-counter (nonprescription) asthma, allergy, sinus, cough, cold, or diet preparations unless you first check with your doctor or pharmacist. Some of these drugs decrease the effectiveness of nitroglycerin.

• The cotton plug should be removed when the bottle is first opened; it should NOT be replaced (the cotton absorbs some of the medication, decreasing its potency).

• Nitroglycerin is highly flammable. Do not use it in places where it might be ignited.

• Be sure to tell your doctor if you are pregnant. Although the systemic form of nitroglycerin appears to be safe, extensive studies in pregnant women have not been conducted. Also, tell your doctor if you are breast-feeding an infant. It is not known whether nitroglycerin passes into breast milk.

nitroglycerin (topical)

BRAND NAMES (Manufacturers)
Deponit (Wyeth)
Nitro-Bid (Marion)
Nitrodisc (Searle)
Nitro-Dur (Key)
nitroglycerin (various manufacturers)
Nitroglycerin Transdermal System (Bolar)
Nitrol (Adria)
Nitrostat (Parke-Davis)
Transderm-Nitro (Ciba)
TYPE OF DRUG
Antianginal
INGREDIENT
nitroglycerin
DOSAGE FORMS
Ointment (2%)
Transdermal system (the patch delivers 0.1 mg, 0.2 mg, 0.3 mg, 0.4 mg, or 0.6 mg per hour)
STORAGE
Nitroglycerin ointment and patches should be stored at room temperature in their original containers. The ointment container should always be tightly capped.

USES
Nitroglycerin is used to prevent angina (chest pain). It is a vasodilator, which relaxes the muscles of the blood vessels, causing an increase in the oxygen supply to the heart. The ointment and patches do not act quickly—they should not be used to treat chest pain that has already started.

TREATMENT
The ointment comes with an applicator with which the prescribed dosage can be easily measured and applied. Before a new dose is applied, the previous dose should be thoroughly removed. Each dose should be applied to a new site on the skin. Do not rub or massage the ointment into the skin. Just spread the ointment in a thin, even layer, covering an area of about the same size each time. Avoid contact of the ointment with other parts of the body, since it is absorbed wherever it touches the skin. Either use plastic or rubber gloves to apply the ointment, or wash your hands immediately after application. Cover the ointment only if directed to do so by your doctor.

The transdermal system (patches) allows controlled, continuous release of nitroglycerin. Patches are convenient and easy to use. For best results, apply the patch to a hairless or clean-shaven area of skin, avoiding scars and wounds. Choose a site (such as the chest or upper arm) that is not subject to excessive movement. It is all right to bathe or shower with a patch in place. In the event that a patch becomes dislodged, discard and replace it. Replace a patch by applying a new unit before removing the old one. This allows for uninterrupted drug therapy, and skin irritation is minimized since the site is changed each time. If redness or irritation develops at the application site, consult your physician. Do not trim or cut the patches. This alters the dose of the medication.

If you miss an application of this medication, apply the missed application as soon as possible, unless it is more than halfway through the interval between doses. In that case, do not apply the missed application at all; just return to your regular dosing schedule. Do not double the next dose.

SIDE EFFECTS
Minor. Dizziness, flushing of the face, headache, light-headedness, nausea, vomiting, or weakness. These side effects should disappear as your body adjusts to the drug.

If you feel dizzy or light-headed, sit or lie down for a while; get up slowly, and be careful on stairs. To avoid dizziness or light-headedness when you stand, contract and relax the muscles of your legs for a few moments before rising. Do this by pushing one foot against the floor while raising the other foot slightly, alternating feet so that you are "pumping" your legs in a pedaling motion.

If you are experiencing headaches acetaminophen may help to relieve them slightly.
Major. Tell your doctor about any side effects that are persistent or particularly bothersome. IT IS ESPECIALLY IMPORTANT TO TELL YOUR DOCTOR about fainting, palpitations, rash, or sweating.

INTERACTIONS
Nitroglycerin can interact with other types of medications:
1. The combination of alcohol and nitroglycerin can lead to dizziness and fainting.
2. Nitroglycerin can increase the side effects of the tricyclic antidepressants.

Before starting to take nitroglycerin, BE SURE TO TELL YOUR DOCTOR about any medications you are currently taking, especially tricyclic antidepressants.

WARNINGS

• Tell your doctor about unusual or allergic reactions you have had to any medications, especially to nitroglycerin or isosorbide dinitrate.

• Before starting to take this medication, be sure to tell your doctor if you now have or if you have ever had anemia, glaucoma, a head injury, low blood pressure, or thyroid disease or if you have recently had a heart attack or have a heart condition.

• If this drug makes you dizzy or light-headed, do not take part in any activity that requires alertness, such as driving a car or operating potentially dangerous machinery. Be especially careful when going up and down stairs.

• Before having surgery or any other medical or dental treatment, be sure to tell your doctor or dentist that you are taking this medication.

• Tolerance to this medication may develop within one to three months. If it seems to lose its effectiveness, contact your doctor.

• You should not discontinue use of nitroglycerin unless you first consult your doctor. Stopping the drug abruptly may lead to further chest pain. Your doctor may, therefore, want to decrease your dosage gradually.

• While taking this medication, do not take any over-the-counter (nonprescription) asthma, allergy, sinus, cough, cold, or diet preparations unless you first check with your doctor or pharmacist. Some of these drugs decrease the effectiveness of nitroglycerin.

• Nitroglycerin is highly flammable. Do not use it in places where it might be ignited.

• Be sure to tell your doctor if you are pregnant. The safety of this drug during pregnancy has not been determined. Although this drug appears to be safe, extensive studies in pregnant women have not yet been conducted. Also, tell your doctor if you are breast-feeding an infant. It is not known whether nitroglycerin passes into breast milk.

Nitroglycerin Transdermal System—see nitroglycerin (topical)

Nitroglyn—see nitroglycerin (systemic)

Nitrol—see nitroglycerin (topical)

Nitrolingual—see nitroglycerin (systemic)

Nitrong—see nitroglycerin (systemic)

Nitrostat—see nitroglycerin (systemic) and nitroglycerin (topical)

Noctec—see chloral hydrate

Nolex LA—see phenylpropanolamine and guaifenesin combination

Nolvadex—see tamoxifen

Nordette—see oral contraceptives

Nordryl—see diphenhydramine

norfloxacin

BRAND NAME (Manufacturer)
Noroxin (Merck Sharp & Dohme)
TYPE OF DRUG
Antibiotic
INGREDIENT
norfloxacin
DOSAGE FORM
Tablets (400 mg)
STORAGE
Norfloxacin should be stored at room temperature in a tightly closed container.

USES

Norfloxacin is an antibiotic that is used to treat bacterial urinary tract infections. It works by interfering with the reproduction of the bacteria. Norfloxacin kills susceptible bacteria but is not effective against viruses, parasites, or fungi.

TREATMENT

In order to obtain the maximum benefit from norfloxacin, it is best to take this drug on an empty stomach (one hour before or two hours after a meal) with a full glass of water. Antacids can decrease the absorption of this medication. Therefore, antacids should not be taken within two hours (before or after) of a dose of norfloxacin, unless otherwise directed by your doctor.

Norfloxacin works best when the level of medicine in your urine is kept constant. It is best, therefore, to take the doses at evenly spaced intervals day and night. For example, if you are to take two doses a day, the doses should be spaced 12 hours apart.

Try not to miss any doses of this medication. If you do miss a dose, take it as soon as you remember. However, if you do not remember to take the missed dose until it is almost time for your next dose, take it; space the following dose about halfway through the regular interval between doses; then continue with your regular dosing schedule.

Take this medication for the entire time prescribed by your doctor (usually five to 14 days), even if the symptoms disappear before the end of that period. If you stop taking the drug too soon, your infection could recur.

SIDE EFFECTS

Minor. Abdominal pain, constipation, diarrhea, dizziness, dry mouth, fatigue, gas, headache, heartburn, nausea, sleeping problems, or vomiting. These side effects should disappear as your body adjusts to this medication.

If you are constipated, increase the amount of fiber in your diet (fresh fruits and vegetables, salads, bran, and whole-grain breads), exercise, and drink more water (unless your doctor directs you to do otherwise).

To reduce mouth dryness, chew sugarless gum or suck on ice chips or hard candy.

If you feel dizzy or light-headed, sit or lie down for a while; get up slowly from a sitting or reclining position, and be careful on stairs.

Major. Tell your doctor about any side effects that are persistent or particularly bothersome. IT IS ESPECIALLY IMPORTANT TO TELL YOUR DOCTOR about depression, difficult or painful urination, rash, visual disturbances, or yellowing of the skin or eyes. Also, if the symptoms of your infection seem to be getting worse rather than improving, contact your doctor.

INTERACTIONS
Norfloxacin can interact with several other types of drugs:
1. Probenecid can block the excretion of norfloxacin into the urinary tract, decreasing its effectiveness in treating infections located there.
2. Antacids can decrease the absorption of norfloxacin from the gastrointestinal tract.
3. Nitrofurantoin may antagonize (act against) the effectiveness of norfloxacin.
   BE SURE TO TELL YOUR DOCTOR about any medications you are currently taking, especially those listed above.

WARNINGS
• Tell your doctor about unusual or allergic reactions you have had to any medications, especially to norfloxacin or to the related antibiotics cinoxacin and nalidixic acid.
• Before starting norfloxacin, tell your doctor if you now have or if you have ever had liver disease or seizures.
• If this drug makes you dizzy, do not take part in any activity that requires alertness, such as driving a car or operating potentially dangerous machinery. Be especially careful when going up and down stairs.
• In order to prevent the formation of crystals in the kidneys, try to drink plenty of fluids (at least eight glasses of water or fruit juice each day) while you are taking this medication (unless your doctor directs you to do otherwise).
• This medication has been prescribed for your current infection only. A subsequent infection, or one that someone else has, may require a different medicine. Do not give your medicine to other people or use it to treat other infections, unless your doctor directs you to do so.
• Be sure to tell your doctor if you are pregnant. Studies in pregnant women have not been conducted. However, lameness has occurred in the immature offspring of animals that received large doses of norfloxacin during pregnancy. Also, tell your doctor if you are breast-feeding an infant. It is not yet known if norfloxacin passes into breast milk.

Norgesic—see orphenadrine, aspirin, and caffeine combination

Norgesic Forte—see orphenadrine, aspirin, and caffeine combination

Norinyl—see oral contraceptives

Norlestrin—see oral contraceptives

Normatane Elixir—see phenylpropanolamine, phenylephrine, and brompheniramine combination

Normatane Expectorant—see phenylephrine, phenylpropanolamine, brompheniramine, and guaifenesin combination

Normodyne—see labetalol

Noroxin—see norfloxacin

Norpace—see disopyramide

Norpace CR—see disopyramide

Norpanth—see propantheline

Norpramin—see desipramine

Nor-Tet—see tetracycline

---

nortriptyline

BRAND NAMES (Manufacturers)
Aventyl (Lilly)
Pamelor (Sandoz)
TYPE OF DRUG
Tricyclic antidepressant
INGREDIENT
nortriptyline
DOSAGE FORMS
Capsules (10 mg, 25 mg, 50 mg, and 75 mg)
Oral solution (10 mg per 5-ml spoonful, with 4% alcohol)
STORAGE
Store at room temperature in a tightly closed container.

USES
Nortriptyline is used to relieve the symptoms of mental depression. It is thought to relieve depression by increasing the concentration of certain chemicals necessary for nerve transmission in the brain.

TREATMENT
This medication should be taken exactly as your doctor prescribes. It can be taken with water or with food to lessen the chance of stomach irritation, unless your doctor tells you to do otherwise.
   If you miss a dose of this medication, take the missed dose as soon as possible, and then return to your regular dosing schedule. However, if the dose you missed was a once-a-day bedtime dose, do not take that dose in the morning; check with your doctor instead. If the dose is taken in the morning, it may cause unwanted side effects. Never double the dose.
   The effects of therapy with this medication may not become apparent for two or three weeks.

SIDE EFFECTS
Minor. Anxiety, blurred vision, confusion, constipation, cramps, diarrhea, dizziness, drowsiness, dry mouth, fatigue, heartburn, insomnia, loss of appetite, nausea, peculiar tastes in the mouth, restlessness, sweating, vomiting, weakness, or weight gain or loss. As your body

adjusts to the medication, these side effects should disappear.

This medication may increase your sensitivity to sunlight. You should, therefore, avoid prolonged exposure to sunlight or sunlamps. Wear protective clothing and use sunscreen.

Dry mouth caused by therapy with this medication can be relieved by chewing sugarless gum or by sucking on ice chips or a piece of hard candy.

To relieve constipation, increase the amount of fiber in your diet (fresh fruits and vegetables, salads, bran, and whole-grain breads), and drink more water (unless your doctor directs you to do otherwise).

To avoid dizziness or light-headedness when you stand, contract and relax the muscles of your legs for a few moments before rising. Do this by pushing one foot against the floor while raising the other foot slightly, alternating feet so that you are "pumping" your legs in a pedaling motion.

Major. Tell your doctor about any side effects that are persistent or particularly bothersome. IT IS ESPECIALLY IMPORTANT TO TELL YOUR DOCTOR about agitation, chest pain, convulsions, difficulty in urinating, enlarged or painful breasts (in both sexes), fainting, fever, fluid retention, hair loss, hallucinations, headaches, impotence, mood changes, mouth sores, nervousness, nightmares, numbness in the fingers or toes, palpitations, ringing in the ears, seizures, skin rash, sleep disorders, sore throat, swelling, tremors, uncoordinated movements or balance problems, unusual bleeding or bruising, or yellowing of the eyes or skin.

INTERACTIONS

Nortriptyline interacts with several other types of medications:

1. Extreme drowsiness can occur when this drug is taken with central nervous system depressants (such as alcohol, antihistamines, barbiturates, benzodiazepine tranquilizers, muscle relaxants, narcotics, pain medications, phenothiazine tranquilizers, and sleeping medications) or other tricyclic antidepressants.

2. Nortriptyline may decrease the effectiveness of antiseizure medications and may block the blood-pressure-lowering effects of clonidine and guanethidine.

3. Birth control pills and estrogen-containing drugs can increase the side effects and reduce the effectiveness of the tricyclic antidepressants (including nortriptyline).

4. Tricyclic antidepressants may increase the side effects of thyroid medication and over-the-counter (nonprescription) cough, cold, asthma, allergy, sinus, and diet medications.

5. The concurrent use of tricyclic antidepressants and monoamine oxidase (MAO) inhibitors should be avoided because the combination may result in fever, convulsions, or high blood pressure. At least 14 days should separate the use of this drug and the use of an MAO inhibitor.

6. Cimetidine can decrease the elimination of nortriptyline from the body, increasing the possibility of side effects.

Before starting to take nortriptyline, BE SURE TO TELL YOUR DOCTOR about any medications you are currently taking, especially any of those listed above.

WARNINGS

• Tell your doctor if you have had unusual or allergic reactions to any medications, especially to nortriptyline or any of the other tricyclic antidepressants (amitriptyline, imipramine, doxepin, trimipramine, amoxapine, protriptyline, desipramine, or maprotiline).

• Tell your doctor if you have a history of alcoholism or if you have ever had asthma, high blood pressure, liver or kidney disease, heart disease, a heart attack, circulatory disease, stomach problems, intestinal problems, difficulty in urinating, enlarged prostate gland, epilepsy, glaucoma, thyroid disease, mental illness, or electroshock therapy.

• If this drug makes you dizzy or drowsy, do not take part in any activity that requires alertness, such as driving a car or operating potentially dangerous machinery.

• Before having surgery or other medical or dental treatment, be sure to tell your doctor or dentist about this drug.

• Do not stop taking this drug suddenly. Abruptly stopping it can cause nausea, headache, stomach upset, fatigue, or a worsening of your condition. Your doctor may want to reduce the dosage gradually.

• The effects of nortriptyline may last as long as seven days after you have stopped taking it, so continue to observe all precautions during that period.

• Be sure to tell your doctor if you are pregnant. Problems in humans have not been reported; however, studies in animals have shown that this type of medication can cause side effects in the fetus when given to the mother in large doses during pregnancy. Also, tell your doctor if you are breast-feeding an infant. Small amounts of this drug can pass into breast milk and may cause unwanted effects, such as irritability or sleeping problems, in nursing infants.

Nortussin with Codeine—see codeine and guaifenesin combination

Novafed A—see pseudoephedrine and chlorpheniramine combination

Novolin—see insulin

Nuprin—see ibuprofen

Nutracort—see hydrocortisone (topical)

Nydrazid—see isoniazid

---

nystatin

BRAND NAMES (Manufacturers)
Mycostatin (Squibb)
Nilstat (Lederle)
nystatin (various manufacturers)
Nystex (Savage)
0-V Statin (Squibb)
TYPE OF DRUG
Antifungal
INGREDIENT
nystatin

DOSAGE FORMS
Oral tablets (500,000 units)
Oral suspension (100,000 units per ml with not more than 1.0% alcohol)
Oral lozenges (200,000 units)
Vaginal tablets (100,000 units)
Topical cream, ointment, and powder (100,000 units per gram)

STORAGE
Nystatin should be stored at room temperature (never frozen) in a tightly closed, light-resistant container.

USES
Nystatin is used to treat fungal infections of the throat, gastrointestinal tract, skin, and vagina. By chemically binding to the cell membranes of fungal organisms, this medication causes the cell contents to leak out, which kills the fungi.

TREATMENT
You can take the oral tablet form of nystatin either on an empty stomach or with food or milk (as directed by your doctor).

The oral suspension should be shaken well just before using each dose. The contents tend to settle, so it is necessary to shake the container to distribute the ingredients evenly and equalize the doses.

Each dose of the oral suspension should then be measured carefully with a specially designed 5-ml measuring spoon. An ordinary kitchen teaspoon is not accurate enough. Place half of the dose in each side of your mouth. Try to hold the suspension in the mouth or swish it through the mouth for as long as possible before swallowing it.

The oral lozenge form should be allowed to dissolve slowly in the mouth.

The vaginal tablets are packaged with instructions and an applicator for inserting the tablets into the vagina. Read the instructions carefully before using this product.

Occasionally, the vaginal tablets are prescribed to be taken orally (to treat mouth or throat infections). The tablets are sucked on to increase contact time with the mouth and throat.

The region where you are to apply the topical cream, ointment, or powder should be washed carefully and patted dry. A sufficient amount of medication should then be applied to the affected area. An occlusive dressing (like kitchen plastic wrap) should NOT be applied over the medication (unless your doctor directs you to do so).

If you are using the powder form to treat a foot infection, sprinkle liberally into your shoes and socks.

Try not to miss any doses of this medication. If you do miss a dose, take (or apply) the missed dose as soon as possible, unless it is almost time for the next dose. In that case, do not take (or apply) the missed dose at all; just return to your regular dosing schedule. Do not double the next dose of this medication.

Take this drug for the entire time prescribed by your doctor (usually seven to 14 days), even if the symptoms disappear before the end of that period. If you stop taking the drug too soon, resistant fungi are given a chance to continue growing, and your infection could recur.

SIDE EFFECTS
Minor. Oral forms: diarrhea, nausea, or vomiting. Topical and vaginal forms: itching. These side effects should disappear as your body adjusts to the drug.
Major. Tell your doctor about any side effects that are persistent or particularly bothersome. IT IS ESPECIALLY IMPORTANT TO TELL YOUR DOCTOR about a rash. Also, if symptoms of your infection seem to be getting worse rather than improving, tell your doctor.

INTERACTIONS
Nystatin should not interact with other medications if it is used according to directions.

WARNINGS
• Tell your doctor about unusual or allergic reactions you have had to any medications, especially to nystatin.
• If you are using this drug to treat a vaginal infection, avoid sexual intercourse or ask your partner to wear a condom until treatment has been completed. These measures help prevent reinfection. Use the vaginal tablets continuously, even during a menstrual period. Unless instructed otherwise by your doctor, do not douche during treatment or until three weeks after you stop using the vaginal tablets. Wear cotton panties, rather than nylon or other nonporous materials, when you are being treated for fungal infections of the vagina. There may be some vaginal drainage while using the vaginal tablets, so you may wish to use a sanitary napkin or panty liner.
• This medication has been prescribed for your current infection only. Another infection later on, or one that someone else has, may require a different medicine. You should not give your medicine to other people or use it for other infections, unless your doctor specifically directs you to do so.
• If the symptoms of infection do not begin to improve two or three days after starting nystatin, CONTACT YOUR DOCTOR. This medication may not be effective against the organism causing your infection.
• Be sure to tell your doctor if you are pregnant. Although nystatin appears to be safe during pregnancy, extensive studies in humans have not been conducted. Also, tell your doctor if you are breast-feeding an infant. It is not known whether this medication passes into breast milk.

Nystex—see nystatin

Nytol—see diphenhydramine

Obalan—see phendimetrazine

Obe-Nix—see phentermine

Obephen—see phentermine

Obermine—see phentermine

Obestin-30—see phentermine

Ocusert Pilo-20—see pilocarpine (ophthalmic)

Ocusert Pilo-40—see pilocarpine (ophthalmic)

omeprazole

BRAND NAME (Manufacturer)
Prilosec (MSD)
TYPE OF DRUG
Gastric acid secretion inhibitor
INGREDIENT
omeprazole
DOSAGE FORM
Delayed-release capsules (20 mg)
STORAGE
Omeprazole should be stored at room temperature in a tightly closed container.

USES

Omeprazole is prescribed to treat peptic ulcer disease, gastroesophageal reflux, and hypersecretory syndromes. This drug suppresses the secretion of acid in the stomach.

TREATMENT

Omeprazole capsules should not be opened, chewed, or crushed. They should be taken with a glass of water on an empty stomach. It is best to take the dose one hour before meals or two hours after meals.

Try to take the medication at the same time(s) each day. If you miss a dose of the medication, take the missed dose as soon as possible, then return to your regular dosing schedule. If it is almost time for the next dose, however, skip the one you missed and return to your regular schedule. Do not double the next dose (unless your doctor directs you to do so) of the medication.

It is important that you take this medication for as long as prescribed by your doctor.

SIDE EFFECTS

Minor. Abdominal pain, burning sensation in mouth, constipation, diarrhea, dizziness, dry mouth, fatigue, headache, or palpitations.

To relieve constipation while you are being treated with this medication, exercise and drink more water, unless your doctor directs you to do otherwise.

To avoid dizziness when you stand, contract and relax the muscles of your legs for a few moments before rising. Do this by pushing one foot against the floor while raising the other foot slightly, alternating feet so that you are "pumping" your legs in a pedaling motion.

To relieve dry mouth, chew sugarless gum or suck on ice chips or a piece of hard candy.
Major. Tell your doctor about any side effects that are persistent or particularly bothersome. IT IS ESPECIALLY IMPORTANT TO TELL YOUR DOCTOR about itching, numbness or tingling of fingers or toes, rash, or yellowing of the eyes and skin.

INTERACTIONS

Omeprazole may increase the effects of diazepam, warfarin, and phenytoin.

Be sure to tell your doctor about any medications you are currently taking, especially any of the ones listed above.

WARNINGS
• Be sure to tell your doctor about unusual reactions you have had to any drugs, especially to omeprazole.
• Tell your doctor if you have ever had thyroid disease, liver disease, Addison's disease, or Cushing's disease.
• This medication may cause dizziness and light-headedness, so use caution while driving a car or operating potentially dangerous equipment.
• Long-term and high-dose treatment with omeprazole has been associated with higher incidences of gastric tumors. Consult your doctor if you need to take high doses of omeprazole for a long time.
• Be sure to tell your doctor if you are pregnant. Adequate human studies have not been conducted with omeprazole. Also, be sure to tell your doctor if you are breast-feeding an infant.

Omnipen—see ampicillin

Ophthacet—see sodium sulfacetamide (ophthalmic)

Optimine—see azatadine

Oragest T.D.—see phenylpropanolamine and chlorpheniramine combination

oral contraceptives

BRAND NAMES (Manufacturers)
Brevicon (Syntex)
Demulen (Searle)
Loestrin (Parke-Davis)
Lo/Ovral (Wyeth)
Modicon (Ortho)
Nordette (Wyeth)
Norinyl (Syntex)
Norlestrin (Parke-Davis)
Ortho-Novum (Ortho)
Ovcon (Mead Johnson)
Ovral (Wyeth)
Tri-Levlen (Berlex)
Tri-Norinyl (Syntex)
Triphasil (Wyeth-Ayerst)
TYPE OF DRUG
Oral contraceptive
INGREDIENTS
estrogens and progestins
DOSAGE FORM
Tablets (in packages of 21 or 28 tablets; when 28 tablets are present, seven of the tablets either are placebos or contain iron)
STORAGE
Oral contraceptives should be stored at room temperature. They should be kept in their original container, which is designed to help you keep track of your dosing schedule.

USES

Oral contraceptives change the hormone balance of the body to prevent pregnancy.

TREATMENT

To avoid stomach irritation, you can take oral contraceptives with food or with a full glass of water or milk.

In order to become accustomed to taking this medication, try to take it at the same time every day.

Use a supplemental method of birth control for the first week after you start taking oral contraceptives (the medication takes time to become fully effective).

Even if you do not start to menstruate on schedule at the end of the pill cycle, begin the next cycle of pills at the prescribed time. Many women taking oral contraceptives have irregular menstruation.

If you miss a dose of this medication and you are on a 21-day schedule, take the missed dose as soon as you remember. If you don't remember until the next day, take the dose of that day plus the one you missed; then return to your regular dosing schedule. If you miss two days' doses, you should take two tablets a day for the next two days; then return to your regular dosing schedule. You should also use another form of birth control during those four days. If you miss your dose three days in a row, you should stop taking this drug and use a different method of birth control until you check with your doctor. Your doctor may want you to start a new package seven days after the last tablet was missed and use an additional method of birth control until the start of your next period. If you are on the 28-day schedule and you miss taking any one of the first 21 tablets, you should follow the instructions for the 21day schedule. If you missed taking any of the last seven tablets, there is no danger of pregnancy, but you should take the first pill of the next month's cycle on the regularly scheduled day.

SIDE EFFECTS

Minor. Abdominal cramps, acne, backache, bloating, change in appetite, changes in sexual desire, diarrhea, dizziness, fatigue, headache, nasal congestion, nausea, nervousness, vaginal irritation, or vomiting. These side effects should disappear as your body adjusts to the medication.

This medication can increase your sensitivity to sunlight. Avoid prolonged exposure to sunlight and sunlamps. Wear protective clothing, and use an effective sunscreen.

If you feel dizzy, sit or lie down for a while.

Major. Tell your doctor about any side effects that are persistent or particularly bothersome. IT IS ESPECIALLY IMPORTANT TO TELL YOUR DOCTOR about abdominal pain; breakthrough vaginal bleeding (spotting); changes in menstrual flow; chest pain; depression; difficult or painful urination; enlarged or tender breasts; hearing changes; increase or decrease in hair growth; migraine headaches; numbness or tingling; pain in your calves; rash; skin color changes; swelling of the feet, ankles, or lower legs; unusual bleeding or bruising; vaginal itching; weight changes; or yellowing of the eyes or skin.

INTERACTIONS

These drugs interact with several other types of drugs:
1. Pain relievers, antimigraine preparations, rifampin, barbiturates, phenylbutazone, phenytoin, primidone, car-

bamazepine, isoniazid, neomycin, griseofulvin, penicillins, tetracycline, chloramphenicol, sulfonamide antibiotics, nitrofurantoin, and ampicillin can decrease the effectiveness of oral contraceptives.
2. Oral contraceptives can reduce the effectiveness of oral anticoagulants (blood thinners, such as warfarin), anticonvulsants, tricyclic antidepressants, antihypertensive agents, oral antidiabetic agents, and vitamins.
3. Oral contraceptives can increase the blood levels of caffeine, diazepam, chlordiazepoxide, metoprolol, propranolol, adrenocorticosteroids (cortisone-like medications), imipramine, clomipramine, phenytoin, and phenylbutazone, which can lead to an increase in side effects.
4. Oral contraceptives can decrease the blood levels and, therefore, the effectiveness of lorazepam and oxazepam.

BE SURE TO TELL YOUR DOCTOR about any medications you are currently taking, especially those listed above.

WARNINGS

• Tell your doctor about unusual or allergic reactions you have had to any medications, especially to estrogens, progestins, or progesterones.

• Before starting to take this medication, be sure to tell your doctor if you now have or if you have ever had asthma, bleeding problems, breast cancer, clotting disorders, diabetes mellitus, endometriosis, epilepsy, gallbladder disease, heart disease, high blood pressure, kidney disease, liver disease, mental depression, migraine headaches, porphyria, strokes, thyroid disease, uterine tumors, vaginal bleeding, or vitamin deficiencies.

• Some women who have used an oral contraceptive have had difficulty becoming pregnant after discontinuing use. Most of these women had had scanty or irregular periods before starting oral contraceptives. Possible subsequent difficulty in becoming pregnant is a matter you should discuss with your doctor before using an oral contraceptive.

• Every prescription comes with a booklet that explains birth control pills. Read this booklet carefully. It contains exact directions on how to use this medicine correctly and describes the risks involved.

• Women over 30 years of age and women who smoke while taking this medication have an increased risk of developing serious heart or blood vessel side effects.

• If this drug makes you dizzy, avoid taking part in any activity that requires alertness, such as driving a car or operating potentially dangerous machinery.

• Before surgery or other medical or dental treatment, tell your doctor or dentist you are taking this drug.

• This type of drug has been suspected of causing cancer. If you have a family history of cancer, you should consult your doctor before taking oral contraceptives.

• Be sure to tell your doctor if you are pregnant. Oral contraceptives have been associated with birth defects in animals and in humans. Because hormones have long-term effects on the body, oral contraceptives should be stopped at least three months prior to becoming pregnant. Another method of birth control should be used for those three months. Also, tell your doctor if you are breast-feeding an infant. This medication passes into breast milk.

Oramide—see tolbutamide

Orasone—see prednisone (systemic)

Oretic—see hydrochlorothiazide

Oreton Methyl—see Methyltestosterone

Orinase—see tolbutamide

Ormazine—see chlorpromazine

Ornade—see phenylpropanolamine and chlorpheniramine combination

---

orphenadrine, aspirin, and caffeine combination

BRAND NAMES (Manufacturers)
Norgesic (Riker)
Norgesic Forte (Riker)
Orphengesic (various manufacturers)
TYPE OF DRUG
Muscle relaxant and analgesic
INGREDIENTS
orphenadrine, aspirin, and caffeine
DOSAGE FORM
Tablets (25 mg orphenadrine, 385 mg aspirin, and 30 mg caffeine {Norgesic}; 50 mg orphenadrine, 770 mg aspirin, and 60 mg caffeine {Norgesic Forte})
STORAGE
This medication should be stored at room temperature in a tightly closed, light-resistant container.

USES
Orphenadrine, aspirin, and caffeine combination drug is used to relax muscles and to relieve the pain of sprains, strains, and other muscle injuries. Orphenadrine acts as a central nervous system (brain and spinal cord) depressant, which blocks reflexes involved in producing and maintaining muscle spasms. It does not act directly on tense muscles. Caffeine is a central nervous system stimulant that acts by constricting the blood vessels in the head. This may help relieve headaches.

TREATMENT
These tablets should be taken with a full glass of water. To avoid stomach irritation, you can also take this medication with food or milk (unless your doctor directs otherwise).

If you miss a dose of this medication and remember within an hour, take the missed dose and then return to your regular dosing schedule. If it has been longer than an hour, do not take the missed dose at all; just return to your regular dosing schedule. Do not double the next dose.

SIDE EFFECTS
Minor. Blurred vision, confusion, constipation, diarrhea, dizziness, drowsiness, dry mouth, headache, indigestion, insomnia, nausea, nervousness, vomiting, or weakness. These side effects should disappear as your body adjusts to the medication.

If you are constipated, increase the amount of fiber in your diet (fresh fruits and vegetables, salads, bran, and whole-grain breads), exercise, and drink more water (unless your doctor directs you to do otherwise).

If you feel dizzy or light-headed, sit or lie down for a while; get up slowly from a sitting or reclining position, and be careful on stairs.

To relieve mouth dryness, suck on ice chips or a piece of hard candy or chew sugarless gum.
Major. Tell your doctor about any side effects that are persistent or particularly bothersome. IT IS ESPECIALLY IMPORTANT TO TELL YOUR DOCTOR about bloody or black, tarry stools; chest tightness; difficulty in breathing; difficulty in urinating; hearing loss; palpitations; rash; ringing in the ears; or severe abdominal pain.

INTERACTIONS
This medication interacts with several other types of drugs:
1. Orphenadrine can cause extreme drowsiness when combined with other central nervous system depressants (such as alcohol, antihistamines, barbiturates, benzodiazepine tranquilizers, phenothiazine tranquilizers, narcotics, and sleeping medications) or with tricyclic antidepressants.
2. Orphenadrine can cause confusion, anxiety, and tremors when combined with propoxyphene.
3. Aspirin can increase the active blood levels of methotrexate, oral antidiabetic agents, and oral anticoagulants (blood thinners, such as warfarin), which can lead to an increase in side effects.
4. The antigout activity of probenecid and sulfinpyrazone are decreased by aspirin.
5. The gastrointestinal side effects of anti-inflammatory medications may be increased by aspirin.

BE SURE TO TELL YOUR DOCTOR about any medications you are currently taking, especially those listed above.

WARNINGS
• Tell your doctor about unusual or allergic reactions you have had to any drugs, especially to orphenadrine, caffeine, aspirin, other salicylates, methyl salicylate, or nonsteroidal anti-inflammatory agents (such as diclofenac, diflunisal, fenoprofen, flurbiprofen, ibuprofen, indomethacin, ketoprofen, meclofenamate, naproxen, oxyphenbutazone, phenylbutazone, piroxicam, sulindac, and tolmetin).
• Tell your doctor if you now have or if you have ever had anemia, bladder obstruction, glaucoma, gout, kidney disease, liver disease, myasthenia gravis, peptic ulcers, enlarged prostate gland, intestinal obstruction, or bleeding problems.
• This medication should not be taken as a substitute for rest, physical therapy, or other measures recommended by your doctor to treat your condition.
• If this medication makes you dizzy or drowsy or blurs your vision, do not take part in any activity that requires alertness, such as driving a car or operating potentially dangerous machinery, while you are taking it.

• Before having surgery or other medical or dental treatment, tell your doctor or dentist about this drug. Treatment with aspirin-containing drugs is usually discontinued several days before any major surgery, to prevent bleeding complications.

• Because this product contains aspirin, additional medications that contain aspirin should not be taken without your doctor's approval. Check the labels on over-the-counter (nonprescription) pain, sinus, allergy, asthma, cough, and cold products to see if they contain aspirin.

• The use of aspirin in children (about 16 years of age or less) with the flu or chicken pox has been associated with a rare, life-threatening condition called Reye's syndrome. Aspirin-containing products should, therefore, not be given to children who are exhibiting signs of infection.

• Diabetic patients should be aware that large doses of aspirin (more than six 385-mg tablets or three 770-mg tablets per day) may interfere with urine sugar testing. Diabetics should, therefore, check with their doctor before changing their insulin dose.

• Be sure to tell your doctor if you are pregnant. Aspirin can prolong labor if it is taken by the mother close to term and can cause heart problems in newborn infants. Also, tell your doctor if you are breast-feeding an infant. It is not known whether orphenadrine passes into breast milk, but small quantities of aspirin and caffeine are able to pass into breast milk.

Orphengesic—see orphenadrine, aspirin, and caffeine combination

Ortega-Otic M—see hydrocortisone, polymyxin B, and neomycin combination (otic)

Ortho-Novum—see oral contraceptives

Orudis—see ketoprofen

Oto—see antipyrine, benzocaine, oxyquinoline, and glycerin combination

Otocort—see hydrocortisone, polymyxin B, and neomycin combination (otic)

Otomycin-Hpn Otic—see hydrocortisone, polymyxin B, and neomycin combination (otic)

Ovcon—see oral contraceptives

Ovral—see oral contraceptives

O-V Statin—see nystatin

oxacillin

BRAND NAMES (Manufacturers)
Bactocill (Beecham)
Prostaphlin (Bristol)
TYPE OF DRUG
Penicillin antibiotic

INGREDIENT
oxacillin
DOSAGE FORMS
Capsules (250 mg and 500 mg)
Oral solution (250 mg per 5-ml spoonful)
STORAGE
Oxacillin capsules should be stored at room temperature in a tightly closed container. The oral solution should be stored in the refrigerator in a tightly closed container. Any unused portion of the solution should be discarded after 14 days. This medication should never be frozen.

USES
Oxacillin is used to treat a wide variety of bacterial infections, especially those involving Staphylococcus bacteria. This medication acts by severely injuring the cell membranes of the infecting bacteria, thereby preventing them from growing and multiplying. Oxacillin kills susceptible bacteria, but it is not effective against viruses, parasites, or fungi.

TREATMENT
Oxacillin should be taken on an empty stomach or with a glass of water one hour before or two hours after a meal. This medication should never be taken with fruit juices or carbonated beverages, because the acidity of these drinks destroys the drug in the stomach.

The oral solution should be measured carefully with a specially designed 5-ml measuring spoon. An ordinary kitchen teaspoon is not accurate enough.

Oxacillin works best when the level of medicine in your bloodstream is kept constant. It is best, therefore, to take the doses at evenly spaced intervals day and night. For example, if you are taking four doses a day, the doses should be spaced six hours apart.

If you miss a dose of this medication, take the missed dose immediately. If you do not remember to take the missed dose until it is almost time for your next dose, take it immediately, space the following dose about halfway through the regular interval between doses, and then return to your regular dosing schedule. Try not to skip any doses.

It is important to continue to take this medication for the entire time prescribed by your doctor (usually seven to 14 days), even if the symptoms of infection disappear before the end of that period. If you stop taking the drug too soon, resistant bacteria are given a chance to continue growing, and the infection could recur.

SIDE EFFECTS
Minor. Diarrhea, heartburn, nausea, or vomiting. These side effects should disappear as your body adjusts to the drug.
Major. Tell your doctor about any side effects that are persistent or particularly bothersome. IT IS ESPECIALLY IMPORTANT TO TELL YOUR DOCTOR about bloating, chills, cough, darkened tongue, difficulty in breathing, difficult or painful urination, fever, irritation of the mouth, muscle aches, rash, rectal or vaginal itching, severe diarrhea, sore throat, or yellowing of the eyes or skin. Also, if your symptoms of infection seem to be getting worse rather than improving, you should contact your doctor.

INTERACTIONS
Oxacillin interacts with other types of medications:
1. Probenecid can increase the blood concentrations of this medication.
2. Oxacillin may decrease the effectiveness of birth control pills, and pregnancy could result. You should, therefore, use another form of birth control while taking this drug. Discuss alternatives with your doctor.

BE SURE TO TELL YOUR DOCTOR about any medications you are currently taking, especially any listed above.

WARNINGS
Tell your doctor about unusual or allergic reactions you have had to any medications, especially to oxacillin, other penicillins, cephalosporin antibiotics, penicillamine, or griseofulvin.

Tell your doctor if you now have or if you have ever had kidney disease, asthma, or allergies.

This medication has been prescribed for your current infection only. Another infection later on, or one that someone else has, may require a different medicine. Therefore, you should not give your medicine to other people or use it for other infections, unless your doctor specifically directs you to do so.

Diabetics taking oxacillin should know that this drug can cause a false-positive sugar reaction with a Clinitest urine glucose test. To avoid this problem while taking oxacillin, you should switch to Clinistix or Tes-Tape to test your urine for sugar.

Be sure to tell your doctor if you are pregnant. Although oxacillin appears to be safe during pregnancy, extensive studies in humans have not been conducted. Also, tell your doctor if you are breast-feeding an infant. Small amounts of this medication pass into breast milk and may temporarily alter the bacterial balance in the intestinal tract of the nursing infant, resulting in diarrhea.

---

oxazepam

BRAND NAME (Manufacturer)
Serax (Wyeth-Ayerst)
TYPE OF DRUG
Benzodiazepine sedative/hypnotic
INGREDIENT
oxazepam
DOSAGE FORMS
Capsules (10 mg, 15 mg, and 30 mg)
Tablets (15 mg)
STORAGE
This medication should be stored at room temperature in a tightly closed, light-resistant container.

USES
Oxazepam is prescribed to treat symptoms of anxiety and sometimes to treat anxiety associated with depression or alcohol withdrawal. It is not clear exactly how this medicine works, but this medication may relieve anxiety by acting as a depressant of the central nervous system (brain and spinal cord). Oxazepam is currently used by many people to relieve nervousness. This medication is very effective for this purpose when used for short periods, however it is important to attempt to remove the cause of the anxiety as well.

TREATMENT
This medication should be taken exactly as directed by your doctor. It can be taken with food or a full glass of water if stomach upset occurs. Do not take oxazepam with a dose of antacids, since they may slow its absorption.

If you are taking this drug regularly and you miss a dose, take the missed dose immediately if remembered within an hour. If more than an hour has passed, skip the dose you missed and wait for the next scheduled dose. Do not double the dose.

SIDE EFFECTS
Minor. Bitter taste in the mouth, constipation, depression, diarrhea, dizziness, drowsiness (after a night's sleep), dry mouth, excessive salivation, fatigue, flushing, headache, heartburn, loss of appetite, nausea, nervousness, sweating, or vomiting. These side effects should disappear as your body adjusts to the medication.

To relieve constipation, increase the amount of fiber in your diet (fresh fruits and vegetables, salads, bran, and whole-grain breads), exercise, and drink more water (unless your doctor directs you to do otherwise).

Dry mouth can be relieved by chewing sugarless gum or by sucking on ice chips.

If you feel dizzy, sit or lie down for a while; get up slowly from a sitting or reclining position, and be careful on stairs.

Major. Tell your doctor about any side effects that are persistent or particularly bothersome. IT IS ESPECIALLY IMPORTANT TO TELL YOUR DOCTOR about blurred or double vision, chest pain, difficulty in urinating, fainting, falling, fever, hallucinations, joint pain, mouth sores, nightmares, palpitations, rash, severe depression, shortness of breath, slurred speech, sore throat, uncoordinated movements, unusual excitement, unusual tiredness, or yellowing of the eyes or skin.

INTERACTIONS
Oxazepam interacts with several other types of medications:
1. To prevent oversedation, this drug should not be taken with alcohol, other sedative drugs, or central nervous system depressants (such as antihistamines, barbiturates, muscle relaxants, pain medicines, narcotics, medicines for seizures, and phenothiazine tranquilizers) or with antidepressants.
2. This medication may decrease the effectiveness of carbamazepine, levodopa, and oral anticoagulants (blood thinners) and may increase the effects of phenytoin.
3. Disulfiram and isoniazid can increase the blood levels of oxazepam, which can lead to toxic effects.
4. Concurrent use of rifampin may decrease the effectiveness of oxazepam.

BE SURE TO TELL YOUR DOCTOR about any medications you are currently taking, especially any listed above.

WARNINGS

- Tell your doctor about unusual or allergic reactions you have had to any medications, especially to oxazepam or other benzodiazepine tranquilizers (such as alprazolam, chlordiazepoxide, clorazepate, diazepam, flurazepam, halazepam, lorazepam, midazolam, prazepam, temazepam, or triazolam).
- Tell your doctor if you have ever had kidney, liver, or lung disease; epilepsy; myasthenia gravis; porphyria; or mental illness or depression.
- This medicine can cause drowsiness. Avoid tasks that require mental alertness, such as driving a car or using potentially dangerous machinery.
- Oxazepam has the potential for abuse and must be used with caution. Tolerance may develop quickly; do not increase the dosage without first consulting your doctor. It is also important not to stop taking this drug suddenly if you have been taking it in large amounts, or if you have used it for several weeks. Your doctor may want to reduce the dosage gradually.
- This is a safe drug when used properly. When it is combined with other sedative drugs or alcohol, however, serious side effects can develop.
- Be sure to tell your doctor if you are pregnant. This medicine may increase the chance of birth defects if it is taken during the first three months of pregnancy. Too much use of this medicine during the last six months of pregnancy may cause the baby to become dependent on it. Use of this medicine during the last weeks of pregnancy may cause unwanted side effects in the newborn. Tell your doctor if you are breast-feeding. Oxazepam may pass into breast milk and cause unwanted side effects in the nursing infant.

oxtriphylline

BRAND NAMES (Manufacturers)
Choledyl (Parke-Davis)
Choledyl SA (Parke-Davis)
oxtriphylline (various manufacturers)
TYPE OF DRUG
Bronchodilator
INGREDIENT
oxtriphylline
DOSAGE FORMS
Tablets (100 mg and 200 mg)
Sustained-release tablets (400 mg and 600 mg)
Oral pediatric liquid (50 mg per 5-ml spoonful)
Oral elixir (100 mg per 5-ml spoonful, with 20% alcohol)
STORAGE
Oxtriphylline tablets, liquid, and elixir should be stored at room temperature in tightly closed containers. This medication should never be frozen.

USES
This medication is used to treat breathing problems (wheezing and shortness of breath) caused by asthma, bronchitis, or emphysema. It relaxes the smooth muscle of the bronchial airways (breathing tubes), which opens the air passages to the lungs and allows air to move in and out more easily.

TREATMENT
Oxtriphylline should be taken on an empty stomach 30 to 60 minutes before or two hours after a meal. If this medication causes stomach irritation, however, you can take it with food or with a full glass of water or milk (unless your doctor directs you to do otherwise).

Antidiarrheal medications prevent the absorption of oxtriphylline. Therefore, at least one hour should separate doses of these two types of medications.

The sustained-release tablets should be swallowed whole (if the tablet is scored for breaking, you can break it along these lines). Chewing, crushing, or crumbling the tablets destroys their sustained-release activity and possibly increases the side effects.

Each dose of the oral liquid should be measured carefully with a specially designed 5-ml measuring spoon. An ordinary kitchen teaspoon is not accurate enough.

Oxtriphylline works best when the level of the medicine in your bloodstream is kept constant. It is best, therefore, to take the doses at evenly spaced intervals day and night. For example, if you are to take four doses a day, the doses should be spaced six hours apart.

Try not to miss any doses of this medication. If you do miss a dose, take the missed dose as soon as possible, unless it is almost time for the next dose. In that case, do not take the missed dose at all; just return to your regular dosing schedule. Do not double the next dose.

SIDE EFFECTS
Minor. Diarrhea, dizziness, flushing, headache, heartburn, increased urination, insomnia, irritability, loss of appetite, nausea, nervousness, stomach pain, or vomiting. These side effects should disappear as your body adjusts to the medication.

If you feel dizzy or light-headed, sit or lie down for a while; get up slowly from a sitting or reclining position.
Major. Tell your doctor about any side effects that are persistent or particularly bothersome. IT IS ESPECIALLY IMPORTANT TO TELL YOUR DOCTOR about bloody or black, tarry stools; confusion; convulsions; difficulty in breathing; fainting; muscle twitches; palpitations; rash; severe abdominal pain; or unusual weakness.

INTERACTIONS
Oxtriphylline interacts with several other types of drugs:
1. It can increase the diuretic effects of furosemide.
2. Reserpine, in combination with oxtriphylline, can cause a rapid heart rate.
3. Beta blockers (acebutolol, atenolol, betaxolol, carteolol, esmolol, labetalol, metoprolol, nadolol, penbutolol, pindolol, propranolol, timolol) can block the effectiveness of oxtriphylline.
4. Phenobarbital and rifampin can increase the elimination of oxtriphylline from the body, decreasing its effectiveness.
5. Cimetidine, erythromycin, oral contraceptives (birth control pills), troleanodomycin, allopurinol, and thiabendazole can decrease the elimination of oxtriphylline from the body, increasing its side effects.

Before you start to take this medication, BE SURE TO TELL YOUR DOCTOR about any medications you are currently taking, especially any of those listed above.

WARNINGS

Tell your doctor about unusual or allergic reactions you have had to any medications, especially to oxtriphylline, aminophylline, caffeine, dyphylline, theophylline, or theobromine.

Tell your doctor if you now have or if you have ever had fibrocystic breast disease, heart disease, kidney disease, low or high blood pressure, liver disease, stomach ulcers, thyroid disease, or an enlarged prostate gland.

Cigarette or marijuana smoking may affect this drug's action. BE SURE TO TELL YOUR DOCTOR if you smoke. Also, do not suddenly stop smoking without informing your doctor.

High fever, diarrhea, the flu, and influenza vaccinations can also affect the actions of this drug. Therefore, tell your doctor about episodes of high fever or prolonged diarrhea. Before having any vaccinations, especially those to prevent the flu, be sure to tell the person administering the vaccine that you are taking this medication.

Avoid drinking large amounts of caffeine-containing beverages (coffee, cocoa, tea, and cola drinks), and avoid eating large amounts of chocolate. These products may increase the side effects of oxtriphylline.

Do not change your diet without first consulting your doctor. The action of this drug may be affected by char-broiled foods or a high-protein, low-carbohydrate diet.

Before having surgery or other medical or dental treatment, be sure to tell your doctor or dentist about this drug.

Before taking any over-the-counter (nonprescription) asthma, allergy, cough, cold, sinus, or diet medication, ask your doctor or pharmacist whether it will interact with oxtriphylline. These products may add to the side effects of oxtriphylline.

Be sure to tell your doctor if you are pregnant. Although oxtriphylline appears to be safe during pregnancy, extensive studies in humans have not been conducted. Also, tell your doctor if you are breast-feeding an infant. Small amounts of oxtriphylline pass into breast milk and may cause irritability, fretfulness, or insomnia in nursing infants.

---

oxybutynin

BRAND NAME (Manufacturer)
Ditropan (Marion)
TYPE OF DRUG
Antispasmodic
INGREDIENT
oxybutynin
DOSAGE FORMS
Tablets (5 mg)
Oral syrup (5 mg per 5-ml spoonful)
STORAGE
Oxybutynin tablets and syrup should be stored at room temperature in tightly closed containers.

USES

Oxybutynin is used to relieve the symptoms associated with urinary incontinence (inability to control the bladder) or urinary frequency.

TREATMENT

Oxybutynin can be taken either on an empty stomach with water only or, to reduce stomach irritation, with food or milk (as directed by your doctor).

Each dose of the oral syrup should be measured carefully with a specially designed 5-ml measuring spoon. An ordinary kitchen teaspoon is not accurate enough.

If you miss a dose of this medication, take the missed dose as soon as possible, unless it is almost time for the next dose. In that case, do not take the missed dose at all; return to your regular dosing schedule. Do not double the dose.

SIDE EFFECTS

Minor. Bloating, blurred vision, constipation, decreased sweating, dizziness, drowsiness, dry mouth, insomnia, nausea, vomiting, or weakness. These side effects should disappear as your body adjusts to the medication.

This medication can also cause increased sensitivity of your eyes to sunlight. Sunglasses may help relieve the discomfort caused by bright lights.

To relieve constipation, increase the amount of fiber in your diet (fresh fruits and vegetables, salads, bran, and whole-grain breads) and exercise (unless your doctor directs you to do otherwise).

If you feel dizzy, sit or lie down for a while; get up slowly from a sitting or reclining position, and be careful on stairs.

To help relieve mouth dryness, chew sugarless gum or suck on ice chips or a piece of hard candy.
Major. Tell your doctor about any side effects that are persistent or particularly bothersome. IT IS ESPECIALLY IMPORTANT TO TELL YOUR DOCTOR about decreased sexual ability, difficult or painful urination, eye pain, itching, palpitations, or skin rash.

INTERACTIONS

Oxybutynin should not interact with other medications if it is used according to directions.

WARNINGS

• Tell your doctor about unusual or allergic reactions you have had to any medications, especially to oxybutynin.
• Before starting to take this medication, be sure to tell your doctor if you now have or if you have ever had bleeding disorders, glaucoma, heart disease, hiatal hernia, high blood pressure, intestinal blockage, kidney disease, liver disease, myasthenia gravis, enlarged prostate gland, thyroid disease, toxemia of pregnancy, ulcerative colitis, or urinary retention.
• If this drug makes you dizzy or blurs your vision, avoid taking part in any activity that requires alertness, such as driving a car or operating potentially dangerous machinery.
• This medication can decrease sweating and heat release from the body. You should, therefore, try not to be-

come overheated (avoid strenuous exercise in hot weather, and do not take hot baths, showers, and saunas). • Be sure to tell your doctor if you are pregnant. Although oxybutynin appears to be safe during pregnancy, extensive studies in humans have not been conducted. Also, tell your doctor if you are breast-feeding. This drug may decrease milk production. It is not known whether oxybutynin passes into breast milk.

oxycodone hydrochloride, oxycodone terephthalate, and aspirin—see aspirin and oxycodone combination

oxycodone hydrochloride with acetaminophen—see acetaminophen and oxycodone combination

Oxydess II—see dextroamphetamine

oxytetracycline

BRAND NAMES (Manufacturers)
E.P. Mycin (Edwards)
oxytetracycline hydrochloride (various manufacturers)
Terramycin (Pfizer)
Uri-Tet (American Urologicals)
TYPE OF DRUG
Tetracycline antibiotic
INGREDIENT
oxytetracycline
DOSAGE FORMS
Tablets (250 mg)
Capsules (250 mg)
STORAGE
Oxytetracycline should be stored at room temperature in a tightly closed, light-resistant container.

USES
Oxytetracycline is used to treat acne and a wide variety of bacterial infections. It acts by inhibiting the growth of bacteria. Bacteria may be partly responsible for the development of acne lesions. Oxytetracycline kills bacteria, but it is not effective against viruses or fungi.

TREATMENT
Ideally, this medication should be taken on an empty stomach one hour before or two hours after a meal. It should be taken with a full glass of water in order to avoid irritation of the throat or esophagus (tube leading to the stomach). If this drug causes stomach upset, however, you can take it with food or water (unless your doctor directs otherwise).

Avoid consuming any dairy products, including milk and cheese, within two hours of any dose of this drug. Avoid taking antacids or laxatives containing aluminum, calcium, or magnesium within an hour or two of a dose. Avoid taking any medication containing iron within three hours of a dose. These products chemically bind oxytetracycline and prevent the drug from being absorbed into the body.

Oxytetracycline works best when the level of medicine in your bloodstream is kept constant. It is best, there-

fore, to take the doses at evenly spaced intervals day and night. For example, if you are to take four doses a day, the doses should be spaced six hours apart.

If you miss a dose of this medication, take the missed dose immediately. However, if you do not remember to take the missed dose until it is almost time for your next dose, take it; space the following dose about halfway through the regular interval between doses; then return to your regular dosing schedule. Try not to skip any doses of this medication.

It is important to continue to take this medication for the entire time prescribed by your doctor, even if the symptoms disappear before the end of that period. If you stop taking the drug too soon, resistant bacteria are given a chance to continue growing, and the infection could recur.

SIDE EFFECTS
Minor. Diarrhea, dizziness, loss of appetite, nausea, stomach cramps and upset, vomiting, or discoloration of the nails. These side effects should disappear as your body adjusts to the medication.

Oxytetracycline can increase your sensitivity to sunlight. You should, therefore, avoid prolonged exposure to sunlight and sunlamps. Wear protective clothing and sunglasses, and use an effective sunscreen.
Major. Tell your doctor about any side effects that are persistent or particularly bothersome. IT IS ESPECIALLY IMPORTANT TO TELL YOUR DOCTOR about darkened tongue, difficulty in breathing, joint pain, mouth irritation, rash, rectal or vaginal itching, sore throat and fever, unusual bleeding or bruising, or yellowing of the eyes or skin. Also, if your symptoms of infection seem to be getting worse rather than improving, contact your doctor.

INTERACTIONS
Oxytetracycline interacts with several other types of drugs:
1. It can increase the absorption of digoxin, which may lead to digoxin toxicity.
2. The gastrointestinal side effects (nausea, vomiting, stomach upset) of theophylline may be increased by oxytetracycline.
3. The dosage of oral anticoagulants (blood thinners, such as warfarin) may need to be adjusted when this medication is started.
4. Oxytetracycline may decrease the effectiveness of oral contraceptives (birth control pills), and pregnancy could result. You should, therefore, use another form of birth control while taking oxytetracycline. Consult your doctor.

BE SURE TO TELL YOUR DOCTOR about any medications you are currently taking, especially any listed above.

WARNINGS
Tell your doctor about unusual or allergic reactions you have had to any medications, especially to oxytetracycline or to tetracycline, doxycycline, or minocycline.

Tell your doctor if you now have or if you have ever had kidney or liver disease.

Oxytetracycline can affect tests for syphilis; tell your doctor you are taking this medication if you are also being treated for this disease.

Make sure that your prescription for oxytetracycline is marked with the expiration date. The drug should be discarded after the expiration date. If the medication is used after it has expired, serious side effects (especially to the kidneys) could result.

This medication has been prescribed for your current infection only. Another infection later on, or one that someone else has, may require a different medicine. Therefore, you should not give your medicine to other people or use it for other infections, unless your doctor specifically directs you to do so.

Be sure to tell your doctor if you are pregnant or if you are breast-feeding an infant. Oxytetracycline crosses the placenta and passes into breast milk. This medication can cause permanent discoloration of the teeth and can inhibit tooth and bone growth if used during their development. In addition, oxytetracycline should not be used for infants or for children less than eight years of age because of the potential risks involved.

oxytetracycline hydrochloride—see oxytetracycline

Pamelor—see nortriptyline

Pamprin-IB—see ibuprofen

Pancrease—see pancrelipase

---

pancreatin

BRAND NAMES (Manufacturers)
Pancreatin Enseals* (Lilly)
Pancreatin Tablets* (Lilly)
*Available over-the-counter (without a prescription)
TYPE OF DRUG
Digestive enzymes
INGREDIENT
Spancreatin, lipase, protease, and amylase
DOSAGE FORMS
Pancreatin Tablets (pancreatin 325 mg; lipase 650 units; protease 8,125 units; amylase 8,125 units)
Pancreatin Enseals (pancreatin 1000 mg; lipase 2000 units; protease 25,000 units; amylase 25,000 units)
STORAGE
Store at room temperature in a tightly closed container.

USES
This medication is a combination of specific digestive (pancreatic) enzymes obtained from pigs or cows. These enzymes aid in the digestion and absorption of fats and starch. Pancreatin is used in the treatment of various pancreatic enzyme deficiencies resulting from conditions such as pancreatitis, cystic fibrosis, or gastrointestinal bypass surgery.

TREATMENT
In order to obtain the maximum benefit from this medication, you should take pancreatin just before or with meals or snacks. The tablets can be crushed and mixed with food.

If you miss a dose of this medication, do not take the missed dose at all; just return to your regular dosing schedule. Do not double the next dose.

SIDE EFFECTS
Minor. Diarrhea, nausea, or stomach cramps. These side effects should disappear as your body adjusts to the medication.
Major. Tell your doctor about any side effects that are persistent or particularly bothersome. IT IS ESPECIALLY IMPORTANT TO TELL YOUR DOCTOR about bloody urine, hives, joint pain, skin rash, or swelling of the feet or legs.

INTERACTIONS
Pancreatin can decrease the absorption of iron from the gastrointestinal tract, which may lead to nutritional deficiency. Your doctor may want to prescribe iron supplements if this becomes a problem. Cimetidine or antacids are often prescribed concurrently with pancreatin in order to maximize its effectiveness. However, calcium- or magnesium-containing antacids should be avoided-they decrease this medication's effectiveness. You should discuss these effects with your doctor.

WARNINGS
Tell your doctor about unusual or allergic reactions you have had to any medications, especially to pancreatin, pancrelipase, or any other digestive enzymes.

Patients who have allergies to pork or beef products may also be allergic to pancreatin, since it is obtained from pigs and cows.

Be sure to tell your doctor if you are pregnant. Although pancreatin appears to be safe during pregnancy, extensive studies have not been conducted. Also, tell your doctor if you are breast-feeding an infant. It is not known whether pancreatin passes into breast milk.

Pancreatin Enseals—see pancreatin

Pancreatin Tablets—see pancreatin

---

pancrelipase

BRAND NAMES (Manufacturers)
Cotazym-S (Organon)
Festal II* (Hoechst-Roussel)
Ilozyme (Adria)
Ku-Zyme HP (Kremers-Urban)
Pancrease (McNeil)
Viokase (Robins)
*Available over-the-counter (without a prescription)
TYPE OF DRUG
Digestive enzymes
INGREDIENT
Slipase, protease, and amylase
DOSAGE FORMS
Tablets (in various strengths)
Capsules (in various strengths)
Powder packets (in various strengths)

STORAGE

Pancrelipase tablets, capsules, and powder should be stored at room temperature in tightly closed containers.

USES

This medication is a combination of digestive (pancreatic) enzymes obtained from pigs. These enzymes aid in the digestion and absorption of starch and fats. Pancrelipase is used to treat pancreatic enzyme deficiencies resulting from conditions such as pancreatitis, cystic fibrosis, or gastrointestinal bypass surgery.

TREATMENT

In order to obtain the maximum benefit, you should take pancrelipase just before or with meals or snacks. The powder can be added to food; the tablets can also be crushed and mixed with food.

If you are taking the capsules containing the enteric-coated microspheres, swallow the capsule whole. Chewing, crushing, or breaking the capsules decreases their effectiveness and increases the side effects. However, if you have difficulty swallowing the capsules, you can open them and sprinkle the contents on a small amount of liquid or soft food, which you should then swallow without chewing. DO NOT mix this medication with alkaline foods (such as dairy products)they can reduce its effectiveness.

If you miss a dose of this medication, do not take the missed dose at all; just return to your regular dosing schedule. Do not double the next dose.

SIDE EFFECTS

Minor. Diarrhea, nausea, or stomach cramps. These side effects should disappear as your body adjusts to the medication.

Major. Tell your doctor about any side effects that are persistent or particularly bothersome. IT IS ESPECIALLY IMPORTANT TO TELL YOUR DOCTOR about bloody urine, hives, joint pain, skin rash, or swelling of the feet.

INTERACTIONS

Pancrelipase can decrease the absorption of iron from the gastrointestinal tract, which may lead to nutritional deficiency. Your doctor may want to prescribe iron supplements if this becomes a problem. Cimetidine or antacids are often prescribed concurrently with pancrelipase, in order to maximize its effectiveness. However, calcium- or magnesium-containing antacids should be avoided-they decrease this medication's effectiveness. You should discuss these effects with your doctor.

WARNINGS

Tell your doctor about unusual or allergic reactions you have had to any medications, especially to pancrelipase, pancreatin, or any other digestive enzymes.

Patients who have allergies to pork products may also be allergic to pancrelipase, since it is obtained from pigs.

The powder form and the powder from opened capsules of this medication can be very irritating to the nose and throat. Avoid inhaling the particles.

Be sure to tell your doctor if you are pregnant. Although pancrelipase appears to be safe during pregnancy, ex-

tensive studies have not been conducted. Also, tell your doctor if you are breast-feeding an infant. It is not known whether pancrelipase passes into breast milk.

Panasol-S—see prednisone (systemic)

Panmycin—see tetracycline

Panwarfin—see warfarin

---

papaverine

BRAND NAMES (Manufacturers)

Cerespan (Rorer)
papaverine hydrochloride (various manufacturers)
Pavabid HP Capsulet (Marion)
Pavabid Plateau (Marion)
Pavacen Cenules (Central)
Pavagen (Rugby)
Pavarine Spancaps (Vortech)
Pavased (Hauck)
Pavatym (Everett)
Paverolan Lanacaps (Lannett)

TYPE OF DRUG

Vasodilator

INGREDIENT

papaverine

DOSAGE FORMS

Tablets (30 mg, 60 mg, 100 mg, 150 mg, 200 mg, and 300 mg)
Sustained-release capsules (150 mg)
Sustained-release tablets (200 mg)

STORAGE

Papaverine should be stored at room temperature in a tightly closed container.

USES

Papaverine is used to treat circulation disorders. It is a vasodilator that acts directly on the muscle tissues of blood vessels to increase blood supply.

TREATMENT

In order to avoid stomach irritation, you can take papaverine with food or with a full glass of water or milk. Ask your doctor if you can take it with an antacid.

The sustained-release capsules should be swallowed whole. Breaking, crushing, or chewing these capsules destroys their sustained-release activity and possibly increases the side effects.

If you miss a dose of this medication, take the missed dose as soon as possible, unless it is almost time for the next dose. In that case, do not take the missed dose at all; just return to your regular dosing schedule. Do not double the next dose.

SIDE EFFECTS

Minor. Abdominal distress, blurred vision, constipation, diarrhea, dizziness, drowsiness, fatigue, flushing, headache, loss of appetite, nausea, or sweating. These side effects should disappear as your body adjusts to the medication.

If you feel dizzy, sit or lie down for a while; get up slowly from a sitting or reclining position.

To relieve constipation, increase the amount of fiber in your diet (fresh fruits and vegetables, salads, bran, and whole-grain breads), exercise, and drink more water (unless your doctor directs you to do otherwise).

Major. Tell your doctor about any side effects that are persistent or particularly bothersome. IT IS ESPECIALLY IMPORTANT TO TELL YOUR DOCTOR about depression, difficulty in breathing, palpitations, rash, unusual bleeding or bruising, or yellowing of the eyes or skin.

INTERACTIONS

Concurrent use of papaverine and levodopa can lead to decreased effectiveness of levodopa.

Before starting to take papaverine, BE SURE TO TELL YOUR DOCTOR about any medications you are currently taking, especially levodopa.

WARNINGS

Tell your doctor about unusual or allergic reactions you have had to any medications, especially to papaverine.

Be sure to tell your doctor if you have ever had angina, glaucoma, heart block, liver disease, low or high blood pressure, a heart attack, or Parkinson's disease.

A government panel has recently reviewed the effectiveness of this medication in the treatment of hardening of the arteries and leg cramps and in the prevention of stroke. This drug may not be as effective as once thought. Before taking any over-the-counter (nonprescription) cough, cold, allergy, asthma, sinus, or diet medication, check with your doctor or pharmacist. Some of these products can decrease the effectiveness of papaverine.

If this drug makes you dizzy or drowsy, do not take part in any activity that requires alertness, such as driving a car or operating potentially dangerous machinery.

The beneficial effects of this medication may be decreased by the nicotine in cigarettes.

To prevent dizziness and fainting while taking this medication, avoid drinking large quantities of alcohol, and try not to get overheated (avoid strenuous exercise in hot weather and do not take hot baths, showers, and saunas).

Be sure to tell your doctor if you are pregnant. Although papaverine appears to be safe, extensive studies in pregnant women have not been conducted. Also, tell your doctor if you are breast-feeding. It is not known whether papaverine passes into breast milk.

Papaverine hydrochloride—see papaverine

Par Glycerol—see codine and iodinated glycerol combination

Parlodel—see bromocriptine

Parlodel SnapTabs—see bromocriptine

Pathocil—see dicloxacillin

Pavabid HP—see papaverine

Pavabid Plateau—see papaverine

Pavacen Cenules—see papaverine

Pavagen—see papaverine

Pavarine Spancaps—see papaverine

Pavased—see papaverine

Pavatym—see papaverine

Paverolan Lanacaps—see papaverine

Paxipam—see halazepam

PCE Dispertab—see erythromycin

PediaCare 2 Liquid—see pseudoephedrine and chlorpheniramine combination

PediaProfen—see ibuprofen

Pediazole—see erythromycin and sulfisoxazole combination

Pedi-Cort V—see hydrocortisone and iodochlorhydroxyquin combination (topical)

pemoline

BRAND NAME (Manufacturer)
Cylert (Abbott)
TYPE OF DRUG
Stimulant
INGREDIENT
pemoline
DOSAGE FORMS
Tablets (18.75 mg, 37.5 mg, and 75 mg)
Chewable tablets (37.5 mg)
STORAGE
Pemoline should be stored at room temperature in a tightly closed container.

USES

Pemoline is a central nervous system (brain and spinal cord) stimulant that is used to treat attention deficit disorders (hyperkinetic syndrome). It is not yet clear how pemoline works to improve behavioral disorders in children, but it seems to decrease hyperactivity and increase attention span.

TREATMENT

Pemoline can be taken either on an empty stomach or with food or milk (as directed by your doctor). The chewable tablet form of this medication can be either chewed or swallowed whole.

If you miss a dose of this medication, take the missed dose as soon as possible, unless it is almost time for the next dose. In that case, do not take the missed dose at all; just return to your regular dosing schedule. Do not double the next dose of this medication.

You may not observe the full therapeutic benefits of this medication for three to four weeks.

SIDE EFFECTS

Minor. Dizziness, drowsiness, headache, insomnia, irritability, loss of appetite, nausea, stomachache, or weight loss. These side effects should disappear as your body adjusts to the drug.

If you feel dizzy, sit or lie down for a while; get up slowly from a sitting or reclining position, and be careful on stairs.

Major. Tell your doctor about any side effects that are persistent or particularly bothersome. IT IS ESPECIALLY IMPORTANT TO TELL YOUR DOCTOR about convulsions; depression; hallucinations; palpitations; skin rash; unusual movements of the tongue, lips, face, hands, or feet; or yellowing of the eyes or skin.

INTERACTIONS

Pemoline should not interact with other medications if it is used according to the directions given to you by your doctor or pharmacist.

WARNINGS

Tell your doctor about unusual or allergic reactions you have had to any medications, especially to pemoline.

Before starting to take this medication, be sure to tell your doctor if you now have or if you have ever had kidney disease, liver disease, or mental disorders.

If this drug makes you dizzy or drowsy, do not take part in any activity that requires alertness, such as driving a car or operating potentially dangerous machinery. Children who are taking this drug should be cautious while playing.

This medication has the potential for abuse and must be used with caution. It should, therefore, not be taken in larger doses or for longer periods than prescribed by your doctor. In addition, you should not stop taking pemoline unless you first check with your doctor. Stopping the drug abruptly can lead to a withdrawal reaction. Your doctor may, therefore, want to reduce the dosage gradually.

Your doctor may want to interrupt pemoline therapy occasionally for short periods ("drug holidays") to see if the symptoms of the attention deficit disorder have disappeared.

Be sure to tell your doctor if you are pregnant. Although pemoline appears to be safe, extensive studies in humans during pregnancy have not been conducted. Also, tell your doctor if you are breast-feeding an infant. It is not known whether pemoline passes into breast milk.

Penecort—see hydrocortisone (topical)

penicillamine

BRAND NAMES (Manufacturers)
Cuprimine (Merck Sharp & Dohme)
Depen Titratable Tablets (Wallace)
TYPE OF DRUG
Chelator and antirheumatic

INGREDIENT
penicillamine
DOSAGE FORMS
Tablets (250 mg)
Capsules (125 mg and 250 mg)
STORAGE
Store at room temperature in a tightly closed container.

USES
This drug is used to treat Wilson's disease (high blood copper levels), severe rheumatoid arthritis, and cystinuria (high urine levels of cystine). Penicillamine binds to copper and cystine, which prevents their harmful effects on the body. It is not clearly understood how penicillamine relieves rheumatoid arthritis.

TREATMENT
In order to obtain the maximum benefit from penicillamine, you should take it on an empty stomach one hour before or two hours after a meal. To ensure maximal absorption of this drug, each dose should be separated from doses of other medications and from food and milk by at least an hour.

If you miss a dose of this drug, take the dose as soon as possible, unless it is almost time for the next dose. In that case, do not take the dose at all; return to your regular dosing schedule. Do not double the dose.

The full benefits of this drug may not become apparent for as long as three months after therapy.

SIDE EFFECTS
Minor. Altered taste sensations, diarrhea, loss of appetite, nausea, stomach upset, or vomiting. These side effects should disappear as your body adjusts to the medication.
Major. Tell your doctor about any side effects that are persistent or particularly bothersome. IT IS ESPECIALLY IMPORTANT TO TELL YOUR DOCTOR about breast enlargement (in both sexes), difficult or painful urination, difficulty in breathing, joint pain, loss of hair, mouth sores, ringing in the ears, skin rash, sore throat, tingling sensations in the fingers or toes, unusual bleeding or bruising, or wheezing.

INTERACTIONS
Penicillamine interacts with several other types of medications:
1. The absorption of penicillamine from the gastrointestinal tract can be decreased by iron or antacids.
2. Penicillamine can decrease the blood levels and beneficial effects of digoxin.
3. Concurrent use of penicillamine and gold salts, hydroxychloroquine, phenylbutazone, oxyphenbutazone, or anticancer drugs can lead to increased side effects to the blood and kidneys.

BE SURE TO TELL YOUR DOCTOR about any medications you are currently taking, especially any of those listed above.

WARNINGS
• Tell your doctor about unusual or allergic reactions you have had to any medications, especially to penicillamine or penicillin or cephalosporin antibiotics.

• Before starting to take this medication, be sure to tell your doctor if you now have or if you have ever had blood disorders or kidney disease.

• Do not stop taking this drug unless you first check with your doctor.

• Penicillamine can decrease the body's ability to repair wounds, so try to avoid injuring yourself while you are taking this medication. This warning is especially important for diabetic patients.

• Before having surgery or any other medical or dental treatment, be sure to tell your doctor or dentist that you are taking this drug.

• Your doctor may want you to take pyridoxine (vitamin B) to prevent some of the side effects (for example, tingling sensations) of penicillamine.

• Be sure to tell your doctor if you are pregnant. Penicillamine has been reported to cause birth defects in both animals and humans. Also, tell your doctor if you are breast-feeding an infant.

penicillin VK

BRAND NAMES (Manufacturers)
Beepen-VK (Beecham)
Betapen-VK (Bristol)
Ledercillin VK (Lederle)
penicillin VK (various manufacturers)
Pen-Vee K (Wyeth)
Robicillin VK (Robins)
Suspen (Circle)
Uticillin VK (Upjohn)
V-Cillin K (Lilly)
Veetids (Apothecon)

TYPE OF DRUG
Penicillin antibiotic

INGREDIENT
penicillin potassium phenoxymethyl

DOSAGE FORMS
Tablets (125 mg, 250 mg, and 500 mg)
Oral solution (125 mg and 250 mg per 5-ml spoonful)

STORAGE
Penicillin VK tablets should be stored at room temperature in a tightly closed container. The oral solution should be stored in the refrigerator in a tightly closed container. Any unused portion of the solution should be discarded after 14 days because the drug loses its potency after that time. This medication should never be frozen.

USES
Penicillin VK is used to treat a wide variety of bacterial infections, including infections of the middle ear, the respiratory tract, and the urinary tract. It acts by severely injuring the cell membranes of infecting bacteria, thereby preventing them from growing and multiplying. Penicillin VK kills susceptible bacteria, but it is not effective against viruses, parasites, or fungi.

TREATMENT
Penicillin VK should be taken on an empty stomach or with a glass of water one hour before or two hours after a meal. This medication should never be taken with fruit juices or carbonated beverages because the acidity of these drinks destroys the drug in the stomach.

The oral solution should be measured carefully with a specially designed 5-ml measuring spoon. An ordinary kitchen teaspoon is not accurate enough.

Penicillin VK works best when the level of medicine in your bloodstream is kept constant. It is best, therefore, to take the doses at evenly spaced intervals day and night. For example, if you are taking four doses a day, the doses should be spaced six hours apart.

If you miss a dose of this medication, take the missed dose immediately. However, if you do not remember to take the missed dose until it is almost time for the next dose, take it; space the following dose about halfway through the regular interval between doses; then return to your regular dosing schedule. Try not to skip any doses.

It is important to continue to take this medication for the entire time prescribed by your doctor (usually seven to 14 days), even if the symptoms of infection disappear before the end of that period. If you stop taking the drug too soon, resistant bacteria are given a chance to continue growing, and the infection could recur.

SIDE EFFECTS
Minor. Diarrhea, heartburn, nausea, or vomiting. These side effects should disappear as your body adjusts to the drug.

Major. Tell your doctor about any side effects that are persistent or particularly bothersome. IT IS ESPECIALLY IMPORTANT TO TELL YOUR DOCTOR about bloating, chills, cough, darkened tongue, difficulty in breathing, fever, irritation of the mouth, muscle aches, rash, rectal or vaginal itching, severe diarrhea, or sore throat. Also, if the infection seems to be getting worse rather than improving, you should contact your physician.

INTERACTIONS
Penicillin VK interacts with several other types of drugs:
1. Probenecid can increase the blood concentrations of this medication.
2. Oral neomycin may decrease the absorption of penicillin from the gastrointestinal tract.
3. Penicillin VK may decrease the effectiveness of oral contraceptives (birth control pills), and pregnancy could result. You should, therefore, use a different or additional form of birth control while taking this medication. Discuss this with your doctor.

BE SURE TO TELL YOUR DOCTOR about any medications you are currently taking, especially any of those listed above.

WARNINGS
• Tell your doctor about unusual or allergic reactions you have had to any medications, especially to penicillin or other penicillin antibiotics (such as ampicillin and amoxicillin), cephalosporin antibiotics, penicillamine, or griseofulvin.

• Tell your doctor if you now have or if you have ever had kidney disease, asthma, or allergies.

• This medication has been prescribed for your current infection only. Another infection later on, or one that someone else has, may require a different medicine. You should not give your medicine to other people or use it for other infections, unless your doctor specifically directs you to do so.

• Diabetics taking penicillin should know that this drug can cause a false-positive sugar reaction with a Clinitest urine glucose test. To avoid this problem while taking penicillin, you should switch to Clinistix or Tes-Tape to test your urine for sugar.

• Be sure to tell your doctor if you are pregnant. Although penicillin appears to be safe during pregnancy, extensive studies in humans have not been conducted. Also, tell your doctor if you are breast-feeding an infant. Small amounts of this medication pass into breast milk and may temporarily alter the bacterial balance in the intestinal tract of a nursing infant, resulting in diarrhea.

pentaerythritol tetranitrate

BRAND NAMES (Manufacturers)
Duotrate Plateau Caps (Jones Medical)
Naptrate (Vortech)
Pentylan (Lannett)
Peritrate (Parke-Davis)
Peritrate SA (Parke-Davis)
P.E.T.N. (various manufacturers)
TYPE OF DRUG
Antianginal
INGREDIENT
pentaerythritol tetranitrate
DOSAGE FORMS
Tablets (10 mg, 20 mg, 40 mg, and 80 mg)
Sustained-release tablets (80 mg)
Sustained-release capsules (30 mg, 45 mg, and 80 mg)
STORAGE
Pentaerythritol tetranitrate should be stored at room temperature in tightly closed containers. This medication loses potency if exposed to heat or moisture.

USES

Pentaerythritol tetranitrate is used to prevent angina (chest pain). It dilates (widens) blood vessels, which increases the oxygen supply to the heart, thereby preventing chest pain. It is not effective in relieving pain once an angina attack has begun.

TREATMENT

To ensure that the maximum amount of medication is absorbed into the bloodstream, you should take pentaerythritol tetranitrate on an empty stomach at least 30 minutes before or one hour after a meal with a glass of water (unless your doctor directs you to do otherwise).

The sustained-release tablets or capsules should be swallowed whole. Chewing, crushing, or breaking these tablets or capsules destroys their sustained-release activity and possibly increases the side effects.

If you miss a dose of this medication and remember within two hours (six hours for the sustained-release tablets or capsules), take the missed dose immediately and then return to your regular dosing schedule. If more than two hours have passed (six hours for the sustained-release tablets or capsules), do not take the missed dose at all; just return to your regular dosing schedule. Never double the dose (unless your doctor specifically directs you to do so).

SIDE EFFECTS

Minor. Dizziness, flushing or redness of the face and neck, headache, light-headedness, nausea, or vomiting. These effects should disappear as your body adjusts to the drug.

If you feel dizzy or light-headed, sit or lie down for a while; get up slowly from a sitting or reclining position, and be careful on stairs.

The use of acetaminophen may help relieve mild headaches that you may experience when taking this drug.

Major. Tell your doctor about any side effects that are persistent or particularly bothersome. IT IS ESPECIALLY IMPORTANT TO TELL YOUR DOCTOR about fainting, palpitations, or skin rash.

INTERACTIONS

Alcohol can increase the blood-pressure-lowering effects of pentaerythritol tetranitrate, which can lead to serious side effects. You should, therefore, avoid drinking alcoholic beverages at any time while taking this medication.

WARNINGS

Tell your doctor about unusual or allergic reactions you have had to any medications, especially to pentaerythritol tetranitrate or to any other nitrate product (such as erythrityl tetranitrate, isosorbide dinitrate, or nitroglycerin).

Before you take this drug, be sure to tell your doctor if you have ever had anemia, a heart attack, or thyroid disease.

If this medication makes you dizzy or light-headed, avoid taking part in any activity that requires alertness, such as driving a car or operating potentially dangerous machinery.

Tolerance to this drug can develop after prolonged use. If you begin to notice a decrease in effectiveness, contact your doctor. Do not increase the dosage of this drug unless you first check with your doctor. Also, stopping the drug abruptly can lead to a worsening in your condition. Your doctor may, therefore, want to reduce your dosage gradually.

Before taking any over-the-counter (nonprescription) cough, cold, allergy, asthma, sinus, or diet preparation, check with your doctor. Some of these products can reduce the effectiveness of pentaerythritol tetranitrate.

If you find whole or partially dissolved sustained-release tablets or capsules in your stool, contact your doctor. This indicates that you are not digesting and absorbing the tablets or capsules completely.

Be sure to tell your doctor if you are pregnant. Although pentaerythritol tetranitrate appears to be safe during pregnancy, extensive studies in humans have not been conducted. Also, tell your doctor if you are breast-feeding an infant. It is not known whether pentaerythritol tetranitrate passes into breast milk.

pentazocine

BRAND NAME (Manufacturer)
Talwin Nx (Winthrop)
TYPE OF DRUG
Analgesic
INGREDIENTS
pentazocine and naloxone
DOSAGE FORM
Tablets (50 mg pentazocine and 0.5 mg naloxone)
STORAGE
Pentazocine tablets should be stored at room temperature in a tightly closed, light-resistant container.

USES
Pentazocine is a narcotic analgesic that acts directly on the central nervous system (brain and spinal cord) to relieve moderate to severe pain. Naloxone is added to this compound to prevent abuse. It is not absorbed from the gastrointestinal tract, but it does block the action of pentazocine if the drug is injected into the body.

TREATMENT
In order to avoid stomach upset, you can take pentazocine with food or with a full glass of milk or water.

This medication works most effectively if you take it at the onset of pain, rather than waiting until the pain becomes intense.

If you are taking this medication on a regular schedule and you miss a dose, take the missed dose as soon as possible, unless it is almost time for your next dose. In that case, do not take the missed dose at all; just return to your regular dosing schedule. Do not double the next dose.

SIDE EFFECTS
Minor. Constipation, dizziness, drowsiness, dry mouth, false sense of well-being, flushing, light-headedness, loss of appetite, nausea, rash, or sweating. These side effects should disappear as your body adjusts to the medication.

If you are constipated, increase the amount of fiber in your diet (fresh fruits and vegetables, salads, bran, and whole-grain breads), exercise, and drink more water (unless your doctor directs you to do otherwise).

Chew sugarless gum or suck on ice chips or a piece of hard candy to reduce mouth dryness.

If you feel dizzy or light-headed, sit or lie down for a while; get up slowly from a sitting or lying position.
Major. Tell your doctor about any side effects that are persistent or particularly bothersome. IT IS ESPECIALLY IMPORTANT TO TELL YOUR DOCTOR about anxiety, difficulty in breathing, excitation, fatigue, painful or difficult urination, palpitations, rash, restlessness, sore throat and fever, tremors, or weakness.

INTERACTIONS
Pentazocine interacts with several other types of drugs:
1. Concurrent use of it with other central nervous system depressants (such as alcohol, antihistamines, barbiturates, benzodiazepine tranquilizers, muscle relaxants, and phenothiazine tranquilizers) or with tricyclic antidepressants can cause extreme drowsiness.

2. A monoamine oxidase (MAO) inhibitor taken within 14 days of this drug can lead to unpredictable side effects.
3. The combination of cimetidine and this medication may cause confusion, disorientation, and shortness of breath.

BE SURE TO TELL YOUR DOCTOR about any medications you are currently taking, especially those listed above.

WARNINGS
• Tell your doctor about unusual or allergic reactions you have had to any medications, especially to pentazocine or to other narcotic analgesics (such as codeine, hydrocodone, hydromorphone, meperidine, methadone, morphine, oxycodone, and propoxyphene).
• Tell your doctor if you now have or if you have ever had acute abdominal conditions, asthma, brain disease, colitis, epilepsy, gallstones or gallbladder disease, head injuries, heart disease, kidney disease, liver disease, lung disease, mental illness, emotional disorders, enlarged prostate gland, thyroid disease, or urethral stricture.
• If this drug makes you dizzy or drowsy, do not take part in any activity that requires alertness, such as driving a car or operating potentially dangerous machinery.
• Before having surgery or any other medical or dental treatment, be sure to tell your doctor or dentist that you are taking this medication.
• Because this product contains pentazocine, it has the potential for abuse and must be used with caution. Usually, it should not be taken on a regular schedule for longer than ten days, unless your doctor directs you to do so. Tolerance develops quickly; do not increase the dosage or stop taking the drug abruptly, unless you first consult your doctor. If you have been taking large amounts of this medication, or have been taking it for long periods, you may experience a withdrawal reaction (muscle aches, diarrhea, gooseflesh, runny nose, nausea, vomiting, shivering, trembling, stomach cramps, sleep disorders, irritability, weakness, excessive yawning, or sweating) when you stop taking it.
• Be sure to tell your doctor if you are pregnant. The effects of this medication during the early stages of pregnancy have not been thoroughly studied in humans. However, pentazocine, used regularly in large doses during the later stages of pregnancy, may result in addiction of the fetus—leading to withdrawal symptoms (irritability, excessive crying, tremors, fever, vomiting, diarrhea, sneezing, or excessive yawning) at birth. Also, tell your doctor if you are breast-feeding an infant. Small amounts of this medication may pass into breast milk and cause excessive drowsiness in the nursing infant.

pentobarbital

BRAND NAMES (Manufacturers)
Nembutal (Abbott)
pentobarbital sodium (various manufacturers)
TYPE OF DRUG
Sedative/hypnotic

INGREDIENT
pentobarbital
DOSAGE FORMS
Capsules (50 mg and 100 mg)
Oral elixir (20 mg per 5-ml spoonful, with 18% alcohol)
Suppositories (30 mg, 60 mg, 120 mg, and 200 mg)
STORAGE
Pentobarbital capsules and oral elixir should be stored at room temperature in tightly closed containers. The suppositories should be stored in the refrigerator. Pentobarbital should never be frozen.

USES
This medication belongs to a group of drugs known as barbiturates, which are central nervous system (brain and spinal cord) depressants. It is used as a sleeping aid in the treatment of insomnia.

TREATMENT
You can take pentobarbital at bedtime. The capsules can be taken with water, food, or milk.

Each dose of the oral elixir form of this medication should be measured carefully with a specially designed 5-ml measuring spoon. An ordinary kitchen teaspoon is not accurate enough. The elixir can be taken by itself or mixed with water, milk, or fruit juice.

To insert the suppository form of this medication, first unwrap it and moisten it slightly with water (if the suppository is too soft to insert, run cold water over it or refrigerate it for 30 minutes before you unwrap it). Lie down on your left side, with your right knee bent. Push the suppository well into the rectum with your finger. Try to avoid having a bowel movement for at least an hour so that the medication can be absorbed.

You should not use this drug as a sleeping aid for more than two weeks. With prolonged use, pentobarbital loses its ability to induce and sustain sleep.

SIDE EFFECTS
Minor. Constipation, diarrhea, dizziness, drowsiness, a "hangover" feeling, headache, nausea, stomach upset, or vomiting. These side effects should disappear as your body adjusts to the medication.

If you feel dizzy or light-headed, sit or lie down for a while; get up slowly from a sitting or reclining position, and be careful on stairs.

To relieve constipation, increase the amount of fiber in your diet (fresh fruits and vegetables, salads, bran, and whole-grain breads), exercise, and drink more water (unless your doctor directs you to do otherwise).

Major. Tell your doctor about any side effects that are persistent or particularly bothersome. IT IS ESPECIALLY IMPORTANT TO TELL YOUR DOCTOR about chest tightness, confusion, depression, difficulty in breathing, excitation, fatigue, feeling faint, hives or itching, loss of coordination, muscle or joint pain, skin rash, slurred speech, sore throat, unusual bleeding or bruising, unusual weakness, or yellowing of the eyes or skin.

INTERACTIONS
Pentobarbital interacts with several other types of drugs:
1. Concurrent use of it with other central nervous system depressants (such as alcohol, antihistamines, benzodiazepine tranquilizers, muscle relaxants, narcotics, pain medications, and phenothiazine tranquilizers) or with tricyclic antidepressants can cause extreme drowsiness.
2. Valproic acid, chloramphenicol, and monoamine oxidase (MAO) inhibitors can prolong the effects of pentobarbital.
3. Pentobarbital can decrease the blood levels and, therefore, the effectiveness of oral anticoagulants (blood thinners, such as warfarin), digitoxin, tricyclic antidepressants, doxycycline, cortisone-like medicines, metronidazole, quinidine, estrogens, birth control pills, phenytoin, acetaminophen, and carbamazepine.
4. The combination of pentobarbital and furosemide can cause low blood pressure and fainting.
5. Pentobarbital can increase the side effects of cyclophosphamide or large doses of acetaminophen.

Before starting to take pentobarbital, BE SURE TO TELL YOUR DOCTOR about any medications you are currently taking, especially any of those listed above.

WARNINGS
Tell your doctor about unusual or allergic reactions you have had to any medications, especially to pentobarbital or to other barbiturates (such as amobarbital, butabarbital, mephobarbital, metharbital, phenobarbital, primidone, and secobarbital).

Before starting to take this medication, be sure to tell your doctor if you now have or if you have ever had acute or chronic (long-term) pain, Addison's disease (an underactive adrenal gland), diabetes mellitus, kidney disease, liver disease, lung disease, mental depression, porphyria, or thyroid disease.

Since this medication makes you drowsy, do not take part in any activity that requires alertness, such as driving a car or operating potentially dangerous machinery.

This drug has the potential for abuse and must be used with caution. Tolerance develops quickly; do not increase the dosage or stop taking this drug without consulting your doctor.

If you have been taking pentobarbital for a long time or have been taking large doses, you may experience anxiety, muscle twitching, tremors, weakness, dizziness, nausea, vomiting, insomnia, or blurred vision when you stop taking it. To avoid this reaction, your doctor may want to reduce your dosage gradually.

Be sure to tell your doctor if you are pregnant. Barbiturates cross the placenta, and there has been an association between birth defects and the use of this class of drugs during pregnancy. Such drugs may also lead to an increase in bleeding complications in the newborn. The risks should be discussed with your doctor. In addition, if pentobarbital is used for prolonged periods during the last three months of pregnancy, there is a chance that the infant will be born addicted to the medication and will experience a withdrawal reaction (convulsions or irritability) at birth. Also, tell your doctor if you are breastfeeding an infant. Small amounts of pentobarbital pass into breast milk and may cause excessive drowsiness or breathing problems in nursing infants.

Pentobarbital Sodium—see pentobarbital

pentoxifylline

BRAND NAME (Manufacturer)
Trental (Hoechst-Roussel)
TYPE OF DRUG
hemorrheologic
INGREDIENT
pentoxifylline
DOSAGE FORM
Controlled-release tablets (400 mg)
STORAGE
Store at room temperature in a tightly closed container.

USES
Pentoxifylline is used to treat intermittent claudication (leg pain caused by poor blood circulation) or peripheral vascular disease.

TREATMENT
To avoid stomach irritation, pentoxifylline should be taken with meals.

The tablets should be swallowed whole; chewing, crushing, or breaking them will destroy the controlled-release activity and increase the risk of side effects.

If you miss a dose of pentoxifylline, take the missed dose as soon as possible, unless it is almost time for the next dose. In that case, do not take the missed dose at all; just wait until the next scheduled dose. Do not double the dose.

The benefits from pentoxifylline may be seen within two to four weeks after starting the medication.

SIDE EFFECTS
Minor. Abdominal pain, altered taste, belching, bloating, constipation, diarrhea, dizziness, drowsiness, dry mouth, excessive salivation, flushing, gas, headache, heartburn, insomnia, nasal congestion, nausea, nosebleeds, trembling of the hands, vomiting, or weight change. As your body adjusts to pentoxifylline, these side effects should disappear.

If you are constipated, increase the amount of fiber in your diet (fresh fruits and vegetables, salads, bran, and whole-grain breads), exercise, and drink more water (unless your doctor directs you to do otherwise).

To reduce mouth dryness, chew sugarless gum.

If you feel dizzy or light-headed, lie or sit down for a while; get up slowly from a sitting or reclining position, and be careful on stairs.
Major. Tell your doctor about any side effects that are persistent or particularly bothersome. IT IS ESPECIALLY IMPORTANT TO TELL YOUR DOCTOR about chest pain, confusion, earache, flu-like symptoms, itching, palpitations, rash, shortness of breath, sore throat, unusual bleeding or bruising, unusual weight gain, visual disturbances, or yellowing of the eyes or skin.

INTERACTIONS
Pentoxifylline interacts with other types of medications:
1. Anticoagulants (blood thinners, such as warfarin) in combination with pentoxifylline can increase the risk of bleeding complications.

2. Pentoxifylline can add to the blood-pressure-lowering effects of antihypertensive medications.

BE SURE TO TELL YOUR DOCTOR about any medications you are currently taking.

WARNINGS
• Before you take this medication, it is important to tell your doctor if you have ever had unusual or allergic reactions to any medications, especially to pentoxifylline or chemically related compounds, such as caffeine, dyphylline, oxtriphylline, theophylline, and aminophylline.
• Tell your doctor if you now have or if you have ever had liver disease, kidney disease, or peptic ulcer disease.
• Before having surgery or any other medical or dental treatment, be sure to tell your doctor or dentist that you are taking this drug. Pentoxifylline can increase bleeding complications.
• If pentoxifylline makes you dizzy or drowsy, do not take part in any activity that requires alertness, such as driving a car or operating dangerous machinery.
• Be sure to tell your doctor if you are pregnant. Although pentoxifylline appears to be safe in animals, studies in pregnant women have not been conducted. Also, tell your doctor if you are breast-feeding an infant. Small amounts of pentoxifylline pass into human breast milk.

Pentylan—see pentaerythritol tetranitrate

Pen-Vee K—see penicillin VK

Pepcid—see famotidine

Percocet—see acetaminophen and oxycodone combination

Percodan—see aspirin and oxycodone combination

Percodan-Demi—see aspirin and oxycodone combination

Periactin—see cyproheptadine

Peridex—see chlorhexidene gluconate

Permitil—see fluphenazine

Peritrate—see pentaerythritol tetranitrate

perphenazine

BRAND NAMES (Manufacturers)
perphenazine (various manufacturers)
Trilafon (Schering)
TYPE OF DRUG
Phenothiazine tranquilizer
INGREDIENT
perphenazine
DOSAGE FORMS
Tablets (2 mg, 4 mg, 8 mg, and 16 mg)
Oral concentrate (16 mg per 5-ml spoonful, with less than 0.1% alcohol)

STORAGE

The tablet forms of this medication should be stored at room temperature in tightly closed, light-resistant containers. The oral concentrate form may be stored in the refrigerator in a tightly closed, light-resistant container. If the oral concentrate turns slightly yellow, the medicine is still effective and can be used. However, if it changes color markedly or has particles floating in it, it should not be used; rather, it should be discarded down the sink. This medication should never be frozen.

USES

Perphenazine is prescribed to treat the symptoms of certain types of mental illness, such as psychosis, the manic phase of manic-depressive illness, and severe behavioral problems in children. This medication is thought to relieve the symptoms of mental illness by blocking certain chemicals involved with the transmission of nerve impulses in the brain.

TREATMENT

To avoid stomach irritation, you can take the tablet form of this medication with a meal or with a glass of water or milk (unless your doctor directs you to do otherwise).

The oral concentrate form of this medication should be measured carefully with the dropper provided, then added to four ounces ($^1/_2$ cup) or more of water, milk, or a carbonated beverage or to applesauce or pudding immediately prior to administration. To prevent possible loss of effectiveness, do not dilute this drug in tea, coffee, or apple juice..

Antacids and antidiarrheal medicines may decrease the absorption of this medication from the gastrointestinal tract. Therefore, at least an hour should separate doses of one of these medicines and perphenazine.

If you miss a dose, take the missed dose as soon as possible, then return to your regular dosing schedule. If it is almost time for the next dose, however, skip the one you missed and return to your regular schedule. Do not double the next dose (unless your doctor directs you to do so).

The full effects of this medication for the control of emotional or mental symptoms may not become apparent for two weeks after you start to take it.

SIDE EFFECTS

Minor. Blurred vision, constipation, decreased sweating, diarrhea, dizziness, drooling, drowsiness, dry mouth, fatigue, jitteriness, menstrual irregularities, nasal congestion, restlessness, vomiting, or weight gain. As your body adjusts to the drug, these side effects should disappear.

Perphenazine can also cause discoloration of the urine—a harmless side effect. The urine may become red, pink, or red-brown.

This medication can cause increased sensitivity to sunlight. It is, therefore, important to avoid prolonged exposure to sunlight and sunlamps. Wear protective clothing and sunglasses, and use an effective sunscreen.

If you are constipated, increase the amount of fiber in your diet (fresh fruits and vegetables, salads, bran, and whole-grain breads), exercise, and drink more water (unless your doctor directs you to do otherwise).

Chew sugarless gum, or suck on ice chips or a piece of hard candy to reduce mouth dryness.

To avoid dizziness or light-headedness when you stand, contract and relax the muscles of your legs for a few moments before rising. Do this by pushing one foot against the floor while raising the other foot slightly, alternating feet so that you are "pumping" your legs in a pedaling motion.

Major. Tell your doctor about any side effects that are persistent or particularly bothersome. IT IS ESPECIALLY IMPORTANT TO TELL YOUR DOCTOR about breast enlargement (in both sexes); chest pain; convulsions; darkened skin; difficulty in swallowing or breathing; fainting; fever; impotence; involuntary movements of the face, mouth, jaw, or tongue; palpitations; rash; sleep disorders; sore throat; tremors; uncoordinated movements; unusual bleeding or bruising; visual disturbances; weakness; or yellowing of the eyes or skin.

INTERACTIONS

Perphenazine interacts with several other types of drugs:
1. It can cause extreme drowsiness when combined with alcohol or other central nervous system (brain and spinal cord) depressants, such as barbiturates, benzodiazepine tranquilizers, muscle relaxants, narcotics, and pain medications or with tricyclic antidepressants.
2. Perphenazine can decrease the effectiveness of amphetamines, guanethidine, anticonvulsants, and levodopa.
3. The side effects of epinephrine, monoamine oxidase (MAO) inhibitors, propranolol, phenytoin, and tricyclic antidepressants may be increased by this medication. At least 14 days should separate the use of this drug and the use of an MAO inhibitor.
4. Lithium may increase the side effects and decrease the effectiveness of this medication.

Before starting to take perphenazine, BE SURE TO TELL YOUR DOCTOR about any medications you are currently taking, especially any of those listed above.

WARNINGS

• Tell your doctor about unusual or allergic reactions you have had to any medications, especially to perphenazine or other phenothiazine tranquilizers (such as chlorpromazine, fluphenazine, mesoridazine, prochlorperazine, promazine, thioridazine, trifluoperazine, and triflupromazine) or to loxapine.

• Tell your doctor if you have a history of alcoholism or if you now have or have ever had blood disease, bone marrow disease, brain disease, breast cancer, blockage in the urinary or digestive tracts, drug-induced depression, epilepsy, high or low blood pressure, diabetes mellitus, glaucoma, heart or circulatory disease, liver disease, lung disease, Parkinson's disease, peptic ulcers, or enlarged prostate gland.

• Tell your doctor about any recent exposure to a pesticide or an insecticide. Perphenazine may increase the side effects from the exposure.

• To prevent oversedation, avoid drinking alcoholic beverages while taking this medication.

• If this drug makes you dizzy or drowsy, do not take part in any activity that requires alertness, such as driving a car or operating dangerous machinery. Be careful on stairs and avoid getting up suddenly from a lying or sitting position.

• Before having surgery or any other medical or dental treatment, be sure to tell your doctor or dentist that you are taking this medication.

• Some of the side effects caused by this drug can be prevented by taking an antiparkinsonism drug. Discuss this with your doctor.

• This medication can decrease sweating and heat release from the body. You should, therefore, try not to get overheated (avoid exercising strenuously in hot weather and taking hot baths, showers, and saunas).

• Do not stop taking this medication suddenly. If the drug is stopped abruptly, you may experience nausea, vomiting, stomach upset, headache, increased heart rate, insomnia, tremors, or a worsening of your condition. Your doctor may want to reduce the dosage gradually.

• If you are planning to have a myelogram or any other procedure in which dye will be injected into your spinal cord, tell your doctor that you are taking this medication.

• Avoid spilling the oral concentrate form on your skin or clothing; it may cause redness and irritation of the skin.

• While taking this medication, do not take any over-the-counter (nonprescription) medications for weight control or for cough, cold, allergy, asthma, or sinus problems without first checking with your doctor.

• Be sure to tell your doctor if you are pregnant. Small amounts of this medication cross the placenta. Although there are reports of safe use of this drug during pregnancy, there are also reports of liver disease and tremors in newborn infants whose mothers received this type of medication close to term. Also, tell your doctor if you are breast-feeding an infant. Small amounts of this medication pass into breast milk and may cause unwanted effects in the nursing infant.

---

perphenazine and amitriptyline combination

BRAND NAMES (Manufacturers)
Etrafon (Schering)
Triavil (Merck Sharp & Dohme)
TYPE OF DRUG
Phenothiazine tranquilizer and tricyclic antidepressant
INGREDIENTS
perphenazine and amitriptyline
DOSAGE FORM
Tablets (2 mg perphenazine and 10 mg amitriptyline; 2 mg perphenazine and 25 mg amitriptyline; 4 mg perphenazine and 10 mg amitriptyline; 4 mg perphenazine and 25 mg amitriptyline; and 4 mg perphenazine and 50 mg amitriptyline)
STORAGE
Store at room temperature in a tightly closed, light-resistant container.

USES
Perphenazine and amitriptyline combination is used to relieve anxiety or depression. Amitriptyline belongs to a group of drugs referred to as tricyclic antidepressants.

These medicines are thought to relieve depression by increasing the concentration of certain chemicals in the brain. Perphenazine is a phenothiazine tranquilizer. It is thought to relieve the symptoms of mental illness by blocking certain chemicals involved with nerve transmission in the brain.

TREATMENT
This medication should be taken exactly as your doctor prescribes. In order to avoid stomach irritation, you can take the tablets with food or with a full glass of water or milk (unless your doctor directs you to do otherwise).

Antacids and antidiarrheal medicines may decrease the absorption of this medication from the gastrointestinal tract. Therefore, at least one hour should separate doses of perphenazine and amitriptyline combination and one of these medicines.

If you miss a dose of this medication, take the missed dose as soon as possible, unless it is within two hours of your next scheduled dose. In that case, do not take the missed dose at all; just return to your regular dosing schedule. Do not double the next dose.

The full benefits of this medication for the control of emotional or mental symptoms may not become apparent for two weeks after you start to take it.

SIDE EFFECTS
Minor. Bloating, blurred vision, constipation, cramps, decreased or increased sweating, diarrhea, dizziness, drowsiness, dry mouth, fatigue, headache, heartburn, insomnia, loss of appetite, nasal congestion, nausea, peculiar tastes in the mouth, restlessness, stomach upset, vomiting, weakness, or weight gain or loss. These side effects should disappear as your body adjusts to the medication.

This medication can increase your sensitivity to sunlight. You should, therefore, avoid prolonged exposure to sunlight and sunlamps. Wear protective clothing and sunglasses, and use an effective sunscreen.

This drug combination may cause a discoloration of the urine. This is a harmless effect.

If you experience dry mouth, you might want to try chewing sugarless gum or sucking on ice chips or a piece of hard candy.

To relieve constipation, increase the amount of fiber in your diet (fresh fruits and vegetables, salads, bran, and whole-grain breads), exercise, and drink more water (unless your doctor directs you to do otherwise).

To avoid dizziness and light-headedness when you stand, contract and relax the muscles of your legs for a few moments before rising. Do this by pushing one foot against the floor while raising the other foot slightly, alternating feet so that you are "pumping" your legs in a pedaling motion.

Major. Tell your doctor about any side effects that are persistent or particularly bothersome. IT IS ESPECIALLY IMPORTANT TO TELL YOUR DOCTOR about agitation, confusion, convulsions, difficult or painful urination, enlarged or painful breasts (in both sexes), fainting, fever, hair loss, hallucinations, chest tightness, impotence, menstrual irregularities, mood changes, mouth sores, nervousness, nightmares, numbness in fingers or toes, palpitations, rash, ringing in the ears, sore throat, tremors, uncoordinated movements or balance problems, unusual bleeding or bruising, or yellowing of the eyes or skin.

INTERACTIONS

This drug interacts with several other types of drugs:

1. Extreme drowsiness can occur if this medication is taken with central nervous system depressants (such as alcohol, antihistamines, barbiturates, benzodiazepine tranquilizers, muscle relaxants, narcotics, pain medications, and sleeping medications) or with other antidepressants.

2. Amitriptyline may decrease the effectiveness of antiseizure medications and block the blood-pressure-lowering effects of clonidine and guanethidine.

3. Estrogens and oral contraceptives (birth control pills) can increase the side effects and reduce the effectiveness of amitriptyline.

4. Amitriptyline may increase the side effects of thyroid medication and of over-the-counter (nonprescription) cough, cold, allergy, asthma, sinus, and diet medications.

5. The concurrent use of this medication with monoamine oxidase (MAO) inhibitors should be avoided, because the combination may result in fever, convulsions, or high blood pressure. At least 14 days should separate the use of this drug and the use of an MAO inhibitor.

6. Perphenazine can decrease the effectiveness of amphetamines, guanethidine, anticonvulsants, and levodopa.

7. The side effects of epinephrine and propranolol may be increased by perphenazine.

Before starting to take this medication, BE SURE TO TELL YOUR DOCTOR about any medications you are currently taking, especially any of those listed above.

WARNINGS

• Tell your doctor about unusual or allergic reactions you have had to any medications, especially to perphenazine or other phenothiazine tranquilizers (such as chlorpromazine, mesoridazine fluphenazine, promazine, thioridazine, and prochlorperazine), or to amitriptyline or other tricyclic antidepressants (such as desipramine, doxepin, imipramine, and nortriptyline).

• Tell your doctor if you have ever had asthma, breast cancer, brain disease, diabetes mellitus, electroshock therapy, epilepsy, glaucoma, heart disease, a heart attack, liver disease, lung disease, kidney disease, thyroid disease, intestinal or urinary tract blockage, low or high blood pressure, Parkinson's disease, peptic ulcers, or enlarged prostate.

• The effects of this medication may last as long as seven days after you have stopped taking it, so continue to observe all precautions during that period.

• To prevent oversedation, avoid drinking alcoholic beverages while taking this medication.

• If this medication makes you dizzy or drowsy, do not take part in any activity that requires alertness, such as driving a car or operating potentially dangerous machinery. Be careful on stairs, and avoid getting up suddenly from a lying or sitting position.

• Prior to having surgery or any other medical or dental treatment, be sure to tell your doctor or dentist that you are taking this medication.

• This medication can decrease sweating and heat release from the body. You should, therefore, try not to get overheated (avoid exercising strenuously in hot weather and taking hot baths, showers, and saunas).

• Do not stop taking this medication suddenly. If the drug is stopped abruptly, you may experience nausea, vomiting, stomach upset, headache, increased heart rate, insomnia, tremors, or a worsening of your condition. Your doctor may, therefore, want to reduce the dosage gradually.

• If you are planning to have a myelogram, or any other procedure in which dye will be injected into your spinal cord, tell your doctor that you are taking this medication.

• While taking this medication, do not take any over-the-counter (nonprescription) medications for weight control or for cough, cold, asthma, allergy, or sinus problems without first checking with your doctor. The combination of these medications with perphenazine and amitriptyline may cause high blood pressure.

• Be sure to tell your doctor if you are pregnant. Small amounts of this medication cross the placenta. Although there are reports of safe use of this drug during pregnancy, there are also reports of liver disease and tremors in newborn infants whose mothers received this type of medication close to term. Also, tell your doctor if you are breast-feeding an infant. Small amounts of this medication pass into breast milk and may cause unwanted effects in the nursing infant.

Persantine—see dipyridamole

Pertofrane—see desipramine

Petitrate SA—see pentaerythritol tetranitrate

P.E.T.N.—see pentaerythritol tetranitrate

Phenameth—see promethazine

Phenaphen-650 with Codeine—see acetaminophen and codeine combination

Phenaphen with Codeine—see acetaminophen and codeine combination

Phenazine VC with Codeine—see phenylephrine, promethazine, and codeine combination

Phenazodine—see phenazopyridine

phenazopyridine

BRAND NAMES (Manufacturers)
Azo-Standard* (Webcon)
Baridium* (Pfeiffer)
Eridium* (Hauck)
Geridium (Goldline)
Phenazodine (Lannett)
phenazopyridine hydrochloride (various manufacturers)
pyridiate (various manufacturers)
pyridium (Parke-Davis)

Urodine (various manufacturers)
Urogesic (Edwards)
*Available (100-mg tablets) without a prescription.
TYPE OF DRUG
Urinary tract analgesic
INGREDIENT
phenazopyridine
DOSAGE FORM
Tablets (100 mg and 200 mg)
STORAGE
Phenazopyridine tablets should be stored at room temperature in a tightly closed, light-resistant container.

USES

Phenazopyridine is used for the symptomatic relief of the burning, pain, and discomfort caused by urinary tract infections or irritations. It is excreted in the urine, where it exerts a topical analgesic effect on the urinary tract. This medication is not useful for other types of pain.

TREATMENT

Phenazopyridine tablets should be taken with a full glass of water, either with meals or immediately after a meal.

If you miss a dose of this medication, take the missed dose as soon as possible, unless it is almost time for the next dose. In that case, do not take the missed dose at all; return to your regular dosing schedule. Do not double the dose.

SIDE EFFECTS

Minor. Dizziness, headache, indigestion, nausea, stomach cramps, or vomiting. These side effects should disappear as your body adjusts to the medication.

This drug causes urine to become orange-red. This is not harmful, but it may stain your clothing. The coloration of the urine will return to normal soon after the drug is discontinued.

If you feel dizzy, sit or lie down for a while; get up slowly from a sitting or reclining position, and be careful on stairs.

Major. Tell your doctor about any side effects that are persistent or particularly bothersome. IT IS ESPECIALLY IMPORTANT TO TELL YOUR DOCTOR about a bluish color of the skin or fingernails, rash, unusual fatigue, or yellowing of the eyes or skin.

INTERACTIONS

Phenazopyridine should not interact with other medications as long as it is used according to directions.

WARNINGS

• Tell your doctor about unusual or allergic reactions you have had to any medications, especially to phenazopyridine.
• Tell your doctor if you have ever had kidney disease or hepatitis.
• If this drug makes you dizzy, do not take part in any activity that requires alertness, such as driving a car.
• Diabetic patients using this medication may get delayed reactions or false-positive readings for sugar or ketones with urine tests. Clinitest is not affected by this medication, but the other urine sugar tests are.

• Be sure to tell your doctor if you are pregnant. Although phenazopyridine appears to be safe in animals, extensive studies in humans have not been conducted. Also, tell your doctor if you are breast-feeding an infant. It is not known whether phenazopyridine passes into breast milk.

phenazopyridine hydrochloride—see phenazopyridine

phendimetrazine

BRAND NAMES (Manufacturers)
Adipost (Ascher)
Adphen (Ferndale)
Anorex (Dunhall)
Bontril PDM (Carnrick)
Bontril Slow-Release (Carnrick)
Dyrexan-OD (Trimen)
Metra (Forest)
Obalan (Lannett)
phendimetrazine tartrate (various manufacturers)
Plegine (Ayerst)
Prelu-2 (Boehringer Ingelheim)
Slyn-LL (Edwards)
Statobex (Lemmon)
Trimcaps (Maynard)
Trimstat (Laser)
Trimtabs (Maynard)
Weh-less (Hauck)
Weightrol (Vortech)
TYPE OF DRUG
Anorectic
INGREDIENT
phendimetrazine
DOSAGE FORMS
Tablets (35 mg)
Capsules (35 mg)
Sustained-release capsules (105 mg)
STORAGE
Phendimetrazine should be stored at room temperature in a tightly closed, light-resistant container.

USES

Phendimetrazine is used as an appetite suppressant during the first few weeks of dieting to help establish new eating habits. This medication is thought to relieve hunger by altering nerve impulses to the appetite control center in the brain. Its effectiveness lasts only for short periods (three to 12 weeks), however.

TREATMENT

You can take phendimetrazine with a full glass of water one hour before meals (unless your doctor directs otherwise).

The sustained-release form of this medication should be swallowed whole. Breaking, chewing, or crushing these capsules destroys their sustained-release activity and may increase the side effects.

In order to avoid difficulty in falling asleep, the last dose of this medication each day should be taken four to six hours (regular tablets) or ten to 14 hours (sustained-release capsules) before bedtime.

If you miss a dose of this medication, take the missed dose as soon as possible, unless it is almost time for your next dose. In that case, do not take the missed dose at all; just return to your regular dosing schedule. Do not double the next dose.

SIDE EFFECTS

Minor. Blurred vision, constipation, diarrhea, dizziness, dry mouth, false sense of well-being, fatigue, insomnia, irritability, nausea, nervousness, restlessness, stomach pain, sweating, unpleasant taste in the mouth, or vomiting. These side effects should disappear as your body adjusts to the medication.

Dry mouth can be relieved by sucking on ice chips or a piece of hard candy or by chewing sugarless gum.

In order to prevent constipation, increase the amount of fiber in your diet (fresh fruits and vegetables, salads, bran, and whole-grain breads), exercise, and drink more water (unless your doctor tells you not to do so).

Major. Tell your doctor about any side effects that are persistent or particularly bothersome. IT IS ESPECIALLY IMPORTANT TO TELL YOUR DOCTOR about changes in sexual desire, chest pain, difficulty in urinating, enlarged breasts (in either sex), fever, hair loss, headaches, impotence, menstrual irregularities, mental depression, mood changes, mouth sores, muscle pains, palpitations, rash, sore throat, tremors, or unusual bleeding or bruising.

INTERACTIONS

Phendimetrazine interacts with several other types of drugs:

1. Use of it within 14 days of a monoamine oxidase (MAO) inhibitor (isocarboxazid, pargyline, phenelzine, tranylcypromine) can result in high blood pressure and other side effects.

2. Phenothiazine tranquilizers (especially chlorpromazine) can antagonize (act against) the appetite-suppressant activity of this medication.

3. Phendimetrazine can decrease the blood-pressure-lowering effects of antihypertensive medications (especially guanethidine) and may alter insulin and oral antidiabetic medication dosage requirements in diabetic patients.

4. The side effects of other central nervous system stimulants, such as caffeine and over-the-counter (nonprescription) cough, allergy, asthma, sinus, diet, or cold preparations, may be increased by this medication.

Before starting to take phendimetrazine, BE SURE TO TELL YOUR DOCTOR about any medications you are currently taking, especially any of those listed above.

WARNINGS

Tell your doctor about unusual or allergic reactions you have had to any medications, especially to phendimetrazine or other appetite suppressants (such as benzphetamine, phenmetrazine, diethylpropion, fenfluramine, mazindol, and phentermine) or to epinephrine, norepinephrine, ephedrine, amphetamines, dextroamphetamine, phenylephrine, phenylpropanolamine, pseudoephedrine, albuterol, metaproterenol, or terbutaline.

Tell your doctor if you have a history of drug abuse or if you have ever had angina, diabetes mellitus, emotional disturbances, glaucoma, heart or cardiovascular disease, high blood pressure, or thyroid disease.

Phendimetrazine can mask the symptoms of extreme fatigue and can cause dizziness or light-headedness. Your ability to perform tasks that require alertness, such as driving a car or operating potentially dangerous machinery, may be decreased.

Before having surgery or other medical or dental treatment, tell your doctor or dentist you are taking this drug.

Phendimetrazine is related to amphetamine and may be habit-forming when taken for long periods of time (both physical and psychological dependence can occur). You should not increase the dosage of this medication or take it for longer than 12 weeks without first consulting your doctor. It is also important that you not stop taking this medication abruptly-fatigue, sleep disorders, mental depression, nausea, vomiting, or stomach cramps or pain could occur. Your doctor may, therefore, want to decrease your dosage gradually.

Be sure to tell your doctor if you are pregnant. Although studies of phendimetrazine in humans have not been conducted, some of the appetite suppressants have been shown to cause side effects in the fetuses of animals that received large doses during pregnancy. Also, tell your doctor if you are breast-feeding an infant. It is not known whether this medication passes into breast milk.

phendimetrazine tartrate—see phendimetrazine

---

phenelzine

BRAND NAME (Manufacturer)
Nardil (Parke-Davis)
TYPE OF DRUG
Monoamine oxidase (MAO) inhibitor
INGREDIENT
phenelzine
DOSAGE FORM
Tablets (15 mg)
STORAGE
Phenelzine should be stored at room temperature in a tightly closed, light-resistant container.

USES

This medication is used to treat depression. Phenelzine belongs to a group of drugs known as monoamine oxidase (MAO) inhibitors. It is not clearly understood how it works, but it is thought to increase the amounts of certain chemicals in the brain that act to relieve depression.

TREATMENT

You can take phenelzine either on an empty stomach or, to avoid stomach irritation, with food or milk (as directed by your doctor).

If you are taking a single daily dose, it is best to take the dose in the morning .

If you miss a dose of this medication and remember within two hours, take the missed dose immediately and then return to your regular dosing schedule. If more than two hours has passed, do not take the missed dose at all; just return to your regular dosing schedule. Do not double the next dose.

The full therapeutic benefits of this medication may not be observed for up to four weeks after you start to take it.

SIDE EFFECTS

Minor. Constipation, diarrhea, dizziness, drowsiness, dry mouth, fatigue, headache, insomnia, nausea, restlessness, stomach upset, sweating, or weakness. These side effects should disappear as your body adjusts to the medication.

Phenelzine can increase your sensitivity to sunlight. Avoid prolonged exposure to sunlight and sunlamps. Wear protective clothing and sunglasses, and use an effective sunscreen.

If you feel dizzy, sit or lie down for a while; get up slowly from a sitting or reclining position, and be careful on stairs.

To relieve constipation, increase the amount of fiber in your diet (fresh fruits and vegetables, salads, bran, and whole-grain breads) and drink more water (unless your doctor directs you to do otherwise).

To relieve mouth dryness, chew sugarless gum or suck on ice chips or a piece of hard candy.

Major. Tell your doctor about any side effects that are persistent or particularly bothersome. IT IS ESPECIALLY IMPORTANT TO TELL YOUR DOCTOR about anxiety, blurred vision, changes in sexual ability, chills, confusion, convulsions, darkened tongue, difficult or painful urination, fainting, false sense of well-being, hallucinations, jitteriness, mental disorders, rapid weight gain (three to five pounds within a week), uncoordinated movements, or yellowing of the eyes or skin.

If you experience a severe headache, stiff neck, chest pains, palpitations, or vomiting while taking this medication, CONTACT YOUR DOCTOR OR AN EMERGENCY ROOM IMMEDIATELY. These symptoms may be the result of a food or drug interaction.

INTERACTIONS

Phenelzine interacts with a number of drugs and foods:

1. Concurrent use of phenelzine with central nervous system depressants (such as alcohol, barbiturates, benzodiazepine tranquilizers, muscle relaxants, narcotics, pain medications, phenothiazine tranquilizers, and sleeping medications) or with tricyclic antidepressants can lead to extreme drowsiness.

2. The dosage of anticonvulsant medications may need to be adjusted when phenelzine is started.

3. The use of phenelzine within 14 days of either another monoamine oxidase inhibitor or carbamazepine, cyclobenzaprine, methyldopa, guanethidine, reserpine, levodopa, meperidine or another narcotic, amphetamines, ephedrine, methylphenidate, phenylpropanolamine, pseudoephedrine, or a tricyclic antidepressant can lead to serious (sometimes fatal) side effects.

4. Tyramine-containing foods and beverages (aged cheeses, sour cream, yogurt, pickled herring, chicken livers, canned figs, raisins, bananas, avocados, soy sauce, broad bean pods, yeast extracts, beer, and certain wines),

excessive amounts of caffeine-containing beverages (coffee, tea, cocoa, and cola), or chocolate can also cause serious reactions in patients on phenelzine therapy.

5. Phenelzine can increase the blood-sugar-lowering effects of insulin and oral antidiabetic medications.

Before starting to take this medication, BE SURE TO TELL YOUR DOCTOR about any medications you are currently taking, especially any of those listed above. Be sure you are aware of the foods that interact with phenelzine.

WARNINGS

Tell your doctor about unusual or allergic reactions you have had to any medications, especially to phenelzine.

Before starting to take this medication, be sure to tell your doctor if you now have or if you have ever had asthma, bronchitis, diabetes mellitus, epilepsy, glaucoma, severe headaches, heart or blood vessel disease, kidney disease, liver disease, mental disorders, Parkinson's disease, pheochromocytoma, or thyroid disease.

If this drug makes you dizzy or drowsy, do not take part in any activity that requires alertness, such as driving a car or operating potentially dangerous machinery.

Before having surgery or any other medical or dental treatment, be sure to tell your doctor or dentist that you are taking this medication.

Check with your doctor or pharmacist before taking any over-the-counter (nonprescription) asthma, allergy, cough, cold, diet, or sinus preparations. Concurrent use of some of these products with phenelzine can lead to serious side effects.

If you also have angina, do not increase your amount of physical activity unless you first check with your doctor. Phenelzine can decrease the symptoms of angina without decreasing the risks of strenuous exercise.

Be sure to tell your doctor if you are pregnant. Studies in animals have shown that phenelzine can cause birth defects if it is taken in high doses during pregnancy. Studies in humans have not been conducted. Also, tell your doctor if you are breast-feeding an infant. Small amounts of phenelzine may pass into breast milk.

Phenergan—see promethazine

Phenergan VC with Codeine—see phenylephrine, promethazine, and codeine combination

Phenergan with Codeine—see promethazine and codeine combination

phenmetrazine

BRAND NAME (Manufacturer)
Preludin Endurets (Boehringer Ingelheim)
TYPE OF DRUG
Anorectic
INGREDIENT
phenmetrazine
DOSAGE FORM
Sustained-release tablets (75 mg)

STORAGE

Phenmetrazine should be stored at room temperature in tightly closed, light-resistant containers.

USES

Phenmetrazine is used as an appetite suppressant during the first few weeks of dieting to help establish new eating habits. This medication is thought to relieve hunger by altering nerve impulses to the appetite control center in the brain. Its effectiveness lasts only for short periods (three to 12 weeks), however.

TREATMENT

You can take phenmetrazine with a full glass of water one hour before meals (unless your doctor directs you to do otherwise).

This medication should be swallowed whole. Breaking, chewing, or crushing these tablets destroys their sustained-release activity and may increase the side effects.

To avoid difficulty in falling asleep, take the last dose of this medication each day ten to 14 hours before bedtime.

If you miss a dose of this medication, take the missed dose as soon as possible, unless it is almost time for your next dose. In that case, do not take the missed dose at all; just return to your regular dosing schedule. Do not double the next dose.

SIDE EFFECTS

Minor. Blurred vision, constipation, diarrhea, dizziness, dry mouth, false sense of well-being, fatigue, insomnia, irritability, nausea, nervousness, restlessness, stomach pain, sweating, unpleasant taste in the mouth, or vomiting. These side effects should disappear as your body adjusts to the drug.

If you experience mouth dryness, try sucking on ice chips or a piece of hard candy or chewing sugarless gum.

In order to prevent constipation, increase the amount of fiber in your diet (fresh fruits and vegetables, salads, bran, and whole-grain breads), exercise, and drink more water (unless your doctor tells you not to do so).

Major. Tell your doctor about any side effects that are persistent or particularly bothersome. IT IS ESPECIALLY IMPORTANT TO TELL YOUR DOCTOR about changes in sexual desire, chest pain, difficulty in urinating, enlarged breasts (in both sexes), fever, hair loss, headaches, impotence, menstrual irregularities, mental depression, mood changes, mouth sores, muscle pains, palpitations, rash, sore throat, tremors, or unusual bleeding or bruising.

INTERACTIONS

Phenmetrazine interacts with several other types of drugs:

1. Use of it within 14 days of a monoamine oxidase (MAO) inhibitor (isocarboxazid, pargyline, phenelzine, or tranylcypromine can result in high blood pressure and other side effects.

2. Tricyclic antidepressants and phenothiazine tranquilizers (especially chlorpromazine) can antagonize (act against) the appetite-suppressant activity of this drug.

3. Phenmetrazine can decrease the blood-pressure-lowering effects of antihypertensive medications (especially guanethidine) and may alter insulin and oral antidiabetic medication dosage requirements in diabetic patients.

4. The side effects of other central nervous system stimulants, such as caffeine or over-the-counter (nonprescription) diet, cough, cold, sinus, asthma, or allergy preparations, may be increased by this medication.

BE SURE TO TELL YOUR DOCTOR about any medications you are currently taking, especially any of those listed above.

WARNINGS

• Tell your doctor about unusual or allergic reactions you have had to any medications, especially to phenmetrazine or other appetite suppressants (such as benzphetamine, phendimetrazine, diethylpropion, fenfluramine, mazindol, and phentermine), or to epinephrine, norepinephrine, ephedrine, amphetamines, dextroamphetamine, phenylephrine, phenylpropanolamine, pseudoephedrine, albuterol, metaproterenol, or terbutaline.

• Tell your doctor if you have a history of drug abuse or if you now have or have ever had angina, diabetes mellitus, emotional disturbances, glaucoma, heart or cardiovascular disease, high blood pressure, or thyroid disease.

• Phenmetrazine can mask the symptoms of extreme fatigue and can cause dizziness or light-headedness. Your ability to perform tasks that require alertness, such as driving a car or operating potentially dangerous machinery, may be decreased. Appropriate caution should, therefore, be taken.

• Before having surgery or any other medical or dental treatment, be sure to tell your doctor or dentist that you are taking this medication.

• Phenmetrazine is related to amphetamine and may be habit-forming when taken for long periods of time (both physical and psychological dependence can occur). Therefore, you should not increase your dosage of this medication or take it for longer than 12 weeks, unless you first consult your doctor. It is also important that you not stop taking this medication abruptly—fatigue, sleep disorders, mental depression, nausea or vomiting, or stomach cramps or pain could occur. Your doctor may, therefore, want to decrease the dosage gradually in order to prevent or minimize these side effects.

• Phenmetrazine 75-mg sustained-release tablets contain the color additive FD&C Yellow No. 5 (tartrazine), which can cause allergic-type reactions (fainting, shortness of breath, or rash) in certain susceptible individuals.

• Be sure to tell your doctor if you are pregnant. Although studies of phenmetrazine in humans have not been conducted, some of the appetite suppressants have been shown to cause side effects in the fetuses of animals that received large doses during pregnancy. Also, tell your doctor if you are breast-feeding an infant. It is not known whether this medication passes into breast milk.

phenobarbital

BRAND NAMES (Manufacturers)
Barbita (Vortech)
phenobarbital (various manufacturers)
Solfoton (Poythress)

TYPE OF DRUG
Barbiturate sedative and anticonvulsant
INGREDIENT
phenobarbital
DOSAGE FORMS
Tablets (8 mg, 16 mg, 32 mg, 65 mg, and 100 mg)
Capsules (16 mg)
Oral liquid (15 mg and 20 mg per 5-ml spoonful, with 13.5% alcohol)
STORAGE
Phenobarbital tablets and capsules should be stored at room temperature in tightly closed containers. The oral liquid should be stored at room temperature in a tightly closed, light-resistant container. Phenobarbital liquid should not be used if the solution becomes cloudy—it is no longer effective. This medication should never be frozen.

USES
Phenobarbital is used to control convulsions, to relieve anxiety or tension, and to promote sleep. Phenobarbital belongs to a group of drugs known as barbiturates. The barbiturates are central nervous system (brain and spinal cord) depressants.

TREATMENT
In order to avoid stomach irritation, you should take phenobarbital with food or with a full glass of water or milk.

The oral liquid should be measured carefully with a specially designed 5-ml measuring spoon. An ordinary kitchen teaspoon is not accurate enough. The liquid dose can be taken by itself or diluted with water, milk, or fruit juice.

If phenobarbital is being taken as a sleeping aid, take it 30 to 60 minutes before you want to go to sleep.

If you are taking this medication for the treatment of seizures, phenobarbital works best when the level of medicine in your bloodstream is kept constant. It is best, therefore, to take the doses at evenly spaced intervals day and night. For example, if you are to take three doses a day, the doses should be spaced eight hours apart.

If you are taking this medication on a regular basis and you miss a dose, take the missed dose as soon as you remember. However, if it is almost time for your next dose, do not take the missed dose at all; just return to your regular dosing schedule. Do not double the next dose. If you are taking this medication to control seizures and you miss more than two doses, be sure to contact your doctor immediately.

SIDE EFFECTS
Minor. Constipation, diarrhea, dizziness, drowsiness, a "hangover" feeling, headache, nausea, stomach upset, or vomiting. These side effects should disappear as your body adjusts to the medication.

If you feel dizzy or light-headed, sit or lie down for a while; get up slowly from a sitting or reclining position, and be careful on stairs.

To relieve constipation, increase the amount of fiber in your diet (fresh fruits and vegetables, salads, bran, and whole-grain breads), exercise, and drink more water (unless your doctor directs you to do otherwise).

Major. Tell your doctor about any side effects that are persistent or particularly bothersome. IT IS ESPECIALLY IMPORTANT TO TELL YOUR DOCTOR about chest tightness, confusion, depression, difficulty in breathing, excitation, fatigue, feeling faint, hives or itching, loss of co-ordination, muscle or joint pain, skin rash, slurred speech, sore throat, unusual bleeding or bruising, unusual weakness, or yellowing of the eyes or skin.

INTERACTIONS
Phenobarbital interacts with other types of medications:
1. Concurrent use of it with other central nervous system depressants (such as alcohol, antihistamines, benzodiazepine tranquilizers, muscle relaxants, narcotics, pain medications, phenothiazine tranquilizers, and sleeping medications) or with tricyclic antidepressants can cause extreme drowsiness.
2. Valproic acid, chloramphenicol, and monoamine oxidase (MAO) inhibitors can prolong the effects of the barbiturates.
3. Phenobarbital can increase the elimination from the body (thereby decreasing the effectiveness) of oral anticoagulants (blood thinners, such as warfarin), digitoxin, tricyclic antidepressants, cortisone-like medications, doxycycline, metronidazole, quinidine, oral contraceptives (birth control pills), estrogen-containing drugs, phenytoin, acetaminophen, and carbamazepine.
4. Phenobarbital can decrease the absorption of griseofulvin from the gastrointestinal tract.
5. The combination of phenobarbital and furosemide can cause low blood pressure and fainting.
6. Phenobarbital can increase the side effects of cyclophosphamide or large doses of acetaminophen.

BE SURE TO TELL YOUR DOCTOR about any medications you are currently taking, especially any listed above.

WARNINGS
• Tell your doctor about unusual or allergic reactions you have had to any medications, especially to phenobarbital or other barbiturates (such as amobarbital, butabarbital, mephobarbital, pentobarbital, primidone, and secobarbital).
• Tell your doctor if you now have or if you have ever had acute or chronic (long-term) pain, Addison's disease (caused by an underactive adrenal gland), diabetes mellitus, kidney disease, liver disease, lung disease, mental depression, porphyria, or thyroid disease.
• Before having surgery or any other medical or dental treatment, tell your doctor or dentist you are taking this drug.
• If this medication makes you dizzy or drowsy, do not take part in any activity that requires alertness, such as driving a car or operating potentially dangerous machinery.
• This drug has the potential for abuse and must be used with caution. Tolerance to the medication develops quickly; do not increase the dosage or stop taking this drug unless you first consult your doctor. If you have been taking this drug for a long time or have been taking large doses of it, you may experience anxiety, muscle twitching, tremors, weakness, dizziness, nausea, vomiting,

insomnia, or blurred vision when you stop taking it. Your doctor may, therefore, want to reduce your dosage of this medication gradually.

• Some of these products contain the color additive FD&C Yellow No. 5 (tartrazine), which can cause allergic-type reactions (rash, fainting, difficulty in breathing) in certain susceptible individuals.

• Be sure to tell your doctor if you are pregnant. Phenobarbital crosses the placenta, and birth defects have been associated with the use of this medication during pregnancy. If phenobarbital is used during the last three months of pregnancy, there is a chance that the infant will be born addicted to the medication and will experience a withdrawal reaction (seizures or irritability) at birth. The infant could also be born with bleeding problems. The risks and benefits of treatment should be discussed with your doctor. Also, tell your doctor if you are breast-feeding an infant. Small amounts of phenobarbital pass into breast milk.

phentermine

BRAND NAMES (Manufacturers)
Adipex-P (Lemmon)
Dapex (Ferndale)
Fastin (Beecham)
Ionamin (Pennwalt)
Obe-Nix (Holloway)
Obephen (Hauck)
Obermine (Forest)
Obestin-30 (Ferndale)
phentermine hydrochloride (various manufacturers)
Phentrol (Vortech)
Wilpowr (Foy)
TYPE OF DRUG
Anorectic
INGREDIENT
phentermine
DOSAGE FORMS
Tablets (8 mg, 30 mg, and 37.5 mg)
Capsules (15 mg, 18.75 mg, 30 mg, and 37.5 mg)
Timed-release capsules (15 mg and 30 mg)
STORAGE
Phentermine should be stored at room temperature in tightly closed, light-resistant containers.

USES
Phentermine is used as an appetite suppressant during the first few weeks of dieting, to help establish new eating habits. This medication is thought to relieve hunger by altering nerve impulses to the appetite control center in the brain. Its effectiveness lasts only for short periods (three to 12 weeks), however.

TREATMENT
You can take phentermine tablets, capsules, or timed-release capsules with a full glass of water one hour before meals (unless your doctor directs you to do otherwise).

The timed-release form of this medication should be swallowed whole. Breaking, chewing, or crushing these

capsules destroys their timed-release activity and may increase side effects.

In order to avoid difficulty in falling asleep, the last daily dose of this medication should be taken four to six hours (regular tablets and capsules) or ten to 14 hours (timed-release capsules) before bedtime.

If you miss a dose of this medication, be sure to take the missed dose as soon as possible, unless it is almost time for your next dose. In that case, do not take the missed dose at all; just return to your regular dosing schedule. Do not double the next dose of the medication.

SIDE EFFECTS
Minor. Blurred vision, constipation, diarrhea, dizziness, dry mouth, false sense of well-being, fatigue, insomnia, irritability, nausea, nervousness, restlessness, stomach pain, sweating, unpleasant taste in the mouth, or vomiting. These side effects should disappear as your body adjusts to the drug.

Dry mouth can be relieved by sucking on ice chips or a piece of hard candy or by chewing sugarless gum.

In order to prevent constipation, increase the amount of fiber in your diet (fresh fruits and vegetables, salads, bran, and whole-grain breads), exercise, and drink more water (unless your doctor tells you not to do so).

Major. Tell your doctor about any side effects that are persistent or particularly bothersome. IT IS ESPECIALLY IMPORTANT TO TELL YOUR DOCTOR about changes in sexual desire, chest pain, difficulty in urinating, enlarged breasts (in both sexes), fever, hair loss, headaches, impotence, menstrual irregularities, mental depression, mood changes, mouth sores, muscle pains, palpitations, rash, sore throat, or tremors.

INTERACTIONS
Phentermine interacts with several other types of medications:

1. Use of it within 14 days of a monoamine oxidase (MAO) inhibitor (isocarboxazid, pargyline, phenelzine, or tranylcypromine can result in high blood pressure and other side effects.

2. Barbiturate medications and phenothiazine tranquilizers (especially chlorpromazine) can antagonize (act against) the appetite-suppressant activity of this medication.

3. Phentermine can decrease the blood-pressure-lowering effects of antihypertensive medications (especially guanethidine) and may alter insulin and oral antidiabetic medication dosage requirements in diabetic patients.

4. The side effects of other central nervous system stimulants, such as caffeine or over-the-counter (nonprescription) cough, cold, sinus, asthma, diet, or allergy preparations, may be increased by this medication.

BE SURE TO TELL YOUR DOCTOR about any medications you are currently taking, especially any of those listed above.

WARNINGS
• Tell your doctor about unusual or allergic reactions you have had to any medications, especially to phentermine or other appetite suppressants (such as benzphet-

amine, phendimetrazine, diethylpropion, fenfluramine, mazindol, and phenmetrazine), or to epinephrine, norepinephrine, ephedrine, amphetamines, dextroamphetamine, phenylephrine, phenylpropanolamine, pseudoephedrine, albuterol, metaproterenol, or terbutaline.
• Tell your doctor if you have a history of drug abuse or if you now have or have ever had angina, diabetes mellitus, emotional disturbances, glaucoma, heart or cardiovascular disease, high blood pressure, or thyroid disease.
• Phentermine can mask the symptoms of extreme fatigue and can cause dizziness or light-headedness. Your ability to perform tasks that require alertness, such as driving a car or operating potentially dangerous machinery, may be decreased. Appropriate caution should, therefore, be taken.
• Before having surgery or other medical or dental treatment, tell your doctor or dentist you are taking this drug.
• Phentermine is related to amphetamine and may be habit-forming when taken for long periods of time (both physical and psychological dependence can occur). You should, therefore, not increase the dosage of this medication or take it for longer than 12 weeks without first consulting your doctor. Do not stop taking this medication abruptly—fatigue, sleep disorders, mental depression, nausea, vomiting, or stomach cramps or pain could occur. Your doctor may, therefore, want to decrease your dosage gradually.
• Be sure to tell your doctor if you are pregnant. Although studies of phentermine in humans have not been conducted, some of the appetite suppressants have been shown to cause side effects in the fetuses of animals that received large doses during pregnancy. Also, tell your doctor if you are breast-feeding an infant. It is not known whether this medication passes into breast milk.

phentermine hydrochloride—see phentermine

Phentrol—see phentermine

phenylbutazone

BRAND NAMES (Manufacturers)
Butazolidin (Geigy)
phenylbutazone (various manufacturers)
TYPE OF DRUG
Nonsteroidal anti-inflammatory analgesic
INGREDIENT
phenylbutazone
DOSAGE FORMS
Tablets (100 mg)
Capsules (100 mg)
STORAGE
Phenylbutazone tablets and capsules should be stored at room temperature in tightly closed containers.

USES
Phenylbutazone is used to reduce inflammation (pain, redness, and swelling) due to arthritis or thrombophlebitis when other anti-inflammatory agents have been unsuc-

cessful. It is not clearly understood how phenylbutazone works, but it is thought to act by interfering with the body's inflammatory mechanism or by decreasing the sensitivity of the body's pain mechanism.

TREATMENT
In order to avoid stomach upset, you can take phenylbutazone with food or with a full glass of water or milk. Ask your doctor if you can take phenylbutazone with an antacid.
Phenylbutazone tablets should be swallowed whole. Do not break or crush them.
If you miss a dose of this medication and you are taking it once or twice a day, take the missed dose as soon as possible, unless it is almost time for the next dose. In that case, do not take the missed dose at all; just return to your regular dosing schedule. Do not double the next dose.
If you are taking phenylbutazone three or more times per day and you miss a dose, take the missed dose right away (if you remember within an hour of the correct time); then take the next dose as scheduled. If more than an hour has passed, however, do not take the missed dose at all; just return to your regular schedule. Do not double the next dose.

SIDE EFFECTS
Minor. Abdominal pain, bloating, constipation, diarrhea, drowsiness, gas, headache, heartburn, indigestion, irritability, nausea, numbness, vomiting, or weakness. These side effects should disappear as your body adjusts to the medication.
You may experience constipation when taking this drug. To relieve constipation, increase the amount of fiber in your diet (fresh fruits and vegetables, salads, bran, and whole-grain breads), exercise, and drink more water (unless your doctor directs you to do otherwise).
Major. Tell your doctor about any side effects that are persistent or particularly bothersome. IT IS ESPECIALLY IMPORTANT TO TELL YOUR DOCTOR about bloody or black, tarry stools; blurred vision; confusion; depression; difficulty in breathing; difficulty in hearing; difficult or painful urination; fatigue; fever; itching; mouth sores; rash; ringing in the ears; severe abdominal pain; sore throat; swelling of the ankles; tremors; unusual bleeding or bruising; weight gain of more than three pounds within a week; or yellowing of the eyes or skin.

INTERACTIONS
Phenylbutazone interacts with several other types of medications:
1. It can increase the kidney side effects of penicillamine; increase skin reactions to chloroquine, gold compounds, and hydroxychloroquine; and increase the effects on the blood of antineoplastic agents (anticancer medicines), chloramphenicol, colchicine, gold compounds, pyrimethamine, and trimethoprim.
2. The gastrointestinal side effects of phenylbutazone analgesic can be increased by the use of alcohol or anti-inflammatory medications.
3. Phenylbutazone can decrease the blood levels and effectiveness of digitoxin, hexobarbital, and cortisone.

4. Cholestyramine can decrease the absorption of phenylbutazone from the gastrointestinal tract, which can decrease its effectiveness.

5. The active blood levels and side effects of oral anticoagulants (blood thinners, such as warfarin), insulin, oral antidiabetic medicines, sulfonamide antibiotics, sodium valproate, methotrexate, sulfonylurea drugs, and phenytoin can possibly be increased by the use of phenylbutazone.

6. Phenylbutazone can decrease the elimination of lithium through the kidneys, which can lead to an increased risk of side effects.

BE SURE TO TELL YOUR DOCTOR about any medications you are currently taking, especially those listed above.

WARNINGS

• Be sure to tell your doctor about unusual or allergic reactions you have had to any medications, especially to phenylbutazone or other nonsteroidal anti-inflammatory medications (such as aspirin, diclofenac, diflunisal, fenoprofen, flurbiprofen, ibuprofen, indomethacin, ketoprofen, meclofenamate, mefenamic acid, naproxen, oxyphenbutazone, sulfinpyrazone, sulindac, or tolmetin).

• Be sure to tell your doctor if you now have or if you have ever had any of the following medical disorders: anemia, blood disorders, heart disease, hypertension, inflamed salivary glands, kidney disease, liver disease, mouth sores, pancreatitis, peptic ulcers, polymyalgia rheumatica, stomach problems, temporal arteritis, or thyroid disease.

• Use of this drug has been associated with leukemia, although there is no definite proof that it causes the disease.

• If phenylbutazone makes you dizzy or drowsy, do not take part in any activity that requires alertness, such as driving a car or operating potentially dangerous machinery. Also, be especially cautious going up and down stairs.

• Because phenylbutazone has been shown to prolong your bleeding time, it is very important that you tell your doctor or dentist that you are taking this medication before having surgery or any other type of medical or dental treatment.

• This medication has been shown to cause serious blood disorders. Therefore, it should never be used for trivial aches or pains.

• This drug should be used for a short time only. Follow your doctor's directions exactly, and never exceed the recommended dosage.

• Some of these products contain the color additive FD&C Yellow No. 5 (tartrazine), which can cause allergic-type reactions (shortness of breath, rash, or fainting) in certain susceptible individuals.

• Be sure to tell your doctor if you are pregnant. Although studies in humans have not been conducted, unwanted effects have been observed in the offspring of animals that received large doses of this drug during pregnancy. If taken late in pregnancy, phenylbutazone can also prolong labor. Also, tell your doctor if you are breast-feeding an infant. Small doses of phenylbutazone pass into breast milk.

phenylephrine, phenylpropanolamine, brompheniramine, and guaifenesin combination

BRAND NAME (Manufacturer)
Normatane Expectorant (Vortech)

TYPE OF DRUG
Adrenergic (decongestant), antihistamine, and expectorant

INGREDIENTS
phenylephrine, phenylpropanolamine, brompheniramine, guaifenesin, and alcohol

DOSAGE FORM
Oral expectorant (5 mg phenylephrine, 5 mg phenylpropanolamine, 2 mg brompheniramine, and 100 mg guaifenesin per 5-ml spoonful, with 3.5% alcohol)

STORAGE
Phenylephrine, phenylpropanolamine, brompheniramine, and guaifenesin combination should be stored at room temperature (never frozen) in a tightly closed container.

USES

This drug combination is used to relieve the coughing and congestion of allergy and the common cold.

Phenylephrine and phenylpropanolamine belong to a group of drugs known as adrenergic agents (decongestants). They act by constricting (narrowing) blood vessels in the nasal passages, thereby reducing swelling and congestion.

Brompheniramine belongs to a group of drugs known as antihistamines, which are used to relieve or prevent symptoms of allergy. Antihistamines block the actions of histamine, which is a chemical released by the body during an allergic reaction.

Guaifenesin is an expectorant, a drug that loosens bronchial secretions.

TREATMENT

In order to avoid stomach upset, you can take phenylephrine, phenylpropanolamine, brompheniramine, and guaifenesin combination with food or with a full glass of milk or water (unless your doctor directs you to do otherwise).

The expectorant should be measured carefully with a specially designed 5-ml measuring spoon. An ordinary kitchen teaspoon is not accurate enough.

If you miss a dose of this medication, take the missed dose as soon as possible, unless it is almost time for your next dose. In that case, do not take the missed dose at all; just return to your regular dosing schedule. Do not double the next dose.

SIDE EFFECTS

Minor. Anxiety; blurred vision; constipation; diarrhea; dizziness; drowsiness; dry mouth, nose, and throat; heartburn; insomnia; irritability; loss of appetite; nasal congestion; nausea; restlessness; reduced sweating; vomiting; or weakness. These side effects should disappear as your body adjusts to the medication.

This medication can increase your sensitivity to sunlight. Avoid prolonged exposure to sunlight and sunlamps, wear protective clothing, and use an effective sunscreen.

If you are constipated, increase the amount of fiber in your diet (fresh fruits and vegetables, salads, bran, and whole-grain breads), exercise, and drink more water (unless your doctor directs you to do otherwise).

Chew sugarless gum or suck on ice chips or a piece of hard candy to reduce mouth dryness.

If you feel dizzy or light-headed, sit or lie down for a while; get up slowly from a sitting or reclining position, and be careful on stairs.

In order to avoid difficulty in falling asleep, take the last dose of this medication several hours before bedtime.

Major. Tell your doctor about any side effects that are persistent or particularly bothersome. IT IS ESPECIALLY IMPORTANT TO TELL YOUR DOCTOR about chest pain, confusion, convulsions, difficult or painful urination, difficulty in breathing, fainting, hallucinations, headaches, loss of coordination, mood changes, nosebleeds, palpitations, rash, severe abdominal pain, sore throat, or unusual bleeding or bruising.

INTERACTIONS

This medication interacts with several other drugs:

1. Concurrent use of it with central nervous system depressants (such as alcohol, barbiturates, benzodiazepine tranquilizers, muscle relaxants, narcotics, pain medications, and phenothiazine tranquilizers) or with tricyclic antidepressants can cause extreme drowsiness.

2. Monoamine oxidase (MAO) inhibitors (isocarboxazid, pargyline, phenelzine, or tranylcypromine and tricyclic antidepressants can increase the side effects of this medication. At least 14 days should separate the use of this drug and the use of an MAO inhibitor.

3. The side effects of the antihistamine part of this medication may be increased by quinidine, procainamide, haloperidol, and phenothiazine tranquilizers, and the side effects of the decongestant component can be increased by digoxin or over-the-counter (nonprescription) diet, allergy, asthma, cough, cold, or sinus preparations.

4. The blood-pressure-lowering effects of guanethidine may be decreased by phenylephrine, phenylpropanolamine, brompheniramine, and guaifenesin combination.

BE SURE TO TELL YOUR DOCTOR about any medications you are currently taking, especially those listed above.

WARNINGS

• Tell your doctor about unusual or allergic reactions you have had to any medications, especially to brompheniramine or other antihistamines (such as azatadine, chlorpheniramine, carbinoxamine, clemastine, cyproheptadine, dexchlorpheniramine, dimenhydrinate, diphenhydramine, diphenylpyraline, doxylamine, hydroxyzine, promethazine, pyrilamine, trimeprazine, tripelennamine, and triprolidine); to phenylpropanolamine,

phenylephrine, or other adrenergic agents (such as albuterol, amphetamines, ephedrine, epinephrine, isoproterenol, metaproterenol, norepinephrine, pseudoephedrine, and terbutaline); or to guaifenesin.

• Tell your doctor if you now have or if you have ever had diabetes mellitus, epilepsy, glaucoma, heart or blood vessel disease, hiatal hernia, high blood pressure, myasthenia gravis, obstructed bladder or intestinal tract, peptic ulcers, enlarged prostate gland, or thyroid disease.

• Because phenylephrine, phenylpropanolamine, brompheniramine, and guaifenesin combination can reduce sweating and heat release from the body, you should avoid excessive work and exercise in hot weather, and do not take hot baths, showers, and saunas.

• While you are taking this drug, drink at least eight glasses of water a day to help loosen bronchial secretions.

• This medication can cause drowsiness. Exercise caution when performing tasks that require alertness.

• Be sure to tell your doctor if you are pregnant. The effects of this medication during pregnancy have not been thoroughly studied in humans. Also, tell your doctor if you are breast-feeding an infant. Small amounts of this medication pass into breast milk and may cause unusual excitement or irritability in nursing infants.

phenylephrine, promethazine, and codeine combination

BRAND NAMES (Manufacturers)
Phenazine VC with Codeine (Halsey)
Phenergan VC with Codeine (Wyeth-Ayerst)
Prometh VC with codeine (various manufacturers)
TYPE OF DRUG
Adrenergic (decongestant), antihistamine, and cough suppressant combination
INGREDIENTS
phenylephrine, promethazine, and codeine
DOSAGE FORM
Oral syrup (5 mg phenylephrine, 6.25 mg promethazine, and 10 mg codeine per 5-ml spoonful, with 7% alcohol)
STORAGE
Phenylephrine, promethazine, and codeine combination should be stored at room temperature (never frozen) in a tightly closed, light-resistant container.

USES

This combination medication is used to provide symptomatic relief of coughs due to colds, minor upper respiratory tract infections, and allergy.

Phenylephrine belongs to a group of drugs known as adrenergic agents (decongestants), which constrict blood vessels in the nasal passages to reduce swelling and congestion.

Promethazine belongs to a group of drugs known as antihistamines, which block the actions of histamine, a chemical released by the body during an allergic reaction. It is used to relieve or prevent symptoms of allergy.

Codeine is a narcotic cough suppressant that acts on the cough reflex center in the brain.

TREATMENT

To avoid stomach upset, take this medication with food, milk, or water (unless your doctor directs otherwise).

The oral syrup should be shaken well just before measuring each dose. The contents tend to settle on the bottom of the bottle, so it is necessary to shake the container to distribute the ingredients evenly and equalize the doses. Each dose should then be measured carefully with a specially designed 5-ml measuring spoon.

If you miss a dose of this medication, take the missed dose as soon as possible, unless it is almost time for your next dose. In that case, do not take the missed dose at all; just return to your regular dosing schedule. Do not double the next dose.

SIDE EFFECTS

Minor. Blurred vision, constipation, diarrhea, dizziness, dry mouth, heartburn, insomnia, loss of appetite, confusion, nasal congestion, nausea, nervousness, rash, restlessness, sweating, vomiting, or weakness. These side effects should disappear as your body adjusts to the medication.

This medication can cause increased sensitivity to sunlight. It is, therefore, important to avoid prolonged exposure to sunlight and sunlamps. Wear protective clothing, and use an effective sunscreen.

If you are constipated, increase the amount of fiber in your diet (fresh fruits and vegetables, salads, bran, and whole-grain breads), exercise, and drink more water (unless your doctor directs you to do otherwise).

Chew sugarless gum or suck on ice chips or a piece of hard candy to reduce mouth dryness.

If you feel dizzy or light-headed, sit or lie down for a while; get up slowly from a sitting or reclining position, and be careful on stairs.

In order to avoid difficulty in falling asleep, check with your doctor to see if you can take the last dose of this medication several hours before bedtime each day.

Major. Tell your doctor about any side effects that are persistent or particularly bothersome. IT IS ESPECIALLY IMPORTANT TO TELL YOUR DOCTOR about convulsions, difficult or painful urination, difficulty in breathing, disturbed coordination, excitation, fainting, headaches, muscle spasms, nightmares, nosebleeds, severe abdominal pain, or sore throat or fever.

INTERACTIONS

This medication interacts with other types of drugs:
1. Concurrent use of this medication with central nervous system depressants (such as alcohol, barbiturates, benzodiazepine tranquilizers, muscle relaxants, narcotics, pain medications, and phenothiazine tranquilizers) or with tricyclic antidepressants can cause extreme drowsiness.
2. This medication can decrease the effectiveness of amphetamines, guanethidine, anticonvulsants, and levodopa.
3. The side effects of monoamine oxidase (MAO) inhibitors (isocarboxazid, pargyline, phenelzine, or tranylcypromine and tricyclic antidepressants may also be in-

creased. At least 14 days should separate the use of this drug and the use of an MAO inhibitor.

BE SURE TO TELL YOUR DOCTOR about any medications you are currently taking, especially those listed above.

WARNINGS

• Tell your doctor about unusual or allergic reactions you have had to any medications, especially to promethazine or other antihistamines (such as azatadine, brompheniramine, carbinoxamine, clemastine, cyproheptadine, chlorpheniramine, dexbrompheniramine, dimenhydrinate, diphenhydramine, diphenylpyraline, doxylamine, hydroxyzine, pyrilamine, trimeprazine, tripelennamine, and triprolidine); to phenothiazine tranquilizers, phenylephrine, or other adrenergic agents (such as albuterol, amphetamines, ephedrine, epinephrine, isoproterenol, metaproterenol, norepinephrine, pseudoephedrine, phenylpropanolamine, and terbutaline); or to codeine or any other narcotic cough suppressant or pain medication.
• Tell your doctor if you now have or if you have ever had asthma, brain disease, blockage of the urinary or digestive tract, diabetes mellitus, colitis, gallbladder disease, glaucoma, heart or blood vessel disease, high blood pressure, kidney disease, liver disease, lung disease, peptic ulcers, enlarged prostate gland, or thyroid disease.
• This medication can cause drowsiness. Your ability to perform tasks that require alertness, such as driving a car or operating potentially dangerous machinery, may be decreased. Appropriate caution should, therefore, be taken.
• Because this product contains codeine, there is a potential for abuse, so it must be used with caution. This medication usually should not be taken for longer than ten days at a time since a tolerance may develop quickly. Do not increase the dosage unless you first consult your doctor.
• Before having surgery or any other medical or dental treatment, be sure to tell your doctor or dentist that you are taking this medication.
• Be sure to tell your doctor if you are pregnant. The effects of this medication during the early stages of pregnancy have not been thoroughly studied in humans. However, regular use of codeine during the later stages of pregnancy may lead to addiction of the fetus, resulting in withdrawal symptoms (irritability, excessive crying, tremors, fever, vomiting, diarrhea, sneezing, or excessive yawning) in the newborn infant. Also, tell your doctor if you are breast-feeding an infant. Small amounts of this medication pass into breast milk and may cause unusual excitement or irritability in nursing infants.

---

phenylpropanolamine and chlorpheniramine combination

BRAND NAMES (Manufacturers)
Allerest 12-Hour* (Fisons)
Condrin-LA (Hauck)

Conex D.A.* (Forest)
Contac 12-Hour* (Smith Kline Consumer)
Dehist* (Forest)
Demazin* (Schering)
Drize (Ascher)
Dura-Vent/A (Dura)
Genamin* (Goldline)
Gencold* (Goldline)
Myminic* (My-K Labs)
Oragest T.D. (Major)
Ornade (Smith Kline & French)
phenylpropanolamine HCl and chlorpheniramine
    maleate (Cord)
Resaid S.R. (Geneva Generics)
Rhinolar-Ex 12 (McGregor)
Ru-Tuss II (Boots)
Triaminic* (Dorsey)
Triaminic-12* (Sandoz)
Trind* (Mead Johnson Nutrition)
Triphenyl (Rugby)
*Available over-the-counter (without a prescription)

TYPE OF DRUG
Adrenergic (decongestant) and antihistamine

INGREDIENTS
phenylpropanolamine and chlorpheniramine

DOSAGE FORMS
Oral tablets (25 mg or 37.5 mg phenylpropanolamine
    and 4 mg chlorpheniramine)
Sustained-release tablets (25 mg phenylpropanolamine
    and 4 mg chlorpheniramine)
Sustained-release capsules (75 mg phenylpropanolamine
    and 4 mg, 8 mg, 10 mg, or 12 mg chlorpheniramine)
Oral syrup (12. 5 mg phenylpropanolamine and 2 mg
    chlorpheniramine per 5-ml spoonful, with 5% or
    7. 5% alcohol)

STORAGE
Store this drug at room temperature in a tightly closed
container.

USES
This drug combination is used to relieve the symptoms
of upper respiratory tract infections, hay fever and other
allergies, and sinusitis (inflammation of the sinuses).

Phenylpropanolamine belongs to a group of drugs
known as adrenergic agents (decongestants). They act by
constricting (narrowing) blood vessels in the nasal passages, thereby reducing swelling and congestion.

Chlorpheniramine belongs to a group of drugs known
as antihistamines, which block the action of histamine,
a chemical released by the body during an allergic reaction. It is used to relieve or prevent symptoms of allergy.

TREATMENT
In order to avoid stomach upset, you can take phenylpropanolamine and chlorpheniramine combination with
food or with a full glass of milk or water (unless your doctor directs you to do otherwise).

The oral syrup form of this medication should be measured carefully with a specially designed 5-ml measuring spoon.

The sustained-release tablets and capsules should be
swallowed whole. Breaking, chewing, or crushing these
tablets or capsules destroys their sustained-release activity and may increase the side effects.

If you miss a dose of this medication, take the missed
dose as soon as possible, unless it is almost time for your
next dose. In that case, do not take the missed dose at
all; just return to your regular dosing schedule. Do not
double the next dose.

SIDE EFFECTS
Minor. Anxiety; blurred vision; constipation; diarrhea;
dizziness; drowsiness; dry mouth, nose, and throat; heartburn; insomnia; irritability; loss of appetite; nasal congestion; nausea; restlessness; decreased sweating; vomiting; or weakness. These side effects should disappear
as your body adjusts to the medication.

This medication can increase your sensitivity to sunlight. Avoid prolonged exposure to sunlight and sunlamps, wear protective clothing, and use a sunscreen.

If you are constipated, increase the amount of fiber in
your diet (fresh fruits and vegetables, salads, bran, and
whole-grain breads), exercise, and drink more water (unless your doctor directs you to do otherwise).

Chew sugarless gum or suck on ice chips or a piece of
hard candy to reduce mouth dryness.

If you feel dizzy, sit or lie down for a while; get up
slowly from a sitting or reclining position, and be careful on stairs.

In order to avoid difficulty in falling asleep, take the
last dose of this medication several hours before bedtime.

Major. Tell your doctor about any side effects that are
persistent or particularly bothersome. IT IS ESPECIALLY
IMPORTANT TO TELL YOUR DOCTOR about chest
pain, convulsions, difficult or painful urination, difficulty
in breathing, fainting, hallucinations, headaches, loss of
coordination, confusion, mood changes, nosebleeds, palpitations, rash, severe abdominal pain, sore throat, or unusual bleeding or bruising.

INTERACTIONS
This drug interacts with several other types of drugs:
1. Concurrent use of it with central nervous system depressants (such as alcohol, barbiturates, benzodiazepine
tranquilizers, muscle relaxants, narcotics, pain medications, and phenothiazine tranquilizers) or with tricyclic
antidepressants can cause extreme drowsiness.
2. Monoamine oxidase (MAO) inhibitors (isocarboxazid,
pargyline, phenelzine, or tranylcypromine and tricyclic
antidepressants can increase the side effects of this medication. At least 14 days should separate the use of this
drug and the use of an MAO inhibitor.
3. The side effects of the antihistamine part of this medication may be increased by quinidine, procainamide,
haloperidol, and phenothiazine tranquilizers; and the
side effects of the decongestant component may be increased by digoxin or over-the-counter (nonprescription)
diet, allergy, asthma, cough, cold, or sinus preparations.
4. The blood-pressure-lowering effects of guanethidine
may be decreased by this medication.

BE SURE TO TELL YOUR DOCTOR about any medications you are currently taking, especially any listed
above.

WARNINGS
• Tell your doctor about unusual or allergic reactions you have had to any medications, especially to chlorpheniramine or other antihistamines (such as azatadine, brompheniramine, carbinoxamine, clemastine, cyproheptadine, dexchlorpheniramine, dimenhydrinate, diphenhydramine, diphenylpyraline, doxylamine, hydroxyzine, promethazine, pyrilamine, trimeprazine, tripelennamine, and triprolidine) or to phenylpropanolamine or other adrenergic agents (such as albuterol, amphetamines, ephedrine, epinephrine, isoproterenol, metaproterenol, norepinephrine, pseudoephedrine, and terbutaline).
• Tell your doctor if you now have or if you have ever had diabetes mellitus, epilepsy, glaucoma, heart or blood vessel disease, hiatal hernia, high blood pressure, myasthenia gravis, obstructed bladder or intestinal tract, peptic ulcers, enlarged prostate gland, or thyroid disease.
• Because this drug can reduce sweating and heat release from the body, avoid excessive work or exercise in hot weather, and do not take hot baths, showers, or saunas.
• This medication can cause drowsiness. Exercise caution when performing tasks that require alertness, such as driving a car or operating potentially dangerous machinery. Be especially careful going up and down the stairs.
• Be sure to tell your doctor if you are pregnant. The effects of this medication during pregnancy have not been thoroughly studied in humans. Also, tell your doctor if you are breast-feeding an infant. Small amounts of this medication pass into breast milk.

phenylpropanolamine and guaifenesin combination

BRAND NAMES (Manufacturers)
Banex-LA (Lu Chem)
Dura-Vent (Dura)
Entex L.A. (Norwich-Eaton)
Guaipax (Vitarine)
Nolex LA (Carnrick)
Rymed-TR (Edwards)
Tega D&E (Ortega)
TYPE OF DRUG
Adrenergic (decongestant) and expectorant
INGREDIENTS
phenylpropanolamine and guaifenesin
DOSAGE FORM
Sustained-release tablets (75 mg phenylpropanolamine and 400 mg or 600 mg guaifenesin)
STORAGE
Phenylpropanolamine and guaifenesin combination tablets and capsules should be stored at room temperature in tightly closed containers.

USES
This drug combination is used to relieve the coughing and congestion associated with colds, sinusitis (inflammation of the sinuses), sore throat, bronchitis, and asthma.

Phenylpropanolamine belongs to a group of drugs known as adrenergic agents (decongestants). They act by constricting (narrowing) blood vessels in the nasal passages, thereby reducing swelling and congestion. Guaifenesin is an expectorant, a drug that loosens bronchial secretions.

TREATMENT
In order to avoid stomach upset, you can take phenylpropanolamine and guaifenesin combination with food or with a full glass of milk or water (unless your doctor directs you to do otherwise).

These sustained-release tablets should be swallowed whole. Breaking, chewing, or crushing them destroys their sustained-release activity and may increase side effects.

If you miss a dose of this medication, take the missed dose as soon as possible, unless it is almost time for your next dose. In that case, do not take the missed dose at all; just return to your regular dosing schedule. Do not double the next dose.

SIDE EFFECTS
Minor. Insomnia, nervousness, or restlessness. These side effects should disappear as your body adjusts to the medication.

In order to help you avoid difficulty in falling asleep, take the last dose of this medication several hours before bedtime.

Major. Tell your doctor about any side effects that are persistent or particularly bothersome. IT IS ESPECIALLY IMPORTANT TO TELL YOUR DOCTOR about fainting, headaches, nosebleeds, or palpitations.

INTERACTIONS
This drug interacts with several other medications:
1. Monoamine oxidase (MAO) inhibitors (isocarboxazid, pargyline, phenelzine, or tranylcypromine can increase the side effects of this medication. At least 14 days should separate the use of this drug and the use of an MAO inhibitor.
2. The blood-pressure-lowering effects of guanethidine may be decreased by this medication.
3. The side effects of the decongestant component of this medication can be increased by digoxin or by over-the-counter (nonprescription) allergy, asthma, cough, cold, diet, or sinus preparations.

BE SURE TO TELL YOUR DOCTOR about any medications you are currently taking, especially any listed above.

WARNINGS
• Tell your doctor about unusual or allergic reactions you have had to any medications, especially to guaifenesin or phenylpropanolamine or to other adrenergic agents (such as albuterol, amphetamines, ephedrine, epinephrine, isoproterenol, metaproterenol, norepinephrine, pseudoephedrine, and terbutaline).
• Tell your doctor if you now have or if you have ever had diabetes mellitus, glaucoma, heart or blood vessel disease, high blood pressure, enlarged prostate, or thyroid disease.

• While you are taking this drug, drink at least eight glasses of water a day to loosen bronchial secretions.
• Be sure to tell your doctor if you are pregnant or if you are breast-feeding an infant.

phenylpropanolamine HCl and chlorpheniramine maleate—see phenylpropanolamine and chlorpheniramine combination

---

phenylpropanolamine, phenylephrine, and brompheniramine combination

BRAND NAMES (Manufacturers)
Bromophen T.D. (Rugby)
brompheniramine, phenylephrine, and phenypropanolamine (Lederle)
Bromtapp Extended Tabs (Blue Cross)
Dimetapp Extentabs* (Robins)
Normatane Elixir (Vortech)
Tamine SR (Geneva Generics)
Veltap Elixir (Lannett)
*Recently reformulated Dimetapp does not contain phenylephrine and is available without a prescription.
TYPE OF DRUG
Adrenergic (decongestant) and antihistamine
INGREDIENTS
phenylpropanolamine, phenylephrine, and brompheniramine
DOSAGE FORMS
Sustained-release tablets (15 mg phenylpropanolamine, 15 mg phenylephrine, and 12 mg brompheniramine; recently reformulated Dimetapp Extentabs contain 75 mg phenylpropanolamine and 12 mg brompheniramine, but no phenylephrine)
Oral elixir (5 mg phenylpropanolamine, 5 mg phenylephrine, 4 mg brompheniramine per 5-ml spoonful, with 2.3% or 3% alcohol)
STORAGE
The tablets and oral elixir should be stored at room temperature in tightly closed, light-resistant containers. This medication should never be frozen.

USES
This drug combination is used to relieve the symptoms of upper respiratory tract infections, hay fever and other allergies, and sinusitis (inflammation of the sinuses).

Phenylpropanolamine and phenylephrine belong to a group of drugs known as adrenergic agents (decongestants). They act by constricting (narrowing) blood vessels in the nasal passages, thereby reducing swelling.

Brompheniramine belongs to a group of drugs known as antihistamines, which block the actions of histamine, a chemical released during an allergic reaction.

TREATMENT
In order to avoid stomach upset, you can take phenylpropanolamine, phenylephrine, and brompheniramine combination with food or with a full glass of milk or water (unless your doctor directs you to do otherwise).

The oral elixir form of this medication should be measured carefully with a specially designed 5-ml measuring spoon. An ordinary kitchen teaspoon is not accurate enough.

The sustained-release tablets should be swallowed whole. Breaking, chewing, or crushing these tablets destroys their sustained-release activity and may increase the side effects.

If you miss a dose of this medication, take it as soon as possible, unless it is almost time for your next dose. In that case, do not take the missed dose at all; just return to your regular dosing schedule. Do not double the next dose.

SIDE EFFECTS
Minor. Anxiety; blurred vision; constipation; diarrhea; dizziness; drowsiness; dry mouth, nose, and throat; heartburn; insomnia; irritability; loss of appetite; nasal congestion; nausea; restlessness; decreased sweating; vomiting; or weakness. These side effects should disappear as your body adjusts to the medication.

If you are constipated, increase the amount of fiber in your diet (fresh fruits and vegetables, salads, bran, and whole-grain breads), and drink more water (unless your doctor directs you to do otherwise).

This medication can increase your sensitivity to sunlight. Avoid prolonged exposure to sunlight and sunlamps, wear protective clothing, and use an effective sunscreen.

If you feel dizzy or light-headed, sit or lie down for a while; get up slowly from a sitting or reclining position, and be careful on stairs.

In order to avoid difficulty in falling asleep, take the last dose of this medication several hours before bedtime.
Major. Tell your doctor about any side effects that are persistent or particularly bothersome. IT IS ESPECIALLY IMPORTANT TO TELL YOUR DOCTOR about chest pain, confusion, convulsions, difficult or painful urination, difficulty in breathing, fainting, hallucinations, headaches, loss of coordination, mood changes, nosebleeds, palpitations, rash, severe abdominal pain, sore throat, or unusual bleeding or bruising.

INTERACTIONS
This drug interacts with several other medications:
1. Concurrent use of it with central nervous system depressants (such as alcohol, barbiturates, benzodiazepine tranquilizers, muscle relaxants, narcotics, pain medications, and phenothiazine tranquilizers) or with tricyclic antidepressants can cause extreme drowsiness.
2. Monoamine oxidase (MAO) inhibitors (isocarboxazid, pargyline, phenelzine, or tranylcypromine and tricyclic antidepressants can increase the side effects of this medication. At least 14 days should separate the use of this drug and the use of an MAO inhibitor.
3. The side effects of the antihistamine part of this medication may be increased by quinidine, procainamide, haloperidol, and phenothiazine tranquilizers; and the side effects of the decongestant component may be in-

creased by digoxin or by over-the-counter (nonprescription) allergy, asthma, cough, cold, diet, or sinus preparations.

4. The blood-pressure-lowering effects of guanethidine may be decreased by this medication.

BE SURE TO TELL YOUR DOCTOR about any medications you are currently taking, especially those listed above.

WARNINGS

• Tell your doctor about unusual or allergic reactions you have had to any medications, especially to brompheniramine, to other antihistamines (such as azatadine, chlorpheniramine, carbinoxamine, clemastine, cyproheptadine, dexchlorpheniramine, dimenhydrinate, diphenhydramine, diphenylpyraline, doxylamine, hydroxyzine, promethazine, pyrilamine, trimeprazine, tripelennamine, and triprolidine), or to phenylpropanolamine, phenylephrine, or other adrenergic agents (such as albuterol, amphetamines, ephedrine, epinephrine, isoproterenol, metaproterenol, norepinephrine, pseudoephedrine, and terbutaline).

• Tell your doctor if you now have or if you have ever had diabetes mellitus, epilepsy, glaucoma, heart or blood vessel disease, hiatal hernia, high blood pressure, myasthenia gravis, obstructed bladder or intestinal tract, peptic ulcers, enlarged prostate gland, or thyroid disease.

• Because this drug can reduce sweating and heat release from the body, avoid excessive work and exercise in hot weather, and do not take hot baths, showers, and saunas.

• This medication can cause drowsiness. Your ability to perform tasks that require alertness, such as driving a car or operating potentially dangerous machinery, may be decreased. Appropriate caution should, therefore, be taken.

• Be sure to tell your doctor if you are pregnant. Also, tell your doctor if you are breast-feeding an infant. Small amounts of this medication pass into breast milk and may cause unusual excitement or irritability in nursing infants.

---

phenylpropanolamine, phenylephrine, chlorpheniramine, and phenyltoloxamine combination

BRAND NAMES (Manufacturers)
Amaril D Spantab (Vortech)
decongestabs (various manufacturers)
Naldecon (Bristol)
naldelate (various manufacturers)
Nalgest (Major)
New-Decongest (Goldline)
Tri-Phen-Chlor (Rugby)

TYPE OF DRUG
Adrenergic (decongestant) and antihistamine

INGREDIENTS
phenylpropanolamine, phenylephrine, chlorpheniramine, and phenyltoloxamine

DOSAGE FORMS
Sustained-release tablets (40 mg phenylpropanolamine, 10 mg phenylephrine, 5 mg chlorpheniramine, and 15 mg phenyltoloxamine)

Sustained-release capsules (50 mg phenylpropanolamine, 25 mg phenylephrine, 12 mg chlorpheniramine, and 30 mg phenyltoloxamine)

Oral syrup (20 mg phenylpropanolamine, 5 mg phenylephrine, 2.5 mg chlorpheniramine, and 7.5 mg phenyltoloxamine per 5-ml spoonful)

Oral pediatric drops (5 mg phenylpropanolamine, 1.25 mg phenylephrine, 0.5 mg chlorpheniramine, and 2 mg phenyltoloxamine per ml)

STORAGE
Store at room temperature in a tightly closed container. This medication should never be frozen.

USES
This drug combination is used to relieve symptoms of upper respiratory tract infections, hay fever and other allergies, and sinusitis (inflammation of the sinuses).

Phenylpropanolamine and phenylephrine belong to a group of drugs known as adrenergic agents (decongestants). They act by constricting (narrowing) blood vessels in the nasal passages, thereby reducing swelling and congestion.

Chlorpheniramine and phenyltoloxamine belong to a group of drugs known as antihistamines, which block the actions of histamine, a chemical released by the body during an allergic reaction. They are, therefore, used to relieve or prevent the symptoms of allergy.

TREATMENT
In order to avoid stomach upset, you can take phenylpropanolamine, phenylephrine, chlorpheniramine, and phenyltoloxamine combination with food or with a full glass of milk or water (unless your doctor directs you to do otherwise).

The oral pediatric drops should be measured carefully.

The oral syrup form of this medication should be measured carefully with a specially designed 5-ml measuring spoon. An ordinary kitchen teaspoon is not accurate enough for measuring your dosage of this medication.

The sustained-release tablets and capsules should be swallowed whole. Breaking, chewing, or crushing them destroys their sustained-release activity and may increase the side effects.

If you miss a dose, take it as soon as possible, unless it is almost time for your next dose. In that case, do not take the missed dose at all; just return to your regular dosing schedule. Do not double the next dose.

SIDE EFFECTS
Minor. Anxiety; blurred vision; constipation; diarrhea; dizziness; drowsiness; dry mouth, nose, and throat; heartburn; insomnia; irritability; loss of appetite; nasal congestion; reduced sweating; restlessness; vomiting; or weakness. These side effects should disappear as your body adjusts to the medication.

This medication can increase your sensitivity to sunlight. Avoid prolonged exposure to sunlight and sunlamps, wear protective clothing, and use an effective sunscreen.

If you are constipated, increase the amount of fiber in your diet (fresh fruits and vegetables, salads, bran, and whole-grain breads), exercise, and drink more water (unless your doctor directs you to do otherwise).

If you experience dry mouth or throat, you should try chewing sugarless gum or sucking on ice chips or a piece of hard candy to reduce mouth dryness.

If you feel dizzy or light-headed, sit or lie down for a while; get up slowly from a sitting or reclining position, and be careful on stairs.

In order to avoid difficulty in falling asleep, take the last dose of this medication several hours before bedtime.

Major. Tell your doctor about any side effects that are persistent or particularly bothersome. IT IS ESPECIALLY IMPORTANT TO TELL YOUR DOCTOR about chest pain, confusion, convulsions, difficult or painful urination, difficulty in breathing, fainting, hallucinations, headaches, loss of coordination, mood changes, nosebleeds, palpitations, rash, severe abdominal pain, sore throat, or unusual bleeding or bruising.

INTERACTIONS

This medication interacts with several other types of drugs:

1. Concurrent use of this medication with central nervous system depressants (such as alcohol, barbiturates, benzodiazepine tranquilizers, muscle relaxants, narcotics, pain medications, and phenothiazine tranquilizers) or with tricyclic antidepressants can cause extreme drowsiness.

2. Monoamine oxidase (MAO) inhibitors (isocarboxazid, pargyline, phenelzine, or tranylcypromine and tricyclic antidepressants can increase the side effects of this medication. At least 14 days should separate the use of this drug and the use of an MAO inhibitor.

3. The side effects of the antihistamine part of this medication may be increased by quinidine, procainamide, haloperidol, and phenothiazine tranquilizers; and the side effects of the decongestant component may be increased by digoxin or by over-the-counter (nonprescription) allergy, asthma, cough, cold, diet, or sinus preparations.

4. The blood-pressure-lowering effects of guanethidine may be decreased by this medication.

BE SURE TO TELL YOUR DOCTOR about any medications you are currently taking, especially any listed above.

WARNINGS

• Tell your doctor about unusual or allergic reactions you have had to any medications, especially to chlorpheniramine, phenyltoloxamine, or any other antihistamine (such as azatadine, brompheniramine, carbinoxamine, clemastine, cyproheptadine, dexchlorpheniramine, dimenhydrinate, diphenhydramine, diphenylpyraline, doxylamine, hydroxyzine, promethazine, pyrilamine, trimeprazine, tripelennamine, and triprolidine), or to phenylpropanolamine, phenylephrine, or any other adrenergic agent (such as albuterol, amphetamines, ephedrine, epinephrine, isoproterenol, metaproterenol, norepinephrine, pseudoephedrine, and terbutaline).

• Tell your doctor if you now have or if you have ever had diabetes mellitus, epilepsy, glaucoma, heart or blood vessel disease, hiatal hernia, high blood pressure, myasthenia gravis, obstructed bladder or intestinal tract, peptic ulcers, enlarged prostate gland, or thyroid disease.

• Because this drug can reduce sweating and heat release from the body, you should avoid excessive work or exercise in hot weather and you should not take hot baths, showers, and saunas while taking this medication.

• This medication can cause drowsiness. Your ability to perform tasks that require alertness, such as driving a car or operating potentially dangerous machinery, may be decreased. Appropriate caution should, therefore, be taken.

• Be sure to tell your doctor if you are pregnant. The effects of this medication during pregnancy have not been thoroughly studied in humans. Also, tell your doctor if you are breast-feeding an infant. Small amounts of this medication pass into breast milk and may cause unusual excitement or irritability in nursing infants.

phenytoin

BRAND NAMES (Manufacturers)
Dilantin (Parke-Davis)
Dilantin Infatab (Parke-Davis)
Dilantin Kapseal (Parke-Davis)
Diphenylan (Lannett)
phenytoin (various manufacturers)

TYPE OF DRUG
Anticonvulsant

INGREDIENT
phenytoin

DOSAGE FORMS
Capsules (30 mg and 100 mg)
Chewable tablets (50 mg)
Oral suspension (30 mg and 125 mg per 5-ml spoonful, with 0.6% alcohol)

STORAGE
Phenytoin capsules, tablets, and oral suspension should be stored at room temperature in tightly closed, light-resistant containers. This medication should never be frozen.

USES

Phenytoin is used to control certain types of convulsions, or seizures. It is not clear exactly how phenytoin works to control convulsions, but it appears to prevent the spread of seizure activity in the brain. Phenytoin may also be used to treat other conditions as determined by your physician.

TREATMENT

To avoid stomach irritation and increase this drug's absorption, take phenytoin with food or with a full glass of water or milk (unless your doctor directs you to do otherwise).

The tablet form of this medication should be chewed before swallowing.

The suspension form of this medication should be shaken well just before measuring each dose. The contents tend to settle on the bottom of the bottle, so it is necessary to shake the container to distribute the ingredients evenly and equalize the doses. Each dose should then be measured carefully with a specially designed 5-ml measuring spoon.

Phenytoin works best when the level of medicine in your bloodstream is kept constant. It is best, therefore, to take the doses at evenly spaced intervals day and night. For example, if you are taking three doses a day, the doses should be spaced eight hours apart.

If you miss a dose of this medication, take the missed dose as soon as possible, unless it is almost time for the next dose. In that case, do not take the missed dose at all; just return to your regular dosing schedule. Do not double the next dose. If you miss two or more doses in a row, contact your doctor.

SIDE EFFECTS

Minor. Constipation, drowsiness (mild), headache, insomnia, nausea, or vomiting. These side effects should disappear as your body adjusts to the medication.

To relieve constipation, increase the amount of fiber in your diet (fresh fruits and vegetables, salads, bran, and whole-grain breads), exercise, and drink more water (unless your doctor directs you to do otherwise).

Major. Tell your doctor about any side effects that are persistent or particularly bothersome. IT IS ESPECIALLY IMPORTANT TO TELL YOUR DOCTOR about blurred vision, chest pain, confusion, dizziness, change in facial features, gum enlargement, increased hair growth, joint pain, muscle twitching, nervousness, numbness, rash, slurred speech, sore throat, swollen glands, uncoordinated movements, unusual bleeding or bruising, change in the color of your urine, or yellowing of the eyes or skin.

INTERACTIONS

Phenytoin interacts with a number of other types of drugs:
1. The effectiveness of phenytoin can be decreased by concurrent use of alcohol, barbiturates, folic acid, tricyclic anti-depressants, reserpine, molindone, benzodiazepine tranquilizers, chloral hydrate, rifampin, phenothiazine tranquilizers, and haloperidol.
2. Phenytoin can decrease the effectiveness of calcifediol, warfarin, quinidine, disopyramide, dexamethasone, doxycycline, levodopa, and oral contraceptives.
3. The active blood levels and side effects of phenytoin can be increased by chloramphenicol, cimetidine, warfarin, disulfiram, isoniazid, oxyphenbutazone, phenylbutazone, ibuprofen, amiodarone, trimethoprim, sulfonamide antibiotics, tolbutamide, chlordiazepoxide, chlorpromazine, diazepam, estrogens, ethosuximide, methylphenidate, and prochlorperazine.
4. Valproic acid can either increase or decrease the effects of phenytoin.
5. The dosage of oral antidiabetic medications may need to be adjusted when phenytoin is started.
6. Phenytoin may decrease the absorption of furosemide from the gastrointestinal tract, decreasing its effectiveness.

7. Antacids, calcium, oxacillin, sucralfate, medicines for diarrhea, and antineoplastics (anticancer drugs) may decrease the gastrointestinal absorption and effectiveness of phenytoin. Do not take phenytoin within two to three hours of taking an antacid or antidiarrheal.

Before starting to take phenytoin, BE SURE TO TELL YOUR DOCTOR about any medications you are currently taking, especially any of those listed above.

WARNINGS

• Tell your doctor about unusual or allergic reactions you have had to any medications, especially to phenytoin, ethotoin, or mephenytoin.
• Before starting to take this medication, be sure to tell your doctor if you now have or if you have ever had blood disorders, diabetes mellitus, or liver disease.
• If this drug makes you dizzy or drowsy, do not take part in any activity that requires alertness, such as driving a car or operating potentially dangerous machinery. Children should be careful while playing.
• Before surgery or other medical or dental treatment, tell your doctor or dentist you are taking phenytoin.
• Do not stop taking this medication unless you first consult your doctor. If this drug is stopped abruptly, you may experience uncontrollable seizures. Your doctor may, therefore, want to reduce your dosage gradually. Be sure you have enough on hand for holidays and vacations.
• Although several generic versions of this drug are available, you should not switch from one brand to another without your doctor's careful assessment and complete approval. If you have your medication refilled and it looks different, be sure to consult with your pharmacist.
• Therapy with phenytoin may cause your gums to enlarge enough to cover your teeth. This can be minimized, at least partially, by frequent brushing and massaging of the gums with the rubber tip of a good toothbrush.
• Be sure to tell your doctor if you are pregnant. Birth defects have been reported more often in infants whose mothers have seizure disorders. It is unclear if the increased risk of birth defects is associated with the seizure disorders or with the anticonvulsant medications, such as phenytoin, that are used to treat them. Discuss this with your doctor. Also, tell your doctor if you are breast-feeding an infant.

Pherazine with Codeine—see promethazine and codeine combination

Phyllocontin—see aminophylline

Pilocar—see pilocarpine (ophthalmic)

pilocarpine (ophthalmic)

BRAND NAMES (Manufacturers)
Adsorbocarpine (Alcon)
Akarpine (Akorn)
Isopto Carpine (Alcon)
Ocusert Pilo-20 (Alza)
Ocusert Pilo-40 (Alza)

Pilocar (Iolab Pharm.)
pilocarpine hydrochloride (various manufacturers)
TYPE OF DRUG
Antiglaucoma ophthalmic solution
INGREDIENT
pilocarpine
DOSAGE FORMS
Ophthalmic drops (0.25%, 0.5%, 1%, 2%, 3%, 4%, 5%, 6%, 8%, and 10%)
Ocular therapeutic system (oval ring of plastic that contains pilocarpine. The ring is placed in the eye, and the drug is released gradually over a period of seven days.)
STORAGE
Pilocarpine eye drops should be stored at room temperature in a tightly closed container. This medication should never be frozen. If it discolors or turns brown, it should be discarded. A color change signifies a loss of potency.

The ocular therapeutic system form of this medication should be stored in the refrigerator in its original container.

USES
Pilocarpine (ophthalmic) is used to reduce the increased pressure in the eye caused by glaucoma or other eye conditions. When pilocarpine is applied to the eye, it constricts the pupil and increases the flow of fluid (aqueous humor) out of the eye, thereby reducing the pressure.

TREATMENT
Wash your hands with soap and water before applying this medication. In order to avoid contamination of the eye drops, be careful not to touch the tube portion of the dropper or let it touch your eye; DO NOT wipe off or rinse the dropper after you use it.

To apply the eye drops, tilt your head back and pull down your lower eyelid with one hand to make a pouch below the eye. Drop the prescribed amount of medicine into this pouch and slowly close your eyes. Try not to blink. Keep your eyes closed, and place one finger at the corner of the eye next to your nose for a minute or two, applying a slight pressure (to prevent loss of medication through the duct that drains fluid from the surface of the eye into the nose and throat). Wipe away any excess with a clean tissue. If you think the medicine did not get into the eye, repeat the process once. Since the drops are somewhat difficult to apply, you may want someone to apply them for you.

If more than one type of eye drop has been prescribed, wait at least five minutes after instilling pilocarpine before using any other eye medicine (this is done in order to give the pilocarpine a chance to work).

The ocular therapeutic system comes packaged with detailed instructions for insertion and removal. Follow these directions carefully. Damaged or deformed ocular therapeutic systems should not be placed or retained in the eye. Use a new system instead.

If you miss a dose of this medication, apply the missed dose as soon as possible, unless it is almost time for the next dose. In that case, do not apply the missed dose at all; just return to your regular dosing schedule. Do not double the next dose.

SIDE EFFECTS
Minor. Blurred vision, browache, headache, or twitching of the eyelids. These side effects should disappear as your body adjusts to the medication.
Major. Tell your doctor about any side effects that are persistent or particularly bothersome. IT IS ESPECIALLY IMPORTANT TO TELL YOUR DOCTOR about diarrhea, difficult or painful urination, flushing, muscle tremors, nausea, nearsightedness, palpitations, shortness of breath, stomach cramps, or sweating.

INTERACTIONS
This medication should not interact with other drugs as long as it is applied according to directions.

WARNINGS
• Tell your doctor about unusual or allergic reactions you have had to any medications, especially to pilocarpine.
• Tell your doctor if you now have or if you have ever had asthma, epilepsy, heart disease, peptic ulcers, thyroid disease, Parkinson's disease, or blockage of the urinary tract.
• This drug can cause difficulty in adjusting to low light levels. Caution should be exercised during night driving and while performing hazardous tasks in poor light.
• Be sure to tell your doctor if you are pregnant. The effects of this drug during pregnancy have not been thoroughly studied in humans, but small amounts of pilocarpine may be absorbed into the bloodstream. Also, tell your doctor if you are breast-feeding an infant.

pilocarpine hydrochloride—see pilocarpine (ophthalmic)

pindolol

BRAND NAME (Manufacturer)
Visken (Sandoz)
TYPE OF DRUG
Beta-adrenergic blocking agent
INGREDIENT
pindolol
DOSAGE FORM
Tablets (5 mg and 10 mg)
STORAGE
Pindolol should be stored at room temperature in a tightly closed, light-resistant container.

USES
Pindolol is used to treat high blood pressure. It belongs to a group of medicines known as beta-adrenergic blocking agents or, more commonly, beta blockers. These drugs work by controlling nerve impulses along certain nerve pathways.

TREATMENT
This medicine can be taken with a glass of water, with meals, immediately following meals, or on an empty stomach (depending on your doctor's instructions). Try to take the medication at the same time(s) each day.

Try not to miss any doses of this medicine. If you do miss a dose, take the missed dose as soon as possible, unless it is within eight hours (if you are taking this medicine once a day) or within four hours (if you are taking this medicine more than once a day) of your next scheduled dose. In that case, do not take the missed dose at all; just return to your regular dosing schedule. Do not double the next dose.

Pindolol does not cure high blood pressure, but it will help to control the condition as long as you take it.

SIDE EFFECTS

Minor. Anxiety; constipation; decreased sexual ability; diarrhea; difficulty in sleeping; drowsiness; dryness of the eyes, mouth, and skin; headache; nausea; tiredness; or weakness. These effects should disappear as you adjust to the drug.

To relieve constipation, increase the amount of fiber in your diet (fresh fruits and vegetables, salads, bran, and whole-grain breads) unless your doctor directs you to do otherwise.

If you are extra-sensitive to the cold, be sure to dress warmly during cold weather.

Plain, nonmedicated eye drops (artificial tears) may help to relieve eye dryness.

Sucking on ice chips or chewing sugarless gum helps to relieve mouth or throat dryness.

Major. Tell your doctor about any side effects that are persistent or bothersome. IT IS ESPECIALLY IMPORTANT TO TELL YOUR DOCTOR about cold hands or feet (due to decreased blood circulation to skin, fingers, and toes), confusion, dizziness, fever and sore throat, hair loss, hallucinations, light-headedness, mental depression, nightmares, numbness or tingling of the fingers or toes, rapid weight gain (three to five pounds within a week), reduced alertness, skin rash, swelling, unusual bleeding or bruising, or wheezing or difficulty in breathing.

INTERACTIONS

Pindolol interacts with a number of other types of drugs:
1. Indomethacin, aspirin, or other salicylates may decrease the blood-pressure-lowering effects of the beta blockers.
2. Concurrent use of beta blockers and calcium channel blockers (diltiazem, nifedipine, or verapamil) or disopyramide can lead to heart failure or very low blood pressure.
3. Cimetidine and oral contraceptives (birth control pills) can increase the blood concentrations of pindolol, which can result in greater side effects.
4. Side effects may also be increased when beta blockers are taken with clonidine, digoxin, epinephrine, phenylephrine, phenylpropanolamine, phenothiazine tranquilizers, prazosin, or monoamine oxidase (MAO) inhibitors. At least 14 days should separate use of a beta blocker and the use of an MAO inhibitor.
5. Beta blockers may antagonize (work against) the effects of theophylline, aminophylline, albuterol, isoproterenol, metaproterenol, and terbutaline.
6. Beta blockers can also interact with insulin or oral antidiabetic agents, raising or lowering blood sugar levels or masking the symptoms of low blood sugar.
7. The concurrent use of pindolol and reserpine can have additive blood-pressure-lowering effects.
8. The action of beta blockers may be increased if they are used with chlorpromazine, furosemide, or hydralazine.
9. Alcohol, barbiturates, and rifampin can decrease the blood concentrations of pindolol, which can result in a decrease in effectiveness.

BE SURE TO TELL YOUR DOCTOR about any medications you are currently taking, especially any listed above.

WARNINGS

• Before starting to take this drug, it is important to tell your doctor if you have ever had unusual or allergic reactions to any beta-blocking medication (acebutolol, atenolol, betaxolol, carteolol, esmolol, labetalol, metoprolol, nadolol, penbutolol, propranolol, or timolol).
• Tell your doctor if you now have or if you have ever had allergies, asthma, hay fever, eczema, slow heartbeat, bronchitis, diabetes mellitus, emphysema, heart or blood vessel disease, kidney disease, liver disease, thyroid disease, or poor circulation in the fingers or toes.
• You may want to check your pulse while taking this medication. If your pulse is much slower than your usual rate (or if it is less than 50 beats per minute), check with your doctor. A pulse rate that is too slow may cause circulation problems.
• This medicine may affect your body's response to exercise. Make sure you discuss with your doctor a safe amount of exercise for your medical condition.
• It is important that you do not stop taking this medicine unless you first check with your doctor. Some conditions may become worse when the medicine is stopped suddenly, and the danger of a heart attack is increased in some patients. Your doctor may want you to reduce gradually the amount of medicine you take before stopping completely. Make sure that you have enough medicine on hand to last through vacations, holidays, and weekends.
• Before having surgery or any other medical or dental treatment, tell your physician or dentist that you are taking pindolol. Often, this medication will be discontinued 48 hours prior to any major surgery.
• Pindolol can cause dizziness, drowsiness, light-headedness, or decreased alertness. Exercise caution while driving a car or using potentially dangerous machinery.
• While taking this medicine, do not use any over-the-counter (nonprescription) allergy, asthma, cough, cold, sinus, or diet preparations unless you first check with your pharmacist or doctor. Some of these medicines can result in high blood pressure if taken in conjunction with a beta blocker.
• Be sure to tell your doctor if you are pregnant. Animal studies have shown that some beta blockers can cause problems in pregnancy when used at very high doses. Adequate studies have not been conducted in humans, but there has been some association between beta blockers used during pregnancy and low birth weight, as well as breathing problems and slow heart rate in newborn infants. However, other reports have shown no effects on newborn infants. Also, tell your doctor if you are breast-feeding. Although pindolol has not been shown

to cause problems in breast-fed infants, some of the medicine may pass into breast milk.

---

piroxicam

BRAND NAME (Manufacturer)
Feldene (Pfizer)
TYPE OF DRUG
Nonsteroidal anti-inflammatory analgesic
INGREDIENT
piroxicam
DOSAGE FORM
Capsules (10 mg and 20 mg)
STORAGE
Store in a tightly closed container at room temperature away from heat and direct sunlight.

USES
Piroxicam is used to treat the inflammation (pain, swelling, and stiffness) of certain types of arthritis, gout, bursitis, and tendinitis. Piroxicam blocks the production of certain body chemicals, called prostaglandins, that may trigger pain. However, it is not fully understood how piroxicam works.

TREATMENT
You should take this medication on an empty stomach 30 to 60 minutes before meals or two hours after meals, so that it gets into your bloodstream quickly. To decrease stomach irritation, your doctor may want you to take the medicine with food or antacids.

It is important to take piroxicam on schedule and not to miss any doses. If you do miss a dose, take the missed dose as soon as possible. However, if you are taking this drug once a day and are six hours late OR if you take this drug twice a day and are two hours late, do not take the missed dose at all; just return to your regular dosing schedule. Do not double the next dose.

If you are taking piroxicam to relieve arthritis, you must take it regularly, as directed by your doctor. It may take up to three months before you feel the full benefits of this medication. Piroxicam does not cure arthritis, but it will help to control the condition as long as you continue to take it.

SIDE EFFECTS
Minor. Abdominal bloating, constipation, difficulty in sleeping, dizziness, drowsiness, headache, heartburn, indigestion, light-headedness, loss of appetite, nausea, nervousness, soreness of the mouth, unusual sweating, or vomiting. As your body adjusts to the drug, these should disappear.

To relieve constipation, increase the amount of fiber in your diet (fresh fruits and vegetables, salads, bran, and whole-grain breads), exercise, and drink more water (unless your doctor directs you to do otherwise).

If you become dizzy, sit or lie down; get up slowly from a sitting or reclining position, and be careful on stairs.
Major. Tell your doctor about any side effects that are persistent or particularly bothersome. IT IS ESPECIALLY

IMPORTANT TO TELL YOUR DOCTOR about bloody or black, tarry stools; blurred vision; confusion; depression; difficult or painful urination; a problem with hearing; palpitations; ringing or buzzing in the ears; skin rash, hives, or itching; stomach pain; swelling of the feet; tightness in the chest; unexplained sore throat and fever; unusual bleeding or bruising; unusual fatigue or weakness; unusual weight gain; wheezing or difficulty in breathing; or yellowing of the eyes or skin.

INTERACTIONS
Piroxicam interacts with several types of medications:
1. Anticoagulants (blood thinners, such as warfarin) can lead to an increase in bleeding complications.
2. Aspirin, salicylates, or other anti-inflammatory medications can increase stomach irritation.
3. Probenecid may increase blood levels of piroxicam, which may increase the risks of side effects.
4. The action of beta blockers may be decreased by this drug.
5. This drug may interact with diuretics (water pills).

BE SURE TO TELL YOUR DOCTOR about any medications you are currently taking, especially any listed above.

WARNINGS
• Before you take this drug, tell your doctor if you have ever had unusual or allergic reactions to piroxicam or any of the other chemically related drugs (including aspirin or other salicylates, diclofenac, diflunisal, fenoprofen, flurbiprofen, ibuprofen, indomethacin, ketoprofen, meclofenamate, mefenamic acid, naproxen, oxyphenbutazone, phenylbutazone, sulindac, and tolmetin).
• Tell your doctor if you have ever had asthma, bleeding problems, colitis, epilepsy, heart disease, high blood pressure, kidney disease, liver disease, mental illness, Parkinson's disease, or stomach ulcers or other stomach problems.
• If this drug makes you dizzy or drowsy, do not take part in any activity that requires alertness, such as driving a car or operating potentially dangerous machinery.
• This drug can prolong bleeding time. Therefore, before having surgery or any other medical or dental treatment, it is important for you to tell your doctor or dentist that you are taking this medication.
• Stomach problems are more likely to occur if you take aspirin regularly or drink alcohol while being treated with this medication. Aspirin and alcohol should, therefore, be avoided (unless your doctor directs you to do otherwise).
• Be sure to tell your doctor if you are pregnant. Although studies in humans have not been conducted, unwanted cardiac (heart) side effects have been observed in the offspring of animals that received this type of drug during pregnancy. If taken late in pregnancy, it can also prolong labor. Also, tell your doctor if you are breast-feeding an infant. Small amounts of piroxicam can pass into breast milk.

Plegine—see phendimetrazine

Poladex—see dexchlorpheniramine

Polaramine—see dexchlorpheniramine

Polaramine Repetabs—see dexchlorpheniramine

Polycillin—see ampicillin

Polymox—see amoxicillin

Poly-Vi-Flor—see vitamins, multiple, with fluoride

Polyvitamins with Fluoride Drops—see vitamins, multiple, with fluoride

Polyvite with Fluoride Drops—see vitamins, multiple, with fluoride

Pondimin—see fenfluramine

Ponstel—see mefenamic acid

Potachlor—see potassium chloride

Potasalan—see potassium chloride

potassium chloride

BRAND NAMES (Manufacturers)
Cena-K (Century)
Kaochlor (Adria)
Kaon (Adria)
Kato (ICN)
Kay Ciel (Forest)
K-Dur (Key)
K-Lor (Abbott)
Klorvess (Sandoz)
Klotrix (Mead Johnson)
K-Lyte/Cl (Mead Johnson)
Kolyum (Pennwalt)
K-Tab (Abbott)
Micro-K (Robins)
Micro-K Extencaps (Robins)
Potachlor (Bay Labs)
Potasalan (Lannett)
potassium chloride (various manufacturers)
Rum-K (Fleming)
Slow-K (Ciba)
TYPE OF DRUG
Potassium replacement
INGREDIENT
potassium chloride
DOSAGE FORMS
Effervescent tablets (20 mEq, 25 mEq, and 50 mEq)
Sustained-release tablets (6.7 mEq, 8 mEq, 10 mEq, and 20 mEq)
Enteric-coated tablets (4 mEq and 13 mEq)
Sustained-release capsules (8 mEq and 10 mEq)
Oral liquid (10 mEq, 15 mEq, 20 mEq, 30 mEq, and 40 mEq per 15-ml spoonful, with alcohol varying from 0% to 5%)
Oral powder (15 mEq, 20 mEq, and 25 mEq per packet)

STORAGE
Store at room temperature in a tightly closed container.

USES
This medication is used to prevent or treat potassium deficiency, especially potassium deficiency that is caused by the use of diuretics (water pills).

TREATMENT
To avoid stomach irritation, take this drug with food or immediately after a meal. Take it at the same time(s) each day.

Each dose of the liquid form of this medication should be measured carefully with a specially designed measuring spoon. An ordinary teaspoon is not accurate enough.

If you are taking the liquid, powder, or effervescent tablet form dilute each dose in at least four ounces ($^1/_2$ cup) of cold water or juice. Be sure the medication has dissolved completely and has stopped fizzing before you drink it. Then sip it slowly. DO NOT use tomato juice to dissolve this medication (unless your doctor directs you to do so). Tomato juice contains a great deal of sodium.

The sustained-release tablets and capsules should be swallowed whole. Chewing, crushing, or breaking these tablets or capsules destroys their sustained-release activity and possibly increases the side effects.

If you miss a dose of this medication, take the missed dose as soon as possible, unless it is within two hours of the next scheduled dose. In that case, do not take the missed dose at all; just return to your regular dosing schedule. Do not double the next dose.

SIDE EFFECTS
Minor. Diarrhea, nausea, stomach pains, or vomiting. These should disappear as your body adjusts to the medicine.
Major. Tell your doctor about any side effects that are persistent or particularly bothersome. IT IS ESPECIALLY IMPORTANT TO TELL YOUR DOCTOR about anxiety; bloody or black, tarry stools; confusion; difficulty in breathing; numbness or tingling in the arms, legs, or feet; palpitations; severe abdominal pain; or unusual weakness.

INTERACTIONS
This drug interacts with several other types of drugs:
1. The combination of potassium chloride with amiloride, spironolactone, or triamterene can lead to hyperkalemia (high levels of potassium in the bloodstream).
2. The combination of digoxin and high doses of potassium chloride can lead to heart problems.

Before starting to take potassium chloride, BE SURE TO TELL YOUR DOCTOR about any medications you are currently taking, especially any of those listed above.

WARNINGS
• Tell your doctor about unusual or allergic reactions you have had to any medications, especially to potassium.
• Before starting to take this medication, be sure to tell your doctor if you now have or if you have ever had

Addison's disease, dehydration, heart disease, heat cramps, hyperkalemia, intestinal blockage, kidney disease, myotonia congenita, or peptic ulcers.
• Ask your doctor about using a salt substitute instead of potassium chloride; salt substitutes are similar, but less expensive and more convenient. However, salt substitutes should only be used with your doctor's approval. Too much potassium can be dangerous.
• If you are taking the sustained-release tablets and you find something that looks like a tablet in your stool, there is no reason for concern. The drug is contained in a wax core that is designed to release the medication slowly. This wax core is eliminated in the stool.
• Some of these products contain the color additive FD&C Yellow No. 5 (tartrazine), which can cause allergic-type reactions (rash, shortness of breath, or fainting) in certain susceptible individuals.
• Be sure to tell your doctor if you are pregnant. Although this drug appears to be safe, extensive studies in pregnant women have not been conducted. Also, tell your doctor if you are breast-feeding an infant.

Pramosone—see hydrocortisone and iodochlorhydroxyquin combination (topical)

prazepam

BRAND NAME (Manufacturer)
Centrax (Parke-Davis)
TYPE OF DRUG
Benzodiazepine sedative/hypnotic
INGREDIENT
prazepam
DOSAGE FORMS
Capsules (5 mg, 10 mg, and 20 mg)
Tablets (10 mg)
STORAGE
This medication should be stored at room temperature in a tightly closed, light-resistant container.

USES
Prazepam is most often prescribed to treat symptoms of anxiety. It is not clear exactly how this medicine works, but prazepam may relieve anxiety by acting as a depressant of the central nervous system. This medication is currently used by many people to relieve nervousness. It is effective for this purpose for short periods, but it is important to attempt to remove the cause of the anxiety as well.

TREATMENT
Prazepam should be taken exactly as directed by your doctor. It can be taken with food or a full glass of water if stomach upset occurs. Do not take this medication with a dose of antacids, since they may retard its absorption.

If you are taking this medication regularly and you miss a dose, take the missed dose immediately if you remember within an hour. If more than an hour has passed, skip the dose you missed and wait for the next scheduled dose. Do not double the next dose.

SIDE EFFECTS
Minor. Bitter taste in mouth, constipation, diarrhea, dizziness, drowsiness (after a night's sleep), dry mouth, excessive salivation, fatigue, flushing, headache, heartburn, loss of appetite, nausea, nervousness, sweating, or vomiting. As your body adjusts to the medicine, these side effects should disappear.

To relieve constipation during therapy with this medication, increase the amount of fiber in your diet (fresh fruits and vegetables, salads, bran, and whole-grain breads), exercise, and drink more water (unless your doctor directs you to do otherwise).

Dry mouth can be relieved by chewing sugarless gum or by sucking on ice chips.

If you feel dizzy, sit or lie down for a while; get up slowly from a sitting or reclining position.
Major. Tell your doctor about any side effects that are persistent or particularly bothersome. IT IS ESPECIALLY IMPORTANT TO TELL YOUR DOCTOR about blurred or double vision, chest pain, depression, difficulty in urinating, fainting, falling, fever, joint pain, hallucinations, mouth sores, nightmares, palpitations, rash, shortness of breath, slurred speech, sore throat, uncoordinated movements, unusual excitement, unusual tiredness, or yellowing of the eyes or skin.

INTERACTIONS
Prazepam interacts with a number of other types of medications:
1. To prevent oversedation, this drug should not be taken with alcohol, other sedative drugs, central nervous system depressants (such as antihistamines, barbiturates, muscle relaxants, pain medicines, narcotics, medicines for seizures, and phenothiazine tranquilizers), or antidepressants.
2. This medication may decrease the effectiveness of levodopa.
3. This drug may increase the effects of phenytoin.
4. Disulfiram, isoniazid, and cimetidine can increase the blood levels of prazepam, which can lead to toxic effects.
5. Concurrent use of rifampin or carbamazepine may decrease the effectiveness of prazepam.

BE SURE TO TELL YOUR DOCTOR about any medications you are currently taking, especially any of those listed above.

WARNINGS
Tell your doctor about any unusual or allergic reactions that you have had to any medications, especially to prazepam or to other benzodiazepine tranquilizers (such as alprazolam, chlordiazepoxide, clorazepate, diazepam, flurazepam, halazepam, lorazepam, oxazepam, temazepam, and triazolam).

Tell your doctor if you now have or if you have ever had liver disease, kidney disease, epilepsy, lung disease, myasthenia gravis, porphyria, mental depression, or mental illness.

This medicine can cause drowsiness. Your ability to perform tasks that require alertness, such as driving a car or using potentially dangerous machinery, may be decreased. Appropriate caution should, therefore, be taken.

Prazepam has the potential for abuse and must be used with caution. Tolerance may develop quickly; do not increase the dosage without first consulting your doctor. It is also important not to stop this drug suddenly if you have been taking it in large amounts or if you have used it for several weeks. Your doctor may reduce the dosage gradually.

This is a safe drug when used properly. When it is combined with other sedative drugs or alcohol, however, serious side effects can develop.

Be sure to tell your doctor if you are pregnant. This type of medicine may increase the chance of birth defects if it is taken during the first three months of pregnancy. In addition, too much use of this medicine during the last six months of pregnancy may result in addiction of the fetus, leading to withdrawal side effects in the newborn. Also, use of this medicine during the last weeks of pregnancy may cause excessive drowsiness, slowed heartbeat, and breathing difficulties in the infant. Tell your doctor if you are breast-feeding an infant. This medicine can pass into the breast milk and cause excessive drowsiness, slowed heartbeat, and breathing difficulties in nursing infants.

prazosin

BRAND NAMES (Manufacturers)
Minipress (Pfizer)
prazosin (various manufacturers)
TYPE OF DRUG
Antihypertensive
INGREDIENT
prazosin
DOSAGE FORM
Capsules (1 mg, 2 mg, and 5 mg)
STORAGE
Prazosin capsules should be stored at room temperature in a tightly closed, light-resistant container.

USES
Prazosin is used to treat high blood pressure. It is a vasodilator that relaxes the muscle tissue of the blood vessels, which in turn lowers blood pressure.

TREATMENT
To avoid stomach irritation, you can take prazosin with food or with a full glass of water or milk. In order to become accustomed to taking this medication, try to take it at the same time(s) each day.

The first dose of this medication can cause fainting. Therefore, it is often recommended that this dose be taken at bedtime.

If you miss a dose of this medication, take the missed dose as soon as possible, unless it is almost time for the next dose. In that case, do not take the missed dose at all; just return to your regular dosing schedule. Do not double the next dose.

Prazosin does not cure high blood pressure, but it will help to control the condition as long as you continue to take the medication.

The effects of this medication may not become apparent for two weeks.

SIDE EFFECTS
Minor. Abdominal pain, constipation, diarrhea, dizziness, drowsiness, dry mouth, frequent urination, headache, impotence, nasal congestion, nausea, nervousness, sweating, tiredness, vomiting, or weakness. These side effects should disappear as your body adjusts to the medication.

To relieve constipation, increase the amount of fiber in your diet (fresh fruits and vegetables, salads, bran, and whole-grain breads), exercise, and drink more water (unless your doctor directs you to do otherwise).

To relieve mouth dryness, chew sugarless gum or suck on ice chips or a piece of hard candy.

If you feel dizzy or light-headed, sit or lie down for a while; get up slowly from a sitting or reclining position, and be careful on stairs. To avoid dizziness or light-headedness when you stand, contract and relax the muscles of your legs for a few moments before rising. Do this by pushing one foot against the floor while raising the other foot slightly, alternating feet so that you are "pumping" your legs in a pedaling motion.

Major. Tell your doctor about any side effects that are persistent or particularly bothersome. IT IS ESPECIALLY IMPORTANT TO TELL YOUR DOCTOR about blurred vision; chest pain; constant erection; depression; difficulty in breathing; difficulty in urinating; fainting; hallucinations; itching; loss of hair; nosebleeds; palpitations; rapid weight gain (three to five pounds within a week); rash; ringing in the ears; swelling of the feet, legs, or ankles; or tingling of the fingers or toes.

INTERACTIONS
Prazosin can interact with other types of medications:
1. The combination of prazosin and alcohol or verapamil can lead to a severe drop in blood pressure and fainting.
2. The severity and duration of the blood-pressure-lowering effects of the first dose of prazosin may be enhanced by a beta blocker.

BE SURE TO TELL YOUR DOCTOR about any medications you are currently taking, especially those listed above.

WARNINGS
• Tell your doctor about unusual or allergic reactions you have had to any medications, especially to prazosin or terazosin.
• Before starting to take this medication, be sure to tell your doctor if you now have or if you have ever had angina (chest pain) or kidney disease.
• Because initial therapy with this drug may cause dizziness or fainting, your doctor will probably start you on a low dosage and increase the dosage gradually.
• If this drug makes you dizzy or drowsy or blurs your vision, do not take part in any activity that requires alertness, such as driving a car or operating potentially dangerous machinery.
• In order to avoid dizziness or fainting while taking this drug, try not to stand for long periods of time, avoid drinking excessive amounts of alcohol, and try not to get over-

heated (avoid exercising strenuously in hot weather and taking hot baths, showers, and saunas).

• Before taking any over-the-counter (nonprescription) sinus, allergy, asthma, cough, cold, or diet preparations, check with your doctor or pharmacist. Some of these products can cause an increase in blood pressure.

• Do not stop taking this medication unless you first check with your doctor. If you stop taking this drug you may experience a rise in blood pressure. Your doctor may, therefore, want to decrease your dosage gradually.

• Be sure to tell your doctor if you are pregnant. Although this drug appears to be safe, there have been only limited studies in pregnant women. Also, tell your doctor if you are breast-feeding an infant.

Prednicen-M—see prednisone (systemic)

prednisolone (systemic)

BRAND NAMES (Manufacturers)
Delta-Cortef (Upjohn)
prednisolone (various manufacturers)
Prelone (Muro)
Sterapred DS (Mayrand)
TYPE OF DRUG
Adrenocorticosteroid hormone
INGREDIENT
prednisolone
DOSAGE FORMS
Tablets (5 mg)
Oral syrup (15 mg per 5-ml spoonful, with 5% alcohol)
STORAGE
Prednisolone tablets and oral syrup should be stored at room temperature (never frozen) in a tightly closed container.

USES

Your adrenal glands naturally produce certain cortisone-like chemicals. These chemicals are involved in various regulatory processes in the body (such as those involving fluid balance, temperature, and reaction to inflammation). Prednisolone belongs to a group of drugs known as adrenocorticosteroids (or cortisone-like medications). It is used to treat a variety of disorders, including endocrine and rheumatic disorders; asthma; blood diseases; certain cancers; eye disorders; gastrointestinal disturbances, such as ulcerative colitis; respiratory diseases; and inflammations, such as arthritis, dermatitis, and poison ivy. How this drug acts to relieve these disorders is not completely understood.

TREATMENT

In order to prevent stomach irritation, you can take prednisolone with food or milk.

Each dose of the oral syrup form should be measured carefully with a specially designed 5-ml measuring spoon. An ordinary kitchen teaspoon is not accurate enough.

If you are taking only one dose of this medication each day, try to take it before 9:00 A.M. This will mimic the body's normal production of this type of chemical.

It is important to try not to miss any doses of prednisolone. However, if you do miss a dose, follow these guidelines:

1. If you are taking it more than once a day, take the missed dose as soon as possible and return to your regular dosing schedule. If it is already time for the next dose, double it.

2. If you are taking this medication once a day, take the dose you missed as soon as possible, unless you don't remember until the next day. In that case, do not take the missed dose at all; just follow your regular dosing schedule. Do not double the next dose.

3. If you are taking this drug every other day, take it as soon as you remember. If you missed the scheduled time by a whole day, take it when you remember, then skip a day before you take the next dose. Do not double the next dose.

If you miss more than one dose of prednisolone, CONTACT YOUR DOCTOR.

SIDE EFFECTS

Minor. Dizziness, false sense of well-being, increased appetite, sweating, indigestion, menstrual irregularities, nausea, reddening of the skin on the face, restlessness, sleep disorders, or weight gain. These effects should disappear as your body adjusts to the medication.

Major. Tell your doctor about any side effects that are persistent or particularly bothersome. IT IS ESPECIALLY IMPORTANT TO TELL YOUR DOCTOR about abdominal enlargement; abdominal pain; acne or other skin problems; back or rib pain; bloody or black, tarry stools; blurred vision; convulsions; eye pain; fever and sore throat; growth impairment (in children); headaches; impaired healing of wounds; increased thirst and urination; mental depression; mood changes; muscle wasting or weakness; rapid weight gain (three to five pounds within a week); rash; shortness of breath; thinning of the skin; unusual bruising or bleeding; or unusual weakness.

INTERACTIONS

Prednisolone interacts with several other types of medications:

1. Alcohol, aspirin, and anti-inflammatory medications (such as diclofenac, diflunisal, fenoprofen, flurbiprofen, ibuprofen, indomethacin, ketoprofen, meclofenamate, mefenamic acid, naproxen, piroxicam, sulindac, and tolmetin) aggravate the stomach problems that are common with use of this medication.

2. The dosage of oral anticoagulants (blood thinners, such as wafarin), oral antidiabetic drugs, or insulin may need to be adjusted when this medication is being taken.

3. The loss of potassium caused by prednisolone can lead to serious side effects in individuals taking digoxin.

4. Thiazide diuretics (water pills) can increase the potassium loss caused by this medication.

5. Phenobarbital, phenytoin, rifampin, or ephedrine can increase the elimination of prednisolone from the body, thereby decreasing its effectiveness.

6. Oral contraceptives (birth control pills) and estrogen-containing drugs may decrease the elimination of this drug from the body, which can lead to an increase in side effects.

7. Prednisolone can increase the elimination of aspirin and isoniazid, thereby decreasing the effectiveness of these two medications.

8. Cholestyramine and colestipol can chemically bind this medication in the stomach and gastrointestinal tract, preventing its absorption.

BE SURE TO TELL YOUR DOCTOR about any medications you are currently taking, especially any listed above.

WARNINGS

• Tell your doctor about unusual or allergic reactions you have had to any medications, especially to prednisolone or other adrenocorticosteroids (such as betamethasone, cortisone, dexamethasone, hydrocortisone, methylprednisolone, prednisone, and triamcinolone).

• Tell your doctor if you now have or if you have ever had bone disease, diabetes mellitus, emotional instability, glaucoma, fungal infections, heart disease, high blood pressure, high cholesterol levels, myasthenia gravis, peptic ulcers, osteoporosis, thyroid disease, tuberculosis, ulcerative colitis, kidney disease, or liver disease.

• To help avoid potassium loss while you are using this medication, you can take your dose of the drug with a glass of fresh or frozen orange juice, or eat a banana each day. The use of a salt substitute also helps prevent potassium loss. Check with your doctor, however, before making any dietary changes or using a salt substitute.

• If you are using this medication for longer than a week, you may need to have your dosage adjusted if you are subjected to stress, which you might experience as a result of serious infections, injury, or surgery. Discuss this with your doctor.

• If you have been taking this drug for more than a week, do not stop taking it suddenly. If it is stopped abruptly, you may experience abdominal or back pain, dizziness, fainting, fever, muscle or joint pain, nausea, vomiting, shortness of breath, or extreme weakness. Your doctor may, therefore, want to reduce the dosage gradually. Never increase the dosage or take the drug for longer than the prescribed time unless you first consult your doctor.

• While you are taking this drug, you should not be vaccinated or immunized. Prednisolone decreases the effectiveness of vaccines and can lead to overwhelming infection if a live-virus vaccine is administered.

• Before having surgery or any other medical or dental treatment, be sure to tell your doctor or dentist that you are taking this medication.

• Because this drug can cause glaucoma and cataracts with long-term use, your doctor may want you to have your eyes examined by an ophthalmologist periodically during treatment.

• If you are taking prednisolone for prolonged periods, you should wear or carry an identification card or notice stating that you are taking an adrenocorticosteroid.

• This medication can raise blood sugar levels in diabetic patients. Blood sugar levels should, therefore, be monitored carefully with blood or urine tests when this medication is being taken.

• Some of these products contain the color additive FD&C Yellow No. 5 (tartrazine), which can cause allergic-type reactions (shortness of breath, wheezing, rash, fainting) in certain susceptible individuals.

• Be sure to tell your doctor if you are pregnant. This drug crosses the placenta, and its safety in humans is not established. Birth defects have been observed in the fetuses of animals who were given large doses of this type of drug during pregnancy. Also, tell your doctor if you are breast-feeding an infant. Small amounts of this drug pass into breast milk and may cause growth suppression or a decrease in natural adrenocorticosteroid hormone production in the nursing infant.

prednisone (systemic)

BRAND NAMES (Manufacturers)
Deltasone (Upjohn)
Liquid Pred (Muro)
Meticorten (Schering)
Orasone (Reid-Rowell)
Panasol-S (Seatrace)
Prednicen-M (Central)
prednisone (various manufacturers)
TYPE OF DRUG
Adrenocorticosteroid hormone
INGREDIENT
prednisone
DOSAGE FORMS
Tablets (1 mg, 2.5 mg, 5 mg, 10 mg, 20 mg, 25 mg, and 50 mg)
Oral syrup (5 mg per 5-ml spoonful, with 5% alcohol)
Oral solution (5 mg per 5-ml spoonful, with 5% alcohol)
Oral intensol solution (5 mg per ml, with 30% alcohol)
STORAGE
Prednisone should be stored at room temperature (never frozen) in a tightly closed container.

USES

Your adrenal glands naturally produce certain cortisone-like chemicals. These chemicals are involved in various regulatory processes in the body (such as those involving fluid balance, temperature, and reaction to inflammation). Prednisone belongs to a group of drugs known as adrenocorticosteroids (or cortisone-like medications). It is used to treat a variety of disorders, including endocrine and rheumatic disorders; asthma; blood diseases; certain cancers; eye disorders; gastrointestinal disturbances, such as ulcerative colitis; respiratory diseases; and inflammations, such as arthritis, dermatitis, and poison ivy. How this drug acts to relieve these disorders is not completely understood.

TREATMENT

In order to prevent stomach irritation, you can take prednisone with food or milk.

If you are taking only one dose of this medication each day, try to take it before 9:00 A.M.

The oral syrup or solution form of this medication should be measured carefully with a specially designed dropper (intensol solution) or 5-ml measuring spoon. An ordinary kitchen teaspoon is not accurate enough.

It is important to try not to miss any doses of prednisone. However, if you do miss a dose, follow these guidelines:

1. If you are taking it more than once a day, take the missed dose as soon as possible and return to your regular dosing schedule. If it is already time for the next dose, double it.

2. If you are taking this medication once a day, take the dose you missed as soon as possible, unless you don't remember until the next day. In that case, do not take the missed dose at all; just follow your regular dosing schedule. Do not double the next dose.

3. If you are taking this drug every other day, take it when you remember. If you missed the scheduled dose by a whole day, take it; then skip a day before you take the next dose. Do not double the dose.

If you miss more than one dose of prednisone, CONTACT YOUR DOCTOR.

SIDE EFFECTS

Minor. Dizziness, false sense of well-being, increased appetite, increased sweating, indigestion, menstrual irregularities, nausea, reddening of the skin on the face, restlessness, sleep disorders, or weight gain. These side effects should disappear as your body adjusts to the medication.

Major. Tell your doctor about any side effects that are persistent or particularly bothersome. IT IS ESPECIALLY IMPORTANT TO TELL YOUR DOCTOR about abdominal enlargement; abdominal pain; acne or other skin problems; back or rib pain; bloody or black, tarry stools; blurred vision; convulsions; eye pain; fever and sore throat; growth impairment (in children); headaches; impaired healing of wounds; increased thirst and urination; mental depression; mood changes; muscle wasting or weakness; rapid weight gain (three to five pounds within a week); rash; shortness of breath; thinning of the skin; unusual bruising or bleeding; or unusual weakness.

INTERACTIONS

Prednisone interacts with several other types of medications:

1. Alcohol, aspirin, and anti-inflammatory medications (such as diclofenac diflunisal, fenoprofen, flurbiprofen, ibuprofen, indomethacin, ketoprofen, meclofenamate, mefenamic acid, naproxen, piroxicam, sulindac, or tolmetin) aggravate the stomach problems that are common with this drug.

2. The dosage of oral anticoagulants (blood thinners, such as warfarin), oral antidiabetic drugs, or insulin may need to be adjusted when this medication is being taken.

3. The loss of potassium caused by prednisone can lead to serious side effects in individuals taking digoxin.

4. Thiazide diuretics (water pills) can increase the potassium loss caused by this medication.

5. Phenobarbital, phenytoin, rifampin, and ephedrine can increase the elimination of prednisone from the body, thereby decreasing its effectiveness.

6. Oral contraceptives (birth control pills) and estrogen-containing drugs may decrease the elimination of this drug from the body, which can lead to an increase in side effects.

7. Prednisone can increase the elimination of aspirin and isoniazid, decreasing the effectiveness of these two drugs.

8. Cholestyramine and colestipol can chemically bind this medication in the stomach and gastrointestinal tract, preventing its absorption.

BE SURE TO TELL YOUR DOCTOR about any medications you are currently taking, especially any listed above.

WARNINGS

• Tell your doctor about unusual or allergic reactions you have had to any medications, especially to prednisone or other adrenocorticosteroids (such as betamethasone, cortisone, dexamethasone, hydrocortisone, methylprednisolone, prednisolone, and triamcinolone).

• Tell your doctor if you now have or if you have ever had bone disease, diabetes mellitus, emotional instability, glaucoma, fungal infections, heart disease, high blood pressure, high cholesterol levels, kidney disease, liver disease, myasthenia gravis, peptic ulcers, osteoporosis, thyroid disease, tuberculosis, or ulcerative colitis.

• To help avoid potassium loss while using this drug, take your dose with a glass of fresh or frozen orange juice or eat a banana each day. The use of a salt substitute also helps prevent potassium loss. Check with your doctor before making any dietary changes.

• If you are using this medication for longer than a week, you may need to have your dosage adjusted if you are subjected to stress, such as serious infections, injury, or surgery.

• If you have been taking this drug for more than a week, do not stop taking it suddenly. If it is stopped abruptly, you may experience abdominal or back pain, dizziness, fainting, fever, muscle or joint pain, nausea, vomiting, shortness of breath, or extreme weakness. Your doctor may therefore want to reduce the dosage gradually. Never increase the dosage or take the drug for longer than the prescribed time unless you first consult your doctor.

• While you are taking this drug, you should not be vaccinated or immunized. This medication decreases the effectiveness of vaccines and can lead to overwhelming infection if a live-virus vaccine is administered.

• Before surgery or other medical or dental treatment, tell your doctor or dentist you are taking this drug.

• Because this drug can cause glaucoma and cataracts with long-term use, your doctor may want you to have your eyes examined by an ophthalmologist during treatment.

• If you are taking this medication for prolonged periods, you should wear or carry an identification card or notice stating that you are taking an adrenocorticosteroid.

• This drug can raise blood sugar levels in diabetic patients. Blood sugar should, therefore, be monitored carefully with blood or urine tests when this drug is started.

• Be sure to tell your doctor if you are pregnant. Birth defects have been observed in the fetuses of animals that were given large doses of this drug during pregnancy. Also, tell your doctor if you are breast-feeding an infant. It has been shown that small amounts of this drug pass into breast milk and may cause growth suppression or a decrease in natural adrenocorticosteroid production in the nursing infant.

Prelone—see prednisolone (systemic)

Prelu-2—see phendimetrazine

Preludin Endurets—see phenmetrazine

Premarin—see estrogens, conjugated

Prilosec—see omeprazole

primidone

BRAND NAMES (Manufacturers)
Myidone (Major)
Mysoline (Wyeth-Ayerst)
primidone (various manufacturers)
TYPE OF DRUG
Anticonvulsant
INGREDIENT
primidone
DOSAGE FORMS
Tablets (50 mg and 250 mg)
Oral suspension (250 mg per 5-ml spoonful)
STORAGE
Primidone tablets and oral suspension should be stored at room temperature in tightly closed containers. This medication should never be frozen.

USES
Primidone is used to treat various seizure disorders. This drug is converted in the body to phenobarbital. It is not clear exactly how primidone or phenobarbital acts to decrease the number of seizures, but both drugs are central nervous system (brain and spinal cord) depressants.

TREATMENT
In order to avoid stomach irritation, you can take primidone with food or with a full glass of water or milk (unless your doctor directs you to do otherwise).

The oral suspension form of this medication should be shaken well just before measuring each dose. The contents tend to settle on the bottom of the bottle, so it is necessary to shake the container to distribute the ingredients evenly and equalize the doses. Each dose should then be measured carefully with a specially designed 5-ml measuring spoon.

Primidone works best when the level of medicine in your bloodstream is kept constant. It is best, therefore, to take the doses at evenly spaced intervals day and night.

It is important to try not to miss any doses of this medication. If you do miss a dose and remember within two hours, take the missed dose immediately. If more than two hours have passed, do not take the missed dose at all; just return to your regular dosing schedule. Do not double the next dose. If you miss two or more consecutive doses, contact your doctor as soon as possible.

SIDE EFFECTS
Minor. Dizziness, drowsiness, fatigue, loss of appetite, nausea, or vomiting. These side effects should disappear as your body adjusts to the medication.

If you feel dizzy, sit or lie down for a while; get up slowly from a sitting or reclining position, and be careful on stairs.

Major. Tell your doctor about any side effects that are persistent or particularly bothersome. TELL YOUR DOCTOR about blurred vision, emotional disturbances, irritability, loss of coordination, or skin rash.

INTERACTIONS
Primidone interacts with several other types of medications:

1. Concurrent use of primidone with other central nervous system depressants (such as alcohol, antihistamines, barbiturates, benzodiazepine tranquilizers, muscle relaxants, narcotics, pain medications, phenothiazine tranquilizers, and sleeping medications) or with tricyclic antidepressants can lead to extreme drowsiness.

2. The blood levels and therapeutic effects of oral anticoagulants (blood thinners, such as warfarin), adrenocorticosteroids (cortisone-like medications), digitoxin, phenytoin, doxycycline, and tricyclic antidepressants can be decreased by primidone.

3. Primidone can decrease the absorption of griseofulvin from the gastrointestinal tract, thereby decreasing its effectiveness.

Before starting to take primidone, BE SURE TO TELL YOUR DOCTOR about any medications you are currently taking.

WARNINGS
• Tell your doctor about unusual or allergic reactions you have had to any medications, especially to primidone, phenobarbital, or other barbiturates (such as amobarbital, butabarbital, mephobarbital, pentobarbital, and secobarbital).

• Before starting to take primidone, be sure to tell your doctor if you now have or if you have ever had asthma, kidney disease, liver disease, or porphyria.

• If this drug makes you dizzy or drowsy, do not take part in any activity that requires alertness, such as driving a car or operating potentially dangerous machinery.

• Before having surgery or any other medical or dental treatment, be sure to tell your doctor or dentist that you are taking primidone.

• Do not stop taking this medication unless you first check with your doctor. Stopping the drug abruptly can lead to a worsening of your condition. Your doctor may therefore want to reduce your dosage gradually or start you on another drug when primidone is stopped.

• Be sure to tell your doctor if you are pregnant. An increased risk of birth defects in infants of mothers with seizure disorders has been reported. It is unclear whether this increased risk is associated with the disorders or with the anticonvulsant medications, such as primidone, that are used to treat them. Such drugs may also lead to bleeding complications in the newborn. The risks and benefits of treatment should be discussed with your doctor. Also, tell your doctor if you are breast-feeding an infant. Primidone passes into breast milk and can cause extreme drowsiness in nursing infants.

Principen—see ampicillin

Prinivil—see lisinopril

Probalan—see probenecid

Pro-Banthine—see propantheline

probenecid

BRAND NAMES (Manufacturers)
Benemid (Merck Sharp & Dohme)
Probalan (Lannett)
probenecid (various manufacturers)
TYPE OF DRUG
Uricosuric (antigout preparation)
INGREDIENT
probenecid
DOSAGE FORM
Tablets (500 mg)
STORAGE
Probenecid should be stored at room temperature in a tightly closed container.

USES
Probenecid is used to prevent gout attacks. It increases the elimination of uric acid (the chemical responsible for the symptoms of gout) through the kidneys. Probenecid is also occasionally used in combination with penicillin or ampicillin to increase the length of time that the antibiotics remain in the bloodstream.

TREATMENT
In order to avoid stomach irritation, you may take probenecid with a full glass of water or milk. You should also drink at least ten to 12 full eight-ounce glasses of liquids (not alcoholic beverages) each day to prevent formation of uric acid kidney stones.

If you miss a dose of this medication, take the missed dose as soon as possible, unless it is almost time for the next dose. In that case, do not take the missed dose at all; just return to your regular dosing schedule. Do not double the next dose.

SIDE EFFECTS
Minor. Dizziness, frequent urination, headache, loss of appetite, nausea, rash, sore gums, or vomiting. These side effects should disappear as your body adjusts to the medication.

If you feel dizzy, sit or lie down for a while; get up slowly from a sitting or reclining position, and be careful on stairs.
Major. Tell your doctor about any side effects that are persistent or particularly bothersome. TELL YOUR DOCTOR about fatigue, fever, flushing, lower back pain, painful or difficult urination, sore throat, unusual bleeding or bruising, or yellowing of the eyes or skin.

INTERACTIONS
Probenecid interacts with several other types of drugs:
1. Aspirin and pyrazinamide antagonize (act against) the antigout effects of probenecid.

2. The blood levels of methotrexate, sulfonamide antibiotics, nitrofurantoin, oral antidiabetic medicines, ketoprofen, naproxen, indomethacin, rifampin, sulindac, dapsone, and clofibrate can be increased by probenecid, which can lead to an increase in side effects.
3. Alcohol, chlorthalidone, ethacrynic acid, furosemide, or thiazide diuretics (water pills) can increase blood uric acid levels, which can decrease the effectiveness of probenecid.

Before starting to take probenecid, BE SURE TO TELL YOUR DOCTOR about any medications you are taking, especially any of those listed above.

WARNINGS
• Tell your doctor about unusual or allergic reactions you have had to any medications, especially to probenecid.
• Before starting to take probenecid, be sure to tell your doctor if you now have or if you have ever had blood diseases, diabetes mellitus, glucose-6-phosphate dehydrogenase (G6PD) deficiency, kidney stones, peptic ulcers, or porphyria.
• Diabetics using Clinitest urine glucose tests may get erroneously high readings of blood sugar levels while they are taking this drug. Temporarily changing to Clinistix or Tes-Tape urine tests will avoid this problem.
• If probenecid makes you dizzy, do not take part in any activity that requires alertness, such as driving a car or operating potentially dangerous machinery.
• Avoid taking large amounts of vitamin C while on probenecid. Vitamin C can increase the risk of kidney stone formation.
• Probenecid is not effective during an attack of gout. It is used to prevent attacks.
• Tell your doctor if you are pregnant. Although probenecid appears to be safe, it does cross the placenta. Extensive studies in pregnant women have not been conducted. Also, tell your doctor if you are breast-feeding an infant. It is not known whether probenecid passes into breast milk.

probucol

BRAND NAME (Manufacturer)
Lorelco (Merrell Dow)
TYPE OF DRUG
Antihyperlipidemic (lipid-lowering drug)
INGREDIENT
probucol
DOSAGE FORM
Tablets (250 mg and 500 mg)
STORAGE
Probucol should be stored at room temperature in a tightly closed, light-resistant container.

USES
This medication is used to treat hypercholesterolemia (high blood cholesterol levels) in patients who have not responded to diet, weight reduction, exercise, and control of blood sugar. It is not clear how probucol lowers blood

cholesterol levels, but it is thought to decrease the body's own production of cholesterol.

TREATMENT
Probucol should be taken with meals, in order to maximize its effectiveness.

If you miss a dose of this medication, take the missed dose as soon as possible, unless it is almost time for the next dose. In that case, do not take the missed dose at all; just return to your regular dosing schedule. Do not double the next dose.

The therapeutic benefits of this medication may not become apparent for up to three months after you begin therapy with this drug.

SIDE EFFECTS
Minor. Diarrhea, dizziness, gas, headache, insomnia, nausea, stomach upset, or vomiting. These side effects should disappear as your body adjusts to the medication.

If you feel dizzy, sit or lie down for a while; get up slowly from a sitting or reclining position, and be careful on stairs. Take special care when operating an automobile or potentially dangerous equipment.
Major. Tell your doctor about any side effects that are persistent or particularly bothersome. IT IS ESPECIALLY IMPORTANT TO TELL YOUR DOCTOR about blurred vision; bloody or black, tarry stools; chest pain; impotence; palpitations; rash; ringing in the ears; sweating; tingling sensations; or unusual bleeding or bruising.

INTERACTIONS
The effectiveness of chenodiol, used to treat gallstone disease, could possibly be decreased by concurrent probucol therapy.

Before starting to take probucol, BE SURE TO TELL YOUR DOCTOR about any medications you are currently taking, especially chenodiol.

WARNINGS
• Tell your doctor about unusual or allergic reactions you may have had to any medications, especially to probucol.
• Before starting this medication, be sure to tell your doctor if you now have or have ever had biliary tract disorders, gallstones or gallbladder disease, heart disease, or liver disease.
• Do not stop taking this medication unless you first check with your doctor. Stopping the medication abruptly may lead to a rapid increase in blood lipid (fats) and cholesterol levels. Your doctor may want to start you on a special diet or another medication when probucol treatment is stopped.
• Be sure to tell your doctor if you are pregnant. Although probucol appears to be safe during pregnancy, extensive studies in humans have not been conducted. If you and your doctor decide that you should stop the medication for a planned pregnancy, some form of birth control should be used for at least six months after probucol therapy is stopped to ensure that the medication has been completely eliminated from the body. Also, tell your doctor if you are breast-feeding an infant. It is not known whether probucol passes into breast milk.

procainamide

BRAND NAMES (Manufacturers)
procainamide hydrochloride (various manufacturers)
Procan-SR (Parke-Davis)
Promine (Major)
Pronestyl (Princeton Pharm)
Rhythmin (Sidmak)
TYPE OF DRUG
Antiarrhythmic
INGREDIENT
procainamide
DOSAGE FORMS
Tablets (250 mg, 375 mg, and 500 mg)
Sustained-release tablets (250 mg, 500 mg, 750 mg, and 1,000 mg)
Capsules (250 mg, 375 mg, 500 mg)
STORAGE
Procainamide tablets and capsules should be stored in tightly closed containers in a cool, dry place. Exposure to moisture causes deterioration of this medication.

USES
Procainamide is used to treat heart arrhythmias. It corrects irregular heartbeats to achieve a more normal rhythm.

TREATMENT
To increase absorption, take procainamide with a full glass of water on an empty stomach one hour before or two hours after a meal. However, if it upsets your stomach, ask your doctor if you can take it with food or milk.

Try to take it at the same time(s) each day. Procainamide works best when the amount of drug in your bloodstream is kept at a constant level. This medication should, therefore, be taken at evenly spaced intervals day and night. For example, if you are to take this medication four times per day, the doses should be spaced six hours apart.

The sustained-release tablets should be swallowed whole. Breaking, chewing, or crushing these tablets destroys their sustained-release activity and possibly increases the side effects.

If you miss a dose of this medication and remember within two hours, take the missed dose immediately. If more than two hours have passed (four hours for the sustained-release tablets), do not take the missed dose; just return to your regular dosing schedule. Do not double the next dose.

SIDE EFFECTS
Minor. Bitter taste in the mouth, diarrhea, dizziness, dry mouth, loss of appetite, nausea, stomach upset, or vomiting. These side effects should disappear as your body adjusts to the medication.

If you feel dizzy, sit or lie down for a while; get up slowly from a sitting or reclining position, and be careful on stairs.

To relieve mouth dryness, chew sugarless gum or suck on ice chips or a piece of hard candy.
Major. Tell your doctor about any side effects that are persistent or particularly bothersome. IT IS ESPECIALLY

IMPORTANT TO TELL YOUR DOCTOR about chest pain, chills, confusion, depression, fainting, fatigue, fever, giddiness, hallucinations, itching, joint pain, palpitations, rash, sore throat, unusual bleeding or bruising, or weakness.

INTERACTIONS

Procainamide interacts with several other types of medications:

1. The combination of digoxin and procainamide can lead to an increase in side effects to the heart.

2. Procainamide can block the effectiveness of neostigmine, pyridostigmine, and prostigmine.

3. Cimetidine, ranitidine, and amiodarone can increase the blood levels of procainamide, which can lead to an increase in side effects.

Before starting to take procainamide, TELL YOUR DOCTOR about any medications you are currently taking.

WARNINGS

• Tell your doctor about unusual or allergic reactions you have had to any medications, especially to procainamide, procaine, lidocaine, benzocaine, or tetracaine.

• Before starting this medication, be sure to tell your doctor if you now have or if you have ever had asthma, heart block, kidney disease, liver disease, myasthenia gravis, or systemic lupus erythematosus.

• If this drug makes you dizzy, do not take part in any activity that requires alertness, such as driving a car or operating potentially dangerous machinery.

• Before having surgery or any other medical or dental treatment, be sure to tell your doctor or dentist that you are taking this medication.

• Do not stop taking this drug without first consulting your doctor. Stopping procainamide abruptly may cause a serious change in the activity of your heart. Your doctor may therefore want to reduce your dosage gradually.

• If you are taking Procan-SR and you occasionally notice something in your stool that looks like a tablet, it does not mean that the drug is not being absorbed. The drug is "held" in a wax core designed to release the medication slowly. The wax core is eliminated in the stool after the drug has been absorbed.

• Some of these products contain the color additive FD&C Yellow No. 5 (tartrazine), which can cause allergic-type symptoms (rash, shortness of breath, fainting) in certain susceptible individuals.

• Be sure to tell your doctor if you are pregnant. Although this drug appears to be safe, extensive studies in pregnant women have not been conducted. Also, tell your doctor if you are breast-feeding an infant. It is not known whether procainamide passes into breast milk.

---

procarbazine

BRAND NAME (Manufacturer)
Matulane (Roche)
TYPE OF DRUG
Antineoplastic (anticancer drug)

INGREDIENT
procarbazine
DOSAGE FORM
Capsules (50 mg)
STORAGE
Procarbazine capsules should be stored at room temperature in a tightly closed, light-resistant container.

USES

This medication belongs to a group of drugs known as alkylating agents. It is used to treat a variety of cancers. Procarbazine is thought to work by binding to the rapidly growing cancer cells, thereby preventing their multiplication and growth.

TREATMENT

In order to prevent stomach irritation, you can take procarbazine with food or milk (unless your doctor directs you to do otherwise).

The timing of the dose of this medication is important. Be sure you completely understand your doctor's instructions on how and when this medication should be taken.

If you miss a dose of this medication and remember within a short period of time, take the missed dose immediately. If more than several hours has passed, check with your doctor to find out when the dose should be taken.

SIDE EFFECTS

Minor. Constipation, diarrhea, dizziness, drowsiness, dry mouth, headache, insomnia, loss of appetite, nausea, or vomiting. These side effects may disappear as your body adjusts to the medication. However, it is important to continue taking this medication despite any nausea and vomiting that occur.

Procarbazine can also cause hair loss (which is reversible when the medication is stopped).

This medication can increase your sensitivity to sunlight. You should, therefore, avoid prolonged exposure to sunlight and sunlamps. Wear protective clothing and sunglasses, and use an effective sunscreen.

To relieve constipation, increase the amount of fiber in your diet (fresh fruits and vegetables, salads, bran, and whole-grain breads), exercise, and drink more water (unless your doctor directs you to do otherwise).

If you feel dizzy, sit or lie down for a while; get up slowly from a sitting or reclining position, and be careful on stairs.

To help relieve mouth dryness, chew sugarless gum or suck on ice chips or a piece of hard candy.

Major. Tell your doctor about any side effects that are persistent or particularly bothersome. IT IS ESPECIALLY IMPORTANT TO TELL YOUR DOCTOR about unusual bleeding or bruising; bloody or black, tarry stools; blurred vision; changes in hearing ability; chest pain; chills; confusion; convulsions; darkening of the skin; depression; difficulty in swallowing; fainting; flushing; fever; hallucinations; itching; joint pain; lethargy; loss of coordination; menstrual irregularities; mouth sores; muscle pains; nervousness; nightmares; skin rash; slurred speech; sore throat; sweating; tingling sensations; tremors; weakness; or yellowing of the eyes or skin.

INTERACTIONS

Procarbazine interacts with several other types of medications:

1. Concurrent use of it with central nervous system depressants (such as alcohol, antihistamines, barbiturates, benzodiazepine tranquilizers, muscle relaxants, narcotics, pain medications, and phenothiazine tranquilizers) or with tricyclic antidepressants can lead to extreme drowsiness.

2. Diabetic patients should know that procarbazine can increase the blood-sugarlowering effects of insulin and oral antidiabetic medications. Dosages of these medications may need to be adjusted when procarbazine is being taken.

3. The combination of procarbazine with guanethidine, levodopa, methyldopa, or reserpine can result in excitation and high blood pressure.

4. Concurrent use of procarbazine with tricyclic antidepressants, monoamine oxidase (MAO) inhibitors, amphetamines, decongestants, or phenothiazine tranquilizers can lead to severe reactions. Tricyclic antidepressants should be stopped seven days before starting procarbazine therapy, and MAO inhibitors should be stopped 14 days prior to starting therapy with procarbazine.

5. Ingestion of alcohol while taking procarbazine can result in fainting, flushing, headache, nausea, vomiting, and weakness.

Before starting to take procarbazine, BE SURE TO TELL YOUR DOCTOR about any medications you are currently taking, especially any of those listed above.

WARNINGS

Tell your doctor about unusual or allergic reactions you have had to any medications, especially to procarbazine.

Before starting to take this medication, be sure to tell your doctor if you now have or if you have ever had blood disorders, chronic or recurrent infections, diabetes mellitus, kidney disease, or liver disease.

If this drug makes you dizzy or drowsy or blurs your vision, avoid taking part in any activity that requires alertness.

Before having surgery or any other medical or dental treatment, be sure to tell your doctor or dentist that you are taking this medication.

You should not receive any immunizations or vaccinations while taking this medication. Procarbazine blocks the effectiveness of vaccines and may result in an overwhelming infection if a live-virus vaccine is administered.

Procarbazine can lower your platelet count, thereby decreasing your body's ability to form blood clots. You should, therefore, be especially careful while brushing your teeth, flossing, or using toothpicks, razors, or fingernail scissors. Try to avoid falls and other injuries.

While you are taking procarbazine, avoid eating foods containing tyramine (certain cheeses, soy sauce, fava beans, chicken liver, avocados, bananas, canned figs, raisins, beer, and certain wines). The combination can lead to severe hypertensive (high blood pressure) reactions.

Procarbazine can decrease fertility in both men and women.

Tell your doctor if you are pregnant. Birth defects have been reported in the offspring of both humans and animals that received procarbazine during pregnancy. The risks should be discussed with your doctor. Also, tell your doctor if you are breast-feeding an infant. It is not known whether procarbazine passes into breast milk.

procainamide hydrochloride—see procainamide

Procan-SR—see procainamide

Procardia—see nifedipine

Procardia XL—see nifedipine

prochlorperazine

BRAND NAMES (Manufacturers)
Compazine (Smith Kline & French)
Compazine Spansules (Smith Kline & French)
prochlorperazine maleate (various manufacturers)
TYPE OF DRUG
Phenothiazine tranquilizer and antiemetic
INGREDIENT
prochlorperazine
DOSAGE FORMS
Tablets (5 mg, 10 mg, and 25 mg)
Sustained-release capsules (10 mg, 15 mg, and 30 mg)
Suppositories (2.5 mg, 5 mg, and 25 mg)
Oral syrup (5 mg per 5-ml spoonful)
STORAGE
The tablet and capsule forms of this medication should be stored at room temperature in tightly closed, light-resistant containers. The oral syrup and suppository forms may be stored in the refrigerator in tightly closed, light-resistant containers. If the oral syrup turns slightly yellow, the medicine is still effective and can be used. However, if it changes color markedly, or has particles floating in it, it should not be used; rather, it should be discarded down the sink. Prochlorperazine should never be frozen.

USES

Prochlorperazine is prescribed to treat the symptoms of certain types of mental illness, such as the emotional symptoms of psychosis, the manic phase of manic-depressive illness, and severe behavioral problems in children. This medication is thought to relieve the symptoms of mental illness by blocking certain chemicals involved with nerve transmission in the brain. Prochlorperazine is also frequently used to treat nausea and vomiting (this medication works at the vomiting center in the brain to relieve nausea and vomiting).

TREATMENT

To avoid stomach irritation, you can take the tablet or capsule form of this medication with a meal or with a glass of water or milk (unless your doctor directs you to do otherwise).

Antacids and antidiarrheal medicines may decrease the absorption of this medication from the gastrointestinal tract. Therefore, at least one hour should separate doses of one of these medicines and prochlorperazine.

The sustained-release capsules should be swallowed whole; do not crush, break, or open them. Breaking the capsules releases the medication all at once, destroying their sustained-release activity.

Measure the oral syrup carefully with a specially designed 5-ml measuring spoon. An ordinary kitchen teaspoon is not accurate enough.

To use the suppository form, remove the foil wrapper (if the suppository is too soft to insert, refrigerate it for half an hour or run cold water over it before removing the wrapper), and moisten the suppository with water. Lie on your left side with your right knee bent. Push the suppository into the rectum, pointed end first. Lie still for a few minutes. Try to avoid having a bowel movement for at least an hour (to give the medication time to be absorbed).

If you miss a dose of this medication, take the missed dose as soon as possible, unless it is almost time for your next dose. In that case, do not take the missed dose at all; just return to your regular schedule. Do not double the dose (unless your doctor directs you to do so).

The full effects of this medication for the control of emotional or mental symptoms may not become apparent for two weeks after you start to take it.

SIDE EFFECTS

Minor. Blurred vision, constipation, decreased sweating, diarrhea, dizziness, drooling, drowsiness, dry mouth, fatigue, jitteriness, menstrual irregularities, nasal congestion, restlessness, vomiting, or weight gain. As your body adjusts to the medication, these side effects should disappear.

Prochlorperazine can also cause discoloration of the urine to red, pink, or red-brown. This is a harmless effect.

This medication can cause increased sensitivity to sunlight. It is, therefore, important to avoid prolonged exposure to sunlight and sunlamps. Wear protective clothing and sunglasses, and use an effective sunscreen.

If you are constipated, increase the amount of fiber in your diet (fresh fruits and vegetables, salads, bran, and whole-grain breads), exercise, and drink more water (unless your doctor directs you to do otherwise).

Chew sugarless gum or suck on ice chips or a piece of hard candy to reduce mouth dryness.

To avoid dizziness or light-headedness when you stand, contract and relax the muscles of your legs for a few moments before rising. Do this by pushing one foot against the floor while raising the other foot slightly, alternating feet so that you are "pumping" your legs in a pedaling motion.

Major. Tell your doctor about any side effects that are persistent or particularly bothersome. IT IS ESPECIALLY IMPORTANT TO TELL YOUR DOCTOR about unusual bleeding or bruising; breast enlargement (in both sexes); chest pain; convulsions; darkened skin; difficulty in swallowing or breathing; fainting; fever; impotence; involuntary movements of the face, mouth, jaw, or tongue; palpitations; rash; sleep disorders; sore throat; tremors; uncoordinated movements; visual disturbances; or yellowing of the eyes or skin.

INTERACTIONS

Prochlorperazine interacts with several other types of medications:

1. It can cause drowsiness when combined with alcohol or central nervous system depressants (drugs that slow the activity of the brain and spinal cord), such as barbiturates, benzodiazepine tranquilizers, muscle relaxants, narcotics, and pain medications, or with tricyclic antidepressants.

2. Prochlorperazine can decrease the effectiveness of amphetamines, guanethidine, anticonvulsants, and levodopa.

3. The side effects of epinephrine, monoamine oxidase (MAO) inhibitors, propranolol, phenytoin, and tricyclic antidepressants may be increased by this medication. At least 14 days should separate the use of this drug and the use of an MAO inhibitor.

4. Lithium may increase the side effects and decrease the effectiveness of this medication.

5. Thiazide diuretics can enhance the blood-pressure-lowering side effects of prochlorperazine.

Before starting to take prochlorperazine, TELL YOUR DOCTOR about any medications you are currently taking.

WARNINGS

• Tell your doctor about unusual reactions you have had to any drugs, especially to prochlorperazine or other phenothiazine tranquilizers (such as chlorpromazine, fluphenazine, mesoridazine, perphenazine, promazine, thioridazine, trifluoperazine, and triflupromazine) or to loxapine.

• Tell your doctor if you have a history of alcoholism or if you now have or have ever had any blood disease, bone marrow disease, brain disease, breast cancer, blockage in the urinary or digestive tracts, drug-induced depression, epilepsy, high or low blood pressure, diabetes mellitus, glaucoma, heart or circulatory disease, liver disease, lung disease, Parkinson's disease, peptic ulcers, or an enlarged prostate gland.

• Tell your doctor about any recent exposure to a pesticide or an insecticide. Prochlorperazine may increase the side effects from the exposure.

• To prevent oversedation, avoid drinking alcoholic beverages while taking this medication.

• If this medication makes you dizzy or drowsy, do not take part in any activity that requires alertness, such as driving a car or operating potentially dangerous machinery. Be careful on stairs, and avoid getting up suddenly from a lying or sitting position.

• Prior to having surgery or any other medical or dental treatment, be sure to tell your doctor or dentist that you are taking this medication.

• Some of the side effects caused by this drug can be prevented by taking an antiparkinsonism drug. Discuss this with your doctor.

• This medication can decrease sweating and heat release from the body. You should therefore try not to get overheated (avoid exercising strenuously in hot weather, and avoid taking hot baths, showers, and saunas).

• Do not stop taking prochlorperazine suddenly if you have been taking it for a prolonged period. If the drug is

stopped abruptly, you may experience nausea, vomiting, stomach upset, headache, increased heart rate, insomnia, tremors, or a worsening of your condition. Your doctor may therefore want to reduce the dosage gradually.
• If you are planning to have a myelogram, or any other procedure in which dye will be injected into your spinal cord, tell your doctor that you are taking this medication.
• Avoid spilling the oral syrup form of this medication on your skin or clothing; it may cause redness and irritation.
• While taking this medication, do not take any over-the-counter medications for weight control or for cough, cold, allergy, asthma, or sinus problems unless you first check with your doctor. The combination of these medications with prochlorperazine may cause high blood pressure.
• Be sure to tell your doctor if you are pregnant. Although there are reports of safe use of this drug during pregnancy, there are also reports of liver disease and tremors in newborn infants whose mothers received this type of medication close to term. Also, tell your doctor if you are breast-feeding an infant.

prochlorperazine maleate—see prochlorperazine

Prolixin—see fluphenazine

Proloprim—see trimethoprim

promazine

BRAND NAME (Manufacturer)
Sparine (Wyeth-Ayerst)
TYPE OF DRUG
Phenothiazine tranquilizer
INGREDIENT
promazine
DOSAGE FORM
Tablets (25 mg, 50 mg, and 100 mg)
STORAGE
This medication should be stored at room temperature in a tightly closed, light-resistant container.

USES
Promazine is prescribed to treat the symptoms of certain types of mental illness, such as emotional symptoms of psychosis, the manic phase of manicdepressive illness, and severe behavioral problems in children. It is thought to relieve symptoms of mental illness by blocking certain chemicals involved with nerve transmission in the brain.

TREATMENT
To avoid stomach irritation, you can take this medication with a meal or with a glass of water or milk (unless your doctor directs you to do otherwise).

If you miss a dose of this medication, take the missed dose as soon as possible, unless it is almost time for your next dose. In that case, do not take the missed dose at all; just return to your regular dosing schedule. Do not

double the dose (unless your doctor directs you to do so).

Antacids and antidiarrheal medicines may decrease the absorption of this medication from the gastrointestinal tract. Therefore, at least one hour should separate doses of one of these medicines and promazine.

The full effects of this medication for the control of emotional or mental symptoms may not become apparent until two weeks after you start to take it.

SIDE EFFECTS
Minor. Blurred vision, constipation, decreased sweating, diarrhea, dizziness, drooling, drowsiness, dry mouth, fatigue, jitteriness, menstrual irregularities, nasal congestion, restlessness, vomiting, or weight gain. As your body adjusts to the medication, these side effects should disappear.

Promazine can also cause discoloration of the urine to red, pink, or red-brown. This is a harmless effect.

This medication can cause increased sensitivity to sunlight. It is, therefore, important to avoid prolonged exposure to sunlight and sunlamps. Wear protective clothing and sunglasses, and use an effective sunscreen.

If you are constipated, increase the amount of fiber in your diet (raw fruits and vegetables, salads, bran, and whole-grain breads), exercise, and drink more water (unless your doctor directs you to do otherwise).

Chew sugarless gum or suck on ice chips or a piece of hard candy to reduce mouth dryness.

To avoid dizziness or light-headedness when you stand, contract and relax the muscles of your legs for a few moments before rising. Do this by pushing one foot against the floor while raising the other foot slightly, alternating feet so that you are "pumping" your legs in a pedaling motion.
Major. Tell your doctor about any side effects that are persistent or particularly bothersome. IT IS ESPECIALLY IMPORTANT TO TELL YOUR DOCTOR about unusual bleeding or bruising; breast enlargement (in both sexes); chest pain; convulsions; darkened skin; difficulty in swallowing or breathing; fainting; fever; impotence; involuntary movements of the face, mouth, jaw, or tongue; palpitations; rash; sleep disorders; sore throat; tremors; uncoordinated movements; visual disturbances; or yellowing of the eyes or skin.

INTERACTIONS
This medication interacts with a number of other types of medications:
1. It can cause extreme drowsiness when combined with alcohol or other central nervous system depressants (drugs that slow the activity of the brain and spinal cord), such as barbiturates, benzodiazepine tranquilizers, muscle relaxants, narcotics, and pain medications, or with tricyclic antidepressants.
2. Promazine can decrease the effectiveness of amphetamines, guanethidine, anticonvulsants, and levodopa.
3. The side effects of epinephrine, monoamine oxidase (MAO) inhibitors, propranolol, phenytoin, and tricyclic antidepressants may be increased by this medication.
4. Lithium may increase the side effects and decrease the effectiveness of this medication.

Before starting to take promazine, BE SURE TO TELL YOUR DOCTOR about any medications you are currently taking, especially any of those listed above.

WARNINGS

Tell your doctor about unusual or allergic reactions you have had to any medications, especially to promazine or other phenothiazine tranquilizers (such as chlorpromazine, fluphenazine, mesoridazine, perphenazine, prochlorperazine, thioridazine, trifluoperazine, and triflupromazine) or to loxapine.

Tell your doctor if you have a history of alcoholism or if you now have or have ever had any blood disease, bone marrow disease, brain disease, breast cancer, blockage in the urinary or digestive tracts, drug-induced depression, epilepsy, high or low blood pressure, diabetes mellitus, glaucoma, heart or circulatory disease, liver disease, lung disease, Parkinson's disease, peptic ulcers, or an enlarged prostate gland.

Tell your doctor about any recent exposure to a pesticide or an insecticide. Promazine may increase the side effects from the exposure.

To prevent oversedation, avoid drinking alcoholic beverages while taking this medication.

If this medication makes you dizzy or drowsy, do not take part in any activity that requires alertness, such as driving a car or operating potentially dangerous machinery. Be careful on stairs, and avoid getting up suddenly from a lying or sitting position.

Prior to having surgery or any other medical or dental treatment, be sure to tell your doctor or dentist that you are taking this medication.

Some of the side effects caused by this drug can be prevented by taking an antiparkinsonism drug. Discuss this with your doctor.

This medication can decrease sweating and heat release from the body. You should, therefore, try not to get overheated (avoid strenuous exercise in hot weather and do not take hot baths, showers, and saunas).

Do not stop taking this medication suddenly. If the drug is stopped abruptly, you may experience nausea, vomiting, stomach upset, headache, increased heart rate, insomnia, tremors, or a worsening of your condition. Your doctor may, therefore, want to reduce the dosage gradually.

If you are planning to have a myelogram, or any other procedure in which dye will be injected into the space surrounding your spinal cord, tell your doctor that you are taking this medication.

While taking this medication, do not take any over-the-counter (nonprescription) medication for weight control or for cough, cold, allergy, asthma, or sinus problems unless you first check with your doctor. The combination of these medications may cause high blood pressure.

Be sure to tell your doctor if you are pregnant. Small amounts of this medication cross the placenta. Although there are reports of safe use of this drug during pregnancy, there are also reports of liver disease and tremors in newborn infants whose mothers received this medication close to term. Also, tell your doctor if you are breast-feeding an infant. Small amounts of this medication pass into breast milk and may cause unwanted effects in nursing infants.

Prometh with Codeine—see promethazine and codeine combination

---

promethazine

BRAND NAMES (Manufacturers)
Phenameth (Major)
Phenergan (Wyeth-Ayerst)
promethazine (various manufacturers)
Prothazine (Vortech)
TYPE OF DRUG
antihistamine and antiemetic
INGREDIENT
promethazine
DOSAGE FORMS
Tablets (12.5 mg, 25 mg, and 50 mg)
Oral syrup (6.25 mg per 5-ml spoonful, with 7% alcohol; 25 mg per 5-ml spoonful, with 1.5% alcohol)
Rectal suppositories (12.5 mg, 25 mg, and 50 mg)
STORAGE
Promethazine tablets and oral syrup should be stored at room temperature (never frozen) in tightly closed, light-resistant containers. The suppositories should be kept in the refrigerator in a tightly closed container.

USES
Promethazine is prescribed for a wide range of conditions. Promethazine belongs to a group of drugs known as antihistamines, which block the action of histamine, a chemical that is released by the body during an allergic reaction. It is, therefore, used to treat or prevent symptoms of allergy or hay fever. Promethazine also (1) works at the vomiting center in the brain and can be used for the prevention or treatment of nausea and vomiting; (2) is a central nervous system (brain and spinal cord) depressant, which produces light sleep or mild sedation; and (3) prevents motion sickness.

TREATMENT
To avoid stomach irritation, you can take the tablet or oral syrup form of this medication with a meal or with a glass of water or milk (unless your doctor directs otherwise).

Measure the oral syrup carefully with a specially designed 5-ml measuring spoon. An ordinary kitchen teaspoon is not accurate enough.

To use the suppository, remove the foil wrapper (if the suppository is too soft to insert, refrigerate it for half an hour or run cold water over it before removing the wrapper), and moisten the suppository with water. Lie on your left side with your right knee bent. Push the suppository into the rectum, pointed end first. Lie still for a few minutes. Try to avoid having a bowel movement for at least an hour (to give the medication time to be absorbed).

If you are taking this medication regularly and you miss a dose, take the missed dose as soon as possible, unless it is almost time for the next dose. In that case, do not take the missed dose at all; just return to your regular schedule. Do not double the next dose (unless your doctor directs you to do so).

SIDE EFFECTS

Minor. Blurred vision, diarrhea, dizziness, drowsiness, dry mouth, light-headedness, nausea, or vomiting. These side effects should disappear as your body adjusts to this drug.

This medication can cause increased sensitivity to sunlight. It is, therefore, important to avoid prolonged exposure to sunlight and sunlamps. Wear protective clothing and sunglasses, and use an effective sunscreen.

To reduce mouth dryness, chew sugarless gum or suck on ice chips or hard candy.

To avoid dizziness or light-headedness when you stand, contract and relax the muscles of your legs for a few moments before rising. Do this by alternately pushing one foot against the floor while raising the other foot slightly, so that you are "pumping" your legs in a pedaling motion.

Major. Tell your doctor about any side effects that are persistent or particularly bothersome. IT IS ESPECIALLY IMPORTANT TO TELL YOUR DOCTOR about confusion; disorientation; involuntary movements of the face, mouth, jaw, or tongue; rash; uncoordinated movements; unusual bleeding or bruising; or yellowing of the eyes or skin.

INTERACTIONS

Promethazine interacts with other types of medications:
1. Promethazine can cause extreme drowsiness when combined with alcohol or other central nervous system depressants (drugs that slow the activity of the brain and spinal cord), such as barbiturates, benzodiazepine tranquilizers, muscle relaxants, narcotics, and pain medications, or with tricyclic antidepressants.
2. Promethazine can decrease the effectiveness of amphetamines, guanethidine, anticonvulsants, and levodopa.
3. The side effects of epinephrine, monoamine oxidase (MAO) inhibitors, propranolol, and tricyclic antidepressants may be increased by this medication. At least 14 days should separate the use of this medication and the use of an MAO inhibitor.

TELL YOUR DOCTOR about any of the medications you are currently taking, especially any of those listed above.

WARNINGS

• Tell your doctor about any unusual or allergic reactions you have had to any medications, especially to promethazine or any chemically related phenothiazine drug (chlorpromazine, fluphenazine, mesoridazine, perphenazine, prochlorperazine, promazine, thioridazine, trifluoperazine, triflupromazine).
• Before starting promethazine, tell your doctor if you now have or if you have ever had asthma, blockage of the urinary or digestive tract, diabetes mellitus, enlarged prostate gland, epilepsy, glaucoma, heart disease, liver disease, peptic ulcers, or sleep apnea.
• To prevent oversedation, avoid drinking alcoholic beverages while taking this medication.

• If this medication makes you dizzy or drowsy, do not take part in any activity that requires alertness, such as driving a car or operating potentially dangerous machinery. Be careful going up and down stairs.
• Prior to having surgery or any other medical or dental treatment, be sure to tell your doctor or dentist that you are taking this medication.
• Be sure to tell your doctor if you are pregnant. Small amounts of this medication cross the placenta. Although there are reports of safe use of this drug during pregnancy, there are also reports of liver disease and tremors in newborns whose mothers received this medication close to term. Also, tell your doctor if you are breast-feeding. Small amounts of this medication pass into breast milk and may cause unwanted effects in nursing infants, such as sudden infant death syndrome (SIDS) or sleep apnea.

promethazine and codeine combination

BRAND NAMES (Manufacturers)
Phenergan with Codeine (Wyeth-Ayerst)
Pherazine with Codeine (Halsey)
Prometh with Codeine (Goldline)
Prothazine DC (Vortech)
TYPE OF DRUG
Antihistamine and cough suppressant
INGREDIENTS
promethazine and codeine
DOSAGE FORM
Oral syrup (6.25 mg promethazine and 10 mg codeine per 5-ml spoonful, with 7% alcohol)
STORAGE
This medication should be stored at room temperature in a tightly closed, light-resistant container. This medication should never be frozen.

USES
This drug combination is used to provide symptomatic relief of coughs due to colds, minor upper respiratory tract infections, or allergy.

Promethazine belongs to a group of drugs known as antihistamines, which block the actions of histamine, a chemical released by the body during an allergic reaction. It is used to relieve or prevent symptoms of allergy.

Codeine is a narcotic cough suppressant that acts at the cough reflex center in the brain.

TREATMENT
To avoid stomach upset, you can take this medication with food or with a full glass of milk or water (unless your doctor directs you to do otherwise).

The oral syrup should be shaken well just before measuring each dose. The contents tend to settle on the bottom of the bottle, so it is necessary to shake the container to distribute the ingredients evenly and equalize the doses. Each dose should then be measured carefully with a specially designed 5-ml measuring spoon. An ordinary kitchen teaspoon is not accurate enough.

If you miss a dose of this medication, take the missed dose as soon as possible, unless it is almost time for your next dose. In that case, do not take the missed dose at all; just return to your regular dosing schedule. Do not double the next dose.

SIDE EFFECTS

Minor. Blurred vision; constipation; diarrhea; dizziness; dry mouth, throat, or nose; irritability; loss of appetite; confusion; nausea; restlessness; stomach upset; or unusual increase in sweating. These side effects should disappear as your body adjusts to the medication.

This medication can cause increased sensitivity to sunlight. Avoid prolonged exposure to sunlight, wear protective clothing and sunglasses, and use an effective sunscreen.

If you are constipated, increase the amount of fiber in your diet (fresh fruits and vegetables, salads, bran, and whole-grain breads), exercise, and drink more water (unless your doctor tells you not to do so).

Chew sugarless gum or suck on ice chips or a piece of hard candy to reduce mouth dryness.

If you feel dizzy or light-headed, sit or lie down for a while; get up slowly from a sitting or reclining position, and be careful on stairs.

Major. Tell your doctor about any side effects that are persistent or particularly bothersome. IT IS ESPECIALLY IMPORTANT TO TELL YOUR DOCTOR about convulsions, difficulty in breathing, difficult or painful urination, disturbed coordination, excitation, fainting, headaches, muscle spasms, nightmares, nosebleeds, palpitations, rash, ringing or buzzing in the ears, severe abdominal pain, sore throat or fever, or yellowing of the eyes or skin.

INTERACTIONS

This medicine interacts with other types of drugs:

1. Concurrent use of it with central nervous system depressants (drugs that slow the activity of the brain and spinal cord), such as alcohol, barbiturates, benzodiazepine tranquilizers, muscle relaxants, narcotics, pain medications, and phenothiazine tranquilizers, or with tricyclic antidepressants can cause extreme drowsiness.

2. This medication can decrease the effectiveness of amphetamines, guanethidine, anticonvulsants, and levodopa.

3. This combination medication can increase the side effects of monoamine oxidase (MAO) inhibitors (isocarboxazid, pargyline, phenelzine, or tranylcypromine) and tricyclic antidepressants. At least 14 days should separate the use of this drug and the use of an MAO inhibitor.

BE SURE TO TELL YOUR DOCTOR about any medications you are currently taking, especially any listed above.

WARNINGS

• Tell your doctor about unusual or allergic reactions you have had to any medications, especially to promethazine or other antihistamines; to phenothiazine tranquilizers; to codeine; or to any other narcotic cough suppressant or pain medication.

• Tell your doctor if you now have or if you have ever had asthma, brain disease, blockage of the urinary or digestive tract, diabetes mellitus, colitis, gallstones or gallbladder disease, glaucoma, heart or blood vessel disease, high blood pressure, kidney disease, liver disease, lung disease, peptic ulcers, enlarged prostate gland, or thyroid disease.

• This medication can cause drowsiness. Your ability to perform tasks that require alertness, such as driving a car or operating potentially dangerous machinery, may be decreased. Appropriate caution should therefore be taken.

• Before having surgery or any other medical or dental treatment, be sure to tell your doctor or dentist that you are taking this medication.

• Because this product contains codeine, it has the potential for abuse and must be used with caution. Usually, it should not be taken on a regular schedule for longer than ten days at a time. Tolerance develops quickly; do not increase the dosage or stop taking the drug abruptly, unless you first consult your doctor. If you have been taking large amounts of this medication or have been taking it for a long period of time, you may experience a withdrawal reaction (muscle aches, diarrhea, gooseflesh, runny nose, nausea, vomiting, shivering, trembling, stomach cramps, sleep disorders, irritability, weakness, excessive yawning, or sweating) when you stop taking it. Your doctor may therefore want to reduce the dosage.

• Be sure to tell your doctor if you are pregnant. The effects of this medication during the early stages of pregnancy have not been thoroughly studied in humans. However, regular use of codeine during the later stages of pregnancy may lead to addiction of the fetus, resulting in withdrawal symptoms (irritability, excessive crying, tremors, fever, vomiting, diarrhea, sneezing, yawning) in the newborn infant. There are also reports of liver disease and tremors in newborns whose mothers received this medication close to term. Also, tell your doctor if you are breast-feeding an infant. Small amounts of this medication pass into breast milk and may cause unusual excitement or irritability in nursing infants as well as sudden infant death syndrome (SIDS) or sleep apnea.

Prometh VC with Codeine—see phenylephrine, promethazine, and codeine combination

Prometh with Codeine—see promethazine and codeine combination

Promine—see procainamide

Pronestyl—see procainamide

Propacet 100—see acetaminophen and propoxyphene combination

---

propantheline

BRAND NAMES (Manufacturers)
Norpanth (Vortech)
Pro-Banthine (Searle)
propantheline bromide (various manufacturers)

TYPE OF DRUG
Anticholinergic (antiulcer drug)

INGREDIENT
propantheline
DOSAGE FORM
Tablets (7.5 mg and 15 mg)
STORAGE
Store at room temperature in a tightly closed container.

USES

Propantheline is used to treat peptic ulcers. It may reduce the amount of acid formed in the stomach. It also relieves cramping and spasms of the gastrointestinal tract and the bladder.

TREATMENT

Take propantheline 30 minutes before meals and at bedtime (unless your doctor directs you to do otherwise).

If you miss a dose of this medication, do not take the missed dose at all; just return to your regular dosing schedule. Do not double the next dose.

SIDE EFFECTS

Minor. Bloating, blurred vision, constipation, decreased sweating, dizziness, drowsiness, dry mouth, headache, increased sensitivity of the eyes to sunlight, nausea, nervousness, taste disorders, or vomiting. These side effects should disappear as your body adjusts to the medication.

To relieve constipation, exercise and drink more water (unless your doctor directs you to do otherwise).

If you feel dizzy, sit or lie down for a while; change positions slowly, and be careful on stairs.

To help relieve mouth dryness, chew sugarless gum or suck on ice chips or a piece of hard candy.

Sunglasses may help to relieve the sensitivity of your eyes to sunlight.

Major. Tell your doctor about any side effects that are persistent or particularly bothersome. IT IS ESPECIALLY IMPORTANT TO TELL YOUR DOCTOR about decreased sexual ability, difficulty in urinating, eye pain, itching, palpitations, or skin rash.

INTERACTIONS

Propantheline interacts with several other types of drugs:
1. Amantadine, antihistamines, disopyramide, haloperidol, monoamine oxidase (MAO) inhibitors, phenothiazine tranquilizers, procainamide, quinidine, and tricyclic antidepressants can increase the side effects of propantheline. At least 14 days should separate the use of this drug and the use of an MAO inhibitor.
2. Antacids and antidiarrheal medications can reduce the absorption of propantheline from the gastrointestinal tract, which can decrease its effectiveness. Therefore, at least two hours should separate doses of one of these types of medications and propantheline.

TELL YOUR DOCTOR about any medications you are currently taking, especially any of those listed above.

WARNINGS

• Tell your doctor about unusual or allergic reactions you have had to any medications, especially to propantheline.
• Before starting this medication, be sure to tell your doctor if you now have or if you have ever had glaucoma,

heart disease, hiatal hernia, high blood pressure, intestinal blockage, kidney disease, liver disease, lung disease, myasthenia gravis, enlarged prostate gland, thyroid disease, ulcerative colitis, or urinary retention.
• This medication can decrease sweating and heat release from the body. You should, therefore, try not to get overheated (avoid strenuous exercise in hot weather, and do not take hot baths, showers, and saunas).
• If this medication makes you dizzy or drowsy or blurs your vision, avoid driving a car or operating potentially dangerous equipment.
• Be sure to tell your doctor if you are pregnant. Although propantheline appears to be safe during pregnancy, extensive studies in humans have not been conducted. Also, tell your doctor if you are breast-feeding an infant. It is not known whether propantheline passes into breast milk.

propantheline bromide—see propantheline

---

propoxyphene

BRAND NAMES (Manufacturers)
Darvon (Lilly)
Darvon-N (Lilly)
Dolene (Lederle)
propoxyphene hydrochloride (various manufacturers)
TYPE OF DRUG
Analgesic
INGREDIENT
propoxyphene
DOSAGE FORMS
Capsules (65 mg)
Tablets (100 mg)
Oral suspension (10 mg per ml)
STORAGE
This medication should be stored at room temperature (never frozen) in tightly closed containers.

USES

Propoxyphene is a narcotic analgesic that acts on the central nervous system (brain and spinal cord) to relieve mild to moderate pain.

TREATMENT

In order to avoid stomach upset, you can take propoxyphene with food or milk.

The suspension form of this medication should be shaken well just before measuring each dose. The contents tend to settle on the bottom of the bottle, so it is necessary to shake the container to distribute the ingredients evenly and equalize the doses. Each dose should be measured carefully with a specially designed 5-ml measuring spoon. An ordinary kitchen teaspoon is not accurate enough.

This medication works best if taken at the first sign of pain. Do not wait for the pain to become severe.

If your doctor has prescribed this medication to be taken on a regular schedule and you miss a dose, take the missed dose as soon as possible, unless it is almost time for your next dose. Do not take the missed dose at all; just return to your regular dosing schedule. Do not double the next dose.

SIDE EFFECTS

Minor. Blurred vision, constipation, dizziness, drowsiness, indigestion, light-headedness, nausea, nervousness, restlessness, vomiting, or weakness. As your body adjusts to the medication, these side effects should disappear.

If you are constipated, increase the amount of fiber in your diet (fresh fruits and vegetables, salads, bran, and whole-grain breads), exercise, and drink more water (unless your doctor directs you to do otherwise).

If you feel dizzy or light-headed, sit or lie down for a while; get up slowly, and be careful on stairs.

Major. Tell your doctor about any side effects that are persistent or particularly bothersome. IT IS ESPECIALLY IMPORTANT TO TELL YOUR DOCTOR about confusion, convulsions, darkening of the urine, depression, difficulty in breathing, hallucinations, palpitations, ringing in the ears, skin rash, yellow stools, or yellowing of the eyes or skin.

INTERACTIONS

Propoxyphene can interact with several types of drugs:
1. Concurrent use of it with other central nervous system depressants (such as antihistamines, barbiturates, tranquilizers, sleeping medications, muscle relaxants, and other pain medications) or with tricyclic antidepressants can cause extreme drowsiness.
2. Propoxyphene can increase carbamazepine blood levels, which in turn can result in greater side effects.
3. A monoamine oxidase (MAO) inhibitor taken within 14 days of this medication can lead to unpredictable and severe side effects.
4. Propoxyphene also interacts with alcohol, increasing its intoxicating effects. You should, therefore, avoid drinking alcoholic beverages while taking this medicine.

TELL YOUR DOCTOR about any medications you are currently taking, especially any of those listed above.

WARNINGS

• Tell your doctor about unusual or allergic reactions you have had to any medications, especially to propoxyphene or to other narcotic analgesics (such as codeine, hydrocodone, hydromorphone, meperidine, methadone, morphine, and oxycodone).
• Tell your doctor if you now have or if you have ever had acute abdominal conditions, asthma, brain disease, colitis, epilepsy, gallstones or gallbladder disease, head injuries, heart disease, kidney disease, liver disease, lung disease, mental illness, emotional disorders, enlarged prostate gland, thyroid disease, or urethral stricture.
• If this drug makes you dizzy or drowsy, do not take part in any activity that requires alertness.
• Before having surgery or any other medical or dental treatment, be sure to tell your doctor or dentist that you are taking this medication.
• Propoxyphene has the potential for abuse and must be used with caution. Usually, you should not take it on a regular schedule for longer than ten days (unless your doctor directs you to do so). Tolerance develops quickly; do not increase the dosage or stop taking the drug abruptly, unless you first consult your doctor. If you have been taking large amounts of this medication or have been taking it for long periods of time, you may experience a withdrawal reaction (muscle aches, diarrhea, gooseflesh, runny nose, nausea, vomiting, shivering, trembling, stomach cramps, sleep disorders, irritability, weakness, excessive yawning, or sweating) when you stop taking it. Your doctor may therefore want to reduce the dosage gradually.
• Be sure to tell your doctor if you are pregnant. The effects of this medication during the early stages of pregnancy have not been thoroughly studied in humans. However, regular use of propoxyphene in large doses during the later stages of pregnancy can result in addiction of the fetus, leading to withdrawal symptoms (irritability, excessive crying, tremors, fever, vomiting, diarrhea, sneezing, or excessive yawning) at birth. Also, tell your doctor if you are breast-feeding an infant. Small amounts of this medication may pass into breast milk and cause excessive drowsiness in the nursing infant.

propoxyphene hydrochloride—see propoxyphene

propoxyphene hydrochloride compound—see aspirin, caffeine, and propoxyphene combination

propoxyphene hydrochloride with acetaminophen—see acetaminophen and propoxyphene combination

propoxyphene napsylate with acetaminophen—see acetaminophen and propoxyphene combination

propranolol

BRAND NAMES (Manufacturers)
Inderal (Wyeth-Ayerst)
Inderal LA (Wyeth-Ayerst)
propranolol (various manufacturers)
TYPE OF DRUG
Beta-adrenergic blocking agent
INGREDIENT
propranolol
DOSAGE FORMS
Tablets (10 mg, 20 mg, 40 mg, 60 mg, 80 mg, and 90 mg)
Extended-release capsules (60 mg, 80 mg, 120 mg, and 160 mg)
Oral solution (4 mg and 8 mg per ml)
Oral concentrated solution (80 mg per ml)
STORAGE
Store at room temperature in a tightly closed, light-resistant container. The solutions should never be frozen.

USES
Propranolol is used to treat high blood pressure, angina pectoris (chest pain), and irregular heartbeats. It is also useful in preventing migraine headaches and preventing additional heart attacks in heart attack patients. Propranolol belongs to a group of medicines known as beta-adrenergic blocking agents or, more commonly,

beta blockers. These drugs work by controlling nerve impulses along certain nerve pathways.

TREATMENT

Propranolol can be taken with a glass of water, with meals, immediately following meals, or on an empty stomach (depending on your doctor's instructions). Try to take the medication at the same time(s) each day.

The extended-release capsules should be swallowed whole. Do not chew or crush them. Breaking the capsule releases the medication all at once—defeating the purpose of extended-release capsules.

The oral solution should be measured with a specially designed 5-ml measuring spoon.

The oral concentrated solution must be mixed in four ounces ($1/2$ cup) of water, juice, or soda before drinking. The cup should be refilled with more of the liquid, which must be drunk to ensure that the entire dose is taken. This form may also be mixed with applesauce or pudding.

It is important to remember that propranolol does not cure high blood pressure, but it will help control the condition as long as you continue to take it.

Try not to miss any doses of this medicine. If you do miss a dose, take the missed dose as soon as possible, unless it is within eight hours (if you are taking this medicine only once a day) or within four hours (if you are taking this medicine more than once a day) of your next scheduled dose. In that case, do not take the missed dose at all; just return to your regular dosing schedule. Do not double the next dose of the medication.

SIDE EFFECTS

Minor. Anxiety; constipation; decreased sexual ability; diarrhea; difficulty in sleeping; drowsiness; dryness of the eyes, mouth, and skin; headache; nausea; nervousness; stomach discomfort; tiredness; or weakness. These side effects should disappear as your body adjusts to the medicine.

To relieve constipation, increase the amount of fiber in your diet (fresh fruits and vegetables, salads, bran, and whole-grain breads) and drink more water (unless your doctor directs you to do otherwise).

If you are extra-sensitive to the cold, be sure to dress warmly during cold weather.

Plain, nonmedicated eye drops (artificial tears) may help to relieve eye dryness.

Sucking on ice chips or chewing sugarless gum helps to relieve mouth and throat dryness.

Major. Tell your doctor about any side effects that are persistent or particularly bothersome. IT IS ESPECIALLY IMPORTANT TO TELL YOUR DOCTOR about breathing difficulty or wheezing, cold hands or feet (due to decreased blood circulation to skin, fingers, and toes), confusion, depression, dizziness, hair loss, hallucinations, light-headedness, nightmares, numbness or tingling of the fingers or toes, rapid weight gain (three to five pounds within a week), reduced alertness, swelling, sore throat and fever, skin rash, or unusual bleeding or bruising.

INTERACTIONS

Propranolol interacts with a number of other types of medications:

1. Indomethacin, aspirin, or other salicylates lessen the blood-pressure-lowering effects of beta blockers.
2. Concurrent use of beta blockers and calcium channel blockers (diltiazem, nifedipine, or verapamil) or disopyramide can lead to heart failure or very low blood pressure.
3. Cimetidine and oral contraceptives (birth control pills) can increase the blood concentrations of propranolol, which can result in greater side effects.
4. Side effects may also be increased when beta blockers are taken with clonidine, digoxin, epinephrine, phenylephrine, phenylpropanolamine, phenothiazine tranquilizers, prazosin, reserpine, or monoamine oxidase (MAO) inhibitors. At least 14 days should separate the use of a beta blocker and an MAO inhibitor.
5. Barbiturates, alcohol, and rifampin can increase the breakdown of propranolol in the body, which can lead to a decrease in its effectiveness.
6. Beta blockers may antagonize (work against) the effects of theophylline, aminophylline, albuterol, isoproterenol, metaproterenol, and terbutaline.
7. Beta blockers can also interact with insulin or oral antidiabetic agents, raising or lowering blood sugar levels or masking the symptoms of low blood sugar.
8. The action of beta blockers may be excessively increased if they are used with chlorpromazine, furosemide, or hydralazine.

BE SURE TO TELL YOUR DOCTOR about any medications you are currently taking, especially any of those listed above.

WARNINGS

• Before starting to take this medication, it is important to tell your doctor if you have ever had unusual or allergic reactions to any beta blocker (acebutolol, atenolol, betaxolol, carteolol, esmolol, labetalol, metoprolol, nadolol, penbutolol, pindolol, propranolol, or timolol).
• Tell your doctor if you now have or if you have ever had allergies, asthma, hay fever, eczema, slow heartbeat, bronchitis, diabetes mellitus, emphysema, heart or blood vessel disease, kidney disease, liver disease, thyroid disease, or poor circulation in the fingers or toes.
• You may want to check your pulse while taking this medication. If your pulse is much slower than your usual rate (or if it is less than 50 beats per minute), check with your doctor. A pulse rate that is too slow may cause circulation problems.
• This medicine may affect your body's response to exercise. Make sure you ask your doctor what an appropriate amount of exercise would be for you, taking into account your medical condition.
• It is important that you do not stop taking this medicine without first checking with your doctor. Some conditions may become worse when the medicine is stopped suddenly, and the danger of a heart attack is increased in some patients. Your doctor may want you to gradually reduce the amount of medicine you take before stopping completely. Make sure that you have enough medicine on hand to last through vacations, holidays, and weekends.
• Before having surgery or any other medical or dental treatment, tell your physician or dentist that you are tak-

ing this medicine. Often, this medication will be discontinued 48 hours prior to any major surgery.

• Propranolol can cause dizziness, drowsiness, lightheadedness, and decreased alertness. Use caution while driving a car or operating dangerous machinery. Be especially careful when going up or down stairs.

• While taking this medicine, do not use any over-the-counter (nonprescription) allergy, asthma, cough, cold, sinus, or diet preparations without first checking with your pharmacist or doctor. The combination of these medicines with a beta blocker can result in high blood pressure.

• Be sure to tell your doctor if you are pregnant. Animal studies have shown that some beta blockers can cause problems in pregnancy when used at very high doses. Adequate studies have not been done in humans, but there has been some association between use of beta blockers during pregnancy and low birth weight, as well as breathing problems and slow heart rate in newborn infants. However, other reports have shown no effects in newborn infants. Also, tell your doctor if you are breast-feeding an infant. Although this medicine has not been shown to cause problems in breast-fed infants, some of the medicine may pass into breast milk, so caution is warranted.

propranolol and hydrochlorothiazide combination

BRAND NAMES (Manufacturers)
Inderide (Wyeth-Ayerst)
Inderide LA (Wyeth-Ayerst)
TYPE OF DRUG
Beta-adrenergic blocking agent and diuretic
INGREDIENTS
propranolol and hydrochlorothiazide
DOSAGE FORMS
Tablets (40 mg propranolol and 25 mg hydrochlorothiazide; 80 mg propranolol and 25 mg hydrochlorothiazide)
Long-acting capsules (80 mg propranolol and 50 mg hydrochlorothiazide; 120 mg propranolol and 50 mg hydrochlorothiazide; and 160 mg propranolol and 50 mg hydrochlorothiazide)
STORAGE
Store at room temperature in a tightly closed, light-resistant container.

USES

This drug is prescribed to treat high blood pressure. Hydrochlorothiazide is a diuretic (water pill), which reduces fluid accumulation in the body by increasing the elimination of salt and water through the kidneys. Propranolol belongs to a group of drugs known as beta-adrenergic blocking agents or, more commonly, beta blockers. They work by controlling nerve impulses along certain nerve pathways.

TREATMENT

This medication can be taken with a glass of water, with meals, immediately following meals, or on an empty stomach (depending on your doctor's instructions).

Try to take the medication at the same time(s) each day. Avoid taking a dose after 6:00 P.M.; otherwise, you may have to get up during the night to urinate.

If you miss a dose of this medication, take the missed dose as soon as possible, unless it is almost time for your next dose. In that case, do not take the missed dose at all; just wait until the next scheduled dose. Do not double the dose.

Propranolol and hydrochlorothiazide combination does not cure high blood pressure, but it will help control the condition as long as you continue to take it.

SIDE EFFECTS

Minor. Anxiety, constipation, cramps, decreased sexual ability, diarrhea, difficulty in sleeping, drowsiness, dizziness, dryness of the eyes and skin, headache, heartburn, loss of appetite, nervousness, stomach discomfort, restlessness, or tiredness. These side effects should disappear as your body adjusts to the medication.

Hydrochlorothiazide can cause increased sensitivity to sunlight. Avoid prolonged exposure to sunlight and sunlamps. Wear protective clothing and use sunscreen.

If you become extra-sensitive to the cold, be sure to dress warmly during cold weather.

To relieve constipation, increase the amount of fiber in your diet (fresh fruits and vegetables, salads, bran, and whole-grain breads) unless your doctor directs you to do otherwise.

Plain, nonmedicated eye drops (artificial tears) may help to relieve eye dryness.

To avoid dizziness or light-headedness when you stand, contract and relax the muscles of your legs for a few moments before rising from a sitting or reclining position. Do this by pushing one foot against the floor while raising the other foot slightly, alternating feet so that you are "pumping" your legs in a pedaling motion.

Major. Tell your doctor about any side effects that are persistent or particularly bothersome. IT IS ESPECIALLY IMPORTANT TO TELL YOUR DOCTOR about blurred vision, cold hands and feet (due to decreased blood circulation to skin, fingers, and toes), confusion, depression, difficulty in breathing, dry mouth, excessive thirst, excessive weakness, fever, hair loss, hallucinations, itching, joint pain, mood changes, muscle spasms, nausea, nightmares, numbness or tingling in the fingers or toes, palpitations, rapid weight gain (three to five pounds within a week), reduced alertness, skin rash, sore throat, swelling, unusual bleeding or bruising, vomiting, or yellowing of the eyes or skin.

INTERACTIONS

This medicine interacts with other types of drugs:
1. Indomethacin, aspirin, and other salicylates may decrease the blood-pressure-lowering effects of beta blockers.
2. Use of propranolol and calcium channel blockers (diltiazem, nifedipine, or verapamil) or disopyramide can lead to heart failure or very low blood pressure.

3. Cimetidine or oral contraceptives (birth control pills) can increase the blood levels of propranolol, which can result in greater side effects. Side effects may also be increased when propranolol is taken with clonidine, digoxin, epinephrine, phenylephrine, phenylpropanolamine, phenothiazine tranquilizers, prazosin, reserpine, or monoamine oxidase (MAO) inhibitors. At least 14 days should separate the use of propranolol and an MAO inhibitor.

4. Barbiturates, alcohol, and rifampin can increase the breakdown of propranolol, which can lead to a decrease in its effectiveness.

5. The action of beta blockers may be increased if they are used with chlorpromazine, furosemide, or hydralazine, which may have a negative effect.

6. Propranolol can antagonize (act against) the effects of theophylline, aminophylline, albuterol, isoproterenol, metaproterenol, and terbutaline.

7. Propranolol can also interact with insulin and oral antidiabetic agents, raising or lowering blood sugar levels and masking the symptoms of low blood sugar.

8. Hydrochlorothiazide can decrease the effectiveness of oral anticoagulants (blood thinners, such as warfarin), antigout medications, and methenamine.

9. Antihypertensive medications may increase the blood-pressure-lowering effects of propranolol and hydrochlorothiazide combination, which can be dangerous.

10. Cholestyramine and colestipol can decrease the absorption of hydrochlorothiazide from the gastrointestinal tract; therefore, hydrochlorothiazide should be taken one hour before or four hours after a dose of cholestyramine or colestipol if one of these medications has also been prescribed for you.

11. Hydrochlorothiazide may increase the side effects of amphotericin B, calcium, cortisone and cortisone-like steroids (such as dexamethasone, hydrocortisone, prednisone, and prednisolone), digoxin, digitoxin, lithium, quinidine, sulfonamide antibiotics, and vitamin D.

TELL YOUR DOCTOR about any medications you are currently taking, especially any of those listed above.

WARNINGS

• Tell your doctor about unusual or allergic reactions you have had to medications, especially to propranolol or any other beta blocker (such as acebutolol, atenolol, betaxolol, carteolol, esmolol, labetalol, metoprolol, nadolol, penbutolol, pindolol, and timolol), to hydrochlorothiazide or other diuretics (such as bendroflumethiazide, benzthiazide, chlorothiazide, chlorthalidone, cyclothiazide, hydroflumethiazide methyclothiazide, metolazone, polythiazide, quinethazone, trichlormethiazide, and furosemide), or to any sulfa drug (oral antidiabetic medication and sulfonamide antibiotic).

• Tell your doctor if you have ever had asthma, diabetes mellitus, heart disease, gout, kidney disease or problems with urination, liver disease, pancreatitis, systemic lupus erythematosus, thyroid disease, or poor circulation in the fingers or toes.

• Hydrochlorothiazide can cause potassium loss. Signs of potassium loss include dry mouth, thirst, weakness, muscle pain or cramps, nausea, and vomiting. If you experience any of these symptoms, call your doctor. To help prevent this problem, your doctor may have blood tests performed periodically to monitor your potassium levels. To help avoid potassium loss, take this medication with a glass of fresh or frozen orange juice or cranberry juice, or eat a banana every day. The use of a salt substitute also helps to prevent potassium loss. Do not change your diet, however, until you discuss it with your doctor. Too much potassium may also be dangerous.

• While you are taking this medication, limit your intake of alcohol, in order to prevent dizziness and light-headedness.

• Do not take any over-the-counter medications for weight control or for allergy, asthma, cough, cold, or sinus problems unless you first check with your doctor.

• To prevent severe water loss (dehydration) while taking this medication, check with your doctor if you have any illness that causes severe or continuous nausea, vomiting, or diarrhea.

• This medication can raise blood sugar levels in diabetic patients. Blood sugar levels should be monitored carefully with blood or urine tests when this medication is being taken.

• You may want to check your pulse while taking this medication. If your pulse is much slower than your usual rate (or if it is less than 50 beats per minute), check with your doctor. A pulse rate that is too slow may cause circulation problems.

• Propranolol can affect your body's response to exercise. Make sure you ask your doctor what an appropriate amount of exercise would be for you, taking into account your medical condition.

• Before having surgery or any other medical or dental treatment, tell your doctor or dentist that you are taking this medicine. Often, this medication will be discontinued 48 hours prior to any major surgery.

• This medication can cause dizziness, drowsiness, light-headedness, or decreased alertness. Therefore, you must exercise caution while driving a car or operating potentially dangerous machinery.

• It is important that you do not stop taking this medicine unless you first check with your doctor. Some conditions worsen when this medicine is stopped suddenly, and the danger of a heart attack is increased in some patients. Your doctor may therefore want you to gradually reduce the amount of medicine you take before stopping completely. Make sure that you have enough medicine on hand to last through vacations, holidays, and weekends.

• A doctor does not usually prescribe a "fixed-dose" drug like this as the first choice in the treatment of high blood pressure. Usually, the patient first receives each ingredient singly. If there is an adequate response to the fixed dose contained in this product, it can then be substituted. The advantage of a combination product is increased convenience and (often) decreased cost.

• Be sure to tell your doctor if you are pregnant. Animal studies have shown that some beta blockers can cause problems in pregnancy when used at very high doses. Adequate studies have not been conducted in humans, but there has been some association between beta blockers used during pregnancy and low birth weight, as well as breathing problems and slow heart rate in newborn infants. However, other reports have shown no such effects in newborn infants. Hydrochlorothiazide has been associated with jaundice, blood problems, and low potassium in the newborn. Also, tell your doctor if you are breast-feeding an infant. Although problems in humans have not been reported, small amounts of propranolol and hydrochlorothiazide pass into breast milk, so caution is warranted.

Prostaphlin—see oxacillin

ProStep—nicotine transdermal patch

Prothazine—see promethazine

Prothazine DC—see promethazine and codeine combination

Protostat—see metronidazole

---

protriptyline

BRAND NAME (Manufacturer)
Vivactil (Merck Sharp & Dohme)
TYPE OF DRUG
Tricyclic antidepressant
INGREDIENT
protriptyline
DOSAGE FORM
Tablets (5 mg and 10 mg)
STORAGE
Store at room temperature in a tightly closed container.

USES
Protriptyline is used to relieve the symptoms of mental depression. This medication belongs to a group of drugs referred to as the tricyclic antidepressants. These medicines are thought to relieve depression by increasing the concentration of certain chemicals necessary for the transmission of nerve impulses in the brain. This drug may also be used in the treatment of certain sleep disorders.

TREATMENT
This medication should be taken exactly as your doctor prescribes. You can take it with water or with food to lessen the chance of stomach irritation, unless your doctor tells you to do otherwise.

If you miss a dose of this medication, take the missed dose as soon as possible, then return to your regular dosing schedule. However, if the dose you missed was a once-a-day bedtime dose, do not take that dose in the morning; check with your doctor instead. If the dose is taken in the morning, it may cause some unwanted side effects. Never double the dose.

The effects of therapy with this medication may not become apparent for two or three weeks.

SIDE EFFECTS
Minor. Anxiety, blurred vision, constipation, cramps, diarrhea, dizziness, drowsiness, dry mouth, fatigue, headache, heartburn, insomnia, loss of appetite, nausea,

peculiar tastes in the mouth, restlessness, sweating, vomiting, weakness, or weight gain or loss. As your body adjusts to the medication, these side effects should disappear.

This medication may increase your sensitivity to sunlight. You should, therefore, avoid prolonged exposure to sunlight and sunlamps. Wear protective clothing, and use an effective sunscreen.

If you experience dry mouth, you should try chewing sugarless gum or sucking on ice chips or a piece of hard candy.

To relieve constipation, increase the amount of fiber in your diet (fresh fruits and vegetables, salads, bran, and whole-grain breads), exercise, and drink more water (unless your doctor directs you to do otherwise).

To avoid dizziness or light-headedness when you stand, contract and relax the muscles of your legs for a few moments before rising. You can accomplish this by pushing one foot against the floor while raising the other foot slightly, alternating feet so that you are ``pumping'' your legs in a pedaling motion.

Major. Tell your doctor about any side effects that are persistent or particularly bothersome. IT IS ESPECIALLY IMPORTANT TO TELL YOUR DOCTOR about agitation, bleeding, chest pain, confusion, convulsions, difficulty in urinating, enlarged or painful breasts (in both sexes), fainting, fever, fluid retention, hair loss, hallucinations, headaches, impotence, mood changes, mouth sores, nervousness, nightmares, nosebleeds, numbness in the fingers or toes, palpitations, ringing in the ears, seizures, skin rash, sleep disorders, sore throat, tremors, uncoordinated movements or balance problems, or yellowing of the eyes or skin.

INTERACTIONS
Protriptyline interacts with a number of other types of medications:

1. Extreme drowsiness can occur when this medicine is taken with central nervous system depressants (medicines that slow the activity of the brain and spinal cord), including alcohol, antihistamines, barbiturates, benzodiazepine tranquilizers, muscle relaxants, narcotics, pain medications, phenothiazine tranquilizers, and sleeping medications, or with other tricyclic antidepressants.

2. Protriptyline may decrease the effectiveness of antiseizure medications and may block the blood-pressure-lowering effects of clonidine and guanethidine.

3. Oral contraceptives (birth control pills) or estrogen-containing drugs can increase the side effects and reduce the effectiveness of tricyclic antidepressants (including protriptyline).

4. Tricyclic antidepressants may increase the side effects of thyroid medication and over-the-counter (nonprescription) cough, cold, allergy, asthma, sinus, and diet medications.

5. The concurrent use of tricyclic antidepressants and monoamine oxidase (MAO) inhibitors should be undertaken very carefully, because the combination may result in fever, convulsions, or high blood pressure.

Before starting to take protriptyline, BE SURE TO TELL YOUR DOCTOR about any medications you are currently taking, especially any of those listed above.

WARNINGS

Tell your doctor if you have had unusual or allergic reactions to any medications, especially to protriptyline or other tricyclic antidepressants (such as amitriptyline, imipramine, doxepin, trimipramine, amoxapine, desipramine, maprotiline, and nortriptyline).

Tell your doctor if you have a history of alcoholism or if you have ever had asthma, high blood pressure, liver or kidney disease, heart disease, a heart attack, circulatory disease, stomach problems, intestinal problems, difficulty in urinating, enlarged prostate gland, epilepsy, glaucoma, thyroid disease, mental illness, or electroshock therapy.

If this drug makes you dizzy or drowsy, do not take part in any activity that requires alertness, such as driving a car or operating potentially dangerous machinery.

Before having surgery or any other medical or dental treatment, be sure to tell your doctor or dentist that you are taking this medication.

Do not stop taking this drug suddenly. Stopping abruptly can cause nausea, headache, stomach upset, fatigue, or a worsening of your condition. Your doctor may want to reduce the dosage gradually.

The effects of this medication may last as long as seven days after you have stopped taking it, so continue to observe all precautions during that period.

Be sure to tell your doctor if you are pregnant. The safe use of this medication in human pregnancy has not been established. Side effects have been observed in the fetuses of animals that received this type of medication in large doses during pregnancy. Also, tell your doctor if you are breast-feeding an infant. Small amounts of this drug can pass into breast milk and may cause unwanted effects, such as irritability or sleeping problems.

Proventil—see albuterol

Provera—see medroxyprogesterone

Prozac—see fluoxetine

Pseudo-Car DM—see pseudoephedrine, carbinoxamine, and dextromethorphan combination

pseudoephedrine and azatadine combination

BRAND NAME (Manufacturer)
Trinalin Repetabs (Schering)
TYPE OF DRUG
Adrenergic (decongestant) and antihistamine
INGREDIENTS
pseudoephedrine and azatadine
DOSAGE FORM
Sustained-release tablets (120 mg pseudoephedrine and 1 mg azatadine)
STORAGE
Pseudoephedrine and azatadine combination tablets should be stored at room temperature in a tightly closed container.

USES

Pseudoephedrine and azatadine combination medication is used to relieve the symptoms of upper respiratory tract infections, hay fever and other allergies, and sinusitis (inflammation of the sinuses).

Pseudoephedrine belongs to a group of drugs known as adrenergic agents (decongestants). They act by constricting (narrowing) blood vessels in the nasal passages to reduce swelling and congestion.

Azatadine belongs to a group of drugs known as antihistamines, which block the action of histamine, a chemical released by the body during an allergic reaction. It is, therefore, used to relieve or prevent symptoms of allergy.

TREATMENT

In order to avoid stomach upset, you can take pseudoephedrine and azatadine combination with food or with a full glass of milk or water unless otherwise directed.

The sustained-release tablets should be swallowed whole. Breaking, chewing, or crushing these tablets destroys their sustained-release activity and may increase the side effects.

If you miss a dose of this medication, take the missed dose as soon as possible, unless it is almost time for your next dose. In that case, do not take the missed dose at all; just return to your regular dosing schedule. Do not double the next dose.

SIDE EFFECTS

Minor. Anxiety; blurred vision; constipation; diarrhea; dizziness; drowsiness; dry mouth, nose, and throat; heartburn; insomnia; irritability; loss of appetite; nasal congestion; nausea; restlessness; decreased sweating; vomiting; or weakness. These side effects should disappear as your body adjusts to the medication.

This medication can increase your sensitivity to sunlight. Avoid prolonged exposure to sunlight and sunlamps.

If you are constipated, increase the amount of fiber in your diet (fresh fruits and vegetables, salads, bran, and whole-grain breads), exercise, and drink more water (unless your doctor directs you to do otherwise).

Chew sugarless gum or suck on ice chips or a piece of hard candy to reduce mouth dryness.

If you feel dizzy or light-headed, sit or lie down for a while; get up slowly from a sitting or reclining position, and be careful on stairs.

In order to avoid difficulty in falling asleep, take this medication several hours before bedtime.

Major. Tell your doctor about any side effects that are persistent or particularly bothersome. TELL YOUR DOCTOR about chest pain, confusion, convulsions, difficult or painful urination, difficulty in breathing, fainting, hallucinations, headaches, loss of coordination, mood changes, nosebleeds, palpitations, rash, severe abdominal pain, sore throat, or unusual bleeding or bruising.

INTERACTIONS

Pseudoephedrine and azatadine combination can interact with several other types of medications:

1. Concurrent use of this medication with central nervous system depressants (drugs that slow the activity of the brain and spinal cord), such as alcohol, barbiturates, benzodiazepine tranquilizers, muscle relaxants, narcotics, pain medications, and phenothiazine tranquilizers, or with tricyclic antidepressants can cause extreme drowsiness.

2. Monoamine oxidase (MAO) inhibitors (isocarboxazid, pargyline, phenelzine, or tranylcypromine) and tricyclic antidepressants can increase the side effects of this drug. At least 14 days should separate the use of this drug and the use of an MAO inhibitor.

3. The action of oral anticoagulants (blood thinners) may be decreased by the antihistamine component of this drug.

4. Procarbazine may interact with the antihistamine component of this drug.

5. The side effects of the antihistamine component of this medication may be increased by quinidine, procainamide, haloperidol, and phenothiazine tranquilizers.

6. The side effects of the decongestant component of this drug may be increased by digoxin or over-the-counter asthma, allergy, cough, cold, diet, or sinus preparations.

7. The blood-pressure-lowering effects of guanethidine may be decreased by this medication.

TELL YOUR DOCTOR about any medications you are currently taking.

WARNINGS

• Tell your doctor about unusual or allergic reactions you have had to any medications, especially to azatadine or other antihistamines (such as brompheniramine, carbinoxamine, chlorpheniramine, clemastine, cyproheptadine, dexchlorpheniramine, dimenhydrinate, dimethindene, diphenhydramine, diphenylpyraline, doxylamine, hydroxyzine, promethazine, pyrilamine, trimeprazine, tripelennamine, and triprolidine) or to pseudoephedrine or other adrenergic agents (such as albuterol, amphetamines, ephedrine, epinephrine, isoproterenol, metaproterenol, norepinephrine, phenylpropanolamine, and terbutaline).

• Be sure to tell your doctor if you now have or if you have ever had diabetes mellitus, epilepsy, glaucoma, heart or blood vessel disease, hiatal hernia, high blood pressure, myasthenia gravis, obstructed bladder or intestinal tract, peptic ulcers, enlarged prostate gland, or thyroid disease.

• This drug can reduce sweating and heat release from the body. Be sure to avoid excessive work and exercise in hot weather, and do not take hot baths, showers, and saunas.

• This medication can cause drowsiness. Your ability to perform tasks that require alertness, such as driving a car or operating potentially dangerous machinery, may be decreased. Appropriate caution should, therefore, be taken.

• Be sure to tell your doctor if you are pregnant. The effects of this medication during pregnancy have not been thoroughly studied in humans. Also, be sure to tell your doctor if you are currently breast-feeding an infant. Small amounts of this medication pass into breast milk and may cause unusual excitement or irritability in nursing infants.

pseudoephedrine and carbinoxamine combination

BRAND NAMES (Manufacturers)
Carbodec (Rugby)
Cardec-S (various manufacturers)
Rondec (Ross)
TYPE OF DRUG
Adrenemine
INGREDIENTS
pseudoephedrine and carbinoxamine
DOSAGE FORMS
Tablets (60 mg pseudoephedrine and 4 mg carbinoxamine)
Oral syrup (60 mg pseudoephedrine and 4 mg carbinoxamine per 5-ml spoonful)
Oral drops (25 mg pseudoephedrine and 2 mg carbinoxamine per ml)
STORAGE
Pseudoephedrine and carbinoxamine combination tablets, oral syrup, and oral drops should be stored at room temperature in tightly closed containers. No form of this medication should ever be frozen.

USES

This drug combination is used to relieve symptoms of upper respiratory tract infections, hay fever and other allergies, and sinusitis (inflammation of the sinuses).

Pseudoephedrine belongs to a group of drugs known as adrenergic agents (decongestants). They act by constricting (narrowing) blood vessels in the nasal passages to reduce swelling and congestion.

Carbinoxamine belongs to a group of drugs known as antihistamines, which block the actions of histamine, a chemical released by the body during an allergic reaction. It is, therefore, used to relieve or prevent symptoms of allergy.

TREATMENT

In order to avoid stomach upset, you can take pseudoephedrine and carbinoxamine combination with food or with a full glass of water (unless your doctor directs you to do otherwise).

The oral drops should be measured carefully with the dropper provided.

The oral syrup form of this medication should be measured carefully with a specially designed 5-ml measuring spoon.

If you miss a dose of this medication, take the missed dose as soon as possible, unless it is almost time for your next dose. In that case, do not take the missed dose at all; just return to your regular dosing schedule. Do not double the next dose.

SIDE EFFECTS

Minor. Anxiety; blurred vision; constipation; diarrhea; dizziness; drowsiness; dry mouth, nose, and throat; heartburn; insomnia; irritability; loss of appetite; nasal congestion; nausea; restlessness; decreased sweating; vomiting; or weakness. These side effects should disappear as your body adjusts to the medication.

This medication can increase your sensitivity to sunlight. You should, therefore, avoid prolonged exposure to sunlight and sunlamps. Wear protective clothing, and use an effective sunscreen.

If you are constipated, increase the amount of fiber in your diet (fresh fruits and vegetables, salads, bran, and whole-grain breads), exercise, and drink more water (unless your doctor directs you to do otherwise).

Chew sugarless gum or suck on ice chips or a piece of hard candy to reduce mouth dryness.

If you feel dizzy or light-headed, sit or lie down for a while; get up slowly from a sitting or reclining position, and be careful on stairs.

In order to avoid difficulty in falling asleep, take the last dose of this medication several hours before bedtime.

Major. Tell your doctor about any side effects that are persistent or particularly bothersome. IT IS ESPECIALLY IMPORTANT TO TELL YOUR DOCTOR about chest pain, confusion, convulsions, difficult or painful urination, difficulty in breathing, fainting, hallucinations, headaches, loss of coordination, mood changes, nosebleeds, palpitations, rash, severe abdominal pain, sore throat, or unusual bleeding or bruising.

INTERACTIONS

Pseudoephedrine and carbinoxamine combination interacts with several other types of medications:

1. Concurrent use of it with central nervous system depressants (drugs that slow the activity of the brain and spinal cord), such as alcohol, barbiturates, benzodiazepine tranquilizers, muscle relaxants, narcotics, pain medications, and phenothiazine tranquilizers, or with tricyclic antidepressants can cause extreme drowsiness.

2. Monoamine oxidase (MAO) inhibitors (isocarboxazid, pargyline, phenelzine, or tranylcypromine) and tricyclic antidepressants can increase the side effects of this drug. At least 14 days should separate the use of this drug and the use of an MAO inhibitor.

3. The action of oral anticoagulants may be decreased by the antihistamine component of this drug.

4. Procarbazine may interact with the antihistamine component of this drug.

5. The side effects of the antihistamine component of this medication may be increased by quinidine, procainamide, haloperidol, and phenothiazine tranquilizers.

6. The side effects of the decongestant component of this drug may be increased by digoxin or over-the-counter asthma, allergy, cough, cold, diet, or sinus preparations.

7. The blood-pressure-lowering effects of guanethidine may be decreased by this medication.

BE SURE TO TELL YOUR DOCTOR about any medications you are currently taking, especially any listed above.

WARNINGS

• Tell your doctor about unusual or allergic reactions you have had to any medications, especially to carbinoxamine or other antihistamines (such as azatadine, chlorpheniramine, clemastine, cyproheptadine, dexchlorpheniramine, dimenhydrinate, dimethindene, diphenhydramine, diphenylpyraline, doxylamine, hydroxyzine, promethazine, pyrilamine, trimeprazine, tripelennamine, and triprolidine) or to pseudoephedrine or other adrenergic agents (such as albuterol, amphetamines, ephedrine, epinephrine, isoproterenol, metaproterenol, norepinephrine, phenylpropanolamine, and terbutaline).

• Tell your doctor if you now have or if you have ever had diabetes mellitus, epilepsy, glaucoma, heart or blood vessel disease, hiatal hernia, high blood pressure, myasthenia gravis, obstructed bladder or intestinal tract, peptic ulcers, enlarged prostate gland, or thyroid disease.

• Because this drug can reduce sweating and heat release from the body, you should avoid excessive work and exercise in hot weather, and do not take hot baths, showers, and saunas.

• This medication can cause drowsiness. Your ability to perform tasks that require alertness, such as driving a car or operating potentially dangerous machinery, may be decreased. Appropriate caution should be taken.

• Be sure to tell your doctor if you are pregnant. The effects of this medication during pregnancy have not been thoroughly studied in humans. Also, tell your doctor if you are breast-feeding an infant. Small amounts of this medication pass into breast milk and may cause unusual excitement or irritability in nursing infants.

pseudoephedrine and chlorpheniramine combination

BRAND NAMES (Manufacturers)
Anamine T.D. (Mayrand)
Brexin L.A. (Savage)
Chlorafed (Half-Strength) (Hauck)
Chlorafed HS Timecelles (Hauck)
Chlor-Trimeton Decongestant* (Schering)
Chlor-Trimeton Decongestant Repetabs* (Schering)
Codimal-L.A. (Central)
Dallergy-D* (Laser)
Deconamine (Berlex)
Deconamine SR (Berlex)
Dorcol Children's Liquid Cold Formula* (Sandoz)
Duralex (American Urologicals)
Fedahist* (Kremers Urban)
Histalet (Reid-Rowell)
Isoclor (Fisons)
Isoclor Timesules* (Fisons)
Kronofed-A Jr. (Ferndale)
Kronofed-A Kronocaps (Ferndale)
Myfedrine Plus* (P.B.I.)
Napril* (Randob)
ND Clear T.D. (Seatrace)
Novafed A (Lakeside)
PediaCare 2 Liquid (McNeil Consumer)
Pseudo-Hist* (Abana)
Ryna* (Wallace)
Sudafed Plus* (Burroughs Wellcome)
T-Dry Jr (T.E. Williams)
*Available over-the-counter (without a prescription)

TYPE OF DRUG
Adrenergic (decongestant) and antihistamine

INGREDIENTS
Pseudoephedrine and chlorpheniramine
DOSAGE FORMS
Tablets (30 mg pseudoephedrine and 4 mg chlorpheniramine; 60 mg pseudoephedrine and 4 mg chlorpheniramine)

Capsules (30 mg pseudoephedrine and 4 mg chlorpheniramine; 30 mg pseudoephedrine and 2 mg chlorpheniramine)

Sustained-release capsules (60 mg pseudoephedrine and 4 mg chlorpheniramine; 65 mg pseudoephedrine and 10 mg chlorpheniramine; 120 mg pseudoephedrine and 8 mg chlorpheniramine; and 120 mg pseudoephedrine and 12 mg chlorpheniramine)

Oral elixir (30 mg pseudoephedrine and 2 mg chlorpheniramine per 5-ml spoonful, with 5% alcohol)

Oral syrup (15 mg pseudoephedrine and 1 mg chlorpheniramine; 15 mg pseudoephedrine and 2 mg chlorpheniramine; 30 mg pseudoephedrine and 2 mg chlorpheniramine; and 45 mg pseudoephedrine and 3 mg chlorpheniramine per 5-ml spoonful)
STORAGE
Pseudoephedrine and chlorpheniramine combination tablets, capsules, elixir, and syrup should be stored at room temperature in tightly closed containers. This medication should never be frozen.

USES
This drug combination is used to relieve the symptoms of upper respiratory tract infections, hay fever and other allergies, and sinusitis (inflammation of the sinuses).

Pseudoephedrine belongs to a group of drugs known as adrenergic agents (decongestants). They act by constricting (narrowing) blood vessels in the nasal passages to reduce swelling and congestion.

Chlorpheniramine belongs to a group of drugs known as antihistamines, which block the actions of histamine, a chemical released by the body during an allergic reaction. It is, therefore, used to relieve or prevent symptoms of allergy.

TREATMENT
In order to avoid stomach upset, you can take pseudoephedrine and chlorpheniramine combination with food or with a full glass of milk or water (unless your doctor directs you to do otherwise).

The oral syrup and elixir forms of this drug should be measured with a specially designed 5-ml measuring spoon.

The sustained-release capsules should be swallowed whole. Breaking, chewing, or crushing these capsules destroys their sustained-release activity and may increase the side effects.

If you miss a dose of this medication, take the missed dose as soon as possible, unless it is almost time for your next dose. In that case, do not take the missed dose at all; just return to your regular dosing schedule. Do not double the next dose.

SIDE EFFECTS
Minor. Anxiety; blurred vision; constipation; diarrhea; dizziness; drowsiness; dry mouth, nose, and throat; heartburn; insomnia; irritability; loss of appetite; nasal congestion; nausea; restlessness; decreased sweating; vomiting; or weakness. These side effects should gradually disappear as your body adjusts to this medication.

This medication can increase your sensitivity to sunlight. You should therefore avoid prolonged exposure to sunlight and sunlamps. Wear protective clothing, and use an effective sunscreen.

If you are constipated, increase the amount of fiber in your diet (fresh fruits and vegetables, salads, bran, and whole-grain breads), exercise, and drink more water (unless your doctor directs you to do otherwise).

Chew sugarless gum or suck on ice chips or a piece of hard candy to reduce mouth dryness.

If you feel dizzy or light-headed, sit or lie down for a while; get up slowly from a sitting or reclining position.

In order to avoid difficulty in falling asleep, take the last dose of this drug several hours before bedtime.

Major. Tell your doctor about any side effects that are persistent or particularly bothersome. IT IS ESPECIALLY IMPORTANT TO TELL YOUR DOCTOR about chest pain, confusion, convulsions, difficult or painful urination, difficulty in breathing, fainting, hallucinations, headaches, loss of coordination, mood changes, palpitations, rash, severe abdominal pain, sore throat, or unusual bleeding or bruising.

INTERACTIONS
Pseudoephedrine and chlorpheniramine combination interacts with several other types of medications:

1. Concurrent use of this medication with central nervous system depressants (drugs that slow the activity of the brain and spinal cord), such as alcohol, barbiturates, benzodiazepine tranquilizers, muscle relaxants, narcotics, pain medications, and phenothiazine tranquilizers, or with tricyclic antidepressants can cause extreme drowsiness.

2. Monoamine oxidase (MAO) inhibitors (isocarboxazid, pargyline, phenelzine, or tranylcypromine) and tricyclic antidepressants can increase the side effects of this medication. At least 14 days should separate the use of this drug and the use of an MAO inhibitor.

3. The action of oral anticoagulants may be decreased by the antihistamine component of this drug.

4. Procarbazine may interact with the antihistamine component of this drug.

5. The side effects of the antihistamine component of this medication may be increased by quinidine, procainamide, haloperidol, or phenothiazine tranquilizers.

6. The side effects of the decongestant component may be increased by digoxin or over-the-counter (nonprescription) asthma, allergy, cough, cold, diet, or sinus preparations.

7. The blood-pressure-lowering effects of guanethidine may be decreased by this medication.

BE SURE TO TELL YOUR DOCTOR about any medications you are currently taking, especially any listed above.

WARNINGS
• Tell your doctor about unusual or allergic reactions you have had to any medications, especially to chlor-

pheniramine or to other antihistamines (such as azata-dine, brompheniramine, carbinoxamine, clemastine, cyproheptadine, dexchlorpheniramine, dimenhydrinate, dimethindene, diphenhydramine, diphenylpyraline, doxylamine, hydroxyzine, promethazine, pyrilamine, trimeprazine, tripelennamine, and triprolidine) or to pseudoephedrine or other adrenergic agents (such as albuterol, amphetamines, ephedrine, epinephrine, isoproterenol, metaproterenol, norepinephrine, phenylpropanolamine, and terbutaline).
• Tell your doctor if you now have or if you have ever had diabetes mellitus, epilepsy, glaucoma, heart or blood vessel disease, hiatal hernia, high blood pressure, myasthenia gravis, obstructed bladder or intestinal tract, peptic ulcers, enlarged prostate gland, or thyroid disease.
• Because this drug can reduce sweating and heat release from the body, you should avoid excessive work or exercise in hot weather, and do not take hot baths, showers, and saunas.
• Pseudoephedrine and chlorpheniramine combination can cause drowsiness. Your ability to perform tasks that require alertness, such as driving a car or operating potentially dangerous machinery.
• Be sure to tell your doctor if you are pregnant. The effects of this medication during pregnancy have not been thoroughly studied in humans. Also, tell your doctor if you are breast-feeding an infant. Small amounts of this medication pass into breast milk and may cause unusual excitement or irritability in nursing infants.

pseudoephedrine, carbinoxamine, and dextromethorphan combination

BRAND NAMES (Manufacturers)
Carbodec DM (Rugby)
Cardec DM (various manufacturers)
Mycadec DM (My-K Labs)
Pseudo-Car DM (Geneva Generics)
Rondec-DM (Ross)
Tussafed (Everett)
TYPE OF DRUG
Adrenergic (decongestant), antihistamine, and cough suppressant
INGREDIENTS
pseudoephedrine, carbinoxamine, and dextromethorphan
DOSAGE FORMS
Oral syrup (60 mg pseudoephedrine, 4 mg carbinoxamine, and 15 mg dextromethorphan per 5-ml spoonful)
Oral drops (25 mg pseudoephedrine, 2 mg carbinoxamine, and 4 mg dextromethorphan per 1-ml dropperful)
STORAGE
Pseudoephedrine, carbinoxamine, and dextromethorphan combination oral syrup and oral drops should be stored at room temperature in a tightly closed, light-resistant glass container. Avoid exposing these medications to excessive heat.

USES
This drug combination is used to relieve coughs and the symptoms of upper respiratory tract infections, hay fever and other allergies, and sinusitis (inflammation of the sinuses).
Pseudoephedrine belongs to a group of drugs known as adrenergic agents (decongestants). They act by constricting (narrowing) blood vessels in the nasal passages to reduce swelling and congestion.
Carbinoxamine belongs to a group of drugs known as antihistamines, which block the actions of histamine, a chemical released by the body during an allergic reaction. It is, therefore, used to relieve or prevent symptoms of allergy.
Dextromethorphan is a cough suppressant, which acts at the cough reflex center in the brain.

TREATMENT
In order to avoid stomach upset, you can take this medicine with food or with a full glass of water (unless your doctor directs you to do otherwise).
The oral drops should be measured carefully with the dropper provided. The oral syrup should be measured carefully with a specially designed 5-ml measuring spoon. An ordinary kitchen teaspoon is not accurate enough.
If you miss a dose of this medication, take the missed dose as soon as possible, unless it is almost time for your next dose. In that case, do not take the missed dose at all; just return to your regular dosing schedule. Do not double the next dose.

SIDE EFFECTS
Minor. Abdominal pain, blurred vision, decreased sweating, diarrhea, dizziness, drowsiness, dry mouth, headache, heartburn, loss of appetite, nausea, nervousness, sleeping problems, vomiting, or weakness. These side effects should disappear as your body adjusts to the medication.
Chew sugarless gum or suck on ice chips or hard candy to reduce mouth dryness.
If you feel dizzy or light-headed, sit or lie down for a while; get up slowly from a sitting or reclining position, and be careful on stairs.
This medication can increase your sensitivity to sunlight. Avoid prolonged exposure to sunlight and sunlamps. Wear protective clothing, and use an effective sunscreen.
In order to avoid difficulty in falling asleep, you should take the last dose of this medication several hours before bedtime.
Major. Tell your doctor about any side effects that are persistent or particularly bothersome, especially chest pain, difficult or painful urination, difficulty in breathing, hallucinations, pallor, palpitations, seizures, or tremors.

INTERACTIONS
This medication can interact with several types of drugs:
1. Concurrent use of it with central nervous system depressants (drugs that slow the activity of the brain and spinal cord), such as alcohol, barbiturates, benzodiazepine tranquilizers, muscle relaxants, narcotics, pain medications, and phenothiazine tranquilizers, or with tricyclic antidepressants can cause extreme drowsiness.

2. Monoamine oxidase (MAO) inhibitors (isocarboxazid, pargyline, phenelzine, or tranylcypromine), beta blockers (acebutolol, atenolol, betaxolol, carteolol, esmolol, labetalol, metoprolol, nadolol, penbutolol, pindolol, propranolol, or timolol), and tricyclic antidepressants can increase the side effects of this drug. At least 14 days should separate the use of this drug and the use of an MAO inhibitor.

3. The side effects of the antihistamine part of this medication may be increased by quinidine, procainamide, haloperidol, and phenothiazine tranquilizers.

4. The side effects of the decongestant component may be increased by digoxin or over-the-counter (nonprescription) asthma, allergy, cough, cold, diet, or sinus preparations.

5. The blood-pressure-lowering effects of guanethidine, methyldopa, and reserpine may be decreased by this drug.

Before starting pseudoephedrine, carbinoxamine, and dextromethorphan combination, TELL YOUR DOCTOR about any medications you are curently taking.

WARNINGS

• Tell your doctor about unusual or allergic reactions you have had to any medications, especially to carbinoxamine or other antihistamines (such as azatadine, chlorpheniramine, clemastine, cyproheptadine, dexchlorpheniramine, dimenhydrinate, dimethindene, diphenhydramine, diphenylpyraline, doxylamine, hydroxyzine, promethazine, pyrilamine, trimeprazine, tripelennamine, and triprolidine), to pseudoephedrine or other adrenergic agents (such as albuterol, amphetamines, ephedrine, epinephrine, isoproterenol, metaproterenol, norepinephrine, phenylpropanolamine, and terbutaline), or to dextromethorphan.

• Tell your doctor if you have ever had diabetes mellitus, glaucoma, heart or blood vessel disease, high blood pressure, myasthenia gravis, obstructed bladder or intestinal tract, peptic ulcers, enlarged prostate, or thyroid disease.

• Because this drug can reduce sweating and heat release from the body, avoid excessive work and exercise in hot weather, and do not take hot baths, showers, and saunas.

• This medication can cause drowsiness. Your ability to perform tasks that require alertness.

•Tell your doctor if you are pregnant. The safe use of this drug in human pregnancy has not been established. Also, tell your doctor if you are breast-feeding an infant. Small amounts of this medication pass into breast milk and may cause unusual excitement or irritability in nursing infants.

pseudoephedrine, triprolidine, and codeine combination

BRAND NAMES (Manufacturers)
Actagen-C Cough Syrup (Goldline)
Actifed with Codeine (Burroughs Wellcome)
Allerfrin with Codeine (Rugby)

Triacin-C (various manufacturers)
Trifed-C (Geneva Generics)

TYPE OF DRUG
Adrenergic (decongestant), antihistamine, and cough suppressant

INGREDIENTS
pseudoephedrine, triprolidine, and codeine

DOSAGE FORM
Oral syrup (30 mg pseudoephedrine, 1.25 mg triprolidine, and 10 mg codeine per 5-ml spoonful, with 4.3% alcohol)

STORAGE
This medication should be stored at room temperature (never frozen) in a tightly closed container.

USES
It is used to provide symptomatic relief of coughs due to colds, minor upper respiratory infections, and allergy.

Pseudoephedrine belongs to a group of drugs known as adrenergic agents (decongestants). They act by constricting (narrowing) blood vessels in the nasal passages, thereby reducing swelling and congestion.

Triprolidine belongs to a group of drugs known as antihistamines, which block the action of histamine, a chemical released by the body during an allergic reaction. It is used to relieve or prevent symptoms of allergy.

Codeine is a narcotic cough suppressant, which acts at the cough reflex center in the brain.

TREATMENT
To avoid stomach upset, you can take this medication with food or with a full glass of milk or water (unless your doctor directs you to do otherwise).

The oral syrup should be measured carefully with a specially designed 5-ml measuring spoon. An ordinary kitchen teaspoon is not accurate enough.

If you miss a dose of this medication, take the missed dose as soon as possible, unless it is almost time for your next dose. In that case, do not take the missed dose at all; just return to your regular dosing schedule. Do not double the next dose.

SIDE EFFECTS
Minor. Blurred vision; constipation; diarrhea; dizziness; dry mouth, throat, or nose; irritability; loss of appetite; nausea; restlessness; stomach upset; unusual increase in sweating; or vomiting. These side effects should disappear as your body adjusts to the medication.

This medication can cause increased sensitivity to sunlight. It is, therefore, important to avoid prolonged exposure to sunlight and sunlamps.

If you are constipated, increase the amount of fiber in your diet (fresh fruits and vegetables, salads, bran, and whole-grain breads), exercise, and drink more water (unless your doctor directs you to do otherwise).

Chew sugarless gum or suck on ice chips or a piece of hard candy to reduce mouth dryness.

If you feel dizzy or light-headed, sit or lie down for a while.

Major. Tell your doctor about any side effects that are persistent or particularly bothersome. IT IS ESPECIALLY IMPORTANT TO TELL YOUR DOCTOR about chest pain, confusion, difficult or painful urination, feeling faint, headaches, palpitations, rash, ringing or buzzing in the ears, severe abdominal pain, sore throat, or unusual bleeding or bruising.

INTERACTIONS

This medicine interacts with several other types of drugs:
1. Concurrent use of it with other central nervous system depressants (drugs that slow the activity of the brain and spinal cord), such as alcohol, barbiturates, benzodiazepine tranquilizers, muscle relaxants, narcotics, pain medications, and phenothiazine tranquilizers, or with tricyclic antidepressants can cause extreme drowsiness.
2. Monoamine oxidase (MAO) inhibitors (isocarboxazid, pargyline, phenelzine, or tranylcypromine) and tricyclic antidepressants can increase the side effects of this medication. At least 14 days should separate the use of this drug and the use of an MAO inhibitor.
3. The action of oral anticoagulants may be decreased by the antihistamine component of this drug.
4. Procarbazine may interact with the antihistamine component of this drug.
5. The side effects of the antihistamine component of this medication may be increased by quinidine, procainamide, haloperidol, or phenothiazine tranquilizers.
6. The blood-pressure-lowering effects of guanethidine, methyldopa, and reserpine may be decreased by this medication.
7. The side effects of the decongestant component of this medication may be increased by digoxin or over-the-counter (nonprescription) allergy, asthma, cough, cold, diet, or sinus preparations.

BE SURE TO TELL YOUR DOCTOR about any medications you are currently taking, especially any of those listed above.

WARNINGS

• Tell your doctor about unusual or allergic reactions you have had to any medications, especially to triprolidine or other antihistamines (such as azatadine, brompheniramine, carbinoxamine, clemastine, cyproheptadine, chlorpheniramine, dexbrompheniramine, dimenhydrinate, dimethindene, diphenhydramine, diphenylpyraline, doxylamine, hydroxyzine, promethazine, pyrilamine, trimeprazine, and tripelennamine), to pseudoephedrine or other adrenergic agents (such as albuterol, amphetamines, ephedrine, epinephrine, isoproterenol, metaproterenol, norepinephrine, phenylephrine, phenylpropanolamine, and terbutaline), or to codeine or any other narcotic cough suppressant or pain medication.
• Tell your doctor if you now have or if you have ever had asthma, brain disease, blockage of the urinary or digestive tract, diabetes mellitus, colitis, gallbladder disease, glaucoma, heart or blood vessel disease, high blood pressure, kidney disease, liver disease, lung disease, peptic ulcers, enlarged prostate gland, or thyroid disease.
• This medicine can cause drowsiness. Exercise caution while performing tasks that require alertness, such as driving a car or operating potentially dangerous machinery.
• While you are taking this medication, drink at least eight glasses of water a day to help loosen bronchial secretions.

• Because this product contains codeine, it has the potential for abuse and must be used with caution. Usually, it should not be taken on a regular schedule for longer than ten days at a time. Tolerance develops quickly; do not increase the dosage or stop taking the drug abruptly, unless you first consult your doctor. If you have been taking large amounts of this medication, or if you have been taking it for long periods of time, you may experience a withdrawal reaction (muscle aches, diarrhea, gooseflesh, runny nose, nausea, vomiting, shivering, trembling, stomach cramps, sleep disorders, irritability, weakness, excessive yawning, or sweating) when you stop taking it. Your doctor may, therefore, want to reduce the dosage gradually.
• Before surgery or other medical or dental treatment, it is very important to tell your doctor or dentist you are taking this drug.
• Tell your doctor if you are pregnant. The effects of this drug during the early stages of pregnancy have not been thoroughly studied in humans. However, the regular use of codeine during the later stages of pregnancy may lead to addiction of the fetus, resulting in withdrawal symptoms (irritability, excessive crying, tremors, fever, vomiting, diarrhea, sneezing, or excessive yawning) in the newborn. Also, tell your doctor if you are breast-feeding. Small amounts of this drug pass into breast milk and may cause unusual excitement or irritability in nursing infants.

Pseudo-Hist—see pseudoephedrine and chlorpheniramine combination

Pyridamole—see dipyridamole

Pyridiate—see phenazopyridine

Pyridium—see phenazopyridine

Questran—see cholestyramine

Questran Light—see cholestyramine

Quibron-T—see theophylline

Quiagen—see theophylline and guaifenesin combination

Quibron—see theophylline and guaifenesin combination

Quibron 300—see theophylline and guaifenesin combination

Quinaglute Dura-Tabs—see quinidine

Quinatime—see quinidine

Quinidex Extentabs—see quinidine

quinidine

BRAND NAMES (Manufacturers)
Cardioquin (Purdue Frederick)
Cin-Quin (Reid-Rowell)

Duraquin (Parke-Davis)
Quinaglute Dura-Tabs (Berlex)
Quinatime (CMC)
Quinidex Extentabs (Robins)
quinidine gluconate (various manufacturers)
quinidine sulfate (various manufacturers)
Quinora (Key)
Quin-Release (Major)

TYPE OF DRUG

Antiarrhythmic

INGREDIENT

quinidine

DOSAGE FORMS

Tablets (100 mg, 200 mg, 275 mg, and 300 mg)
Sustained-release tablets (300 mg, 324 mg, and 330 mg)
Capsules (200 mg and 300 mg)

STORAGE

Quinidine tablets and capsules should be stored at room temperature in tightly closed, light-resistant containers.

USES

Quinidine is used to treat heart arrhythmias. It corrects irregular heartbeats and helps to achieve a more normal rhythm.

TREATMENT

To increase absorption of the drug, take quinidine on an empty stomach with a full glass of water one hour before or two hours after a meal. To lessen stomach upset, ask your doctor if you can take it with food or milk.

Take it at the same time(s) each day. Quinidine works best when the amount in your bloodstream is kept constant. This medication should, therefore, be taken at evenly spaced intervals day and night. For example, if you take quinidine four times per day, the doses should be six hours apart.

The sustained-release tablets should be swallowed whole.

If you miss a dose of this medication and remember within two hours, take the missed dose immediately and then return to your regular dosing schedule. If more than two hours have passed (four hours for the sustained-release tablets), do not take the missed dose at all; just return to your regular dosing schedule. Do not double the next dose.

SIDE EFFECTS

Minor. Abdominal pain, bitter taste in mouth, confusion, cramping, diarrhea, flushing, headache, loss of appetite, nausea, restlessness, or vomiting. These side effects should disappear as your body adjusts to the medication.

Major. Tell your doctor about any side effects that are persistent or particularly bothersome. IT IS ESPECIALLY IMPORTANT TO TELL YOUR DOCTOR about blurred vision, difficulty in breathing, dizziness, fainting, fever, headache, light-headedness, palpitations, rash, ringing in the ears, sore throat, or unusual bleeding or bruising.

INTERACTIONS

Quinidine interacts with several foods and medications:
1. It can increase the effects of warfarin, which can lead to bleeding complications.

2. Acetazolamide, cimetidine, thiazide diuretics (water pills), sodium bicarbonate, antacids, and citrus fruit juices can increase the blood levels and thus the possibility of side effects of quinidine.
3. Nifedipine, phenobarbital, phenytoin, and rifampin can decrease blood levels of quinidine.
4. The combination of quinidine and phenothiazine tranquilizers, reserpine, nifedipine, amiodarone, or other antiarrhythmic agents can lead to cardiac side effects that can be very harmful.
5. Quinidine can increase blood levels of digoxin, leading to serious side effects.

BE SURE TO TELL YOUR DOCTOR about any medications you are currently taking, especially any listed above.

WARNINGS

• Tell your doctor about unusual or allergic reactions you have had to any drugs, especially to quinidine or quinine.

• Before starting to take this medication, be sure to tell your doctor if you have ever had heart block, hypokalemia (low blood levels of potassium), kidney disease, liver disease, lung disease, myasthenia gravis, psoriasis, or thyroid disease.

• Although many quinidine products are on the market, they are not all bioequivalent; that is, they may not all be absorbed into the bloodstream at the same rate or have the same overall pharmacologic activity. Do not change brands of this drug without consulting your doctor or pharmacist.

• Do not take any over-the-counter (nonprescription) products for asthma, allergy, sinus, cough, cold, or weight reduction unless you first check with your doctor or pharmacist.

• If this drug makes you dizzy or light-headed, do not take part in any activity that requires alertness, such as driving a car or operating potentially dangerous machinery.

• Before having surgery or other medical or dental treatment, tell your doctor or dentist you are currently taking this medication.

• Do not stop taking this drug without first consulting your doctor. Stopping quinidine abruptly may cause a serious change in the activity of your heart. Your doctor may, therefore, want to reduce your dosage gradually.

• Be sure to tell your doctor if you are pregnant. Although this drug appears to be safe, extensive studies in pregnant women have not been conducted. Also, tell your doctor if you are breast-feeding an infant. Small amounts of quinidine pass into breast milk.

quinidine gluconate—see quinidine

quinidine sulfate—see quinidine

Quinora—see quinidine

Quin-Release—see quinidine

Racet—see hydrocortisone and iodochlorhydroxyquin combination (topical)

ranitidine

BRAND NAMES (Manufacturers)
Zantac (Glaxo)
Zantac (Roche)
TYPE OF DRUG
Gastric acid secretion inhibitor (decreases stomach acid)
INGREDIENT
ranitidine
DOSAGE FORMS
Tablets (150 mg and 300 mg)
Oral syrup (15 mg per ml)
STORAGE
Ranitidine should be stored at room temperature in a tightly closed, light-resistant container.

USES

Ranitidine is used to treat duodenal and gastric ulcers. It is also used in the long-term treatment of excessive stomach acid secretion, in the prevention of recurrent ulcers, and in the treatment of reflex esophagitis (inflammation of the esophagus). Ranitidine works by blocking the effects of histamine on the stomach, thereby reducing stomach acid secretion.

TREATMENT

You can take ranitidine either on an empty stomach or with food or milk.

Antacids can block the absorption of ranitidine. If you are taking antacids as well as ranitidine, at least one hour should separate doses of the two medications.

If you miss a dose of this medication, take the missed dose as soon as possible, unless it is almost time for the next dose. In that case, do not take the missed dose at all; just return to your regular dosing schedule. Do not double the next dose.

SIDE EFFECTS

Minor. Constipation, diarrhea, dizziness, headache, nausea, or stomach upset. These side effects should disappear as your body adjusts to the medication.

To relieve constipation, exercise and drink more water (unless your doctor directs you to do otherwise).

If you feel dizzy while taking this medication, sit or lie down for a while.
Major. Tell your doctor about any side effects that are persistent or particularly bothersome. IT IS ESPECIALLY IMPORTANT TO TELL YOUR DOCTOR about confusion, decreased sexual ability, unusual bleeding or bruising, or weakness.

INTERACTIONS

Ranitidine can interact with other types of medications:
1. Ranitidine may increase the blood-sugar-lowering effects of glipizide.
2. Ranitidine can decrease the elimination of warfarin from the body, which can increase the risk of bleeding complications.
3. Ranitidine can increase blood levels of procainamide.
4. Ranitidine may cause a false positive result with the Multistix urine protein test.

BE SURE TO TELL YOUR DOCTOR about any medications you are currently taking, especially any listed above.

WARNINGS

• Tell your doctor about unusual or allergic reactions you have had to any medications, especially to ranitidine.
• Tell your doctor if you now have or if you have ever had kidney or liver disease.
• Ranitidine should be taken continuously for as long as your doctor prescribes. Stopping therapy early may be a cause of ineffective therapy.
• Cigarette smoking may block the beneficial effects of ranitidine.
• If this drug makes you dizzy, do not take part in any activity that requires alertness.
• Be sure to tell your doctor if you are pregnant. Ranitidine appears to be safe during pregnancy; however, extensive testing has not been conducted. Also, tell your doctor if you are breast-feeding an infant. Small amounts of ranitidine pass into breast milk.

Rectacort—see hydrocortisone, benzyl benzoate, bismuth resorcin compound, bismuth subgallate, zinc oxide, and Peruvian balsam combination (topical)

Reglan—see metoclopramide

Rela—see carisoprodol

Relaxadon—see atropine, scopolamine, hyoscyamine, and phenobarbital combination

Renoquid—see sulfonamide antibiotics (oral)

Reposans-10—see chlordiazepoxide

Resaid S.R.—see phenylpropanolamine and chlorpheniramine combination

reserpine

BRAND NAMES (Manufacturers)
reserpine (various manufacturers)
Serpalan (Lannett)
Serpasil (Ciba)
TYPE OF DRUG
Antihypertensive
INGREDIENT
reserpine
DOSAGE FORM
Tablets (0.1 mg, 0.25 mg, and 1 mg)
STORAGE
Reserpine tablets should be stored at room temperature in tightly closed, light-resistant containers.

USES

Reserpine is used to treat high blood pressure. It works by depleting certain chemicals from the nervous system that are responsible for maintaining high blood pressure.

TREATMENT

To avoid stomach irritation, you can take reserpine with food or with a full glass of water or milk (unless your doctor directs otherwise). Try to take reserpine at the same time(s) each day, to become accustomed to taking it.

Reserpine does not cure hypertension, but it will help to control the condition as long as you continue to take it.

If you miss a dose of this medication, take the missed dose as soon as possible, unless it is almost time for the next dose. Do not take the missed dose at all; just return to your regular dosing schedule. Do not double the next dose.

SIDE EFFECTS

Minor. Abdominal pain, constipation, diarrhea, dizziness, dry mouth, headache, impotence, loss of appetite, nasal congestion, nausea, nosebleeds, vomiting, or weight gain. These side effects should disappear as your body adjusts to the medication.

To relieve constipation, increase the amount of fiber in your diet (fresh fruits and vegetables, salads, bran, and whole-grain breads), exercise, and drink more water (unless your doctor directs you to do otherwise).

If you feel dizzy, sit or lie down for a while; get up slowly from a sitting or reclining position, and be careful on stairs.

To relieve mouth dryness, chew sugarless gum or suck on ice chips or a piece of hard candy.

Major. Tell your doctor about any side effects that are persistent or particularly bothersome. IT IS ESPECIALLY IMPORTANT TO TELL YOUR DOCTOR about anxiety; black, tarry stools; chest pain; decrease in sexual desire; depression; difficulty in urinating; drowsiness; enlarged breasts (in both sexes); fainting; fatigue; flushing of the skin; hearing loss; itching; muscle aches; nervousness; nightmares; palpitations; pinpoint pupils of eyes; rapid weight gain (three to five pounds within a week); rash; severe dizziness; shortness of breath; tremors; unusual bleeding or bruising; or weakness.

INTERACTIONS

Reserpine interacts with several other types of medications:

1. Concurrent use of reserpine with central nervous system depressants, such as alcohol, antihistamines, barbiturates, benzodiazepine tranquilizers, muscle relaxants, narcotics, pain medications, phenothiazine tranquilizers, and sleeping medications, or with tricyclic antidepressants can cause extreme drowsiness.

2. Reserpine can increase the side effects of digoxin, beta blockers, and quinidine and can decrease the effectiveness of levodopa.

3. Methotrimeprazine can increase the blood-pressure-lowering effects of reserpine, which can be dangerous.

4. Tricyclic antidepressants can decrease the blood-pressure-lowering effects of reserpine.

5. Concurrent use of reserpine and monoamine oxidase (MAO) inhibitors can lead to severe side effects. At least 14 days should separate the use of this drug and the use of an MAO inhibitor.

Before starting reserpine, TELL YOUR DOCTOR about any drugs you are taking, especially those listed above.

WARNINGS

• Tell your doctor about unusual or allergic reactions you have had to any medications, especially to reserpine or to any rauwolfia alkaloids.

• Before starting to take this medication, be sure to tell your doctor if you now have or if you have ever had arrhythmias, epilepsy, gallstones or gallbladder disease, heart disease, kidney disease, lung disease, mental depression, Parkinson's disease, peptic ulcers, pheochromocytoma, or ulcerative colitis.

• Reserpine should not be used within two weeks of electroshock therapy.

• If this drug makes you dizzy or drowsy, do not take part in any activity that requires alertness, such as driving a car or operating potentially dangerous machinery.

• Before having surgery or any other medical or dental procedure, tell your doctor or dentist you are taking this drug.

• Before taking any over-the-counter (nonprescription) cough, cold, sinus, asthma, allergy, or diet medications, consult your doctor or pharmacist. Some of these products may increase your blood pressure.

• Be sure to tell your doctor if you are pregnant. Reserpine has been reported to cause birth defects in infants whose mothers received the drug during pregnancy. Also, tell your doctor if you are breast-feeding. Reserpine can pass into breast milk and cause side effects in the nursing infant.

Respbid—see theophylline

Restoril—see temazepam

Retin-A—see tretinoin

Retrovir—see zidovudine

Rhinolar-Ex 12—see phenylpropanolamine and chlorpheniramine combination

Rhythmin—see procainamide

Ridaura—see auranofin

Rifadin—see rifampin

---

rifampin

BRAND NAMES (Manufacturers)
Rifadin (Marion Merrell Dow)
Rimactane (Ciba)
TYPE OF DRUG
Antibiotic
INGREDIENT
rifampin
DOSAGE FORM
Capsules (150 mg and 300 mg)
STORAGE
Rifampin should be stored at room temperature in a tightly closed, light-resistant container.

USES

Rifampin is an antibiotic that is used to treat tuberculosis and to prevent meningococcal meningitis. Rifampin works by preventing the growth and multiplication of susceptible bacteria. Rifampin, however, is not effective against viruses, parasites, or fungi.

TREATMENT

Rifampin should be taken with a full glass of water on an empty stomach one hour before or two hours after a meal. If this medication causes stomach irritation, however, check with your doctor to see if you can take it with food.

Try not to miss any doses of this medication. If you do miss a dose, take the missed dose as soon as possible, unless it is almost time for your next dose. In that case, do not take the missed dose at all; just return to your regular dosing schedule. Do not double the next dose.

Continue to take this medication for the entire time prescribed by your doctor (which may be months to years), even if the symptoms disappear before the end of that period. If you stop taking the drug too soon, resistant bacteria will continue to grow, and your infection could recur.

SIDE EFFECTS

Minor. Diarrhea, dizziness, drowsiness, gas, headache, heartburn, loss of appetite, nausea, stomach irritation, or vomiting. These side effects should disappear as your body adjusts to the medication.

If you feel dizzy, sit or lie down for a while; get up slowly from a sitting or reclining position.
Major. Tell your doctor about any side effects that are persistent or particularly bothersome. IT IS ESPECIALLY IMPORTANT TO TELL YOUR DOCTOR about confusion, difficult or painful urination, fatigue, fever, flushing, itching, muscle weakness, numbness, skin rash, uncoordinated movements, visual disturbances, or yellowing of the eyes or skin. Also, if your symptoms of infection seem to be worsening rather than improving, tell your doctor.

INTERACTIONS

Rifampin interacts with several other types of medications:
1. Concurrent use with paminosalicylic acid may decrease the blood levels and effectiveness of rifampin.
2. Rifampin can decrease the blood levels and effectiveness of metoprolol, propranolol, verapamil, aminophylline, theophylline, oxtriphylline, quinidine, adrenocorticosteroids (cortisone-like medicines), progestins, clofibrate, methadone, oral anticoagulants (blood thinners, such as warfarin), oral antidiabetic medicines, barbiturates, benzodiazepine tranquilizers, dapsone, digitoxin, and trimethoprim.
3. Concurrent use of rifampin with alcohol or isoniazid can lead to an increased risk of liver damage.
4. Rifampin may decrease the effectiveness of oral contraceptives (birth control pills), and pregnancy could result. You should use a different or additional form of birth control while taking rifampin. Discuss this with your doctor.

BE SURE TO TELL YOUR DOCTOR about any medications you are currently taking.

WARNINGS

• Tell your doctor about unusual or allergic reactions you have had to any medications, especially to rifampin.
• Before starting to take this medication, be sure to tell your doctor if you have a history of alcoholism or liver disease.
• Rifampin has been prescribed for your current infection only. Another infection later on, or one that someone else has, may require a different medicine. You should not give your medicine to other people or use it for other infections, unless your doctor specifically directs you to do so.
• If this drug makes you dizzy or drowsy, do not take part in any activity that requires alertness, such as driving a car or operating potentially dangerous machinery.
• Rifampin can cause reddish-orange to reddish-brown discoloration of your urine, feces, saliva, sputum, sweat, and tears. This is a harmless effect. The drug may also permanently discolor soft contact lenses. You might want to stop wearing them while you are taking this medication. Discuss this with your ophthalmologist.
• Do not stop taking this medication unless you first check with your doctor. Stopping the drug and restarting it at a later time can lead to an increase in side effects.
• Be sure to tell your doctor if you are pregnant. Although rifampin appears to be safe in humans, birth defects have been reported in the offspring of animals that received large doses of the drug during pregnancy. Also, tell your doctor if you are breast-feeding an infant. Small amounts of rifampin pass into breast milk.

Rimactane—see rifampin

Ritalin—see methylphenidate

Ritalin-SR—see methylphenidate

---

ritodrine

BRAND NAME (Manufacturer)
Yutopar (Astra)
TYPE OF DRUG
Beta-adrenergic receptor agonist (labor inhibitor)
INGREDIENT
ritodrine
DOSAGE FORM
Tablets (10 mg)
STORAGE
Ritodrine should be stored at room temperature in a tightly closed container.

USES

Ritodrine is used to prevent premature labor. It belongs to a group of drugs called beta-adrenergic nerve receptor stimulants. It prevents premature labor by relaxing uterine muscle, thus decreasing the strength and frequency of uterine contractions.

TREATMENT

Ritodrine treatment is usually begun intravenously. Once the contractions stop, the medication is generally continued orally (in tablet form).

Ritodrine tablets can be taken either on an empty stomach or with food or milk (as directed by your doctor).

BE SURE YOU UNDERSTAND YOUR DOCTOR'S INSTRUCTIONS on how this medication should be taken.

It is important to try not to miss any doses of this medication. If you do miss a dose and remember within an hour, take the missed dose immediately. If more than an hour has passed, do not take the missed dose at all; just return to your regular dosing schedule. Do not double the next dose of the medication.

SIDE EFFECTS

Minor. Nausea or jitteriness. These side effects should disappear as your body adjusts to the medication.
Major. Tell your doctor about any side effects that are persistent or particularly bothersome. IT IS ESPECIALLY IMPORTANT TO TELL YOUR DOCTOR about palpitations, shortness of breath, skin rash, tremors, or vomiting.

INTERACTIONS

This medication interacts with a number of other types of medications:
1. Beta blockers (acebutolol, atenolol, betaxolol, carteolol, esmolol, labetalol, metoprolol, nadolol, penbutolol, pindolol, propranolol, timolol) decrease the effectiveness of ritodrine.
2. Concurrent use of ritodrine and adrenocorticosteroids (cortisone-like medicines) can lead to additional side effects in the mother or newborn.

BE SURE TO TELL YOUR DOCTOR about any medications you are currently taking, especially any of those listed above.

WARNINGS

Be sure to tell your doctor about any unusual or allergic reactions that you have had to any medications, especially to ritodrine.

Before starting to take ritodrine, be sure to tell your doctor if you now have or if you have ever had diabetes mellitus, eclampsia or pre-eclampsia, heart disease, high blood pressure, pulmonary hypertension, or thyroid disease.

Do not take any over-the-counter (nonprescription) cough, cold, allergy, asthma, sinus, or diet medication, unless you first check with your doctor or pharmacist. Some of these products decrease the effectiveness of ritodrine.

You should CHECK WITH YOUR DOCTOR IMMEDIATELY for further instructions if your contractions begin again or if your water bag breaks while you are taking this medication.

RMS—see morphine

Robaxin—see methocarbamol

Robicillin VK—see penicillin VK

Robimycin—see erythromycin

Robitet Robicaps—see tetracycline

Robitussin A-C—see codeine and guaifenesin combination

Rocaltrol—see calcitriol

Rogaine—see minoxidil (topical)

Rondec—see pseudoephedrine and carbinoxamine combination

Rondec-DM—see pseudoephedrine, carbinoxamine, and dextromethorphan combination

Roxanol—see morphine

Roxanol SR—see morphine

Rufen—see ibuprofen

Rum-K—see potassium chloride

Ru-Tuss II—see phenylpropanolamine and chlorpheniramine combination

Ru-Vert-M—see meclizine

Rymed-TR—see phenylpropanolamine and guaifenesin combination

Ryna—see pseudoephedrine and chlorpheniramine combination

Sandimmune—see cyclosporine

Sanorax—see mazindol

S.A.S.-500—see sulfasalazine

Satric—see metronidazole

Scabene—see lindane

scopolamine (transdermal)

BRAND NAME (Manufacturer)
Transderm-Scop (Ciba)
TYPE OF DRUG
Antiemetic and antivertigo
INGREDIENT
scopolamine
DOSAGE FORM
Transdermal system (the patch delivers 0.5 mg of scopolamine over three days)
STORAGE
The scopolamine (transermal) patches should be stored at room temperature in their original containers. Always try to keep these containers away from direct heat and light.

USES

Scopolamine is used to prevent nausea and vomiting associated with motion sickness. Transdermal scopolamine is a small patch that is applied to the skin. Transdermal application (i.e. application of medicine through the skin) delivers reduced doses of scopolamine, which decreases the risk of adverse side effects.

TREATMENT

The transdermal system (patches) allows controlled continuous release of scopolamine. Patches are easy to use and convenient. For best results, wash and dry hands thoroughly before handling. Apply the disc to the hairless area of the skin behind the ear at least four hours before the antiemetic effect is required. Do not place over any cuts or irritations. Wash hands thoroughly after handling the disc to prevent direct contact of the medication with the eyes. The medication should last up to three days. If treatment is needed for more than three days, discard the used disc, and replace with a new disc behind the other ear. It is all right to bathe or shower with a patch in place. If the disc becomes displaced at any time during treatment, it should be discarded, and a fresh one placed on the hairless area behind the other ear. If redness or irritation develops at the application site, consult your physician. Do not trim or cut the patches.

SIDE EFFECTS

Minor. Blurred vision and enlargement of pupils; drowsiness; or dryness of mouth, nose, and throat.

   To relieve mouth dryness, chew sugarless gum or suck on ice chips or hard candy.

   If you feel dizzy or light-headed, sit or lie down for a while.

Major. Tell your doctor about any side effects that are persistent or particularly bothersome. IT IS ESPECIALLY IMPORTANT TO TELL YOUR DOCTOR ABOUT blurred vision (severe); confusion (severe); convulsions; difficulty in breathing; dizziness; drowsiness (severe); dry mouth, nose, or throat (severe); eye pain (severe); fast heart beat; fever; rash; slurred speech; unusual excitement or restlessness; unusual warmth; dryness; or flushing of the skin.

INTERACTIONS

Scopolamine can interact with other types of medications:

1. It can cause additive drowsiness when combined with alcohol or other central nervous system depressants (such as antihistamines, barbiturates, benzodiazepine tranquilizers, muscle relaxants, narcotics, and pain medications) or with tricyclic antidepressants.

2. It can cause additive anticholinergic effects (such as dryness of mouth, nose, and throat, or difficulty in urinating) when combined with drugs such as belladonna alkaloids, antidepressants, and antihistamines.

   Before starting to take scopolamine, BE SURE TO TELL YOUR DOCTOR about any medications you are currently taking, especially any of those listed above.

WARNINGS

• Tell your doctor about unusual or allergic reactions you have had to any medications, especially to scopolamine.

• Tell your doctor if you now have or if you have ever had blockage of the urinary tract, stomach, or intestinal tract.

• Tell your doctor if you now have or if you have ever had metabolic, liver, or kidney disease.

• Tell your doctor if you have glaucoma (increased pressure in the eyeball).

• This medication may cause drowsiness or blurred vision. Make sure you know how you react to this medication before you attempt activities such as driving a car or operating potentially dangerous equipment.

• Patients who use the patch for more than three days are more likely to experience dizziness, headache, nausea, or vomiting for a short time following discontinuation.

• Do not use the transdermal system on children.

• Elderly patients may be especially susceptible to the central nervous system effects (confusion, sedation, memory impairment, unusual excitement) of scopolamine.

• Be sure to tell your doctor if you are pregnant. Extensive studies in pregnant women have not been conducted. Also, tell your doctor if you are breast-feeding. It is not known whether scopolamine passes into breast milk.

---

secobarbital

BRAND NAMES (Manufacturers)
secobarbital sodium (various manufacturers)
Seconal (Lilly)
TYPE OF DRUG
Barbiturate sedative/hypnotic
INGREDIENT
secobarbital
DOSAGE FORMS
Tablets (100 mg)
Capsules (50 mg and 100 mg)
STORAGE
Secobarbital tablets and capsules should be stored at room temperature in tightly closed containers.

USES

Secobarbital belongs to a group of drugs known as barbiturates, which are central nervous system depressants (drugs that slow the activity of the brain and spinal cord). This medication is used as a sleeping aid in the treatment of insomnia.

TREATMENT

You can take secobarbital at bedtime. The tablets and capsules can be taken with water, food, or milk.

   You should not use this drug as a sleeping aid for more than two weeks. With prolonged use, secobarbital loses its ability to induce and sustain sleep.

SIDE EFFECTS

Minor. Constipation, diarrhea, dizziness, drowsiness, a "hangover" feeling, headache, nausea, nightmares, stomach upset, or vomiting. These side effects should disappear as your body adjusts to the medication.

If you feel dizzy or light-headed, sit or lie down for a while; get up slowly from a sitting or reclining position, and be careful on stairs.

To relieve constipation, increase the amount of fiber in your diet (fresh fruits and vegetables, salads, bran, and whole-grain breads), exercise, and drink more water (unless your doctor directs you to do otherwise).

Major. Tell your doctor about any side effects that are persistent or particularly bothersome. IT IS ESPECIALLY IMPORTANT TO TELL YOUR DOCTOR about chest tightness, confusion, depression, difficulty in breathing, excitation, fatigue, feeling faint, fever, hives or itching, loss of coordination, muscle or joint pain, skin rash, slurred speech, sore throat, unusual bleeding or bruising, unusual weakness, or yellowing of the eyes or skin.

INTERACTIONS

Secobarbital interacts with several other types of medications:

1. Concurrent use of this barbiturate medication with other central nervous system depressants (such as alcohol, antihistamines, benzodiazepine tranquilizers, muscle relaxants, narcotics, pain medications, and phenothiazine tranquilizers) or with tricyclic antidepressants can cause extreme drowsiness.

2. Valproic acid, chloramphenicol, and monoamine oxidase (MAO) inhibitors can prolong the effects of secobarbital.

3. Secobarbital can decrease the blood levels and effectiveness of oral anticoagulants (blood thinners, such as warfarin), digoxin, tricyclic antidepressants, cortisone-like medicines, doxycycline, quinidine, estrogens, oral contraceptives (birth control pills), phenytoin, acetaminophen, and carbamazepine.

4. The combination of secobarbital and furosemide can cause low blood pressure and fainting.

5. Secobarbital can increase the side effects of cyclophosphamide or large doses of acetaminophen.

Before starting secobarbital, BE SURE TO TELL YOUR DOCTOR about any medications you are currently taking, especially any of those listed above.

WARNINGS

Tell your doctor about unusual or allergic reactions you have had to any medications, especially to secobarbital or to other barbiturates (such as amobarbital, butabarbital, mephobarbital, metharbital, pentobarbital, phenobarbital, and primidone).

Tell your doctor if you now have or if you have ever had acute or chronic (longterm) pain, Addison's disease (caused by an underactive adrenal gland), diabetes mellitus, kidney disease, liver disease, lung disease, mental depression, porphyria, or thyroid disease.

If this medication makes you dizzy or drowsy during the day, do not take part in any activity that requires alertness, such as driving a car or operating potentially dangerous machinery.

Children, the elderly, and very ill patients are more likely to experience unusual excitement, confusion, or mental depression.

Secobarbital has the potential for abuse and must be used with caution. Tolerance to the medication develops quickly; do not increase the dosage or stop taking this drug unless you first consult your doctor. If you have been taking secobarbital for a long time or have been taking large doses, you may experience anxiety, muscle twitching, tremors, weakness, dizziness, nausea, vomiting, insomnia, or blurred vision when you stop taking it. To avoid or minimize this reaction, your doctor may want to reduce your dosage gradually.

Be sure to tell your doctor if you are pregnant. Barbiturates cross the placenta, and there has been an association between birth defects and the use of this class of drugs during pregnancy. Such drugs may also lead to bleeding complications in the newborn. The risks involved with secobarbital therapy should be discussed with your doctor. In addition, if secobarbital is used for long periods during the last three months of pregnancy, there is a chance that the infant will be born addicted to the medication and will experience a withdrawal reaction (convulsions, irritability) at birth. Also, tell your doctor if you are breast-feeding an infant. Small amounts of secobarbital pass into breast milk and may cause excessive drowsiness and breathing problems in nursing infants.

secobarbital sodium—see secobarbital

Seconal—see secobarbital

Sectral—see acebutolol

Seldane—see terfenadine

---

selegiline

BRAND NAME (Manufacturer)
Eldepryl (Somerset)
TYPE OF DRUG
Antiparkinson agent
INGREDIENT
selegiline
DOSAGE FORM
Tablets (5 mg)
STORAGE
Selegilene should be stored at room temperature in a tightly closed container.

USES

This medication is used either alone or in combination with levodopa or levodopa/carbidopa to treat the symptoms of Parkinson's disease. This drug helps to increase and extend the beneficial effects of levodopa. Recent studies suggest that selegiline may help to slow the progression of Parkinson's disease when taken early in the course of the disease. This drug has also been used to treat depression.

TREATMENT

This drug should be taken exactly as your doctor prescribes. You can take it with food to lessen the chance of irritation, unless your doctor tells you otherwise.

If you miss a dose of this medication, take the missed dose as soon as possible, then return to your regular dosing schedule. However, if you do not remember the missed dose until late afternoon or evening, skip the missed dose. If the drug is taken late in the afternoon, it may cause some unwanted side effects. Never double the dose.

The full effects of this medication may not be apparent for two to three days. At that time, your doctor may change your dose of levodopa or levodopa/carbidopa.

SIDE EFFECTS

Minor. Dizziness, drowsiness, dryness of mouth, headache, heartburn, light-headedness, nausea, nervousness, restlessness, stomach pain, trouble sleeping, or vomiting. These side effects should lessen or disappear as your body adjusts to the medication.

Dry mouth can be relieved by chewing sugarless gum or by sucking on ice chips or a piece of hard candy.

To avoid dizziness or light-headedness when you stand, contract and relax the muscles of your legs for a few moments before rising. Do this by pushing one foot against the floor while raising the other foot slightly, alternating feet so that you are "pumping" your legs in a pedaling motion.

Major. Tell your doctor about any side effects that are persistent or particularly bothersome. IT IS ESPECIALLY IMPORTANT TO TELL YOUR DOCTOR about blood in your urine; chest pain; convulsions; dark or tarry stools; difficulty in breathing; difficulty in speaking; difficulty in urination; fast heartbeat; feelings of euphoria; hallucinations; mood changes; persistent restlessness; severe stomach pain; stiff neck; or uncontrolled movements of your arms, legs, or face.

INTERACTIONS

When taken in the recommended dose at the times directed by your doctor, selegiline should not interact with many types of medications or foods.

Tell your doctor if you have taken the drug meperidine in the two to three weeks before starting selegiline therapy.

Be sure to tell your doctor about any medications, including over-the-counter products, you are currently taking.

WARNINGS

• Tell your doctor if you have had unusual or allergic reactions to any medications, especially to selegiline or to any monoamine oxidase (MAO) inhibitors (such as tranylcypromine, phenelzine, and isocarboxazid).
• Tell your doctor if you have a history of stomach problems, intestinal problems, asthma, high blood pressure, or seizure disorders.
• If this drug makes you dizzy or drowsy, do not take part in any activity that requires alertness, such as driving a car or operating potentially dangerous equipment.
• Before having surgery or any other medical or dental treatment, tell your doctor or dentist you are taking this drug.
• Your doctor may give you a list of foods that you should either avoid or limit in your diet. These foods or beverages may include those containing caffeine (coffee, tea, cola, or chocolate) or those containing a substance called tyramine (found in certain cheeses and meats).
• Be sure to tell your doctor if you are pregnant. This drug has not caused adverse effects to the fetuses in animal studies, and problems in humans have not been reported. Also, tell your doctor if you are breast-feeding an infant.

Septra—see sulfamethoxazole and trimethoprim combination

Septra DS—see sulfamethoxazole and trimethoprim combination

Ser-A-Gen—see hydralazine, hydrochlorothiazide, and reserpine combination

Seralazide—see hydralazine, hydrochlorothiazide, and reserpine combination

Ser-Ap-Es—see hydralazine, hydrochlorothiazide, and reserpine combination

Serax—see oxazepam

Serentil—see mesoridazine

Serophene—see clomiphene

Serpalan—see reserpine

Serpasil—see reserpine

Serpazide—see hydralazine, hydrochlorothiazide, and reserpine combination

Sinequan—see doxepin

Sleep-Eze 3—see diphenhydramine

Slo-bid Gyrocaps—see theophylline

Slo-Phyllin—see theophylline

Slo-Phyllin GG—see theophylline and guaifenesin combination

Slow-K—see potassium chloride

Slyn-LL—see phendimetrazine

Sodium Sulamyd—see sodium sulfacetamide (ophthalmic)

sodium sulfacetamide (ophthalmic)

BRAND NAMES (Manufacturers)
AK-Sulf (Akorn)
AK-Sulf Forte (Akorn)

Bleph-10 (Allergan)
Cetamide (Alcon)
Isopto Cetamide (Alcon)
Ophthacet (Vortech)
Sodium Sulamyd (Schering)
sodium sulfacetamide (various manufacturers)
Sulf-10 (Iolab Pharm.)
Sulfair 15 (Pharmafair)
Sulten-10 (Bausch & Lomb)

TYPE OF DRUG
Ophthalmic antibiotic

INGREDIENT
sodium sulfacetamide

DOSAGE FORMS
Ophthalmic drops (10%, 15%, and 30%)
Ophthalmic ointment (10%)

STORAGE
Sodium sulfacetamide drops and ointment should be stored at room temperature in tightly closed containers. This medication should never be frozen. If the eye drops discolor or turn brown, they should be discarded.

USES
Sodium sulfacetamide is used to treat bacterial eye infections and corneal ulcers. Sodium sulfacetamide is an antibiotic that is effective against a wide range of bacteria. It acts by preventing production of the nutrients that are required for growth of the infecting bacteria. This medication, however, is not effective against infections that are caused by viruses or fungi.

TREATMENT
Wash your hands with soap and water before applying this medication. To avoid contamination of the eye drops or ointment, be careful not to touch the tube of the dropper or the tip of the ointment tube or let them touch your eyes; DO NOT wipe off or rinse the dropper after use.

To apply the drops, tilt your head back and pull down the lower eyelid with one hand to make a pouch below the eye. Drop the prescribed amount of medicine into this pouch and slowly close your eyes. Try not to blink. Keep your eyes closed, and place one finger at the corner of the eye next to your nose for a minute or two, applying a slight pressure (this is done to prevent loss of medication through the duct that drains fluid from the surface of the eye into the nose and throat). Then wipe away any excess with a clean tissue.

To apply the ointment, tilt the head back, pull down the lower lid to form a pouch below the eye, and squeeze a small amount of ointment (approximately $1/8$ to $1/4$ inch) in a line along the pouch. Close the eyes, and place your finger at the corner of the eye next to your nose for a minute or two. Do not rub your eyes. Wipe off excess ointment with a clean tissue.

Since this medication is somewhat difficult to apply, you may want to have someone else apply it for you.

It is important to continue to take this medication for the entire time prescribed by your doctor, even if the symptoms disappear before the end of that period. If you stop applying the drug too soon, resistant bacteria are given a chance to continue growing, and the infection could recur.

If you miss a dose of this medication, apply the missed dose as soon as possible, unless it is almost time for your next dose. In that case, do not apply the missed dose at all; just return to your regular dosing schedule. Do not use twice as much medication at the next dose.

SIDE EFFECTS
Minor. Sodium sulfacetamide may cause blurred vision or burning or stinging in the eyes immediately after it is applied (especially the 30% solution). This effect should last only a few minutes.

Major. Tell your doctor about any side effects that are persistent or particularly bothersome. IT IS ESPECIALLY IMPORTANT TO TELL YOUR DOCTOR about signs of irritation in the eyes (such as redness, swelling, or itching) that last more than several minutes, chills, fever, itching, or difficulty in breathing. If your symptoms of infection are getting worse rather than improving, contact your doctor.

INTERACTIONS
This drug should not be used concurrently with preparations containing silver, such as silver nitrate opthalmic. Be sure to tell your doctor about any medications you are currently taking.

WARNINGS
• Tell your doctor about unusual or allergic reactions you have had to any medications, especially to sodium sulfacetamide or to any other sulfa medication (diuretics, oral antidiabetic medications, sulfonamide antibiotics).

• This medication may cause allergic-type symptoms, such as hives, itching, wheezing, or anaphylaxis, in sulfite-sensitive patients.

• Sodium sulfacetamide may cause eye sensitivity to bright light; wearing sunglasses may help to lessen this problem.

• This medication has been prescribed for your current infection only. Another infection later on, or one that someone else has, may require a different medicine. You should not give your medicine to other people or use it for other infections, unless your doctor specifically directs you to do so.

• In order to allow your eye infection to clear, do not apply makeup to the affected eye.

• If there is no change in your condition two or three days after starting to take this medication, contact your doctor.

• Be sure to tell your doctor if you are pregnant. The safe use of this medication in human pregnancy has not been established. Although an ophthalmic, if large amounts of this drug are applied for prolonged periods, some of it may be absorbed into the bloodstream. Also, tell your doctor if you are breast-feeding an infant. If this drug is absorbed, small amounts may pass into the breast milk and may temporarily alter the bacterial balance in the intestinal tract of the nursing infant, resulting in diarrhea.

Sodol—see carisoprodol

Sofarin—see warfarin

Solfoton—see phenobarbital

Soma—see carisoprodol

Sominex 2—see diphenhydramine

Somophyllin—see aminophylline

Somophyllin-DF—see aminophylline

Somophyllin-T—see theophylline

Sonazine—see chlorpromazine

Soprodol—see carisoprodol

Sorbitrate—see isosorbide dinitrate

Sorbitrate SA—see isosorbide dinitrate

Spancap No. 1—see dextroamphetamine

Sparine—see promazine

Spasmolin—see atropine, scopolamine, hyoscyamine, and phenobarbital combination

Spasmophen—see atropine, scopolamine, hyoscyamine, and phenobarbital combination

Spasquid—see atropine, scopolamine, hyoscyamine, and phenobarbital combination

Spironazide—see spironolactone and hydrochlorothiazide combination

---

spironolactone

BRAND NAMES (Manufacturers)
Alatone (Major)
Aldactone (Searle)
spironolactone (various manufacturers)
TYPE OF DRUG
Diuretic and antihypertensive
INGREDIENT
spironolactone
DOSAGE FORM
Tablets (25 mg, 50 mg, and 100 mg)
STORAGE
Spironolactone should be stored at room temperature in a tightly closed, light-resistant container.

USES
This drug is used to treat high blood pressure. It is also used to reduce fluid accumulation in the body caused by conditions such as heart failure, cirrhosis of the liver, kidney disease, and the long-term use of some drugs.

Spironolactone reduces fluid accumulation by increasing the elimination of salt and water through the kidneys. It may be used in combination with other diuretics to prevent potassium loss. Since spironolactone

blocks the effects of a chemical (aldosterone) released from the adrenal gland, it can also be used to diagnose and treat an overactive adrenal gland.

TREATMENT
To decrease stomach irritation, you can take spironolactone with a glass of milk or with a meal (unless your doctor directs you to do otherwise). Try to take it at the same time every day. Avoid taking a dose after 6:00 P.M.; otherwise, you may have to get up during the night to urinate.

This medication does not cure high blood pressure, but it will help to control the condition as long as you continue to take it.

If you miss a dose of this medication, take the missed dose as soon as possible, unless it is almost time for the next dose. In that case, do not take the missed dose at all; just wait until the next scheduled dose. Do not double the dose.

SIDE EFFECTS
Minor. Cramping, diarrhea, dizziness, drowsiness, dry mouth, headache, increased urination, nausea, rash, restlessness, vomiting, or weakness. As your body adjusts to the medication, these side effects should disappear.

Dry mouth can be relieved by chewing sugarless gum.

To avoid dizziness or light-headedness when you stand, contract and relax the muscles of your legs for a few moments before rising. Do this by pushing one foot against the floor while raising the other foot slightly, alternating feet so that you are "pumping" your legs in a pedaling motion.

Major. Tell your doctor about any side effects that are persistent or particularly bothersome. IT IS ESPECIALLY IMPORTANT TO TELL YOUR DOCTOR about anxiety; clumsiness; confusion; deepening of the voice (in women); enlarged breasts (in both sexes); fever; impotence; increased hair growth; menstrual disturbances; muscle cramps; numbness or tingling in the hands, feet, or lips; palpitations; postmenopausal bleeding; rapid weight gain (three to five pounds within a week); stomach cramps; uncoordinated movements; or unusual tiredness or weakness.

INTERACTIONS
Spironolactone interacts with several foods and medications:

1. Concurrent use of spironolactone with amiloride, captopril, triamterene, potassium salts, low-salt milk, salt substitutes, or laxatives can cause serious side effects such as hyperkalemia (high levels of potassium in the blood).

2. Spironolactone may increase the side effects of lithium, digoxin, digitoxin, and ammonium chloride.

3. The effectiveness of oral anticoagulants (blood thinners, such as warfarin) may be decreased by this medication.

4. Aspirin may decrease the diuretic effects of spironolactone.

Before starting to take spironolactone, BE SURE TO TELL YOUR DOCTOR about any medications you are currently taking, especially any of those listed above.

WARNINGS

• Tell your doctor about unusual or allergic reactions you have had to any medications, especially to spironolactone or to any other diuretic.

• Tell your doctor if you now have or if you have ever had kidney or urination problems, heart disease, hyperkalemia (high blood levels of potassium), liver disease, menstrual abnormalities, breast enlargement, or diabetes mellitus.

• Spironolactone can cause hyperkalemia. Signs of hyperkalemia include palpitations; confusion; numbness or tingling in the hands, feet, or lips; anxiety; or unusual tiredness or weakness. However, do not alter your diet in an effort to avoid this problem, unless your doctor tells you to do so. Elderly patients may be more susceptible to hyperkalemia.

• There are several "generic brands" of this drug. Consult your pharmacist about these items; some of them are not equivalent to the brand-name medications.

• Limit your intake of alcoholic beverages to prevent dizziness and light-headedness while taking this drug.

• Do not take any over-the-counter (nonprescription) medications for weight control or for allergy, asthma, cough, cold, or sinus problems unless you first check with your doctor.

• To prevent severe water loss (dehydration) while taking this medication, check with your doctor if you have any illness that causes severe or continuous nausea, vomiting, or diarrhea.

• Be sure to tell your doctor if you are pregnant. This drug crosses the placenta, and its safety in human pregnancy has not been established. Adverse effects have been observed in the fetuses of animals that were given large doses of this drug during pregnancy. Also, tell your doctor if you are breast-feeding an infant.

spironolactone and hydrochlorothiazide combination

BRAND NAMES (Manufacturers)
Alazide (Major)
Aldactazide (Searle)
Spironazide (Henry Schein)
spironolactone and hydrochlorothiazide
    (various manufacturers)
Spirozide (Rugby)
TYPE OF DRUG
Diuretic and antihypertensive
INGREDIENTS
spironolactone and hydrochlorothiazide
DOSAGE FORM
Tablets (25 mg spironolactone and 25 mg hydrochlorothiazide; 50 mg spironolactone and 50 mg hydrochlorothiazide)
STORAGE
Store at room temperature in a tightly closed, light-resistant container.

USES
Spironolactone and hydrochlorothiazide combination is prescribed to treat high blood pressure. It is also used to reduce fluid acccumulation in the body caused by conditions such as heart failure, cirrhosis of the liver, kidney disease, and the long-term use of some medications. This medication reduces fluid accumulation by increasing the elimination of salt and water through the kidneys. Spironolactone is combined with hydrochlorothiazide to prevent potassium loss from the body.

TREATMENT
To decrease stomach irritation, you can take this medication with a glass of milk or with a meal (unless your doctor directs you to do otherwise). Try to take it at the same time every day. Avoid taking a dose after 6:00 P.M.

This medication does not cure high blood pressure, but it will help to control the condition as long as you continue to take it.

If you miss a dose of this medication, take the missed dose as soon as possible, unless it is almost time for the next dose. In that case, do not take the missed dose at all; just wait until the next scheduled dose. Do not double the dose.

SIDE EFFECTS
Minor. Constipation, cramping, diarrhea, dizziness, headache, increased urination, loss of appetite, lack of energy, light-headedness, restlessness, or unusual sweating. These side effects should disappear as your body adjusts to this medication.

This medication can increase your sensitivity to sunlight. You should, therefore, avoid prolonged exposure to sunlight and sunlamps. Wear protective clothing, and use an effective sunscreen.

To relieve constipation, increase the amount of fiber in your diet (fresh fruits and vegetables, salads, bran, and whole-grain breads) and exercise more (unless your doctor directs you to do otherwise).

To avoid dizziness or light-headedness when you stand, contract and relax the muscles of your legs for a few moments before rising. Do this by pushing one foot against the floor while raising the other foot slightly, alternating feet so that you are "pumping" your legs in a pedaling motion.

Major. Tell your doctor about any side effects that are persistent or particularly bothersome. IT IS ESPECIALLY IMPORTANT TO TELL YOUR DOCTOR about anxiety; blurred vision; breast tenderness or enlargement (in both sexes); clumsiness; confusion; deepening of the voice (in women); drowsiness; dry mouth; impotence; increased hair growth; irregular menstrual periods or vaginal bleeding; joint pain; mood changes; muscle cramps; nausea; numbness or tingling in the hands, feet, or lips; palpitations; rapid weight gain (three to five pounds within a week); rash; sore throat and fever; swelling; thirst; unusual bleeding or bruising; unusual tiredness or weakness; vomiting; or yellowing of the eyes or skin.

INTERACTIONS
Spironolactone and hydrochlorothiazide combination interacts with several foods and medications:

1. Concurrent use of it with amiloride, captopril, certain antihypertensives such as enalapril and lisinopril, triamterene, potassium salts, low-salt milk, salt substitutes, or laxatives can cause serious side effects from hyperkalemia (high levels of potassium in the blood).

2. This drug may decrease the effectiveness of oral anticoagulants, antigout medications, insulin, oral antidiabetic medicines, and methenamine.

3. Fenfluramine may increase the blood-pressure-lowering effects of this drug.

4. Indomethacin and aspirin may decrease the blood-pressure-lowering effects of this drug.

5. Cholestyramine and colestipol can decrease the absorption of this medication from the gastrointestinal tract. Therefore, spironolactone and hydrochlorothiazide combination should be taken one hour before or four hours after a dose of cholestyramine or colestipol if either of these medications has also been prescribed for you.

6. Spironolactone and hydrochlorothiazide may increase the side effects of calcium, cortisone and cortisone-like steroids (such as dexamethasone, hydrocortisone, and prednisolone), digoxin, digitoxin, digitalis, lithium, quinidine, sulfonamide antibiotics, and vitamin D.

BE SURE TO TELL YOUR DOCTOR about any medications you are currently taking, especially those listed above.

WARNINGS

• Tell your doctor about unusual or allergic reactions you have had to any medications, especially to spironolactone or hydrochlorothiazide or to any other sulfa drug, including other diuretics (water pills), oral antidiabetic medications, or sulfonamide antibiotics.

• Before you start taking this medication, tell your doctor if you now have or if you have ever had kidney disease or problems with urination, diabetes mellitus, gout, liver disease, asthma, pancreas disease, systemic lupus erythematosus, hyperkalemia, menstrual abnormalities, breast enlargement, acidosis, or hypercalcemia.

• The hydrochlorothiazide component of this drug can occasionally cause potassium loss from the body. Signs of potassium loss include dry mouth, muscle pain or cramps, nausea, thirst, vomiting, and weakness. If you experience any of these symptoms, call your doctor.

• The spironolactone component of this drug can cause hyperkalemia, or increased potassium levels in the body. Signs of hyperkalemia include anxiety; confusion; numbness or tingling in the hands, feet, or lips; palpitations; or unusual tiredness or weakness. Do not alter your diet in an attempt to avoid this problem unless you first consult your doctor. Elderly patients may be more susceptible to hyperkalemia.

• There are several "generic brands" of this drug. Products made by different companies may not work in exactly the same way. Before switching brands, consult you doctor or pharmacist.

• Limit your intake of alcoholic beverages to prevent dizziness and lightheadedness while taking this drug.

• Do not take any over-the-counter (nonprescription) medications for weight control or for allergy, asthma, cough, cold, or sinus problems unless you check with your doctor.

• To prevent severe water loss (dehydration), check with your doctor if you develop any illness that causes severe or continuous nausea, vomiting, or diarrhea.

• This drug can raise blood sugar levels in diabetic patients. Blood sugar should be monitored carefully with blood or urine tests when this drug is being taken.

• A doctor does not usually prescribe a "fixed-dose" drug like this as the first choice in the treatment of high blood pressure. Usually, the patient first receives each ingredient singly. If there is an adequate response to the fixed dose contained in this product, it can then be substituted. The advantages of a combination product are increased convenience and (often) decreased cost.

• Be sure to tell your doctor if you are pregnant. This drug crosses the placenta, and its safety in human pregnancy has not been established. Adverse effects have been observed in the fetuses of animals that were given large doses of this drug during pregnancy. Also, tell your doctor if you are breast-feeding an infant.

Spirozide—see spironolactone and hydrochlorothiazide combination

S-P-T—see thyroid hormone

Statobex—see phendimetrazine

Stelazine—see trifluoperazine

Sterapred DS—see prednisolone (systemic)

StuartNatal 1+1—see vitamins, prenatal

---

succimer

BRAND NAME (Manufacturer)
Chemet (McNeil Consumer Products)
TYPE OF DRUG
Oral chelator (remover) for lead
INGREDIENT
succimer
DOSAGE FORM
Capsules (100mg)
STORAGE
Succimer capsules should be stored at room temperature in a tightly closed, light-resistent container.

USES

Succimer is used to remove excess lead in the body. Although patients with excess lead levels may not look or act sick, the lead may cause learning difficulties if left untreated over time. Succimer binds to the excess lead in the bloodstream. The combination of lead and succimer is removed from the body when the patient urinates.

TREATMENT

In order to avoid stomach upset, succimer capsules can be taken whole with food or with a glass of milk (unless your doctor directs you to do otherwise)

If succimer is prescribed for a young child who cannot swallow capsules, you may open the capsule and sprinkle the contents on a spoonful of soft food such as applesauce, ice cream, or pudding.

SIDE EFFECTS

Minor. Bad or metallic taste in mouth, diarrhea, loss of appetite, or vomiting. These side effects should disappear as your body adjusts to the medication.

Major. Tell your doctor about any side effects that are persistent or particularly bothersome. IT IS ESPECIALLY IMPORTANT TO TELL YOUR DOCTOR about skin rash, severe abdominal pain, severe headaches, tingling in the arms or legs, or yellowing of the skin or eyes.

INTERACTIONS

It is not known at this time whether or not succimer interacts with other medication.

WARNINGS

• It is important to tell your doctor if you have ever had an unusual or allergic reaction to succimer or any other medication.

• It is important that you drink plenty of fluids while taking succimer.

• Succimer may cause your breath or urine to have a bad odor. This is a harmless effect.

• This medication has been prescribed for your current condition only. Do not give this medication to other people or use it for any other purpose than that prescribed by your doctor.

• Your doctor may want you to have regular blood tests to make sure that this medication is working properly.

• Be sure to tell your doctor if you are pregnant or if you are breast-feeding an infant. The safe use of this medication during human pregnancy or breast-feeding has not been established.

sucralfate

BRAND NAME (Manufacturer)
Carafate (Marion Merrel Dow)
TYPE OF DRUG
Antiulcer
INGREDIENT
sucralfate
DOSAGE FORM
Tablets (1 g)
STORAGE
Sucralfate should be stored at room temperature in a tightly closed container.

USES

Sucralfate is used for the short-term treatment of ulcers. This medication binds to the surface of the ulcer, thereby protecting it from stomach acid and promoting healing.

TREATMENT

In order to obtain maximum benefit from this drug, you should swallow it whole with a full glass of water. Take it on an empty stomach one hour before or two hours after a meal and at bedtime. Do not take antacids within 30 minutes before or one hour after taking sucralfate.

Continue to take sucralfate for the full length of time prescribed by your doctor, even if your symptoms disappear. Your ulcer may not yet be healed. However, do not take it for more than eight weeks without your doctor's authorization.

If you miss a dose of this medication, take the missed dose as soon as possible, unless it is almost time for the next dose. In that case, do not take the missed dose at all; just return to your regular dosing schedule. Do not double the next dose.

SIDE EFFECTS

Minor. Back pain, constipation, diarrhea, dizziness, drowsiness, dry mouth, indigestion, nausea, or stomach pain. These side effects should disappear as your body adjusts to the medication.

To relieve constipation, exercise and drink more water (unless your doctor directs you to do otherwise).

If you feel dizzy, sit or lie down for a while; get up slowly from a sitting or reclining position, and be careful on stairs.

To relieve mouth dryness, chew sugarless gum or suck on ice chips or a piece of hard candy.

Major. Tell your doctor about any side effects that are persistent or particularly bothersome. IT IS ESPECIALLY IMPORTANT TO TELL YOUR DOCTOR about itching or rash. Also, if your condition does not improve or seems to be getting worse, you should contact your doctor.

INTERACTIONS

1. Sucralfate may prevent the absorption of tetracycline, digoxin, phenytoin, ranitidine, and fat-soluble vitamins (vitamins A, D, E, and K) from the gastrointestinal tract. At least one hour should separate doses of any of these medications and sucralfate.

2. Sucralfate may increase stomach absorption of ciprofloxacin and norfloxacin. At least two hours should separate doses of these medications and sucralfate.

BE SURE TO TELL YOUR DOCTOR about any medications you are currently taking, especially any listed above.

WARNINGS

• Tell your doctor about unusual or allergic reactions you have had to any medications, especially to sucralfate.

• Tell your doctor if you now have or if you have ever had kidney disease.

• If sucralfate makes you dizzy or drowsy, do not take part in any activity that requires alertness, such as driving a car or operating potentially dangerous machinery.

• Be sure to tell your doctor if you are pregnant. Although sucralfate appears to be safe, extensive studies in pregnant women have not been conducted. Also, tell your doctor if you are breast-feeding an infant. It is not known whether sucralfate passes into breast milk.

Sudafed Plus—see pseudoephedrine and chlorpheniramine combination

Sulf-10—see sodium sulfacetamide (ophthalmic)

sulfacytine—see sulfonamide antibiotics (oral)

sulfadiazine—see sulfonamide antibiotics (oral)

Sulfa-Gyn—see sulfathiazole, sulfacetamide, and sulfabenzamide combination

Sulfair 15—see sodium sulfacetamide (ophthalmic)

sulfamethizole—see sulfonamide antibiotics (oral)

sulfamethoxazole—see sulfonamide antibiotics (oral)

---

sulfamethoxazole and phenazopyridine combination

BRAND NAME (Manufacturer)
Azo Gantanol (Roche)
TYPE OF DRUG
Antibiotic and urinary tract analgesic
INGREDIENTS
sulfamethoxazole and phenazopyridine
DOSAGE FORM
Tablets (500 mg sulfamethoxazole and 100 mg phenazopyridine)
STORAGE
Sulfamethoxazole and phenazopyridine combination tablets should be stored at room temperature in a tightly closed, light-resistant container.

USES
This medication is used to treat painful infections of the urinary tract. Sulfamethoxazole acts by preventing production of the nutrients that are required for growth of the infecting bacteria. Phenazopyridine is excreted in the urine, where it exerts a topical analgesic (pain-relieving) effect on the urinary tract. This medication is not useful for any pain other than that of a urinary tract infection.

TREATMENT
It is best to take this medication with a full glass of water on an empty stomach, either one hour before or two hours after a meal. However, if it causes stomach upset, check with your doctor to see if you can take it with food or milk.

This medication works best when the level of medicine in your blood and urine is kept constant. It is best, therefore, to take the doses at evenly spaced intervals day and night. For example, if you are to take two doses a day, the doses should be spaced 12 hours apart.

If you miss a dose of this medication, take the missed dose immediately. However, if you do not remember to take the missed dose until it is almost time for your next dose, take the missed dose immediately; space the following dose about halfway through the regular interval between doses; and then return to your regular dosing schedule. Try not to skip any doses.

It is important to continue to take this medication for the entire time prescribed by your doctor (usually seven to 14 days), even if the symptoms disappear before the end of that period. If you stop taking the drug too soon, resistant bacteria are given a chance to continue growing and the infection could recur.

SIDE EFFECTS
Minor. Abdominal pain, diarrhea, dizziness, headache, indigestion, insomnia, loss of appetite, nausea, or vomiting. These side effects should disappear as your body adjusts to the medication.

Sulfamethoxazole can cause increased sensitivity to sunlight. It is, therefore, important to avoid prolonged exposure to sunlight and sunlamps. Wear protective clothing and sunglasses, and use an effective sunscreen. However, a sunscreen containing para-aminobenzoic acid (PABA) interferes with the antibacterial activity of this medication and should NOT be used.

Phenazopyridine causes your urine to become orange-red in color. This is not harmful. However, it may stain your clothing. The urine will return to its normal color soon after the drug is discontinued.

If you feel dizzy during treatment with this drug, sit or lie down for a while.

Major. Tell your doctor about any side effects that are persistent or particularly bothersome. IT IS ESPECIALLY IMPORTANT TO TELL YOUR DOCTOR about aching joints and muscles, back pain, bloating, blood in the urine, chest pain, chills, confusion, convulsions, depression, difficult or painful urination, difficulty in breathing, difficulty in swallowing, fever, hallucinations, hives, itching, loss of coordination, pale skin, rash or peeling skin, ringing in the ears, sore throat, swelling of the front part of the neck, swollen ankles, unusual bleeding or bruising, unusual tiredness, or yellowing of the eyes or skin. Also, if your symptoms of infection seem to be getting worse rather than improving, you should contact your doctor.

INTERACTIONS
This medicine interacts with other types of drugs:
1. Sulfamethoxazole can increase the blood levels of oral anticoagulants (blood thinners, such as warfarin), oral antidiabetic agents, aspirin, methotrexate, and phenytoin, which can lead to serious side effects.
2. Methenamine can increase the side effects to the kidneys caused by sulfamethoxazole.
3. Probenecid, phenylbutazone, oxyphenbutazone, and sulfinpyrazone can increase the blood levels of sulfamethoxazole, which can lead to an increase in side effects.

Before starting to take this medication, BE SURE TO TELL YOUR DOCTOR about any medications you are currently taking, especially any of those listed above.

WARNINGS
• Tell your doctor about unusual or allergic reactions you have had to any medications, especially to phenazopyridine, sulfamethoxazole, or any other sulfa drug (other sulfonamide antibiotics, diuretics, dapsone, sulfoxone, oral antidiabetic medications, oral antiglaucoma medication, or acetazolamide).

• Tell your doctor if you now have or if you have ever had glucose-6-phosphate dehydrogenase (G6PD) deficiency, kidney disease, liver disease, or porphyria.

• This medication has been prescribed for your current infection only. Another infection later on, or one that someone else has, may require a different medicine. You should not give your medicine to other people or use it for other infections, unless your doctor specifically directs you to do so.

• This medication should be taken with plenty of water in order to avoid kidney stone formation.

• If this drug makes you dizzy or drowsy, do not take part in any activity that requires alertness, such as driving a car or operating potentially dangerous machinery.

• Diabetic patients using this medication (phenazopyridine) may get delayed reactions or false-positive readings for sugar or ketones with urine tests. Clinitest is not affected by this medication.

• If there is no improvement in your condition several days after starting this medication, check with your doctor. This medication may not be effective against the particular type of bacteria causing your infection.

• Before having surgery or any other medical or dental treatment, be sure to tell your doctor or dentist that you are taking this medication.

• Be sure to tell your doctor if you are pregnant. Small amounts of sulfamethoxazole cross the placenta. Although this medication appears to be safe during pregnancy, extensive studies in humans have not been conducted. Tell your doctor if you are breast-feeding an infant. Small amounts of this drug pass into breast milk and may temporarily alter the bacterial balance in the intestinal tract of the nursing infant, resulting in diarrhea. This drug should not be used in an infant less than two months of age.

sulfamethoxazole and trimethoprim combination

BRAND NAMES (Manufacturers)
Bactrim (Roche)
Bactrim DS (Roche)
Bethaprim DS (Major)
Cotrim (Lemmon)
Cotrim DS (Lemmon)
Cotrim Pediatric (Lemmon)
Septra (Burroughs Wellcome)
Septra DS (Burroughs Wellcome)
sulfamethoxazole and trimethoprim (various manufacturers)
Sulfatrim (various manufacturers)
Sulfatrim DS (various manufacturers)
TYPE OF DRUG
Antibiotic
INGREDIENTS
sulfamethoxazole and trimethoprim
DOSAGE FORMS
Tablets (400 mg sulfamethoxazole and 80 mg trimethoprim) Double-strength (DS) tablets (800 mg sulfamethoxazole and 160 mg trimethoprim)

Oral suspension (200 mg sulfamethoxazole and 40 mg trimethoprim per 5-ml spoonful)
STORAGE
Sulfamethoxazole and trimethoprim combination tablets and oral suspension should be stored at room temperature in tightly closed, light-resistant containers. The oral suspension does not need to be refrigerated. This medication should never be frozen.

USES
Sulfamethoxazole and trimethoprim combination is used to treat a broad range of infections, including urinary tract infections, certain respiratory and gastrointestinal infections, and otitis media (middle ear infection). Sulfamethoxazole and trimethoprim acts by preventing production of the nutrients that are required for growth of the infecting bacteria.

TREATMENT
It is best to take this medication with a full glass of water on an empty stomach, either one hour before or two hours after a meal. However, if it causes stomach upset, check with your doctor to see if you can take it with food or milk.

The oral suspension form of this medication should be shaken well just before measuring each dose. The contents tend to settle on the bottom of the bottle, so it is necessary to shake the container to distribute the ingredients evenly and equalize the doses. Each dose should then be measured carefully with a specially designed 5-ml measuring spoon. An ordinary kitchen teaspoon is not accurate enough.

This medication works best when the level of medicine in your bloodstream (and urine) is kept constant. It is best, therefore, to take the doses at evenly spaced intervals day and night. For example, if you are to take two doses a day, the doses should be spaced 12 hours apart. Try not to skip any doses.

If you miss a dose of this medication, take the missed dose immediately. However, if you do not remember to take the missed dose until it is almost time for your next dose, take the missed dose immediately; space the following dose about halfway through the regular interval between doses (wait about six hours if you are taking two doses a day); and then return to your regular dosing schedule.

It is important to continue to take this medication for the entire time prescribed by your doctor (usually seven to 14 days), even if the symptoms disappear before the end of that period. If you stop taking the drug too soon, resistant bacteria are given a chance to continue growing, and the infection could recur.

SIDE EFFECTS
Minor. Abdominal pain, diarrhea, dizziness, headache, loss of appetite, nausea, sore mouth, or vomiting. These side effects should disappear as your body adjusts to the drug.

Sulfamethoxazole can cause increased sensitivity to sunlight. It is, therefore, important to avoid prolonged exposure to sunlight and sunlamps. Wear protective clothing and sunglasses, and use an effective sunscreen.

However, a sunscreen containing para-aminobenzoic acid (PABA) interferes with the antibacterial activity of this medication and should NOT be used.

If you feel dizzy, sit or lie down for a while; get up slowly from a sitting or reclining position, and be careful on stairs.

Major. Tell your doctor about any side effects that are persistent or particularly bothersome. IT IS ESPECIALLY IMPORTANT TO TELL YOUR DOCTOR about bloody urine, convulsions, difficult or painful urination, difficulty in breathing, difficulty in swallowing, fever, hallucinations, itching, joint pain, lower back pain, pale skin, rash, ringing in the ears, sore throat, swelling of the front part of the neck, swollen or inflamed tongue, tingling in the hands or feet, unusual bleeding or bruising, unusual fatigue, or yellowing of the eyes or skin. Also, if your infection seems to be getting worse rather than improving, contact your doctor.

INTERACTIONS
This medicine interacts with other types of drugs:

1. Sulfamethoxazole can increase the blood levels of oral anticoagulants (blood thinners, such as warfarin), oral antidiabetic agents, methotrexate, aspirin, and phenytoin, which can lead to serious side effects.

2. Methenamine can increase the side effects to the kidneys caused by sulfamethoxazole.

3. Probenecid, phenylbutazone, oxyphenbutazone, and sulfinpyrazone can increase the blood levels of sulfamethoxazole, which can lead to an increase in side effects.

4. Rifampin can increase the elimination of trimethoprim from the body, decreasing its antibacterial effects.

5. Concurrent use of trimethoprim with antineoplastic agents (anticancer drugs) can increase the risk of developing blood disorders.

6. Trimethoprim can decrease the elimination of phenytoin from the body and increase the chance of side effects.

BE SURE TO TELL YOUR DOCTOR about any medications you are currently taking, especially any listed above.

WARNINGS
• Tell your doctor about unusual or allergic reactions you have had to any medications, especially to trimethoprim, sulfamethoxazole, or other sulfa drugs (other sulfonamide antibiotics, diuretics, dapsone, sulfoxone, oral antidiabetic medications, oral antiglaucoma medication, or acetazolamide).

• Tell your doctor if you now have or if you have ever had glucose-6-phosphate dehydrogenase (G6PD) deficiency, kidney disease, liver disease, porphyria, or megaloblastic anemia (folate-deficiency anemia).

• This medication has been prescribed for your current infection only. Another infection later on, or one that someone else has, may require a different medicine. You should not give your medicine to other people or use it for other infections, unless your doctor specifically directs you to do so.

• This medication should be taken with plenty of water in order to avoid kidney stone formation.

• If this drug makes you dizzy or drowsy, do not take part in any activity that requires alertness.

• If there is no improvement in your condition several days after starting to take this medication, check with your doctor. This medication may not be effective against the bacteria causing your infection.

• Before having surgery or any other medical or dental treatment, tell your doctor or dentist you are taking this drug.

• Be sure to tell your doctor if you are pregnant. Small amounts of sulfamethoxazole and trimethoprim cross the placenta. Although these drugs appear to be safe during pregnancy, extensive studies in humans have not been conducted. Trimethoprim has been shown to cause birth defects in the offspring of animals that received very large doses during pregnancy. Tell your doctor if you are breastfeeding. Small amounts of sulfamethoxazole pass into breast milk and may temporarily alter the bacterial balance in the intestinal tract of the nursing infant, resulting in diarrhea. Also, small amounts of trimethoprim pass into breast milk, and there is a chance that it may cause anemia in the nursing infant. This combination medication should not be used in an infant less than two months of age (to avoid side effects involving the liver).

sulfasalazine

BRAND NAMES (Manufacturers)
Azaline (Major)
Azulfidine (Pharmacia)
Azulfidine EN-tabs (Pharmacia)
S.A.S.-500 (Rowell)
sulfasalazine (various manufacturers)
TYPE OF DRUG
Sulfonamide and anti-inflammatory
INGREDIENT
sulfasalazine
DOSAGE FORMS
Tablets (500 mg)
Enteric-coated tablets (500 mg)
Oral suspension (250 mg per 5-ml spoonful)
STORAGE
Store at room temperature in a tightly closed, light-resistant container. This medication should never be frozen.

USES
This medication is used to treat inflammatory bowel disease (regional enteritis or ulcerative colitis). In the intestine, sulfasalazine is converted to 5-aminosalicylic acid, an aspirin-like drug, which acts to relieve inflammation.

TREATMENT
In order to avoid stomach irritation while you are being treated with this medication, you should take your doses with a full glass of water, with food, or after meals (unless your doctor directs you to do otherwise).

The enteric-coated tablets should be swallowed whole. The enteric coating is added to lessen stomach irritation. Chewing, breaking, or crushing these tablets destroys the coating.

The suspension form of this medication should be shaken well just before measuring each dose. The contents tend to settle on the bottom of the bottle, so it is necessary to shake the container to distribute the ingredients evenly and equalize the doses. Each dose should then be measured carefully with a specially designed 5-ml measuring spoon. An ordinary kitchen teaspoon is not accurate enough.

If you miss a dose of this medication, take the missed dose as soon as possible, unless it is almost time for the next dose. In that case, do not take the missed dose at all; just return to your regular dosing schedule. Do not double the next dose.

SIDE EFFECTS

Minor. Diarrhea, dizziness, drowsiness, insomnia, loss of appetite, mild headache, nausea, stomach upset, or vomiting. These should disappear as your body adjusts to the drug.

This medication can increase your sensitivity to sunlight. Avoid prolonged exposure to sunlight and sunlamps. Wear protective clothing, and use an effective sunscreen. However, a sunscreen containing para-aminobenzoic acid (PABA) interferes with this drug and should not be used.

Sulfasalazine can discolor contact lenses. You may want to stop wearing them while taking this medication. Discuss this with your ophthalmologist.

Sulfasalazine can cause your urine to change to an orange-yellow color. This is a harmless effect.

If you feel dizzy, sit or lie down for a while; get up slowly from a sitting or reclining position, and be careful on stairs.

Major. Tell your doctor about any side effects that are persistent or particularly bothersome. IT IS ESPECIALLY IMPORTANT TO TELL YOUR DOCTOR about blood in the urine, convulsions, depression, difficulty in swallowing, difficult or painful urination, fatigue, fever, hallucinations, hearing loss, itching, joint pain, lower back pain, mouth sores, pale skin, rash or peeling skin, ringing in the ears, severe headache, sore throat, swelling of the front part of the neck, tingling sensations, unusual bleeding or bruising, or yellowing of the eyes or skin.

INTERACTIONS

Sulfasalazine interacts with several other types of drugs:
1. It can increase the side effects of oral anticoagulants (blood thinners, such as warfarin), oral antidiabetic agents, methotrexate, aspirin, and phenytoin.
2. The blood levels and effectiveness of digoxin and folic acid are decreased by concurrent use of sulfasalazine.
3. Probenecid, oxyphenbutazone, phenylbutazone, methenamine, and sulfinpyrazone can increase the blood levels and side effects of sulfasalazine.

BE SURE TO TELL YOUR DOCTOR about any medications you are currently taking, especially any listed above.

WARNINGS

• Tell your doctor about unusual or allergic reactions you have had to any medications, especially to sulfasalazine, aspirin or other salicylates, or any sulfa drug (diuretics, oral antidiabetic medications, sulfonamide antibiotics, oral antiglaucoma medication, acetazolamide, sulfoxone, dapsone).
• Before starting to take this medication, be sure to tell your doctor if you now have or if you have ever had blood disorders, blockage of the urinary tract or intestine, glucose-6-phosphate dehydrogenase (G6PD) deficiency, kidney disease, liver disease, or porphyria.
• To help prevent the formation of kidney stones, try to drink at least eight to 12 glasses of water or fruit juice each day while you are taking this medication (unless your doctor directs you to do otherwise).
• Before having surgery or other medical or dental treatment, tell your doctor or dentist you are taking this drug.
• If your condition does not improve within a month or two after starting to take sulfasalazine, check with your doctor. It may be necessary to change your medication.
• Be sure to tell your doctor if you are pregnant. Although sulfasalazine appears to be safe during most of pregnancy, extensive studies in humans have not been conducted. There is also concern that if this drug is taken during the ninth month of pregnancy, it may cause liver or brain disorders in the infant. Also, tell your doctor if you are breast-feeding an infant. Small amounts of sulfasalazine pass into breast milk.

sulfathiazole, sulfacetamide, and sulfabenzamide combination

BRAND NAMES (Manufacturers)
Sulfa-Gyn (Mayrand)
Sultrin Triple Sulfa (Ortho)
Triple Sulfa (vaginal) (various manufacturers)
Trysul (Savage)
TYPE OF DRUG
Antibiotic
INGREDIENTS
sulfathiazole, sulfacetamide, and sulfabenzamide
DOSAGE FORMS
Vaginal tablets (172.5 mg sulfathiazole, 143.75 mg sulfacetamide, and 184 mg sulfabenzamide)
Vaginal cream (3.42% sulfathiazole, 2.86% sulfacetamide, and 3.7% sulfabenzamide)
STORAGE
This medication should be stored at room temperature (never frozen) in tightly closed, light-resistant containers.

USES

Sulfathiazole, sulfacetamide, and sulfabenzamide are sulfonamide antibiotics used to treat vaginal infections. They work by blocking production of nutrients needed by the infecting bacteria, thus killing the bacteria.

TREATMENT

This product is packaged with instructions and an applicator. Read the instructions carefully before inserting the vaginal cream or tablets. Wash the applicator with warm water and soap, and dry it thoroughly after each use.

It is important to continue to take this medication for the entire time prescribed by your doctor, even if your symptoms disappear before the end of that period. If you stop taking the medication too soon, your infection could recur.

If you miss a dose of this medication, insert the missed dose as soon as possible, unless it is almost time for the next dose. In that case, do not insert the missed dose; return to the regular dosing schedule. Do not double the dose.

SIDE EFFECTS

Minor. This medication combination can cause a mild, temporary burning or stinging sensation after each of the first few applications. As your body adjusts to this medication combination, this side effect should disappear.
Major. Tell your doctor about any side effects that are persistent or particularly bothersome. IT IS ESPECIALLY IMPORTANT TO TELL YOUR DOCTOR about itching, rash, redness, swelling, or any other signs of irritation that were not present before you started taking this medication.

INTERACTIONS

Sulfathiazole, sulfacetamide, and sulfabenzamide combination should not interact with other medications if it is used according to your doctor's directions.

WARNINGS

• Tell your doctor about unusual or allergic reactions you have had to any medications, especially to sulfathiazole, sulfacetamide, sulfabenzamide, or any other sulfa drug, including sulfonamide antibiotics, diuretics (water pills), oral antidiabetic medicines, oral antiglaucoma medication, dapsone, sulfone, and sulfoxone.
• Before starting to take this medication, tell your doctor if you now have or if you have ever had kidney disease.
• You should not use tampons while using this medication.
• During intercourse, your partner should wear a condom to prevent reinfection. Ask your doctor if your partner needs to be treated at the same time as you.
• This medication combination has been prescribed for your current infection only. Another infection later on, or one that someone else has, may require a different medicine. You should not give your medicine to other people or use it for other infections, unless your doctor directs you to do so.
• If symptoms do not begin to improve within several days after starting this medication, CONTACT YOUR DOCTOR. This medication may not be effective for your infection.
• If you are pregnant or breast-feeding, ASK YOUR DOCTOR if you should continue to use this medication.

Sulfatrim—see sulfamethoxazole and trimethoprim combination

Sulfatrim DS—see sulfamethoxazole and trimethoprim combination

sulfinpyrazone

BRAND NAMES (Manufacturers)
Anturane (Ciba)
sulfinpyrazone (various manufacturers)
TYPE OF DRUG
Antigout and antiplatelet
INGREDIENT
sulfinpyrazone
DOSAGE FORMS
Tablets (100 mg)
Capsules (200 mg)
STORAGE
Sulfinpyrazone tablets and capsules should be stored at room temperature in tightly closed containers.

USES

Sulfinpyrazone is used to treat gout. It acts by increasing the elimination of uric acid (the chemical responsible for gout) through the kidneys. This medication is also used to prevent further heart attacks in patients who have had a recent attack by preventing the formation of certain types of blood clots.

TREATMENT

In order to prevent stomach irritation, you should take sulfinpyrazone with food, milk, or antacids (unless your doctor directs you to do otherwise).

Sulfinpyrazone does not cure gout, but it will help to control blood levels of uric acid as long as you continue to take the medication.

If you miss a dose of this medication, take the missed dose as soon as possible, unless it is almost time for your next dose. In that case, do not take the missed dose at all; just return to your regular dosing schedule. Do not double the next dose.

SIDE EFFECTS

Minor. Nausea, stomach upset, or vomiting. These side effects should disappear as you adjust to the medication.
Major. Tell your doctor about any side effects that are persistent or particularly bothersome. IT IS ESPECIALLY IMPORTANT TO TELL YOUR DOCTOR about back pain; bloody or black, tarry stools; convulsions; diarrhea; difficult or painful urination; fever; sore throat; skin rash; or unusual bleeding or bruising.

INTERACTIONS

Sulfinpyrazone interacts with other types of medications:
1. Aspirin can increase uric acid levels, thereby decreasing the therapeutic effects of sulfinpyrazone.
2. Sulfinpyrazone can increase the side effects of sulfonamide antibiotics, oral antidiabetic medications, oral anticoagulants (blood thinners, such as warfarin), and nitrofurantoin.
3. Alcohol, pyrazinamide, and diuretics (water pills) can increase the blood levels of uric acid, thereby decreasing the effectiveness of sulfinpyrazone.

Before starting to take this medication, BE SURE TO TELL YOUR DOCTOR about any medications you are currently taking, especially any of those listed above.

WARNINGS

• Tell your doctor about unusual or allergic reactions you have had to any medications, especially to sulfinpyrazone, oxyphenbutazone, or phenylbutazone.
• Before starting to take this drug, tell your doctor if you have ever had blood disorders, kidney disease, peptic ulcers, or stomach or intestinal inflammation.
• Before taking any over-the-counter (nonprescription) medication, check the label to see if it contains aspirin. Aspirin can decrease the effectiveness of sulfinpyrazone.
• Sulfinpyrazone is not an analgesic (pain reliever) and does not relieve an acute gout attack. It is used to prevent future gout attacks.
• In order to prevent the formation of kidney stones, try to drink at least eight to 12 glasses of water or fruit juice each day while taking this medication (unless your doctor directs you to do otherwise).
• Before having surgery or other medical or dental treatment, tell your doctor or dentist you are taking this drug. Treatment with sulfinpyrazone is usually discontinued several days prior to surgery, to prevent bleeding complications.
• Tell your doctor if you are pregnant.Extensive studies in humans have not been conducted. Also, tell your doctor if you are breast-feeding an infant.

sulfisoxazole—see sulfonamide antibiotics (oral)

sulfisoxazole and phenazopyridine combination

BRAND NAMES (Manufacturers)
Azo Gantrisin (Roche)
Azo-Sulfisoxazole (various manufacturers)
TYPE OF DRUG
Antibiotic and urinary tract analgesic
INGREDIENTS
sulfisoxazole and phenazopyridine
DOSAGE FORM
Tablets (500 mg sulfisoxazole and 50 mg phenazopyridine)
STORAGE
Sulfisoxazole and phenazopyridine combination tablets should be stored at room temperature in a tightly closed, light-resistant container.

USES

Sulfisoxazole and phenazopyridine combination is used to treat painful infections of the urinary tract. Sulfisoxazole is a sulfonamide antibiotic, which acts by preventing production of nutrients that are required for growth of infecting bacteria. Phenazopyridine is excreted in the urine, where it exerts a topical analgesic (pain-relieving) effect on the urinary tract. This medication is not useful for any pain other than that of a urinary tract infection.

TREATMENT

It is best to take this medication with a full glass of water on an empty stomach, either one hour before or two hours after a meal. However, if it causes stomach upset, check with your doctor to see if you can take it with food or milk.

This medication works best when the level of medication in your blood and urine is kept constant. It is best, therefore, to take the doses at evenly spaced intervals day and night. For example, if you are to take two doses a day, the doses should be spaced 12 hours apart.

If you miss a dose of this medication, take the missed dose immediately. However, if you do not remember to take the missed dose until it is almost time for your next dose, take the missed dose immediately; space the following dose about halfway through the regular interval between doses; and then return to your regular dosing schedule. Try not to skip any doses.

It is important to continue to take this medication for the entire time prescribed by your doctor (usually seven to 14 days), even if your symptoms disappear before the end of that period. If you stop taking the drug too soon, resistant bacteria are given a chance to continue growing, and the infection could recur.

SIDE EFFECTS

Minor. Abdominal pain, diarrhea, dizziness, headache, indigestion, insomnia, loss of appetite, nausea, or vomiting. These side effects should disappear as your body adjusts to the medication.

Sulfisoxazole can cause increased sensitivity to sunlight. It is, therefore, important to avoid prolonged exposure to sunlight and sunlamps. Wear protective clothing and sunglasses, and use an effective sunscreen. However, a sunscreen containing para-aminobenzoic acid (PABA) interferes with the antibacterial activity of this medication and should NOT be used.

Phenazopyridine causes your urine to become orange-red in color. This is not harmful; however, it may stain your clothing. The urine will return to its normal color soon after the drug is discontinued.

If you feel dizzy, sit or lie down for a while; get up slowly from a sitting or reclining position, and be careful on stairs.

Major. Tell your doctor about any side effects that are persistent or particularly bothersome. IT IS ESPECIALLY IMPORTANT TO TELL YOUR DOCTOR about aching joints and muscles, back pain, bloating, blood in the urine, chest pain, chills, confusion, convulsions, depression, difficulty in breathing, difficulty in swallowing, difficult or painful urination, fever, hallucinations, hives, itching, loss of coordination, pale skin, rash or peeling skin, ringing in the ears, sore throat, swelling of the front part of the neck, swollen ankles, unusual bleeding or bruising, unusual tiredness, or yellowing of the eyes or skin. Also, if your symptoms of infection seem to be getting worse rather than improving, you should contact your doctor.

INTERACTIONS

This drug interacts with several types of drugs:
1. Sulfisoxazole can increase the blood levels of oral anticoagulants (blood thinners, such as warfarin), oral antidiabetic agents, methotrexate, aspirin, thiopental, and phenytoin, which can lead to serious side effects.

2. Methenamine can increase the side effects to the kidneys caused by sulfisoxazole.

3. Probenecid, oxyphenbutazone, phenylbutazone, and sulfinpyrazone can increase the side effects of sulfisoxazole.

BE SURE TO TELL YOUR DOCTOR about any medications you are currently taking, especially those listed above.

WARNINGS

• Tell your doctor about any reactions you have had to drugs, especially to phenazopyridine, sulfisoxazole, or any other sulfa drug (other sulfonamide antibiotics, diuretics, dapsone, sulfoxone, oral antidiabetic medications, oral antiglaucoma medications, or acetazolamide).

• Tell your doctor if you now have or if you have ever had glucose-6-phosphate dehydrogenase (G6PD) deficiency, kidney disease, liver disease, or porphyria.

• This medication has been prescribed for your current infection only. Another infection later on, or one that someone else has, may require a different medicine. You should not give your medicine to other people or use it for other infections, unless your doctor specifically directs you to do so.

• This medication should be taken with plenty of water in order to prevent kidney stone formation.

• If this drug makes you dizzy or drowsy, it is especially important that do not take part in any activity that requires alertness, such as driving a car or operating potentially dangerous machinery.

• Diabetic patients using this medication, which contains phenazopyridine, may get delayed reactions or false-positive readings for sugar or ketones with urine tests. Clinitest is not affected by this medication, but the other urine sugar tests may be. Discuss this with your doctor or pharmacist.

• If there is no improvement in your condition several days after starting to take this medication, check with your doctor. This medication may not be effective against the bacteria causing your infection.

• Before having surgery or any other medical or dental treatment, be sure to tell your doctor or dentist that you are taking this medication.

• Be sure to tell your doctor if you are pregnant. Small amounts of sulfisoxazole cross the placenta. Although this medication appears to be safe during pregnancy, extensive studies in humans have not been conducted. Also, tell your doctor if you are breast-feeding. Small amounts of this medication pass into breast milk and may temporarily alter the bacterial balance in the intestinal tract of a nursing infant, resulting in diarrhea. This medication should not be used in an infant less than two months of age (in order to avoid side effects involving the liver).

---

sulfonamide antibiotics (oral)

BRAND NAMES (Manufacturers)
Gantanol (Roche)
Gantrisin (Roche)
Gulfasin (Major)

Microsulfon (CMC)
multiple sulfonamides (various manufacturers)
Neotrizine (Lilly)
Renoquid (Glenwood)
sulfacytine (various manufacturers)
sulfadiazine (various manufacturers)
sulfamethizole (various manufacturers)
sulfamethoxazole (various manufacturers)
sulfisoxazole (various manufacturers)
Terfonyl (Squibb)
Thiosulfil Forte (Ayerst)
Triple Sulfa (systemic) (various manufacturers)
Urobak (Shionogi USA)

TYPE OF DRUG
Anti-infective

INGREDIENTS AND DOSAGE FORMS
sulfacytine (Renoquid)
Tablets (250 mg)
sulfadiazine (Microsulfon)
Tablets (500 mg)
sulfamethiazole (Proklar, Thiosulfil Forte)
Tablets (250 mg and 500 mg)
sulfamethoxazole (Gamazole, Gantanol, Gantanol DS, Urobak)
Tablets (500 mg and 1 g)
Suspension (500 mg per 5-ml spoonful)
sulfisoxazole (Gantrisin, Gulfasin, Lipo-Gantrisin)
Tablets (500 mg)
Syrup (500 mg per 5-ml spoonful)
Pediatric suspension (500 mg per 5-ml spoonful)
Emulsion, long-acting (1 g per 5-ml spoonful)
multiple sulfonamides (Neotrizine, Sul-Trio MM #2, Terfonyl, Triple Sulfa)
Tablets (167 mg sulfadiazine, 167 mg sulfamerazine, and 167 mg sulfamethazine)
Suspension (167 mg sulfadiazine, 167 mg sulfamerazine, and 167 mg sulfamethazine per 5-ml spoonful, with 2% alcohol)

STORAGE
Store at room temperature in the original container.

USES
Sulfonamide antibiotics are a family of related drugs that have activity against many types of bacteria. This group of medications is often used to treat urinary tract infections, as well as other infections. These medications kill the bacteria responsible for the infection.

TREATMENT
Sulfonamide antibiotics should be taken with a full glass of water on an empty stomach (either one hour before or two hours after a meal). Several additional glasses of water should also be taken every day (unless your doctor directs you to do otherwise). Sulfonamide antibiotics work best when the level of the medicine in your bloodstream is kept constant. It is best, therefore, to take the doses at evenly spaced intervals day and night. For example, if you are to take four doses a day, the doses should be spaced about six hours apart.

If the liquid suspension or emulsion form of the sulfonamides has been prescribed for you, be sure to shake the bottle well. The contents tend to settle on the bottom of the bottle, so it is necessary to shake the container to distribute the ingredients evenly and equalize the doses. Be sure to use specially marked droppers or spoons to accurately measure the correct amount of liquid. Household teaspoons vary in size and may not give you the correct dosage.

If you miss a dose, take the missed dose as soon as possible, unless it is almost time for your next dose. In that case, if you are taking two doses a day, space the missed dose and the following dose five to six hours apart; if you are taking three or more doses a day, space the missed dose and the following dose two to four hours apart, or double the next dose. Then return to your regular dosing schedule.

It is very important to continue to take these medications for the entire time prescribed by your doctor (usually ten days), even if the symptoms disappear before the end of that period. If you stop taking the drug too soon, resistant bacteria are given a chance to continue growing, and your infection could recur.

SIDE EFFECTS

Minor. Diarrhea, dizziness, headache, loss of appetite, nausea, or vomiting. As your body adjusts to the medication, these side effects should disappear.

These drugs can increase your sensitivity to sunlight. You should, therefore, avoid prolonged exposure to sunlight and sunlamps. Wear protective clothing and sunglasses; and use an effective sunscreen, but not one that contains para-aminobenzoic acid (PABA). PABA interferes with the antibacterial activity of this medication.
Major. Tell your doctor about any side effects that are persistent or particularly bothersome. IT IS ESPECIALLY IMPORTANT TO TELL YOUR DOCTOR about aching of joints and muscles; blood in the urine; difficulty in swallowing; itching; lower back pain; pain while urinating; pale skin; redness, blistering, or peeling of the skin; skin rash; sore throat and fever; swelling of the front part of the neck; unusual bleeding or bruising; unusual tiredness; or yellowing of the eyes or skin. Also, if your symptoms of infection seem to be getting worse rather than improving, you should contact your doctor.

INTERACTIONS

Sulfonamides interact with several types of drugs:
1. Para-aminobenzoic acid products (sunscreens) can decrease the effectiveness of the sulfonamides.
2. The activity and side effects of anticoagulants (blood thinners, such as warfarin), oral antidiabetic medications, methotrexate, aspirin, phenytoin, and thiopental may be increased when sulfonamides are also taken.
3. Oxyphenbutazone, phenylbutazone, methenamine, probenecid, and sulfinpyrazone can increase the toxicity of the sulfonamides.

BE SURE TO TELL YOUR DOCTOR about any medications you are currently taking, especially any of those listed above.

WARNINGS

• Before starting to take this medication, tell your doctor about any unusual or allergic reactions you have had to any medications, especially to sulfonamide antibiotics

or other sulfa drugs, including diuretics (water pills), dapsone, sulfoxone, oral antidiabetics, and oral antiglaucoma medication.
• Tell your doctor if you now have or if you have ever had glucose-6-phosphate dehydrogenase (G6PD) deficiency, liver disease, porphyria, or kidney disease.
• Before having surgery or any other medical or dental treatment, be sure to tell your doctor or dentist that you are taking a sulfonamide antibiotic.
• This medication has been prescribed for your current infection only. Another infection later on, or one that someone else has, may require a different medicine. You should not give your medicine to other people, and you should not use it for other infections, unless your doctor specifically directs you to do so.
• Be sure to tell your doctor if you are pregnant. These medications, if given to a woman late in pregnancy, can be toxic to the fetus. Also, tell your doctor if you are breast-feeding an infant. Sulfonamides can pass into breast milk and may cause side effects in a small number of nursing infants—those who have glucose-6-phosphate dehydrogenase (G6PD) deficiency. In addition, you should not give sulfonamides to an infant less than one month of age, unless your doctor specifically directs you to do so.

---

sulindac

BRAND NAME (Manufacturer)
Clinoril (Merck Sharp & Dohme)
TYPE OF DRUG
Nonsteroidal anti-inflammatory analgesic
INGREDIENT
sulindac
DOSAGE FORM
Tablets (150 mg and 200 mg)
STORAGE
This medication should be stored in a closed container at room temperature away from heat and direct sunlight.

USES

Sulindac is used to treat the inflammation (pain, swelling, and stiffness) of certain types of arthritis, gout, bursitis, and tendinitis. Sulindac has been shown to block the production of certain body chemicals, called prostaglandins, that may trigger pain. However, it is not fully understood how sulindac works.

TREATMENT

To decrease stomach irritation, your doctor may want you to take this medication with food or antacids.

It is important to take sulindac on schedule and not to miss any doses. If you do miss a dose, take it as soon as possible, unless it is almost time for your next dose. In that case, do not take the missed dose at all; just return to your regular dosing schedule. Do not double the next dose.

If you are taking sulindac to relieve arthritis, you must take it regularly, as directed by your doctor. It may take up to three weeks for you to feel the full benefits of this medication. Sulindac does not cure arthritis, but it will help to control the condition as long as you continue to take it.

SIDE EFFECTS

Minor. Bloating, constipation, diarrhea, difficulty in sleeping, dizziness, drowsiness, headache, heartburn, indigestion, light-headedness, loss of appetite, nausea, nervousness, soreness of the mouth, unusual sweating, or vomiting. As you adjust to the medication, these side effects should stop.

To relieve constipation, increase the amount of fiber in your diet (fresh fruits and vegetables, salads, bran, and whole-grain breads), exercise, and drink more water (unless your doctor directs you to do otherwise).

If you become dizzy or light-headed while taking this drug, sit or lie down for a while; get up slowly from a sitting or reclining position; and be careful on stairs. Also, be especially careful when driving an automobile or operating potentially dangerous equipment.

Major. Tell your doctor about any side effects that are persistent or particularly bothersome. IT IS ESPECIALLY IMPORTANT TO TELL YOUR DOCTOR about bloody or black, tarry stools; blurred vision; chills; confusion; depression; difficulty in breathing; difficulty in hearing; difficult or painful urination; palpitations; ringing or buzzing in the ears; skin rash, hives, or itching; stomach pain; swelling; tightness in the chest; unexplained sore throat and fever; unusual bleeding or bruising; unusual fatigue or weakness; unusual weight gain; vaginal bleeding; wheezing; or yellowing of the eyes or skin.

INTERACTIONS

Sulindac interacts with several types of medications:
1. The combination of anticoagulants (blood thinners, such as warfarin) and sulindac can lead to an increase in bleeding complications.
2. Aspirin, salicylates, or other anti-inflammatory medications can cause an increase in stomach irritation.
3. Probenecid can increase the amount of sulindac in the bloodstream when the drugs are taken concurrently.
4. The blood-pressure-lowering effects of beta blockers may be decreased by this drug.
5. This medication may interact with diuretics (water pills) and cause an increase in the effects of the diuretic.

BE SURE TO TELL YOUR DOCTOR about any medications you are currently taking, especially any of those listed above.

WARNINGS

• Be sure to tell your doctor if you have ever had unusual or allergic reactions to sulindac or any of the other chemically related medications (including aspirin and other salicylates, diclofenac, diflunisal, etodoloc, fenoprofen, flurbiprofen, ibuprofen, indomethacin, ketoprofen, meclofenamate, mefenamic acid, nabumetone, naproxen, oxyphenbutazone, phenylbutazone, piroxicam, and tolmetin).
• Be sure to tell your doctor if you have ever had asthma, bleeding problems, colitis, stomach ulcers or other stomach problems, epilepsy, heart disease, high blood pressure, kidney disease, liver disease, mental illness, or Parkinson's disease.

• If sulindac makes you dizzy or drowsy, do not take part in any activity that requires alertness, such as driving a car or operating potentially dangerous machinery.
• Be sure to tell your doctor or dentist that you are taking this medication before having surgery or any other type of medical or dental treatment.
• Stomach problems are more likely to occur if you take aspirin or other salicylates regularly or drink alcoholic beverages while being treated with this medication. These should be avoided (unless your doctor directs you to do otherwise).
• Be sure to tell your doctor if you are pregnant. The safe use of this medication in human pregnancy has not been established. Side effects have been observed in the development of bones and organs in the offspring of animals that received sulindac during pregnancy. If taken late in pregnancy, this type of drug can also prolong labor. Also, tell your doctor if you are currently breast-feeding an infant. Small amounts of sulindac have been shown to pass into breast milk.

Sulten-10—see sodium sulfacetamide (ophthalmic)

Sultrin Triple Sulfa—see sulfathiazole, sulfacetamide, and sulfabenzamide combination

Sumycin—see tetracycline

Surmontil—see trimipramine

Susano—see atropine, scopolamine, hyoscyamine, and phenobarbital combination

Suspen—see penicillin VK

Sustaire—see theophylline

Symadine—see amantadine

Symmetrel—see amantadine

Synacort—see hydrocortisone (topical)

Synalar—see fluocinolone (topical)

Synalar-HP—see fluocinolone (topical)

Synalgos-DC—see aspirin, caffeine, and dihydrocodeine combination

Synemol—see fluocinolone (topical)

Synophylate-GG—see theophylline and guaifenesin combination

Synthroid—see levothyroxine

Tagamet—see cimetidine

Talwin Nx—see pentazocine

Tamine SR—see phenylpropanolamine, phenylephrine, and brompheniramine combination

tamoxifen

BRAND NAME (Manufacturer)
Nolvadex (ICI)
TYPE OF DRUG
Antiestrogen and antineoplastic (anticancer drug)
INGREDIENT
tamoxifen
DOSAGE FORM
Tablets (10 mg)
STORAGE
Tamoxifen should be stored at room temperature in a tightly closed, light-resistant container.

USES

This medication is used in the treatment of advanced breast cancer in postmenopausal women. Tamoxifen is a nonsteroidal antiestrogen drug. It is not yet fully understood how tamoxifen works, but it is possible that the drug acts to block estrogen from binding to the breast tissue, this action would work to inhibit further tumor growth.

TREATMENT

Tamoxifen can be taken either on an empty stomach or with food or a glass of milk, unless your doctor directs you to do otherwise.

If you miss a dose of this medication, take the missed dose as soon as possible, unless it is almost time for the next dose. In that case, do not take the missed dose at all; just return to your regular dosing schedule. Do not double the next dose.

SIDE EFFECTS

Minor. Distaste for food, dizziness, headache, hot flashes, light-headedness, nausea, vaginal itching, or vomiting. These side effects should disappear as your body adjusts to the medication.

It is extremely important that you continue to take this medication in spite of any nausea or vomiting that you may experience. If you vomit immediately after taking a dose, call your doctor; it may be necessary for you to repeat the dose.

It is possible that you may experience an increase in bone and tumor pain when your treatment with tamoxifen is first started. The pain generally subsides rapidly but may require the temporary use of analgesics (pain relievers). Be sure to consult your doctor if you experience any unusual pain after starting tamoxifen.

If you feel dizzy or light-headed, sit or lie down for a while; get up slowly from a sitting or reclining position.
Major. Tell your doctor about any side effects that are persistent or particularly bothersome. IT IS ESPECIALLY IMPORTANT TO TELL YOUR DOCTOR about blurred vision, chills, depression, fever, rapid weight gain (three to five pounds within a week), rash, sore throat, unusual weakness, or vaginal bleeding or discharge.

INTERACTIONS

The activity and anticoagulant (blood-thinning) effects of drugs such as warfarin can be increased when they are taken at the same time as tamoxifen. Be sure to tell your doctor if you are taking an anticoagulant.

WARNINGS

• Be sure to tell your doctor about any unusual or allergic reactions you have had to any medications, especially to tamoxifen.
• Before starting to take this medication, be sure to tell your doctor if you now have or if you have ever had blood disorders or visual disturbances.
• Before starting to take this medication, it is very important for you to tell your doctor if you are pregnant. Although there have been no studies done on the effects of this medication in pregnant women, isolated reports of problems have been documented when pregnant women have been using tamoxifen. Also be sure to tell your doctor if you are breast-feeding.

Taractan—see chlorprothixene

Tavist—see clemastine

Tavist-1—see clemastine

T-Dry Jr.—see pseudoephedrine and chlorpheniramine combination

Tebamide—see trimethobenzamide

Tega D&E—see phenylpropanolamine and guaifenesin combination

Tegopen—see cloxacillin

Tegretol—see carbamazepine

Tegretol Chewable—see carbamazepine

temazepam

BRAND NAMES (Manufacturers)
Restoril (Sandoz)
temazepam (various manufacturers)
TYPE OF DRUG
Benzodiazepine sedative/hypnotic
INGREDIENT
temazepam
DOSAGE FORM
Capsules (15 mg and 30 mg)
STORAGE
This medication should be stored at room temperature in a tightly closed, light-resistant container.

USES

Temazepam is prescribed to treat insomnia, including problems with falling asleep, waking during the night, and early morning wakefulness. It is not clear exactly how this medicine works, but it may relieve insomnia by acting as a depressant of the central nervous system (brain and spinal cord).

TREATMENT

This medicine should be taken 30 to 60 minutes before bedtime. It can be taken with food or a full glass of water if stomach upset occurs. Do not take this medication with antacids, since they may retard its absorption from the gastrointestinal tract.

If you are taking this medication regularly and you miss a dose, take the missed dose immediately if you remember within an hour. If more than an hour has passed, do not take the missed dose at all; just wait for the next scheduled dose. Do not double the dose.

SIDE EFFECTS

Minor. Bitter taste in the mouth, constipation, diarrhea, dizziness, drowsiness (after a night's sleep), dry mouth, excessive salivation, fatigue, flushing, headache, heartburn, loss of appetite, nausea, nervousness, sweating, or vomiting. As your body adjusts to the medication, these side effects should disappear.

To relieve constipation, increase the amount of fiber in your diet (fresh fruits and vegetables, salads, bran, and whole-grain breads), exercise, and drink more water (unless your doctor directs you to do otherwise).

Dry mouth can be relieved by chewing sugarless gum or by sucking on ice chips.

If you feel dizzy, sit or lie down for a while; get up slowly from a sitting or reclining position, and be careful on stairs.

Major. Tell your doctor about any side effects that are persistent or particularly bothersome. IT IS ESPECIALLY IMPORTANT TO TELL YOUR DOCTOR about blurred or double vision, chest pain, depression, difficulty in urinating, fainting, falling, fever, joint pain, hallucinations, mouth sores, nightmares, palpitations, rash, severe depression, shortness of breath, slurred speech, sore throat, uncoordinated movements, unusual excitement, unusual tiredness, or yellowing of the eyes or skin.

INTERACTIONS

Temazepam interacts with several other types of drugs:
1. To prevent oversedation, this drug should not be taken with alcohol, other sedative drugs, or central nervous system depressants (such as antihistamines, barbiturates, muscle relaxants, pain medications, narcotics, antiseizure medications, and phenothiazine tranquilizers) or with antidepressants.
2. Temazepam may decrease the effectiveness of carbamazepine, levodopa, and oral anticoagulants (blood thinners) and may increase the effects of phenytoin.
3. Disulfiram, cimetidine, oral contraceptives (birth control pills), and isoniazid may increase the blood levels of temazepam, which can lead to toxic effects.
4. Concurrent use of rifampin may decrease the effectiveness of temazepam.

BE SURE TO TELL YOUR DOCTOR about any medications you are currently taking, especially those listed above.

WARNINGS

• Tell your doctor about unusual or allergic reactions you have had to any medications, especially to temazepam or other benzodiazepine tranquilizers (such as alprazolam, chlordiazepoxide, clorazepate, diazepam, flurazepam, halazepam, lorazepam, oxazepam, prazepam, and triazolam).
• Tell your doctor if you now have or if you have ever had liver disease, kidney disease, epilepsy, lung disease, myasthenia gravis, porphyria, mental depression, or mental illness.
• This medicine can cause drowsiness. Avoid tasks that require alertness, such as driving a car.
• Temazepam has the potential for abuse and must be used with caution. Tolerance may develop quickly; do not increase the dosage without first consulting your doctor. It is also important not to stop taking this drug suddenly if you have been taking it in large amounts or if you have used it for several weeks. Your doctor may want to reduce the dosage gradually.
• This is a safe drug when used properly. When it is combined with other sedative drugs or alcohol, however, serious side effects may develop.
• Be sure to tell your doctor if you are pregnant. This type of medicine may increase the chance of birth defects if it is taken during the first three months of pregnancy. In addition, use of this medicine during the last six months of pregnancy may result in addiction of the fetus, leading to withdrawal side effects in the newborn. Also, use of this medicine during the last weeks of pregnancy may cause excessive drowsiness, slowed heartbeat, and breathing difficulties in the infant. Tell your doctor if you are breast-feeding. This medicine can pass into breast milk and cause unwanted side effects in nursing infants.

Tenoretic—see atenolol and chlorthalidone combination

Tenormin—see atenolol

Tenuate—see diethylpropion

Tenuate Dospan—see diethylpropion

Tepanil—see diethylpropion

Tepanil Ten-Tab—see diethylpropion

terbutaline

BRAND NAMES (Manufacturers)
Brethaire (Geigy)
Brethine (Geigy)
Bricanyl (Lakeside)
TYPE OF DRUG
Bronchodilator
INGREDIENT
terbutaline
DOSAGE FORMS
Tablets (2.5 mg and 5 mg)
Inhalation aerosol (each spray delivers 0.2 mg)
STORAGE
Terbutaline tablets should be stored at room temperature in a tightly closed, light-resistant container. The inhalation

aerosol should be stored at room temperature away from excessive heat; the contents are pressurized and can explode if heated. Discard any outdated medication.

USES

Terbutaline is used to relieve wheezing and shortness of breath caused by lung diseases such as asthma, bronchitis, and emphysema. This drug acts directly on the muscles of the bronchi (breathing tubes) to relieve bronchospasm (muscle contractions of the bronchi), which in turn reduces airway resistance and allows air to move more freely to and from the lungs—making breathing easier.

TREATMENT

In order to lessen stomach upset, you can take terbutaline with food (unless your doctor directs you to do otherwise).

The inhalation aerosol form of this medication is usually packaged with an instruction sheet. Read the directions carefully before using the medication. The contents should be shaken well just before each use. The contents tend to settle on the bottom, so it is necessary to shake the bottle to distribute the ingredients evenly and equalize the doses. If more than one inhalation is necessary, wait at least one full minute between doses in order to receive the full benefit of the first dose.

If you miss a dose of this medication and remember within an hour, take the missed dose immediately and then return to your regular schedule. If more than an hour has passed, do not take the missed dose at all; just return to your regular dosing schedule. Do not double the next dose.

SIDE EFFECTS

Minor. Anxiety, bad taste in mouth, dizziness, headache, flushing, irritability, insomnia, loss of appetite, nausea, nervousness, restlessness, sweating, vomiting, or weakness. These side effects should disappear as your body adjusts to the medication.

To prevent dryness or irritation of the mouth or throat, rinse your mouth with water after each dose.

In order to avoid difficulty in falling asleep, check with your doctor to see if you can take the last dose of this medication several hours before bedtime each day.

If you feel dizzy, sit or lie down for a while; get up from a sitting or lying position slowly, and be careful on stairs.

Major. Tell your doctor about any side effects that are persistent or particularly bothersome. IT IS ESPECIALLY IMPORTANT TO TELL YOUR DOCTOR about bluish coloration of the skin, chest pain, difficult or painful urination, increased wheezing or difficulty in breathing, muscle cramps, palpitations, or tremors.

INTERACTIONS

Terbutaline interacts with other types of medications:
1. The beta blockers (acebutolol, atenolol, betaxolol, carteolol, esmolol, labetalol, metoprolol, nadolol, penbutolol, pindolol, propranolol, or timolol) antagonize (act against) this medication, decreasing its effectiveness.
2. Monoamine oxidase (MAO) inhibitors; tricyclic anti-

depressants; antihistamines; levothyroxine; and over-the-counter (nonprescription) cough, cold, allergy, asthma, diet, and sinus medications may increase the side effects of terbutaline. At least 14 days should separate the use of this drug and the use of an MAO inhibitor.
3. There may be a change in the dosage requirements of insulin or oral antidiabetic medications when terbutaline is started.
4. The blood-pressure-lowering effects of guanethidine may be decreased by this medication.
5. The use of terbutaline with other bronchodilator drugs (either oral or inhalant drugs) can have additive side effects. Discuss this with your doctor.

BE SURE TO TELL YOUR DOCTOR about any medications you are currently taking, especially those listed above.

WARNINGS

• Tell your doctor about unusual or allergic reactions you have had to any medications, especially to terbutaline or any related drug (albuterol, amphetamines, ephedrine, epinephrine, isoproterenol, norepinephrine, phenylephrine, phenylpropanolamine, pseudoephedrine, or metaproterenol).
• Tell your doctor if you now have or if you have ever had diabetes, glaucoma, high blood pressure, epilepsy, heart disease, enlarged prostate gland, or thyroid disease.
• This medication can cause dizziness. Your ability to perform tasks that require alertness, such as driving a car may be decreased. Appropriate caution should be taken.
• Before having surgery or any other medical or dental treatment, tell your doctor or dentist you are taking this drug.
• Avoid allowing the aerosol inhalation to come in contact with eyes.
• Do not puncture, break, or burn the aerosol inhalation container. The contents are under pressure and may explode.
• Do not exceed the recommended dosage of this medication; excessive use may lead to an increase in side effects or a loss of effectiveness. Contact your doctor if you do not respond to the usual dose of this medication. It may be a sign of worsening asthma, which may require additional therapy.
• Tell your doctor if you are pregnant. Terbutaline should only be administered during pregnancy if the benefits to the mother clearly outweigh potential risks to the fetus. Also, tell your doctor if you are breast-feeding. Small amounts of terbutaline pass into breast milk.

terfenadine

BRAND NAME (Manufacturer)
Seldane (Marion Merrell Dow)
TYPE OF DRUG
Antihistamine
INGREDIENT
terfenadine
DOSAGE FORM
Tablets (60 mg)

STORAGE

Terfenadine should be stored at room temperature in a tightly closed container. The tablets should not be exposed to high temperatures (above 104°F), direct sunlight, or moisture during storage.

USES

Terfenadine is used to treat the symptoms of allergy, including sneezing, runny nose, itching, and tearing. It belongs to a group of drugs known as antihistamines, which acts by blocking the action of histamine, a chemical that is released by the body during an allergic reaction.

TREATMENT

Terfenadine can be taken either on an empty stomach or with food or milk (unless your doctor directs otherwise).

Terfenadine should be taken only as needed to control the symptoms of allergy.

If you miss a dose of this medication and you are taking it on a regular schedule, take the missed dose as soon as possible, unless it is almost time for your next dose. In that case, do not take the missed dose at all; just return to your regular dosing schedule. Do not double the next dose.

SIDE EFFECTS

Minor. Abdominal pain; cough; dizziness; drowsiness; dry mouth, nose, or throat; fatigue; headache; increased appetite; insomnia; nausea; nervousness; nosebleeds; sore throat; sweating; vomiting; or weakness. These side effects should disappear as your body adjusts to this medication.

To reduce mouth dryness, chew sugarless gum or suck on ice chips or hard candy.

If you feel dizzy or light-headed, sit or lie down for a while; get up slowly from a sitting or reclining position, and be careful on stairs.

Major. Tell your doctor about any side effects that are persistent or particularly bothersome. IT IS ESPECIALLY IMPORTANT TO TELL YOUR DOCTOR about depression, hair loss, itching, menstrual disorders, muscle or bone pain, nightmares, palpitations, shortness of breath, tingling of your fingers or toes, tremors, urinary frequency, visual disturbances, or yellowing of the skin or eyes.

INTERACTIONS

Terfenadine interacts with the following medications:

1. The combination of terfenadine and ketocorcizole can result in increased adverse effects.

2. The combination of terfenadine and certain antibiotics, such as erythromycin and troleandomycin, can result in increased adverse effects.

BE SURE TO TELL YOUR DOCTOR about any medications you are currently taking, especially any listed above.

WARNINGS

• Tell your doctor about unusual or allergic reactions you have had to any medications, especially to terfenadine.

• Before starting terfenadine, tell your doctor if you now have or if you have ever had asthma.

• Terfenadine causes less drowsiness than other antihistamines. However, until you see how it affects you, be cautious about performing tasks that require alertness, such as driving a car or operating potentially dangerous machinery.

• Be sure to tell your doctor if you are pregnant. This drug's safety in human pregnancy has not been established. Also, tell your doctor if you are breast-feeding. The effects of terfenadine on nursing infants are not yet known.

Terfonyl—see sulfonamide antibiotics (oral)

Terramycin—see oxytetracycline

Testred—see methyltestosterone

Tetracap—see tetracycline

tetracycline

BRAND NAMES (Manufacturers)
Achromycin V (Lederle)
Nor-Tet (Vortech)
Panmycin (Upjohn)
Robitet Robicaps (Robins)
Sumycin (Squibb)
Tetracap (Circle)
tetracycline hydrochloride (various manufacturers)
Tetracyn (Pfizer)
Tetralan (Lannett)
Tetram (Dunhall)
TYPE OF DRUG
Tetracycline antibiotic
INGREDIENT
tetracycline
DOSAGE FORMS
Tablets (250 mg and 500 mg)
Capsules (100 mg, 250 mg, and 500 mg)
Oral suspension (125 mg per 5-ml spoonful)
STORAGE
Tetracycline tablets, capsules, and oral suspension should be stored at room temperature in tightly closed, light-resistant containers. Any unused portion of the suspension should be discarded after 14 days because the drug loses its potency after that period. Discard any medication that is outdated or no longer needed. This medication should never be frozen.

USES

Tetracycline is used to treat acne (bacteria may be partly responsible for the development of acne lesions) and a wide variety of bacterial infections. It acts by inhibiting the growth of bacteria. Tetracycline kills susceptible bacteria, but it is not effective against viruses or fungi.

TREATMENT

Ideally, this medication should be taken on an empty stomach one hour before or two hours after a meal. It should be taken with a full glass of water in order to avoid irritating the throat or esophagus (swallowing tube). If this drug causes stomach upset, however, you can take it with food (unless your doctor directs you to do otherwise).

Avoid consuming dairy products (milk, cheese, etc.) within two hours of any dose of this drug. Avoid taking antacids and laxatives that contain aluminum, calcium, or magnesium within an hour or two of a dose. Avoid taking any medication containing iron within three hours of a dose. These products, including vitamins, chemically bind tetracycline in the stomach and gastrointestinal tract, preventing the drug from being absorbed into the body.

The oral suspension form of this medication should be shaken well just before measuring each dose. The contents tend to settle on the bottom of the bottle, so it is necessary to shake the container to distribute the ingredients evenly and equalize the doses. Each dose should then be measured carefully with a specially designed 5-ml measuring spoon. An ordinary kitchen teaspoon is not accurate enough. The oral suspension form of this medication should not be mixed with any other substance, unless your doctor says so.

Tetracycline works best when the level of medicine in your bloodstream is kept constant. It is best, therefore, to take the doses at evenly spaced intervals day and night. For example, if you are to take four doses a day, the doses should be spaced six hours apart.

If you miss a dose of this medication, take the missed dose immediately. However, if you do not remember to take the missed dose until it is almost time for your next dose, take it; space the following dose about halfway through the regular interval between doses; and then return to your regular dosing schedule.

It is important to continue to take this medication for the entire time prescribed by your doctor, even if the symptoms disappear before the end of that period. If you stop taking the drug too soon, resistant bacteria are given a chance to continue growing, and the infection could recur.

SIDE EFFECTS
Minor. Diarrhea, discoloration of the nails, dizziness, loss of appetite, nausea, stomach cramps and upset, or vomiting. These side effects should disappear as your body adjusts to the medication.

Tetracycline can increase your sensitivity to sunlight. You should, therefore, avoid prolonged exposure to sunlight or sunlamps. Wear protective clothing and sunglasses, and use an effective sunscreen.

Major. Tell your doctor about any side effects that are persistent or particularly bothersome. IT IS ESPECIALLY IMPORTANT TO TELL YOUR DOCTOR about darkened tongue, difficulty in breathing, joint pain, mouth irritation, rash, rectal or vaginal itching, sore throat and fever, unusual bleeding or bruising, or yellowing of the eyes or skin. Also, if your symptoms of infection seem to be getting worse rather than improving, you should contact your doctor.

INTERACTIONS
Tetracycline interacts with other types of medications:
1. It can increase the absorption of digoxin, which may lead to digoxin toxicity.

2. The gastrointestinal side effects (nausea, vomiting, or stomach upset) of theophylline may be increased by tetracycline.
3. The dosage of oral anticoagulants (blood thinners, such as warfarin) may need to be adjusted when this medication is started.
4. Tetracycline may decrease the effectiveness of oral contraceptives (birth control pills), and pregnancy could result. You should, therefore, use a different or additional form of birth control while taking tetracycline. Discuss this with your doctor.

BE SURE TO TELL YOUR DOCTOR about any medications that you are currently taking, especially any of the medications that are listed above.

WARNINGS
• Tell your doctor about unusual or allergic reactions you have had to any medications, especially to tetracycline or to oxytetracycline, doxycycline, or minocycline.
• Tell your doctor if you now have or if you have ever had kidney or liver disease.
• Tetracycline can affect tests for syphilis; tell your doctor you are taking this drug if you are being treated for syphilis.
• Make sure that your prescription for this drug is marked with the expiration date. The drug should be discarded after the expiration date. If tetracycline is used after it has expired, serious side effects (especially to the kidneys) could result.
• This medication has been prescribed for your current infection only. Another infection later on, or one that someone else has, may require a different medicine. You should not give your medicine to other people or use it for other infections unless your doctor specifically directs you to do so.
• Be sure to tell your doctor if you are pregnant or if you are breast-feeding. Tetracycline crosses the placenta and passes into breast milk. If used during tooth development, this drug can cause permanent tooth discoloration. It can also inhibit tooth and bone growth in the fetus. It should not be used in pregnant or nursing women, infants, or children less than eight years of age.

tetracycline hydrochloride—see tetracycline

Tetracyn—see tetracycline

Tetralan—see tetracycline

Tetram—see tetracycline

Texacort—see hydrocortisone (topical)

T-Gen—see trimethobenzamide

T-Gesic—see acetaminophen and hydrocodone combination

Thalitone—see chlorthalidone

Theo-24—see theophylline

Theobid—see theophylline

Theochron—see theophylline

Theoclear—see theophylline

Theocolate—see theophylline and guaifenesin combination

Theo-Dur—see theophylline

Theolair—see theophylline

Theolate—see theophylline and guaifenesin combination

Theon—see theophylline

theophylline

BRAND NAMES (Manufacturers)
Accurbron (Merrell Dow)
Aerolate (Fleming)
Aquaphyllin (Ferndale)
Asmalix (Century)
Bronkodyl (Breon)
Constant-T (Geigy)
Elixomin (Cenci)
Elixophyllin (Berlex)
Lanophyllin (Lannett)
Quibron-T (Mead Johnson)
Respbid (Boehringer Ingelheim)
Slo-bid Gyrocaps (Rorer)
Slo-Phyllin (Rorer)
Somophyllin-T (Fisons)
Sustaire (Pfipharmics)
Theo-24 (Searle)
Theobid (Glaxo)
Theochron (Forest)
Theoclear (Central)
Theo-Dur (Key)
Theolair (Riker)
Theon (Bock)
theophylline (various manufacturers)
Theospan (Laser)
Theostat (Laser)
Theo-Time (Major)
Theovent (Schering)
Uniphyl (Purdue Frederick)

TYPE OF DRUG
Bronchodilator

INGREDIENT
theophylline

DOSAGE FORMS
Tablets (100 mg, 125 mg, 200 mg, 225 mg, 250 mg, and 300 mg)
Capsules (100 mg, 200 mg, and 250 mg)
Sustained-release tablets and capsules (50 mg, 60 mg, 65 mg, 75 mg, 100 mg, 125 mg, 130 mg, 200 mg, 250 mg, 260 mg, 300 mg, 400 mg, and 500 mg)
Oral liquid (80 mg, 150 mg, and 160 mg per 15-ml spoonful, some with alcohol of varying amounts, including 1%, 7. 5%, and 20%)
Oral suspension (300 mg per 15-ml spoonful)

STORAGE
Theophylline tablets, capsules, liquid, and suspension should be stored at room temperature. It should also be kept in tightly closed, light-resistant containers. This medication should never be frozen. Discard any outdated medication.

USES
Theophylline is prescribed to treat breathing problems (wheezing and shortness of breath) caused by asthma, bronchitis, or emphysema. It relaxes the smooth muscle of the bronchial airways (breathing tubes), which opens the air passages to the lungs and allows air to move in and out more easily.

TREATMENT
Theophylline should be taken on an empty stomach 30 to 60 minutes before a meal or two hours after a meal. If this medication causes stomach irritation, however, you can take it with food or with a full glass of water or milk (unless your doctor directs you to do otherwise).

Antidiarrheal medications and some antacids prevent the absorption of theophylline from the gastrointestinal tract. Therefore, at least one hour should separate doses of one of these medications and theophylline.

The sustained-release tablets and capsules should be swallowed whole. Chewing, crushing, or crumbling the tablets or capsules destroys their sustained-release activity and possibly increases the side effects. If the tablet is scored for breaking, you can break it along these lines. If the regular capsules are too large to swallow, they can be opened and the contents mixed with jam, jelly, or applesauce. The mixture should then be swallowed without chewing.

The theophylline sprinkle capsules can also be taken whole, or the capsule can be opened and the beads sprinkled on a spoonful of soft food, such as applesauce or pudding. The sprinkles should be swallowed immediately without chewing the beads. The contents of the capsule should not be subdivided in order to ensure equal doses.

If you are using the suspension form of this medication, the bottle should be shaken well just before measuring each dose. The contents tend to settle on the bottom of the bottle, so it is necessary to shake the container to distribute the medication evenly and equalize the doses. Each dose of the oral liquid or suspension should be measured carefully with a 5-ml measuring spoon or a dose cup designed for that purpose. Ordinary kitchen spoons are not accurate enough to ensure that you receive the proper dose.

Theophylline works best when the level of the medicine in your bloodstream is kept constant. It is best, therefore, to take it at evenly spaced intervals day and night. For example, if you are to take four doses a day, the doses should be spaced six hours apart. Try to take your medication at the same time(s) each day.

Try not to miss any doses of this medication. If you do miss a dose, take the missed dose as soon as possible, unless it is almost time for the next dose. In that case, do not take the missed dose at all; just return to your regular dosing schedule. Do not double the next dose.

SIDE EFFECTS

Minor. Diarrhea, dizziness, flushing, headache, heartburn, increased urination, insomnia, irritability, loss of appetite, nausea, nervousness, stomach pain, or vomiting. These side effects should disappear as your body adjusts to the medication.

If you feel dizzy or light-headed, sit or lie down for a while; get up slowly from a sitting or reclining position, and be careful on stairs.

Major. Tell your doctor about any side effects that are persistent or particularly bothersome. IT IS ESPECIALLY IMPORTANT TO TELL YOUR DOCTOR about black, tarry stools; confusion; convulsions; difficulty in breathing; fainting; muscle twitches; palpitations; rash; severe abdominal pain; or unusual weakness.

INTERACTIONS

Theophylline interacts with several other types of drugs:

1. It can increase the diuretic effect of furosemide.

2. Concurrent use of reserpine and theophylline can cause a rapid heart rate.

3. Beta blockers (acebutolol, atenolol, betaxolol, carteolol, esmolol, labetalol, metoprolol, nadolol, penbutolol, pindolol, propranolol, or timolol) can decrease the effectiveness of theophylline.

4. Theophylline can increase the side effects of over-the-counter (nonprescription) sinus, cough, cold, asthma, allergy, and diet products; digoxin; and oral anticoagulants (blood thinners, such as warfarin).

5. Theophylline can decrease the effectiveness of phenytoin and lithium.

6. Phenobarbital, carbamazepine, and rifampin can increase the elimination of theophylline from the body, decreasing its effectiveness.

7. Cimetidine, ciprofloxacin, erythromycin, norfloxacin, troleandomycin, oral contraceptives (birth control pills), allopurinol, and thiabendazole can decrease the elimination of theophylline from the body and increase its side effects.

8. Verapamil can cause an increase in the effects of theophylline.

Before you start to take this medication, BE SURE TO TELL YOUR DOCTOR about any medications you are currently taking, especially any of those listed above.

WARNINGS

• Tell your doctor about unusual or allergic reactions you have had to any medications, especially to theophylline, aminophylline, caffeine, dyphylline, oxtriphylline, or theobromine.

• Tell your doctor if you now have or if you have ever had an enlarged prostate gland, fibrocystic breast disease, heart disease, kidney disease, low or high blood pressure, liver disease, stomach ulcers, or thyroid disease.

• Cigarette or marijuana smoking may affect this drug's action. BE SURE TO TELL YOUR DOCTOR if you smoke. Also, do not quit smoking without informing your doctor.

• High fever, diarrhea, flu, and influenza vaccinations can affect the action of this drug. Therefore, be sure to tell your doctor if you experience any episodes of high fever or prolonged diarrhea while taking this drug. Before having any vaccinations, especially those to prevent the flu, BE SURE TO TELL YOUR DOCTOR that you are taking this medication.

• Avoid drinking large amounts of caffeine-containing beverages (coffee, cocoa, tea, or cola drinks), and avoid eating large amounts of chocolate. These products may increase the side effects of theophylline.

• Do not change your diet without first consulting your doctor. A high-protein, low-carbohydrate diet or charbroiled foods may affect the action of this drug.

• Before having surgery or any other medical or dental treatment, be sure to tell your doctor or dentist that you are taking this medication.

• Before taking any over-the-counter (nonprescription) asthma, allergy, cough, cold, sinus, or diet products, ask your doctor or pharmacist. These products may add to the side effects of theophylline.

• Do not change brands or dosage forms of this medication without your doctor's permission. If your medication refill looks different, check with your doctor.

• The elderly and young children may be more sensitive to the effects of theophylline.

• Your doctor may require you to have periodic blood tests to be sure your medication is working properly.

• Be sure to tell your doctor if you are pregnant. Although theophylline appears to be safe during pregnancy, extensive studies in humans have not been conducted. Also, tell your doctor if you are breast-feeding an infant. Small amounts of theophylline pass into breast milk and may cause irritability, fretfulness, or insomnia in nursing infants.

theophylline and guaifenesin combination

BRAND NAMES (Manufacturers)
Asbron G (Sandoz)
Bronchial (various manufacturers)
Glyceryl-T (Rugby)
Lanophyllin-GG (Lannett)
Quiagen (Goldline)
Quibron (Bristol Labs)
Quibron 300 (Bristol Labs)
Slo-Phyllin GG (Rorer)
Synophylate-GG (Central)
Theocolate (My-K Labs)
Theolate (various manufacturers)

TYPE OF DRUG
Bronchodilator and expectorant

INGREDIENT
Stheophylline and guaifenesin

DOSAGE FORMS
Tablets (137 mg or 138 mg theophylline and 100 mg guaifenesin)
Capsules (150 mg theophylline and 90 mg guaifenesin; 300 mg theophylline and 180 mg guaifenesin)
Oral liquid (100 mg theophylline and 100 mg guaifenesin; 137 mg theophylline and 100 mg guaifenesin;

and 150 mg theophylline and 90 mg guaifenesin per 15-ml spoonful, some with alcohol {10% or 15%})

STORAGE

Theophylline and guaifenesin combination tablets, capsules, and oral liquid should be stored at room temperature in tightly closed containers. This medication should never be frozen. Discard any outdated medication or medication that is no longer needed.

USES

Theophylline and guaifenesin combination medication is prescribed to treat breathing problems (wheezing and shortness of breath) caused by asthma, bronchitis, or emphysema. Theophylline relaxes the smooth muscle of the bronchial airways (breathing tubes), which opens up the air passages, allowing air to move more easily to and from the lungs. Guaifenesin is an expectorant that is used to loosen phlegm, thin bronchial secretions, and promote discharge of mucus from the respiratory tract.

TREATMENT

Theophylline and guaifenesin should be taken on an empty stomach 30 to 60 minutes before a meal or two hours after a meal. If this medication causes stomach irritation, however, you can take it with food or with a full glass of water or milk (unless your doctor directs you to do otherwise).

Antidiarrheal medications and some antacids prevent the absorption of theophylline. Therefore, at least one hour should separate doses of these two types of medication.

The dose of the oral liquid should be measured carefully with a 5-ml measuring spoon or a dose cup designed for that purpose. An ordinary kitchen teaspoon is not accurate enough.

Theophylline works best when the concentration of medicine in your bloodstream is kept constant. It is best, therefore, to take the doses at evenly spaced intervals day and night. For example, if you are to take four doses a day, the doses should be spaced six hours apart.

Try not to miss any doses of this medication. If you do miss a dose, take the missed dose as soon as possible, unless it is almost time for the next dose. Do not take more than the recommended dose.

SIDE EFFECTS

Minor. Diarrhea, dizziness, flushing, headache, heartburn, increased urination, insomnia, irritability, loss of appetite, nausea, nervousness, paleness, stomach pain, or vomiting. These side effects should disappear as your body adjusts to the medication.

If you feel dizzy or light-headed, sit or lie down for a while; get up slowly from a sitting or reclining position, and be careful on stairs.

This medication may cause you to cough more frequently. Coughing is your body's way of discharging the mucus from the respiratory tract. This medication loosens and thins the mucus in your respiratory tract, making your cough more productive.

Major. Tell your doctor about any side effects that are persistent or particularly bothersome. IT IS ESPECIALLY IMPORTANT TO TELL YOUR DOCTOR about black,

tarry stools; confusion; convulsions; difficulty in breathing; fainting; muscle twitches; palpitations; rash; severe abdominal pain; or unusual weakness.

INTERACTIONS

Theophylline interacts with several other types of drugs:
1. It can increase the effects (diuresis, or increased urination) of furosemide.
2. Concurrent use of reserpine and theophylline can cause a rapid heart rate.
3. Beta blockers (acebutolol, atenolol, betaxolol, carteolol, esmolol, labetalol, metoprolol, nadolol, penbutolol, pindolol, propranolol, timolol) can decrease the effectiveness of theophylline.
4. Theophylline can increase the side effects of over-the-counter (nonprescription) sinus, cough, cold, asthma, allergy, and diet products; digoxin; and oral anticoagulants (blood thinners, such as warfarin).
5. Theophylline can decrease the effectiveness of phenytoin and lithium.
6. Phenobarbital, carbamazepine, and rifampin can increase the elimination of theophylline from the body, decreasing its effectiveness.
7. Cimetidine, erythromycin, troleandomycin, oral contraceptives (birth control pills), allopurinol, and thiabendazole can decrease the elimination of theophylline from the body and increase its side effects.

Before starting to take this medication, BE SURE TO TELL YOUR DOCTOR about any medications you are currently taking, especially any of those listed above.

WARNINGS

Tell your doctor about unusual or allergic reactions you have had to any medications, especially to theophylline, aminophylline, caffeine, dyphylline, oxtriphylline, theobromine, or guaifenesin.

Tell your doctor if you now have or if you have ever had an enlarged prostate gland, fibrocystic breast disease, heart disease, kidney disease, low or high blood pressure, liver disease, stomach ulcers, or thyroid disease.

Cigarette or marijuana smoking may affect this drug's action. BE SURE TO TELL YOUR DOCTOR if you smoke. Also, do not suddenly stop smoking without informing your doctor.

High fever, diarrhea, the flu, or an influenza vaccination can also affect the action of this drug. You should tell your doctor about episodes of high fever or prolonged diarrhea. Before having any vaccinations, especially those to prevent the flu, BE SURE TO TELL YOUR DOCTOR that you are taking this medication.

Avoid drinking large amounts of caffeine-containing beverages (coffee, cocoa, tea, or cola drinks), and avoid eating large amounts of chocolate. These products may increase the side effects of theophylline.

While you are taking this medication, drink at least eight glasses of water a day to help loosen bronchial secretions (unless your doctor directs you to do otherwise).

Do not change brands of this medication without your doctor's permission. If you receive a refill, and the medication looks different, consult your doctor or pharmacist.

Do not change your diet without first consulting your doctor. A high-protein, low-carbohydrate diet or char-broiled foods can affect the action of this drug.

Before having surgery or any other medical or dental treatment, be sure to tell your doctor or dentist that you are taking this medication.

Your doctor may want you to have regular blood tests done to make sure this medication is working properly.

Elderly patients and young children are more sensitive to the effects of this medication.

Be sure to tell your doctor if you are pregnant. Although theophylline appears to be safe during pregnancy, extensive studies in humans have not been conducted. Also, tell your doctor if you are breast-feeding. Small amounts of theophylline pass into breast milk and may cause irritability, fretfulness, and insomnia in nursing infants.

Theospan—see theophylline

Theostat—see theophylline

Theo-Time—see theophylline

Theovent—see theophylline

thioridazine

BRAND NAMES (Manufacturers)
Mellaril (Sandoz)
Millazine (Major)
thioridazine hydrochloride (various manufacturers)
TYPE OF DRUG
Phenothiazine tranquilizer
INGREDIENT
thioridazine
DOSAGE FORMS
Tablets (10 mg, 15 mg, 25 mg, 50 mg, 100 mg, 150 mg, and 200 mg)
Oral concentrate (30 mg and 100 mg per ml, with 3% and 4.2% alcohol, respectively)
Oral suspension (25 mg and 100 mg per 5-ml spoonful)
STORAGE
The tablet form of this medication should be stored at room temperature in a tightly closed, light-resistant container. The oral concentrate and oral suspension forms of this medication should be stored in the refrigerator in tightly closed, light-resistant containers. If the oral concentrate or suspension turns slightly yellowish, the medication is still effective and can be used. However, if it changes color markedly or has particles floating in it, it should not be used; rather, it should be discarded down the sink. This medication should never be frozen.

USES
Thioridazine is prescribed to treat the symptoms of certain types of mental illness, such as emotional symptoms of psychosis, the manic phase of manic-depressive illness, and severe behavioral problems in children. It may also be used for moderate to marked depression or sleep disturbances in adults. This medication is thought to relieve the symptoms of mental illness by blocking certain chemicals involved with nerve transmission in the brain. Thioridazine may also be used to treat anxiety.

TREATMENT
In order to avoid stomach irritation, you can take this medication with a meal or with a glass of water or milk (unless your doctor directs you to do otherwise).

Antacids and antidiarrheal medicines may decrease the absorption of this medication from the gastrointestinal tract. Therefore, at least one hour should separate doses of one of these medicines and thioridazine.

The oral suspension form of this medication should be shaken well just before measuring each dose. The contents tend to settle on the bottom of the bottle, so it is necessary to shake the container to distribute the ingredients evenly and equalize the doses. Each dose should then be measured carefully with a specially designed 5-ml measuring spoon. An ordinary kitchen teaspoon is not accurate enough.

The oral concentrate form of this medication should be measured carefully with the dropper provided, then added to four ounces ($^1/_2$ cup) or more of water, milk, or a carbonated beverage or to applesauce or pudding immediately prior to administration. To prevent possible loss of effectiveness, the medication should not be diluted in tea, coffee, or apple juice.

If you miss a dose of this medication, take the missed dose as soon as possible, unless it is almost time for your next dose. In that case, do not take the missed dose at all; just return to your regular dosing schedule. Do not double the next dose (unless your doctor directs you to do so).

The full effects of this medication for the control of emotional or mental symptoms may not become apparent for at least two weeks after you start to take it.

SIDE EFFECTS
Minor. Blurred vision, constipation, decreased sweating, diarrhea, dizziness, drowsiness, dry mouth, fatigue, jitteriness, menstrual irregularities, nasal congestion, restlessness, vomiting, and weight gain. As your body adjusts to the medication, these side effects should disappear.

This medication can cause increased sensitivity to sunlight. It is, therefore, important to avoid prolonged exposure to sunlight and sunlamps. Wear protective clothing and sunglasses, and use an effective sunscreen.

Thioridazine can also cause discoloration of the urine to red, pink, or red-brown. This is a harmless effect.

If you are constipated, increase the amount of fiber in your diet (fresh fruits and vegetables, salads, bran, and whole-grain breads), exercise, and drink more water (unless your doctor directs you to do otherwise).

Chew sugarless gum or suck on ice chips or a piece of hard candy to reduce mouth dryness.

To avoid dizziness or light-headedness when you stand, contract and relax the muscles of your legs for a few moments before rising. Do this by pushing one foot against the floor while raising the other foot slightly, alternating feet so that you are "pumping" your legs in a pedaling motion.

Major. Tell your doctor about any side effects that are persistent or particularly bothersome. IT IS ESPECIALLY IMPORTANT TO TELL YOUR DOCTOR about breast enlargement (in both sexes); chest pain; convulsions; darkened skin; difficulty in swallowing or breathing; drooling; fainting; fever; impotence; involuntary movements of the face, mouth, jaw, or tongue; palpitations; rash; sleep disorders; sore throat; tremors; uncoordinated movements; unusual bleeding or bruising; visual disturbances; or yellowing of the eyes or skin.

INTERACTIONS

Thioridazine interacts with several other medications:

1. It can cause extreme drowsiness when combined with alcohol or other central nervous system depressants (drugs that slow the activity of the brain and spinal cord), such as barbiturates, benzodiazepine tranquilizers, muscle relaxants, narcotics, and pain medications, or with tricyclic antidepressants.

2. Thioridazine can decrease the effectiveness of amphetamines, guanethidine, anticonvulsants, and levodopa.

3. The side effects of epinephrine, monoamine oxidase (MAO) inhibitors, metoprolol, propranolol, phenytoin, and tricyclic antidepressants may be increased by this medication. At least 14 days should separate the use of this drug and the use of an MAO inhibitor.

4. Lithium may increase the side effects and decrease the effectiveness of this medication.

5. False-positive pregnancy tests may occur. If you think you may be pregnant, call your doctor.

BE SURE TO TELL YOUR DOCTOR about any medications you are currently taking, especially those listed above.

WARNINGS

• Tell your doctor about unusual or allergic reactions you have had to any medications, especially to thioridazine or any other phenothiazine tranquilizers (such as chlorpromazine, fluphenazine, mesoridazine, perphenazine, prochlorperazine, promazine, trifluoperazine, and triflupromazine) or to loxapine.

• Tell your doctor if you have a history of alcoholism or if you now have or have ever had any blood disease, bone marrow disease, brain disease, breast cancer, blockage in the urinary or digestive tracts, drug-induced depression, epilepsy, high or low blood pressure, diabetes mellitus, glaucoma, heart or circulatory disease, liver disease, lung disease, Parkinson's disease, peptic ulcers, or enlarged prostate gland.

• Tell your doctor about any recent exposure to a pesticide or an insecticide. Thioridazine may increase the side effects from the exposure.

• To prevent oversedation, avoid drinking alcoholic beverages while taking this medication.

• If this medication makes you dizzy or drowsy, do not take part in any activity that requires alertness, such as driving a car or operating potentially dangerous machinery. Be careful on stairs, and avoid getting up suddenly from a lying or sitting position.

• Prior to having surgery or any other medical or dental treatment, be sure to tell your doctor or dentist that you are taking thioridazine.

• Some of the side effects caused by this drug can be prevented by taking an antiparkinsonism drug. Discuss this with your doctor.

• This medication can decrease sweating and heat release from the body. You should, therefore, try not to become overheated (avoid exercising strenuously in hot weather, and do not take hot baths, showers, and saunas).

• Do not stop taking this medication suddenly. If the drug is stopped abruptly, you may experience nausea, vomiting, stomach upset, headache, increased heart rate, insomnia, tremors, or a worsening of your condition. Your doctor may want to reduce the dosage gradually.

• If you are planning to have a myelogram, or any other procedure in which dye will be injected into your spinal cord, tell your doctor that you are taking this medication.

• Avoid spilling the oral concentrate or suspension form of this medication on your skin or clothing; either may cause redness and irritation of the skin.

• While taking this medication, do not take any over-the-counter (nonprescription) drugs for weight control or for cough, cold, allergy, asthma, or sinus problems unless you first check with your doctor. Concurrent use of any of these drugs and thioridazine may cause high blood pressure.

• Your doctor may schedule regular office visits for your first few months of therapy with this medication in order to monitor your progress and possibly adjust your dosage.

• Your doctor may want to schedule you for an eye examination if you take thioridazine for longer than a year. Prolonged use of this drug can cause visual disturbances.

• Be sure to tell your doctor if you are pregnant. Small amounts of this medication cross the placenta. Although there are reports of safe use of this drug during pregnancy, there are also reports of liver disease and tremors in newborn infants whose mothers received this type of medication close to term. Also, tell your doctor if you are breast-feeding. Small amounts of this medication pass into breast milk and may cause unwanted effects in nursing infants.

thioridazine hydrochloride—see thioridazine

Thiosulfil Forte—see sulfanomide antibiotics (oral)

---

thiothixene

BRAND NAMES (Manufacturers)
Navane (Roerig)
thiothixene (various manufacturers)
TYPE OF DRUG
Antipsychotic
INGREDIENT
thiothixene
DOSAGE FORMS
Capsules (1 mg, 2 mg, 5 mg, 10 mg, and 20 mg)
Oral concentrate (5 mg per ml, with 7% alcohol)
STORAGE
Thiothixene capsules should be stored at room temperature in a tightly closed, light-resistant container. The oral concentrate should be stored in the refrigerator in a tightly

closed, light-resistant container. This medication should never be frozen. Discard any medication that is outdated or no longer needed.

USES
Thiothixene is prescribed to treat the symptoms of certain types of mental illness, such as emotional symptoms of psychosis.

TREATMENT
To avoid stomach irritation, you can take the capsule form of thiothixene with a meal or with a glass of water or milk (unless your doctor directs you to do otherwise).

The oral concentrate form of this medication should be measured carefully with the dropper provided and then added to eight ounces of water, milk, or a carbonated beverage, or to applesauce or pudding immediately prior to administration. To prevent possible loss of effectiveness, this medication should not be diluted in tea, coffee, or apple juice.

Antacids and antidiarrheal medicines decrease the absorption of this medication from the gastrointestinal tract. Therefore, at least one hour should separate doses of one of these medicines and thiothixene.

If you miss a dose of this medication, take the missed dose as soon as possible and then return to your regular dosing schedule. If it is almost time for the next dose, however, skip the one you missed and return to your regular schedule. Do not double the dose (unless so directed by your doctor).

The full effects of this medication for the control of emotional or mental symptoms may not become apparent for at least two weeks after you start to take it.

SIDE EFFECTS
Minor. Blurred vision, constipation, decreased sweating, diarrhea, dizziness, drowsiness, dry mouth, fatigue, jitteriness, menstrual irregularities, nasal congestion, restlessness, vomiting, or weight gain. As your body adjusts to the medication, these side effects should disappear.

This medication can cause increased sensitivity to sunlight. It is, therefore, important to avoid prolonged exposure to sunlight and sunlamps. Wear protective clothing, and use an effective sunscreen.

Thiothixene can cause discoloration of the urine to red, pink, or red-brown. This is a harmless effect.

If you are constipated, increase the amount of fiber in your diet (fresh fruits and vegetables, salads, bran, and whole-grain breads), exercise, and drink more water (unless your doctor directs you to do otherwise).

To reduce mouth dryness, chew sugarless gum or suck on ice chips or a piece of hard candy.

To avoid dizziness or light-headedness when you stand, contract and relax the muscles of your legs for a few moments before rising. Do this by pushing one foot against the floor while raising the other foot slightly, alternating feet so that you are "pumping" your legs in a pedaling motion.

Major. Tell your doctor about any side effects that are persistent or particularly bothersome. IT IS ESPECIALLY IMPORTANT TO TELL YOUR DOCTOR about breast enlargement (in both sexes); chest pain; convulsions; darkened skin; difficulty in swallowing or breathing; drooling; fainting; fever; impotence; involuntary movements of the face, mouth, jaw, or tongue; palpitations; rash; sleep disorders; sore throat; tremors; uncoordinated movements; unusual bleeding or bruising; visual disturbances; or yellowing of the eyes or skin.

INTERACTIONS
Thiothixene interacts with other types of medications:
1. It can cause extreme drowsiness when combined with alcohol or other central nervous system depressants (drugs that slow the activity of the brain and spinal cord), such as barbiturates, benzodiazepine tranquilizers, muscle relaxants, narcotics, and pain medications, or with tricyclic antidepressants.
2. Thiothixene can decrease the effectiveness of amphetamines, guanethidine, anticonvulsants, and levodopa.
3. The side effects of epinephrine, monoamine oxidase (MAO) inhibitors, and tricyclic antidepressants may be increased by this medication. At least 14 days should separate the use of this drug and the use of an MAO inhibitor.
4. Lithium may increase the side effects and decrease the effectiveness of thiothixene.
5. False-positive pregnancy tests may occur. If you think you may be pregnant, call your doctor.

BE SURE TO TELL YOUR DOCTOR about any medications you are currently taking, especially any of those listed above.

WARNINGS
• Tell your doctor about unusual or allergic reactions you have had to any medications, especially to thiothixene, chlorprothixene, or any phenothiazine tranquilizer.
• Tell your doctor if you have a history of alcoholism or if you now have or have ever had blood disease, bone marrow disease, brain disease, breast cancer, blockage in the urinary or digestive tract, drug-induced depression, epilepsy, high or low blood pressure, diabetes mellitus, glaucoma, heart or circulatory disease, liver disease, lung disease, Parkinson's disease, peptic ulcers, or enlarged prostate gland.
• Avoid drinking alcoholic beverages while taking this medication, in order to prevent oversedation.
• If this drug makes you dizzy or drowsy, do not take part in any activity that requires alertness, such as driving a car or operating potentially dangerous machinery.
• Prior to having surgery or any other medical or dental treatment, be sure to tell your doctor or dentist that you are taking this medication.
• Some of the side effects caused by this drug can be prevented by taking an antiparkinsonism drug. Discuss this with your doctor.
• This medication can decrease sweating and heat release from the body. You should, therefore, try not to become overheated (avoid exercising strenuously in hot weather, and do not take hot baths, showers, and saunas).
• Do not stop taking this medication suddenly. If the drug is stopped abruptly you may experience nausea, vomiting, stomach upset, headache, increased heart rate, insomnia, tremors, or worsening of your condition. Your doctor may want to reduce the dosage gradually.

• If you are planning to have a myelogram, or any other procedure in which dye is injected into the space surrounding the spinal cord, tell your doctor that you are taking this medication.

• Avoid spilling the oral concentrate form of this medication on your skin or clothing; it can cause redness and irritation of the skin.

• While taking this medication, do not take any over-the-counter (nonprescription) medications for weight control or for cough, cold, allergy, asthma, or sinus problems unless you first check with your doctor. The combination of these medications may cause high blood pressure.

• Your doctor may schedule regular office visits during your first few months of therapy with this medication in order to monitor your progress.

• Be sure to tell your doctor if you are pregnant. Small amounts of this medication cross the placenta. Although there are reports of safe use of this drug during pregnancy, there are also reports of liver disease and tremors in newborn infants whose mothers received this type of medication close to term. Also, tell your doctor if you are breast-feeding. Small amounts of this medication pass into breast milk and may cause unwanted effects in nursing infants.

Thiuretic—see hydrochlorothiazide

Thorazine—see chlorpromazine

Thorazine Spansules—see chlorpromazine

Thor-Prom—see chlorpromazine

Thyrar—see thyroid hormone

thyroid hormone

BRAND NAMES (Manufacturers)
Armour Thyroid (USV)
S-P-T (Fleming)
Thyrar (USV)
Thyroid Strong (Marion Merrel Dow)
thyroid USP (various manufacturers)
TYPE OF DRUG
Thyroid hormone
INGREDIENT
thyroid hormone
DOSAGE FORMS
Tablets (15 mg, 30 mg, 60 mg, 90 mg, 120 mg, 180 mg, 240 mg, and 300 mg)
Sugar-coated tablets (30 mg, 60 mg, 120 mg, and 180 mg)
Capsules (60 mg, 120 mg, 180 mg, and 300 mg)
Note that 15 mg=$^1/_4$ grain (gr); 30 mg=$^1/_2$ gr; 60 mg=1 gr; 90 mg=1 $^1/_2$ gr; 120 mg=2 gr; 180 mg=3 gr; 240 mg=4 gr; and 300 mg=5 gr.
STORAGE
Store at room temperature in a tightly closed, light-resistant container. Discard outdated medication.

USES
This medication is prescribed to replace natural thyroid hormones that are absent because of a thyroid gland disorder. This product is obtained from animal thyroid glands.

TREATMENT
Thyroid hormone tablets should be taken on an empty stomach with a full glass of water. If this medication upsets your stomach, however, you can check with your doctor to see if you can take the medication with food or milk.

In order to get used to taking this medication, try to take it at the same time each day. Try not to miss any doses. If you do miss a dose of this medication, take it as soon as you remember, unless it is almost time for the next dose. In that case, do not take the missed dose at all; just return to your regular dosing schedule. Do not double the next dose. If you miss more than one or two doses of this medication, check with your doctor.

SIDE EFFECTS
Minor. Constipation, dry puffy skin, fatigue, headache, listlessness, muscle aches, or weight gain. These side effects should disappear as your body adjusts to the medication.

To relieve constipation, increase the amount of fiber in your diet (fresh fruits and vegetables, salads, bran, and whole-grain breads), exercise, and drink more water (unless your doctor directs you to do otherwise).
Major. Tell your doctor about any side effects that are persistent or particularly bothersome. Most of the major side effects associated with this drug are the result of too large a dose. The dosage of this medication may need to be adjusted if you experience any of the following side effects: chest pain, diarrhea, fever, heat intolerance, insomnia, irritability, leg cramps, menstrual irregularities, nervousness, palpitations, shortness of breath, sweating, trembling, or weight loss. If you experience any of these effects, CHECK WITH YOUR DOCTOR.

INTERACTIONS
Thyroid hormone interacts with other types of medications:
1. Dosing requirements for digoxin, insulin, or oral antidiabetic agents may change when this medication is used.
2. The effects of oral anticoagulants (blood thinners, such as warfarin) may be increased by thyroid hormone, which could lead to bleeding complications.
3. Cholestyramine and colestipol chemically bind thyroid hormone in the gastrointestinal tract, preventing its absorption. Therefore, at least four hours should separate doses of thyroid hormone and one of these medications.
4. Oral contraceptives (birth control pills) and estrogen-containing drugs may change your dosing requirements for thyroid hormone.
5. Phenobarbital may decrease the effectiveness of thyroid hormone.
6. Phenytoin, tricyclic antidepressants, and over-the-counter (nonprescription) allergy, asthma, cough, cold,

sinus, or diet medications may increase the side effects of thyroid hormone.

BE SURE TO TELL YOUR DOCTOR about any medications you are currently taking, especially any listed above.

WARNINGS

• Tell your doctor about unusual or allergic reactions you have had to any medications, especially to thyroid hormone or to beef or pork products.
• Tell your doctor if you now have or if you have ever had angina pectoris, diabetes mellitus, heart disease, high blood pressure, kidney disease, or an underactive adrenal or pituitary gland.
• If you have an underactive thyroid gland, you may need to take this medication for life. You should not stop taking it unless you first check with your doctor.
• Patients with certain heart diseases may experience chest pain or shortness of breath while on this medication. Check with your doctor if you experience such effects. Do not overdo physical work or exercise.
• Before having surgery or any other medical or dental treatment, be sure to tell your doctor or dentist that you are taking thyroid hormone.
• Over-the-counter (nonprescription) allergy, asthma, cough, cold, sinus, and diet medications can increase the side effects of thyroid hormone. Therefore, be sure to check with your doctor or pharmacist before taking ANY of these preparations.
• Although many thyroid products are on the market, they are not all bioequivalent—that is, they may not all be absorbed into the bloodstream at the same rate or have the same overall activity. DO NOT CHANGE BRANDS of this drug without first consulting your doctor or pharmacist to make sure you are receiving an equivalent product.
• Be sure to tell your doctor if you are pregnant. Thyroid hormone does not readily cross the placenta, and the drug appears to be safe during pregnancy. However, your dosing requirements of thyroid hormone may change during pregnancy. Also, tell your doctor if you are breast-feeding. Small amounts of thyroid hormone pass into breast milk.

Thyroid Strong—see thyroid hormone

thyroid USP—see thyroid hormone

Tigan—see trimethobenzamide

Timolide—see timolol and hydrochlorothiazide combination

timolol (ophthalmic)

BRAND NAME (Manufacturer)
Timoptic (Merck Sharp & Dohme)
TYPE OF DRUG
Antiglaucoma ophthalmic solution
INGREDIENT
timolol

DOSAGE FORM
Ophthalmic drops (0.25% and 0.5%)
STORAGE
Timolol ophthalmic drops should be stored at room temperature in a tightly closed container. This medication should never be frozen. If this medication discolors or turns brown, it should be discarded—a color change indicates a loss of potency.

USES
Timolol (ophthalmic) is used to reduce pressure in the eye caused by glaucoma or other eye conditions. This medication belongs to a group of drugs known as beta blockers. When applied to the eye, timolol reduces pressure within the eye by decreasing eye fluid (aqueous humor) production and perhaps by increasing the outflow of fluid from the eye.

TREATMENT
Be sure to wash your hands with soap and water before applying this medication. In order to avoid contamination of the eye drops, be careful not to touch the tube portion of the dropper or let it touch your eye, and do not wipe off or rinse the dropper after you use it.

To apply the ophthalmic drops, tilt your head back and pull down your lower eyelid with one hand to make a pouch below the eye. Drop the prescribed amount of medicine into this pouch and slowly close your eyes. Try not to blink. Keep your eyes closed, and place one finger at the corner of the eye next to your nose for a minute or two, applying a slight pressure (this is done to prevent loss of medication through the duct that drains fluid from the surface of the eye into the nose and throat). Then wipe away any excess medication with a clean tissue. Since applying the medication is somewhat difficult to do, you may want to have someone else apply the ophthalmic drops for you.

If you miss a dose of this medication, apply the missed dose as soon as possible, unless it is almost time for your next dose. In that case, do not apply the missed dose at all; just return to your regular dosing schedule. If the medication is used only once a day, and you do not remember missing a dose until the next day, skip the missed dose. Do not double the next dose.

SIDE EFFECTS
Minor. When you first apply this medication, you may have a stinging sensation your eyes. This should stop in a few minutes.
Major. Be sure to tell your doctor about any side effects that are persistent or particularly bothersome. IT IS ESPECIALLY IMPORTANT TO TELL YOUR DOCTOR about itching, skin rash, hives, or irritation of the eye that lasts more than a few minutes after application. Major side effects are rare when this product is administered correctly. However, rare occurrences of anxiety, confusion, depression, dizziness, drowsiness, generalized rash, indigestion, loss of appetite, nausea, weakness, and a slight reduction of the resting heart rate have been observed in some users of this medication. If you have any of these symptoms, it is important that you contact your doctor as soon as possible.

INTERACTIONS

Timolol (ophthalmic) may increase the side effects of reserpine and oral beta blockers.

Before starting to take timolol (ophthalmic), BE SURE TO TELL YOUR DOCTOR about any medications you are currently taking.

WARNINGS

• Tell your doctor about unusual or allergic reactions you have had to any medications, especially to timolol or to any other beta blockers (acebutolol, atenolol, betaxolol, carteolol, esmolol, labetalol, metoprolol, nadolol, penbutolol, pindolol, or propranolol).
• Tell your doctor if you now have or if you have ever had asthma, diabetes mellitus, heart disease, or myasthenia gravis.
• Your doctor should check your eye pressure regularly to be sure the glaucoma is under control.
• Tell your doctor if you are pregnant. Small amounts of timolol may be absorbed into the bloodstream, and its safety in pregnancy has not been established. Birth defects have been observed in the fetuses of animals that were given large doses of this drug during pregnancy. Also, tell your doctor if you are breast-feeding. If this drug reaches the bloodstream and passes into the breast milk, it can cause a slowed heart rate in the nursing infant.

---

timolol and hydrochlorothiazide combination

BRAND NAME (Manufacturer)
Timolide (Merck Sharp & Dohme)
TYPE OF DRUG
Beta-adrenergic blocking agent and diuretic
INGREDIENT
Stimolol and hydrochlorothiazide
DOSAGE FORM
Tablets (10 mg timolol and 25 mg hydrochlorothiazide)
STORAGE
Timolol and hydrochlorothiazide combination tablets should be stored at room temperature in a tightly closed, light-resistant container.

USES

Timolol and hydrochlorothiazide combination is prescribed to treat high blood pressure. Hydrochlorothiazide is a diuretic, which reduces fluid accumulation in the body by increasing the elimination of salt and water through the kidneys. Timolol belongs to a group of medicines known as beta-adrenergic blocking agents or, more commonly, beta blockers. They work by controlling impulses along certain nerve pathways.

TREATMENT

This medication can be taken with a glass of water, with meals, immediately following meals, or on an empty stomach—depending on your doctor's instructions.

Try to take the medication at the same time(s) each day. Avoid taking a dose after 6:00 P.M.; otherwise, you may have to get up during the night to urinate.

If you miss a dose of this medication, take the missed dose as soon as possible, unless it is almost time for your next dose. In that case, do not take the missed dose at all; just wait until the next scheduled dose. Do not double the dose.

Timolol and hydrochlorothiazide combination does not cure high blood pressure, but it will help to control the condition as long as you continue to take it.

SIDE EFFECTS

Minor. Abdominal pain, constipation, diarrhea, dizziness, drowsiness, dryness of the eyes and skin, headache, heartburn, loss of appetite, or tiredness. These side effects should disappear as your body adjusts to the medication.

If you become extra-sensitive to the cold, be sure to dress warmly during cold weather.

Plain, nonmedicated eye drops (artificial tears) may help to relieve eye dryness.

Sucking on ice chips or chewing sugarless gum helps to relieve mouth and throat dryness.

To relieve constipation, increase the amount of fiber in your diet (fresh fruits and vegetables, salads, bran, and whole-grain breads) and drink more water unless your doctor directs you to do otherwise.

To avoid dizziness or light-headedness when you stand, contract and relax the muscles of your legs for a few moments before rising. Do this by pushing one foot against the floor while raising the other foot slightly, alternating feet so that you are "pumping" your legs in a pedaling motion.

Hydrochlorothiazide can cause increased sensitivity to sunlight. Avoid prolonged exposure to sunlight and sunlamps, wear protective clothing and sunglasses, and use an effective sunscreen.

Major. Tell your doctor about any side effects that are persistent or particularly bothersome. IT IS ESPECIALLY IMPORTANT TO TELL YOUR DOCTOR about blurred vision, chest pain, cold hands or feet (due to decreased blood circulation to skin, fingers, and toes), confusion, decreased sexual ability, depression, difficulty in breathing, dry mouth, fever, hair loss, hallucinations, itching, joint pain, mood changes, muscle pain or cramps, nausea, numbness or tingling in your fingers or toes, palpitations, rapid weight gain (three to five pounds within a week), ringing in the ears, skin rash, sore throat, thirst, unusual bleeding or bruising, vomiting, weakness, or yellowing of the eyes or skin.

INTERACTIONS

This medicine interacts with other types of medications:
1. Indomethacin, aspirin, and other salicylates may decrease the blood-pressure-lowering effects of beta blockers.
2. Concurrent use of timolol and disopyramide or calcium channel blockers (diltiazem, nifedipine, verapamil) can lead to heart failure or very low blood pressure.
3. Side effects can be increased when timolol is taken with cimetidine, clonidine, digoxin, epinephrine, phenyle-

phrine, phenylpropanolamine, phenothiazine tranquilizers, prazosin, reserpine, chlorpromazine, furosemide, hydralazine, oral contraceptives (birth control pills), or monoamine oxidase (MAO) inhibitors. At least 14 days should separate the use of timolol and the use of an MAO inhibitor.

4. Timolol can antagonize (act against) the effects of theophylline, aminophylline, albuterol, isoproterenol, metaproterenol, and terbutaline.

5. Timolol can also interact with insulin and oral antidiabetic agents, raising or lowering blood sugar levels and masking the symptoms of low blood sugar.

6. Alcohol, barbiturates, and rifampin can decrease the blood concentrations of beta blockers, which can result in a decrease of effectiveness.

7. Hydrochlorothiazide can decrease the effectiveness of oral anticoagulants (blood thinners, such as warfarin), antigout medications, and methenamine.

8. Fenfluramine may increase the blood-pressure-lowering effects of this drug, which can be dangerous.

9. Cholestyramine and colestipol can decrease the absorption of hydrochlorothiazide from the gastrointestinal tract. This medication should, therefore, be taken one hour before or four hours after a dose of cholestyramine or colestipol (if you have also been prescribed one of these medications).

10. Hydrochlorothiazide may increase the side effects of amphotericin B, calcium, cortisone and cortisone-like steroids (such as dexamethasone, hydrocortisone, prednisone, and prednisolone), digoxin, digitalis, lithium, quinidine, sulfonamide antibiotics, and vitamin D.

Before starting to take timolol and hydrochlorothiazide combination, BE SURE TO TELL YOUR DOCTOR about any medications you are currently taking, especially any of the medications that are listed above.

WARNINGS

• Be sure to tell your doctor about unusual or allergic reactions you have had to any medications, especially to timolol or any other beta blockers (acebutolol, atenolol, betaxolol, carteolol, esmolol, labetalol, metoprolol, nadolol, penbutolol, pindolol, propranolol), hydrochlorothiazide or other diuretics (such as bendroflumethiazide, benzthiazide, chlorothiazide, chlorthalidone, cyclothiazide, hydroflumethiazide, methyclthiazide, metolazone, polythiazide, quinethazone, trichlormethiazide, and furosemide), or to any other sulfa drug (oral antidiabetic medication, or sulfonamide antibiotic).

• Be sure to tell your doctor if you now have or if you have ever had any of the following: asthma, diabetes mellitus, heart disease, gout, kidney disease or problems with urination, liver disease, pancreatitis, systemic lupus erythematosus, thyroid disease, or poor circulation in the fingers or toes.

• Hydrochlorothiazide can cause potassium loss. Signs of potassium loss include dry mouth, thirst, weakness, muscle pain or cramps, nausea, and vomiting. If you experience any of these symptoms, call your doctor. To help prevent this problem, your doctor may have blood tests performed periodically to monitor your potassium levels. To help avoid potassium loss, take this medication with a glass of fresh or frozen orange juice or cran-

berry juice, or eat a banana every day. The use of a salt substitute also helps to prevent potassium loss. Do not change your diet, however, until you discuss it with your doctor. Too much potassium can also be dangerous.

• While taking this medication, you should limit your intake of alcoholic beverages in order to prevent dizziness and light-headedness.

• While taking this medication, do not take any over-the-counter (nonprescription) medication for weight control or for allergy, asthma, cough, cold, or sinus problems unless you first check with your doctor.

• To prevent severe water loss (dehydration) while taking this medication, check with your doctor if you have any illness that causes severe or continuous nausea, vomiting, or diarrhea.

• This medication can raise blood sugar levels in diabetic patients. Blood sugar levels should be monitored carefully with blood or urine tests when this medication is being taken.

• You may want to check your pulse while taking this medication. If your pulse is much slower than your usual rate (or if it is less than 50 beats per minute), check with your doctor. A pulse rate that is too slow may cause circulation problems.

• Timolol can affect your body's response to exercise. Make sure you ask your doctor what an appropriate amount of exercise would be for you, taking into account your medical condition.

• Before having surgery or any other medical or dental treatment, tell your doctor or dentist that you are taking this medicine. Often, this medication will be discontinued 48 hours prior to any major surgery.

• This medication can cause dizziness, drowsiness, light-headedness, or decreased alertness. Therefore, you should exercise caution while driving a car or operating potentially dangerous machinery.

• A doctor does not usually prescribe a "fixed-dose" drug like this as the first choice in the treatment of high blood pressure. Usually, the patient first receives each ingredient singly. If there is an adequate response to the fixed dose contained in this product, it can then be substituted. The advantages of a combination product are increased convenience and (often) decreased cost.

• It is important that you do not stop taking this medicine unless you first check with your doctor. Some conditions worsen when this medicine is stopped suddenly, and the danger of a heart attack is increased in some patients. Your doctor may, therefore, want you to gradually reduce the amount of medicine you take before stopping completely. Make sure that you have enough medicine on hand to last through weekends, holidays, and vacations.

• Be sure to tell your doctor if you are pregnant. Animal studies have shown that some beta blockers can cause problems in pregnancy when used at very high doses. Extensive studies have not been conducted in humans, but there has been some association between beta blockers used during pregnancy and low birth weight, as well as breathing problems and slow heart rate in newborn infants. However, some other reports have shown this type of medication to have no effects on newborn infants. Also, tell your doctor if you are breast-feeding an infant. Although problems in humans have not yet been reported, small amounts of timolol and hydrochlorothiazide may pass into breast milk, so caution is warranted.

Timoptic—see timolol (ophthalmic)

Tipramine—see imipramine

---

timolol maleate (systemic)

BRAND NAMES (Manufacturers)
Blocadren (Merck Sharp & Dohme)
timolol maleate (various manufacturers)
TYPE OF DRUG
Beta-adrenergic blocking agent
INGREDIENT
timolol
DOSAGE FORM
Tablets (5 mg, 10 mg, and 20 mg)
STORAGE
Timolol should be stored at room temperature in a tightly closed, light-resistant container.

USES
Timolol is used to treat high blood pressure and to prevent additional heart attacks in heart attack patients. This drug belongs to a group of medicines known as beta-adrenergic blocking agents or, more commonly, beta blockers. These drugs work by controlling nerve impulses along certain nerve pathways.

TREATMENT
Timolol tablets can be taken with a glass of water, with meals, immediately following meals, or on an empty stomach, depending on your doctor's instructions for taking your medication. You should try to take your dose(s) of the medication at the same time(s) each day.

Try not to miss any doses of this medication. If you do miss a dose, take the missed dose as soon as possible. However, if the next scheduled dose is within eight hours (if you are taking this medicine only once a day) or within four hours (if you are taking this medicine more than once a day), do not take the missed dose at all; just return to your regular dosing schedule. Do not double the next dose that you take of this medication.

It is important to remember that timolol does not cure high blood pressure, but it will help to control the condition as long as you continue to take it.

SIDE EFFECTS
Minor. Anxiety; constipation; decreased sexual ability; diarrhea; difficulty in sleeping; drowsiness; dryness of the eyes, mouth, and skin; headache; nausea; nervousness; stomach discomfort; tiredness; or weakness. These side effects should disappear during treatment, as your body adjusts to the medicine.

If you are extra-sensitive to the cold, be sure to dress warmly during cold weather.

To relieve constipation, increase the fiber in your diet (fresh fruits and vegetables, salads, bran, and whole-grain breads) unless your doctor directs otherwise.

Plain, nonmedicated eye drops (artificial tears) may help to relieve eye dryness.

Sucking on ice chips or chewing sugarless gum helps to relieve mouth and throat dryness.

Major. Tell your doctor about any side effects that are persistent or particularly bothersome. IT IS ESPECIALLY IMPORTANT TO TELL YOUR DOCTOR about cold hands or feet (due to decreased blood circulation to skin, fingers, and toes), confusion, depression, dizziness, fever and sore throat, hair loss, hallucinations, light-headedness, nightmares, numbness or tingling of the fingers or toes, rapid weight gain (three to five pounds within a week), reduced alertness, skin rash, swelling, unusual bleeding or bruising, or wheezing or difficulty in breathing.

INTERACTIONS
Timolol may interact with several other types of drugs:
1. Indomethacin has been shown to decrease the blood-pressure-lowering effects of the beta blockers. This may also happen with aspirin or other salicylates.
2. Concurrent use of beta blockers and calcium channel blockers (diltiazem, nifedipine, or verapamil) or disopyramide can lead to heart failure or very low blood pressure.
3. Cimetidine and oral contraceptives (birth control pills) can increase the blood concentrations of timolol, which can result in greater side effects.
4. Side effects may also be increased when beta blockers are taken with clonidine, digoxin, epinephrine, phenylephrine, phenylpropanolamine, phenothiazine tranquilizers, prazosin, reserpine, or monoamine oxidase (MAO) inhibitors. At least 14 days should separate the use of a beta blocker and the use of an MAO inhibitor.
5. Alcohol, barbiturates, and rifampin can decrease the blood concentrations of beta blockers, which can result in a decrease in effectiveness.
6. Beta blockers may antagonize (work against) the effects of theophylline, aminophylline, albuterol, isoproterenol, metaproterenol, and terbutaline.
7. Beta blockers can also interact with insulin or oral antidiabetic agents, raising or lowering blood sugar levels or masking the symptoms of low blood sugar.
8.The action of beta blockers may be increased if they are used with chlorpromazine, furosemide, or hydralazine.

BE SURE TO TELL YOUR DOCTOR about any medications you are currently taking, especially any of those listed above.

WARNINGS
• Before starting to take this medication, it is important to tell your doctor if you have ever had unusual or allergic reactions to timolol or to any beta blocker (acebutolol, atenolol, betaxolol, carteolol, esmolol, labetalol, metoprolol, nadolol, penbutolol, pindolol, or propranolol).
• Tell your doctor if you now have or if you have ever had allergies, asthma, hay fever, eczema, slow heartbeat, bronchitis, diabetes mellitus, emphysema, heart or blood vessel disease, kidney disease, liver disease, thyroid disease, or poor circulation in the fingers or toes.
• You may want to check your pulse while taking this medication. If your pulse is much slower than your usual

rate (or if it is less than 50 beats per minute), check with your doctor. A pulse rate that is too slow may cause circulation problems.

• This medicine may affect your body's response to exercise. Be sure you discuss with your doctor how much exercise is safe for you, taking into account your medical condition.

• It is important that you do not stop taking this medicine unless you first check with your doctor. Some conditions may become worse when the medicine is stopped suddenly, and the danger of a heart attack is increased in some patients. Your doctor may want you to gradually reduce the amount of medicine you take before stopping completely. Make sure that you have enough medicine on hand to last through weekends, vacations, and holidays.

• Before having surgery or any other medical or dental treatment, tell your doctor or dentist that you are taking this medication. Often, this medication will be discontinued 48 hours prior to major surgery.

• This medication can cause dizziness, drowsiness, lightheadedness, or decreased alertness. Exercise caution while driving a car or using any potentially dangerous machinery.

• While taking this medicine, do not use any over-the-counter (nonprescription) allergy, asthma, cough, cold, sinus, or diet preparations unless you first check with your pharmacist or doctor. Some of these medicines can result in high blood pressure when combined with timolol.

• Be sure to tell your doctor if you are pregnant. Animal studies have shown that some beta blockers can cause problems in pregnancy when used at very high doses.There has been some association between use of beta blockers during pregnancy and low birth weight, as well as breathing problems and slow heart rate in newborn infants. However, other reports have shown no effects on newborn infants. Also, tell your doctor if you are breast-feeding. Small amounts of timolol may pass into breast milk.

Timoptic—see timolol (ophthalmic)

Tipramine—see imipramine

tobramycin (ophthalmic)

BRAND NAME (Manufacturer)
Tobrex (Alcon)
TYPE OF DRUG
Ophthalmic antibiotic
INGREDIENT
tobramycin
DOSAGE FORMS
Ophthalmic drops (0.3% tobramycin)
Ophthalmic ointment (0.3% tobramycin)
STORAGE
The ophthalmic solution and ointment should be stored at room temperature in tightly closed containers. Discard any medication that is outdated or no longer needed.

USES
Tobramycin ophthalmic is used for the short-term treatment of bacterial infections of the eyes. Tobramycin is an aminoglycoside antibiotic, which acts to prevent the growth and multiplication of infecting bacteria.

TREATMENT
Wash your hands with soap and water before using this medication. In order to prevent contamination of the medicine, be careful not to touch the tube portion of the dropper and do not let it touch the eye.

Note that the bottle of the eye drops is not completely full—this is to allow control of the number of drops used.

To apply the drops, tilt your head back and pull down the lower eyelid with one hand to make a pouch below the eye. Drop the prescribed amount of medicine into the pouch and slowly close your eyes. Try not to blink. Keep your eyes closed, and place one finger at the corner of the eye next to your nose for a minute or two, applying a slight pressure (this is done to prevent loss of medication through the duct that drains fluid from the surface of the eye into the nose and throat). Then wipe away any excess with a clean tissue. If you think that the medicine did not get into your eye, repeat the process once. If you are using more than one type of eye drop, wait at least five minutes between doses of the two types of medication.

Follow the same general procedure for applying the ointment. Tilt your head back, pull down the lower eyelid, and squeeze the prescribed amount of ointment in a line along the pouch below the eye. Close your eyes, and place your finger at the corner of the eye, near the nose, for a minute or two. Do not rub your eyes. Wipe off excess ointment and the tip of the tube with clean tissues.

Since applying the medication is somewhat difficult to do, you may want someone else to administer the drops or ointment for you.

If you miss a dose of this drug, insert the drops or apply the ointment as soon as possible, unless it is almost time for the next application. In that case, do not use the missed dose at all; just return to your regular dosing schedule.

It is important to continue to take this medication for the entire time prescribed by your doctor, even if the symptoms of infection disappear before the end of that period. If you stop applying the medication too soon, resistant bacteria are given a chance to continue growing, and the infection could recur.

SIDE EFFECTS
Minor. Blurred vision, burning, or stinging. These side effects should disappear as your body adjusts to the drug.
Major. Tell your doctor about any side effects that are persistent or particularly bothersome. IT IS ESPECIALLY IMPORTANT TO TELL YOUR DOCTOR about disturbed or reduced vision; eye pain, itching, or swelling; severe irritation; or rash.

INTERACTIONS
This medication should not interact with other medication as long as it is used according to directions.

WARNINGS

• Tell your doctor about any reactions you have had to drugs, especially to tobramycin or to any other aminoglycoside antibiotic (amikacin, gentamicin, kanamycin, neomycin, netilmicin, paromomycin, streptomycin, or viomycin).

• Before starting tobramycin (ophthalmic), tell your doctor if you now have or if you have ever had fungal or viral infections of the eye, kidney disease, or myasthenia gravis.

• If there is no change in your condition two or three days after starting to take this drug, contact your doctor. The drug may not be effective for your infection.

• This medication has been prescribed for your current infection only. A subsequent infection, or one that someone else has, may require a different medicine. You should not give your medicine to other people or use it to treat other infections, unless your doctor specifically directs you to do so.

• In order to allow your eye infection to clear, do not apply makeup to the affected eye.

• Be sure to tell your doctor if you are pregnant. Extensive studies in pregnant women have not been conducted. Also, tell your doctor if you are breast-feeding an infant. Small amounts of tobramycin may pass into the breast milk.

Tobrex—see tobramycin (ophthalmic)

---

tocainide

BRAND NAME (Manufacturer)
Tonocard (Merck Sharp & Dohme)
TYPE OF DRUG
Antiarrhythmic
INGREDIENT
tocainide
DOSAGE FORM
Tablets (400 mg and 600 mg)
STORAGE
Store at room temperature in a tightly closed container.

USES

Tocainide is used to treat heart arrhythmias. It suppresses irregular heartbeats and helps to achieve a more normal rhythm.

TREATMENT

To decrease stomach irritation, you can take tocainide with a glass of milk or with food (unless your doctor directs you to do otherwise).

Try to take the drug at the same time(s) every day. Tocainide works best when the amount of drug in your bloodstream is kept constant. This medication should, therefore, be taken at evenly spaced intervals day and night. For example, if you are to take tocainide three times per day, the doses should be spaced eight hours apart.

Try not to miss any doses of tocainide. If you do miss a dose, take the missed dose as soon as possible. However, if the next scheduled dose is within four hours (if you are taking tocainide three times daily) or within six hours (if you are taking it twice daily), do not take the missed dose at all; just return to your regular dosing schedule. Do not double the next dose.

SIDE EFFECTS

Minor. Abdominal pain, altered taste, anxiety, constipation, diarrhea, difficulty in swallowing, dizziness, drowsiness, dry mouth, fatigue, headache, heartburn, hot or cold feelings, increased thirst, light-headedness, loss of appetite, nausea, restlessness, sweating, or vomiting. These side effects should disappear as your body adjusts to this medication.

If you feel dizzy or light-headed, sit or lie down for a while; get up slowly from a sitting or reclining position, and be careful on stairs.

If you experience mouth dryness, chew sugarless gum or suck on ice chips or a piece of hard candy.

To relieve constipation, increase the amount of fiber in your diet (fresh fruits and vegetables, salads, bran, and whole-grain breads), exercise, and drink more water (unless your doctor directs you to do otherwise).

Major. Tell your doctor about any side effects that are persistent or particularly bothersome. IT IS ESPECIALLY IMPORTANT TO TELL YOUR DOCTOR about chest pain, chills, confusion, coughing, depression, disorientation, earache, fever, hair loss, hallucinations, hearing loss, incoordination, itching, leg cramps, mental changes, mood changes, mouth sores, muscle or joint pain, neck pain, palpitations, rash, ringing in the ears, seizures, shakiness, shortness of breath, sleep disorders, slurred speech, sore throat, tingling in the fingers or toes, unsteadiness, unusual bleeding or bruising, urination problems, visual disturbances, weakness, wheezing, or yellowing of the skin or eyes.

INTERACTIONS

The concurrent use of tocainide and metoprolol can have additive negative effects on the heart.

BE SURE TO TELL YOUR DOCTOR about any medications you are currently taking, especially metoprolol.

WARNINGS

• Be sure to tell your doctor about any unusual or allergic reactions you have had to any medications, especially to tocainide or any other chemically related local anesthetic or antiarrhythmic, such as bupivacaine, dibucaine, etidocaine, lidocaine, mepivacaine, or prilocaine.

• Before starting tocainide, be sure to tell your doctor if you now have or if you have ever had blood disorders, bone marrow disease, heart block, heart failure, kidney disease, or liver disease.

• Before surgery or other medical or dental treatment, tell your doctor or dentist you are taking this drug.

• If this drug makes you dizzy or drowsy, do not take part in any activity that requires alertness, such as driving a car or operating potentially dangerous machinery.

• During the first three months of tocainide therapy, your doctor may schedule periodic blood counts. It is important for you to have these blood tests done to monitor for possible side effects on the bone marrow.

• Tell your doctor if you are pregnant. Studies in pregnant women have not been conducted. However, adverse effects have occurred in the offspring of animals that were given large doses of tocainide. Also, tell your doctor if you are breast-feeding an infant. It is not yet known if tocainide passes into human breast milk.

Tofranil—see imipramine

Tofranil-PM—see imipramine

---

tolazamide

BRAND NAMES (Manufacturers)
tolazamide (various manufacturers)
Tolinase (Upjohn)
TYPE OF DRUG
Oral antidiabetic
INGREDIENT
tolazamide
DOSAGE FORM
Tablets (100 mg, 250 mg, and 500 mg)
STORAGE
This medication should be stored at room temperature in a tightly closed container. Discard any outdated medication.

USES
Tolazamide is used for the treatment of diabetes mellitus (sugar diabetes) that appears in adulthood and cannot be managed by control of diet alone. This type of diabetes is known as non-insulin-dependent diabetes (also called maturity-onset or Type II diabetes). Tolazamide lowers the blood sugar level by increasing the release of insulin.

TREATMENT
In order for this medication to work correctly, it must be taken as directed by your doctor. It is best to take this medicine at the same time each day in order to maintain a constant blood sugar level. It is, therefore, important to try not to miss any doses of tolazamide. If you do miss a dose, take it as soon as possible, unless it is almost time for the next dose. In that case, do not take the missed dose at all; just return to your regular dosing schedule. Do not double the next dose. Tell your doctor if you feel any side effects from missing a dose of this drug.

SIDE EFFECTS
Minor. Diarrhea, headache, heartburn, loss of appetite, nausea, stomach discomfort, stomach pain, or vomiting. These side effects usually disappear as your body adjusts to the drug.

Tolazamide may increase your sensitivity to sunlight. You should, therefore, avoid prolonged exposure to sunlight and sunlamps. Wear protective clothing and sunglasses, and use an effective sunscreen.

Major. Tell your doctor about any side effects that are persistent or particularly bothersome. IT IS ESPECIALLY IMPORTANT TO TELL YOUR DOCTOR about dark urine, fatigue, itching of the skin, light-colored stools, sore throat and fever, unusual bleeding or bruising, or yellowing of the eyes or skin.

INTERACTIONS
Tolazamide interacts with several other types of drugs:
1. Chloramphenicol, guanethidine, fenfluramine, sulfinpyrazone, insulin, monoamine oxidase (MAO) inhibitors, oxyphenbutazone, oxytetracycline, phenylbutazone, probenecid, aspirin or other salicylates, and sulfonamide antibiotics, when combined with tolazamide, can lower blood sugar levels—sometimes to dangerously low levels. At least 14 days should separate the use of this drug and the use of an MAO inhibitor.
2. Thyroid hormones, dextrothyroxine, epinephrine, phenytoin, thiazide diuretics (water pills), and cortisone-like medications (such as dexamethasone, hydrocortisone, and prednisone), combined with tolazamide, can actually increase blood sugar levels—just what you are trying to avoid.
3. Rifampin can decrease the blood concentrations of tolazamide, which can lead to a decrease in its effectiveness.
4. Oral antidiabetic medications can increase the effects of warfarin, which can lead to bleeding complications.
5. Beta-blocking medications (acebutolol, atenolol, betaxolol, carteolol, esmolol, labetalol, metoprolol, nadolol, penbutolol, pindolol, propranolol, or timolol) combined with tolazamide can result in either high or low blood sugar levels. Beta blockers can also mask the symptoms of low blood sugar, which can be dangerous.

BE SURE TO TELL YOUR DOCTOR about any medications you are currently taking, especially those listed above.

WARNINGS
• It is important to tell your doctor if you have ever had unusual or allergic reactions to tolazamide or to any other sulfa medication (sulfonamide antibiotics, diuretics [water pills], or other oral antidiabetics).
• It is also important to tell your doctor if you now have or if you have ever had kidney disease, liver disease, severe infections, or thyroid disease.
• Avoid drinking alcoholic beverages while taking this medication (unless otherwise directed by your doctor). Some patients who take this medicine suffer nausea, vomiting, dizziness, stomach pain, pounding headache, sweating, and redness of the face and skin when they drink alcohol. Also, large amounts of alcohol can lower your blood sugar concentration to a dangerously low level.
• Follow the special diet that your doctor gave you. This is an important part of controlling your blood sugar and is necessary in order for this medicine to work properly.
• Before having surgery or any other medical or dental treatment, be sure to tell your doctor or dentist that you are taking this medicine.
• Test for sugar in your urine as directed by your doctor. It is a convenient way to determine whether your diabetes is being controlled by this medicine.
• Eat or drink something containing sugar right away if you experience any symptoms of hypoglycemia (low blood sugar), such as anxiety, chills, cold sweats, cool

or pale skin, drowsiness, excessive hunger, headache, nausea, nervousness, rapid heartbeat, shakiness, or unusual tiredness or weakness. It is important that your family and friends know the symptoms of low blood sugar and what to do if they observe any of these symptoms in you.

Even if the hypoglycemic symptoms seem to disappear after you eat or drink a sugar-containing product, it is important to contact your doctor as soon as possible. The blood-sugar-lowering effects of tolazamide can last for hours, and your symptoms may return during this period. Good sources of sugar are orange juice, corn syrup, honey, sugar cubes, and table sugar. You are at greatest risk of developing low blood sugar if you skip or delay meals, exercise more than usual, are unable to eat because of nausea or vomiting, or drink large amounts of alcohol.

• You may need to be switched to insulin if you suffer diabetic coma, have a severe infection, are scheduled for major surgery, or become pregnant.

• Be sure to tell your doctor if you are pregnant. Your dosing requirements for tolazamide may change during pregnancy. Although extensive studies in humans have not been conducted, adverse effects have been observed in the fetuses of animals that received this type of medication during pregnancy. Also, be sure to tell your doctor if you are breast-feeding an infant. Small amounts of tolazamide may pass into breast milk.

tolbutamide

BRAND NAMES (Manufacturers)
Oramide (Major)
Orinase (Upjohn)
tolbutamide (various manufacturers)
TYPE OF DRUG
Oral antidiabetic
INGREDIENT
tolbutamide
DOSAGE FORM
Tablets (250 mg and 500 mg)
STORAGE
This medication should be stored at room temperature in a tightly closed container. Discard any outdated medication.

USES
Tolbutamide is used for the treatment of diabetes mellitus (sugar diabetes) that appears in adulthood and cannot be managed by control of diet alone. This type of diabetes is known as non-insulin-dependent diabetes (also called maturity-onset or Type II diabetes). Tolbutamide lowers blood sugar by increasing the release of insulin from the pancreas.

TREATMENT
In order for this medication to work correctly, it must be taken as directed by your doctor. It is best to take this medicine at the same time(s) each day, in order to maintain a constant blood sugar level. It is, therefore, important

to try not to miss any doses of tolbutamide. If you do miss a dose, take it as soon as possible, unless it is almost time for the next dose. In that case, do not take the missed dose at all; just return to your regular dosing schedule. Do not double the next dose. Tell your doctor if you feel any side effects from missing a dose of this drug.

SIDE EFFECTS
Minor. Diarrhea, headache, heartburn, loss of appetite, nausea, stomach discomfort, stomach pain, or vomiting. These side effects usually disappear during treatment, as your body adjusts to the medication.

Tolbutamide may increase your sensitivity to sunlight. You should, therefore, avoid prolonged exposure to sunlight and sunlamps. Wear protective clothing and sunglasses, and use an effective sunscreen.
Major. Tell your doctor about any side effects that are persistent or particularly bothersome. IT IS ESPECIALLY IMPORTANT TO TELL YOUR DOCTOR about dark urine, fatigue, itching of the skin, light-colored stools, sore throat and fever, unusual bleeding or bruising, or yellowing of the eyes or skin.

INTERACTIONS
Tolbutamide interacts with a number of other types of drugs:

1. The combination of tolbutamide and chloramphenicol, guanethidine, insulin, fenfluramine, sulfinpyrazone, monoamine oxidase (MAO) inhibitors, oxyphenbutazone, oxytetracycline, phenylbutazone, probenecid, aspirin or other salicylates, or sulfonamide antibiotics can lower blood sugar levels—sometimes to dangerously low levels. At least 14 days should separate the use of this drug and the use of an MAO inhibitor.

2. Thyroid hormones, dextrothyroxine, epinephrine, phenytoin, thiazide diuretics (water pills), and cortisone-like medications (such as dexamethasone, hydrocortisone, and prednisone), combined with tolbutamide, can actually increase blood sugar levels—just what you are trying to avoid.

3. Rifampin can decrease the blood concentrations of tolbutamide, which can lead to a decrease in its effectiveness.

4. Oral antidiabetic medications can increase the effects of blood thinners, such as warfarin, which can lead to bleeding complications.

5. The combination of tolbutamide and beta-blocking medications (acebutolol, atenolol, betaxolol, carteolol, esmolol, labetalol, metoprolol, nadolol, penbutolol, pindolol, propranolol, or timolol) can result in either high or low blood sugar levels. Beta blockers can also mask the symptoms of low blood sugar, which can be dangerous.

BE SURE TO TELL YOUR DOCTOR about any medications you are currently taking, especially those listed above.

WARNINGS
• It is important to tell your doctor if you have ever had unusual or allergic reactions to tolbutamide or to any other sulfa medication (sulfonamide antibiotics, diuretics [water pills], or other oral antidiabetics).

• It is also important to tell your doctor if you now have or if you have ever had kidney disease, liver disease, severe infection, or thyroid disease.

• Be sure to avoid drinking alcoholic beverages while taking this medication (unless otherwise directed by your doctor). Some patients who take this medicine suffer nausea, vomiting, dizziness, stomach pain, pounding headache, sweating, and redness of the face and skin when they drink alcohol. Also, large amounts of alcohol can lower your blood sugar concentration to a dangerously low level.

• Follow the special diet that your doctor gave you. This is an important part of controlling your blood sugar levels and is necessary in order for this medicine to work properly.

• Before having surgery or any other medical or dental treatment, be sure to tell your doctor or dentist about this drug.

• It is very important to test for sugar in your urine as directed by your doctor. This is a convenient way to determine whether your diabetes is being controlled by this medicine.

• Eat or drink something containing sugar right away if you experience any symptoms of hypoglycemia (low blood sugar), such as anxiety, chills, cold sweats, cool or pale skin, drowsiness, excessive hunger, headache, nausea, nervousness, rapid heartbeat, shakiness, or unusual tiredness or weakness). It is important that your family and friends know the symptoms of low blood sugar and what to do if they observe any of these symptoms in you.

Even if the hypoglycemic symptoms seem to disappear after you eat or drink a sugar-containing product, it is important to contact your doctor as soon as possible. The blood-sugar-lowering effects of tolbutamide can last for hours, and your symptoms may return during this period. Good sources of sugar are orange juice, corn syrup, honey, sugar cubes, and table sugar. You are at greatest risk of developing low blood sugar if you skip or delay meals, exercise more than usual, are unable to eat because of nausea or vomiting, or drink large amounts of alcohol.

• You may need to be switched to insulin if you have a severe infection, are scheduled for major surgery, suffer diabetic coma, or become pregnant.

• Be sure to tell your doctor if you are pregnant. Your dosing requirements for tolbutamide may change during pregnancy, or you may be switched to insulin. Although extensive studies in humans have not been conducted, adverse effects have been observed in the fetuses of animals that received the drug tolbutamide during pregnancy. Also, tell your doctor if you are breast-feeding an infant. Since small amounts of tolbutamide may pass into breast milk, cautious use is warranted.

Tolectin—see tolmetin

Tolectin DS—see tolmetin

Tolectin-600—see tolmetin

Tolinase—see tolazamide

tolmetin

BRAND NAMES (Manufacturers)
Tolectin (McNeil)
Tolectin DS (McNeil)
Tolectin-600 (McNeil)
TYPE OF DRUG
Nonsteroidal anti-inflammatory analgesic
INGREDIENT
tolmetin
DOSAGE FORMS
Tablets (200 mg and 600 mg)
Capsules (400 mg)
STORAGE
This medication should be stored in tightly closed containers at room temperature away from heat and direct sunlight.

USES
Tolmetin is used to treat the inflammation (pain, swelling, and stiffness) of certain types of arthritis, gout, bursitis, and tendinitis. Tolmetin has been shown to block the production of certain body chemicals that may trigger pain. However, it is not yet fully understood how tolmetin works.

TREATMENT
You should take this medication on an empty stomach 30 to 60 minutes before meals or two hours after meals, so that it gets into your bloodstream quickly. However, to decrease stomach irritation, your doctor may want you to take the medicine with food or antacids.

If you are taking tolmetin to relieve arthritis, you must take it regularly, as directed by your doctor. It may take up to two weeks before you feel the full benefits of this medication.

Tolmetin does not cure arthritis, but it will help to control the condition as long as you continue to undergo treatment with the medication.

It is important to take tolmetin on schedule and not to miss any doses. If you do miss a dose, take it as soon as possible, unless it is almost time for your next dose. In that case, do not take the missed dose at all; just return to your regular dosing schedule. Do not double the next dose.

SIDE EFFECTS
Minor. Bloating, constipation, diarrhea, difficulty in sleeping, dizziness, drowsiness, headache, heartburn, indigestion, light-headedness, loss of appetite, nausea, nervousness, soreness of the mouth, unusual sweating, or vomiting. As your body adjusts to the drug, these side effects should disappear.

To relieve constipation, increase the amount of fiber in your diet (fresh fruits and vegetables, salads, bran, and whole-grain breads), exercise, and drink more water (unless your doctor directs you to do otherwise).

If you become dizzy or light-headed, sit or lie down for a while; get up slowly from a sitting or reclining position, and be careful on stairs.

Major. Tell your doctor about any side effects that are persistent or particularly bothersome. IT IS ESPECIALLY

IMPORTANT TO TELL YOUR DOCTOR about bloody or black, tarry stools; blurred vision; confusion; depression; difficult or painful urination; difficulty in hearing; palpitations; ringing or buzzing in the ears; skin rash, hives, or itching; stomach pain; swelling of the feet; tightness in the chest; unexplained sore throat and fever; unusual bleeding or bruising; unusual fatigue or weakness; unusual weight gain; wheezing or difficulty in breathing; or yellowing of the eyes or skin.

INTERACTIONS
Tolmetin interacts with several types of medications:
1. Anticoagulants (blood thinners, such as warfarin) in combination with tolmetin can lead to an increase in bleeding complications.
2. Aspirin, salicylates, or other anti-inflammatory medications can increase the stomach irritation caused by tolmetin.
3. Probenecid may increase blood levels of tolmetin, which may increase the risk of side effects.
4. The action of beta blockers may be decreased by this drug.
5. This drug can interact with diuretics (water pills).

BE SURE TO TELL YOUR DOCTOR about any medications you are currently taking, especially any listed above.

WARNINGS
• Before you take this medication, it is important to tell your doctor if you have ever had unusual or allergic reactions to tolmetin or any of the other chemically related drugs (including aspirin, other salicylates, diclofenac, diflunisal, etodolac, fenoprofen, flurbiprofen, ibuprofen, ketoprofen, meclofenamate, mefenamic acid, nabumetone, naproxen, oxyphenbutazone, phenylbutazone, piroxicam, sulindac, and indomethacin).
• Tell your doctor if you have ever had asthma, bleeding problems, colitis, stomach ulcers or other stomach problems, epilepsy, heart disease, high blood pressure, kidney disease, liver disease, mental illness, or Parkinson's disease.
• If this drug makes you dizzy or drowsy, do not take part in any activity that requires alertness, such as driving a car or operating potentially dangerous machinery.
• Because this drug can prolong your bleeding time, it is important to tell your doctor or dentist that you are taking this drug before having surgery or any other medical or dental treatment.
• Stomach problems are more likely to occur if you take aspirin regularly or drink alcohol while being treated with this medication. These should, therefore, be avoided (unless your doctor directs you to do otherwise).
• Be sure to tell your doctor if you are pregnant. The safe use of this medicine in human pregnancy has not been established. Side effects have been observed in the offspring of animals that received this type of medication during pregnancy. If taken late in pregnancy, tolmetin can prolong labor. Also, tell your doctor if you are breastfeeding an infant. Small amounts of tolmetin can pass into breast milk.

Tonocard—see tocainide

Torganic-DM—see dextromethorphan and iodinated glycerol combination

Totacillin—see ampicillin

Trandate—see labetalol

Transderm-Nitro—see nitroglycerin (topical)

Transderm-Scop—see scopolamine (transdermal)

Tranxene-SD—see clorazepate

Tranxene T-Tabs—see clorazepate

---

trazodone

BRAND NAMES (Manufacturers)
Desyrel (Mead Johnson)
Desyrel Dividose (Mead Johnson)
trazodone (various manufacturers)
TYPE OF DRUG
Antidepressant
INGREDIENT
trazodone
DOSAGE FORM
Tablets (50 mg, 100 mg, 150 mg, and 300 mg)
STORAGE
Trazodone tablets should be stored at room temperature in a tightly closed, light-resistant container.

USES
Trazodone is used to relieve the symptoms of mental depression. It is thought to relieve depression by increasing the concentration of certain chemicals involved with nerve transmission in the brain.

TREATMENT
Trazodone should be taken exactly as your doctor prescribes. It can be taken with water, milk, or food to lessen stomach irritation (unless your doctor tells you to do otherwise).

If you miss a dose of this medication, take the missed dose as soon as possible, and then return to your regular dosing schedule. If, however, the dose you missed was a once-a-day bedtime dose, do not take that dose in the morning; check with your doctor instead. If the dose is taken in the morning, it may cause some unwanted side effects. Never double the next dose.

The benefits of therapy with this medication may not become apparent for two to four weeks.

SIDE EFFECTS
Minor. Blurred vision, constipation, diarrhea, dizziness, drowsiness, dry mouth, gas, headache, heartburn, lightheadedness, nausea, sleep disorders, vomiting, or weight gain or loss. These side effects should disappear as your body adjusts to the medication.

This medication can cause increased sensitivity to sunlight. It is, therefore, important to avoid prolonged exposure to sunlight and sunlamps. Wear protective clothing and sunglasses, and use an effective sunscreen.

Dry mouth can be relieved by chewing sugarless gum or by sucking on ice chips or a piece of hard candy.

To relieve constipation, increase the amount of fiber in your diet (fresh fruits and vegetables, salads, bran, and whole-grain breads), exercise, and drink more water (unless your doctor directs you to do otherwise).

To avoid dizziness and light-headedness when you stand, contract and relax the muscles of your legs for a few moments before rising. Do this by pushing one foot against the floor while raising the other foot slightly, alternating feet so that you are "pumping" your legs in a pedaling motion.

Major. Tell your doctor about any side effects that are persistent or particularly bothersome. IT IS ESPECIALLY IMPORTANT TO TELL YOUR DOCTOR about chest tightness, confusion, difficult or painful urination, hallucinations, loss of coordination, mood changes, muscle aches or pains, palpitations, prolonged or inappropriate erection of the penis, rash, ringing in the ears, shortness of breath, tingling in the fingers or toes, tremors, unusual bleeding or bruising, or unusual tiredness or weakness.

INTERACTIONS

Trazodone interacts with several other types of medications:

1. Extreme drowsiness can occur when trazodone is taken with central nervous system depressants (drugs that slow the activity of the brain and spinal cord), including alcohol, antihistamines, barbiturates, benzodiazepine tranquilizers, muscle relaxants, narcotics, pain medications, phenothiazine tranquilizers, and sleeping medications, or with tricyclic antidepressants.

2. The concurrent use of trazodone and monoamine oxidase (MAO) inhibitors should be avoided because the combination can result in fever, convulsions, or high blood pressure. At least 14 days should separate the use of this drug and the use of an MAO inhibitor.

3. Trazodone may increase the blood levels of digoxin and phenytoin, which can lead to increased side effects.

4. Blood-pressure-lowering effects of antihypertensives may be increased by trazodone, which can be dangerous.

BE SURE TO TELL YOUR DOCTOR about any medications you are currently taking, especially any listed above.

WARNINGS

• Tell your doctor if you have had unusual or allergic reactions to any medications, especially to trazodone.

• Tell your doctor if you have a history of alcoholism or if you ever had electroshock therapy, heart disease, a heart attack, kidney disease, or liver disease.

• If this drug makes you dizzy or drowsy, do not take part in any activity that requires alertness, such as driving a car or operating potentially dangerous machinery.

• Before having surgery or any other medical or dental treatment, be sure to tell your doctor or dentist that you are taking this medication.

• Do not stop taking this drug suddenly. Stopping this medication abruptly may cause nausea, headache, stom-

ach upset, fatigue, or worsening of your condition. Your doctor may, therefore, want to reduce the dosage gradually.

• The effects of this medication may last as long as seven days after you have stopped taking it, so continue to observe all precautions during this period.

• Be sure to tell your doctor if you are pregnant. The safe use of this medication in pregnancy has not been established. Side effects have been observed in the offspring of animals that were given this medication in large doses during pregnancy. Also, tell your doctor if you are breast-feeding an infant. Small amounts of this drug pass into breast milk and may cause unwanted effects, such as irritability or sleeping problems, in nursing infants.

Trendar—see ibuprofen

Trental—see pentoxifylline

tretinoin

BRAND NAME (Manufacturer)
Retin-A (Ortho)
TYPE OF DRUG
Acne preparation
INGREDIENT
tretinoin (retinoic acid; vitamin A acid)
DOSAGE FORMS
Cream (0.025%, 0.05%, and 0.1%)
Gel (0.025% and 0.01%, with 90% alcohol)
Liquid (0.05%, with 55% alcohol)
STORAGE
Tretinoin cream, gel, and liquid should be stored at room temperature in tightly closed, light-resistant containers. This medication should never be frozen.

USES

Tretinoin is used topically (on the skin) to treat acne vulgaris. It appears to work by increasing the turnover (death and replacement) of skin cells.

TREATMENT

This product is packaged with instructions for the patient. Read them carefully before applying tretinoin.

Wash your skin with a mild or hypoallergenic soap and warm water. Pat dry with a clean towel. Then wait about 30 minutes before applying tretinoin cream, gel, or liquid. The medication should be applied once a day just before going to bed. Apply it only to the skin where the acne lesions appear, unless you are directed to do otherwise by your doctor. Be sure to cover the entire affected area LIGHTLY. You may use a fingertip, gauze pad, or cotton swab to apply the liquid. To avoid applying too much medication, be careful not to oversaturate the gauze pad or cotton swab. To avoid contamination, use a gauze pad or cotton swab only once and then throw it away.

During the early weeks of treatment with this drug, there may be an apparent increase in skin lesions. This is usually not a reason to discontinue its use. However, your doctor may want to change the concentration of the drug. Benefits may be noted within two to three weeks, although more than six weeks may be required before definite benefits are observed.

If you miss a dose of this medication, apply the missed dose as soon as possible, and then return to your regular dosing schedule. However, if you do not remember until the following day, do not apply the missed dose at all; just return to your regular dosing schedule.

SIDE EFFECTS

Minor. Immediately after applying tretinoin to your skin, you may experience a sensation of warmth or a mild stinging sensation, or your skin may become reddened. After a few days of treatment with this medication, some peeling of the skin is to be expected. You may also find that you have a heightened sensitivity to sunlight, wind, or cold.

If this drug does increase your sensitivity to sunlight, you should try to avoid prolonged exposure to sunlight and sunlamps. Also, you should wear protective clothing, and use an effective sunscreen.

Major. Tell your doctor about any side effects that are persistent or particularly bothersome. IT IS ESPECIALLY IMPORTANT TO TELL YOUR DOCTOR about blistering, crusting, severe redness, severe burning, swelling, or marked darkening or lightening of the skin.

INTERACTIONS

Tretinoin interacts with several other products:

1. Abrasive or medicated soaps or cleaners.
2. Other acne preparations (particularly peeling agents containing sulfur, resorcinol, benzoyl peroxide, or salicylic acid).
3. Cosmetics that have a strong drying effect.
4. Locally applied products containing high amounts of alcohol, spices, or lime.

These products should be used with caution during treatment with tretinoin, since they can increase the irritation caused by this medication.

WARNINGS

• Tell your doctor about unusual or allergic reactions you have had to any drugs, especially to tretinoin or vitamin A.
• Before starting to take this medication, be sure to tell your doctor if you have eczema.
• This medication should not be used if you are sunburned; it may increase the irritation.
• Keep tretinoin away from the eyes, the mouth, the creases on either side of the nose, open cuts, and mucous membranes; it can severely irritate these sensitive areas.
• Avoid washing your face too often while using tretinoin. Be sure to use a mild or hypoallergenic soap.
• Normal use of nonmedicated cosmetics is permissible, but the skin should be cleaned thoroughly before tretinoin is applied.
• This medication has been prescribed for your current condition only. Do not give this medication to other people or use it for any other purpose than that prescribed by your doctor.

• Be sure to tell your doctor if you are pregnant. The safe use of this medication in human pregnancy or during breast-feeding has not been established.

Triacet—see triamcinolone (topical)

Triacin-C—see pseudoephedrine, triprolidine, and codeine combination

---

triamcinolone (systemic)

BRAND NAMES (Manufacturers)
Aristocort (Lederle)
Kenacort (Squibb)
triamcinolone (various manufacturers)
TYPE OF DRUG
Adrenocorticosteroid hormone
INGREDIENT
triamcinolone
DOSAGE FORMS
Tablets (1 mg, 2 mg, 4 mg, and 8 mg)
Oral syrup (2 mg and 4 mg per 5-ml spoonful)
STORAGE
Triamcinolone tablets and oral syrup should be stored at room temperature in tightly closed containers. Discard any outdated medication or any medication that is no longer needed.

USES
Your adrenal glands naturally produce certain cortisone-like chemicals. These chemicals are involved in various processes in the body (such as maintenance of fluid balance, regulation of temperature, and reaction to inflammation). Triamcinolone belongs to a group of drugs known as adrenocorticosteroids (or cortisone-like medications). It is used to treat a variety of disorders, including endocrine and rheumatic disorders; asthma; blood diseases; certain cancers; eye disorders; gastrointestinal disturbances, such as ulcerative colitis; respiratory diseases; and inflammations such as arthritis, dermatitis, and poison ivy. How this drug acts to relieve these disorders is not completely understood.

TREATMENT
In order to prevent stomach irritation, you can take triamcinolone with food or milk (unless your doctor directs you to do otherwise).

To help avoid potassium loss while using this drug, take your dose with a glass of fresh or frozen orange juice, or eat a banana each day. The use of a salt substitute also helps prevent potassium loss. Check with your doctor.

If you are taking only one dose of this medication each day, try to take it before 9:00 A.M.

The oral syrup form of this medication should be measured carefully with a specially designed 5-ml measuring spoon. An ordinary kitchen teaspoon is not accurate enough.

It is important to try not to miss any doses of triamcinolone. If you do miss a dose of this medication, follow these guidelines:

1. If you are taking it more than once a day, take the missed dose as soon as possible, and then return to your regular dosing schedule. If it is already time for the next dose, double the dose.

2. If you are taking this medication once a day, take the dose you missed as soon as possible, unless you do not remember until the next day. In that case, do not take the missed dose at all; just follow your regular dosing schedule. Do not double the next dose.

3. If you are taking this drug every other day, take it as soon as you remember. If you miss the dose by a whole day, take it when you remember, and then skip a day before you take the next dose. Do not double the dose.

If you miss more than one dose of triamcinolone, CONTACT YOUR DOCTOR.

SIDE EFFECTS

Minor. Dizziness, false sense of well-being, increased appetite, increased sweating, indigestion, nausea, reddening of the skin on the face, restlessness, sleep disorders, or weight gain. These side effects should disappear as your body adjusts to the medication.

Major. Tell your doctor about any side effects that are persistent or particularly bothersome. IT IS ESPECIALLY IMPORTANT TO TELL YOUR DOCTOR about abdominal enlargement; abdominal pain; acne or other skin problems; back or rib pain; bloody or black, tarry stools; blurred vision; convulsions; difficulty in breathing; eye pain; fatigue; fever and sore throat; filling out of the face; growth impairment (in children); headaches; impaired healing of wounds; increased thirst and urination; menstrual irregularities; mental depression; mood changes; muscle wasting or weakness; nightmares; rapid weight gain (three to five pounds within a week); rash; thinning of the skin; unusual bleeding or bruising; or unusual weakness.

INTERACTIONS

Triamcinolone interacts with several other types of medications:

1. Alcohol, aspirin, and anti-inflammatory medications (such as diflunisal, ibuprofen, indomethacin, ketoprofen, meclofenamate, mefenamic acid, naproxen, piroxicam, sulindac, and tolmetin) aggravate the stomach problems that are common with use of this medication.

2. There may be a change in the dosage requirements of oral anticoagulants, oral antidiabetic drugs, or insulin when this medication is started or stopped.

3. The loss of potassium caused by triamcinolone can lead to serious side effects in individuals taking digoxin.

4. Thiazide diuretics (water pills) can increase the potassium loss caused by triamcinolone.

5. Phenobarbital, phenytoin, rifampin, and ephedrine can increase the elimination of triamcinolone from the body, thereby decreasing its effectiveness.

6. Oral contraceptives (birth control pills) and estrogen-containing drugs may decrease the elimination of this drug from the body, which can lead to an increase in side effects.

7. Triamcinolone can increase the elimination of aspirin and isoniazid from the body, thereby decreasing the effectiveness of these two medications.

8. Cholestyramine and colestipol can chemically bind this medication in the stomach and gastrointestinal tract, preventing its absorption.

BE SURE TO TELL YOUR DOCTOR about any medications you are currently taking, especially any of those listed above.

WARNINGS

Tell your doctor about unusual or allergic reactions you have had to any medications, especially to triamcinolone or other adrenocorticosteroids (such as betamethasone, cortisone, dexamethasone, hydrocortisone, methylprednisolone, paramethasone, prednisolone, and prednisone).

Tell your doctor if you now have or if you have ever had bone disease, diabetes mellitus, emotional instability, glaucoma, fungal infections, heart disease, high blood pressure, high cholesterol levels, myasthenia gravis, peptic ulcers, osteoporosis, thyroid disease, tuberculosis, ulcerative colitis, kidney disease, or liver disease.

If you are using this medication for longer than a week, you may need to receive higher doses if you are subjected to stress, such as serious infections, injury, or surgery. Discuss this with your doctor.

If you have been taking this drug for more than a week, do not stop taking it suddenly. If it is stopped abruptly, you may experience abdominal or back pain, difficulty in breathing, dizziness, fainting, fever, muscle or joint pain, nausea, vomiting, or extreme weakness. Your doctor may, therefore, want to reduce the dosage gradually. Never increase the dosage or take the drug for longer than the prescribed time, unless you first consult your doctor.

While you are taking this drug, you should not be vaccinated or immunized. This medication decreases the effectiveness of vaccines and can lead to overwhelming infection if a live-virus vaccine is administered.

Before having surgery or any other medical or dental treatment, be sure to tell your doctor or dentist that you are taking this medication.

Because this drug can cause glaucoma and cataracts with long-term use, your doctor may want you to have your eyes examined by an ophthalmologist periodically.

If you are taking this medication for prolonged periods, you should wear or carry an identification card or notice stating that you are taking an adrenocorticosteroid.

This medication can raise blood sugar levels in diabetic patients. Blood sugar levels should, therefore, be monitored carefully with blood or urine tests when this medication is being taken.

Some of these products contain the color additive FD&C Yellow No. 5 (tartrazine), which can cause allergic-type reactions (wheezing, rash, fainting, difficulty in breathing) in certain susceptible individuals.

Be sure to tell your doctor if you are pregnant. This drug crosses the placenta, and its safety in human pregnancy is not established. Birth defects have been observed in the offspring of animals given large doses of this type of drug during pregnancy. Also, tell your doctor if you are breast-feeding. Small amounts of this drug pass into breast milk and may cause growth suppression or a decrease in natural adrenocorticosteroid production in the nursing infant.

triamcinolone (topical)

BRAND NAMES (Manufacturers)
Aristocort (Fujisawa)
Aristocort A (Fujisawa)
Flutex (Syosset)
Kenalog (Westwood/Squibb)
Kenalog-H (Westwood/Squibb)
Triacet (various manufacturers)
triamcinolone acetonide (various manufacturers)
Triderm (Del-Rey)
Trymex (Savage)

TYPE OF DRUG
Adrenocorticosteroid hormone

INGREDIENT
triamcinolone

DOSAGE FORMS
Ointment (0.025%, 0.1%, and 0.5%)
Cream (0.025%, 0.1%, and 0.5%)
Lotion (0.025% and 0.1%)
Paste (0.1%)
Aerosol (two seconds of spray delivers approximately 0.2
   mg of drug, with 10.3% alcohol)

STORAGE
Triamcinolone ointment, cream, lotion, and paste should be stored at room temperature in tightly closed containers. This medication should never be frozen.

The spray (foam) form of this medication is packed under pressure. It should not be stored near heat or an open flame or in direct sunlight, and the container should never be punctured.

USES
Your adrenal glands naturally produce certain cortisone-like chemicals. These chemicals are involved in various processes in the body (such as maintenance of fluid balance, regulation of temperature, and reaction to inflammation). Triamcinolone belongs to a group of drugs known as adrenocorticosteroids (or cortisone-like medications). It is used to relieve the skin inflammation (redness, swelling, itching, and discomfort) associated with conditions such as dermatitis, eczema, and poison ivy. How this drug acts to relieve these disorders is not completely understood.

TREATMENT
Before applying this medication, wash your hands. Then, unless your doctor gives you different instructions, gently wash the area of the skin where the medication is to be applied. With a clean towel, pat the area almost dry; it should be slightly damp when you put the medicine on.

If you are using the lotion form of this medication, shake it well before pouring. The contents tend to settle on the bottom of the bottle, so it is necessary to shake the container to distribute the ingredients evenly and equalize the doses.

Apply a small amount of the medication to the affected area in a thin layer. Do not bandage the area unless your doctor tells you to do so. If you are to apply an occlusive dressing (like kitchen plastic wrap), be sure you understand the instructions. Wash your hands again after application.

If you are using the aerosol spray form of this medication, shake the can in order to disperse the medication evenly. Hold the can upright six to eight inches from the area to be sprayed, and spray the area for one to three seconds. DO NOT SMOKE while you are using the aerosol spray.

If you miss a dose of this medication, apply the dose as soon as possible, unless it is almost time for the next application. In that case, do not apply the missed dose; just return to your regular dosing schedule. Do not put twice as much of the medication on your skin at the next application.

SIDE EFFECTS
Minor. Acne, burning sensation, irritation of the affected area, or skin dryness.

If the affected area is extremely dry or scaling, the skin may be moistened by soaking in water or by applying water with a clean cloth before applying the medication. The ointment form is probably better for dry skin.

A mild, temporary stinging sensation may occur after this medication is applied. If this persists, contact your doctor.

Major. Tell your doctor about any side effects that are persistent or particularly bothersome. IT IS ESPECIALLY IMPORTANT TO TELL YOUR DOCTOR about blistering, increased hair growth, itching, loss of skin color, rash, secondary infection in the area being treated, or thinning of the skin with easy bruising.

INTERACTIONS
This medication should not interact with other medications as long as it is used according to the directions given to you by your doctor or pharmacist.

WARNINGS
• Tell your doctor about unusual or allergic reactions you have had to any medications, especially to triamcinolone or other adrenocorticosteroids (such as amcinonide, betamethasone, clocortolone, cortisone, desonide, desoximetasone, dexamethasone, diflorasone, flumethasone, fluocinolone, fluocinonide, fluorometholone, flurandrenolide, halcinonide, hydrocortisone, methylprednisolone, prednisolone, and prednisone).
• Tell your doctor if you now have or if you have ever had blood vessel disease, chicken pox, diabetes mellitus, fungal infection, peptic ulcers, shingles, tuberculosis of the lungs or skin, vaccinia, or any other type of infection, especially at the site currently being treated.
• If any kind of irritation develops while you are using this drug, you should immediately discontinue its use and notify your doctor.
• This product is intended for topical use only. It is not for use in the eyes or on the mucous membranes; contact may result in side effects.
• Do not use this product with an occlusive wrap unless your doctor directs you to do so. Systemic absorption of this drug is increased if extensive areas of the body are treated, particularly if occlusive bandages are used. If it is necessary for you to use this drug under a wrap, follow your doctor's instructions exactly; do not leave the wrap in place longer than specified.

• If you are using this medication on a child's diaper area. It is important to not put tight-fitting diapers or plastic pants on the child. This may lead to increased systemic absorption of the medication and an increase in side effects.

• In order to avoid freezing skin tissue when using the aerosol form of triamcinolone, it is important that you are sure you do not spray for more than three seconds, and be sure to hold the container at least six inches away from the skin.

• To prevent side effects when using the aerosol form of this medication on the face, cover your eyes, and do not inhale the spray.

• Do not use this medication for longer than the time prescribed by your doctor.

• It is very important that you tell your doctor if you are pregnant. If large amounts of triamcinolone are applied for prolonged periods, some of it will be absorbed and may cross the placenta. Although extensive studies in humans have not yet been conducted, birth defects have been observed in the offspring of animals that were given large oral doses of this type of drug during pregnancy. Also, tell your doctor if you are currently breast-feeding an infant. If absorbed through the skin, small amounts of triamcinolone pass into breast milk and may cause growth suppression or a decrease in natural adrenocorticosteroid hormone production in the nursing infant.

triamcinolone acetonide—see triamcinolone (topical)

triamcinolone, neomycin, gramicidin, and nystatin combination (topical)—see triamcinolone, neomycin, nystatin, and gramicidin combination (topical)

---

triamcinolone, neomycin, nystatin, and gramicidin combination (topical)

BRAND NAMES (Manufacturers)
Myco Triacet (various manufacturers)
triamcinolone, neomycin, gramicidin, and nystatin combination (topical) (various manufacturers)
TYPE OF DRUG
Adrenocorticosteroid and anti-infective
INGREDIENTS
triamcinolone, neomycin, nystatin, and gramicidin
DOSAGE FORMS
Cream (0.1% triamcinolone; 2.5 mg neomycin; 100,000 units nystatin; and 0.25 mg gramicidin per gram)
Ointment (0.1% triamcinolone; 2.5 mg neomycin; 100,000 units nystatin; and 0.25 mg gramicidin per gram)
STORAGE
The cream and ointment should be stored at room temperature (never frozen) in tightly closed containers. Discard any outdated medicine or medicine no longer needed.

USES
Your adrenal glands naturally produce certain cortisone-like chemicals. These chemicals are involved in various processes in the body (such as maintenance of fluid balance, regulation of temperature, and reaction to inflammation). Triamcinolone belongs to a group of medications known as adrenocorticosteroids (or cortisone-like medications). It is used to relieve the skin inflammation (redness, swelling, itching, and discomfort) associated with conditions such as dermatitis, eczema, and poison ivy. How this medication acts to relieve these disorders is not completely understood. Neomycin and gramicidin are antibiotics, which act to prevent the growth and multiplication of infecting bacteria. Nystatin is an anti-infective agent that is active against the fungus *Candida albicans*.

TREATMENT
Before applying this medication, wash your hands. Then, unless your doctor gives you different instructions, gently wash the area of skin where the medication is to be applied. With a clean towel, pat the area almost dry; it should be slightly damp when you apply this particular medication.

Apply a small amount of this medication to the affected area in a thin layer. Do not bandage the area unless your doctor specifically tells you to do so. If you are to apply an occlusive dressing (like kitchen plastic wrap), be sure that you understand the instructions. Wash your hands again after application.

If you miss a dose of this medication, apply the dose as soon as possible, unless it is almost time for the next application. In that case, do not apply the missed dose at all; just return to your regular dosing schedule. Do not put twice as much of the medication on your skin at the next application.

Use this medication for the full length of time prescribed by your doctor; do not take the medication for longer than the prescribed period.

SIDE EFFECTS
Minor. Acne, burning sensation, irritation of the affected area, or skin dryness.

If the affected area is extremely dry or scaling, the skin may be moistened by soaking in water or by applying water with a clean cloth before applying the medication. The ointment form is probably better for dry skin.

A mild, temporary stinging sensation may occur after this medication is applied. If this persists, contact your doctor.

Major. Tell your doctor about any side effects that are persistent or particularly bothersome. IT IS ESPECIALLY IMPORTANT TO TELL YOUR DOCTOR about blistering, increased hair growth, itching, loss of skin color, rash, secondary infection in the area being treated, or thinning of the skin with easy bruising. Also, if your symptoms of infection seem to be getting worse rather than improving, you should contact your doctor.

INTERACTIONS
This medication should not interact with other medications, as long as it is used according to directions.

WARNINGS

• Tell your doctor about unusual or allergic reactions you have had to any medications, especially to triamcinolone or other adrenocorticosteroids (such as amcinonide, betamethasone, clocortolone, cortisone, desonide, desoxi-metasone, dexamethasone, diflorasone, flumethasone, fluocinolone, fluocinonide, fluorometholone, flurandrenolide, halcinonide, hydrocortisone, methylprednisolone, prednisolone, and prednisone) or to neomycin, nystatin, or gramicidin.

• Tell your doctor if you now have or if you have ever had circulation problems, chicken pox, diabetes mellitus, peptic ulcers, shingles, tuberculosis of the lungs or skin, vaccinia, or viral or fungal infections of the skin in addition to a *Candida* infection.

• If any kind of irritation develops while you are using this drug, you should immediately discontinue its use and notify your doctor.

• Do not use in the eyes; contact may result in side effects.

• This medication should not be used in the external ear canal of people with perforated eardrums.

• Do not use this product with an occlusive wrap unless your doctor directs you to do so. Systemic absorption of this drug is increased when extensive areas of the body are treated, particularly if occlusive bandages are used. If it is necessary for you to use this drug under a wrap, follow your doctor's instructions exactly, and do not leave the wrap in place longer than specified.

• If you are using this medication on a child's diaper area, do not put tight-fitting diapers or plastic pants on the child. This may lead to increased systemic absorption of the drug and an increase in side effects.

• Be sure to tell your doctor if you are pregnant. If large amounts of this medication are applied for prolonged periods, some of it will be absorbed and may cross the placenta. Although studies in humans have not been conducted, birth defects have been observed in the offspring of animals that were given large oral doses of this type of medication during pregnancy. Also, tell your doctor if you are breast-feeding an infant. If absorbed through the skin, small amounts of this medication pass into breast milk and may cause growth suppression or a decrease in natural adrenocorticosteroid hormone production in the nursing infant.

Triaminic—see phenylpropanolamine and chlorpheniramine combination

Triaminic-12—see phenylpropanolamine and chlorpheniramine combination

triamterene

BRAND NAME (Manufacturer)
Dyrenium (Smith Kline Beecham)
TYPE OF DRUG
Diuretic and antihypertensive
INGREDIENT
triamterene

DOSAGE FORM
Capsules (50 mg and 100 mg)
STORAGE
Triamterene should be stored at room temperature in a tightly closed, light-resistant container.

USES

Triamterene is prescribed to treat high blood pressure. It is also used to reduce fluid accumulation in the body caused by conditions such as heart failure, cirrhosis of the liver, kidney disease, and the long-term use of some medications. Triamterene reduces fluid accumulation by increasing the elimination of salt and water through the kidneys. It may also be used in combination with other diuretics to prevent potassium loss.

TREATMENT

To decrease stomach irritation, you can take triamterene with a glass of milk or with a meal (unless your doctor directs you to do otherwise). Try to take it at the same time(s) every day. Avoid taking a dose after 6:00 P.M.; otherwise, you may have to get up during the night to urinate.

This medication does not cure high blood pressure, but it will help to control the condition as long as you take it.

If you miss a dose of this medication, take the missed dose as soon as possible, unless it is almost time for the next dose. In that case, do not take the missed dose at all; just wait until the next scheduled dose. Do not double the dose.

SIDE EFFECTS

Minor. Diarrhea, dizziness, drowsiness, dry mouth, headache, increased thirst, increased urination, nausea, tiredness, upset stomach, or vomiting. As your body adjusts to triamterene, these side effects from this medication should disappear.

This medication can cause increased sensitivity to sunlight. It is, therefore, important to avoid prolonged exposure to sunlight and sunlamps while you are taking this medication. Wear protective clothing, and use an sunscreen.

Triamterene may cause the urine to turn bluish; this is a harmless side effect.

Dry mouth can be relieved by sucking on ice chips or a piece of hard candy or by chewing sugarless gum.

To avoid dizziness or light-headedness when you stand, contract and relax the muscles of your legs for a few moments before rising. Do this by pushing one foot against the floor while raising the other foot slightly, alternating feet so that you are "pumping" your legs in a pedaling motion.

Major. Tell your doctor about any side effects that are persistent or particularly bothersome. IT IS ESPECIALLY IMPORTANT TO TELL YOUR DOCTOR about anxiety; back or flank (side) pain; confusion; cracking at the corners of the mouth; difficulty in breathing; extreme weakness; fever; mouth sores; numbness or tingling in the hands, feet, or lips; painful urination; palpitations; rash; a red or inflamed tongue; sore throat; unusual bleeding or bruising; or unusual tiredness.

INTERACTIONS

Triamterene interacts with several foods and medications:

1. Concurrent use of it with antihypertensives such as benazepril, fusinopril, lisinopril, and ramipril, or with spironolactone, amiloride, potassium salts, low-salt milk, salt substitutes, captopril, enalapril, or laxatives can cause serious side effects from hyperkalemia (high levels of potassium in the blood).

2. Triamterene may decrease the effectiveness of antigout medications, insulin, and oral antidiabetic medications.

3. It may increase the side effects of lithium.

4. Indomethacin may decrease the diuretic effects of triamterene.

Before starting to take triamterene, BE SURE TO TELL YOUR DOCTOR about any medications you are currently taking, especially any of those listed above.

WARNINGS

• Before starting to take triamterene, be sure to tell your doctor if you have ever had unusual or allergic reactions to any medications, especially to triamterene or to any other diuretic.

• Be sure to tell your doctor if you now have or if you have ever had kidney disease, kidney stones, urination problems, hyperkalemia, diabetes mellitus, liver disease, acidosis, or gout.

• Triamterene can cause hyperkalemia (high blood levels of potassium). Signs of hyperkalemia include palpitations; confusion; numbness or tingling in the hands, feet, or lips; anxiety; or unusual tiredness or weakness. In order to avoid this problem, it is important that you not alter your diet, and do not use salt substitutes unless your doctor tells you to do so.

• You should limit your intake of alcoholic beverages while taking this drug in order to prevent dizziness and light-headedness.

• Do not take any over-the-counter (nonprescription) medications for weight control or for allergy, asthma, cough, cold, or sinus problems unless you first check with your doctor. Some of these products can lead to an increase in blood pressure.

• It is possible that treatment with this medication can cause severe water loss (dehydration). In order to prevent this, be sure to check with your doctor if you have any illness that causes severe or continuous nausea, vomiting, or diarrhea.

• If you are taking quinidine (an antiarrhythmia heart medication), it is important to know that triamterene may interfere with the laboratory determination of your blood quinidine concentration. Before you undergo this type of test, be sure to tell your doctor that you are also taking the drug triamterene.

• Your doctor may schedule regular office visits to monitor your progress and possibly adjust your dosage.

• Be sure to tell your doctor if you are pregnant. This medication crosses the placenta, and its safety in human pregnancy has not been thoroughly investigated. However, effects have been reported in the fetuses of animals that received large doses of this medication during pregnancy. Also, be sure to tell your doctor if you are breast-feeding an infant. It has been established that small amounts of triamterene pass into breast milk.

triamterene and hydrochlorothiazide combination

BRAND NAMES (Manufacturers)

Dyazide (Smith Kline Beecham)
Maxzide (Lederle)
triamterene and hydrochlorothiazide (various manufacturers)

TYPE OF DRUG

Diuretic and antihypertensive

INGREDIENTS

triamterene and hydrochlorothiazide

DOSAGE FORMS

Capsules (50 mg triamterene and 25 mg hydrochlorothiazide) Tablets (37.5 mg triamterene and 25 mg hydrochlorothiazide, and 75 mg triamterene and 50 mg hydrochlorothiazide)

STORAGE

This medication should be stored at room temperature in a tightly closed, light-resistant container.

USES

Triamterene and hydrochlorothiazide combination is prescribed to treat high blood pressure. It is also used to reduce fluid accumulation in the body caused by conditions such as heart failure, cirrhosis of the liver, kidney disease, and the long-term use of some medications. It reduces fluid accumulation by increasing the elimination of salt and water through the kidneys. Triamterene is combined with hydrochlorothiazide to prevent potassium loss.

TREATMENT

To decrease stomach irritation, you can take this medication with a glass of milk or with a meal (unless your doctor directs you to do otherwise). Try to take it at the same time every day. Avoid taking a dose after 6:00 P.M.; otherwise, you may have to get up during the night to urinate.

This drug does not cure high blood pressure but will help to control the condition as long as you continue to take it.

If you miss a dose of this medication, take the missed dose as soon as possible, unless it is almost time for the next dose. In that case, do not take the missed dose at all; just wait until the next scheduled dose. Do not double the dose.

SIDE EFFECTS

Minor. Constipation, cramps, diarrhea, dizziness, drowsiness, headache, increased urination, loss of appetite, restlessness, tiredness, or upset stomach. These side effects should disappear as your body adjusts to the medication.

This medication can cause increased sensitivity to sunlight. It is, therefore, important to avoid prolonged exposure to sunlight and sunlamps. Wear protective clothing, and use an effective sunscreen.

Triamterene can cause the urine to turn bluish; this is a harmless side effect.

To relieve constipation, increase the amount of fiber in your diet (fresh fruits and vegetables, salads, bran, and whole-grain breads) and exercise more (unless your doctor directs you to do otherwise).

If you experience dryness of the mouth, you might want to try sucking on ice chips or a piece of hard candy or chewing sugarless gum.

To avoid dizziness or light-headedness when you stand, contract and relax the muscles of your legs for a few moments before rising. Do this by pushing one foot against the floor while raising the other foot slightly, alternating feet so that you are "pumping" your legs in a pedaling motion.

Major. Tell your doctor about any side effects that are persistent or particularly bothersome. IT IS ESPECIALLY IMPORTANT TO TELL YOUR DOCTOR about anxiety; back or flank (side) pain; confusion; cracking at the corners of the mouth; difficulty in urinating; difficulty in breathing; dry mouth; fever; itching; mood changes; mouth sores; muscle cramps or spasms; nausea; painful urination; palpitations; rash; red or inflamed tongue; sore throat; thirst; tingling or numbness in the hands, feet, or lips; unusual bleeding or bruising; unusual tiredness or weakness; vomiting; or yellowing of the eyes or skin.

INTERACTIONS

Triamterene and hydrochlorothiazide combination interacts with several foods and medications:

1. Concurrent use of it with antihypertensives, such as benazepril, fusinopril, lisinopril, and ramipril, or with spironolactone, amiloride, potassium salts, low-salt milk, salt substitutes, captopril, enalapril, or laxatives can cause serious side effects from hyperkalemia (high levels of potassium in the blood).

2. This drug may decrease the effectiveness of oral anticoagulants, antigout medications, insulin, oral antidiabetic medicines, and methenamine.

3. Fenfluramine may increase the blood-pressure-lowering effects of this drug (which can be dangerous).

4. Indomethacin may decrease the effectiveness of this medication.

5. Cholestyramine and colestipol can decrease the absorption of this medication from the gastrointestinal tract. Therefore, triamterene and hydrochlorothiazide combination should be taken one hour before or four hours after a dose of cholestyramine or colestipol if one of these medications has also been prescribed.

6. This medication may increase the side effects of amphotericin B, calcium, cortisone and cortisone-like steroids (such as dexamethasone, hydrocortisone, prednisone, and prednisolone), digoxin, digitalis, lithium, quinidine, sulfonamide antibiotics, and vitamin D.

BE SURE TO TELL YOUR DOCTOR about any medications you are currently taking, especially any of those listed above.

WARNINGS

• Tell your doctor about unusual or allergic reactions you have had to any medications, especially to triamterene or hydrochlorothiazide or to any other sulfa drugs, including other diuretics, oral antidiabetic medications, and sulfonamide antibiotics.

• Before you start to take triamterene and hydrochlorothiazide combination, tell your doctor if you now have or if you have ever had kidney disease, kidney stones, problems with urination, diabetes mellitus, gout, liver disease, asthma, acidosis, pancreatic disease, systemic lupus erythematosus, anemia, blood disease, hypercalcemia, or hyperkalemia.

• This drug can occasionally cause potassium loss from the body. Signs of potassium loss include dry mouth, thirst, weakness, muscle pain or cramps, nausea, and vomiting. If you experience any of these symptoms, call your doctor.

• Triamterene can cause hyperkalemia (high levels of potassium in the blood). Signs of hyperkalemia include palpitations; confusion; numbness or tingling in the hands, feet, or lips; anxiety; or unusual tiredness or weakness. In order to avoid this problem, do not alter your diet, and do not use salt substitutes unless you first consult your doctor.

• If you are taking quinidine (an antiarrhythmia heart medication), it is important to know that triamterene may interfere with the laboratory determination of your blood quinidine concentration. Before you undergo such a test, be sure to tell your doctor that you are also taking triamterene and hydrochlorothiazide combination.

• Limit your intake of alcoholic beverages while taking this medication, in order to prevent dizziness and light-headedness.

• Do not take any over-the-counter (nonprescription) medications for weight control or for allergy, asthma, cough, cold, or sinus problems unless you first check with your doctor. Some of these products can lead to an increase in blood pressure.

• Do not change brands of this medication without consulting your doctor.

• To prevent severe water loss (dehydration) while taking this medication, check with your doctor if you have any illness that causes severe or continuous nausea, vomiting, or diarrhea.

• This medication can raise blood sugar levels in diabetic patients. Therefore, blood sugar should be monitored carefully with blood or urine tests when this medication is being taken.

• A doctor does not usually prescribe a "fixed-dose" medication like triamterene and hydrochlorothiazide combination as the first choice in the treatment of high blood pressure. Usually, the patient will first receive each ingredient singly. If there is an adequate response to the fixed dose contained in an individual product, it can then be substituted. The advantages of a combination product include increased convenience and (often) decreased cost to the consumer.

• Your doctor may schedule regular office visits in order to monitor your progress and possibly adjust the dosage of this medication.

• Be sure to tell your doctor if you are pregnant. This drug crosses the placenta, and its safety in human pregnancy has not been established. Adverse effects have been observed in the fetuses of animals that received large doses of this type of drug during pregnancy. Also, tell your doctor if you are breast-feeding an infant. Small amounts of this drug pass into breast milk.

Triavil—see perphenazine and amitriptyline combination

---

triazolam

BRAND NAME (Manufacturer)
Halcion (Upjohn)
TYPE OF DRUG
Benzodiazepine sedative/hypnotic
INGREDIENT
triazolam
DOSAGE FORM
Tablets (0.125 mg)
STORAGE
This medication should be stored at room temperature in a tightly closed, light-resistant container.

USES
Triazolam is prescribed to treat insomnia, including problems with falling asleep, waking during the night, and early morning wakefulness. It is not clear exactly how this medicine works, but it may relieve insomnia by acting as a depressant of the central nervous system (brain and spinal cord).

TREATMENT
This medicine should be taken 30 to 60 minutes before bedtime. It can be taken with a full glass of water or with food if stomach upset occurs. Do not take this medication with a dose of antacids, since they may slow its absorption.

If you are taking this medication regularly and you miss a dose, take the missed dose immediately if you remember within an hour. If more than an hour has passed, skip the dose you missed and wait for the next scheduled dose. Do not double the dose.

SIDE EFFECTS
Minor. Bitter taste in mouth, constipation, diarrhea, dizziness, drowsiness (after a night's sleep), dry mouth, excessive salivation, fatigue, flushing, headache, heartburn, loss of appetite, nausea, nervousness, sweating, or vomiting. As your body adjusts to the medication, these should disappear.

To relieve constipation, increase the amount of fiber in your diet (fresh fruits and vegetables, salads, bran, and whole-grain breads), exercise, and drink more water (unless your doctor directs you to do otherwise).

Dry mouth can be relieved by chewing sugarless gum or by sucking on ice chips.

If you feel dizzy, sit or lie down for a while; get up slowly from a sitting or reclining position, and be careful on stairs.

Major. Tell your doctor about any side effects that are persistent or particularly bothersome. IT IS ESPECIALLY IMPORTANT TO TELL YOUR DOCTOR about blurred or double vision, chest pain, depression, difficulty in urinating, fainting, falling, fever, hallucinations, joint pain, mouth sores, nightmares, palpitations, rash, shortness of breath, slurred speech, sore throat, uncoordinated movements, unusual excitement, unusual tiredness, or yellowing of the eyes or skin.

INTERACTIONS
Triazolam interacts with a number of other types of drugs:
1. To prevent oversedation, it should not be taken with alcohol, other sedative drugs, central nervous system depressants (such as antihistamines, barbiturates, muscle relaxants, pain medicines, narcotics, medicines for seizures, and phenothiazine tranquilizers), or with antidepressants.
2. Triazolam may decrease the effectiveness of carbamazepine, levodopa, and oral anticoagulants (blood thinners, such as warfarin) and may increase the side effects of phenytoin.
3. Disulfiram, oral contraceptives (birth control pills), isoniazid, and cimetidine can increase the blood levels of triazolam, which can lead to toxic effects.
4. Concurrent use of rifampin may decrease the effectiveness of triazolam.

BE SURE TO TELL YOUR DOCTOR about any medications you are currently taking, especially those listed above.

WARNINGS
• Tell your doctor about unusual or allergic reactions you have had to any medications, especially to triazolam or other benzodiazepine tranquilizers (such as alprazolam, chlordiazepoxide, clorazepate, diazepam, flurazepam, halazepam, lorazepam, prazepam, and temazepam).
• Tell your doctor if you now have or if you have ever had liver disease, kidney disease, epilepsy, lung disease, myasthenia gravis, porphyria, mental depression, or mental illness.
• This medicine can cause drowsiness. Avoid tasks that require mental alertness, such as driving a car or operating potentially dangerous machinery.
• Triazolam has the potential for abuse and must be used with caution. Tolerance may develop quickly; do not increase the dosage unless you first consult your doctor. It is also important not to stop taking this drug suddenly if you have been taking it in large amounts or if you have used it for several weeks. Your doctor may want to reduce the dosage gradually.
• This is a safe drug when used properly. When it is combined with other sedative drugs or with alcohol, however, serious side effects can develop.
• Be sure to tell your doctor if you are pregnant. This type of medicine may increase the chance of birth defects if it is taken during the first three months of pregnancy. In addition, use of too much of this medicine during the last six months of pregnancy may lead to addiction of the fetus, resulting in withdrawal side effects in the newborn. Also, use of this medicine during the last weeks of pregnancy may cause excessive drowsiness, slowed heartbeat, and breathing difficulties in the infant. Tell your doctor if you are breast-feeding an infant. This medicine can pass into breast milk and cause unwanted side effects in nursing infants.

Trichlorex—see trichlormethiazide

trichlormethiazide

BRAND NAMES (Manufacturers)
Diurese (American Urologicals)
Metahydrin (Merrell Dow)
Naqua (Schering)
Niazide (Major)
Trichlorex (Lannett)
trichlormethiazide (various manufacturers)
TYPE OF DRUG
Diuretic and antihypertensive
INGREDIENT
trichlormethiazide
DOSAGE FORM
Tablets (2 mg and 4 mg)
STORAGE
This medication should be stored at room temperature in a tightly closed container.

USES
Trichlormethiazide is prescribed to treat high blood pressure. It is also used to reduce fluid accumulation in the body caused by conditions such as heart failure, cirrhosis of the liver, and kidney disease and by the long-term use of some medications. This medication reduces fluid accumulation by increasing the elimination of sodium and water through the kidneys.

TREATMENT
To decrease stomach irritation, you can take this medication with a glass of milk or with a meal (unless your doctor directs you to do otherwise). Try to take it at the same time every day. Avoid taking a dose after 6:00 P.M.; otherwise, you may have to get up during the night to urinate.

If you miss a dose of this medication, take the missed dose as soon as possible, unless it is almost time for the next dose. In that case, do not take the missed dose at all; just wait until the next scheduled dose. Do not double the next dose.

This medication does not cure high blood pressure, but will help control the condition as long as you continue to take it.

SIDE EFFECTS
Minor. Constipation, cramps, diarrhea, dizziness, drowsiness, headache, heartburn, loss of appetite, nausea, restlessness, or upset stomach. As your body adjusts to the medication, these side effects should disappear.

This medication can cause increased sensitivity to sunlight. It is, therefore, important to avoid prolonged exposure to sunlight and sunlamps. Wear protective clothing, and use an effective sunscreen.

To avoid dizziness or light-headedness when you stand, contract and relax the muscles of your legs for a few moments before rising. Do this by pushing one foot against the floor while raising the other foot slightly, alternating feet so that you are "pumping" your legs in a pedaling motion.

Major. Tell your doctor about any side effects that are persistent or particularly bothersome. IT IS ESPECIALLY IMPORTANT TO TELL YOUR DOCTOR about blurred vision, confusion, difficulty in breathing, dry mouth, excessive thirst, excessive weakness, fever, itching, joint pain, mood changes, muscle pain or spasms, nausea, palpitations, skin rash, sore throat, tingling in the fingers or toes, vomiting, or yellowing of the eyes or skin.

INTERACTIONS
Trichlormethiazide interacts with other types of medications:

1. It may decrease the effectiveness of oral anticoagulants, antigout medications, insulin, oral antidiabetic medicines, and methenamine.

2. Fenfluramine can increase the blood-pressure-lowering effects of trichlormethiazide (which can be dangerous).

3. Indomethacin can decrease the blood-pressure-lowering effects of trichlormethiazide, thereby counteracting the desired effects.

4. Cholestyramine and colestipol decrease the absorption of this medication from the gastrointestinal tract. Trichlormethiazide should, therefore, be taken one hour before or four hours after a dose of cholestyramine or colestipol if one of these medications has also been prescribed.

5. Trichlormethiazide may increase the side effects of amphotericin B, calcium, cortisone and cortisone-like steroids (such as dexamethasone, hydrocortisone, prednisone, prednisolone), digoxin, digitalis, lithium, quinidine, sulfonamide antibiotics, and vitamin D.

BE SURE TO TELL YOUR DOCTOR about any medications you are currently taking, especially any of those listed above.

WARNINGS
Tell your doctor about unusual or allergic reactions you have had to any medications, especially to trichlormethiazide or to other sulfa drugs, including other diuretics, oral antidiabetic medications, and sulfonamide antibiotics.

Before you start taking trichlormethiazide, tell your doctor if you now have or if you have ever had kidney disease or problems with urination, diabetes mellitus, gout, liver disease, asthma, pancreatic disease, or systemic lupus erythematosus.

Trichlormethiazide can cause potassium loss. Signs of potassium loss include dry mouth, thirst, weakness, muscle pain or cramps, nausea, and vomiting. If you experience any of these symptoms, call your doctor. To help avoid potassium loss, take this drug with a glass of fresh or frozen orange or cranberry juice, or eat a banana every day. The use of a salt substitute also helps to prevent potassium loss. Do not change your diet, however, before discussing it with your doctor; too much potassium can also be dangerous. Your doctor may want to have blood tests performed periodically in order to monitor your potassium levels.

In order to prevent dizziness and light-headedness, limit your intake of alcoholic beverages while taking this drug.

Do not take any over-the-counter (nonprescription) medications for weight control or for allergy, asthma, cough, cold, or sinus problems unless directed to do so by your doctor.

To prevent dehydration (severe water loss) while taking this medication, check with your doctor if you have any illness that causes severe or continuous nausea, vomiting, or diarrhea.

This medication can raise blood sugar levels in diabetic patients. Therefore, blood sugar should be carefully monitored with blood or urine tests when this medication is being taken.

Some of these products contain the color additive FD&C Yellow No. 5 (tartrazine), which can cause allergic-type reactions (wheezing, rash, fainting, difficulty in breathing) in certain susceptible individuals.

The elderly may be more likely to experience dizziness, light-headedness, and too much potassium loss as a result of therapy with this drug.

Be sure to tell your doctor if you are pregnant. This drug is able to cross the placenta. Safety in human pregnancy has not been established. Adverse effects have been observed in the fetuses of animals that received large doses of this type of drug during pregnancy. Also, tell your doctor if you are breast-feeding an infant. Although problems in humans have not been reported, small amounts of this drug can pass into breast milk, so caution is warranted.

Triderm—see triamcinolone (topical)

Trifed-C—see pseudoephedrine, triprolidine, and codeine combination

---

trifluoperazine

BRAND NAMES (Manufacturers)
Stelazine (Smith Kline Beecham)
trifluoperazine (various manufacturers)
trifluoperazine hydrochloride
TYPE OF DRUG
Phenothiazine tranquilizer
INGREDIENT
trifluoperazine
DOSAGE FORMS
Tablets (1 mg, 2 mg, 5 mg, and 10 mg)
Oral concentrate (10 mg per ml)
STORAGE
The tablet form of this medication should be stored at room temperature in a tightly closed, light-resistant container. The oral concentrate form should be stored in the refrigerator (never frozen) in a tightly closed, light-resistant container. If the oral concentrate turns slightly yellowish, the medicine is still effective and can be used. However, if it changes color markedly or has particles floating in it, it should not be used; instead, it should be discarded down the sink. Discard any outdated medication.

USES

Trifluoperazine is prescribed to treat the symptoms of certain types of mental illness, such as emotional symptoms of psychosis, the manic phase of manic-depressive illness, and severe behavioral problems in children. This medication is thought to relieve the symptoms of mental illness by blocking certain chemicals involved with nerve transmission in the brain.

TREATMENT

In order to avoid stomach irritation, you can take the tablet form of this medication with a meal or with a glass of water or milk (unless your doctor directs you to do otherwise).

The oral concentrate form of this medication should be measured carefully with the dropper provided and then added to four ounces (cup) or more of water, milk, or a carbonated beverage or to applesauce or pudding immediately prior to administration. The medication should not be diluted with tea, coffee, or apple juice.

Antacids and antidiarrheal medications may decrease the absorption of this medication from the gastrointestinal tract. Therefore, at least one hour should separate doses of one of these medicines and trifluoperazine.

If you miss a dose of this medication, take the missed dose as soon as possible, unless it is almost time for the next dose. In that case, do not take the missed dose at all; just return to your regular dosing schedule. Do not double the next dose (unless your doctor directs you to do so).

The full effects of this medication for the control of emotional or mental symptoms may not become apparent for at least two weeks after you start to take it.

SIDE EFFECTS

Minor. Blurred vision, constipation, decreased sweating, diarrhea, dizziness, drowsiness, dry mouth, fatigue, jitteriness, menstrual irregularities, nasal congestion, restlessness, vomiting, or weight gain. As your body adjusts to the medication, these side effects should disappear.

This medication can cause increased sensitivity to sunlight. It is, therefore, important to avoid prolonged exposure to sunlight and sunlamps. Wear protective clothing, and use an effective sunscreen.

Trifluoperazine can also cause discoloration of the urine to red, pink, or red-brown. This is a harmless effect.

If you are constipated, increase the amount of fiber in your diet (fresh fruits and vegetables, salads, bran, and whole-grain breads), exercise, and drink more water (unless your doctor directs you to do otherwise).

Chew sugarless gum or suck on ice chips or a piece of hard candy to reduce mouth dryness.

To avoid dizziness or light-headedness when you stand, contract and relax the muscles of your legs for a few moments before rising. Do this by pushing one foot against the floor while raising the other foot slightly, alternating feet so that you are "pumping" your legs in a pedaling motion.

Major. Tell your doctor about any side effects that are persistent or particularly bothersome. IT IS ESPECIALLY IMPORTANT TO TELL YOUR DOCTOR about breast enlargement (in both sexes); chest pain; convulsions; darkened skin; difficulty in swallowing or breathing; drooling; fainting; fever; impotence; involuntary movements of the face, mouth, jaw, or tongue; palpitations; rash; sleep disorders; sore throat; suicidal tendencies; tremors;

uncoordinated movements; unusual bleeding or bruising; visual disturbances; or yellowing of the eyes or skin.

INTERACTIONS

Trifluoperazine interacts with several other types of medications:

1. It can cause extreme drowsiness when combined with alcohol or other central nervous system depressants (drugs that slow the activity of the brain and spinal cord), such as barbiturates, benzodiazepine tranquilizers, muscle relaxants, narcotics, and pain medications, or with tricyclic antidepressants.

2. Trifluoperazine can decrease the effectiveness of amphetamines, guanethidine, anticonvulsants, and levodopa.

3. The side effects of epinephrine, monoamine oxidase (MAO) inhibitors, propranolol, phenytoin, and tricyclic antidepressants may be increased by this medication. At least 14 days should separate the use of this drug and the use of an MAO inhibitor.

4. Lithium may increase the side effects and decrease the effectiveness of this medication.

5. Trifluoperazine used with methyldopa may increase blood pressure.

6. False-positive pregnancy tests may occur. If you think you may be pregnant, call your doctor.

BE SURE TO TELL YOUR DOCTOR about any medications you are currently taking, especially those listed above.

WARNINGS

• Tell your doctor about unusual or allergic reactions you have had to any medications, especially to trifluoperazine or other phenothiazine tranquilizers (such as chlorpromazine, fluphenazine, mesoridazine, perphenazine, prochlorperazine, promazine, thioridazine, and triflupromazine) or to loxapine.

• Tell your doctor if you have a history of alcoholism or if you now have or have ever had blood disease, bone marrow disease, brain disease, breast cancer, blockage of the urinary or digestive tract, drug-induced depression, epilepsy, high or low blood pressure, diabetes mellitus, glaucoma, heart or circulatory disease, liver disease, lung disease, Parkinson's disease, peptic ulcers, or enlarged prostate gland.

• Tell your doctor about any recent exposure to a pesticide or an insecticide. Trifluoperazine may increase the side effects from the exposure.

• To prevent oversedation, avoid drinking alcoholic beverages while taking this medication.

• If this drug makes you dizzy or drowsy, avoid any activity that requires alertness, such as driving a car or operating dangerous machinery. Be careful on stairs, and avoid getting up suddenly from a lying or sitting position.

• Prior to surgery or other medical or dental treatment, tell your doctor or dentist you are taking this drug.

• Some of the side effects caused by this drug can be prevented by taking an antiparkinsonism drug. Discuss this with your doctor.

• This medication can decrease sweating and heat release from the body. You should, therefore, try not to get overheated (avoid exercising strenuously in hot weather, and do not take hot baths, showers, and saunas).

• Do not stop taking this drug suddenly. If the drug is stopped abruptly, you may experience nausea, vomiting, stomach upset, headache, increased heart rate, insomnia, tremors, or a worsening of your condition. It is important to let your doctor know you have stopped taking this drug. Your doctor may want to reduce the dosage gradually.

• If you are planning to have a myelogram or any other procedure in which dye will be injected into your spinal cord, be sure to tell your doctor that you are undergoing treatment with this medication.

• Avoid spilling the oral concentrate form of this drug on your skin or clothing; it may cause redness and skin irritation.

• While taking this drug, do not take any over-the-counter (nonprescription) medications for weight control or for cough, cold, allergy, asthma, or sinus problems unless you first check with your doctor. The combination of these medications with trifluoperazine may cause high blood pressure.

• Tell your doctor if you are pregnant. Small amounts of this drug cross the placenta. Although there are reports of safe use of this drug during pregnancy, there are also reports of liver disease and tremors in newborn infants whose mothers received this drug close to term. Also, be sure to tell your doctor if you are breast-feeding an infant. Small amounts of this drug pass into breast milk, which may result in unwanted effects in nursing infants.

trifluoperazine hydrochloride—see trifluoperazine

Trihexane—see trihexyphenidyl

Trihexy—see trihexyphenidyl

---

trihexyphenidyl

BRAND NAMES (Manufacturers)
Artane (Lederle)
Artane Sequels (Lederle)
Trihexane (Rugby)
Trihexy (Geneva Generics)
trihexyphenidyl hydrochloride (various manufacturers)
TYPE OF DRUG
Antiparkinsonism agent
INGREDIENT
trihexyphenidyl
DOSAGE FORMS
Tablets (2 mg and 5 mg)
Sustained-release capsules (5 mg)
Oral elixir (2 mg per 5-ml spoonful, with 5% alcohol)
STORAGE
Store at room temperature in a tightly closed container. This medication should never be frozen.

USES

Trihexyphenidyl is used to treat the symptoms of Parkinson's disease or to control the side effects of phenothiazine tranquilizers. It is thought to act by balancing certain chemicals in the brain.

TREATMENT

In order to reduce stomach irritation, you should take trihexyphenidyl with food or just after a meal.

Antacids and antidiarrheal medications prevent the absorption of this medication from the gastrointestinal tract, so at least one hour should separate doses of trihexyphenidyl and one of these medicines.

The oral elixir form of this medication should be measured carefully with a specially designed 5-ml measuring spoon.

The sustained-release capsules should be swallowed whole. Chewing, crushing, or breaking the capsules destroys their sustained-release activity and possibly increases the side effects.

If you miss a dose of this medication, take the missed dose as soon as possible, unless it is within two hours of the next dose of the tablets or oral elixir or within eight hours of the next dose of the sustained-release capsules. In that case, do not take the missed dose at all; just return to your regular dosing schedule. Do not double the next dose.

SIDE EFFECTS

Minor. Bloating; blurred vision; constipation; decreased sweating; dizziness; drowsiness; dry mouth, throat, and nose; false sense of well-being; headache; increased sensitivity of the eyes to light; muscle cramps; nausea; nervousness; and weakness. These side effects should disappear as your body adjusts to the medication.

If you are constipated, increase the amount of fiber in your diet (fresh fruits and vegetables, salads, bran, whole-grain breads), exercise, and drink more water (unless your doctor directs you to do otherwise).

Chew sugarless gum or suck on ice chips or a piece of hard candy to reduce mouth dryness.

Wear sunglasses if you find that your eyes have become sensitive to light.

If you feel dizzy, sit or lie down for a while; get up slowly from a sitting or reclining position, and be careful on stairs.

Major. Tell your doctor about any side effects that are persistent or particularly bothersome. IT IS ESPECIALLY IMPORTANT TO TELL YOUR DOCTOR about confusion, depression, difficulty in urinating, hallucinations, involuntary muscle movements, numbness or tingling of the fingers or toes, palpitations, or unusual excitement.

INTERACTIONS

Trihexyphenidyl interacts with other types of medications:

1. It can cause extreme drowsiness when combined with alcohol or other central nervous system depressants (drugs that slow the activity of the brain and spinal cord), such as antihistamines, barbiturates, benzodiazepine tranquilizers, muscle relaxants, narcotics, and pain medications, or with tricyclic antidepressants.

2. Amantadine, antihistamines, haloperidol, monoamine oxidase (MAO) inhibitors, phenothiazine tranquilizers, procainamide, quinidine, and tricyclic antidepressants can increase the side effects of trihexyphenidyl. At least 14 days should separate the use of this drug and the use of an MAO inhibitor.

3. Trihexyphenidyl can decrease the effectiveness of chlorpromazine.

4. Trihexyphenidyl can decrease the effectiveness of the drug levodopa.

BE SURE TO TELL YOUR DOCTOR about any medications you are currently taking.

WARNINGS

• Tell your doctor about unusual reactions you have had to any medications, especially to trihexyphenidyl.

• Tell your doctor if you now have or if you have ever had achalasia, glaucoma, heart disease, myasthenia gravis, blockage of the intestinal or urinary tract, enlarged prostate gland, stomach ulcers, or thyroid disease.

• If this drug makes you dizzy or drowsy, avoid any activity that requires alertness.

• This medication can decrease sweating and heat release from the body. You should, therefore, try not to get overheated (avoid exercising strenuously in hot weather, and do not take hot baths, showers, or saunas).

• Your doctor may recommend periodic eye exams to check pressure in your eyes.

• Be sure to tell your doctor if you are pregnant. Although trihexyphenidyl appears to be safe during pregnancy, extensive studies have not been conducted. Also, tell your doctor if you are breast-feeding an infant. Small amounts of this medication may pass into breast milk.

trihexyphenidyl hydrochloride—see trihexyphenidyl

Tri-Hydroserpine—see hydralazine, hydrochlorothiazide, and reserpine combination

Trilafon—see perphenazine

Tri-Levlen—see oral contraceptives

Trimcaps—see phendimetrazine

---

trimethobenzamide

BRAND NAMES (Manufacturers)
Tebamide (G & W)
T-Gen (Goldline)
Tigan (Beecham)
trimethobenzamide (various manufacturers)
TYPE OF DRUG
Antiemetic (antinauseant)
INGREDIENT
trimethobenzamide
DOSAGE FORMS
Capsules (100 mg and 250 mg)
Suppositories (100 mg and 200 mg)
STORAGE
Trimethobenzamide should be stored at room temperature in a tightly closed container.

USES
This drug is used to control nausea and vomiting. It is thought to act directly on the vomiting center in the brain.

TREATMENT

Trimethobenzamide capsules can be taken with a full glass of water.

The suppository form of this medication should be inserted into the rectum (if the suppository is too soft to insert, run it under cold water or put it in the refrigerator for 30 minutes). To insert it, remove the foil wrapper, moisten the suppository with a little water, and then lie down on your left side with your right knee bent. Push the suppository into your rectum with your finger. Remain lying down for a few minutes. Try to avoid having a bowel movement for an hour or longer after inserting the suppository in order to allow time for the drug to be absorbed.

If you miss a dose of this medication, take the missed dose as soon as possible, unless it is almost time for the next dose. In that case, do not take the missed dose at all; return to your regular dosing schedule. Do not double the dose.

SIDE EFFECTS

Minor. Diarrhea, dizziness, drowsiness, headache, or muscle cramps. These side effects should disappear as your body adjusts to the medication.

If you feel dizzy or light-headed, sit or lie down for a while; get up slowly from a sitting or reclining position, and be careful on stairs.

Major. Tell your doctor about any side effects that are persistent or particularly bothersome. IT IS ESPECIALLY IMPORTANT TO TELL YOUR DOCTOR about back pain, blurred vision, convulsions, depression, disorientation, mouth sores, rash, tremors, unusual bleeding or bruising, unusual hand or face movements, or yellowing of the eyes or skin.

INTERACTIONS

Concurrent use of trimethobenzamide with central nervous system depressants (drugs that slow the activity of the brain and spinal cord), such as alcohol, antihistamines, barbiturates, benzodiazepine tranquilizers, muscle relaxants, narcotics, pain medications, phenothiazine tranquilizers, and sleeping medications, or with tricyclic antidepressants can cause extreme drowsiness.

BE SURE TO TELL YOUR DOCTOR about any medications you are currently taking, especially those listed above.

WARNINGS

• Tell your doctor about unusual or allergic reactions you have had to any medications, especially to trimethobenzamide (or to benzocaine or other local anesthetics if you are using the suppository form).
• Be sure to tell your doctor if you now have or if you have ever had acute fever, dehydration, electrolyte imbalance, intestinal infection, or viral infections.
• If this drug makes you dizzy or drowsy, do not take part in any activity that requires alertness, such as driving a car or operating potentially dangerous machinery.
• Be sure to tell your doctor if you are pregnant. Safe use in pregnancy has not been established. Extensive studies in pregnant women have not been conducted. Also, tell your doctor if you are breast-feeding an infant. It is not known whether trimethobenzamide passes into breast milk.

trimethoprim

BRAND NAMES (Manufacturers)
Proloprim (Burroughs Wellcome)
trimethoprim (various manufacturers)
Trimpex (Roche)
TYPE OF DRUG
Antibiotic
INGREDIENT
trimethoprim
DOSAGE FORM
Tablets (100 mg and 200 mg)
STORAGE
Trimethoprim tablets should be stored in a dry place at room temperature in a tightly closed, light-resistant container.

USES

This antibiotic is used in the treatment of uncomplicated urinary tract infections. It acts by preventing production of the nutrients that are required for the growth of infecting bacteria. Trimethoprim kills a wide range of bacteria, but it is not effective against viruses or fungi.

TREATMENT

You can take trimethoprim tablets on an empty stomach or, to avoid stomach upset, with food or milk.

This medication works best when the level of the medicine in your urine is kept constant. It is best, therefore, to take the doses at evenly spaced intervals day and night. For example, if you are to take two doses a day, the doses should be spaced 12 hours apart.

If you miss a dose of this medication, take the missed dose immediately. However, if you do not remember to take the missed dose until it is almost time for your next dose, space the missed dose and the following dose ten to 12 hours apart if you are taking one dose a day or five to six hours apart if you are taking two doses a day. Then return to your regular dosing schedule. Try not to skip any doses.

It is important to continue to take this medication for the entire time prescribed by your doctor (usually seven to 14 days), even if the symptoms disappear before the end of that period.

SIDE EFFECTS

Minor. Abdominal pain, diarrhea, headache, loss of appetite, nausea, unusual taste in the mouth, or vomiting. These should disappear as your body adjusts to the drug.

Major. Tell your doctor about any side effects that are persistent or particularly bothersome. IT IS ESPECIALLY IMPORTANT TO TELL YOUR DOCTOR about itching, skin rash, sore throat and fever, swollen or inflamed tongue, unusual bleeding or bruising, unusual fatigue, or unusually pale skin. Also, if your symptoms of infection seem to be getting worse rather than improving, contact your doctor.

INTERACTIONS

Trimethoprim interacts with several other types of drugs:

1. Rifampin can increase the elimination of trimethoprim from the body and thus decrease its antibacterial effectiveness.

2. Concurrent use of trimethoprim with antineoplastic agents (anticancer drugs) can increase the risk of developing blood disorders.

3. Trimethoprim can decrease the elimination of phenytoin from the body and may, therefore, lead to an increase in the risk of side effects.

Before starting to take this medication, BE SURE TO TELL YOUR DOCTOR about any medications you are currently taking, especially any of those listed above.

WARNINGS

• Tell your doctor about unusual or reactions you have to any medications, especially to trimethoprim.

• Tell your doctor if you now have or if you have ever had megaloblastic anemia (folate-deficiency anemia), kidney disease, or liver disease.

• This medication has been prescribed for your current infection only. Another infection later on, or one that a family member or friend has, may require a different medicine. You should not give your medicine to other people or use it for other infections, unless your doctor specifically directs you to do so.

• If there is no improvement in your condition several days after starting this medication, check with your doctor. Trimethoprim may not be effective.

• Before having surgery or any other medical or dental treatment, be sure to tell your doctor or dentist that you are taking this drug.

• Be sure to tell your doctor if you are pregnant. Although there are reports of safe use of trimethoprim during pregnancy, extensive studies in humans have not been conducted. In addition, this medication has been shown to cause birth defects in the offspring of animals that received very large doses of it during pregnancy. Also, tell your doctor if you are breast-feeding an infant. Small amounts of the drug pass into breast milk, and there is a chance that it may cause anemia in the nursing infant.

trimipramine

BRAND NAME (Manufacturer)
Surmontil (Wyeth-Ayerst)
TYPE OF DRUG
Tricyclic antidepressant
INGREDIENT
trimipramine
DOSAGE FORM
Capsules (25 mg, 50 mg, and 100 mg)
STORAGE
This medication should be stored at room temperature in a tightly closed container.

USES

Trimipramine is used to relieve the symptoms of mental depression. This medication belongs to a group of drugs referred to as the tricyclic antidepressants. These medicines are thought to relieve depression by increasing the concentration of certain chemicals necessary for nerve transmission in the brain.

TREATMENT

This medication should be taken exactly as your doctor prescribes. You can take it with water or with food to lessen the chance of stomach irritation, unless your doctor tells you to do otherwise.

If you miss a dose of this medication, take the missed dose as soon as possible, then return to your regular dosing schedule. However, if the dose you missed was a once-a-day bedtime dose, do not take that dose in the morning; check with your doctor instead. If the dose is taken in the morning, it may cause unwanted side effects. Never double the dose.

The effects of therapy with this medication may not become apparent for at least two or three weeks.

SIDE EFFECTS

Minor. Agitation, anxiety, blurred vision, confusion, constipation, cramps, diarrhea, dizziness, drowsiness, dry mouth, fatigue, heartburn, insomnia, loss of appetite, nausea, peculiar tastes in the mouth, restlessness, sweating, vomiting, weakness, or weight gain or loss. As your body adjusts to the medication, these side effects should disappear.

This drug may cause increased sensitivity to sunlight. Avoid prolonged exposure to sunlight and sunlamps, wear protective clothing and sunglasses, and use an effective sunscreen.

Dry mouth can be relieved by chewing sugarless gum or by sucking on ice chips or a piece of hard candy.

To relieve constipation, increase the amount of fiber in your diet (fresh fruits and vegetables, salads, bran, and whole-grain breads), exercise, and drink more water (unless your doctor directs you to do otherwise).

To avoid dizziness or light-headedness when you stand, contract and relax the muscles of your legs for a few moments before rising. Do this by pushing one foot against the floor while raising the other foot slightly, alternating feet so that you are "pumping" your legs.

Major. Tell your doctor about any side effects that are persistent or particularly bothersome. IT IS ESPECIALLY IMPORTANT TO TELL YOUR DOCTOR about chest pain, convulsions, difficulty in urinating, enlarged or painful breasts (in both sexes), fainting, fever, hair loss, hallucinations, headaches, impotence, mood changes, mouth sores, nervousness, nightmares, numbness or tingling in the fingers or toes, palpitations, rapid weight gain or loss (three to five pounds within a week), ringing in the ears, seizures, skin rash, sleep disorders, sore throat, tremors, uncoordinated movements or balance problems, unusual bleeding or bruising, or yellowing of the eyes or skin.

INTERACTIONS

Trimipramine interacts with several other types of medications:

1. Extreme drowsiness can occur when it is taken with central nervous system depressants (drugs that slow the activity of the brain and spinal cord), including alcohol, antihistamines, barbiturates, benzodiazepine tranquilizers, muscle relaxants, narcotics, pain medications, phenothiazine tranquilizers, and sleeping medications, or with other tricyclic antidepressants.

2. Trimipramine may decrease the effectiveness of antiseizure medications and may block the blood-pressure-lowering effects of clonidine and guanethidine.

3. Oral contraceptives (birth control pills) and estrogen-containing drugs can increase the side effects and reduce the effectiveness of the tricyclic antidepressants (including trimipramine).

4. Tricyclic antidepressants may increase the side effects of thyroid medication and over-the-counter (nonprescription) cough, cold, allergy, asthma, sinus, and diet medications.

5. The concurrent use of tricyclic antidepressants and monoamine oxidase (MAO) inhibitors should be avoided because the combination may result in fever, convulsions, or high blood pressure. At least 14 days should separate the use of this drug and the use of a MAO inhibitor.

Before starting to take trimipramine, BE SURE TO TELL YOUR DOCTOR about any medications you are currently taking, especially any of those listed above.

WARNINGS

• Tell your doctor if you have had unusual or allergic reactions to any medications, especially to trimipramine or other tricyclic antidepressants (such as amitriptyline, imipramine, doxepin, amoxapine, protriptyline, desipramine, maprotiline, and nortriptyline).

• Tell your doctor if you have a history of asthma, high blood pressure, liver or kidney disease, heart disease, heart attack, circulatory disease, stomach problems, intestinal problems, alcoholism, difficulty in urinating, enlarged prostate gland, epilepsy, glaucoma, thyroid disease, or mental illness or have ever received electroshock therapy.

• If this drug makes you dizzy or drowsy, do not take part in any activity that requires alertness.

• Before having surgery or any other medical or dental treatment, be sure to tell your doctor or dentist that you are taking this medication.

• Do not stop taking this drug suddenly. Stopping it abruptly can cause nausea, headache, stomach upset, fatigue, or a worsening of your condition.

• The effects of this medication may last as long as seven days after you have stopped taking it, so continue to observe all precautions during that period.

• Be sure to tell your doctor if you are pregnant. The use of this medication in human pregnancy has not been established. Also, tell your doctor if you are breast-feeding an infant. Small amounts of this drug can pass into breast milk and may cause unwanted effects, such as irritability or sleeping problems, in nursing infants.

Trimox—see amoxicillin

Trimpex—see trimethoprim

Trimstat—see phendimentrazine

Trimtabs—see phendimentrazine

Trinalin Repetabs—see pseudoephedrine and azatadine combination

Trind—see phenylpropanolamine and chlorpheniramine combination

Tri-Norinyl—see oral contraceptives

Triphasil—see oral contraceptives

Tri-Phen-Chlor—see phenylpropanolamine, phenylephrine, chlorpheniramine, and phenyltoloxamine combination

Triphenyl—see phenylpropanolamine and chlorpheniramine combination

Triple Antibiotic with HC—see hydrocortisone, polymyxin B, neomycin, and bacitracin combination (ophthalmic)

Triple-Gen—see hydrocortisone, polymyxin B, neomycin, and bacitracin combination (ophthalmic)

Triple Sulfa (systemic)—see sulfonamide antibiotics (oral)

Triple Sulfa (vaginal)—see sulfathiazole, sulfacetamide, and sulfabenzamide combination

Triple-Vita-Flor—see vitamins A, D, and C with fluoride

Tri-Vi-Flor—see vitamins A, D, and C with fluoride

Tri-Vitamin with Fluoride Drops—see vitamins A, D, and C with fluoride

Truphylline—see aminophylline

Trymex—see triamcinolone (topical)

Trysul—see sulfathiazole, sulfacetamide, and sulfabenzamide combination

Tussafed—see pseudoephedrine, carbinoxamine, and dextromethorphan combination

Tusside—see dextromethorphan and iodinated glycerol combination

Tussi-Organidin—see codeine and iodinated glycerol combination

Tussi-Organidin DM—see dextromethorphan and iodinated glycerol combination

Tussi-R-Gen—see codeine and iodinated glycerol

Tussi-R-Gen DM—see dextromethorphan and iodinated glycerol combination

Tusstat—see diphenhydramine

Twilite—see diphenhydramine

Tylenol with Codeine—see acetaminophen and codeine combination

Tylox—see acetaminophen and oxycodone combination

Ty-tabs—see acetaminophen and codeine combination

Unipen—see nafcillin

Ultracef—see cefadroxil

Uniphyl—see theophylline

Unipres—see hydralazine, hydrochlorothiazide, and reserpine combination

Unisom Nighttime Sleep Aid—see diphenhydramine

Urabeth—see bethanechol

Urecholine—see bethanechol

Urex—see methenamine

Uri-Tet—see oxytetracycline

Urobak—see sulfonamide antibiotics (oral)

Urodine—see phenazopyridine

Urogesic—see phenazopyridine

Uticillin VK—see penicillin VK

Utimox—see amoxicillin

Valisone—see betamethasone valerate (topical)

Valisone Reduced Strength—see betamethasone valerate (topical)

Valium—see diazepam

valproic acid

BRAND NAMES (Manufacturers)
Depakene (Abbott)
Depakote* (Abbott)
Myproic acid (My-K Labs)
valproic acid (various manufacturers)
*Note: Divalproex sodium, sold under the brand name Depakote, is chemically and therapeutically similar to valproic acid. It has been formulated as an enteric-coated tablet in order to prolong its effects and to decrease stomach irritation.
TYPE OF DRUG
Anticonvulsant
INGREDIENT
valproic acid

DOSAGE FORMS
Capsules (250 mg)
Enteric-coated tablets (125 mg, 250 mg, and 500 mg)
Oral syrup (250 mg per 5-ml spoonful)
Sprinkle capsule (125 mg)
STORAGE
Valproic acid should be stored at room temperature in tightly closed containers. This medication should never be frozen.

USES
Valproic acid is used to treat various seizure disorders. It prevents seizures or convulsions by increasing concentrations of a certain chemical (gamma-aminobutyric acid) in the brain.

TREATMENT
In order to avoid stomach irritation, you should take valproic acid with food or milk (unless your doctor directs you to do otherwise).

The capsules or enteric-coated tablets should be swallowed whole. Chewing or opening the capsules before swallowing releases their contents, which may cause irritation of the mouth and throat.

Each dose of valproic acid oral syrup should be measured carefully with a specially designed 5-ml measuring spoon. An ordinary kitchen teaspoon is not accurate enough to ensure that you receive the proper dose.

Only the specially designed sprinkle capsules should be opened before swallowing. The entire content of the sprinkle capsule should be placed on a teaspoonful of applesauce or pudding and swallowed immediately. Do not chew the food-drug mixture.

Valproic acid works best when the level of medication in the bloodstream is kept constant. It is best, therefore, to take the doses at evenly spaced intervals day and night. For example, if you are to take four doses a day, the doses should be spaced six hours apart.

It is important to try not to miss any doses of this medication. If you do miss a dose and remember within six hours, take the missed dose immediately. If more than six hours has passed, do not take the missed dose at all; just return to your regular dosing schedule. Do not double the next dose of this medication. If you miss two or more consecutive doses of valproic acid, contact your doctor as soon as possible for further instructions.

SIDE EFFECTS
Minor. Constipation, diarrhea, dizziness, drowsiness, hair loss, headache, increased or decreased appetite, insomnia, nausea, stomach upset, vomiting, or weight gain or loss. These side effects should disappear as your body adjusts to the medication.

To relieve constipation, increase the amount of fiber in your diet (fresh fruits and vegetables, salads, bran, and whole-grain breads), exercise, and drink more water (unless your doctor directs you to do otherwise).

If you feel dizzy, sit or lie down for a while; get up slowly from a sitting or reclining position, and be careful on stairs.
Major. Tell your doctor about any side effects that are persistent or particularly bothersome. IT IS ESPECIALLY

IMPORTANT TO TELL YOUR DOCTOR about blurred vision, cramps, depression, facial edema (swelling), loss of coordination, menstrual disorders, mental disorders, skin rash, tremors, unusual bleeding or bruising, weakness, or yellowing of the eyes or skin.

INTERACTIONS

Valproic acid interacts with several other types of drugs:
1. Concurrent use of it with other central nervous system depressants (drugs that slow the activity of the brain and spinal cord), such as alcohol, antihistamines, barbiturates, muscle relaxants, narcotics, pain medications, phenothiazine tranquilizers, and sleeping medications, or with tricyclic antidepressants can lead to drowsiness.
2. Valproic acid can lead to bleeding complications when combined with oral anticoagulants (blood thinners, such as warfarin), aspirin, dipyridamole, or sulfinpyrazone.
3. Valproic acid can increase the blood levels and side effects of phenobarbital and primidone.
4. The combination of valproic acid and clonazepam or phenytoin can lead to an increase in seizure activity.
5. Aspirin may interfere with the metabolism of valproic acid, which may result in increased toxicity and increased side effects.

Before beginning treatment with valproic acid,BE SURE TO TELL YOUR DOCTOR about any medications that you are currently taking, especially any of those medications listed above.

WARNINGS

• Tell your doctor about unusual or allergic reactions you have had to any medications, especially to valproic acid, sodium valproate, or divalproex sodium.
• Be sure to tell your doctor if you now have or if you have ever had blood disorders, kidney disease, or liver disease.
• If this drug makes you dizzy or drowsy, do not take part in any activity that requires alertness, such as driving a car or operating potentially dangerous machinery.
• Before having surgery or any other medical or dental treatment, be sure to tell your doctor or dentist that you are taking this medication.
• Do not stop taking this medication unless you first check with your doctor. Stopping the drug abruptly may lead to a worsening of your condition. Your doctor may want to reduce your dosage gradually or start you on another medication when valproic acid is discontinued. Make sure you have enough medication on hand to last through weekends, holidays, and vacations.
• Diabetic patients should know that valproic acid can interfere with urine tests for ketones. You should, therefore, check with your doctor before adjusting your insulin dose to determine if changes are necessary.
• Be sure to tell your doctor if you are pregnant. Valproic acid has been shown to cause birth defects in the offspring of animals that received large doses of the drug during pregnancy. It has also been associated with spinal cord birth defects in humans when used during the first three months of pregnancy. The risks and benefits of treatment should be discussed with your doctor. Also, tell your doctor if you are breast-feeding an infant. Small amounts of valproic acid pass into breast milk.

Valrelease—see diazepam

Vasoderm—see fluocinonide (topical)

Vasoderm E—see fluocinonide (topical)

Vasotec—see enalapril

Vazepam—see diazepam

V-Cillin K—see penicillin VK

Veetids—see penicillin VK

Velosef—see cephradine

Velosulin—see insulin

Veltane—see brompheniramine

Veltap Elixir—see phenylpropanolamine, phenylephrine, and brompheniramine combination

Ventolin—see albuterol

---

verapamil

BRAND NAMES (Manufacturers)
Calan (Searle)
Calan SR (Searle)
Isoptin (Knoll)
Isoptin SR (Knoll)
verapamil (various manufacturers)
Verelan (Lederle)
TYPE OF DRUG
Antianginal (calcium channel blocker) and antihypertensive
INGREDIENT
verapamil
DOSAGE FORMS
Tablets (40 mg, 80 mg, and 120 mg)
Sustained-release tablets (180 mg and 240 mg)
Sustained-release capsules (120 mg, 180 mg, and 240 mg)
STORAGE
Store at room temperature in a tightly closed container.

USES

Verapamil is used to treat angina pectoris (chest pain) and high blood pressure. It belongs to a group of drugs known as calcium channel blockers. It is not clearly understood how verapamil works, but it is thought to increase the blood supply to the heart. It is also a vasodilator that relaxes the muscle tissue of the blood vessels, thereby lowering blood pressure.

TREATMENT

Verapamil can be taken either on an empty stomach or with meals, as directed by your doctor or pharmacist. The sustained-release tablets should not be crushed or chewed, but swallowed whole.

If you miss a dose of this medication, take the missed dose as soon as possible, unless it is almost time for the next dose. In that case, do not take the missed dose at all; just return to your regular dosing schedule. Do not double the next dose.

This medication does not cure high blood pressure, but it will help to control the condition as long as you continue to take it.

SIDE EFFECTS

Minor. Abdominal pain, blurred vision, constipation, dizziness, headache, muscle cramps, nausea, sleeplessness, or sweating. These side effects should disappear as your body adjusts to the medication.

To relieve constipation, increase the amount of fiber in your diet (fresh fruits and vegetables, salads, bran, and whole-grain breads), and drink more water (unless your doctor directs you to do otherwise).

Major. Tell your doctor about any side effects that are persistent or particularly bothersome. IT IS ESPECIALLY IMPORTANT TO TELL YOUR DOCTOR about changes in menstruation, confusion, depression, fainting, fatigue, hair loss, itching, loss of balance, palpitations, rapid weight gain (three to five pounds within a week), shortness of breath, swelling of the hands or feet, tremors, or unusual weakness.

INTERACTIONS

This drug interacts with a number of other types of drugs:
1. The concurrent use of alcohol, quinidine, or prazosin and verapamil can cause a severe drop in blood pressure and result in fainting.
2. Beta blockers (acebutolol, atenolol, betaxolol, carteolol, esmolol, labetalol, metoprolol, nadolol, penbutolol, pindolol, propranolol, or timolol) and digoxin should be used cautiously with verapamil, because side effects to the heart may be increased.
3. Disopyramide should not be taken within 48 hours of verapamil; the combination of these medications could lead to heart failure.
4. Cimetidine can decrease the elimination of verapamil from the body, which can lead to an increased risk of side effects.
5. Sulfinpyrazone and rifampin can increase the elimination of verapamil from the body, which can lead to a decrease in its effectiveness.
6. Verapamil can cause an increase in the effects of the drug theophylline.

BE SURE TO TELL YOUR DOCTOR about any medications you are currently taking.

WARNINGS

• Tell your doctor about unusual or allergic reactions you have had to any medications, especially to verapamil.
• Before starting therapy with this medication, be sure that you inform your doctor if you have ever had any type of heart disease, kidney disease, liver disease, low blood pressure, or a slowed heartbeat.
• Your doctor may want you to check your pulse while you are taking this drug. If your heart rate drops below 50 beats per minute, contact your doctor.

• Verapamil is not effective for an attack of chest pain that has already started; this medication is only effective in preventing attacks from occurring.
• It is extremely important that you do not stop taking this medication without first consulting your doctor. Stopping abruptly may lead to a worsening of your chest pain. Your doctor may, therefore, want to reduce your dosage gradually or have you switch to another similar medication when verapamil is discontinued.
• In order to prevent dizziness or fainting while taking this medication, try not to stand for long periods of time, avoid drinking alcoholic beverages, and try not to become overheated (avoid exercising strenuously in hot weather, and do not take hot baths, showers, and saunas).
• Be sure to tell your doctor if you are pregnant. Extensive studies in pregnant women have not been conducted. Also, be sure to tell your doctor if you are breast-feeding an infant. Small amounts of verapamil pass into breast milk and may cause unwanted side effects in the nursing infant.

Verelan—see verapamil

Vibramycin Hyclate—see doxycycline

Vibra Tabs—see doxycycline

Vicodin—see acetaminophen and hydrocodone combination

Vi-Daylin F—see vitamins, multiple, with fluoride

Vi-Daylin F ADC Drops—see vitamins A, D, and C with fluoride

Vioform-Hydrocortisone—see hydrocortisone and iodochlorhydroxyquin combination (topical)

Viokase—see pancrelipase

Virilon—see methyltestosterone

Visken—see pindolol

Vistaril—see hydroxyzine

Vitamin D—see ergocalciferol (vitamin D)

vitamin K

BRAND NAME (Manufacturer)
Mephyton (Merck Sharp & Dohme)
TYPE OF DRUG
vitamin K supplement
INGREDIENT
phytonadione
DOSAGE FORM
Tablets (5 mg)
STORAGE
Vitamin K tablets should be stored at room temperature in a tightly closed, light-resistant container.

USES

Vitamin K is required by the body to produce the blood clots that are necessary for wound healing and the day-to-day repair of body tissues. Normally, bacteria present in the gastrointestinal tract produce large quantities of the vitamin, which is then absorbed into the bloodstream. Some vitamin K is also absorbed directly from the foods we eat (leafy green vegetables, meats, and dairy products). This medication is used as a supplement for those patients who cannot, for various reasons (for example, gastrointestinal bypass surgery, malnutrition, antibiotic therapy), absorb sufficient vitamin K from their gastrointestinal tracts. This supplement, therefore, prevents the blood clotting disorders that would result from vitamin K deficiency.

TREATMENT

Vitamin K can be taken either on an empty stomach or, to avoid stomach irritation, with food or milk (unless your doctor directs you to do otherwise).

If you miss a dose of this medication, take the missed dose as soon as possible, unless it is almost time for the next dose. In that case, do not take the missed dose of the medication at all; just return to your regular dosing schedule. Do not double the next dose of medication. Be sure to tell your doctor about any missed doses.

SIDE EFFECTS

Minor. Alterations in taste, headache, nausea, stomach upset, or vomiting. These side effects should disappear as your body adjusts to the medication.

Major. Tell your doctor about any side effects that are persistent or particularly bothersome. IT IS ESPECIALLY IMPORTANT TO TELL YOUR DOCTOR about itching, shortness of breath, or skin rash.

INTERACTIONS

Vitamin K interacts with a number of other types of medications:

1. Antibiotics, quinine, quinidine, aspirin, oral antidiabetic medications, cholestyramine, colestipol, and mineral oil can increase the dosage requirements of vitamin K.

2. Vitamin K can reduce the effectiveness of oral anticoagulants (blood thinners, such as warfarin).

BE SURE TO TELL YOUR DOCTOR about any medications you are currently taking, especially any of those listed above.

WARNINGS

• Be sure to tell your doctor about any unusual or allergic reactions you have had to any medication, especially to vitamin K supplements.

• Be sure to tell your doctor if you now have or if you have ever had glucose-6-phosphate dehydrogenase (G6PD) deficiency or liver disease.

• Before having surgery or any other medical or dental treatment, be sure to tell your doctor or dentist that you are taking this medication.

• Be sure to tell your doctor if you are pregnant. Extensive studies in humans have not been conducted. Also, tell your doctor if you are breast-feeding an infant. It is not known whether vitamin K passes into breast milk.

vitamins A, D, and C with fluoride

BRAND NAMES (Manufacturers)
Triple-Vita-Flor (P.B.I)
Tri-Vi-Flor (Mead Johnson)
Tri-Vitamin with Fluoride Drops (Rugby)
Vi-Daylin F ADC Drops (Ross)

TYPE OF DRUG
Multivitamin and fluoride supplement

INGREDIENTS
vitamin A, vitamin D, vitamin C, and fluoride

DOSAGE FORMS
Chewable tablets (2,500 IU {international units} vitamin A; 400 IU vitamin D; 60 mg vitamin C; and 1 mg fluoride)

Oral drops (1,500 IU vitamin A; 400 IU vitamin D; 35 mg vitamin C; and 0.25 mg or 0.5 mg fluoride per ml)

STORAGE
The chewable tablets should be stored at room temperature in a tightly closed, light-resistant container. The oral drops should be stored at room temperature in the original plastic container (glass containers interact with and destroy the fluoride in the solution). A slight darkening in the color of the drops does not indicate a loss in potency of the vitamins or fluoride; the solution can still be used safely. This medication should never be frozen.

USES
Multivitamins with fluoride are used to protect against tooth decay and vitamin deficiencies in children. Fluoride has been found to be helpful in preventing cavities.

TREATMENT
The tablets should be chewed or crushed before being swallowed. To provide maximum protection, the tablets should be given at bedtime after the teeth have been brushed. To allow the fluoride to work on the teeth, nothing should be eaten for at least 15 minutes after chewing the tablets.

The oral drop form of this multivitamin and fluoride supplement can be taken directly or can be mixed with juice or foods. The dose should be measured carefully with the dropper provided.

Milk prevents the absorption of fluoride from the gastrointestinal tract. Therefore, this product should not be taken with milk or other dairy products.

If your child misses a dose of this medication, administer the missed dose as soon as possible, unless it is almost time for the next dose. In that case, do not give the missed dose at all; just return to the child's regular dosing schedule. Do not double the next dose.

SIDE EFFECTS
Minor. This product seldom causes side effects, but can occasionally cause constipation, diarrhea, drowsiness, fatigue, loss of appetite, nausea, vomiting, and weakness. These side effects should disappear as the body adjusts to the medication.

To relieve constipation, increase the amount of fiber in your child's diet (fresh fruits and vegetables, salads, bran, and whole-grain breads) and encourage the child to drink more water (unless your doctor directs you to do otherwise).

Major. Tell your doctor about any side effects that are persistent or particularly bothersome. IT IS ESPECIALLY IMPORTANT TO TELL YOUR DOCTOR about bloody or black, tarry stools; difficulty in swallowing; discoloration of the teeth; excessive drooling; excitation; mouth sores; rash; stomach cramps; or tremors.

INTERACTIONS

This product should not interact with other medications if it is used according to directions.

WARNINGS

• Tell your doctor about unusual or allergic reactions your child has had to vitamins, fluoride, or any medications.

• Tell your doctor if your child now has or has ever had bone, heart, kidney, or thyroid disease.

• The chewable tablets should not be used if the fluoride content of your drinking water is 0.7 part per million or more. The oral drops should not be used by children less than three years of age in areas where the drinking water contains 0.3 part per million or more of fluoride. If you are unsure of the fluoride content of your drinking water, ask your doctor or call the county health department.

• Vitamins with fluoride are often prescribed for infants who are not being given any source of fluorinated water. Once your infant is given fluorinated water consistently, ask your doctor if you should continue this medication.

• You should NEVER refer to this medication as "candy" or "candy-flavored vitamins." Your child may take you literally and swallow too many.

---

vitamins, multiple, with fluoride

BRAND NAMES (Manufacturers)
Florvite (Everett)
Multi-Vita Drops with Fluoride (P.B.I)
Poly-Vi-Flor (Mead Johnson)
Polyvitamins with Fluoride Drops (Rugby)
Polyvite with Fluoride Drops (Geneva Generics)
Vi-Daylin F (Ross)
TYPE OF DRUG
Multivitamin and fluoride supplement
INGREDIENTS
vitamins A, D, E, C, B_6, B_{12}, folic acid, riboflavin, niacin, fluoride, and thiamine
DOSAGE FORMS
Chewable tablets (2,500 IU {international units} vitamin A; 400 IU vitamin D; 15 IU vitamin E; 60 mg vitamin C; 0.3 mg folic acid; 1.0 mg thiamine; 1.2 mg riboflavin; 13.5 mg niacin; 1.0 mg vitamin B_6; 4.5 mcg vitamin B_{12}; and 0.5 mg or 1.0 mg fluoride)
Oral drops (1,500 IU vitamin A; 400 IU vitamin D; 4. 1 or 5 IU vitamin E; 35 mg vitamin C; 0.5 mg thiamine; 0.6 mg riboflavin; 8 mg niacin; 0.4 mg vitamin B_6; 2 mcg vitamin B_{12}; and 0.25 mg or 0.5 mg fluoride per ml)
STORAGE
The chewable tablets should be stored at room temperature in a tightly closed, light-resistant container. The oral drops should be stored at room temperature in the original plastic container (glass containers interact with and destroy the fluoride in the solution). A slight darkening in the color of the drops does not indicate a loss in potency of the vitamins or fluoride; the solution can still be used safely. This medication should never be frozen.

USES

Multivitamins with fluoride are used to protect against tooth decay and vitamin deficiencies in children. Fluoride has been found to be helpful in preventing cavities.

TREATMENT

The tablets should be either chewed or crushed before being swallowed. To provide maximum protection, the tablets should be given at bedtime after the teeth have been brushed. Nothing should be eaten for at least 15 minutes after chewing the tablets to allow the fluoride to work on the teeth.

The oral drop form of this medication can be taken directly, or can be mixed with juice or foods. The dose should be measured carefully with the dropper provided.

Milk prevents the absorption of fluoride from the gastrointestinal tract. Therefore, this product should not be taken with milk or other dairy products.

If your child misses a dose, administer the missed dose as soon as possible, unless it is almost time for the next dose. In that case, do not give the missed dose at all; return to the child's regular dosing schedule. Do not double the dose.

SIDE EFFECTS

Minor. Occasionally, this product causes constipation, diarrhea, drowsiness, fatigue, loss of appetite, nausea, vomiting, or weakness. These side effects should disappear as the body adjusts to the medication.

To relieve constipation, increase the amount of fiber in your child's diet (fresh fruits and vegetables, salads, bran, and whole-grain breads) and encourage your child to drink more water (unless your doctor directs you to do otherwise).

Major. Tell your doctor about any side effects that are persistent or particularly bothersome. IT IS ESPECIALLY IMPORTANT TO TELL YOUR DOCTOR about bloody or black, tarry stools; difficulty in swallowing; discoloration of the teeth; excessive drooling; excitation; mouth sores; rash; stomach cramps; or tremors.

INTERACTIONS

This product should not interact with other medications if it is used according to directions.

WARNINGS

• Tell your doctor about unusual or allergic reactions your child has had to vitamins, fluoride, or any medications.

• Be sure to tell your doctor if your child now has or has ever had any of the following: bone, heart, kidney, or thyroid disease.

• The chewable tablets should not be used if the fluoride content of your drinking water is 0.7 part per million or more. The oral drops should not be used by children less than three years of age in areas where the drinking water contains 0.3 part per million or more of fluoride. If you are unsure of the fluoride content of your drinking water, ask your doctor or call the county health department.

• Vitamins with fluoride are often prescribed for infants who are not being given any source of fluorinated water. Once your infant is given fluorinated water consistently, ask you doctor if you should continue this medication.

• NEVER call this medication "candy" or "candy-flavored vitamins." Your child may take you literally and swallow too many.

vitamins, prenatal

BRAND NAME (Manufacturer)
StuartNatal 1+1 (Stuart)
TYPE OF DRUG
Multivitamin and mineral supplement
INGREDIENTS
Calcium, iron, folic acid, zinc, copper, niacin, riboflavin, thiamine, and vitamins A, D, E, B_6, B_{12}, and C
DOSAGE FORM
Tablets (200 mg calcium; 65 mg iron; 1.0 mg folic acid; 4,000 IU {international units} vitamin A; 400 IU vitamin D; 11 IU vitamin E; 1.5 mg thiamine; 3 mg riboflavin; 20 mg niacin; 10 mg vitamin B_6; 12 mcg vitamin B_{12}; 120 mg vitamin C; 25 mg zinc; 2 mg copper)
STORAGE
These tablets should be stored at room temperature in a tightly closed, light-resistant container.

USES

This product is a multivitamin and mineral supplement for use during pregnancy and nursing.

TREATMENT

In order to avoid stomach irritation, you can take this product with food or with a full glass of water or milk.

If you miss a dose of this medication, take the missed dose as soon as possible, unless it is almost time for the next dose. In that case, do not take the missed dose at all; just return to your regular dosing schedule. Do not double the next dose.

SIDE EFFECTS

Minor. Constipation, diarrhea, nausea, stomach upset, or vomiting. These side effects should disappear as your body adjusts to the medication.

To relieve constipation, increase the amount of fiber in your diet (fresh fruits and vegetables, salads, bran, and whole-grain breads), exercise, and drink more water (unless your doctor directs you to do otherwise).

Black stools are a normal consequence of iron therapy and do not indicate a problem.
Major. Tell your doctor about any side effects that are persistent or particularly bothersome. IT IS ESPECIALLY IMPORTANT TO TELL YOUR DOCTOR about bloody or tarry stools or severe abdominal pain.

INTERACTIONS

This product should not interact with other medications if it is used according to directions.

WARNINGS

• Tell your doctor about unusual or allergic reactions you have had to any medications, especially to any vitamins, minerals, or iron.

• Be sure to tell your doctor if you have ever had bone disease, liver disease, kidney disease, or stomach ulcers.

• Because this product may mask the symptoms of pernicious anemia, it should be used only under a doctor's supervision.

Vivactil—see protriptyline

Voltaren—see diclofenac

Vytone—see hydrocortisone and iodochlorhydroxyquin combination (topical)

warfarin

BRAND NAMES (Manufacturers)
Coumadin (DuPont)
Panwarfin (Abbott)
Sofarin (Lemmon)
warfarin sodium (various manufacturers)
TYPE OF DRUG
Anticoagulant
INGREDIENT
warfarin
DOSAGE FORM
Tablets (2 mg, 2.5 mg, 5 mg, 7.5 mg, and 10 mg)
STORAGE
Warfarin should be stored at room temperature in a tightly closed, light-resistant container.

USES

Warfarin is used to prevent blood clot formation. It acts by decreasing the production of blood clotting substances by the liver.

TREATMENT

You can take warfarin with a full glass of water. In order to become accustomed to taking this medication, try to take it at the same time each day.

If you miss a dose of this medication, take the missed dose as soon as possible, unless it is almost time for the next dose. In that case, do not take the missed dose at all; just return to your regular dosing schedule. Do not double the next dose. If you miss more than two doses in a row of this medication, contact your doctor.

SIDE EFFECTS

Minor. Blurred vision, cramps, decreased appetite, diarrhea, or nausea. These side effects should disappear as your body adjusts to the medication. Warfarin may produce a red-orange discoloration of urine.

Major. Tell your doctor about any side effects that are persistent or particularly bothersome. IT IS ESPECIALLY IMPORTANT TO TELL YOUR DOCTOR about bloody or black, tarry stools; blood in sputum; fever; heavy bleeding from cuts; internal bleeding (signs of internal bleeding include abdominal pain or swelling and vomiting of blood or material that resembles coffee grounds); loss of hair; mouth sores; nosebleeds; nausea; rash; red urine; severe bruising; severe headache; swelling of joints; unusually heavy menstrual bleeding; or yellowing of the eyes or skin.

INTERACTIONS

Warfarin interacts with several other types of drugs:

1. Alcohol, allopurinol, amiodarone, anabolic steroids, antibiotics, chloral hydrate, chloramphenicol, chlorpropamide, cimetidine, clofibrate, danazol, disulfiram, erythromycin, glucagon, isoniazid, ketoconazole, methyldopa, methylphenidate, metronidazole, monoamine oxidase (MAO) inhibitors, nalidixic acid, phenylbutazone, propoxyphene, quinidine, quinine, salicylates, sulfamethoxazole and trimethoprim combination, sulfinpyrazone, sulfonamides, sulindac, tetracycline, thyroid hormones, and tolbutamide can increase the effects of warfarin, which can be dangerous.

2. Azathioprine, barbiturates, carbamazepine, cholestyramine, colestipol, estrogens, ethchlorvynol, griseofulvin, oral contraceptives (birth control pills), phenytoin, propylthiouracil, rifampin, sucralfate, and vitamin K can decrease the effectiveness of warfarin.

3. Adrenocorticosteroids (cortisone-like medications), anticancer drugs, aspirin, diflunisal, dipyridamole, fenoprofen, ibuprofen, indomethacin, oxyphenbutazone, phenylbutazone, potassium, quinidine, quinine, and salicylates can increase the bleeding complications of warfarin.

4. Warfarin can increase the side effects of oral antidiabetic agents and phenytoin.

5. Diuretics (water pills) may either increase the effects or decrease the effectiveness of warfarin. Ask your doctor about concurrent use of diuretics and warfarin.

Before starting to take warfarin, BE SURE TO TELL YOUR DOCTOR about any medications (both prescription and nonprescription) you are currently taking, especially any of those listed above.

WARNINGS

• Tell your doctor about unusual or allergic reactions you have had to any medications, especially to warfarin.
• Before starting to take this medication, BE SURE TO TELL YOUR DOCTOR if you now have or if you have ever had any condition for which bleeding is an added risk—an aneurysm, blood disorders, cancer, diabetes mellitus, congestive heart failure, edema, endocarditis, high blood pressure, indwelling catheters, intestinal infections, kidney or liver disease, malnutrition, menstrual difficulties, pericarditis, surgery, thyroid disease, tuberculosis, ulcers, vasculitis, or wounds and injuries.

• Before having surgery or any other medical or dental treatment, BE SURE TO TELL YOUR DOCTOR OR DENTIST THAT YOU ARE TAKING WARFARIN.
• Do not take any aspirin-containing products or any over-the-counter products while you are on warfarin, unless you first check with your doctor or pharmacist. Aspirin can increase the risk of bleeding complications from warfarin.
• Avoid any activity, such as a contact sport, that might lead to physical injury. Tell your doctor about any fall or blow that occurs. Warfarin can cause HEAVY bleeding from cuts.
• Use an electric razor while shaving to reduce the risk of cutting yourself, and be especially careful while brushing your teeth.
• Since factors such as travel, diet, the environment, and your health can affect your body's response to warfarin, your dosage level should be carefully monitored.
• Do not stop taking warfarin unless you first consult your doctor. If you stop taking this drug abruptly, you may experience blood clotting. Your doctor may, therefore, want to reduce your dosage gradually.
• Do not change brands of this medication without consulting your doctor.
• Some of these products contain the color additive FD&C Yellow No. 5 (tartrazine), which can cause allergic-type reactions in certain susceptible individuals.
• Be sure to tell your doctor if you are pregnant. Warfarin has been associated with birth defects and bleeding complications in fetuses. Also, tell your doctor if you are breast-feeding an infant.

warfarin sodium—see warfarin

Weh-less—see phendimetrazine

Wehvert—see meclizine

Weightrol—see phendimetrazine

Wellbutrin—see bupropion

Westcort—see hydrocortisone (topical)

Wigraine—see ergotamine and caffeine combination

Wilpowr—see phentermine

Wyamycin S—see erythromycin

Wygesic—see acetaminophen and propoxyphene combination

Wymox—see amoxicillin

Wytensin—see guanabenz

Xanax—see alprazolam

Yutopar—see ritodrine

Zantac—see ranitidine

Zarontin—see ethosuximide

Zaroxolyn—see metolazone

Zestril—see lisinopril

---

zidovudine (AZT)

BRAND NAME (Manufacturer)
Retrovir (Burroughs Wellcome)
TYPE OF DRUG
antiviral
INGREDIENT
azidothymidine (AZT)
DOSAGE FORMS
Capsules (100 mg)
Syrup (50 mg per ml)
STORAGE
Zidovudine capsules and syrup should be stored at room temperature in tightly closed, light-resistant containers. This drug should not be frozen.

USES

Zidovudine is used in the treatment of human immunodeficiency virus (HIV) infection. HIV is the virus that causes AIDS. Zidovudine works by inhibiting the reproduction, or growth, of the virus, which slows down the progression of AIDS. Zidovudine does not cure AIDS but may delay the onset of other infections and diseases caused by AIDS.

TREATMENT

This medication works best when the level of medicine in your bloodstream is kept constant. It is best to take the drug at evenly spaced intervals throughout the day.

If you are using the zidovudine syrup, use a special measuring spoon to measure the doses.

If you miss a dose of this medication, take it as soon as possible. However, if it is almost time for your next dose, skip the missed dose and go back to your regular dosing schedule. Do not double the doses.

SIDE EFFECTS

Minor. Blue or brown bands on nails, difficulty sleeping, headache, muscle soreness, or nausea. Some of these side effects may go away during treatment as your body adjusts to the medicine.
Major. Abdominal discomfort, chills, confusion, convulsions, fever, loss of appetite, mania, muscle tenderness or weakness, pale skin, sore throat, or unusual tiredness.

INTERACTIONS

Zidovudine interacts with several other drugs.
1. Concurrent use of some other antibiotic, antifungal, or antiviral agents may increase toxicity of zidovudine.
2. Methadone can interfere with your body's ability to eliminate zidovudine and may increase toxicity of zidovudine.
3. Zidovudine can alter the level of phenytoin in your body.

Be sure to tell your doctor about any medication you are currently taking, especially any of those listed above.

WARNINGS

• Tell your doctor about unusual or allergic reactions you have had to any medications, especially zidovudine. Also tell your doctor about any allergic reaction you have had to any foods, preservatives, or dyes.
• You may require periodic blood sample checks at your physician's office to monitor the effects of zidovudine.
• Be sure to tell your doctor if you have anemia, liver disease, or vitamin deficiencies.
• Before having surgery or any other medical or dental treatment, tell your doctor or dentist that you are taking this drug.
• If you are infected with HIV, it is best to avoid any sexual activity involving an exchange of body fluids with other people. If you do have vaginal, anal or oral sex, always wear (or have your partner wear) a latex condom.
• If you inject drugs, do not share needles with anyone.
• Be sure to tell your doctor if your are pregnant. Tell your doctor if your are breast-feeding an infant. It is not known if zidovudine passes into breast milk, but HIV or the AIDS virus can be transmitted through breast milk.

Zithromax—see azithromycin

ZORprin—see aspirin

Zovirax—see acyclovir

Zurinol—see allopurinol

Zydone—see acetaminophen and hydrocodone combination

Zyloprim—see allopurinol

Canadian Brand Names

Following is a list of commonly prescribed Canadian brand-name medications and their manufacturers. Also listed are the profile names under which you can find information about each brand-name drug. Please note that in Canada acetaminophen is known as paracetamol, albuterol is known as salbutamol, metaproterenol is known as orciprenaline, and meperidine is known as pethidine.

BRAND NAME (Manufacturer) Profile

Brand Name (Manufacturer)	Profile
Acet-Am® (Organon)	**theophylline**
Acetazolam® (ICN)	**acetazolamide**
Alloprin® (ICN)	**allopurinol**
Amersol® (Horner)	**ibuprofen**
Ampicin® (Bristol)	**ampicillin**
Ampilean® (Organon)	**ampicillin**
Ansaid® (Upjohn)	**flurbiprofen**
Antazone® (ICN)	**sulfinpyrazone**
Anturan® (Geigy)	**sulfinpyrazone**
Aparkane® (ICN)	**trihexyphenidyl**
Apo-Ampi® (Apotex)	**ampicillin**
Apo-Pen-VK® (Apotex)	**penicillin VK**
Athrombin-K® (Purdue Frederick)	**warfarin**
Bactopen® (Beecham)	**cloxacillin**
Bensylate® (ICN)	**benztropine**
Bentylol® (Merrell)	**dicyclomine**
Benuryl® (ICN)	**probenecid**
Betaloc® (Astra)	**metoprolol**
Bonamine® (Pfizer)	**meclizine**
Canesten® (Miles)	**clotrimazole (vaginal)**
Carbolith® (ICN)	**lithium**
Ceporex® (Glaxo)	**cephalexin**
Chlorpromanyl® (Technilab)	**chlorpromazine**
Claripex® (ICN)	**clofibrate**
Clavulin® (Beecham)	**amoxicillin and clavulanic acid combination**
Corium® (ICN)	**chlordiazepoxide and clidinium combination**
Coronex® (Ayerst)	**isosorbide dinitrate**
Corophyllin® (Beecham)	**aminophylline**
Cytotec® (Searle)	**misoprostol**
Dalacin C® (Upjohn)	**clindamycin (systemic)**
Depen® (Horner)	**penicillamine**
Detensol® (Desbergers)	**propranolol**
Dimelor® (Lilly)	**acetohexamide**
Diuchlor H® (Medic)	**hydrochlorothiazide**
Dixarit® (Boehringer Ingelheim)	**clonidine**
Dopamet® (ICN)	**methyldopa**

BRAND NAME (Manufacturer) Profile

Brand Name (Manufacturer)	Profile
Eltroxin® (Glaxo)	**levothyroxine**
Emex® (Beecham)	**metoclopramide**
E-Pam® (ICN)	**diazepam**
Erythromid® (Abbott)	**erythromycin**
Euglucon® (Boehringer Mannheim)	**glyburide**
Fivent® (Fisons)	**cromolyn sodium (inhalation)**
Froben® (Organon)	**flurbiprofen**
Hibidel 1:2000 (Ayerst)	**chlorhexidine gluconate**
Hibitane® Gluconate 20% (Ayerst)	**chlorhexidine gluconate**
Hibitane® Skin Cleanser 2% and 4% (Ayerst)	**chlorhexidine gluconate**
Hip-Rex® (Riker)	**methenamine**
Hismanal® (Janssen)	**astemizole**
Impril® (ICN)	**imipramine**
Indocid® (MSD)	**indomethacin**
Intrabutazone® (Organon)	**phenylbutazone**
Kwellada® (R & C)	**lindane**
Largactil® (Rh|one-Poulenc)	**chlorpromazine**
Lenoltec with codeine No. 4® (Technilab)	**acetaminophen and codeine combination**
Levate® (ICN)	**amitriptyline**
Lidemol® (Syntex)	**fluocinonide (topical)**
Lithane® (Pfizer)	**lithium**
Lithizine® (Maney)	**lithium**
Loxapac® (Lederle)	**loxapine**
Maxeran® (Nordic)	**metoclopramide**
Mazepine® (ICN)	**carbamazepine**
Medilium® (Medic)	**chlordiazepoxide**
Megacillin® (Frosst)	**penicillin G**
Meval® (Medic)	**diazepam**
Minestrin 1/20® (P.D.)	**oral contraceptives**
Min-Ovral® (Wyeth)	**oral contraceptives**
Mobenol® (Horner)	**tolbutamide**
Moduret® (MSD)	**amiloride and hydrochlorothiazide combination**
Myclo® (Boehringer Ingelheim)	**clotrimazole (topical), clotrimazole (vaginal)**
Nadopen-V® (Nadeau)	**penicillin VK**
Natrimax® (Trianon)	**hydrochlorothiazide**
Naxen® (SynCare)	**naproxen**
Neo-Codema® (Neolab)	**hydrochlorothiazide**
Neo-Metric® (Neolab)	**metronidazole**
Nephronex® (Cortunon)	**nitrofurantoin**
Nobesine® (Rougier)	**diethylpropion**
Novamoxin® (Novopharm)	**amoxicillin**
Novobutamide® (Novopharm)	**tolbutamide**
Novobutazone® (Novopharm)	**phenylbutazone**
Novocimetine® (Novopharm)	**cimetidine**
Novocloxin® (Novopharm)	**cloxacillin**
Novodipam® (Novopharm)	**diazepam**

BRAND NAME (Manufacturer)	Profile
Novodoparil® (Novopharm)	**methyldopa and hydrochlorothiazide combination**
Novofibrate® (Novopharm)	**clofibrate**
Novoflupam® (Novopharm)	**flurazepam**
Novoflurazine® (Novopharm)	**trifluoperazine**
Novofuran® (Novopharm)	**nitrofurantoin**
Novohexidyl® (Novopharm)	**trihexyphenidyl**
Novohydrazide® (Novopharm)	**hydrochlorothiazide**
Novolexin® (Novopharm)	**cephalexin**
Novomedopa® (Novopharm)	**methyldopa**
Novomethacin® (Novopharm)	**indomethacin**
Novonaprox® (Novopharm)	**naproxen**
Novonidazole® (Novopharm)	**metronidazole**
Novopen G® (Novopharm)	**penicillin G**
Novopen-VK® (Novopharm)	**penicillin VK**
Novopoxide® (Novopharm)	**chlordiazepoxide**
Novopramine® (Novopharm)	**imipramine**
Novopranol® (Novopharm)	**propranolol**
Novoprofen® (Novopharm)	**ibuprofen**
Novopropamide® (Novopharm)	**chlorpropamide**
Novopropoxyn® (Novopharm)	**propoxyphene**
Novopurol® (Novopharm)	**allopurinol**
Novopyrazone® (Novopharm)	**sulfinpyrazone**
Novoridazine® (Novopharm)	**thioridazine**
Novosemide® (Novopharm)	**furosemide**
Novosorbide® (Novopharm)	**isosorbide dinitrate**
Novospiroton® (Novopharm)	**spironolactone**
Novospirozine® (Novopharm)	**spironolactone and hydrochlorothiazide combination**
Novotetra® (Novopharm)	**tetracycline**
Novothalidone® (Novopharm)	**chlorthalidone**
Novotriamzide® (Novopharm)	**triamterene and hydrochlorothiazide combination**
Novotrimel® (Novopharm)	**sulfamethoxazole and trimethoprim combination**
Novotriptyn® (Novopharm)	**amitriptyline**
Nyaderm® (TARO)	**nystatin**
Orbenin® (Ayerst)	**cloxacillin**
Oxpam® (ICN)	**oxazepam**
Oxycocet® (Technilab)	**acetaminophen and oxycodone combination**
Oxycodan® (Technilab)	**aspirin and oxycodone combination**
Penbritin® (Ayerst)	**ampicillin**
Peptol® (Horner)	**cimetidine**
Peridol® (Technilab)	**haloperidol**
Pertofrane® (Geigy)	**desipramine**
Phenazo® (ICN)	**phenazopyridine**
Ponderal® (Servier)	**fenfluramine**
Proavil® (Pro Doc)	**perphenazine and amitriptyline combination**

BRAND NAME (Manufacturer)	Profile
Procytox® (Horner)	**cyclophosphamide**
Purinol® (Horner)	**allopurinol**
PVF® (Frosst)	**penicillin VK**
Reserfia® (Medic)	**reserpine**
Rhythmodan® (Roussel)	**disopyramide**
Rival® (Riva)	**diazepam**
Rivotril® (Roche)	**clonazepam**
Rofact® (ICN)	**rifampin**
Rogaine™ Topical Solution (Upjohn)	**minoxidil (topical)**
Roubac® (Rougier)	**sulfamethoxazole and trimethoprim combination**
Rouhex®-G 2% and 4% (Rougier)	**chlorhexidine**
Rounox® with Codeine (Rougier)	**acetaminophen and codeine combination**
Rynacrom® (Fisons)	**cromolyn sodium (nasal)**
Salazopyrin® (Pharmacia)	**sulfasalazine**
Solazine® (Horner)	**trifluoperazine**
Solium® (Horner)	**chlordiazepoxide**
Somnol® (Horner)	**flurazepam**
Som-Pam® (ICN)	**flurazepam**
Stemetil® (May & Baker)	**prochlorperazine**
Stieva-A® (Stiefel)	**tretinoin**
Sulcrate® (Nordic)	**sucralfate**
Tecnal® (Technilab)	**aspirin, caffeine, and butalbital combination**
Terfluzine® (ICN)	**trifluoperazine**
Transderm-V (Ciba-Geigy)	**scopolamine (transdermal)**
Triadapin® (Fisons)	**doxepin**
Uridon® (ICN)	**chlorthalidone**
Uritol® (Horner)	**furosemide**
Urozide® (ICN)	**hydrochlorothiazide**
Vivol® (Horner)	**diazepam**
Voltaren® (Geigy)	**diclofenac (sodium)**
Warfilone® (Frosst)	**warfarin**
Winpred® (ICN)	**prednisone (systemic)**

INDEX

Prescription Drugs are listed alphabetically in this book starting on page 428

A